ESSENTIALS OF FAMILY MEDICINE

SIXTH EDITION

PHILIP D. SLOANE, MD, MPH
Elizabeth and Oscar Goodwin Distinguished Professor
Department of Family Medicine
University of North Carolina at Chapel Hill
Chapel Hill, North Carolina

LISA M. SLATT, MEd
Associate Professor
Associate Director, Medical Student Programs
Department of Family Medicine
University of North Carolina at Chapel Hill
Chapel Hill, North Carolina

MARK H. EBELL, MD, MS
Associate Professor, Department of Epidemiology and Biostatistics
College of Public Health
The University of Georgia
Editor-in-chief, *Essential Evidence*
Deputy Editor, *American Family Physician*

MINDY A. SMITH, MD
Professor, Department of Family Medicine
Michigan State University College of Human Medicine
East Lansing, Michigan
Associate Editor, *FP Essentials*™

DAVID V. POWER, MB, MPH
Associate Professor, Director of Medical Student Education
Department of Family Medicine and Community Health
University of Minnesota Medical School
Minneapolis, Minnesota

ANTHONY J. VIERA, MD, MPH
Assistant Professor
Department of Family Medicine
University of North Carolina at Chapel Hill
Chapel Hill, North Carolina

Wolters Kluwer | Lippincott Williams & Wilkins
Health

Philadelphia • Baltimore • New York • London
Buenos Aires • Hong Kong • Sydney • Tokyo

Acquisitions Editor: Susan Rhyner
Product Managers: Catherine Noonan
Marketing Manager: Joy Fisher-Williams
Vendor Manager: Alicia Jackson
Manufacturing Manager: Margie Orzech
Designer: Holly McLaughlin
Compositor: Aptara, Inc.

Sixth Edition

351 West Camden Street
Baltimore, MD 21201

Two Commerce Square, 2001 Market Street
Philadelphia, PA 19103

Printed in China

9 8 7 6 5 4 3 2 1

Library of Congress Cataloging-in-Publication Data

Essentials of family medicine / [edited by] Philip D. Sloane ... [et al.]. – 6th ed.
p. ; cm.
Includes bibliographical references and index.
Summary: "Perhaps more remarkable is how much hasn't changed in the past quarter century. The patient-centered encounter remains the backbone of effective care, whether in the office, on the telephone or online. In these encounters, attentiveness to the interaction between biological, socioeconomic, and psychological factors is as crucial and relevant as ever. Family medicine residency programs continue to provide excellent preparation for physicians interested in caring for individuals of all ages and their families within a broad range of practice settings, styles, and populations. Primary medical care continues to be recognized as the cornerstone of an effective health care system, although integration of primary care into the broader US system remains far from ideal" – Provided by publisher.
ISBN 978-1-60831-655-7
1. Family medicine. I. Sloane, Philip D.
[DNLM: 1. Family Practice. WB 110]
RC46.E88 2012
616—dc22

2011003428

To purchase additional copies of this book, call our customer service department at **(800) 638-3030** or fax orders to **(301) 223-2320.** International customers should call **(301) 223-2300.**

Visit Lippincott Williams & Wilkins on the Internet: http://www.lww.com. Lippincott Williams & Wilkins customer service representatives are available from 8:30 am to 6:00 pm, EST.

CCS0411

To the family physicians in practice nationwide who, despite ever-increasing work demands, continue to teach and mentor students. And to Sheryl, my wife, partner, and inspiration.

P. S.

To my husband, Alan Spanos

L. M. S.

To my wife, Laura Bierema and my late son, Lukas Willem

M. H. E.

To the many students, residents, and fellows who I have been privileged to learn from and teach.

M. A. S.

To my family: Dianna, Rhetta, Oran

D. V. P.

To my wife, Julie and our daughters, Kaitlyn and Kristen

A. J. V.

ABOUT THE EDITORS

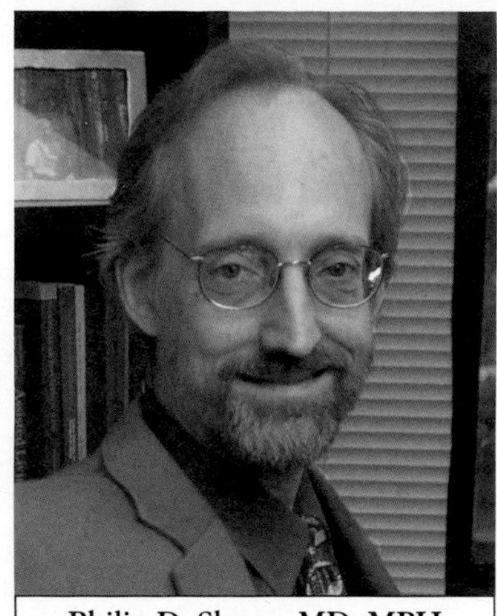
Philip D. Sloane, MD, MPH

Philip D. Sloane, MD, MPH, is the Elizabeth and Oscar Goodwin Distinguished Professor of Family Medicine at the University of North Carolina at Chapel Hill. Jointly certified in family medicine and geriatric medicine, he continues to see patients of all ages in multiple settings and has published over 200 articles and 15 books.

Lisa M. Slatt, MEd, is Associate Professor in the Department of Family Medicine at the University of North Carolina at Chapel Hill. Her interests focus on competency-based education and assessment.

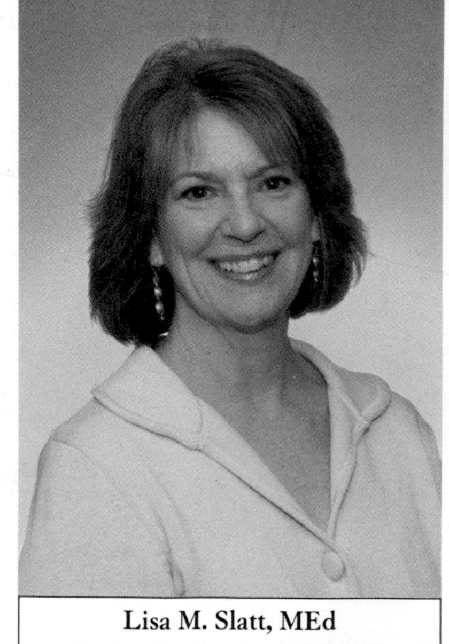
Lisa M. Slatt, MEd

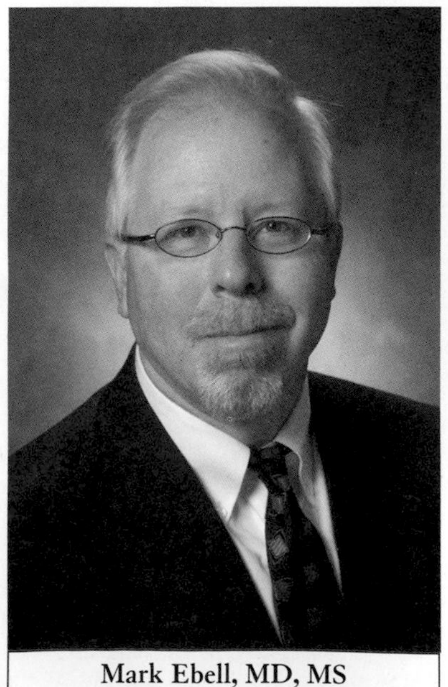
Mark Ebell, MD, MS

Mark Ebell, MD, MS, is Associate Professor in the Department of Epidemiology and Biostatistics in the College of Public Health at the University of Georgia. He is Editor-in-Chief of *Essential Evidence* and Deputy Editor of *American Family Physician*.

Mindy A. Smith, MD, MS, is Professor in the Department of Family Medicine at Michigan State University (MSU), College of Human Medicine; Associate Medical Editor of the *American Academy of Family Physician FP Essentials*™; and Deputy Editor of *Essential Evidence*. Teaching is one of her passions, and she currently teaches research and writing skills to faculty fellows in the MSU Primary Care Faculty Development Program and chair's the mock study section portion of the Grant Generating Project.

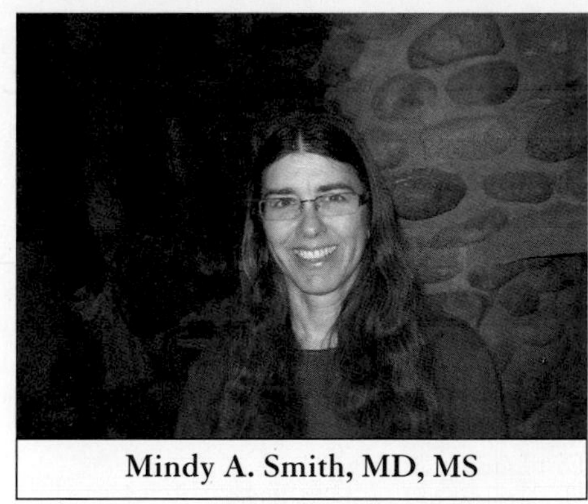

Mindy A. Smith, MD, MS

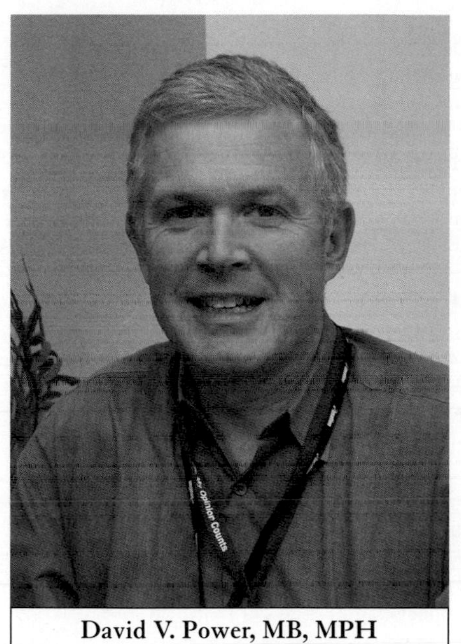

David V. Power, MB, MPH

David V. Power, MB, MPH, is Clerkship Director, Director of Medical Student Education, and an Associate Professor in the Department of Family Medicine and Community Health, University of Minnesota Medical School. He has received a number of teaching awards including a 2009 Leonard Tow Humanism in Medicine award and has published widely on medical student-related and various clinical and international health topics.

Anthony J. Viera, MD, MPH, is an Assistant Professor in the Department of Family Medicine and an Associate Director of the MD-MPH Program at the University of North Carolina at Chapel Hill. In addition to practicing full-scope family medicine and conducting cardiovascular disease prevention research, he is passionate about teaching medical students, graduate students, and residents.

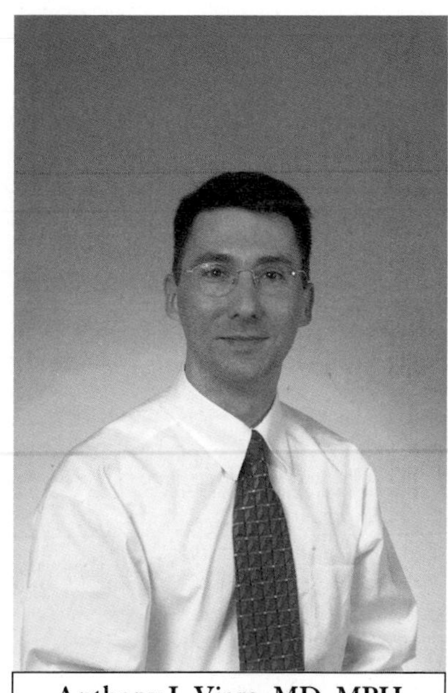

Anthony J. Viera, MD, MPH

CONTRIBUTING AUTHORS

Cathleen Abbott, MD
Assistant Professor, Department of Family Medicine
Michigan State University
East Lansing, Michigan
Department of Family Medicine
Sparrow Hospital
Lansing, Michigan

Albert Asante, MD, MPH
Physician (Resident), Department of Gynecology and Obstetrics
Emory University Hospital
Atlanta, Georgia

Henry C. Barry, MD, MS
Associate Professor, Department of Family Medicine
Michigan State University College of Human Medicine
East Lansing, Michigan

Timothy J. Benton, MD
Program Director and Associate Professor,
Department of Family Medicine
Texas Tech University Health Sciences Center
Amarillo, Texas

George R. Bergus, MD, MA(Ed)
Professor, Department of Family Medicine
University of Iowa
Staff Physician, Department of Family Medicine
University of Iowa Hospital & Clinics
Iowa City, Iowa

Larissa S. Bucculo, MD
HCA Physician Services
Jacksonville, Florida

Elizabeth A. Burns, MD, MA
Professor of Family Medicine
Dean, President and CEO
Michigan State University/Kalamazoo Center of Medical Studies
Kalamazoo, MI

Beth Choby, MD, FAAFP
Associate Professor, Clerkship Director Department of Family Medicine
University of Tennessee College of Medicine-Chattanooga
Chattanooga, TN

Sandra C. Clark, MD
Family Physician/Provider
Piedmont Health Services
Carrboro, North Carolina
Adjuvant Attending, Department of Family Medicine
University of North Carolina Hospitals
Chapel Hill, North Carolina

Molly Cohen-Osher, MD
Assistant Professor, Department of Family Medicine
Tufts University School of Medicine
Boston, Massachusetts
Faculty Physician, Department of Family Medicine
Tufts University Family Medicine Residency Program at Cambridge Health Alliance
Malden, Massachusetts

Timothy P. Daaleman, DO, MPH
Professor and Vice Chair, Department of Family Medicine
University of North Carolina at Chapel Hill
Attending Physician, Department of Family Medicine
University of North Carolina Hospitals
Chapel Hill, North Carolina

Amy C. Denham, MD, MPH
Assistant Professor, Department of Family Medicine
University of North Carolina at Chapel Hill,
Chapel Hill, North Carolina

Philip M. Diller, MD, PhD
Professor & Interim Chair, Department of Family & Community Medicien
University of Cincinnati
Chief, Department of Family Medicine
The Christ Hospital
Cincinnati, Ohio

Katrina E. Donahue, MD, MPH
Associate Professor, Department of Family Medicine
University of North Carolina at Chapel Hill
Chapel Hill, North Carolina

Marguerite Duane, MD, MHA, FAAFP
Adjunct Associate Professor, Department of Family Medicine
Georgetown University
Washington, D.C.

Brian R. Forrest, MD
Adjunct Associate Professor, Department of Family Medicine
University of North Carolina at Chapel Hill
Chapel Hill, North Carolina

Linda French, MD
Professor and Chair, Department of Family Medicine
University of Toledo
Chief, Department of Family Medicine
University of Toledo Medical Center
Toledo, Ohio

Stephen H. Gamboa, MD, MPH
Adjunct Assistant Professor, Department of Family Medicine
University of North Carolina at Chapel Hill
Staff Physician, Department of Emergency Medicine
University of North Carolina
Chapel Hill, North Carolina

Frank Ganzhorn, MD
Department of Pulmonary Medicine
Salinas Valley Memorial Hospital
Salinas, California

David L. Gaspar, MD, MPH
Director, Medical Student Education
Department of Family Medicine
University of Colorado School of Medicine
Aurora, Colorado

Christina Gillespie, MD, MPH
Assistant Professor, Department of Family Medicine
Georgetown University
Program Director, Family Medicine Residency
Providence Hospital
Washington, D.C.

John R. Gimpel, DO, MEd
President
National Board of Osteopathic Medical Examiners
Conshohocken, Pennsylvania
Attending Physician, Department of Family Medicine
The Bryn Mawr Hospital
Byrn Mawr, Pennsylvania

Adam Oliver Goldstein, MD, MPH
Professor, Department of Family Medicine
University of North Carolina at Chapel Hill
Chapel Hill, North Carolina

Mark Duane Goodman, MD
Associate Professor and Interim Chair, Department of Family Medicine
Creighton University School of Medicine
Omaha, Nebraska

Gary R. Gray, DO
Associate Clinical Professor, Department of Family and Community Medicine
University of California, San Francisco
San Francisco, California
Chief Medical Officer
Natividad Medical Center
Salinas, California

Larry A. Green, MD
Epperson Zorn Chair for Innovation in Family Medicine and Primary Care
Department of Family Medicine
University of Colorado Denver
Denver, Colorado

Lee Green, MD, MPH
Professor, Department of Family Medicine
University of Michigan
Ann Arbor, Michigan

Robert E. Gwyther, MD, MBA
Professor of Family Medicine, Department of Family Medicine
University of North Carolina at Chapel Hill
Chapel Hill, North Carolina

Peter S. Ham, MD
Assistant Professor, Department of Family Medicine
University of Virginia
Clinical Faculty, Department of Family Medicine
University of Virginia Health System
Charlottesville, Virginia

Steven W. Harrison, MD
Service Chief, Department of Family Practice and Assistant Director
Medicine Residency Program
Natividad Medical Center
Salinas, California

Parul Harsora, MD
Assistant Professor, Department of Family Medicine
University of Texas Southwestern Medical Center
Dallas, Texas

Caryl J. Heaton, DO
Associate Professor, Department of Family Medicine
New Jersey Medical School-UMDNJ
Vice Chair, Department of Family Medicine
University Hospital
Newark, New Jersey

Iryna Sophia Hepburn, MD
Fellow
Gastroenterology and Hepatology, Department of Medicine
Medical College of Georgia
Augusta, Georgia

William Y. Huang, MD
Associate Professor, Department of Family and Community Medicine
Baylor College of Medicine
Houston, Texas

William J. Hueston, MD
Professor and Chair, Department of Family Medicine
Medical University of South Carolina
Charleston, South Carolina

Robert Jackman, MD
Assistant Professor of Family Medicine
Associate Director/Clinical Medical Director
Cascades East Family Medicine
Oregon Health & Science University
Staff, Department of Family Medicine
Skylakes Medical Center
Klamath Falls, Oregon

Anila Jamal, MD
Chief Resident, Department of Family Medicine
Medical College of Georgia
Augusta, Georgia

Robert J. Johnson, MD
Professor, Department of Family Medicine and Community Health
University of Minnesota
Fellowship Director of Sports Medicine
Department of Family Medicine
Hennepin County Medical Center
Minneapolis, Minnesota

Mollie L. Kane, MD, MPH
Assistant Professor, Department of Pediatrics
University of Wisconsin
Department of Pediatrics
University of Wisconsin Hospitals
Madison, Wisconsin

Daniel I. Kaufer, MD
Associate Professor and Division Chief, Cognitive Neurology & Memory Disorders
Department of Neurology
University of North Carolina at Chapel Hill
Chapel Hill, North Carolina

Jennifer Keehbauch, MD, FAAFP
Assistant Professor, Department of Family Medicine
Loma Linda University School of Medicine
Loma Linda, California
Director Woman's Health Fellowship
Graduate Medical Education
Florida Hospital
Orlando, Florida

Jennifer B. Kessman, MD
Staff Physician, Department of Family Medicine
Medical Clinics of North Texas
Dallas, Texas

Christine Mazzola Khandelwal, DO
Clinical Assistant Professor, Department of Family Medicine
University of North Carolina at Chapel Hill
University of North Carolina Hospitals at Chapel Hill
Chapel Hill, North Carolina

Scott Kinkade, MD, MSPH
Associate Professor, Department of Family Medicine and Community Medicine
University of Missouri School of Medicine
Columbia, MO

Kathleen Klink, MD
Director, Division of Medicine and Dentistry
HRSA, Bureau of Health Professions
Rockville, Maryland

Charles Kodner, MD
Associate Professor, Department of Family and Geriatric Medicine
University of Louisville School of Medicine
Louisville, Kentucky

Caroline Jane LeClair, DO
Senior Instructor, Department of Family Medicine
University of Colorado Denver
Faculty, Department of Family Medicine
University of Colorado Hospital
Denver, Colorado

Arch G. Mainous III, PhD
Professor, Department of Family Medicine
Medical University of South Carolina
Charleston, South Carolina

Otto R. Maarsingh, MD, PhD
Family Physician and Researcher, Department of Family Practice
VU University Medical Center
Amsterdam, The Netherlands

Ranit Mishori, MD, MHS
Assistant Professor, Department of Family Medicine
Georgetown University School of Medicine
Staff Physician, Department of Obstetrics and Gynecology/Family Medicine
Georgetown University Hospital, MedStar Health
Washington, D.C.

Donald E. Nease, Jr., MD
Associate Professor, Department of Family Medicine
University of Michigan
Associate Professor, Department of Family Medicine
University of Michigan Health System
Ann Arbor, Michigan

Warren Polk Newton, MD, MPH
Vice Dean for Medical Education
William Aycock Distinguished Professor & Chair of Family Medicine
University of North Carolina at Chapel Hill
Chapel Hill, North Carolina

Mary B. Noel, MPH, PhD, RD
Professor and Senior Associate Chair, Department of Family Medicine
College of Human Medicine, Michigan State University
East Lansing, Michigan

James T. Pacala, MD, MS
Distinguished Teaching Professor and Associate Head
Department of Family Medicine & Community Health
University of Minnesota and Community Health
Minneapolis, Minnesota

Louise Parent-Stevens, PharmD, BCPS
Clinical Assistant Professor, Department of Pharmacy Practice
College of Pharmacy, University of Illinois
Clinical Pharmacist, Family Medicine C enter
University of Illinois at Chicago Medical Center
Chicago, Illinois

Vinod Patel, MBBS
Jefferson Family Medicine
Buffalo, New York

Katharine Miles Patsakham, MPH, CTTS
Social Clinical Research Specialist, Department of Family Medicine
University of North Carolina at Chapel Hill
Chapel Hill, North Carolina

Janey M. Purvis, MD
Adjunct Assistant Clinical professor, Department of Family Medicine
Oregon Health & Sciences University
Portland, Oregon
Clinic Physician, Cascades East Family Medicine Residency Program
Klamath Falls, Oregon

Allen B. Radner, MD
Associate Clinical Professor of Family and Community Medicine
Department of Family and Community Medicine
University of California, San Francisco School of Medicine
San Francisco, California
Medical Director Infectious Diseases, Department of Infectious Diseases and Internal Medicine
Natividad Medical Center
Salinas, California

Jeri R. Reid, MD
Associate Professor, Department of Family and Geriatric Medicine
University of Louisville
Louisville, Kentucky

Carol E. Ripley-Moffitt, MDiv
Research Specialist, Department of Family Medicine
University of North Carolina at Chapel Hill
Chapel Hill, North Carolina

Philip E. Rodgers, MD
Assistant Professor, Department of Family Medicine
University of Michigan
Attending Physician, Department of Family Medicine
University of Michigan Hospitals
Ann Arbor, Michigan

Mary W. Roederer, PharmD, BCPS, CPP
Research Assistant Professor
Institute of Pharmacogenomics and Indivualized Therapy
Eshelman School of Pharmacy
Clinical Assistant Professor, Department of Family Medicine
University of North Carolina at Chapel Hill
Chapel Hill, North Carolina

Michelle A. Roett, MD, MPH, FAAFP
Associate Professor, Department of Family Medicine
Georgetown University Medical Center
Washington, D.C.
Medical Director, Interim Associate Program Director
Georgetown University-Providence Hospital Family Medicine Residency Program
Fort Lincoln Family Medicine Center
Colmar Manor, Maryland

Rebecca L. Rosen, MD
Attending Faculty/Assistant Clinical Professor, Department of Family Medicine
Natividad Medical Center Family Medicine Residency
UCSF Affiliate
Attending Faculty, Department of Family Medicine
Natividad Medical Center
Salinas, California

Thomas C. Rosenthal, MD
Professor and Chair, Department of Family Medicine
University at Buffalo
Buffalo, New York

Steven E. Roskos, MD
Associate Professor, Department of Family Medicine
Michigan State University, College of Human Medicine
East Lansing, Michigan

Hemant K. Satpathy
Fellow, Division of MFM, Department of Obstetrics & Gynecology
Emory University School of Medicine
Atlanta, Georgia

Robert R. Schade, MD
Professor of Medicine, Section of Gastroenterology and Hepatology
Georgia Health Sciences University – Medical College of Georgia
Chief, Section of Gastroenterology and Hepyatology
Department of Medicine
MCG Medical Center
Augusta, Georgia

Kendra Schwartz, MD, MSPH
Professor, Department of Family Medicine & Public Health
Wayne State University
Detroit, Michigan

Vani Selvan, MD
Board Certified in Family Medicine
India

Allen F. Shaughnessy, PharmD
Professor, Department of Family Medicine
Tufts University
Boston, Massachusetts
Director, Master Teacher Fellowship
Tufts University Family Medicine Residency
Cambridge Health Alliance
Malden, Massachusetts

Leslie A. Shimp, PharmD, MS
Professor, College of Pharmacy
University of Michigan
Clinical Pharmacist – Ambulatory Care
University of Michigan Health System
Ann Arbor, Michigan

Evaron Rose Sigmon, FNP, CDE
Family Nurse Practitioner, Department of Family Medicine
University of North Carolina at Chapel Hill
Chapel Hill, North Carolina

David C. Slawson, MD
Professor of Family Medicine, Department of Family Medicine
University of Virginia
Charlottesville, Virginia

Douglas R. Smucker, MD
Adjunct Professor, Department of Family & Community Medicine
University of Cincinnati
Cincinnati, Ohio

Kurt C. Stange, MD, PhD
Professor of Family Medicine, Epidemiology & Biostatistics, Oncology and Sociology
Case Western Reserve University
Cleveland, Ohio

Beat D. Steiner, MD, MPH
Professor, Department of Family Medicine
University of North Carolina at Chapel Hill
Chapel Hill, North Carolina

J. Herbert Stevenson, MD
Director, Sports Medicine Fellowship, Department of Family & Community Medicine
University of Massachusetts Medical School
UMass Memorial Health Care
Worcester, Massachusetts

Margaret E. Thompson, MD
Associate Professor, Community Associate Dean
Department of Family Medicine
Michigan State University College of Human Medicine
Grand Rapids, Michigan

Richard P. Usatine, MD
Professor
Department of Family & Community Medicine
Department of Dermatology and Cutaneous Surgery
University of Texas Health Science Center at San Antonio
Medical Director
Skin Clinic
University Health System
San Antonio, Texas

Gregg K. VandeKieft, MD, MA
Clinical Associate Professor, Department of Family Medicine
University of Washington School of Medicine
Seattle, Washington
Medical Director, Palliative Care Program
Providence St. Peter Hospital
Olympia, Washington

Dorothy E. Vura-Weiss, MD, MPH
Staff Physician, Assistant Health Officer
San Mateo County Health Department
San Mateo, California

William C. Wadland, MD, MS
Professor and Chair, Department of Family Medicine
Michigan State University
East Lansing, Michigan

Samuel Stucker Weir, MD
Associate Professor, Department of Family Medicine
University of North Carolina at Chapel Hill
Medical Director, Ambulatory Care Excellence
University of North Carolina Healthcare
Chapel Hill, North Carolina

David P. Weismantel, MD, MS
Associate Professor, Department of Family Practice
Michigan State University College of Human Medicine
East Lansing, Michigan

Thad Wilkins, MD
Associate Professor, Department of Family Medicine
Medical College of Georgia
Faculty, Department of Family Medicine
Medical College of Georgia
Augusta, Georgia

Vince J. WinklerPrins, MD, FAAFP
Associate Professor, Department of Family Medicine
College of Human Medicine
Michigan State University
Faculty, Department of Family Medicine
Sparrow Hospital
Lansing, Michigan

Adam J. Zolotor, MD, MPH
Assistant Professor, Department of Family Medicine
University of North Carolina Hospitals
Chapel Hill, North Carolina

PREFACE

Much has changed in primary care in the 25 years since our first edition of *Essentials of Family Medicine*. We have considerably more scientific evidence on which to base our clinical decision making and far greater access to the tools that allow us to incorporate that evidence into daily care. Our role in prevention has become increasingly important and complex, demanding that practices be organized and work in teams more than ever before. We have an ever greater role in assisting our patients with complex chronic disease management, as diabetes and obesity have joined (and possibly overtaken) hypertension and heart disease as the leading chronic conditions that family physicians must prevent and treat.

Perhaps more remarkable is how much hasn't changed in the past quarter century. The patient-centered encounter remains the backbone of effective care, whether in the office, on the telephone, or online. In these encounters, attentiveness to the interaction between biological, socioeconomic, and psychological factors is as crucial and relevant as ever. Family medicine residency programs continue to provide excellent preparation for physicians interested in caring for individuals of all ages and their families within a broad range of practice settings, styles, and populations. Primary medical care continues to be recognized as the cornerstone of an effective health care system, although integration of primary care into the broader U.S. system remains far from ideal.

Essentials of Family Medicine is intended as a practical and comprehensive overview of the specialty. It can be read from cover to cover or used as a basic daily reference by primary care providers, students, and residents. It is suitable for medical students completing their third- and fourth-year clerkships in family medicine. Other professionals, including specialists in other fields, physician assistants, and nurse practitioners, may read it as an introduction to the field or use the many algorithms and tables for quick reference at the point-of-care. We hope our readers continue to find it useful and easy to read.

In this sixth edition, we cover the key elements of family medicine while attempting to keep the book short, the content interesting, and the writing style informal. Among the key features of this edition are:

- Extensive updating of every chapter, with addition of several new ones
- Continued emphasis on preventive care and the management of common problems, using a biopsychosocial approach
- An evidence-based format, in which, whenever possible, we grade the strength of scientific evidence behind diagnostic and therapeutic recommendations
- Generous incorporation of figures and tables, making the material readily accessible to the reader
- A more streamlined format, including posting of references to a Web site, to keep the book small enough to easily fit into a bookbag or backpack.

As always, we welcome comments, corrections, and suggestions for the next edition. Please address them to Philip Sloane or Lisa Slatt in care of Department of Family Medicine, Aycock Building, CB# 7595, University of North Carolina, Chapel Hill, NC 27599.

Finally, we'd like to thank the people who have helped put this edition together. The list must include, first and foremost, our author–colleagues who drafted chapters while pursuing busy clinical and academic lives. Special recognition goes to Linda Allred, who expertly coordinated development of the manuscripts. We would also like to acknowledge the assistance of Catherine Feaga, who, as a fourth-year medical student, helped edit the early stages of several of the manuscripts. In addition, key assistance has been provided by our editorial team at Lippincott Williams & Wilkins, including Susan Rhyner, Senior Acquisitions Editor, and Catherine Noonan, Associate Product Manager.

Philip D. Sloane
Lisa M. Slatt
Mark H. Ebell
Mindy A. Smith
David V. Power
Anthony J. Viera

CONTENTS

Principles of Family Medicine

CHAPTER 1

Primary Care and the Evolving US Health Care System

Philip D. Sloane, Larry Green, Warren P. Newton, and Kurt Stange

CLINICAL OBJECTIVES

1. To present evidence supporting the role of primary care in an effective health care system.
2. To describe the principles of good primary care.
3. To describe how primary care is evolving to provide higher quality care, and the innovations within health care that are fostering this evolution.

US HEALTH CARE: HIGH COSTS, MIXED RESULTS

The US health care system is "fundamentally flawed" according to the Institute of Medicine (1). These flaws, and the unsustainable rate of growth of health care spending in relation to our gross domestic product, present new opportunities for reforming US health care with a solid base of primary care (2).

Several reports have compared US health care with that of other developed countries (3,4). Data comparing selected health indicators for the United States, five industrialized countries, and Mexico (a typical developing country), are displayed in Table 1.1. Among the points that can be made about these comparisons are the following:

- US health care is expensive, consuming 16% of our gross domestic product. Switzerland, which has the second most expensive health care system in the world, spends 61% as much as we do per capita.
- In spite of the money we spend, the United States lags behind every one of these comparison nations except Mexico in the key health care outcome indicators of life expectancy and infant mortality.
- Our increased health care costs are not due to having too many doctors or using hospitals too much. The United States is in the middle of the pack in both measures of health care resources; in fact, our hospital utilization is less than that of Germany, France, Switzerland, and the United Kingdom.
- One contributing factor to the high cost of US medicine appears to be overemphasis on technology, and the potential for its use to be influenced by financial interests (3). Compared with most other industrialized nations, the US excels in performance of computerized tomography scans, magnetic resonance imaging studies, cardiac catheterizations, percutaneous coronary interventions, knee replacements, and dialysis.
- Another contributing factor appears to be the fragmentation and administrative complexity and resultant inefficiencies of the US health care system, with little continuity or coordination of care, which has been implicated not only in higher costs of care but also in the high frequency of medical errors (5).

Atul Gawande, in a provocative 2009 essay, tried to look within the United States for factors influencing health care costs. He did this by comparing two adjacent counties in Texas that had similar populations and similar health outcomes but vastly different per capita health care costs. He concluded that physician behavior was the biggest determinant of health care costs. "The most expensive piece of medical equipment," he concluded, "is a doctor's pen," and physicians play a key role in determining both health outcomes and health costs (6).

Physicians do not operate in a vacuum, however, and their behavior is greatly influenced by the incentives and disincentives of the system in which they work. In a landmark report issued in 2001, the Institute of Medicine posited that the US health care system was poorly equipped to meet the evolving needs of our population and the rapid progress of medical research. The report called for redesign of the system to be more safe, effective, patient-centered, timely, efficient, and equitable (5).

These factors have led to an intense reexamination of the US health care system and, during the past decade, have put in motion factors that are changing and will continue to change the way medicine is practiced in the future. Some of these forces were embodied in the Affordable Care ("health care reform") Act of 2010; many others are moving forward with corporate, governmental, or health care provider sponsorship. As a result, these are dynamic and exciting times in US medicine. The rapidly evolving nature of health care today does, however, underscore the need for today's health care students and professionals to learn about, participate in, and provide leadership as the health system evolves.

ROLE OF PRIMARY CARE IN A WELL-FUNCTIONING HEALTH CARE SYSTEM

Primary care physicians play a key role in the world's most cost-effective health care systems. This is also true within the

TABLE 1.1 Health System Resource Use and Outcome Indicators for Seven Countries

Indicator	United States	United Kingdom	Canada	Germany	France	Switzer-land	Mexico
Indicators of Health System Resources and Utilization							
Total per capita expenditures for health care (2008)*	$7,538	$3,129	$4,029	$3,737	$3,696	$4,627	$852
Percent of gross domestic product spent on health care (2008)*	16.0	8.7	10.4	10.5	11.2	10.7	5.9
Percent of total health costs borne out-of-pocket (2006)*	12.1	11.1	14.7	13.0	7.4	30.8	49.3
Number of practicing physicians per 1000 population (2008)*	2.58	2.61	2.27	3.89	3.34	3.88	2.00
Number of hospitalizations per 1000 population (2006)*	12.6	13.4	8.5	22.0	27.6	16.1	5.4
Average hospital length of stay (2007)*	5.5	7.2	7.5	7.8	5.3	7.8	3.8
Number of computed tomography scans performed per 1000 population (2006–2008)*	228	—	103	—	130	—	—
Percent of population age 65+ who received flu shots (2007)*	67	74	67	56	70	56	35
Health Outcome Indicators							
Life expectancy at birth (2007)*	77.9	79.7	80.7	80.0	80.9	81.9	75.0
Life expectancy at age 65, men (2007)*	17.1	17.6	18.1	17.4	18.0	18.6	16.8
Life expectancy at age 65, women (2007)*	19.8	20.2	21.3	19.9	20.7	22.2	18.2
Infant mortality (2006)*	6.7	5.0	5.0	3.8	3.8	4.4	16.2
Obesity, percent of population†	30.6	23.0	14.3	12.9	9.4	7.7	24.2

*Most recent figures available as of 2010 were used for each indicator. Source: Organisation for Economic Co-Operation and Development (OECD) Health Data 2010. *http://www.oecd.org/document/16/0,3343,en_2649_34631_2085200_1_1_1_1,00.html.* Accessed July 12, 2010.

†Obesity is defined as a body mass index >30 kg/m^2. Data from 2005. Source: *http://www.nationmaster.com/graph/hea_obe-health-obesity.* Accessed July 12, 2010.

United States. Starfield et al. at the Johns Hopkins University School of Public Health showed this in an analysis of 15 years of health data from all 50 states. The higher the ratio of primary care physicians to subspecialists, they concluded, the better the outcomes and the lower the cost. "Regardless of the year," they wrote, "after variable lag periods between the assessment of primary care and health outcomes, levels of analysis (state, county, or local area), or type of outcome as measured by all-cause mortality, infant mortality, low birth weight, life expectancy, and self-rated health. . . . The magnitude of improvement associated with an increase of one primary care physician per 10,000 population (a 12.6 percent increase over the current average supply) averaged 5.3 percent." Furthermore, "the supply of primary care physicians was significantly associated with lower all-cause mortality, whereas a greater supply of subspecialty physicians was associated with higher mortality" (7,8). In contrast, subspecialist-focused care tends to lead to higher costs and poorer health outcomes. This is portrayed graphically in Figure 1.1.

How does a greater emphasis on primary care lead to better, more cost-effective overall health care? There are several answers. When patients have a primary care physician as the regular source of care (7,9–12):

- care is integrated, personalized, and prioritized;
- preventive services are more consistently delivered;
- chronic diseases, such as asthma, cardiovascular disease, and diabetes, are better managed;
- acute problems are diagnosed and treated earlier;
- people with low incomes tend to have greater access to care and, concomitantly, fewer disparities in health outcomes; and
- primary care physicians tend to be active at a community level to improve health care resources and attitudes for both healthy patients and those with chronic diseases.

As a result, people get sick less often. And when they do get sick, they get treated before it becomes severe enough to land them in the hospital. And when they do have a severe episode leading to hospitalization, the after-hospital care they

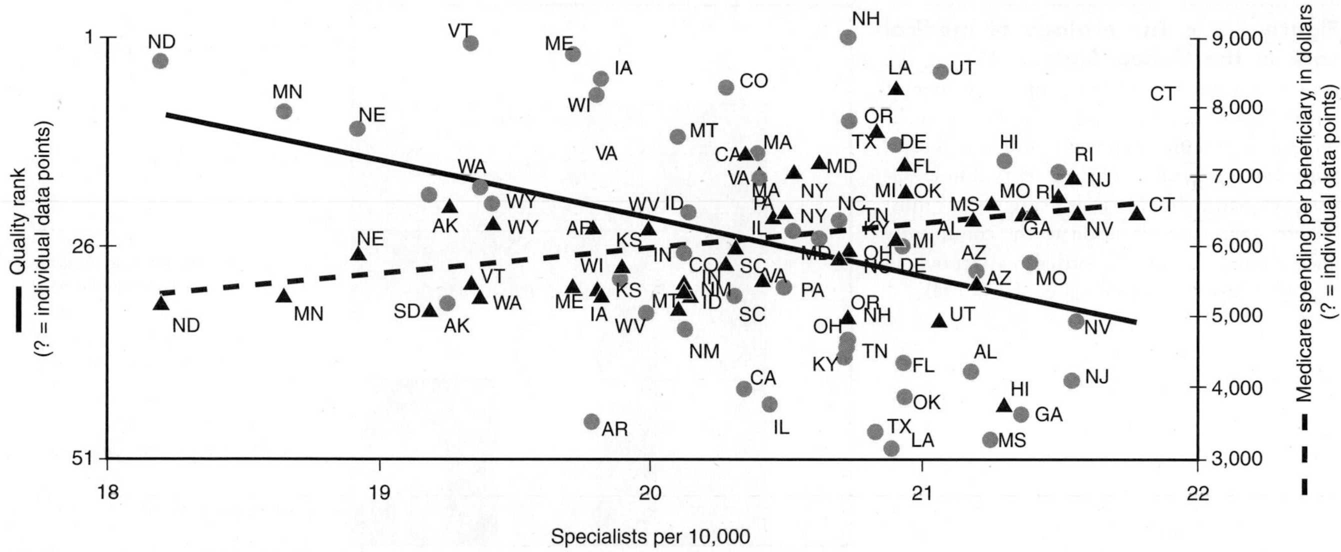

Figure 1.1 • The relationship between provider mix and quality, by state, United States, 2000. These data document that as the number of medical specialists in a state increases, the cost of care increases, and the quality of care decreases. Key: ● = state rank in Medicare indicators of quality of care (smaller values indicate better quality); ▲ = state rank in dollars spent per Medicare beneficiary. Smaller values indicate lower cost per patient. Source: Baicker & Chandra, 2004 (42).

receive reduces readmission rates. Consequently, overall health is better.

When patients go to subspecialists for their care without having a primary care provider, their care tends to be fragmented and discontinuous (10). Furthermore, treatment focused on one body system can have unintended adverse impacts in other areas; more and more care is not necessarily best for patients. On the other hand, when access to subspecialists is severely restricted, patients often suffer symptoms for months or years without getting available treatments.

Therefore, a well-functioning health care system needs both primary care providers and subspecialists. In the United States, that balance is currently tilted toward specialty care. As a result, a 2008 analysis in the *Annals of Internal Medicine* concluded that "investment in primary and preventive care can result in better health outcomes, reduce costs," and recommended that "the nation's workforce policy must focus on ensuring an adequate supply of primary and principal care physicians trained to manage care for the whole patient" (4).

The role of primary care in the overall health care system is illustrated in Figure 1.2. It shows that only a small minority of people are affected by specialized health care. Thus, to affect population health overall—particularly those who are at risk for having serious health problems—the health care system must focus significant care efforts on the community level. It also implies that prevention-oriented primary care must reach out to the community at large, because many people with illness and risk factors for illness do not seek medical care at all.

Defining and Describing Primary Care

Primary care is defined as "integrated, accessible health care services by clinicians who are accountable for addressing a large majority of personal health care needs, developing a sustained partnership with patients, in the context of family and community" (13). Primary care providers include family physicians; general internists; general pediatricians; family, adult care, and pediatric nurse practitioners; some physician assistants; and some gynecologists. Because they provide care that is aimed at preventing adverse, costly events such as hospitalizations and further morbidity, primary care physicians are well positioned to address national health priorities.

To find out what primary care physicians actually do, a comprehensive study of the activities of family physicians directly observed 4,454 patient visits to 138 family physicians in 84 practices. Among the findings of that study follows (14).

- An extensive variety of common, rare, and undifferentiated problems are managed in primary care. Often, management includes a process in which the patient presents with new symptoms and leaves with a new or provisional diagnosis.
- Prevention is practiced broadly in primary care visits, and not just during "physicals." During 32% of illness visits, the family physician delivers at least one service recommended by the US Preventive Services Task Force. Health habit messages are tailored toward high-risk patients and teachable moments; for example, smoking counseling is more often given in the context of smoking-related illness visits.
- Mental health problems present frequently and are often managed without referral. For example, in 18% of visits, family physicians either diagnose or provide counseling related to depression or anxiety.
- Patient education is a major part of primary care practice. Fully 90% of office visits, and 19% of visit time overall, involve patient education or health habit advice.
- Care is often provided in the context of family. Seventy percent of patients have another family member seeing the same physician. In 18% of visits, care is provided to another family member in addition to the identified patient.

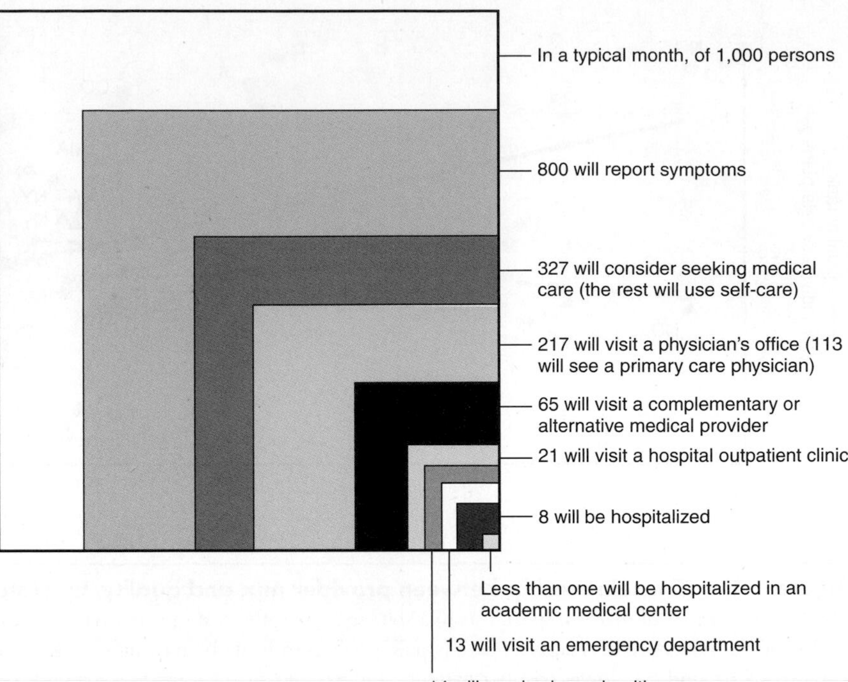
In a typical month, of 1,000 persons
800 will report symptoms
327 will consider seeking medical care (the rest will use self-care)
217 will visit a physician's office (113 will see a primary care physician)
65 will visit a complementary or alternative medical provider
21 will visit a hospital outpatient clinic
8 will be hospitalized
Less than one will be hospitalized in an academic medical center
13 will visit an emergency department
14 will receive home health care

Figure 1.2 • The ecology of medical care in the United States. During the course of a month, 80% of people have one or more symptoms, but only a minority seeks medical attention, and fewer than 1% are hospitalized in academic medical centers. These statistics explain why the health care system must devote significant attention to the community and primary care level in order to affect overall health. Adapted from Green et al., 2001 (4).

- Coordination of care is common. During 10% of office visits, a referral is made to a medical specialist, mental health provider, physical therapist, social worker, or other health professional.

The study also showed that family physicians have to prioritize among a broad agenda of competing opportunities, taking a patient-centered approach. By developing relationships over time, problems are addressed gradually, over many visits.

In summary, primary care practice involves a broad series of activities that include early diagnosis, chronic disease management, acute care, mental health care, prevention, family care, and attention to community (11,13,15,16). These activities occur because of ongoing relationships between the patient and a personal physician who knows and is trusted by the patient. It is not surprising, then, that costs are lower and health outcomes better when primary care is the cornerstone of a health care system (17).

Principles of Good Primary Care

The principles of good primary care are embodied in the principles of family medicine (Table 1.2). They include: access to care; continuity of care; team-based, comprehensive care; coordination of services; community orientation; prevention focus; evidence-based practice; a biopsychosocial, life-cycle perspective; and family orientation. Each is described briefly below.

- **Access to Care.** Primary care should be readily available. Open access is one way of helping assure this. It is a system of organizing a medical practice that keeps slots open for same-day appointments, uses telephone protocols to triage patients by urgency of need, and organizes schedules to correspond with consumer demand (18). Online scheduling allows patients to pick a time that is most convenient for them rather than that which is most conveniently offered by a receptionist. Access to a quick response to questions is also important. A 24-hour call service for patients and secure email correspondence can save time and facilitate closer monitoring. One example is providing day-to-day insulin adjustments in a newly diagnosed diabetic.
- **Continuity of Care.** The average family medicine patient visits the same practice 20 times in 5 years (14). Seeing the same provider over time is called *continuity of care*. Several evidence-based reviews have identified numerous favorable outcomes from continuity of care (Table 1.3) (19–22). In addition, it is associated with fuller, more satisfying relationships for both the doctor and the patient. However, because no physician can be available all the time, continuity of care can be enhanced by using a comprehensive, shared medical record (continuity of information) and by organizing a large practice into small teams.
- **Team-based, Comprehensive, Personalized Care.** A family physician manages without referral between 85% and 90%

TABLE 1.2 Principles of Family Medicine

Access to care
Continuity of care
Team-based, comprehensive, personalized care
Coordination of care
Community orientation
Prevention focus
Patient self-empowerment and self-management
Evidence-based practice
Family orientation
Biopsychosocial, life-cycle perspective

TABLE 1.3 Relationship between Continuity of Care and Patient Outcomes (12–15)

Outcome Affected	Statistical Finding	Strength of Recommendation*
Frequency of preventive visits	Increased likelihood during a year (OR=3.41)	B
Referral of diabetics for eye examinations	Increased likelihood (OR = 2.89)	B
Hospitalization rate	Reduced from 9.1 days/year to 5.7 days/year	B
Annual cost of health care	33%–36% lower	B
Patient satisfaction with care	Increased in 19 of 22 studies	B
Trust in provider	Higher (several studies)	B

*A = consistent, good-quality patient-oriented evidence; B = inconsistent or limited quality patient-oriented evidence; C = consensus, disease-oriented evidence, usual practice, expert opinion, or case series.
For information about the Strength of Recommendation Taxonomy evidence rating system, see *http://www.aafp.org/afpsort.xml.*

of patient problems. In doing so, a wide range of services are provided, including acute care, chronic disease care, preventive care, and care for biomedical and psychosocial problems, and they are tailored to the personal needs and priorities of the patient (14). This provision of a wide variety of services, covering the majority of patient needs, is termed *comprehensiveness of care*. It is convenient for the patient, as there is no need to go to multiple providers to get service. However, as health care has become more complex, primary care offices are increasingly using multidisciplinary teams and electronic health records to enhance their ability to provide comprehensive care. Team-based services can include onsite behavioral counseling on such issues as smoking and diet, a pharmacy, dental services, physical therapy, and a variety of complementary/alternative health providers. Electronic health records enhance comprehensiveness (and quality) of care by providing ready access to clinically useful information, such as practice guidelines, standardized order sets, evidence summaries, disease tracking, prevention reminders, and drug interaction data.

- **Coordination of Care.** Primary care providers help their patients negotiate the complex health care system by serving as coordinators of care. This process of coordination includes being aware of the variety of services available, making appropriate requests for consultation or referral, collecting and interpreting results of studies and specialist visits, and advising when additional care is and is not warranted. It also involves helping patients comprehend what is happening to them, by helping them integrate what are often disparate messages into a coherent whole (23).
- **Community Orientation.** Although most of the physician's work is at the patient level, good primary care physicians also seek to improve the broader health of the community. In working with patients, they are aware of the many community resources, both formal and informal, that are available to help patients manage their medical and psychosocial needs, often relying on other health care team members (such as nurses or social workers) to help link patients to community resources. As part of this community orientation, primary care physicians are often active in a variety of volunteer activities. Examples include serving on a local school board, active participation in church service projects, acting as advisor to the local health department, lobbying for improved pollution controls in a local factory, advocating for better snacks in school vending machines, providing medical oversight for a free clinic or homeless shelter, organizing preparticipation screening for children, and standing at the sidelines as team physician during high school football games.
- **Prevention Focus.** Preventive care is the most common reason patients visit a family physician's office. Examples of preventive visits include prenatal care, adult physicals, well-baby checkups, well child examinations, preemployment physicals, visits in preparation for international travel, and checkups before participation in sports or summer camp. Among the facets of preventive care are measures to reduce disease risk, such as assistance with smoking cessation; immunizations; measures to prevent morbidity in people who have established disease, such as prescription of aspirin for people with coronary artery disease; and minimization of disability through such services as therapeutic exercises for people with arthritis or rehabilitation for someone who has suffered a stroke. The actual delivery of prevention has for years been impaired by the large numbers of uninsured patients in the United States and by the lack of third-party reimbursement for many preventive services. Addressing this problem has been one of the main targets of the recent health care reform legislation, and hopefully over time prevention will be able to receive even more emphasis in primary care.
- **Patient Self-empowerment and Self-management.** Effective chronic illness care requires a partnership in which medical providers help the patient acquire the knowledge, skills, and self-empowerment to manage risk factors, monitor the illness, and make adjustments in their care. For example, literature has shown that asthmatics who are able to independently adjust their medications when symptoms change have better symptom relief and fewer acute attacks (24); similarly, diabetics who have been educated in self-management

achieve better hemoglobin A1c levels (25). One of the recent innovations in self-management training in primary care has been the use of group visits for people with chronic diseases such as diabetes. Such visits use provider time efficiently, reduce costs, provide longer contact time for patient education, and foster peer support (26–28).

- **Evidence-based Practice.** Exemplary primary care is evidence-based. By this we mean that the primary care physician has access to and uses effectively what is available in the literature to guide practice. In line with the principle of evidence-based care, this textbook teaches (see Chapter 2) and provides evidence-based guidance whenever possible. Unfortunately, the majority of clinical questions that arise in family medicine practice do not have adequate empirical data to be answered in a wholly "evidence-based" manner. As a result, primary care physicians must integrate different kinds of evidence, depending on logic, clinical intuition, and knowledge of the patient, family, and community to arrive at the best decisions (23).
- **Family Orientation.** Quality primary care must take into account the family context. By family we mean the entire range of relationships—whether or not by blood or marriage—that can comprise a patient's close social network (29,30). Being oriented to the family context is important in medical care because most health behaviors and illness episodes involve some connection with the patient's social support network. The pregnant woman who has entwined her life with both the father and the child, and who will, because of this, see her relationship with her mother change; the man who develops a chronic illness that will require him to eat differently and take medications that may affect his mood or sexual drive; even the healthy young athlete who twists her ankle, needs crutches, and has to be driven around for several days. These are examples of situations that present in primary care settings in which the care of patient involves consideration of the family. Many tools are available to assess and treat families, though most family physicians do the majority of their history-taking and therapeutic work with families informally. A genogram (formal family tree) can at times be helpful in understanding family relationships in complex systems. Another simple tool—the family circle—is illustrated in the case example that follows.
- **Biopsychosocial, Life-cycle Perspective.** Effective primary care physicians view patients from a broad perspective, taking into account physiology, physical illness, emotional health, and the social, occupational, and environmental context within which the person lives. Such a biopsychosocial approach is important because health and illness behavior are strongly colored by the personality and environment of the patient. For example, whether or not a patient will actually take a prescribed medicine will depend on many factors, such as the medication's cost, the experience of the person and others he or she knows with similar medical treatment, and the interaction between side effects and the person's needs.

Case Example

To illustrate how many of the principles of family medicine described previously can be applied to the care of patients, we will describe the real case of a woman who did not have a primary care physician, and how lack of application of these principles compromised her care. Cases such as this remain disturbingly frequent in the United States and around the world (31).

The patient was a 36-year-old named Mary, who was hospitalized for asthma. This was her sixth admission in 3 years, all for severe asthma. On the most recent three admissions, the asthma had required intensive care, and she was near death on one occasion. One of the major frustrations of the resident who admitted Mary was her lack of adherence with medication regimens. As she had a few months beforehand, she presented to the hospital severely ill and admitted to not having followed her prescribed regimen.

Mary lived 30 miles from the hospital and did not have health insurance. Primary care was sporadic and occurred in the hospital emergency department and outpatient clinics. Nowhere in her hospital chart could the name of a primary care physician be found. Each time she was transferred from the intensive care unit back to the regular floor, her physician changed. Various specialists cared for her from time to time. A review of outpatient and inpatient records revealed little communication between her respective physicians. Many of the tests ordered in one setting had been repeated in another, thus increasing the cost of care. This lack of continuity, communication, and coordination places a tremendous burden on the health care system, as well as on the patient and family.

Mary had excellent hospital care for her biological problems. There were pulmonary function tests, blood chemistries, and so on. However, the chart did not discuss her psychological status, her occupation, or the condition of her home. Physicians assumed that dust was present in the environment. Home health nurse and social services referrals had been ordered, but no report was available in the hospital record. The hospital and outpatient clinic records consisted entirely of acute and post-hospitalization visits, and did not provide information on whether and when Pap smears had been done, influenza vaccination had been given, or the role of diet and exercise had been discussed as prevention of osteoporosis, heart disease, and cancer. In summary, her record provided a good example of care of the disease rather than care of the patient.

To learn more about her home situation and its possible relationship to her illness, a visiting physician asked Mary to tell her about her family. She explained that she was married to Jeff, and they had three children. Of the children, the two girls were healthy and the boy had mild asthma. Both of Mary's parents were deceased, and her father had been an alcoholic. Jeffs parents were both living; his mother had dementia and his father was an alcoholic. Jeff's parents had moved into the family's two-bedroom home 3 years before.

Next, Mary was asked to draw a family circle—a brief assessment technique in which a patient is asked to graphically represent the relationships between individuals in his or her family. The physician drew a large circle on a blank piece of paper and instructed Mary to draw her family members within or outside the circle, representing the relationships between them by how large she made the individuals and how close to each other she placed them.

Mary quickly drew her own family circle (see Fig. 1.3). On one side was Jeff (J). Behind him were his mother and father. At the other side was Mary (M), with the three children behind her.

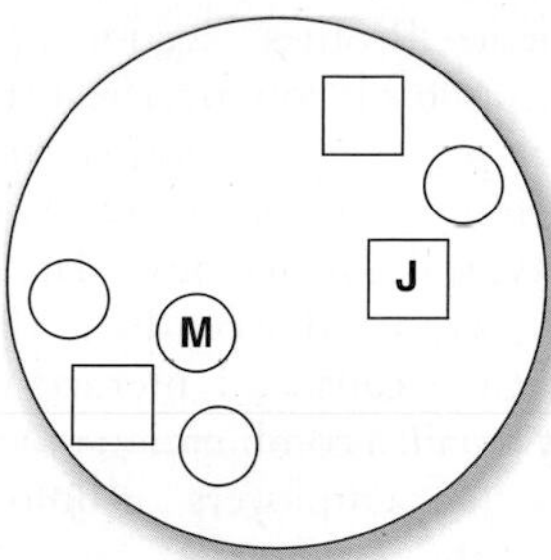

Figure 1.3 • Maria's family circle. On one side is Maria, with her three children behind her; on the other is Jeff, with his parents behind him. See text for interpretation.

The physician asked Mary for an interpretation, and she began to tell her story.

> Jeff and his father would begin drinking and start to pick on the son, and on occasion would beat him. Mary would become upset, and she would begin to wheeze. As her story unfolded, it became evident why her asthma had worsened 3 years before, when Jeff's family moved in, and that every one of Mary's attacks had been triggered by drinking in the family. Once Mary became severely ill, her illness protected her children, because it shifted attention away from her son and onto herself. It only protected them for awhile, however, and she expressed deep worry about what was happening to the children when she was not there to protect them.

This case exemplifies a truism in medicine: Most problems encountered in a physician's office have both medical and psychological components. Although addressing the medical issues can at times lead to resolution, more often than not—and especially in severe or chronic disease—psychosocial issues also need to be addressed. To most effectively apply a biopsychosocial approach requires continuity of care, a family and community orientation, comprehensiveness, and application of the other principles of family medicine. In the case of Mary, the unfolding of her story led to a family conference, a comprehensive management plan, more attention to developing a relationship with a single provider, and, ultimately, much better management of her asthma.

PRIMARY CARE IN EVOLUTION: THE CHANGING NATURE OF 21ST-CENTURY PRACTICE

It is a time of crisis, change, and challenge for the US health care system. As noted previously, medical costs in the United States are the highest in the world, but outcomes lag behind those of many other countries. Furthermore, rising medical costs are stressing the budgets of individuals, employers, and governments; the proportion of individuals without health insurance has been growing; and prominent racial and socioeconomic disparities in health outcomes exist. At the same time, scientific advances continue to occur at a rapid pace, as does generation of new knowledge through research.

Because of these pressures, several processes have been set in motion that will shape the provision of primary care in the coming decade. The most publicized of these—the Patient Protection and Affordable Care Act of 2010 ("health care reform")—strengthens movements and changes that were already beginning to occur, in response to rising costs and concerns about quality. These changes will accelerate in the coming years, resulting in more dynamic, better supported, and higher quality primary care. The remaining sections of this chapter present some of these key trends, with the final section discussing the primary care-relevant aspects of the health care reform legislation.

Quality Monitoring and Improvement

Two reports by the Institute of Medicine crystallized concerns about problems with quality of care, including medical errors (1,32). The response to these and other concerns about quality has been major efforts to monitor and improve quality, and to make care more consistent with the research evidence. "Guidelines" for care are ubiquitous, and physicians are increasingly expected to adhere to them. Research results are being made accessible to the practitioner, and consequently, providers are increasingly expected to be up-to-date.

The combined concerns about cost and quality have led to a drive toward outcome-based reimbursement, in which third-party payers monitor selected health care outcomes and reward providers based on their performance. In primary care office practice, this movement began by addressing "hard," easily measurable outcomes for which considerable evidence existed regarding their impact on health. The prototypical outcome indicator in these "pay-for-performance" systems is the hemoglobin A1c test; others are rates of delivery of preventive health services (e.g., mammography in women ages 50 to 75).

The Patient-centered Medical Home

The patient-centered medical home (PCMH) is a model of health care delivery system reform that incorporates virtually all of the principles of family medicine elucidated previously. The PCMH has four cornerstones: 1) comprehensive, coordinated primary care delivered by a team of providers led by the patient's personal physician; 2) patient-centered care, tailored to individual needs and preferences; 3) a high-tech practice model that includes patient registries, quality monitoring and improvement, point-of-care decision support, and electronic health records; and 4) a reimbursement system that includes payment for care coordination and for achievement of quality of care benchmarks, as well as fee-for-service and case-mix adjustments for practices serving patients with complex chronic illnesses and multiple comorbid conditions (33,34).

The concept of the PCMH initiated in pediatrics and was refined and promulgated by a series of reports from a task force on the future of family medicine (35,36). Several major events in the past few years have provided impetus for growth of the PCMH:

- It has been embraced and championed by a broad coalition of employers, consumers, and providers. In 2005, IBM concluded that US health care was failing to deliver adequate care for its employees because of the way primary care was financed. They joined with several other large national employers and reached out to the American Academy of Family Physicians, the American College of Physicians, and other primary care groups to advocate for the PCMH model as the cornerstone of health care in American. The movement grew to include more than 600 organizations, including employers, consumer groups, patient quality organizations, health plans, labor unions, hospitals, and clinicians, and has had a strong influence on development of PCMH incentives by insurance companies, and on inclusion of components of the PCMH in the 2010 health care reform act (37).

- The National Center for Quality Assurance, the nation's most respected resource on quality and quality improvement standards in medical practice, developed standards for and began certifying practices as PCMHs. Following their lead, numerous major insurance companies have begun to provide primary care practices with increased reimbursement if they meet National Center for Quality Assurance standards for certification as a PCMH (38).
- By 2009, numerous funding agencies, including the American Academy of Family Physicians and the US Centers for Medicare and Medicaid Services, had initiated more than 22 demonstration pilot projects to develop, field test, and evaluate PCMH models (39–41).
- PCHM concepts were included in the 2010 health care reform bill (see the following sections).

Community Health Centers

Community health centers (CHCs) are a large, growing provider of primary care, especially for poor, minority, and uninsured Americans. As of 2010, more than 1,200 CHCs in 6,000 sites were providing primary medical care for an estimated 17 million Americans, providing access to quality services for a population that is 60% minority and 40% uninsured. CHCs receive federal funding to provide primary care as a major component of the "safety net" for people with limited financial resources. Federal funds for CHC growth were expanded in 2009–2010, and consequently CHCs are projected to serve 30 million people by 2015 (41).

CHCs are increasingly using electronic medical records; engaging in quality monitoring and improvement programs; and employing comprehensive health teams including physicians, nurse practitioners, physician assistants, dentists, nutrition counselors, social workers, nurses, and others. Studies have shown that people residing in communities with CHCs have considerably better access to care (42), and CHCs have been credited with helping narrow the black/white and Latino/white health gap in key areas, such as infant mortality, prenatal care, and tuberculosis death rates.

Low Overhead Practice Models

Overhead expenses from support staff devour around two-thirds of a primary care practice's revenue. By reducing this overhead to as low as 20% of revenue by operating on a cash-only basis with limited office staff, low overhead practices can see fewer patients per day and charge far less per visit. Patients find them appealing because the total cost of care is often no more than they would expend as the co-pay under traditional insurance. Physicians find them appealing because they are able to spend more time with patients and generate a similar income to that of more traditional practices. Because concerns about efficiency and the need for patient co-pays will not disappear, even under health care reform, low overhead practice models are likely to continue growing in the foreseeable future.

One low overhead family physician, for example, schedules two patients per hour and reports an annual income considerably higher than the median for primary care physicians (43). See the "Practice Profiles" section at the end of this chapter for a description his low-overhead practice. Another low overhead office practice, Qliance, started in 2007 in the Seattle area and within 3 years was operating three clinics with 13 providers. The typical Qliance physician carries a panel of 800 patients and in a typical day conducts 10 patient care visits, handles 3 to 10 phone calls, and interacts with between one and five patients by email; a combination of low visit costs paid directly by patients, their employers, or unions, plus a modest monthly fee, support the services (44).

Another rapidly growing form of low-overhead practice is the home care or nursing home practice. In these practices, one or more physicians work out of a car or van, supported by a lean infrastructure of staff that schedule visits, phone patients for follow-up, and manage administrative paperwork. The majority of patients in these practices are homebound elderly, assisted living residents, and nursing home residents. Some home care practices are partly subsidized by hospitals, because they reduce emergency department use. As one home care physician wrote, "I can deliver high-quality medical care to patients in comfort and privacy at a reasonable cost to them and with a reasonable income for me" (45). Some home care practices are cash only; those that focus on assisted living or nursing home patients receive most of their reimbursement from Medicare.

INTEGRATED HEALTH CARE SYSTEMS THAT EMPHASIZE PRIMARY CARE

Medical and surgical specialists are increasingly recognizing the value of working in health care settings where primary care and specialty services are well integrated, and where primary care is at the center of health system design. As a result, some of the nation's oldest and most respected private health care systems, including the Mayo Clinic, the Geisinger Health System, and Group Health Cooperative, have been structured around strong primary care programs. These primary care-based integrated health systems serve large populations of patients of all socioeconomic groups, providing high quality health care to millions at remarkably low per capita costs (6). Recently, several integrated health care systems have been among the leading organizations in developing and implementing the patient-centered medical home (46–49).

Health Care Reform and Primary Care

One of the forces most strongly shaping the direction of health care in this decade will be implementation of the Patient Protection and Affordable Care Act of 2010 ("health care reform" bill). Through a series of measures aimed at improving access, providing incentives to the provision of quality care, emphasizing prevention, and more closely regulating insurance companies, health care reform is projected to reduce by more than half the number of uninsured patients in the United States, reduce the annual growth rate of health care expenditures, and save the federal budget $143 billion over 10 years (50).

A key feature of health care reform is investment in an improved primary care system. According to a summary of the health care reform act prepared by the Commonwealth Fund, "a strong network of primary care physicians is central to a high performance health system that works for everyone . . . . Health care reform will test a new model of care that changes the way health care is organized. Patients can enroll in a patient-centered medical home, which is accountable for ensuring that patients get all recommended care. By offering care on nights and weekends, by using information technology and office systems to remind patients about preventive care, and by assisting them with obtaining needed specialty care, medical homes provide high-quality, coordinated care. . . . Financial incentives will help these practices succeed" (51).

Among the legislative provisions of health care reform and related congressional initiative are the following, which directly impact primary care:

- increased payments for primary care under Medicare and Medicaid,
- incentives for practices to meet the requirements for certification as medical homes,
- improved access to care for low-income and uninsured people through expansion of community health centers and the National Health Service Corps,
- a requirement that insurance plans provide free preventive care for services that have sufficient evidence supporting their effectiveness
- investment in primary care training, and
- special financial incentives for practices to adopt electronic medical records and to use them to monitor and report quality indicators.

As a result, the coming decade will be one of rapid growth and evolution in primary care, incorporating many of the principles and innovations described in this chapter.

KEY POINTS

- Health care systems that are based on available, high-quality primary care have lower costs and better overall health outcomes than systems that are specialty-focused.
- The principles of family medicine (and of quality primary care) include access to care; continuity of care; team-based, comprehensive care; coordination of services; community orientation; prevention focus; patient self-empowerment; evidence based practice; family centeredness; and a biopsychosocial, life cycle perspective.
- Between 2010 and 2020 primary care will expand and evolve at a rapid rate, due to innovations such as the patient-centered medical home, private initiatives to improve primary care, and provisions included in the health care reform act.

APPENDIX

1.1

A Career in Family Medicine: A World of Opportunities

Philip D. Sloane, Catherine C. Feaga, and Harold Gutmann

Training in family medicine opens up a wide array of career options; in this appendix, we provide a glimpse of some of those options. Possible career paths include outpatient and inpatient care, rural or urban settings, community or academic medicine, international health care, travel medicine, maternal–child health, sports medicine, geriatrics, health system leadership, and research. What all these career paths share is a commitment to deliver excellent, patient-oriented primary care across the range of organ systems, using a biopsychosocial approach to care. In the succeeding sections, we profile a few examples of the range of careers available within family medicine.

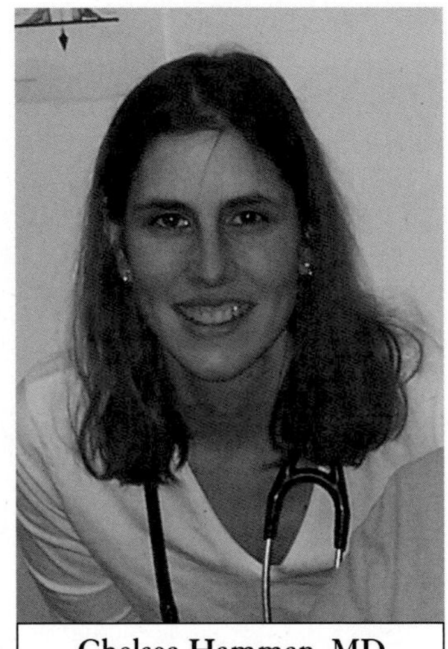
Chelsea Hamman, MD

One such option is rural practice. Dr. Chelsea Hamman-practices in Marion, VA, a town of 6000 nestled between the Appalachian and Blue Ridge Mountains. Along with her husband—a Lutheran pastor—and three children, she has 20 chickens and goats on their 58-acre farm. "This is a great place for a family," Hamman said. "My daughter loves riding horses, so we're planning on adding a horse to the menagerie. It's a lot of fun. If you had asked me 10 years ago if I would have this, I would have never thought it possible." Hamman chose rural medicine because it provided a healthy balance between work and family. She begins her day at 8:30 a.m. and finishes all her paperwork by 5 p.m. She sees 18 to 25 patients per day and shares an office with three other family physicians. Each helps the other if someone is overbooked or needs a day off. "The variety is good. You never know what will be behind the door."

Being a doctor in a small town offers many blessings and some unique challenges. "Most people respect your boundaries. Sometimes they don't though and they try to run me down in Wal-Mart because they need a refill on a prescription."

Hamman gets two Fridays off per month, except for once every 8 weeks when she is on hospital duty. "It's obvious what an important role family physicians play in the health-care system here. We're available to fill in for pediatrics, [emergency room] and the hospitalists."

Resort communities are often quite rural as well, so they too are perfect settings for the broad skills of a family physician. On a typical day, Dr. James Kennedy, who practices in Winter Park, CO, will see a patient with bursitis, another with a broken finger, one with depression and anxiety, another for an allergy injection, someone with back pain, and one with acute shortness of breath, plus two well-child checkups and an adult physical. "People feel pretty comfortable coming here for most anything," he said. "The only thing we don't do is obstetrics, and that's because there isn't a hospital (in town)."

Kennedy chose Winter Park because he can go skiing between seeing patients and he's able to work alongside his daughter, Dr. Kelly Glancey. Kennedy and Glancey manage everything themselves and have no support staff. Maintaining low overhead allows Kennedy to break even on just two patients per day. "That frees up our time for walk-ins, and allows us to do the billing, answer phones, answer questions, do prescription refills—all of the things patients like a physician to do." It is also much more efficient because there are no information handoffs. "I can handle the refill before the patient is off the phone."

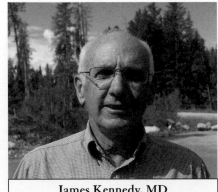
James Kennedy, MD

Exploring new ways of practicing medicine is common in family medicine. One leader in innovation is Dr. Brian Forrest, of Apex, NC. Forrest's low-overhead model of practice allows him to break even on four patients per day. He charges much less than usual ($49 for a full physical), has more autonomy, and takes home more than $250,000 a year. Most visits are 30 to 50 minutes, virtually always with the same provider, decreasing waste and inefficiencies.

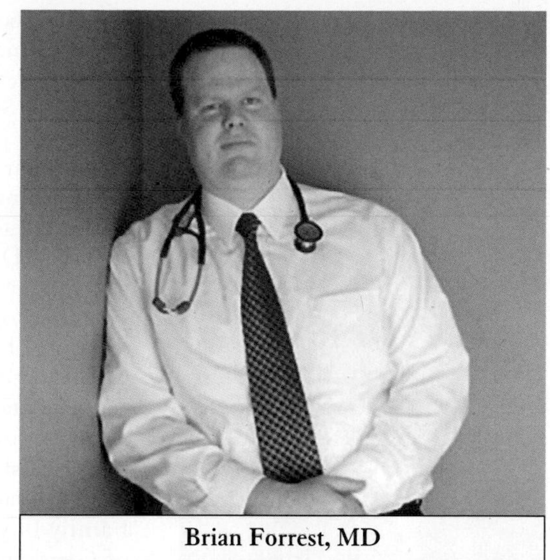
Brian Forrest, MD

During residency, Forrest was struck by the viscous cycle of high overhead, declining reimbursement, and increasing productivity demands that plagued many practices. He was also alarmed that patients who were paying out of pocket were charged the most. To address these issues, he decided to eliminate the insurance "middle men." This allowed him to reduce his overhead to 24% (vs. 65–70% for the typical practice) and pass the savings on to the patient. "I post a price list of services out front so there is total transparency and patients can figure out the cost of their bill before they even see me. People pay at the time of service, and my collection rate is 99.8%. It's efficient."

Dr. Forrest draws blood, runs the electrocardiograms, administers vaccinations, and even takes out the trash. That translates to savings for the practice, but it also leads to increased patient satisfaction. "People enjoy having their doctor's undivided attention rather than being passed off to support personnel."

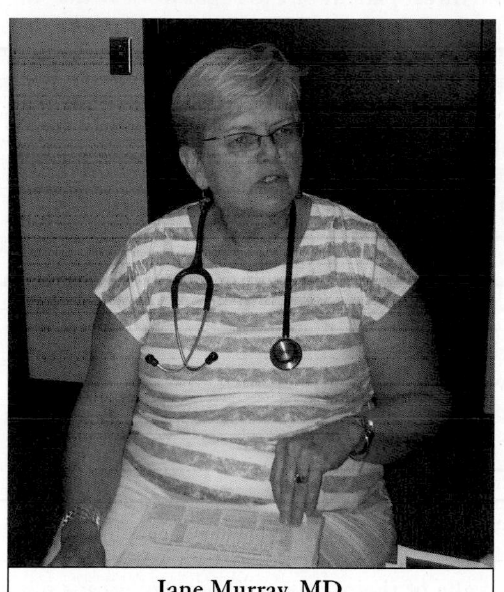
Jane Murray, MD

Trailblazing new, improved health care delivery models seem to be in the blood of many family physicians. When Dr. Jane Murray had enough of the academic world (as department chairman at the University of Kansas), she founded the Sastun Center of Integrative Healthcare in Kansas City to create a positive environment for patients and practitioners.

Besides Murray, the clinic staff includes a family nurse practitioner, a psychiatrist, a psychologist, two naturopathic physicians, a Chinese medicine practitioner, a bodywork practitioner, an energy worker, a nutritionist, a pharmacist and a yoga instructor. "I wanted to be part of something that addressed a person's totality of needs," Murray said. "Medicine is more than just giving someone a pill."

Murray feels that the need for physicians who approach a patient holistically is growing. "Patients are interested in education, and our goal is to empower them. Sastun holds regular yoga classes and informational seminars taught by practitioners, and Murray's goal is to have the classroom going constantly.

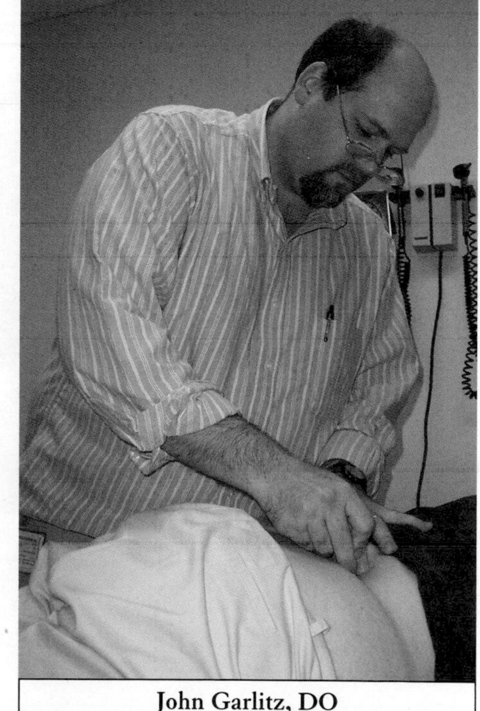
John Garlitz, DO

Murray no longer does obstetrics or consults in hospitals, but she does carry a pager at all times. "The interesting thing is that when people are empowered, they know how to take care of themselves. I usually get only three calls a week." Murray's schedule at Sastun has her seeing patients from 9 a.m. to noon and from 2 to 5 p.m. 4 days per week, often in 30- to 60-minute appointment slots. "I love working with people in a way that allows me to be present with them. I'm able to really listen and put everything together from the ground up."

For osteopathic physicians, a career in family medicine helps blend traditional medicine with a complementary medicine tradition. John Garlitz was motivated to pursue a career as a Doctor of Osteopathy by a boyhood experience with successful osteopathic treatment of refractory back spasms, and seeing his chronically ill mother in need of coordinated care. "I wanted to focus on keeping my patients out of the hospital, and the only way to do that was to understand the root causes of their symptoms." Osteopaths are trained to look for causes and manifestations of disease on the physical, mental, emotional, and spiritual levels. Although family physicians comprised only 14% of practicing MDs in 2004, they represented 41% of DOs. "There have been times I've been able to help a patient because I knew what was going on with the rest of the family," said Garlitz, a physician, teacher, and course administrator at West Virginia School of Osteopathic Medicine.

As an osteopath, he tries to think holistically about each patient. "For example, rather than putting a patient with [gastrointestinal reflux disease] on a [proton pump inhibitor], which treats the symptom and not the root cause (which is often obesity), I talk with them about lifestyle changes and decreasing weight, reducing the need for the drug. That's great because decreased stomach acidity can lead to calcium and B12 absorption problems. So instead of treating a symptom, we're trying to find the root of the cause and correct it."

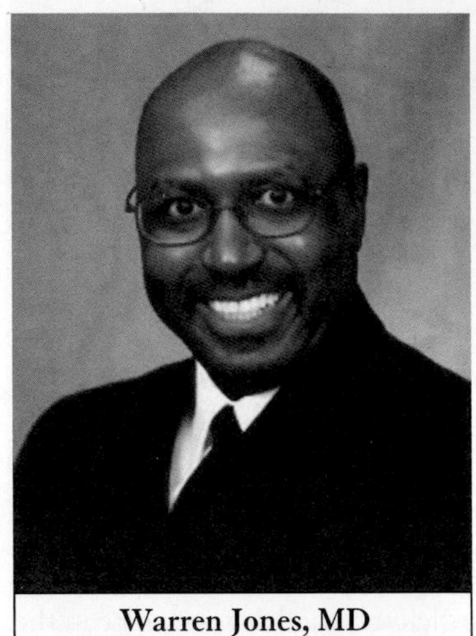

Warren Jones, MD

Military medicine is built around family physicians, and has recently adopted the Patient-centered Medical Home as a cornerstone of service provision. In the military, family doctors often find themselves rising to high leadership positions quickly. For example, Dr. Warren Jones rose from being a general medical officer in the Navy to become the medical director of the more than 10 million member TRICARE Military Health Program. Jones credits his generalist perspective for his success. The understanding of individual, family, community, and environmental health that he developed in the practice of family medicine enabled him to expand and apply solutions on regional and national levels. "As family doctors, we're taught to look at the big picture while not overlooking the things on which you can stub your toe. A lot of people don't have that skill," Jones said.

He was also the first African-American president of the American Academy of Family Physicians and later developed the Mississippi Institute for the Improvement of Geographical Minority Health to empower underserved communities across the state.

Jones has delivered more than 2200 babies and practiced in the air, at sea, and in foreign lands. Though he officially retired from direct patient care to begin work with community, state, and national health care issues, he still identifies himself first and foremost as a family physician. "Being a doctor is more than being able to write a prescription. It's to help a community heal itself. I do that by teaching. *Doctore* in Latin means 'to teach,' and that's what I do every day and I love it."

American's chief health teacher is also a family doctor—Dr. Regina Benjamin, who recently became the 18th Surgeon General of the United States. She started out as the only doctor in Bayou La Batre, AL, a shrimping village with approximately 2,500 residents. There she established a family medicine that allowed her to treat the area's uninsured, often taking a pickup truck to make house calls on isolated or immobile patients.

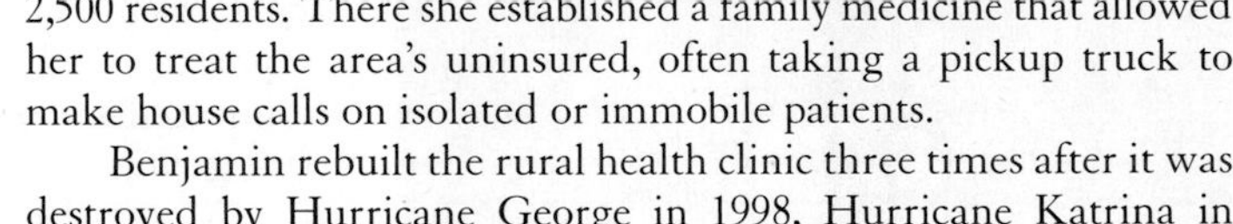

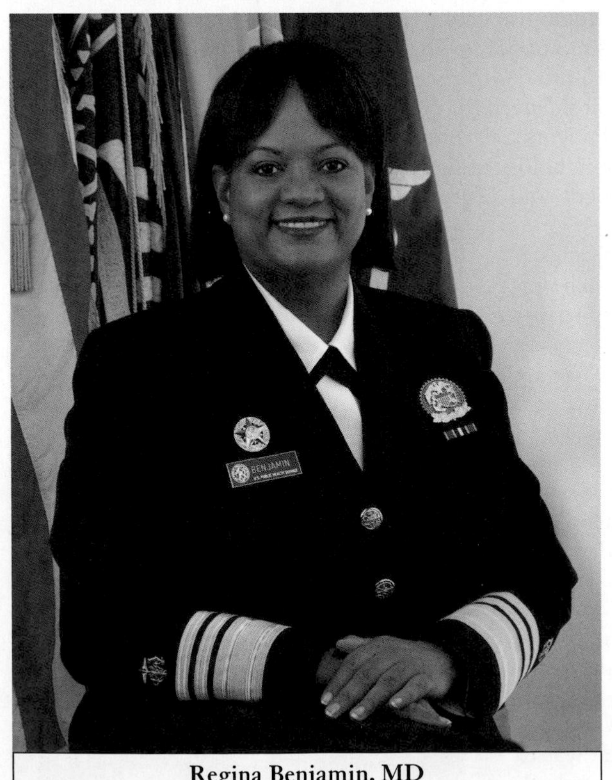

Regina Benjamin, MD

Benjamin rebuilt the rural health clinic three times after it was destroyed by Hurricane George in 1998, Hurricane Katrina in 2005, and a devastating fire in 2006. Benjamin also became the first African-American woman to head a state medical society when she was named president of the Medical Association of the State of Alabama.

Her efforts were commended by President Barack Obama, who nominated Benjamin to be "America's Doctor" on July 13, 2009. "(Benjamin) represents what's best about health care in America," Obama said. "Doctors and nurses who give and care and sacrifice for the sake of their patients; those Americans who would do anything to heal a fellow citizen . . . . When people couldn't pay, she didn't charge them. When the clinic wasn't making money, she didn't take a salary for herself. When Hurricane George destroyed the clinic in 1998, she made house calls to all her patients while it was rebuilt. When Hurricane Katrina destroyed it again and left most of her town homeless, she mortgaged her house and maxed out her credit cards to rebuild the clinic for a second time."

Serving the underserved extends beyond national boundaries, and again family medicine skills are often what's needed. That is what Dr. Stephanie Van Dyke decided, and why she entered a rural family medicine training program in Oregon. As an undergraduate, she had become very interested in a community in Uganda, so much so that, while at Albany Medical College, she returned three times, bringing physicians, residents, and other students with her. When her grandmother passed away, she used her small inheritance to establish the Engeye Health Clinic.

Reflecting on what she would need to lead the clinic, Van Dyke realized that family medicine would be the most useful training, because it was the only specialty that would prepare her to care for young and old patients and focus on the outpatient setting that was so relevant in Uganda. Specialists are often not readily available in the hospital where she chose to train. "So it forces us to do a lot of our own work," she noted. "If there's a lumbar puncture, we're it. If I have a patient with an infection, there is no infectious disease consult service, so I have to learn it and treat it myself. This type of program forces a resident to gain the competence and confidence she will need to handle things on her own afterwards."

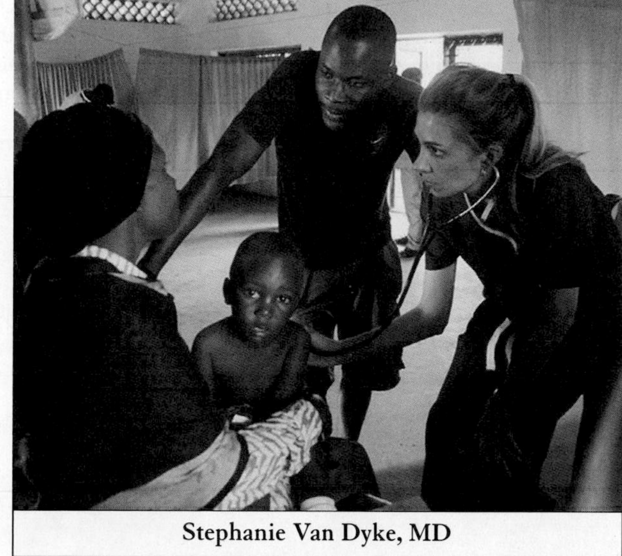

Stephanie Van Dyke, MD

Another family physician who is making an international impact is Dr. Jeffrey Heck, a professor of family medicine and also the founder and director of Shoulder to Shoulder (Hombro a Hombro), a nonprofit, nongovernmental organization that seeks to improve the health of more than 60,000 Hondurans under its care in its service area of approximately 300 square miles. Shoulder to Shoulder operates two medical centers, provides a range of dentistry services, makes home visits to elderly and chronically ill patients, maintains an electronic medical record system, holds regional health seminars and training sessions for village midwives and health promoters, provides scholarships to the brightest and poorest children, and provides entrepreneurial opportunities to help empowers girls in the area. "It is so easy to get burned out in our current health care system," Heck notes. "But I have seen thousands of medical students, residents, doctors and nurses come to Shoulder to Shoulder and leave with a renewed sense of purpose and vision as to why they are in the healthcare profession. It's transformative."

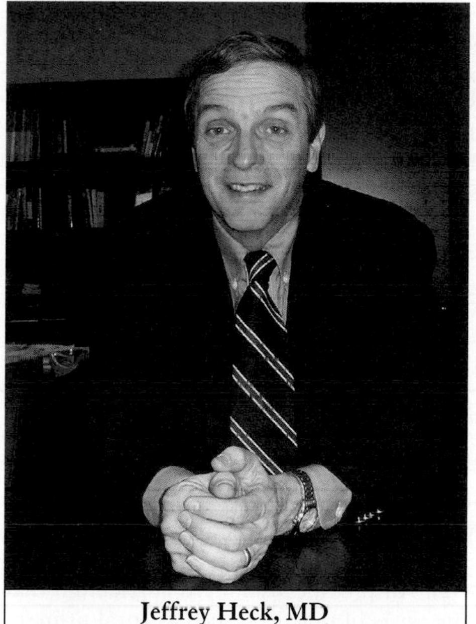

Jeffrey Heck, MD

"The great thing about being a family doctor is that you can grow with your patients. When I was a young guy in a small town, I was known as 'the kid doctor' and most of my practice was obstetrics and pediatrics. As I've gotten older, I found myself really attracted to older people. The medicine is interesting and complex and tends to draw upon the skills of an older, more experienced physician."

—Jeffrey Heck, MD

Family doctors often also work in sports medicine, and even at the Olympics. Indeed, one of the most memorable moments in Olympic diving history had family physician James Puffer right in the middle of it. It was 1988, at the Seoul Olympics, during the preliminary competition. Defending champion Greg Louganis of the United States hit his head against the diving board and splashed into the water. Louganis had only 35 minutes before his next dive, so as head physician for the US Olympic team Puffer gave the bloodied star four temporary stitches on the top of his head. "We had a limited period of time during which to care for him," Puffer said. "I remember searching for the gloves I was sure I had restocked in my medical kit that morning, but could not find them. I went ahead and sutured his scalp without the gloves and got him back in time to make his next dive that secured his place in the finals. He competed and won the gold medal the next day."

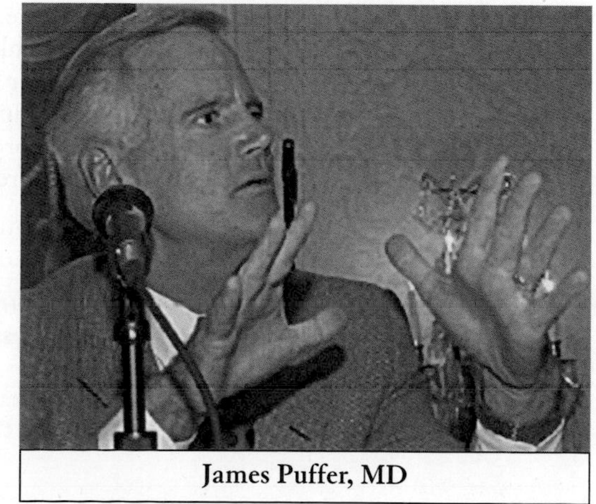

James Puffer, MD

Having won two national championships in water polo at UCLA, Puffer gravitated to sports medicine as a fourth-year medical student. "I realized the need in athletics for care provided by physicians with broad primary care training." Shortly after Puffer finished his residency, US Water Polo approached him and asked if he would put together their sports medicine program. Working his way up through the volunteer

Olympic Physician process, he helped to care for the 1984 US Winter Olympic Team in Sarajevo and was chosen as head physician in Seoul, South Korea. Dr. Puffer is now Executive Director of the American Board of Family Medicine.

Another family physician that has incorporated personal interests into his career is Dr. Jon Hallberg. "Being a generalist means I have lots of options," Hallberg remarks, and he seems to have taken advantage of all of them. He is a team doctor for the Minnesota Twins, attending their preseason training camp in Florida. He has also taken weeklong trips to Scandinavia and Eastern Europe with the St. Paul Chamber Orchestra. He acts as a public health analyst on Minnesota Public Radio, a position only appropriate for a generalist.

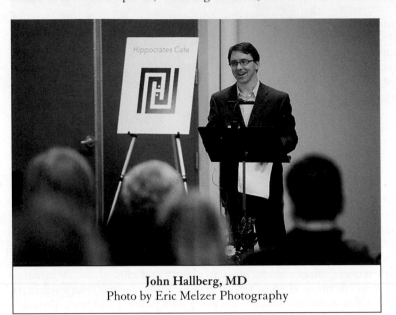

John Hallberg, MD
Photo by Eric Melzer Photography

Because of his interests in theater and community medicine, Hallberg created Hippocrates Café. "I wanted a way to bring people together—patients, neighbors, colleagues, students—and I couldn't think of anything in our professional lives that did that." The Café creates and offers performances centered on medical topics that are designed to create discussions between audience members. "We're planning one for this April on leprosy because of the heavy metaphorical aspect of the disease. I want to challenge people to think about who the lepers in our society are today. Are they the homeless, the schizophrenics, the alcoholics, those who have been disfigured? We would also like to do something to commemorate the 30th anniversary of HIV/AIDS."

Hallberg's enthusiasm for family medicine is obvious. "For me, it has always been the liberal arts approach to medicine. Family medicine justifies my broad interests, and I know I am a better physician because of it."

TRAINING OPPORTUNITIES AND RESOURCES

For students who are considering a career in family medicine, training opportunities include:

- Medical student electives. A good way for students to learn more about the range of family medicine practice is to take one or more electives sponsored by university departments of family medicine. Typically, these include a wide range of settings and practice styles.
- A residency in family medicine. As of 2009, there were 457 accredited programs (52). All provide a standard curriculum that prepares trainees to practice quality primary care. For students interested in specific types of practices, such as rural primary care, international medicine, or inner city practice, there are residencies with special concentrations in those areas.
- Postresidency fellowship training. Several fellowship training opportunities are available for family physicians who have finished residency and desire additional training, including practitioners who want to change the focus of their practice. Among the types of fellowships available to family physicians include geriatric medicine, sports medicine, preventive medicine, hospitalist care, maternal–child health, sleep medicine, adolescent medicine, and hospice and palliative medicine.
- A master's degree in public health. For people thinking of a career that would include administration or public policy work, including working in a public health department or for a state or federal agency, or for international work, a master's degree in public health or an equivalent discipline can be very valuable. Programs tailored toward physicians allow completion of the degree in a year. Preventive medicine fellowship training programs—two year programs aimed at training public health-oriented physicians—typically include obtaining a master's degree as part of their curriculum.

A good source of information is faculty within family medicine departments in medical schools. In addition, here are a few internet-based resources that are helpful to students and others considering career opportunities in family medicine:

- The Virtual Family Medicine Interest Group: *http://fmignet.aafp.org/online/fmig/index.html*
- The AAFP Directory of Family Medicine Residency Training Programs: *http://www.aafp.org/online/en/home/ membership/directories/residencyprograms.html*
- The American Board of Family Medicine residency information: *https://www.theabfm.org/residency/index.aspx*
- The American Association of Medical Colleges Careers in Medicine Page: *http://www.aamc.org/students/cim/pub_fp.htm*

CHAPTER

2

Information Mastery: Basing Care on the Best Available Evidence

Molly Cohen-Osher, Mark H. Ebell, David C. Slawson, and Allen F. Shaughnessy

CLINICAL OBJECTIVES

1. Define the role of relevance, validity, and work in determining the usefulness of an information source.
2. Distinguish the importance of secondary point-of-care resources and tools to keep up with the relevant medical literature.
3. Identify the uses and limitations of other information sources including review articles, practice guidelines, original research journals, clinical experience, lectures, experts, internet searches, controlled circulation journals, and pharmaceutical representatives.
4. Recognize key factors to consider when evaluating the relevance and validity and interpreting the results of original research on therapy.
5. Comprehend the value of sensitivity, specificity, predictive values, and likelihood ratios when evaluating diagnostic tests.

The prevailing focus in many areas of medicine is practicing "evidence-based medicine." This style of medical practice involves "an acknowledgment that there is a hierarchy of evidence and that conclusions related to evidence from controlled experiments are accorded greater credibility than conclusion grounded in other sorts of evidence" (1).

Many clinicians believe that they have always practiced in this way. However, too often decisions are actually based on local custom, habit, the clinician's experience with a single case, or the teaching of experts. An evidence-based approach means that the clinician has made the effort to identify the strongest, most valid studies, is able to change his or her mind when the evidence supports a change in practice, and acknowledges when the evidence available for making a decision is less than ideal. Sometimes we have good, clear evidence to support medical practices, whereas at other times we have relatively little information to help guide care. The trick is to know the strength of evidence available to support one's current practice, to acknowledge that level of evidence when making decisions, and to use this information to help patients choose the best approaches among valid competing alternatives.

Much of the current evidence in medicine addresses narrow questions in highly selected patients. Although this is good science, it means that data are lacking on some of the most challenging aspects of family medicine: the patient with multiple problems, and patients with vague symptoms such as fatigue and dizziness. Another limitation is that the majority of research has been conducted in referral settings and may not be applicable to primary care populations. Finally, it is worth noting that because much research funding is provided by the pharmaceutical industry, far more clinical trials have been conducted of pharmaceutical products than of alternative therapies. Thus, the absence of evidence is not evidence of absence of an effect.

The bottom line with evidence-based medicine is that the patient—not pathophysiologic reasoning, schools of thought, or specialty-specific approaches—should be the center of all care decisions. Patient outcomes that matter—decreased symptoms, better quality of life, lower mortality, and cost—should supersede tradition, anecdote, turf, authority, mental gymnastics, and other approaches that have plagued the practice of medicine.

INFORMATION MASTERY

During a typical day of patient care, a family physician generates about 15 to 20 clinical questions (2). Studies have shown that approximately two-thirds of these go unanswered. In one study, doctors' unanswered questions were submitted to medical librarians, who answered them and returned them to the physicians. Physicians reported that approximately half of the answers would have impacted their practice (3). Although most physicians want to provide evidence-based care, and want to further their own understanding and abilities, there are many reasons that these questions are never answered. They include lack of time, lack of resources, lack of the ability to find the answer, or the physician's perception that there is no good answer to their clinical question (4).

When physicians do spend the time to answer their own clinical questions, they most frequently get their answers from textbooks or colleagues. Although they may get their questions answered, textbooks are quickly outdated, and colleagues are subject to their own biases. A main concept of information mastery involves using sources that give you the highest yield of relevant and valid information with the least amount of work. This is the concept of "usefulness."

Determining Usefulness

The first key concept of information mastery is to recognize that not all sources of information are equal, but that they differ with regard to their usefulness. This useful information has three attributes: it must be relevant to our practice; it must be correct (valid); and it must take little work to obtain. These three factors can be conceptually related in the following manner:

$$\text{Usefulness of information} = \frac{\text{Relevance} \times \text{Validity}}{\text{Work}}$$

- *Relevance* refers to the applicability of the information to practice.
- *Validity* refers to the extent to which the information is scientifically based and free of bias.
- *Work* refers to the time and energy required to get the answer to your question.

Each of these concepts is discussed in more detail in the sections that follow.

RELEVANCE

When determining relevance, we need to consider whether the information is patient-oriented evidence that matters (POEM). Three questions will help you determine whether information is relevant.

1. *Did the study evaluate an outcome patients care about?* The first criterion for a POEM is that the outcome of the study be something that patients care about or is patient-oriented evidence. For example, a patient may care about symptoms, morbidity, or mortality. At first glance, you might think that all studies evaluate patient-oriented outcomes. However, if you contrast this with studies that look at disease-oriented evidence (DOEs) you will understand the distinction. A DOE study measures outcomes that are physiologic markers for disease such as blood pressure, peak flow, bacteriologic cure, or serum creatinine. Although this information is crucial to researchers in medicine, it does not always translate to clinical medicine. Disease-oriented information assumes a chain of causality that may look convincing, but links are often found to be missing or broken when the topic is studied with patient-oriented outcomes. For example, studies have shown that intensive glucose lowering can decrease hemoglobin A1c levels in patients with diabetes. This disease-oriented outcome has affected the way that we treat patients with diabetes by following a fairly convincing chain of causality—if intense glucose control lowers the A1c, it must help prolong life by decreasing myocardial infarctions, strokes, and renal failure. However, recent studies have shown that intensive glucose lowering does not decrease the patient-oriented outcome of mortality and may actually increase it (5,6). Sometimes DOEs support POEMs (e.g., treatment of hypertension with a diuretic reduces the risk of myocardial infarction and death); in other cases, the POEM disproves a therapy that had been promising based on DOEs. See Table 2.1 for more examples of disagreement between DOEs and POEMs.
2. *Did the study evaluate a condition, disease, or issue that is relevant to your practice?* The next idea in determining whether a study is a POEM is to determine if the patient-oriented outcome matters. When evaluating whether the study matters you want to consider if the problem is common and the intervention feasible. For example, a recent study might have shown that a new medication can lower strokes in patients with atrial fibrillation (a patient-oriented outcome); however, the medication is not available in the United States where you practice.

TABLE 2.1 Comparison of Disease-Oriented Evidence (DOE) with Patient-Oriented Evidence that Matters (POEM) for Common Conditions

Disease or Condition	DOE Evidence	POEM Evidence
Doxazosin for blood pressure (16)	Reduces blood pressure	Increases mortality in African-Americans
Antiarrhythmic medication following acute myocardial infarction (17)	Suppresses arrhythmias	Increases mortality
Sleeping infants on their stomach or side (18)	Anatomy and physiology suggest this will decrease aspiration	Increased risk of sudden infant death syndrome
Vitamin E to prevent for heart disease (19)	Reduces levels of free radicals	No change in mortality
Histamine antagonists and proton pump inhibitors for non-ulcer dyspepsia (20)	Significantly reduce gastric pH levels	Little or no improvement in symptoms in patients with non-gastrointestinal reflux disease, non-ulcer dyspepsia
Hormone replacement therapy to prevent heart disease (21)	Reduced low-density lipoprotein cholesterol, increased high-density lipoprotein cholesterol	No decrease in cardiovascular or all-cause mortality and an increase in cardiovascular events
β-blockers for heart failure (22)	Reduced cardiac output	Reduced mortality in moderate to severe disease

3. *If the information is true, would the findings require you to change the way you practice?* The final step in determining whether a study is a POEM is if the study results are true, will it require you to change your practice? Let's say that a recent new study shows that using estrogen in postmenopausal women is not helpful in decreasing myocardial infarctions. The study looks at a patient-oriented outcome (decreased myocardial infarctions) and the intervention is feasible (not to give estrogen). However, this is an example of patient-oriented evidence that doesn't matter because most clinicians already know that estrogen therapy for postmenopausal women does not decrease myocardial infarction, so there is no need to change their practice.

VALIDITY

Assessing the validity of research is time-consuming and difficult without formal training and a great deal of practice. In addition, after these skills are learned, busy clinicians must not only stay current with important clinical content, but also with changes in critical appraisal techniques. Several secondary sources have been created to evaluate the validity of studies and list it in a way that is transparent and easy to evaluate. These sources remove the time-consuming step of evaluating the validity of each study for you. We will discuss this more when we review point-of-care resources.

THE IDEA OF WORK

Think about the last time you did a PubMed search to find the answer to a clinical question. How long did it take you to find relevant articles? Then how long did it take you to determine whether the article or articles were based on valid study design? This can take a lot of time and energy and therefore increases the amount of work. Now think about asking an attending or a specialist for the answer to a question. How much time and energy does this take? How about looking for an answer in a textbook? What about looking on the internet? The more work you have to do to get your answer, the less useful a source is.

So why wouldn't you always want to do something quick like call an expert or use an online search engine? To answer this, you need to look at the other parts of the usefulness equation: the relevance and the validity. If you used an online search engine to look for an answer for treatment of pediatric asthma and it brings you to a parent's blog that might answer your specific question, the answer may require little work but has a good chance of not being scientifically valid. A textbook might have helpful information, but it could be outdated. Remember that relevance and validity are multiplied: if the information is not valid, its usefulness equals zero.

INFORMATION SOURCES

Now that we have discussed the concepts of why it is so important to answer clinical questions, why they are so often unanswered, and what useful information is, we need to discuss how to find the answers to our questions in the most "useful" way. Numerous sources of medical information are available, each with its advantages and disadvantages. The main ones are discussed in this section.

Strength of Recommendation Taxonomy (SORT)

Strength of recommendation	*Basis for recommendation*
A	Consistent, good-quality patient-oriented evidence
B	Inconsistent or limited-quality patient-oriented evidence
C	Consensus, disease-oriented evidence, usual practice, expert opinion, or case series for studies of diagnosis, treatment, prevention, or screening

Figure 2.1 • The Strength of Recommendation Taxonomy (SORT).

Secondary Point-of-Care Resources (Hunting Tools)

There are multiple point-of-care resources that have been developed to organize all of the relevant medical literature (i.e., those involving POEMs) and synthesize the information into a searchable database. The more useful of these sources grade the validity of an individual study and the strength of the evidence of a recommendation based on a body of research. Most grading systems focus primarily on validity, although the Strength of Recommendations Taxonomy (SORT) (Fig. 2.1) also incorporates relevance into its grading scheme. These systems are important because they give you a quick way to judge the usefulness of the information you are reading. Figure 2.1 presents the SORT taxonomy.

In addition to grading the validity, the more useful point-of-care resources are *transparent*, meaning that they describe the process that they use to gather their evidence, the inclusion and exclusion criterion for information, and any conflicts of interest with study sponsors.

Medical students are generally taught the skills to evaluate relevance and understand the validity of research studies. However, with more than 20,000 original research articles and 200 to 300 POEMs published annually in the top 100 clinical journals, it is impractical to do it all yourself. Instead, you should familiarize yourself with one or more independent sources that survey the literature, evaluate relevance (ideally using the POEMs criteria described previously), assess the article for validity and bias, and summarize it in a concise, structured format for you. Sources are even available that automatically download the latest summaries to your handheld computer. Such sources are summarized in Table 2.2.

Keeping up with the Literature (Foraging Tools)

To remain an effective clinician you need a source (or sources) of information for answering clinical questions, but you also need a source (or sources) of information to keep current. New important research with patient-oriented evidence that matters is being generated at a rapid pace, but unless you know that this new information exists, you would not know that there is a need to change your practice. Therefore, it is imperative that students and physicians develop a system to keep up with the

TABLE 2.2 Web-based Sources of Evidence-Based Clinical Information

Site	Web Address	Comment
Free		
Centre for Evidence-Based Medicine	*http://cebm.jr2.ox.ac.uk/*	This site has useful tools and resources, including the "official" table of levels of evidence
Netting the Evidence	*http://www.shef.ac.uk/~scharr/ir/netting*	An extensive list of sites
Bandolier	*http://www.jr2.ox.ac.uk/Bandolier/index.html*	Popular British site, includes essays and features a good sense of humor
National Guidelines Clearinghouse	*www.guidelines.gov*	Repository for practice guidelines. Note that not all are evidence based
Subscription		
Essential Evidence Plus	*www.essentialevidenceplus.com*	Source of POEMs, Cochrane abstracts, guidelines, and decision support software
Gwent/Turning Research Into Practice (TRIP)	*http://www.tripdatabase.com*	Lets you search over a dozen evidence-based sites at once
The Cochrane Library	*http://www.updateusa.com/clibhome/clib.htm*	The Cochrane Library contains the Cochrane Database of Systematic Reviews, the Database of Abstracts of Reviews of Effectiveness, and The Cochrane Controlled Trials Register
ACP Journal Club	*http://www.acpjc.org/*	Abstracts of adult medicine studies with commentary
Dynamed	*http://www.dynamic medical.com/*	A medical information database with clinical topic summaries as well as weekly updates

patient-oriented evidence that matters. The most useful foraging tools are transparent, clearly describing their criterion for inclusion and exclusion, methods, and affiliations or conflicts of interest. E-mail services such as Daily POEMs or Dynamed Weekly Updates present information filtered for relevance and validity in bite-sized pieces. The *Prescriber's Letter* offers updates in short paragraphs, with more information online for readers wanting more information. *The ACP Journal Club, Bandolier, Journal Watch, FP-IM Database*, and others, provide abstracts and sometimes commentary on articles of interest to family physicians. Review services, such as *The Medical Letter* and *Primary Care Reports*, AAFP Home Study course, as well as audiotape subscription services such as the *Audio-Digest* series focus on one or a few issues each month. As with any source of information, consider the relevance (how the articles are selected for the newsletter) and validity (how they are evaluated).

Increasingly, audio digests and newsletters are being offered as podcasts. They automate the updating process, are often free, and can be listened to while exercising or driving. Remember, though, to look for relevance and validity in these low-work sources.

Other Information Sources

Although the electronic products mentioned previously should often be used first to answer clinical questions at the point-of-care, there are times when other resources can be valuable. These include review articles, practice guidelines, controlled circulation journals, lectures, clinical experience, experts, internet searches, and pharmaceutical representatives. Each of these can and should be evaluated for relevance and validity.

REVIEW ARTICLES

There are two types of medical review articles: systematic reviews/meta analyses and summary reviews.

Systematic reviews and meta analyses focus on only one or two clinical questions. A good systematic review has four steps: 1) identification of one or two highly focused clinical questions; 2) an exhaustive search of the world's medical literature; 3) evaluation of the quality of each article, with inclusion of only those that meet criteria for quality; and 4) synthesis of the data. The synthesis can be qualitative (a textual description of the bottom line) or quantitative (using specific statistical methods to combine the data from different studies into a single summary measure of effect, a technique called meta-analysis, a technique that can only be done when the outcome measures from different studies are generally the same and their study designs are similar). Systematic reviews and meta-analyses can be powerful tools because they have an increased ability to draw valid conclusions over single articles. For example, 19 of 23 trials of the use of β-blockers after myocardial infarction did not show a statistically significant benefit to this therapy. However, when all of the trial results were analyzed together, β-blocker therapy was associated with a 23% relative reduction of the risk of death (7).

One of the best sources of this type of high quality review is the Cochrane Library (*http://www.updateusa.com/clibhome/clib.htm*). It includes the Cochrane Database of Systematic Reviews. Each review is aimed at answering a specific question (e.g., "Are antibiotics effective in the treatment of acute bronchitis in adults?"). The methods used to identify all relevant research on this question are outlined in the review. Only results of randomized, controlled trials—the strongest form of clinical research—are used in the reviews. The Cochrane Library also includes the Database of Abstracts of Reviews of Effectiveness, a compilation of systematic reviews from other sources that meet the Cochrane's rigorous standards for systematic reviews. The Cochrane Controlled Trials Register is a database of more than 260,000 individual controlled clinical trials and their abstracts, many of which are not found in Medline.

Summary reviews cover a lot of ground, making in-depth discussion of individual points impossible. As a result, it is difficult to assess the validity of the information behind the conclusion, and bias, often unrecognized by the author, can creep into these reviews. A recent analysis of review articles on type II diabetes examined the methodological rigor of both relevance and validity assessments. It found that the average score was 1 of a possible high score of 15, with the best score being only 5 (8). In 1993, Oxman et al. identified 36 summary review articles and had them evaluated by professionals trained to critique review articles for methodological rigor using 10 criteria (9). What they found was that reviews written by experts in a particular field consistently received lower scores than those written by nonexperts.

Summary reviews may not be current, especially in rapidly changing areas of medicine. For example, 6 years elapsed between publication of a meta-analysis showing a pronounced decrease in mortality by thrombolytic therapy for myocardial infarction and when the majority of reviews recommended its general use (10), and even longer before it was routinely recommended in medical textbooks.

Textbooks such as this one can be thought of as collections of summary reviews. They usually present the bottom line and are sometimes hard to evaluate for validity. One thing that distinguishes this textbook is the focus on an evidence-based approach to care, which means providing detailed information to support each recommendation. Because textbooks gradually become outdated, textbooks of the future will increasingly use electronic methods to update themselves.

PRACTICE GUIDELINES

The goal of practice guidelines (also called policies, consensus reports, or practice parameters) is to help clinicians improve the quality of care that they deliver and reduce inappropriate variation in practice. Although some guidelines come from a careful synthesis of all of the available evidence, others are developed by simply polling experts for their consensus opinion. The latter may reduce inappropriate variation in practice, but do not necessarily improve the quality of care. When evaluating a guideline, look for a description of how the evidence was assembled, and make sure that the authors rate the strength of key recommendations. The best use of clinical guidelines is as a suggestion to help govern most practice most of the time, and not as an inviolable protocol. Like a master chef, you will learn to use these cookbooks as the guides that they are designed to be, taking each recipe and varying it to meet the needs of the moment.

ORIGINAL RESEARCH JOURNALS

Research journals can help us to find answers to specific questions as well as to stay abreast of new medical developments. However, reviewing original research can be time-consuming. It can also be difficult to find the most relevant article, and original research articles are usually not quick reading. Examples of original research journals include *JAMA, Annals of Family Medicine, BMJ,* and at least 4,000 others.

Research studies published in knowledge-creation journals can be quickly skimmed for relevance by reading the title of the article and the abstract. This initial screen should focus on the three questions that we used to determine relevance for POEMs previously:

- Is the problem studied one that is common to my practice and is the intervention feasible?
- Did the authors study an outcome that patients would care about?
- Will this information, if true, require me to change my current practice?

This simple screening method will help you quickly eliminate most of the articles in research journals (11,12).

CLINICAL EXPERIENCE

Clinical experience is often given short shrift in discussions of evidence-based medicine and information mastery. This is unfortunate, because clinical experience and clinical skills are central to the effective, compassionate practice of medicine. Information mastery does not tell us how to listen to a patient, take a comprehensive history, perform a physical examination, communicate effectively with patients, help them make decisions that are best for them, or deal with ethical issues. However, information mastery does help us make the best use of the information that we gather from patients, helps us streamline our clinical examination to focus on the most important elements, and helps us present the best possible array of options to our patients. The synthesis of information mastery and clinical experience is "clinical jazz," because it melds the structure and rhythm of the scientific method with the improvisation and skill of clinical practice.

LECTURES

Clinicians often leave a continuing medical education (CME) lecture feeling they have learned something. However, a large body of research has shown that practice habits are rarely influenced by CME presentations. This has been called "Chinese dinner memory dysfunction," which is a temporary feeling of satiety derived from "learning something" that is quickly followed by an inability to remember or apply information (13). To evaluate the usefulness of a CME presentation, ask yourself: Is the topic common or important in your practice? Is the speaker focusing on patient-oriented outcomes or disease-oriented outcomes? Does the speaker cite the strength of supporting evidence for key recommendations, or does the talk appear to be based on anecdote, habit, and custom? Does the speaker refer to key evidence-based sources, such as the

Cochrane Database, systematic reviews, and evidence-based guidelines, or is the survey of the literature more selective? Do not assume that the speaker is an expert who is beyond reproach. The next section should give you some insight into why experts can and must be questioned.

EXPERTS

We often turn to someone with greater experience and knowledge in a particular area when we have a question. These people are content experts. Information from a content expert tends to be quite subjective; even in narrowly focused specialties, experts have a tough time agreeing. The experts cannot be faulted for these discrepancies, for all of medicine has built-in imprecision, and the toughest areas are often the ones involving human interpretation. Furthermore, experts will often have diagnostic or therapeutic approaches that they believe in, for which the evidence is not as strong as their opinion. All of these issues make expert opinion questionable, though unquestionably also quite useful.

There is another type of expert, the clinical scientist. These experts in methodology may be physicians, pharmacists, epidemiologists, or librarians who are expert at evaluating information for validity but are not necessarily content experts. They are able to give an objective assessment of the quality of information, unencumbered by the bias of experience and training, but are at times unable to interpret the validity or clinical usefulness of the literature.

INTERNET SEARCHES

Using internet search engines is a way that many physicians use to find answers to clinical questions. Now think about a search engine such as Google, and relate it to the usefulness equation. What do you think about the work, reliability and validity? A search engine such as Google often decreases your work—it is quick and brings you to many sources. However, the sources that Google brings you to all have differing reliability and validity which may be very difficult to determine.

CONTROLLED CIRCULATION JOURNALS

Also called translation journals, these are journals delivered without charge to physicians, supported solely by pharmaceutical company or device manufacturer advertising. They consist mainly of expert reviews or opinion. *Patient Care, Emergency Medicine, Hospital and Staff Physician*, and many others are in this category. Articles in these publications are generally fun to read and are useful for review or for rapidly refamiliarizing yourself with a topic. The downside of these articles is that too often there is no real quality control to ensure the information is correct. Unlike systematic reviews, these articles generally are written backwards, meaning the author writes his or her conclusions and then finds data to support this viewpoint, rather than looking at all of the data and arriving at a conclusion. Some journals, such as *American Family Physician*, have greatly improved the "evidence-basedness" of their articles in recent years by providing evidence summaries to authors and requiring strength of evidence labeling.

PHARMACEUTICAL REPRESENTATIVES

These well-dressed, polite individuals present their information in an easy-to-understand fashion. The relevance and validity of their information, as with any other source, should be carefully evaluated, however, pharmaceutical representatives have a job to do, and that job is to sell specific medications. As a result, speaking to pharmaceutical representatives is a highly inefficient method of getting information and should generally be minimized. If you do speak with sales representatives, keep in mind: (a) the common sales techniques they employ (Table 2.3), and (b) the STEPS mnemonic, which stands for five characteristics of a drug that determine its

TABLE 2.3 Sales Techniques Often Used to Promote Pharmaceuticals

Technique	Example
Appeal to authority: Using the opinion of an authority, not the evidence, to support a particular medication	"Dr. Knowitall, the famous cardiologist from Atlanta, prescribes our drug a lot!"
The Bandwagon appeal: Using the popularity of a medication to support its superiority	"Cephakillitall is the most widely prescribed antibiotic in the United States!"
The red herring appeal: Using factual but irrelevant information (disease-oriented evidence) to support a medication.	"Our antibiotic achieves the highest minimum inhibitory concentration in the respiratory epithelium!"
The appeal to pity: Basing a decision on emotions (pity, wishful thinking) instead of the evidence	"You've got to help me out here—our sales are really suffering this year!"
Appeal to curiosity: Similar to the red herring appeal, it is the use of a demonstration or highlighting of a nonclinical uniqueness to captivate your mind	"Our pill has a unique shape that's easy to remember!
Error of omission: Not mentioning useful information. The STEPS acronym (see text) can help identify omissions.	"Really? A recent study showed it's no more effective than hydrochlorothiazide? I'll look into that, doctor!"

usefulness: Safety, Tolerability, Effectiveness, Price, and Simplicity. Also, remember to focus on patient-oriented rather than disease-oriented outcomes. If you don't hear any, don't be afraid to ask for it.

DECIPHERING RESEARCH REPORTS

Reading an original research study can be a challenge: the language is often stilted, the articles are filled with acronyms, and the statistics can be intimidating. In the next section, we will help you understand how to interpret research results.

Therapy

There are many biases that can invalidate the results of a study of therapy. The best way to overcome these biases is to randomize, double blind, control, and have concealed allocation. *Randomization* means that patients are randomly assigned to one arm of the study or another; this increases the likelihood that the only difference between groups is the treatment intervention. *Double blind* means that both patients and investigators don't know who is a treatment or control subject. Having a *placebo* or better yet *active comparison group* (one that receives current "best practice" treatment) also improves the validity of the study. *Concealing allocation* prevents the researcher who is recruiting subjects from knowing to which group the patient will be assigned, precluding inadvertent or deliberate selective enrollment of subjects based on this knowledge.

As described previously, the most valid research about a therapy comes from randomized controlled double-blinded studies. However, there are many other types of study design that are frequently used to evaluate therapies. Case-control and cohort studies are not randomized; they may mistakenly find an association between a treatment and a favorable outcome (or harm) because they are unable to adjust for unknown confounding variables (14).

The next thing to consider when you are reviewing a study on therapy is how to interpret the results. Interpretation of study results usually starts with the p-value, the probability that a difference between two groups was simply by chance. A p value of 0.05 (the usual criterion for "statistical significance") tell us there is only a 5% chance that the findings represent chance rather than a real effect of the intervention on the outcome. However, this means that there is still a 1-in-20 chance that the difference in treatment is actually due to chance. The lower the p value is, the more certain you can be that the difference between the groups was not simply due to chance.

Once we know that a difference is statistically significant, we need to understand the magnitude of benefit. This is where it gets really tricky, because we can easily be influenced by how the data are presented. For example, studies have shown that statins will decrease the likelihood of a heart attack or stroke, but summary results can be expressed in many ways. Here are some of the ways one can present the same benefit of statin therapy in a high risk patient (one with a 10% risk of a heart attack or stroke over 10 years):

- The risk decreases from 10% to 8% (absolute risk)
- The risk reduction is 20% (relative risk reduction)
- The risk decreases by 2 percentage points (absolute risk reduction)
- One heart attack or stroke is prevented among 50 high-risk people who are treated for 10 years (number needed to treat [NNT])
- For every 50 high-risk people treated with a statin, 49 will not receive benefit (NNT, negative spin)
- For every 50 high-risk people treated with a statin, 48 will be healthy regardless of treatment, 1 will experience a heart attack or stroke despite treatment, and 1 will be prevented from having a heart attack or stroke (NNT, expanded)

Graphic representations can also give us a different feel for the data (Figs. 2.2a–d). The advantage of using number needed to treat or the graphic depiction of smiley faces (Fig. 2.2d) is that it is often easier to understand, especially when comparing the effect of different interventions, and facilitates communication with patients about risk and benefit. When the likelihood of an outcome is low, NNTs will be high. NNTs will decrease as either the likelihood of the outcome increases or as the benefit of the treatment increases. Table 2.4 presents some NNTs for various medical interventions.

Diagnosis

Often, a study will describe the accuracy of a diagnostic test. Tests can include history and physical examination maneuvers, clinical decision rules such as the Ottawa Ankle Rules, blood tests, and imaging studies. It is important to evaluate the overall benefit of using a new diagnostic test. Does the test change diagnosis? Does it change treatment? Does it change patient-oriented outcomes? Is it cost effective? These questions can only be answered in clinical trials where the new diagnostic test is used in one population of patients (the intervention group) and not in another (the control group).

The accuracy of a diagnostic test can be expressed in several ways. Designers of diagnostic tests evaluate the accuracy using sensitivity and specificity, since these statistics do not change based on the prevalence of disease. *Sensitivity* is the proportion of patients with disease who have a positive test, while *specificity* is the proportion of patients without disease who have a negative test.

$$\text{Sensitivity} = \frac{\text{\# with a true positive test}}{\text{\# persons with disease}}$$

$$\text{Sensitivity} = \frac{\text{\# with a true negative test}}{\text{\# persons without disease}}$$

In many cases, sensitivity and specificity can be used in clinical practice using the Spin and Snout mnemonics. When positive, tests with a very high specificity can rule in disease (Spin), whereas tests with a very high sensitivity, if negative, can rule out disease (Snout). This rule works for many tests when the prevalence of disease is neither very high nor very low.

Positive (PPV) and *negative predictive values (NPV)* are more useful to clinicians because they reflect diagnostic test performance at different degrees of prevalence of disease (pretest probability). The PPV is the proportion of patients with a positive test who actually have disease, whereas the

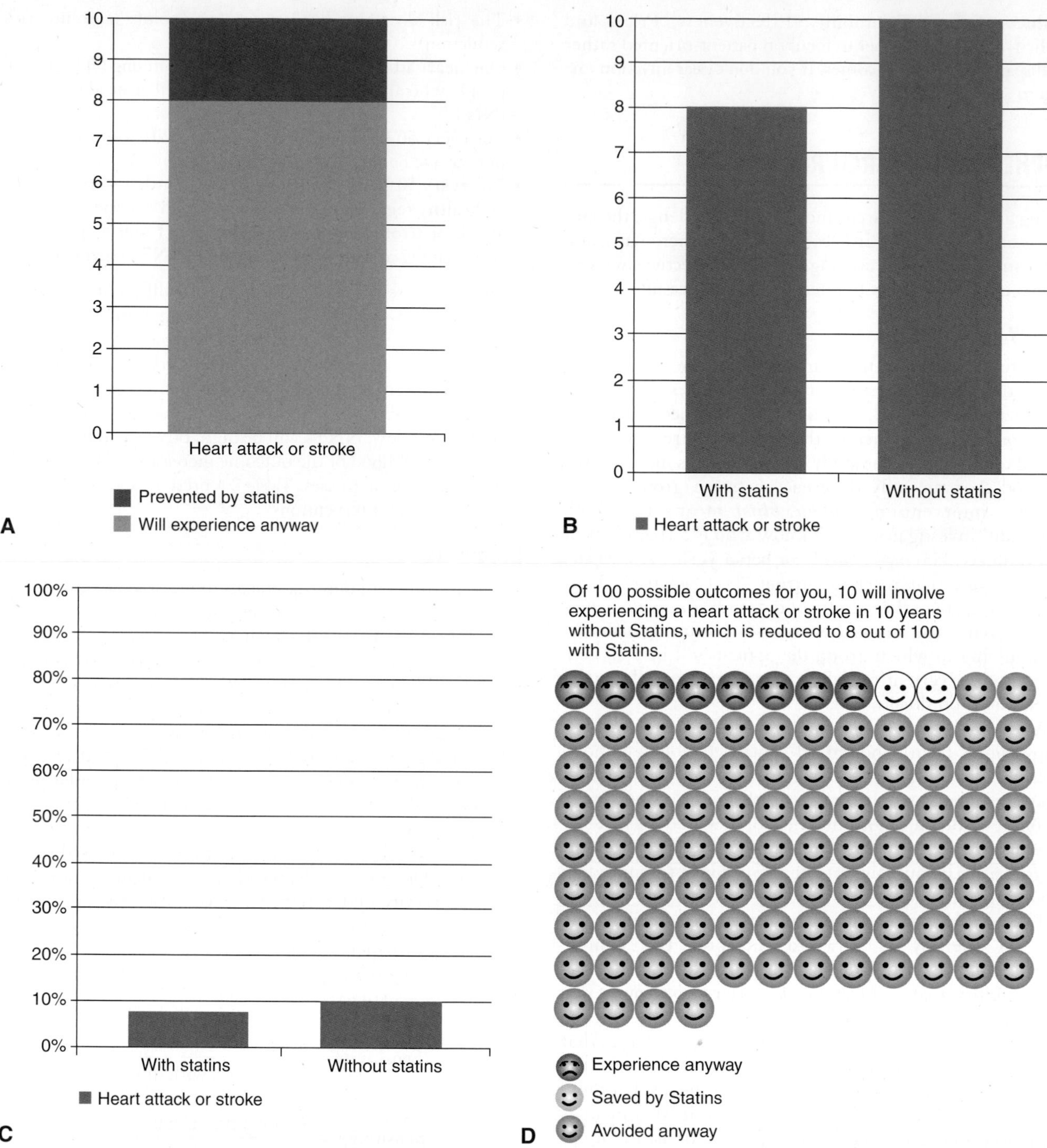

Figure 2.2 • Four ways of illustrating the same result involving the effect of taking statins for more than 10 years for patients at high risk of heart attack and stroke. Figure 2.2a displays the relative risk reduction; Figure 2.2b compares the relative risk; Figure 2.2c compares the absolute risk among statin users and nonusers; and Figure 2.2d uses a smiley face representation to demonstrate the number needed to treat. (*Source*: 2,845 ways to spin the risk. Available at: *http://understandinguncertainty.org/node/233*)

NPV is the proportion of patients with a negative test who are actually free of disease.

$$PPV = \frac{\text{\# of true-positive test results}}{(\text{\# of true-positive results}) + (\text{number of false-positive results})}$$

$$= \frac{(\text{sensitivity}) \times (\text{prevalence})}{[(\text{sensitivity}) \times (\text{prevalence}) + (1\text{-specificity})\,(1\text{-prevalence})]}$$

$$NPV = \frac{\text{\# of true-negative test results}}{(\text{\# of true-negative results}) + (\text{numbe of false-negative results})}$$

$$= \frac{(\text{specificity}) \times (1\text{-prevalence})}{[(\text{specificity})(1\text{-prrevalence}) + (1\text{-sensitivity})\,(\text{prevalence})]}$$

USING PREDICTIVE VALUES: THE STORY OF BABY JEFF JR.

Jeff Jr. was the first born baby to a family medicine resident, Dr. Jeff, and his wife after years of difficulty conceiving. As you could imagine, the new parents were thrilled. A new screening test for all male newborns had been implemented at the hospital where Baby Jeff was born a few weeks before his arrival that boasted a sensitivity of 100% and a specificity of 99.98% for detecting muscular dystrophy with a heel stick CPK. Much to everyone's dismay, Baby Jeff's CPK test was abnormal. Mom and Dr. Jeff called the neonatologist to ask what the likelihood was that Baby Jeff had muscular dystrophy and they were told that it was unfortunately very high (what with the high sensitivity and specificity of the test) and that they should start preparing themselves for this. To confirm the diagnosis, however, Baby Jeff would need a gastrocnemius biopsy, but he would have to wait a few weeks to get this done. Mom, Dad, and their whole family were devastated. Mom couldn't stop crying and Dr. Jeff was distraught that he had made this baby his namesake.

A few weeks later, Baby Jeff went for the biopsy and the results were negative! Everybody was relieved. So, the question is—did Baby Jeff's parents get lucky? Was he the rare negative?

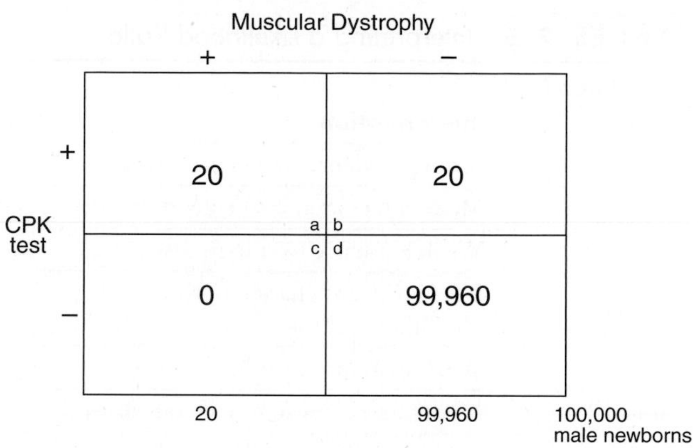

Figure 2.3 • Two-by-two table illustrating that the predictive value of a positive predictive value (PPV) in the case of Jeff Jr. is 50%. In a population of 100,000 people with a prevalence of muscular dystrophy of 1 in 5,000 (0.02%), 20 will have muscular dystrophy (100,000 × 0.0002). Because the test has a sensitivity of 100%, the test will correctly identify all 20 babies that have the disease. 100,000 of the sample minus 20 male newborns who truly have muscular dystrophy is 99,980 males in the sample who truly do not have muscular dystrophy. The specificity of the test is 99.98%, which leaves 99,960 of the males without muscular dystrophy who will test negative (99,980 × 0.9998). Subtracting 99,960 from 99,980 identifies that 20 males who do not have muscular dystrophy will have a positive screening test, or a PPV of 50% (15).

To answer this, we need to determine what Baby Jeff's probability of having muscular dystrophy was just based on the screening test. The prevalence of muscular dystrophy at birth ranges from 1 in 3,500 to 1 in 15,000 male births. Using a conservative and easy estimate to calculate prevalence—1 in 5,000 males or 0.02%—we can calculate the predictive value to be only 50%. So the likelihood that Baby Jeff actually had muscular dystrophy before he had the biopsy was only 50-50 (15). This is illustrated in Figure 2.3.

TABLE 2.4 Examples of Numbers Needed to Treat (NNT)*

Therapy	Event Prevented	Length of Follow-up	NNT
Helicobacter pylori eradication in duodenal ulcer	Ulcer at 1 year	1 year	1.1
Finasteride for benign prostatic hypertropy	Need for one operation	2 years	39
Streptokinase and aspirin for acute myocardial infarction	One death	5 weeks	20
Enalapril for Class I or II chronic heart failure	One death	1 year	100
Lipid lowering in patients with congestive heart disease	One myocardial infarction or stroke-related death	5 years	16
Treatment of mild hypertension	One myocardial infarction, stroke, or death	1 year	700
Treatment of severe hypertension	One myocardial infarction, stroke, or death	1 year	15

*The number of patients that would need to be treated to prevent one adverse clinical event during the follow-up period.

TABLE 2.5 Interpreting a Likelihood Ratio

Likelihood Ratio	Interpretation
>10	Strong evidence to rule in disease
5–10	Moderate evidence to rule in disease
2–5	Weak evidence to rule in disease
0.5–2	No significant change in the likelihood of disease
0.2–0.5	Weak evidence to rule out disease
0.1–0.2	Moderate evidence to rule out disease
<0.1	Strong evidence to rule out disease

The story of Baby Jeff teaches us an important lesson about the utility of sensitivity and specificity. Sensitivity and specificity only tell us the usefulness of the test in identifying positive and negative test results, not necessarily in determining the disease in a person. This can only be answered by factoring in the prevalence of the disease and using PPV and NPV, or by using a more clinically useful measure called the likelihood ratio.

LIKELIHOOD RATIOS

Likelihood ratios have the advantage of not changing when the likelihood of disease changes. The likelihood ratio describes the degree that a positive or negative test result increases or decreases the likelihood of having the disease. Every test has its own likelihood ratio. A likelihood ratio >1 indicates an increased likelihood of disease, whereas a likelihood ratio <1 reduces the likelihood of disease. The further the likelihood ratio is from 1, the more likely the test will signify the presence or absence of disease. A likelihood ratio between 0.2 and 5.0 means that the test result has only a small effect on the likelihood of disease. Likelihood ratios of >5.0 and <0.2 are associated with a greater likelihood of detecting the presence or absence of disease.

Table 2.5 gives some general guidelines on how to interpret likelihood ratios. Using the nomogram on the inside cover of this book, you can use likelihood ratios to convert a pretest probability to a posttest probability. Another important aspect of likelihood ratios is that they can be used to describe the accuracy of tests with multiple outcomes, such as a test that categorizes patients as low, moderate, high, and very high risk.

USING INFORMATION TO CHANGE YOUR PRACTICE WITH CONFIDENCE

As a physician, you should continuously reflect on your performance, learn to value the clinical questions that arise in daily practice, and make an effort to answer them with the best available evidence. The best physician asks more questions, not fewer.

Develop a system for yourself to keep track of your clinical questions. Familiarize yourself with useful (low work, valid, reliable, and transparent) resources that you feel comfortable using in order to answer your questions either during the point-of-care or soon after. Find high-quality foraging tools that help keep you up to date.

Finally, remember that good evidence is available to support only about half of what we do as physicians. This leaves much room to include personal experience, reasoning, and the preferences of patients in the decision-making process. Seek to combine clinical experience with information mastery to provide evidenced based, patient-centered care.

KEY POINTS

- Not all information resources are of equal value. Think about the relevance, validity, work, and transparency of your sources.
- Familiarize yourself with different point-of-care resources and tools to keep up with the relevant medical literature. Choose a few that you like best and develop a system to integrate new information into your practice.
- Evaluating original research can be a lot of work. If you choose to do it, remember the tools you can use to evaluate relevance, validity, study results, and diagnostic tests.

II

Preventive Care

CHAPTER 3

Overview of Prevention and Screening

Anthony J. Viera and David V. Power

CLINICAL OBJECTIVES

1. Define primary, secondary, and tertiary prevention.
2. Understand the elements that constitute a useful screening test.
3. Appreciate that not all available screening tools or prevention strategies improve health.
4. Access up-to-date resources on prevention.

This chapter is an introduction to the preventive care section of this book. In many ways, the family physician is the most ideally placed of all physicians to recommend preventive care to his or her patients, given the continuous relationships over time that are developed with patients and families. In this chapter, we will review the general topic of prevention, present definitions, and outline a broad approach to applying prevention in practice, irrespective of patient age. We will review general principles and present links to useful resources to allow you to stay current with evidence-based recommendations for preventive care. Each subsequent chapter in this section will address specific elements of prevention as they relate to particular populations or age groups.

WHAT IS PREVENTION?

The goal of preventive medicine is to protect, promote, and maintain health and well-being and prevent disease, disability, and premature death. Prevention has traditionally been divided into three different categories designated primary, secondary, and tertiary prevention. With *primary prevention*, efforts are directed at healthy individuals to avoid the development of disease. Recommendations to maintain an ideal body weight, never commence smoking cigarettes, and eat a balanced diet are examples of primary preventive strategies. *Secondary prevention* efforts are those aimed at detecting early disease so that further morbidity or symptoms can be reduced. An example is screening for elevated fasting blood glucose in hypertensive patients before they have developed any symptoms of diabetes. *Tertiary prevention* refers to efforts intended to improve both the health outcomes of people with a diagnosed disease and preventing further morbidity from that condition. An example is taking an antithrombotic agent to prevent recurrent stroke in those who have suffered a cerebrovascular accident. Much of the work of family physicians falls into one of these categories of prevention. Every patient encounter is an opportunity to think about health risks and consider how to prevent adverse outcomes, whereas specific health care maintenance clinic visits allow greater time to address prevention.

WHEN SHOULD PREVENTION BE CONSIDERED?

As a clinician, it is important to approach prevention with a clear understanding of what health problem or adverse event you are trying to prevent. Keep in mind that the goal of prevention is to help people live longer or have better quality of life, not merely to detect disease early. We must also recognize that not every health problem can be prevented. An important initial criterion for deciding whether a health problem should be included in routine preventive care is the burden of suffering caused by the problem. Burden of suffering is determined not only by the prevalence of the health problem in the population, but also by the seriousness of the health problem. Seriousness of the health problem can be thought of in terms of the "6 Ds": death, disease, disability, discomfort, dissatisfaction, and destitution. The more of these the problem causes, the more serious it is. Another useful way to think about seriousness of the health problem is in terms of disability-adjusted life years (DALYs). DALYs for a health problem are calculated as the sum of the years of life lost from premature mortality from that problem and the years lost from disability for incident cases of that health problem. The sum of DALYs across a population can be thought of as a measurement of the gap between current health status and an ideal health situation in which the entire population lives to an advanced age, free of disease and disability.

A second—but critical—criterion that must be met before incorporating prevention into clinical practice is that there must be an effective and safe intervention that improves outcomes. In primary prevention, the intervention must work to delay or prevent the health problem. In secondary prevention (screening), there must be an effective treatment that prevents disease from advancing, and it must be more effective when applied at the time asymptomatic disease is found than if applied at the time the patient would have presented with symptoms. Obviously, any preventive intervention must have low potential for causing harm. Remember that clinical prevention means that we are offering something to people who have no symptoms. Because most prevention interventions must be offered to many people for only a few to benefit, we must ensure that the benefits clearly outweigh any potential harm.

A third criterion is cost-effectiveness. It is often assumed that prevention always saves the health care system money.

Although this is true for a few interventions, most preventive interventions actually add cost. The question that must be asked is whether the preventive intervention is worth the cost in terms of lives saved, disability prevented, or quality of life gained. Cost-effectiveness is a particular consideration when there is more than one intervention that could be used to prevent a given health problem. For example, before statins became available generically, it was more cost-effective to offer aspirin alone to people at moderate risk for coronary heart disease (1).

A final but important general comment is that prevention should be thought of as a population-level activity. That is, many patients must participate for the effects to be seen. Also, all preventive measures can provide have benefits, harms, and costs. Typically, a prevention intervention yields large benefits only for a very small number of participants. A large number of participants will be caused minor harms, inconveniences, and expenses; and more substantial harms and costs will accrue to a variable number. For example, of 1,900 women ages 40 to 49 years who are screened for 10 years by mammography, one woman will not die of breast cancer who otherwise would have. She is the one who benefits. All 1,900 women undergo the minor harm of an uncomfortable test, and many undergo the more substantial harms of biopsy, worry about a false positive, and even unnecessary treatment of overdiagnosed breast cancers. All 1,900 of the women also have the cost (or cost-share) of mammography, and some have the costs of further evaluation and treatment.

WHAT IS SCREENING?

Screening is testing for a health problem or risk factor when there are no recognized signs or symptoms that would indicate the presence of that problem or risk factor. It is important to remember that the goal of screening is not merely to *find* problems, however. The goal of screening is to identify asymptomatic people for whom an intervention will help reduce the progression of early disease or prevent an adverse health event. An example of screening is sampling the ectocervix (performing a Pap smear) on asymptomatic sexually active adult women with the goal of detecting early cervical cancer. When early precancerous or cancerous changes are discovered, treatment effectively reduces a woman's risk of cervical cancer and reduces mortality (2). Remember that performing tests in patients who already have symptoms is not screening. For example, a Pap smear for a woman with abnormal bleeding, lower abdominal pain, and weight loss would instead be a diagnostic test performed as part of a workup.

Recognize that not all screening tests are laboratory tests. Any question you ask an asymptomatic patient on a review of systems can be considered a screening "test." Physical examination maneuvers performed on asymptomatic patients (e.g., during a "routine physical") are all screening interventions. Questionnaires, radiology studies, and various procedures are all used in certain instances as screening tests. Screening can be the initial intervention that results in a cascade of subsequent events that ultimately can help a person by preventing disease progression or adverse health outcomes. Alternatively, though, the cascade of events started by screening could yield no benefit, or in some cases, could even lead to harm. For example, teaching of self-breast examination leads to more breast imaging and unnecessary breast biopsies, but with an end result of no increase in either early detection of breast cancer or reduced mortality from breast cancer (3).

TABLE 3.1 Criteria to Guide Evaluation of a Screening Program

- Significant burden of suffering of the target health problem
- Detectable preclinical phase exists
- Adequate sensitivity, specificity, and predictive value of available screening test
- Intervention that when administered in the detectable preclinical phase is more effective than if given when symptoms develop
- Screening procedure is acceptable
- Program is cost-effectiveness and benefit exceeds harm for the population screened

There are several characteristics of a screening program that must be considered when evaluating its effectiveness (Table 3.1). The significance and prevalence of the health problem, existence of an effective intervention, and cost-effectiveness were discussed above. Other features pertinent to screening are that: (1) the health condition must have a detectable preclinical phase, (2) the screening test must perform well, and (3) the screening test must be acceptable to patients.

Detectable Preclinical Phase

The condition that screening is to identify must have a preclinical (asymptomatic or latent) phase that can be detected by the screening test. A health problem that causes symptoms immediately or relatively soon after its onset would not be a candidate for a screening program. Influenza, for example, is a common illness for which prevention is valuable to reduce morbidity and mortality. However, there is no preclinical phase during which "pre-influenza" is detectable. Prevention efforts for influenza must therefore use alternative primary prevention strategies such as immunization, hand-washing, and masks. It is worth reiterating that a screening program's effectiveness ultimately hinges on whether an intervention given during the detectable preclinical phase works better than an intervention given after the patient becomes symptomatic and is diagnosed clinically. The most commonly used measures of the effectiveness of screening are improved quality of life and reduced mortality. Prostate cancer is a good example of a disease that often has a long preclinical phase but for which treatment during that phase has not been shown to necessarily improve outcomes (see Chapter 30).

Performance of Test

The screening test itself must perform well. It is important for screening tests to have high sensitivity as well as adequate specificity. Recall that the predictive value of a test is intimately tied to the prevalence of the disease or condition being considered (Fig. 3.1). With screening tests, the prevalence of the condition being sought is usually very low, often even among so-called "high-risk" groups. Therefore, a highly sensitive test is

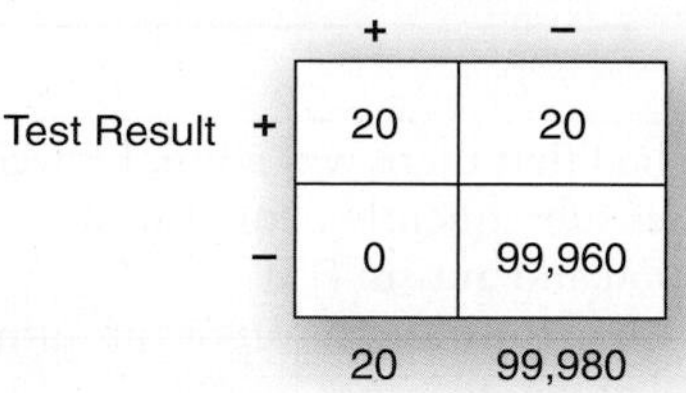

Presence of Disease (MD)
+
−
Test Result
+
−
20
20
0
99,960
20
99,980

Figure 3.1 • Calculating positive predictive value. Consider a screening test for muscular dystrophy (MD) that has a sensitivity of 100% and a specificity of 99.98% and would be used to screen newborn males for the condition. A conservative estimate of the prevalence of MD is 1 in 5000 newborn males. Of a hypothetical population of 100,000 newborn males, 20 will therefore have disease. This information can be used to fill in a 2 × 2 table as shown. Because the test has 100% sensitivity, all 20 of the newborn males with MD will be detected (there will be no false negatives). With a 99.98% specificity, 99,960 (0.9998 × 99,980) of the babies who do not have MD will be correctly identified; however, 20 babies who do NOT have MD will test positive. The positive predictive value (PPV) of the test is calculated as the proportion of those who test positive who truly have disease (true positives/all positives). Thus, the PPV is 20/40, or 50%. This means that there is a 50% chance that the baby has MD., or that one of every two diagnostic workups will be for a false-negative screening test. (Adapted from: Slawson DC, Shaughnessy AF. Teaching information mastery: the case of Baby Jeff and the importance of Bayes' theorem. *Fam Med* 2002;34(2):140–142.)

needed so that after performing it on large numbers of patients, the test does not miss the few cases of disease that are actually present (few false negatives). A screening test also needs to have high specificity to avoid additional testing ("workups") or treatments for people who do not have the disease (few false positives). Still, even with a highly sensitive and highly specific screening test, many workups for falsely assigned test results will occur.

Acceptability to Patients

The screening procedure should be well tolerated by the patient. Blood tests (e.g., lipid assays) and short questionnaires (e.g., PHQ2 depression screening tool) are generally quite acceptable to patients. When tests are acceptable, screening rates tend to be much higher. Colonoscopy is a good example of an effective screening test that is not acceptable to some patients. Even fecal occult blood testing, which requires patients to collect and submit three samples of stool, may be unacceptable to some people. The lower acceptability of these tests may be one reason for the current relatively low colorectal cancer screening rates.

APPROACHES TO PREVENTING DISEASE

In addition to screening, clinicians use three other main approaches to prevention: immunizations, chemoprophylaxis, and counseling.

Immunizations

Immunizations are one of the most effective prevention strategies ever introduced. Diseases such as smallpox, measles, and polio—not long ago responsible for much morbidity and mortality—have either been eradicated or are under much improved control as a result of widespread vaccination (Table 3.2). In addition to being extremely effective, immunizations are also one of the most cost-effective of all primary prevention activities.

TABLE 3.2 Prevaccine Era and Current Estimated Morbidity for Vaccine-Preventable Diseases

Disease	20th-Century Annual Morbidity	2005 Annual Morbidity	Percent Decrease
Smallpox	48,164	0	100
Diphtheria	175,885	0	100
Measles	503,282	66	>99
Mumps	152,209	314	>99
Pertussis	147,271	25,616	83
Polio (paralytic)	16,316	1*	>99
Rubella	47,745	11	>99
Congenital rubella syndrome	823	1	>99
Tetanus	1,314	27	98
Haemophilus influenza, type b and unknown (<5 years of age)	20,000	226	99

*Vaccine-associated paralytic polio.
Sources: CDC. MMWR 1999;48:242–264; CDC. MMWR 2006;55:880–893.

TABLE 3.3 Some Common Misconceptions about Vaccines

Misconception	Context and Possible Physician Response
Children can get autism from vaccines	A case-series published in *Lancet* in 1998 implied that there was a link between MMR vaccine and autism (12). Several studies subsequently demon strated consistently that there is no association between vaccination and autism (13). In 2010, *Lancet* formally fully retracted the 1998 study as a result of the author's dishonesty in reporting and other ethical violations (12).
Vaccines can cause the disease they are supposed to prevent	A common example is the myth that influenza vaccine causes the flu. Some people may have had viral symptoms (flu or non-flu) developing at the time they received influenza vaccine, but it was only coincidence. Others may have side effects (mild aches, low-grade fever) that might be perceived as "the flu." The fact is that most vaccines manufactured today are made from killed virus, so the virus cannot reproduce and cause infection. Even vaccines made from live viruses or bacteria are made with only part of the virus or bacteria. You can't get the flu from the flu vaccine, because the vaccine is made from a killed virus.
Vaccines can cause mercury poisoning	Thimerosal, which is used in development of some vaccines, contains mercury. The amount of mercury actually present in thimerosal is minute, does not accumulate in the body, and is much less toxic than other forms of mercury. Today, influenza vaccine is the only immunization that contains thimerosal, and preservative-free (thimeros al-free) influenza is available for young children.
Vaccines are dangerous and not tested	Vaccine development and manufacturing follows standard protocols. Before being released, vaccines are carefully tested. After release, vaccine safety is carefully monitored.

Despite the fact that many vaccine-preventable diseases of childhood have been virtually eliminated from the United States, it remains important to continue to strongly promote immunization of the US population. First, globally, the prevalence of some infections remains moderately high, and the increasing frequency of international travel brings can bring American patients into contact with infected individuals. For example, China reported 131,441 measles cases (98.4 per million) in 2008 and a large outbreak in Japan resulted in more than 18,000 (140.7 per million) reported cases in 2007 (4). Immunization confers protection in the case of individual exposures. Second, the concept of *herd immunity* applies, whereby high levels of immunization in a population protect the few unimmunized persons from infection. When individuals decline to vaccinate themselves or their family, the degree of herd immunity decreases so that unimmunized persons are more likely to become infected and the risk of an epidemic of infection increases. You should be prepared to respond to patients' and parents' common misconceptions about vaccines (Table 3.3). A good source of information is the Centers for Disease Control and Prevention (CDC) website (*http://www.cdc.gov/vaccines/*).

Chemoprophylaxis

Chemoprophylaxis, also called chemoprevention, is the use of a medication to prevent disease or an adverse health outcome. Examples are shown in Table 3.4 (5,6). Many interventions commonly referred to as "treatment" are actually chemoprevention. For example, statins offered to people with elevated cholesterol are really given to reduce the risk of cardiovascular events. Bisphosphonates, offered to patients with osteoporosis, are really given in hopes of preventing fragility fractures.

TABLE 3.4 Examples of Chemoprevention

Medication	Preventive Use(s)	Potential Harms
Aspirin	Reduce risk of myocardial infarction in men 45 to 79 years; reduce risk of ischemic stroke in women 55 to 79 years	Gastrointestinal bleeding, hemorrhagic stroke
Folic acid	Reduce risk of neural tube defects in women of childbearing age	None
Tamoxifen and raloxifene	Reduce risk of breast cancer in women at high risk	Pulmonary embolism, deep venous thrombosis, hot flashes, endometrial cancer

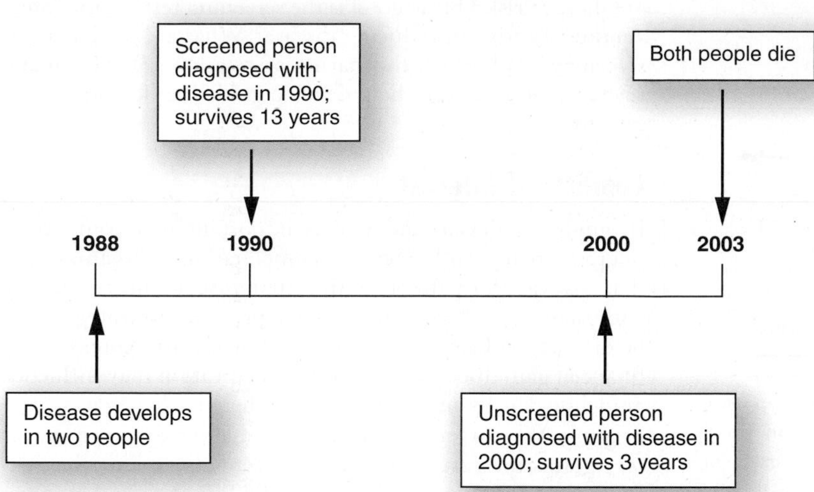

Figure 3.2 • Lead time bias. Screening gives the appearance that the person diagnosed in 1990 survived longer, when in fact both people lived 13 years after they developed disease. Adapted from: Bhatnagar V, Kaplan RM. Treatment options for prostate cancer: evaluating the evidence. *Am Fam Physician.* 2005; 71(10): 1915–1922.

When considering any chemoprevention, it is important to balance the potential risk reduction against the potential for harm and attendant costs.

Counseling

Clinicians' efforts to counsel people to exercise, eat healthier, lose weight, and limit alcohol intake are examples of preventive interventions to encourage individuals to change behavior. The effectiveness of such counseling should be subjected to the same scrutiny as other prevention interventions. A successful intervention supported by evidence is tobacco cessation counseling (7). Even brief advice given by a clinician to a smoker to quit smoking leads to greater cessation attempts and greater cessation rates. Use of the "Five As" (see Chapter 47, "Addictions") is one technique that can help clinicians counsel patients to engage in healthier behaviors. Intensive counseling is effective for some patients with other conditions (e.g., weight loss for obese patients).

THE PERIODIC HEALTH EXAM

Historically, an "annual physical exam" was recommended for all patients irrespective of their age or risk factors. The effectiveness of such annual physicals for all is generally not supported by evidence. Instead, "periodic health exams" (PHE) are considered more appropriate where the periodicity is determined by the age and risk factors of each patient. Therefore, a 24-year-old healthy male medical student who exercises regularly and who does not smoke may not need a PHE more often than every 3 to 5 years, whereas a 51-year-old male smoker who has already had a myocardial infarction may need his preventive care addressed at least annually. The focus of PHEs should be on offering and performing prevention services that are supported by evidence.

EVIDENCE FOR SCREENING AND PREVENTION

It is commonly assumed that any preventive intervention is good and that there are few if any downsides. Demonstrating people's enthusiasm for cancer screening, one study found that approximately three of four US women 40 years and older and men 50 years and older would rather have a full-body computed tomography scan than $1000 cash (8). Further, when it comes to screening, people seem to minimize the undue harm endured caused by false-positive tests. In the same study, 38% of people experienced at least one false-positive screening test, more than 40% of whom described the experience as "very scary" or the "scariest time of [their] life." Still, 98% were glad they had the screening test.

Contrary to the public's general perception, the importance of having evidence for clinical prevention services cannot be overstated. First, clinicians need to be certain that a preventive service will not do more harm than good. Overdiagnosis (finding disease that did not need to be treated), labeling as diseased, unnecessary confirmatory tests, side effects of treatment, and even death are all possible harms of a preventive intervention. Second, after a preventive intervention is introduced and undergoes widespread adoption, it is difficult to reverse clinician and patient behavior related to the service. For example, changing patient and physician behavior pertaining to prostate cancer screening is difficult. Such screening was adopted and promoted based on observational studies before better quality evidence existed. Unfortunately, observational designs are problematic when it comes to studying screening.

Sources of Bias in Studies of Screening

Observational studies of the effects of screening generally suffer from two major biases: lead-time bias and length-time bias. Lead-time bias occurs when people whose disease was diagnosed by screening *appear* to have longer survival than those whose disease was diagnosed because of symptoms or signs, even if actual years of life were not prolonged (Fig. 3.2). This apparent discrepancy occurs because "survival" is measured from time of diagnosis. Hence, a person who is screened may be diagnosed earlier than a person who is not screened but will not live any longer in absolute lifespan. Length-time bias occurs because screening tends to detect more indolent cases of disease (e.g., slow-growing cancer), whereas rapidly advancing disease (e.g., aggressive cancer) is less likely to be

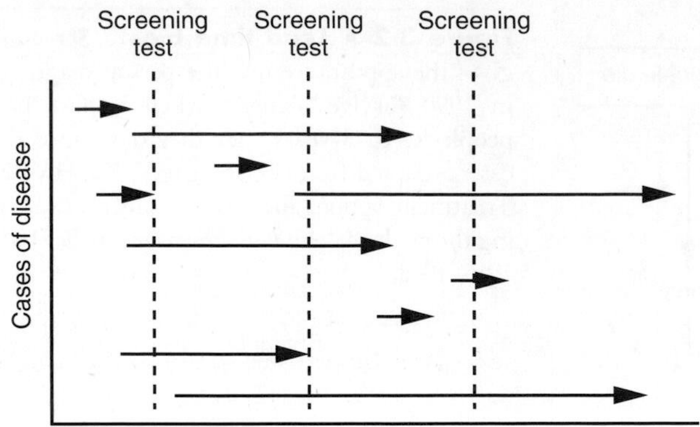

Figure 3.3 • Length-time bias. Aggressive diseases (short arrows) are less likely to be detected by screening than slowly advancing diseases (long arrows). Thus, screening appears favorable because it detects diseases that have a more favorable prognosis. (Adapted from: Kramer BS, Croswell JM. Cancer screening: the clash of science and intuition. *Annu Rev Med.* 2009;60: 125–137.)

detected by screening because it has a much shorter presymptomatic phase (Fig. 3.3). Therefore, people who are screened will *appear* to have a better prognosis because they have disease that inherently has a better prognosis. The way to mitigate these two important biases is to perform randomized controlled trials of screening that report mortality as the primary outcome (not 5-year survival). Adequate randomization will ensure that there is a balance of people with indolent and aggressive disease in both groups (screened and unscreened). In addition, the point at which people are randomized marks an equivalent starting time in both groups, so that lead time is avoided.

Overdiagnosis can be thought of as an extreme form of length-time bias. Overdiagnosis is not the same as false-positive tests. In overdiagnosis, histologic cancer is actually detected, but the cancer is one that would never have become clinically relevant. That is, the patient would have lived just as long without ever having had the cancer detected and treated. Some people use the term "pseudodisease" to describe these indolent forms of cancer (9). Overdiagnosis is one likely explanation why current screening programs for breast and prostate cancer have failed to reduce mortality (10). Only by finding and adequately reducing the mortality from the aggressive cancers will screening make a difference. At the same time, it is important to develop strategies to reduce the unnecessary treatments for people whose screen-detected disease has little or no true malignant potential.

Systematic Reviews

Because a single study rarely answers the question of whether the evidence is sufficient to adopt a clinical preventive service, a systematic evidence review is helpful for preventive strategies. The review is systematic because it uses a prespecified, scientifically based plan to identify all relevant research addressing the question at hand. For reviewing the evidence of a preventive strategy, it may take several systematic reviews because there are several questions to be addressed (e.g., Who are those at risk? How good is the screening test? Is the intervention effective in reducing disease? What are the harms of screening? What are the harms of treatment?). Systematic reviews can be used to help develop guidelines for preventive services.

Conflicts of Interest

In guideline development, it is important that conflicts of interest do not influence recommendations. Organizations that advocate for patients with certain diseases may be overly enthusiastic about recommending a prevention strategy, even before the evidence is sufficient. Similarly, the potential for financial gain due to from a test or medication may influence guideline development and needs to be guarded against. For example, the current guidelines on whether to screen adults for glaucoma are notably different between the US Preventive Services Task Force (USPSTF) and the American Academy of Ophthalmology (AAO) (11). The USPSTF concluded that the evidence is insufficient, whereas the AAO recommends that adults be screened as part of comprehensive eye care. Whether these differences are due to vested interest or different interpretations of the evidence is difficult to know.

Guidelines and Resources

The USPSTF is an independent panel of prevention experts, including family physicians, who conduct rigorous, impartial assessments of the scientific evidence for the effectiveness of a broad range of clinical preventive services, including screening, counseling, and chemoprevention. Because of their rigor, explicit methods, and impartiality, the USPSTF recommendations are considered by many to be the "gold standard" for clinical preventive services. The USPSTF regularly updates its recommendations as new evidence accumulates. Its recommendations, systematic reviews, and evidence summaries (also published in peer-reviewed journals) are available at their website (*http://www.ahrq.gov/CLINIC/uspstfix.htm*). The USPSTF provides several user-friendly and patient-friendly options to guide preventive decision-making. The CDC website (*http://www.cdc.gov/vaccines/*) is a good source for information on current immunization recommendations. There are also local organizations that review the evidence to support various preventive strategies and make recommendations to their members about best practices. One such well-regarded organization is the Institute for Clinical Systems Improvement. (*www.icsi.org*).

When Guidelines Conflict

Unfortunately, guidelines about preventive services will sometimes conflict, leaving the clinician and patient in somewhat of a quandary. In most cases, such conflicts will arise when the evidence is simply insufficient. The USPSTF often will classify services lacking good quality evidence in this way. As a clinician, you should become familiar with the issues about the service that are controversial, and where the evidence is weak, it is recommended that you consider using a strategy of shared decision making with patients. That is, you discuss the preventive service and its potential for helping the patient as well as its potential risks. The goal is to reach a mutually agreeable decision that reflects the health preferences of the patient; that is, to individualize the preventive recommendation in the absence of consensus.

AN APPROACH TO APPLYING PREVENTIVE CARE IN CLINICAL PRACTICE

The ***RISE*** mnemonic is one approach to help you remember to apply the principles of preventive medicine in daily clinical practice. First identify the particular **R**isks of this patient; consider recommended **I**mmunizations (and chemoprophylaxis); review recommended **S**creening with this patient; and address appropriate **E**ducation or counseling. Where applicable, we will continue to use this mnemonic in the following chapters to categorize an approach to providing preventive care in specific age groups and specific populations.

SYSTEMS OF CARE

Preventive care is improved by its incorporation into systems of health delivery. Many elements of prevention do not necessarily need to be provided directly by the family physician. For example, reminders can be automatically mailed to patients when their mammogram or colonoscopy is due. Office staff can be trained to identify patients deficient in their recommended preventive care needs, and these patients' charts can be flagged for physician review. They can also help implement screening programs, such as the 5 As, for all patients who use tobacco. Electronic record systems particularly allow for more ease of tracking preventive care than previous paper charts. However, any system requires flexibility given the frequent updates and changes in recommendations that may occur as new evidence of effectiveness emerges or new technologies become available to enhance earlier detection.

KEY POINTS

- Clinical preventive services include immunizations, counseling (e.g., to stop smoking), screening, and chemoprophylaxis (i.e., taking a medicine to prevent adverse health outcome).
- Immunizations are one of the most effective prevention strategies ever introduced; family physicians need to be prepared to address patient and parental concerns regarding vaccine safety and reasons for immunizing.
- The goal of screening is not merely to find problems but rather to identify asymptomatic persons for whom an intervention will reduce progression of early disease or prevent an adverse health event.
- When considering any chemoprophylaxis strategy (e.g., aspirin to prevent myocardial infarction), it is important to balance the potential risk reduction against the potential for harm.
- Effectiveness of a prevention activity should be demonstrated before implementing it widely in clinical practice. Most prevention interventions also have the potential for causing harm.

CHAPTER

4

Prenatal Care

Beth A. Choby

CLINICAL OBJECTIVES

1. Describe the best means of accurately determining the gestational age of a pregnancy.
2. Cite when prenatal vitamins or supplements are indicated during pregnancy.
3. Summarize when and how you should screen a pregnant woman for neural tube defects, gestational diabetes, or Down syndrome.
4. Demonstrate how a history of prior cesarean delivery influences delivery options.

Prenatal care introduces many women into the medical system. It allows physicians to address nonobstetric issues such as baseline health status and immunization history. It may positively influence the treatment of certain obstetric conditions. Prenatal care likely benefits both maternal and infant health by encouraging long-term health maintenance and increasing the likelihood that infants receive timely care.

Family physicians' knowledge, scope of practice, and comprehensive training makes them uniquely suited to provide prenatal care for women and their families. Bonds formed during maternity care often translate into lifelong relationships with families. Prenatal care is a highly rewarding part of family medicine because of this special type of continuity.

Family physicians care for pregnant women in a variety of settings. A large percentage of family physicians provide prenatal care or see pregnant women during routine office visits. Twenty-four percent of family physicians perform deliveries as a regular part of their practice, 18% perform vacuum extraction, 6.4% do forceps deliveries, and 6.5% offer trial of labor after cesarean delivery (TOLAC) (1). Although only 7.3% of family physicians who deliver babies perform cesarean deliveries, in the east south central United States, 18.5% of these doctors perform them (1). This chapter explores evidence-based prenatal care, medical and psychosocial issues in pregnancy, and the role of family physicians as maternity care providers.

THE PRECONCEPTION VISIT

A preconception visit can be used to maximize the expectant parents' health, safety, and well-being before conception, and to maximize fetal health in the early months of pregnancy. The consultation ideally occurs 3 to 6 months before conception and covers health promotion, risk assessment, and medical intervention. Opportunities for informal preconception guidance include well-woman exams, Pap smears, visits for contraception or a negative pregnancy test, and follow-up visits after poor birth outcomes.

Among the issues that can be covered in a preconception visit are:

- *Minimizing occupational risks.* Environmental exposures that adversely affect the fetus include solvents (e.g., pesticides, paint thinner/strippers, fertilizers), heavy metals (e.g., lead, mercury, arsenic), anesthetic gases (which may reduce fertility in settings where gas-scavenging equipment is not available), ionizing radiation, chemotherapeutic agents, and misoprostol.
- *Prescribing folic acid.* Children of women who consume at least 400 mcg (0.4 mg) of folic acid in early pregnancy have a threefold overall decrease in the risk of neural tube defects (NTD) (2). Leafy green vegetables and fortified whole grains are good dietary sources of folic acid; though if a pregnancy is planned the simplest way to assure adequate intake is to prescribe a prenatal vitamin at the preconception visit.
- *Maximizing chronic illness care.* Infants of mothers with diabetes mellitus are at a fourfold increased risk for congenital malformations and elevated maternal blood glucose levels increase the likelihood of anomalies, especially during the first trimester. The recommended range for fasting blood glucose is 4 to 7 mmol/L (72 to 126 mg/dL) and hemoglobin A1C should be <6%; a metaanalysis of preconception care in diabetes reported fewer major and minor anomalies in women receiving preconception diabetes care (2.4% vs. 7.7%, respectively) (3).
- *Improving health habits.* A review of tobacco, alcohol, and illicit substance use is important during the preconception visit. Smoking is associated with many adverse effects including placental abruption, sudden infant death syndrome, intrauterine growth restriction, and stillbirth; smoking cessation is estimated to result in an 11% reduction in stillbirth and 5% reduction in neonatal deaths (4). The CAGE questionnaire (see Chapter 47) can be used to screen women for alcohol use during a preconception visit. Binge drinking (consuming more than five drinks in one sitting) is more dangerous to fetal neurologic development than non-binge usage. Disulfiram (Antabuse) should not be used during pregnancy because of an association with fetal anomalies. Because no safe amount of drinking is known, abstinence is suggested (see Chapter 47 for interventions).
- *Review current medications and assess safety.* Use of all prescription and over-the-counter drugs, herbal supplements,

and vitamins should be reviewed and documented at the preconception visit. If a woman requires a drug with teratogenic potential, informed consent and a discussion about safer options is necessary. Switching to an alternative with a better-known safety profile is prudent, especially during organogenesis.

Genetic Screening and Counseling

The risk for genetic disorders is increased in several ethnic groups and certain heritable genetic diseases are best diagnosed in individuals before becoming pregnant (Table 4.1). The goals of preconception genetic counseling are twofold. Individuals who are at risk for a fetal anomaly or genetic disorder can be counseled about risk in a future pregnancy and couples can be informed about available screening tests. Specific questionnaires for genetic screening are available from the American Congress of Obstetricians and Gynecologists (ACOG) at *http://www.acog.org*.

In patients with known familial disorders, genetic testing allows for carrier testing. For example, screening the partner of a woman with sickle cell disease is recommended to estimate risks for a planned pregnancy. Routine screening for thalassemia in pregnancy is not recommended and most cases of thalassemia in pregnancy are mild. However, newborns with the most severe form of alpha-thalassemia (Bart hemoglobin) usually deliver stillborn at 28 to 30 weeks. Cases number

TABLE 4.1 Preconception Screening Recommendations for Specific Diseases

Disease	Cause	Heritability	Epidemiology	Screening Available	Recommendations for Screening
Tay Sachs	Deficiency of the enzyme hexosaminidase A	Recessively inherited	1:30 carrier risk in Ashkenazi Jewish heritage; Cajuns and French Canadian carriers	Enzyme assay for hexosaminidase A	Routine preconception screening for those at risk*
Sickle cell anemia	Amino acid substitution of valine for glutamic acid on the HBB gene of chromosome 11	Autosomal recessive	10% African-American carriers; increased risk among Indo-Pakistani and Arab ethnic groups	Hemoglobin electrophoresis	Preconception screening for women at risk; partner screening for women with sickle cell trait (50% chance of affected fetus if both carriers)*
Thalassemia alpha and beta type	Abnormality in hemoglobin production with inadequate oxygen carrying capability and anemia	Autosomal recessive	1:12 carrier rate in people of Asian or Mediterranean descent	DNA testing for women with low MCV, normal hemoglobin electrophoresis	Preconception screening for women at risk and partners of women with abnormal hemoglobin genes (25% risk if both carriers)
CF	Mutations in the CF transmembrane conductance regulator	Autosomal recessive	1:29 carrier risk in whites of Northern European heritage	DNA testing	Preconception screening if family history of CF and partners of women with CF (25% risk if both carriers*,†,‡
Diabetes mellitus	Fourfold increased risk for congenital malformations	Multifactorial	1.2% of pregnancies in Caucasians; higher if Asian descent	Fasting blood glucose (normal 4–7 mmol/L) or glucose test	Early Glucola in patients at risk for diabetes

CF = cystic fibrosis; MCV = mean corpuscular volume.
*Recommended by American Congress of Obstetricians and Gynecologists (ACOG).
†Recommended by American College of Medical Genetics.
‡Recommended by the National Institutes of Health (NIH).

14,000 to 28,000 annually, and preconception screening in couples at risk may decrease the number of affected pregnancies (5).

Immunizations

The preconception visit is a useful time to update immunization status. Screening all women for rubella susceptibility by history of previous vaccination or serology is recommended during the initial preconception encounter. Nonimmune women should be immunized with the measles mumps rubella (MMR) vaccine. Vaccination on or after the first year of life, proof of immunity via serology, or physician diagnosed measles implies immunity. While women have historically been counseled not to conceive within 3 months of MMR immunization, the likelihood of the fetus developing congenital rubella syndrome is largely theoretical. In one study, 683 women inadvertently given MMR within 3 months of conception or during pregnancy had no increased incidence of fetal anomalies or congenital rubella syndrome (6).

Immunity to varicella (chicken pox) should be documented during the preconception visit. Although uncommon during pregnancy, congenital varicella in the newborn and maternal varicella pneumonia cause significant morbidity and mortality. Eighty-five to 90% of adults who deny having had varicella are actually immune. A negative history of varicella can be confirmed through titers. Women who are not immune should receive immunization with varicella vaccine (Varivax) before conception.

PRENATAL CARE

The goals of prenatal care are confirming the pregnancy, assessing and modifying risk, screening for and managing conditions that arise, and providing patient education and support.

Diagnosing and Dating the Pregnancy

Amenorrhea, nausea, fatigue, and breast tenderness are the most common symptoms of early pregnancy. Combinations of symptoms have increased predictive value over single symptoms.

Physical signs of pregnancy include alterations in the skin and mucous membranes. Nonspecific skin changes of pregnancy are linea nigra (hyperpigmented streak appearing below the umbilicus) and chloasma (reddish hyperpigmentation over the bridge of the nose and cheeks). Women taking oral contraceptives occasionally develop chloasma. The changes observed on vaginal examination are Hegar sign (softened consistency of the cervix and uterus) and Chadwick sign (bluish discoloration of the cervix, vulva, and vagina caused by vascular engorgement) have high specificity (94%) but low sensitivity (18%) for diagnosing pregnancy (7).

A detailed menstrual history is obtained to accurately determine the first day of the most recent menstrual cycle for calculating the estimated date of delivery (EDD). For women with reliable menstrual histories, Naegele's rule can be used to estimate the EDD using the following formula: EDD = (LMP − 3 months) + 7 days. The rule is most useful in women who have regular 28-day cycles followed by an abrupt cessation of menses.

Pregnancy tests use urine or serum to check for beta human chorionic gonadotropin (β-HCG). β-HCG is detectable in the blood almost immediately after conception. It is an accurate marker for pregnancy and is the assay of choice for most qualitative (urine) and quantitative (serum) pregnancy tests. Urine tests are generally positive around the time of the first missed period. β-HCG concentrations in the range of 25 to 50 mIU/mL are detectible on qualitative urine samples. Serum pregnancy tests detect β-HCG at levels as low as 10 to 15 mIU/mL.

Mean serum β-HCG levels correspond closely with gestational age during the first trimester. In healthy gestations, β-HCG levels double every 1.4 to 2 days. A minimum increase of 66% is expected every 48 hours. β-HCG levels increase exponentially until the fetus is 8 to 10 weeks old. Levels then plateau and decline somewhat, remaining steady for the duration of the pregnancy. An appropriate rise in β-HCG levels on two quantitative (serum) pregnancy tests drawn 48 hours apart is reassuring for normal pregnancy.

Transvaginal ultrasound is the best diagnostic choice for women with abnormal bleeding or abdominal pain and a positive pregnancy test. Sonographic landmarks such as the gestational sac and fetal pole correlate strongly with specific HCG levels. The gestational sac is generally seen when the HCG level is >1,000 mIU/mL and the pregnancy is 4.5 to 5 weeks along. The double decidual sign is the thick, hyperechoic (white) ring that surrounds the gestational sac. The yolk sac is the early nourishment for the embryo, seen at 6 weeks when HCG levels are >2,500 mIU/mL. The fetal pole is seen at 7 weeks' gestation and with HCG levels higher than 5,000 mIU/mL. Ultrasound measurements of the gestational sac and the crown to rump length of the fetus are a very accurate means of establishing the EDD. First trimester transvaginal ultrasound confirms gestational age within ±4 days.

Risk Assessment

OBSTETRIC HISTORY

Documentation of the obstetric history includes gravidity (the total number of pregnancies) and parity (the number of pregnancies carried beyond 20 weeks' gestation). Gravidity includes the current pregnancy along with prior gestations. Parity is further divided into four categories including the number of pregnancies carried to term, the number delivered preterm (<37 weeks' gestation), the number of fetal losses (included elective abortions), and the total number of living children. Multiple gestations (i.e., twins, triplets, etc.) count as one pregnancy, but the number of infants delivered is described by the parity.

If there is a history of spontaneous or elective abortion, document the gestational age at the time of loss. Method of delivery with previous pregnancies identifies women with a scarred uterus or previous operative vaginal delivery (vacuum or forceps). Record the weights and sex of previous newborns, in addition to any complications during the labor or delivery. History of poor obstetric outcome includes stillbirth (fetal death at term) and preterm delivery. The greatest risk factor for preterm delivery in the current pregnancy is a history of preterm delivery. Women with a history of gestational hypertension or diabetes, grand multiparity (more than five deliveries), multiple gestations, and isoimmunization are also at increased risk for complications.

CURRENT MEDICAL AND SURGICAL HISTORY

A detailed medical history should be obtained. Asthma, diabetes, hypertension, cardiac conditions, thyroid and renal disease, and certain infectious diseases can have an adverse effect on pregnancy. Surgical history of importance includes any procedure involving the reproductive tract, including previous cesarean, tubal surgery for ectopic pregnancy or infertility, and cervical or vaginal surgery. The type of skin incision (i.e., Pfannenstiel) does not guarantee a low-transverse entry to the uterus with a previous cesarean delivery. An operative report should be reviewed to confirm the type of uterine scar. For women considering TOLAC, this information is critical. Women with prior abdominal surgery (e.g., cholecystectomy, appendectomy) may have adhesions that make future surgery more difficult.

FAMILY HISTORY

Family history of interest includes any mental retardation, birth defects, or genetic conditions in either parents or family members.

HEALTH HABITS AND OCCUPATIONAL RISKS

Social history includes tobacco, alcohol, and drug use. Expectant women who smoke less than one pack per day are most successful quitting when offered a 5- to 15-minute counseling session and repeat discussions at subsequent prenatal visits that employs the 5As approach (see Chapter 47) (8). The use of pharmaceuticals and nicotine replacement for smoking cessation during pregnancy and lactation has not been studied sufficiently (9). Use of nicotine gum, patches, inhalers, and antidepressants (bupropion) to reduce withdrawal symptoms during pregnancy and lactation should be considered only after nonpharmacologic therapies and counseling have failed. When benefits outweigh risks, products with intermittent dosages such as nicotine gum and inhalers should be tried first.

Occupational risks should be documented (see Preconception Care).

Immunization and Chemoprophylaxis

Immunization history should be documented. Although ideally assessed before pregnancy (see preconception immunization section), you should obtain serology for women who do not report previous vaccination for rubella. Nonimmune women should be advised to avoid contact with individuals with a known outbreak of rubella and be vaccinated with the MMR vaccine in the postpartum period. If vaccination is inadvertently given during pregnancy, abortion is not indicated because there is no evidence for teratogenicity although evidence of fetal infection has been reported (10). Although live vaccines (e.g., MMR, poliomyelitis) are contraindicated in pregnancy, inactivated vaccines (e.g., influenza, hepatitis, pneumococcus) may be given during pregnancy if indicated (10).

Additional nutrients needed during pregnancy include folic acid, iron, and calcium. Folic acid was discussed in preconception care. The US Centers for Disease Control and Prevention recommends that pregnant women take 30 mg of ferrous iron supplements daily. A Cochrane review concluded that pregnant women taking iron or iron and folic acid are less likely to have anemia or iron deficiency at term; however, no significant reduction in adverse maternal or neonatal outcomes were found (11).

Recommended daily intake of calcium is 1,000 to 1,300 mg per day. Milk products (300 mg calcium per 8-ounce serving of milk), tofu (434 mg per half-cup serving) and Swiss cheese (272 mg per 1-ounce serving) are excellent sources, although women with lactose intolerance may require supplements. Routine calcium supplementation may benefit women at risk for gestational hypertension. Elevated blood pressure in pregnancy is a major cause of maternal death and a frequent cause of preterm delivery and fetal death. A recent Cochrane review suggests that calcium supplementation during pregnancy is both cost-effective and safe for decreasing the risk of preeclampsia in those at risk and in women with inadequate calcium intake (12). In addition, calcium supplementation reduced the rare occurrence of death or serious problems in women who developed preeclampsia (12). Research is needed to determine the ideal dose of calcium and confirm safety. The need for other nutrients during pregnancy is unclear, and although routine use of prenatal vitamins is not recommended by ACOG, many women have marginal nutritional status and may benefit from supplements.

Screening as Part of Prenatal Care

In the United States, family physicians, obstetrician/gynecologists, midwives, or nurse practitioners are the usual prenatal care providers. Nurses, nutritionists, geneticists, and social workers are also often involved. Continuity of care during pregnancy by one provider or a small team seems to benefit women. Women receiving prenatal care from a single physician are likely to receive more prenatal care, which has been correlated with increased maternal weight gain and infant birth weights (13). A Cochrane review concluded that low-risk prenatal care provided by family physicians, obstetricians, and midwives is equally effective, although women seem to be more satisfied with care provided by family physicians and midwives (14).

Women in the United States have an average of 14 prenatal appointments. The first appointment generally is at 6 to 8 weeks' gestation, with return visits monthly until 28 weeks. From 28 to 36 weeks, appointments are usually scheduled every 2 weeks. After 36 weeks, weekly visits ensue, with many providers scheduling biweekly visits after 40 to 41 weeks' gestation. The current visit schedule is more tradition based than evidence based. A Cochrane review shows that a model with fewer prenatal visits is not likely to increase maternal or fetal risk compared with the traditional model. A benefit of the abbreviated system is decreased cost, although women may be less satisfied with fewer visits (15).

First Trimester Prenatal Care

The first 13 weeks of pregnancy are the most critical period in fetal development. The majority of organogenesis occurs during this time and the embryo/fetus is most susceptible to environmental and teratogenic insults.

PHYSICAL EXAMINATION

The following are part of the prenatal physical exam:

- *Blood pressure measurement*. This is likely the best screening strategy for detecting hypertension in pregnancy. Levels

TABLE 4.2 Institute of Medicine Recommendations for Weight Gain in Pregnancy by Body Mass Index

Pre-pregnancy BMI	Institute of Medicine Weight Gain (lb)
<19.8 (low)	28–40
19.8–26.0 (normal)	25–35
26.1–29.0 (overweight)	15–25
>29.0 (obese)	11–20

http://www.iom.edu/en/Reports/2009/Weight-Gain-During-Pregnancy-Reexamining-the-Guidelines.aspx

higher than 140 mm Hg systolic or 90 mm Hg diastolic recorded on two occasions more than 6 hours apart indicate hypertension. At a gestational age of <20 weeks, blood pressure elevation is usually attributed to chronic hypertension unless trophoblastic (molar) disease or multiple gestations is present. Gestational hypertension is defined as hypertension after 20 weeks of pregnancy that not is associated with proteinuria.

- *Height and weight measurement.* Used to calculate the patient's body mass index (weight (kg)/[height (m)]^2) so that a recommended weight gain during pregnancy can be determined based on the woman's prepregnancy body mass index (Table 4.2).
- *The head, eyes, ears, nose and throat (HEENT) exam.* Of importance is examination of the thyroid and dentition. The thyroid increases in size by 15%, although not clinically noticeable. Any goiter or nodule warrants evaluation. Poor dentition, specifically gingival disease, increases the risk of preterm delivery. A recent case-control multicenter study found a significant association between generalized periodontitis and induced preterm birth for preeclampsia (adjusted odds ratio 2.46 [95% CI 1.58–3.830]) (16).
- *Cardiopulmonary exam.* Increased splitting of the first and second heart sounds and an S3 gallop is often audible on cardiac exam in pregnancy. Dyspnea may be confused with the fatigue and decreased aerobic tolerance that affects women in early pregnancy.
- *Patellar and ankle reflexes.* These are checked and documented because preeclampsia often manifests with hyperreflexia.
- *Clinical breast exam.* Used to detect abnormalities such as cancer or fibrocystic disease. Randomized controlled trials (RCTs) do not show that any intervention influences success with breastfeeding and suggest discontinuing exam of the nipples for inversion.
- *Pelvic exam.* Used to detect anatomic defects of the reproductive tract and screen for sexually transmitted infections (STI) (see Chapter 32). The perineum and external genitalia should be inspected for any abnormalities, including herpetic lesions, genital lesions, or condyloma. Cervical length, dilation, effacement, and position should be documented during the initial exam. Routinely examining the cervix is not an effective method for predicting preterm birth and should be discouraged. The bimanual exam is useful for evaluating the adnexa and estimating uterine size.

Clinical pelvimetry has traditionally been recommended to estimate pelvic adequacy for delivery. The pelvic planes (pelvic inlet, midpelvis, and pelvic outlet) are measured digitally on bimanual exam to provide an estimate of pelvic size and contour. Both clinical pelvimetry and X-ray are no longer recommended because of low predictive value for inability to deliver vaginally and an association with increased cesarean rates (17–19).

LABORATORY TESTING

Table 4.3 lists the laboratory tests that are routinely performed during prenatal care. Sensitivity, specificity, positive and negative likelihood ratios, and levels of evidence are provided comparing the currently available guidelines.

Identifying blood group, D (Rh) factor, and red cell antibodies and administration of Rho (D) immune globulin (RhoGAM) to Rh negative pregnant women helps prevent hemolytic disease of the newborn and identify problems with transfusions (18). Fifteen percent of women are D (Rh) negative. Incompatibility (i.e., D-negative woman carrying a D-positive fetus) occurs in 10% of pregnancies.

Repeat antibody testing for D(Rh) is recommended in all un-sensitized women at 28 weeks' gestation, with a 300-mcg RhoGAM dose given to antibody negative women. A postpartum dose of RhoGAM is also given within 72 hours of delivery if the infant's blood type is D-positive. Situations that result in maternal–fetal blood exchange (i.e. amniocentesis, abruptio placenta, trauma, threatened pregnancy loss and elective termination) necessitate RhoGAM in Rh(D) negative women.

Iron supplements (30 mg elemental iron daily) are indicated for women with hemoglobin <11 g/dL in the first or third trimester or <10.5 g/dL in the second trimester, although data are inconclusive that iron supplementation improves outcomes (11).

Syphilis is an STI caused by *Treponema pallidum*. Women at increased risk for syphilis include sex-trade workers and intravenous drug users and screening and treatment recommendations are discussed in Chapter 32.

Women who are rubella non-immune should be counseled about the risks of rubella during pregnancy (Table 4.3). Nearly all fetuses exposed in the first trimester have rubella sequelae.

For women at risk of hepatitis B, vaccination is safe in pregnancy. Newborns of mothers who are HBsAg positive should receive hepatitis B vaccination and hepatitis B immunoglobin immediately after delivery. The hepatitis C infection transmission rate to infants born to hepatitis C virus–positive mothers is about 5% (20). The American Academy of Family Physicians (AAFP), ACOG, and the United States Preventive Services Task Force (USPSTF) do not recommend routine hepatitis C virus serologic testing of pregnant women. Screening should be offered to women with risk factors (e.g., injection drug users; women with multiple sexual partners, tattoos, or elevated liver functions; prison inmates; women with HIV; and women with exposure to blood or blood products).

Routine universal screening for gonorrhea and chlamydia is not recommended by most guidelines but should be performed in women at risk for sexually transmitted infections (see Chapter 32). Potential risks are shown in Table 4.3.

TABLE 4.3 Routine Laboratory Tests Performed During Routine Prenatal Care

Test	Reasons for Testing	Positive Likelihood Ratio	Negative Likelihood Ratio	Strength of Recommendation
ABO type, Rh, and antibody screen	If Rh negative, RhoGAM prevents isoimmunization. Without treatment, one-third of fetuses develop hemolytic anemia and hyperbilirubinemia and one-fourth develop hydrops resulting in death	99	0.01	A
Hemoglobin/ hematocrit	Test for anemia, most commonly iron deficiency	1.6	0.23	B: first visit C: repeat testing in asymptomatic low risk women
RPR/VDRL for syphilis	Premature delivery 20% and vertical transmission 70% to 100% Congenital syphilis causes fetal anemia, hepatosplenomegaly, pneumonia, and nonimmune hydrops	2.1	0.54	A: rescreen in third trimester if high risk
Rubella titer	Congenital rubella causes sensorineural deafness, microphthalmia, encephalopathy, cataracts, and cardiac abnormalities	3.3	0.11	B: screen pregnant women by vaccination history or serology
Hepatitis B surface antigen (HBsAg)	A 70% to 90% chance of vertical transmission if mother is positive for HBsAg or e-antigen; 85 to 90% of infants become chronic carriers (33). Infected infant carriers develop cirrhosis, chronic active hepatitis, or hepatocellular carcinoma	49	0.02	A: rescreen in third trimester if high risk
Gonorrhea	Infection strongly linked with preterm delivery and fetal infection can result in spontaneous abortion and stillbirth Neonatal infection causes gonococcal ophthalmia, arthritis, and sepsis	80	0.2	B: high risk C: universal screening
Chlamydia	Increased preterm delivery and intrauterine growth restriction Neonatal infection can cause pneumonia and ophthalmia neonatorum	7	0.31	B: high risk C: universal screening
Papanicolaou smear	To detect cervical dysplasia or cancer	6	0.44	A
Urine culture	Asymptomatic bacteriuria in pregnancy is a risk factor for pyelonephritis and preterm delivery and low birth weight	16.5	0.02	A: 12–16 weeks' gestation
HIV	Maternal treatment with zidovudine reduces vertical transmission of HIV from 25.5% to 8.3% (37)	190	0.05	A: high risk C: universal screening
Gestational diabetes	Associated with preeclampsia and increased fetal weight and perinatal morbidity	6	0.024	C: selective screening for high risk^ with 1-hour Glucola (<130–140 mg/dL normal)

Low risk is defined as meeting all of the following criteria: age less than 25 years, pre-pregnancy BMI less than 25, no family history of diabetes, no personal history of GDM or abnormal glucose tolerance, and not belonging to a high-risk ethnic group (i.e., Native American, Hispanic, African American, Asian, and Pacific Islander).

Papanicolaou (Pap) smear specimens should be obtained using a spatula and cytobrush, or a broom if liquid-based cytology is used. Testing may cause minimal spotting, but there is no association with adverse outcomes.

Screening for asymptomatic bacteriuria is performed through urine culture rather than urine dipstick testing because of a 50% false-negative rate and failure to identify certain microbes such as group B streptococcus (Table 4.3).

Bacterial vaginosis (BV) is believed to result from an imbalance of the *Lactobacillus* bacteria that normally colonize the vagina and anaerobic species overgrowth. BV is a common cause of vaginal discharge during pregnancy with rates ranging from 6.1% in Asian-Pacific Islander women to 22.7% in black women (21); about 50% is asymptomatic. The USPSTF and ACOG recommend against screening women at average risk for preterm delivery because screening and treating all pregnant women with BV does not appear to prevent preterm delivery (22). Women with a history of preterm delivery may benefit from BV screening/treatment, but it is unknown whether there is a benefit to neonates (22).

All pregnant women should receive education and counseling regarding HIV as part of routine pregnancy care. HIV testing is voluntary, and informed consent is necessary. Pretest counseling includes a discussion of risk factors, the risk of HIV transmission to the fetus, and therapies known to reduce this risk. An RCT shows that maternal treatment with zidovudine started by 14 to 34 weeks' gestation and continued until 6 weeks postpartum reduces vertical transmission of HIV from 25.5 to 8.3% (23). Other combinations of medications also reduce transmission (lamivudine [Epivir], zidovudine [Retrovir], and nevirapine [Viramune]). Although elective cesarean may decrease the risk of HIV transmission, recent US studies show no benefit beyond that of use of highly active antiretroviral therapy (24).

ULTRASOUND

Ultrasound at 18 to 20 weeks' gestation is standard of care in many localities. Current evidence, however, fails to correlate routine ultrasound screening in pregnancy with improved outcomes, including perinatal mortality (25). A Cochrane review concluded that routine ultrasound before 24 weeks allows for improved dating of gestational age and decreased need for postdate induction. Although ultrasound allows for earlier diagnosis of multiple gestations and fetal malformations at a time when termination is an option, no significant differences in clinical outcomes are evident (12).

The National Institutes of Health and ACOG recommend ultrasound for specific indications rather than routinely in low-risk pregnancies. Table 4.4 lists specific indications for ultrasound. ACOG and the American Institute of Ultrasound in Medicine have endorsed a policy that use of ultrasound for nonmedical purposes such as creating keepsake photos, videos, or for gender determination is considered "contrary to responsible medical practice" (27).

TABLE 4.4 Indications for Ultrasound During Pregnancy

Estimation of gestational age
Unsure dates
Planned scheduled elective repeat cesarean delivery
Planned induction or elective termination of pregnancy
Vaginal bleeding
Evaluation of fetal growth
Evaluation for placentation/multiple gestation pregnancy
Suspected hydatidiform mole
Suspected ectopic pregnancy
Size/dates discrepancy
Suspected polyhydramnios or oligohydramnios
Evaluation of abnormal genetic screening tests
Fetal anomaly assessment
History of previous fetal anomaly/congenital defects

Reference: American College of Radiology. ACR practice guidelines for the performance of antepartum obstetrical ultrasound. In: ACR practice guidelines and technical standards, 2003. Philadelphia, PA: ACR; 2003;625–631.

Genetic Testing

Screening methods available to detect fetal structural and chromosomal anomalies include ultrasound and maternal serum screening. The goal of screening is to identify fetal anomalies that are not compatible with life, are associated with long-term disability and morbidity, are amenable to intrauterine treatment, or require specific therapy at birth. The risks and benefits of all screening tests must be thoroughly discussed and documented, including a plan for what happens if screening is abnormal.

Serum markers available for first-trimester Down syndrome screening include β-HCG and pregnancy-associated plasma protein A (PAPP-A). This combination of tests is comparable in sensitivity and specificity to the second-trimester triple screen, with a detection rate for Down syndrome of 63% and false-positive rate of 5% (28). First-trimester serum testing does not detect NTDs.

Nuchal translucency (NT) of the fetal neck using ultrasound is often combined with β-HCG and PAPP-A for first trimester Down syndrome screening (called first trimester combined test). NT is the measurement of the subcutaneous space between the skin and the cervical spine of the fetus. Fetuses with increased nuchal thickness may be at risk for Down syndrome.

Women with an abnormal first-trimester genetic screening can be offered chorionic villus sampling (CVS) between 10 and 12 weeks' gestation or amniocentesis between 15 and 20 weeks' gestation. Placental tissue is obtained using ultrasound-guided needle biopsy of the placental villi. Samples can be collected transabdominally or transcervically and used for chromosomal, DNA, or metabolic studies. The risk of pregnancy loss with CVS is 1% to 2%; this is 0.5% to 1.0% higher than with amniocentesis. In addition, CVS cannot be used to diagnose neural tube defects. CVS results are available earlier than with amniocentesis, but the increased risk of loss must be weighed against having an earlier diagnosis.

Second and Third Trimester Prenatal Care

Traditional components of the subsequent prenatal visit include measurement of weight, blood pressure, fundal height, fetal heart tones, and a urine dipstick for protein and glucose. Different low-risk prenatal guidelines lack consensus but most recommend routine measurement of maternal weight, blood pressure, fundal height, and fetal heart tones.

PHYSICAL EXAMINATION

- *Weight assessment.* Inadequate weight gain is associated with low birth weight, preterm delivery, and intrauterine growth restriction. For morbidly obese women, weight gain of more than 25 pounds is associated with large for gestation infants (29). Because weight gain information may not change clinical management and may create undue anxiety, weight measurements may only be needed for women for whom nutrition is a concern (e.g., underweight, overweight, obese).
- *Blood pressure measurement.* Continued screening for gestational hypertensive disorders.
- *Fundal height measurement.* In the second or third trimester, fundal height is a good estimate of uterine size and gestational age. Fundal height is measured as the distance in centimeters between the superior edge of the pubic symphysis and the top of the uterine fundus. At 20 weeks' gestation, the fundus should be at the level of the umbilicus. During each week between 20 and 36 weeks' gestation, the fundal height increases by about 1 cm. Measurements deviating by more than 2 cm may indicate problems with fetal growth.
- *Auscultation of the fetal heart rate (FHR).* Generally performed at all follow-up visits, normal fetal heart rate ranges from 110 to 160 beats per minute. Although hearing the fetal heart confirms that the fetus is alive, well-being is harder to evaluate because decelerations or poor variability are rarely noted during this rapid check. Although guidelines differ in recommendations for FHR, they do suggest measuring FHR on patient request (18,19).

LABORATORY TESTING

Routine urine dipstick tests for protein and glucose are no longer recommended during prenatal visits. They are unreliable in detecting the moderate or variable elevations of albumin that occur with preeclampsia. As discussed in the section on genetic screening, the quadruple screen is recommended between 16 and 18 weeks' gestation.

Diabetes Screening

Gestational diabetes mellitus (GDM) is one of the most common obstetric complications, with incidence ranging from 3 to 10% in developed countries. There is currently a lack of consensus in the medical literature regarding screening for GDM because data fail to show that universal screening for GDM benefits the population.

Selective screening exempts women considered at low risk for GDM (Table 4.3). ACOG states that although universal screening is the most sensitive means of detection, certain low risk women may benefit from selective screening (SOR = C). The American Diabetes Association (ADA) also endorses selective screening, generally performed at 24 to 28 weeks' gestation with a 1-hour test (blood glucose measured 1 hour after oral ingestion of 50 g glucose in 150 mL fluid). The test is performed either fasting or nonfasting, although fasting may increase the chances of a false-positive screen. Women at higher risk for GDM (Table 4.3) can be screened at the initial prenatal visit, with follow-up testing done at 24 to 28 weeks if the first test is normal.

If the 1-hour test is abnormal, a 3-hour glucose challenge test should be administered. The test is performed after an overnight fast. A 100-g glucose load is given orally, with blood drawn before ingestion and hourly for three consecutive samples. A diet containing at least 150 g of carbohydrates must be consumed for 3 days before testing. Carbohydrate depletion causes spuriously high glucose levels on the glucose challenge test. A diagnosis of GDM is made when elevation occurs with either the fasting glucose alone or with two or more of the 3-hour measurements.

Specific treatment including dietary advice and insulin for GDM reduces the risk of maternal preeclampsia and perinatal morbidity (composite outcome of death, shoulder dystocia, bone fracture, and nerve palsy). However, it is associated with higher risk of labor induction (30). Intensive insulin therapy is associated with lower rates of macrosomia and need for cesarean, but increased risks for both maternal and neonatal hypoglycemia. Sulfonylureas (glipizide and glyburide) and metformin (Glucophage) are being used in women with preexisting type 2 diabetes, especially when polycystic ovarian disease is present.

Rh Screening

An antibody screen for isoimmunization in women who are Rh negative is done at 28 weeks' gestation. Rho(D) immune globulin is given to Rh-negative women with a negative screen. Women with a positive antibody screen do not benefit from Rho(D) injection and should be evaluated for Rh hemolytic disease.

Screening for Anemia

Retesting for anemia with a hematocrit or hemoglobin at 28 weeks' gestation is appropriate because the maternal blood volume expands during the second trimester. Dietary counseling and supplements are prescribed for pregnant women found to be anemic.

Infectious Disease Screening

In the third trimester, both ACOG and USPSTF recommend repeat screening for hepatitis B, syphilis, gonorrhea, and chlamydia in high-risk populations (Chapter 32). Patients and their partners should be asked about a history of genital and orolabial herpes simplex virus infection (HSV). Herpes outbreaks are classified as primary, nonprimary (first infection with herpes simplex type 2 in a woman with previous type 1 outbreak) or recurrent. Rates of vertical transmission at delivery are 50% in primary HSV infections and 33% in nonprimary first episodes. Transmission risk for recurrent infection is 0 to 3% (31). Genital herpes infection during pregnancy does not increase the risk of neonatal HSV infection as long as seroconversion is complete before labor begins.

The manifestations of neonatal herpes vary from localized disease causing lesions on the neonate's face, eyes, and mouth to more severe infection involving the central nervous system; disseminated HSV infection causes 57% mortality in neonates (32). ACOG recommends antiviral therapy (acyclovir) for women with primary HSV infections and those at risk for recurrent infections after 36 weeks' gestation

(SOR = C). Delivery by cesarean is recommended for women who have active genital lesions present at the time of delivery. Pregnant women should avoid sexual contact if either partner has lesions.

Group B streptococcus (GBS), *Streptococcus agalactiae,* is a leading cause of neonatal morbidity and mortality. GBS exists in the genital and gastrointestinal tract of pregnant women, affecting 6.6 to 20% of mothers in the United States. The CDC, ACOG, and the American Academy of Pediatrics all recommend that women be offered screening for GBS at 35 to 37 weeks' gestation. Specimens are collected using two swabs: one is collected from the lower vagina and posterior fourchette, and the second from the rectum. Studies show that women can reliably collect their own specimens when given appropriate instructions.

Women who are culture positive for GBS should receive antibiotic prophylaxis when in labor except for those who have an elective cesarean delivery done before onset of labor or rupture of membranes. The antibiotic of choice is intravenous penicillin G in nonallergic women at 5 million units followed by 2.5 million units every 4 hours starting at rupture of membranes or active labor and continuing until delivery. Ampicillin can also be used. Sensitivity testing of GBS isolates is recommended in women with a penicillin allergy. Erythromycin and clindamycin are indicated for susceptible isolates, with vancomycin given for resistant cultures. Women with GBS urinary tract infections should be treated both when diagnosed and again at delivery because GBS bacteriuria indicates very heavy colonization.

Women who miss GBS screening because of no prenatal care or unavailable results should be managed according to a risk-based protocol when in labor. Women meeting any of the following criteria require antibiotic prophylaxis.

- Ruptured membranes for >18 hours
- Fever
- Less than 37 weeks' gestation
- History of GBS bacteruria with the current pregnancy
- History of previous infant with invasive GBS disease

Genetic Screening

Second trimester genetic screening includes maternal serum tests and amniocentesis. The quadruple screen is replacing the triple screen as recommended second trimester screening. The quadruple test combines the serum markers of maternal serum alpha-fetoprotein (MSAFP), estriol (uE3), β-HCG, and inhibin A. The quadruple test detects 86% of infants with Down syndrome (trisomy 21) with a false-positive rate of 8.2% (19). The combination of markers also identifies fetuses at risk for NTDs and trisomy 18 (Edward syndrome).

Accurate dating of the pregnancy is important because the marker levels are time sensitive. Testing is possible between weeks 15 through 22 of gestation, with the optimal time being 16 to 18 weeks. Information about maternal weight, race, and the presence of insulin-dependent diabetes mellitus or multifetal pregnancy is required for interpretation of the quadruple test.

MSAFP is the marker in the quadruple screen used to diagnose NTDs. The marker also detects 80% of cases of open spina bifida and 90% of cases of anencephaly. One percent to 5% of women have an elevated MSAFP on the initial quadruple test. 90- to 99% of these women deliver healthy infants, with most abnormal tests from incorrect dating. Confirmation of gestational age by ultrasound is indicated when MSAFP is abnormal.

The risk of Down syndrome increases with maternal age. The odds of having an infant with Down syndrome at age 20 are approximately 1:1,440, increasing to 1:338 at age 35 and 1:32 at 45 years of age (17). All pregnant women 35 years or older at the time of delivery should be offered genetic counseling and CVS or amniocentesis for the diagnosis of genetic abnormalities. Other indications include an abnormal quadruple screen, an abnormal ultrasound, or a parent who carries a balanced translocation. 35 years is the threshold for offering amniocentesis because this is the age when the risk of having a fetus with a chromosomal defect equals the rate of fetal loss from amniocentesis.

PATIENT EDUCATION AND PSYCHOSOCIAL SUPPORT

When expectant parents do not have preconception care, first-trimester visits are an opportunity to discuss common pregnancy topics. Counseling on dietary recommendations, lifestyle changes, and safety issues is best addressed during these initial visits.

Diet and Dietary Supplements

Recommended weight gain is based on the prepregnancy body mass index (SOR = C) (see Table 4.2). Women are encouraged to eat a varied diet during pregnancy. Most pregnant women need 1,900 to 2,800 calories daily, with an additional 150 calories needed during the first trimester and 300 to 500 extra calories in the second and third trimesters. Fifty to sixty percent of the diet should be from carbohydrates and 30% from fats. High-protein supplementation during pregnancy is not beneficial and may be harmful to the fetus according to a Cochrane review (33).

Pregnant women are at risk from certain foods during pregnancy. Consumption of monkfish, swordfish, shark, king mackerel, tilefish, and tuna is linked to mercury exposure. Mercury may adversely affect fetal neurologic development, and the Food and Drug Administration advises pregnant women to consume no more than 12 ounces of tuna weekly (34). Oysters, certain types of sushi, and raw shellfish may harbor *Vibrio cholera, Vibrio parahaemolyticus*, hepatitis A, or parasites and are best avoided during pregnancy. *Escherichia coli* (*E. coli*) food poisoning can result from eating beef that is not thoroughly cooked. Listeriosis is a bacterial infection associated with milk, fruit juice, cheese, or dairy products that are not pasteurized. Listeriosis is associated with chorioamnionitis, preterm delivery, and fetal demise. Recent outbreaks of listeriosis are linked to delicatessen cold cuts. Pregnant women should avoid soft, unpasteurized cheeses such as brie and camembert, and all varieties of pâté.

Lifestyle Topics

Lifestyle changes are a source of questions for many expectant couples. Most couples can safely continue normal sexual relations. Sexual intercourse is contraindicated with placenta previa, preterm labor, and cervical insufficiency. Barrier contraception (condoms) is advised if exposure to STI is a possibility.

When traveling by car, pregnant women should wear seat belts. Motor vehicle accidents are a leading cause of death and disability in pregnant women. Three-point restraints should be worn when driving or riding as a passenger. The lap belt should be worn under the uterus and across the hips, never over the fundus, and the shoulder belt worn above the fundus and between the breasts.

Strong evidence suggests that exercise in pregnancy is safe and beneficial. Regular exercise improves maternal fitness and well-being, reduces musculoskeletal complaints, and moderates maternal weight gain. In the absence of medical or obstetric contraindications, most women who are active before pregnancy can continue their usual activities. Thirty minutes or more of moderate exercise is recommended daily. Walking, swimming, and water aerobics are good forms of exercise for pregnant women, individualized based on prepregnancy fitness level.

Medication Use

Prescribing medications during pregnancy involves balancing maternal benefit with potential risks to the fetus. Unfortunately, only a small number of drugs have well-established safety profiles in pregnancy. Guidelines for drug use in pregnancy are available from several sources. The Food and Drug Administration categorizes drugs based on risk of birth defects (Table 4.5), ACOG classifies antimicrobial safety, and the American Academy of Pediatrics ranks drug safety in lactation. A history should be obtained listing any drug taken currently or prior to conception, including over-the-counter, herbal, and health food supplements. Medication use is advised only when necessary, and after the first trimester when possible. Women who require drugs with known risk should be transitioned to medication with less risk when possible, especially during organogenesis. Explaining risks and benefits and obtaining informed consent from the patient is necessary.

Nearly half of all women use complementary and alternative therapies (CAM). Several including evening primrose oil (EPO), raspberry leaf (*Rubus idaeus*), and ginger have been examined in studies of clinical safety during pregnancy. EPO, a prostaglandin precursor, is a commonly used herb recommended by some midwives for labor induction. Initial studies demonstrated an increased incidence of prolonged rupture of membranes with EPO use and no current RCTs support its use for labor induction (35). Red raspberry leaf in tea or capsule form is also purported to stimulate labor. Ginger is thought to reduce nausea and vomiting in early pregnancy by blocking 5-HT3 receptors, and suppressing the neural pathway between the emetic center in the medulla and the stomach. Although neither raspberry leaf nor ginger is associated with adverse pregnancy outcomes in current research, raspberry leaf has not demonstrated benefit (17).

TABLE 4.5 Categorization of Drug Safety Classifications in Pregnancy and Lactation

Food and Drug Administration Categories on Potential Fetal Risk

Class	Description	Examples
A	Controlled human studies show no fetal risk in first trimester; no evidence of risk in later pregnancy; fetal harm remote	
B	Animal studies show no risk/there are no controlled studies in pregnant women; or animal studies show adverse affect not confirmed in first trimester human studies; no evidence of risk in later trimesters	Acetaminophen, diphenhydramine, azithromycin, cephalosporins, penicillin, low molecular weight heparin, bupropion, methyldopa, loratadine, metoclopramide, sucralfate, H2 antagonists
C	Use only when benefit outweighs risk; animal studies with teratogenic or embryocidal effects and no controlled human studies available; or no research available	Tramadol, ibuprofen*, ketorolac, trimethoprim, clarithromycin, heparin, amitriptyline, venlafaxine, calcium channel blockers, clonidine, albuterol, promethazine, disulfiram, ethosuximide, gabapentin, lamotrigine, vancomycin
D	Documented human fetal risk; use only if benefit is clearly acceptable despite risk; no safer alternatives available	Most benzodiazepines, sulfonamides (third trimester), tetracyclines, most anticonvulsants, ACE inhibitors, ARBs, lithium, nicotine patches, spray and inhalers
X	Contraindicated in women who are or may become pregnant; fetal risk/known abnormalities in humans	Warfarin flurazepam, temazepam, HMG-CoA reductase inhibitors, isotretinoin, oral contraceptives, methotrexate, Cytotec, ergotamines

ACE = angiotensin-converting enzyme; ARB = angiotensin receptor blocker; HMG-CoA = 3-hydroxy-3-methylglutaryl coenzyme A.
*Risk category D in third trimester.

Intimate Partner Violence

Intimate partner violence affects up to 20% of pregnant women (see Chapter 31). Abuse often intensifies during pregnancy, and women who are abused may be less likely to obtain prenatal care. Trauma to the mother or fetus, abruption, low birth weight, fetal loss, and postpartum depression are all associated with intimate partner violence. Women should be asked about safety at home confidentially and privately. Women who are in an abusive situation should be counseled on community services, including shelters, child care, and legal services.

Common Problems

Subsequent visits are an appropriate time for talking with couples about issues related to normal pregnancy. Women experience numerous physiologic changes, most of which are benign and resolve after delivery. Reassuring women that these changes are normal, common, and transient is important. Common problems include heartburn, genitourinary concerns, and pain.

- *Heartburn.* Heartburn is common because of relaxation of the lower esophageal sphincter due to increased progesterone. Eating smaller meals and avoiding greasy foods often improves symptoms. Antacids containing calcium carbonate or magnesium hydroxide are indicated for severe heartburn.
- *Urinary concerns.* Frequency and stress incontinence (urine loss after coughing, sneezing, or laughing) occur in the first and third trimesters and generally resolve after pregnancy. Women are encouraged to do Kegel exercises to strengthen their pelvic floor muscles.
- *Hemorrhoids.* Hemorrhoids worsen in pregnancy because of increased venous congestion in the rectal vascular plexus. Topical treatments, such as witch hazel pads, external hemorrhoid cream, and sitz baths may help and prophylactic stool softeners such as docusate sodium (Colace) can be tried.
- *Backache.* This is common in later pregnancy because of compensatory lordosis from the enlarging uterus and relaxin causing loosening of ligaments in the pubic symphysis, back, and pelvis. Wearing flat-heeled shoes and maintaining good posture can counter changes in the center of gravity.
- *Round ligament pain.* Spasm of the round ligaments produces a sharp, stabbing, sporadic pain in the inguinal area that is not harmful to the fetus. Pain is worse in multiparas. Exercise, warm baths, a pregnancy girdle, and acetaminophen sometimes help with symptoms.
- *Leukorrhea.* Vaginal secretions in pregnancy are heavier than usual and whitish. The discharge results from increased vaginal blood flow and high estrogen levels. Reassurance is helpful, because women often assume it is caused by infection.

Large amounts of information are available during pregnancy through books, videos, and the internet and many women have specific ideas about what they want during labor. Women desiring "natural childbirth" need to be questioned about what this means to them. Use of epidural, breastfeeding, infant rooming-in versus nursery care, pacifier use, and circumcision can all be addressed as part of the birth plan. Discussing the planned course early allows the physician flexibility in accommodating the couples' wishes while ensuring the highest standards of maternity care. The benefit of formal classes is unclear, although observational studies demonstrate improved performance in labor in expectant women who attend childbirth classes.

The World Health Organization recommends that all infants be fed with breast milk exclusively from birth to at least age 6 months. Babies who are breastfed are less likely to develop otitis media, gastroenteritis, upper respiratory infections, and urinary tract infections. A recent Cochrane review found that two to four short (10 to 15 minutes) breastfeeding education sessions with a lactation consultant provided to low income women two to four times during prenatal care resulted in a significant increase in the women's duration of breastfeeding (36).

TOLAC

Discussing plans for delivery in women with a previous cesarean delivery is best done starting in the late second trimester. For many women, TOLAC is preferred over elective repeat cesarean delivery. The total cesarean rate has increased from 5.5% in 1970 to 31.8% in 2007, making it the 11th consecutive year of increase and another record high in the United States (37). In 2002, 12.4% of women elected to attempt TOLAC, down from a high of 28.3% of women in 1996.

Both ACOG and AAFP have issued guidelines for women considering TOLAC. Women with one previous cesarean delivery with a low transverse uterine incision are candidates for and should be offered a trial of labor. Several factors influence the likelihood of success of a vaginal birth after cesarean (VBAC). Positive factors include maternal age younger than 40 years, having a prior vaginal delivery or VBAC, a favorable cervix, spontaneous labor, and a nonrecurrent indication that was the reason for the prior cesarean delivery (i.e., breech). Factors that decrease the likelihood of successful VBAC include a history of multiple surgical deliveries, gestational age older than 40 weeks, fetal weight over 4,000 g, and the need for labor augmentation or induction (38).

Prostaglandins (Prepidil, Cervidil) are not recommended for cervical ripening or induction because their use is associated with higher rates of uterine rupture. ACOG and AAFP differ on recommendations as to facilities in which TOLAC should be attempted. ACOG recommends that TOLAC be restricted to facilities in which surgical teams are physically present throughout labor. The AAFP states that there is not good evidence available that having a surgical team standing by results in improved outcomes, and that a clinically appropriate plan for uterine rupture or any emergency requiring rapid surgical delivery must be documented for any woman attempting TOLAC. Providers should discuss all issues pertinent to a woman's decision, including recovery time, safety, and prior birth experiences. Unfortunately, no evidence-based recommendation is currently available regarding the best method for presenting risks and benefits of TOLAC to patients.

SPECIAL TOPICS

Early Pregnancy Loss and Ectopic Pregnancy

Family physicians will encounter women with abnormal pregnancies. 10- to 15% of clinically recognized pregnancies end in fetal loss. Risk factors for pregnancy loss include increased age, previous spontaneous abortion, smoking, certain infectious diseases, and immunologic dysfunction.

Vaginal bleeding is common during pregnancy and approximately one quarter of women experience bleeding during the first trimester. Half of these women have uneventful prenatal courses. Cramping and abdominal pain increase the likelihood of spontaneous pregnancy loss (spontaneous abortion). If the cervix is dilated or products of conception are seen in the vagina, the prognosis is poor. If the cervical os is closed, transvaginal ultrasound and serial β-HCG levels help in the assessment of viability.

It is critical to rule out ectopic pregnancy in cases of first trimester bleeding. Risk factors for ectopic pregnancy include previous pelvic inflammatory disease, history of ectopic pregnancy, tubal surgery, assisted reproductive technology, and current use of an intrauterine device. Diagnosing ectopic pregnancy can be challenging. Patients may have first trimester bleeding or be asymptomatic. Pelvic pain begins insidiously or suddenly, is usually lateralized, and can be mild or severe. The uterine size may be smaller than expected and an adnexal mass may be present. Ultrasound may show a fetal pole or heartbeat visible outside the uterine cavity or a thick-walled adnexal mass without a yolk sac or fetal pole that is separate from the ovary.

Early diagnosis of an ectopic pregnancy is augmented using quantitative β-HCG (increase by at least 66% over 48 hours expected) and transvaginal ultrasound. Prompt identification and timely treatment are critical, as ectopic gestation occurs in 2% of total pregnancies and is the leading cause of maternal mortality during the first trimester.

Postdates Pregnancy

One-tenth of pregnancies continue to at least 42 weeks' gestation and are considered postdates. Maternal risks associated with postdates pregnancy include dystocia, postpartum hemorrhage, emergent surgical delivery, and cephalopelvic disproportion. Fetal risks include asphyxia, meconium aspiration, septicemia, and death. The perinatal mortality rate (stillbirths and neonatal deaths) is 2 to 3 per 1,000 at term, doubles by 42 weeks, and is four to six times greater by 44 weeks' gestation (39).

Management of pregnancy beyond 40 weeks' gestation depends on the accurate assessment of gestational age. The most common cause of postterm pregnancy is inaccurate dating. Elective induction of pregnancies before 42 weeks is advocated to reduce risks of adverse maternal and fetal outcomes. A Cochrane review of 19 RCTs found that routine labor induction at 41 weeks or later is associated with fewer perinatal deaths, although the absolute risk is extremely small. Women induced at 37 to 40 completed weeks' gestation were more likely to have a cesarean delivery than those who underwent labor induction at 41 weeks (40). No difference between groups was noted for meconium aspiration syndrome or other neonatal morbidity, but infants in the expectant management group more frequently had meconium stained amniotic fluid.

There is not a current consensus on the management of postdates pregnancy. The Society of Obstetricians and Gynecologists of Canada recommends routine induction of labor at 41 weeks' gestation. ACOG does not define an upper gestational age at which induction is suggested, but does recommend fetal assessment beginning at 42 weeks' gestation. When a physician and patient elect to manage a postterm pregnancy expectantly, fetal monitoring is indicated. A combination of twice-weekly non-stress testing, amniotic fluid index or biophysical profile is used, although evidence of benefit is unclear and no single test is better than another (Table 4.6).

TABLE 4.6 Testing Methods for Postdates Pregnancy Surveillance

Nonstress Testing

Result	Criteria
Category 1 (normal-previously "reactive")	Two or more fetal heart rate accelerations over a 20-minute period; each acceleration must be at least 15 beats above the baseline heart rate and last at least 15 seconds; testing may be extended to 40 minutes to account for fetal sleep–wake cycles
Category 2 (equivocal)	Further testing required
Category 3 (previously nonreactive [abnormal])	No accelerations seen over a 40-minute period; if strip does not normalize, consider delivery

Biophysical Profile Parameters

Subsets	Score of 0	Score of 2
Fetal movement	Absent, abnormal, or insufficient	Three or more discrete body or limb movements within 30 minutes
Fetal tone	Abnormal, absent, or insufficient	At least one extension of extremity with return to flexion; opening or closing of hand
Fetal breathing	Abnormal, absent, or insufficient	One episode of fetal breathing movements lasting 30 seconds or more within 30 minutes
Amniotic fluid volume	Largest vertical pocket 2 cm or less	Single vertical pocket >2 cm
Nonstress test	Nonreactive	Reactive

Adapted from: ACOG practice bulletin. Antepartum fetal surveillance. Number 9, October 1999. Clinical management guidelines for obstetrician-gynecologists. Int J Gynaecol Obstet 2000;68:175–185; ACOG Practice Bulletin No. 106: Intrapartum fetal heart rate monitoring: nomenclature, interpretation, and general management principles. Obstetrics and Gynecology 2009;114(1):192–202.

TABLE 4.7 Summary of Evidence-based Recommendations

Preconception Careod

Recommendation	Strength of Recommendation*	Reference
Women considering becoming pregnant and pregnant women should be counseled that dietary supplementation with folic acid (400 mcg) before conception and during the first trimester decreases the risk of neural tube defects in the fetus	A	4
Intensive preconception glycemic control in women with diabetes prevents major congenital anomalies in offspring	A	4
Women with epilepsy planning to conceive should be changed to monotherapy or less teratogenic medications when possible, and advised to take at least 1 mg of folic acid daily before conception	B	4
Smoking cessation should be advised for all women who anticipate becoming pregnant because of decreases in neonatal morbidity and mortality	A	17

Pregnancy Care

Recommendation	Strength of Recommendation*	References
The traditional visit schedule can be abbreviated without an increase in adverse maternal or neonatal outcomes. The abbreviated schedule is less expensive, but women may be less satisfied with the decreased number of visits	A	10
Women with a continuity provider more likely attend prenatal education, discuss concerns, require less analgesia in labor, and feel prepared for delivery and infant care	A	9
Maternal weight and height should be measured at the fist antenatal appointment in order to calculate the body mass index (BMI)	B	17, 18
Blood pressure measurement is recommended at each prenatal visit	C	18
Routine breast examination during antenatal care is not recommended for the promotion of postpartum breast feeding	A	17
Routine cervical examination is not effective for predicting preterm birth and should not be offered unless clinically indicated	A	17
Pregnant women should be offered fundal height measurements at each prenatal visit to detect small or large for gestation fetuses	B	17
Routine ultrasound before 24 weeks allows for better estimation of gestational age and decreased need for labor induction for postdate pregnancy. No significant difference in clinical outcomes is apparent	A	25

Pregnant women older than age 35 or with an abnormal screening test (triple screen, quadruple screen) should be offered screening for Down syndrome. The screening test should have a detection rate >60% and a false-positive rate <5%. These tests fulfill these criteria:
• 11–14 weeks:
  • nuchal translucency (NT)
  • the combined test (NT, human chorionic gonadotropin [HCG], and pregnancy-associated plasma protein A)
• 14–20 weeks:
  • the triple test (HCG, estriol [uE3], and alpha-fetoprotein [AFP])
  • the quadruple test (HCG, uE3, AFP, and inhibin A)
	B	17

Healthy, pregnant women are encouraged to participate in mild to moderate exercise three or more times weekly	A	18
Individualized exercise programs should consider each pregnant woman's pre-pregnancy activity and fitness levels	B	18
Pregnant women should be counseled as to the proper use and positioning of seat belts (three-point restraints located across the hips and above the fundus)	B	17
Sexual intercourse during pregnancy is not associated with harmful effects in the absence of obstetric contraindications	B	17

*A, consistent, good-quality patient-oriented evidence; B, inconsistent or limited-quality patient-oriented evidence; C, consensus, disease-oriented evidence, usual practice, expert opinion, or case series. For information about the SORT evidence rating system, see *http://www.aafp.org/afpsort.xml.*

The interpretation of non-stress testing has recently been revised and is shown in Table 4.6. A Category 1 NST has a negative predictive value for stillbirth of 99.8%, and a positive predictive value of 10%. The biophysical profile has a negative predictive rate of 99.9%, whereas an abnormal study has a PPV of 40% (41).

Family Physicians' Approach to Maternity Care

Family medicine is the only specialty that emphasizes longitudinal, comprehensive care for families without regard to age, sex, or disease condition. Family physicians view pregnancy as a normal, healthy life event. Providing prenatal and infant care as part of an ongoing family relationship allows for continuity that is so often lacking in the modern healthcare system. Family physicians who deliver babies are more likely to earn higher incomes, be more psychologically satisfied with work, perform more procedures, and have a younger practice than those who do not do obstetrics (42).

Family physicians who provide maternity care have a broad range of practice patterns. Some provide prenatal care only, while others perform cesarean deliveries and share call with obstetrician-gynecologists. Family physicians are well trained to provide independent, evidence-based maternity care for women and competently manage low risk pregnancies. Family physicians with advanced fellowship training are capable of managing higher acuity pregnancy care.

Family Physicians and Obstetric Consultants

Family physicians work closely with their obstetric consultants in caring for pregnant women who require higher acuity care. When the consultation process works effectively, the patient benefits from a specialty opinion while maintaining the continuity relationship with the primary physician. The AAFP-ACOG liaison committee has published guidelines for consultations between family physicians and obstetrician gynecologists (43). Family physicians are encouraged to request consults in a timely fashion, clearly discuss the reasons for consultation, and maintain collegial relationships with physicians who provide backup. Physicians who provide backup for family physicians should see the patient in a timely fashion, and be a collaborative part of the care team. Family physicians who act as consultants for obstetrician-gynecologists for medical referrals should also strive to provide timely and evidence-based care. Evidence-based recommendations for prenatal care are found in Table 4.7.

KEY POINTS

- The preconception visit is used to maximize the expectant parents' health and well being prior to conception and covers health promotion (e.g., smoking cessation, immunizations), risk assessment (e.g., occupational exposure, genetic screening, medical comorbidity, substance use), and medical intervention (e.g., folic acid supplementation, medication adjustment). It is likely the most important prenatal visit for the prevention of birth defects.
- Clinical information useful for diagnosing pregnancy includes a detailed menstrual history, symptom review (most commonly amenorrhea, nausea, fatigue, and breast tenderness), physical signs (e.g., softening and bluish cervical discoloration), and a urine or serum pregnancy test. Transvaginal ultrasound is the best diagnostic choice for women with abnormal bleeding or abdominal pain and a positive pregnancy test and sonographic landmarks (e.g., gestational sac) assist in dating the pregnancy.
- Additional nutrients needed during pregnancy include folic acid (400 mcg (0.4 mg) starting at least 1 month prior to conception), iron (30 mg of ferrous iron), and calcium (1,000 to 1,300 mg per day).
- Screening for Down syndrome can be performed with a first trimester combined test (nuchal translucency using ultrasound combined with β-HCG and PAPP A) or with the quadruple test (serum markers of maternal serum alpha fetoprotein (MSAFP), estriol (uE3), β-HCG, and inhibin A); the latter detects 86% of infants with Down syndrome. Selective screening for gestational diabetes (exempts women considered at low risk) is generally performed at 24 to 28 weeks' gestation using a 1 hour blood glucose test after oral ingestion of 50 g glucose.
- Discussing plans for delivery in women with a previous cesarean delivery is best done starting in the late second trimester. For many women, trial of labor after cesarean (TOLAC) is preferred over elective repeat cesarean delivery.
- There is lack of consensus on the management of post dates pregnancy; options include elective induction at 41 weeks (results in lower perinatal mortality) or expectant management with monitoring using biweekly non stress tests and modified or full biophysical profiles until 42 weeks followed by induction.

CHAPTER

5

Well-child and Adolescent Care

Beat Steiner

CLINICAL OBJECTIVES

1. Describe preventive care tailored to pediatric and adolescent patients.
2. List which screening tests are most recommended for a child who comes for a well-child visit.
3. Discuss what information should be provided to patients and parents when considering the risks and benefits of immunizations that are given to a child.
4. Describe which health-related behaviors physicians can expect to influence most when seeing adolescent patients in the office.

PROVIDING EFFECTIVE PREVENTIVE CARE TO CHILDREN AND ADOLESCENTS: AN OVERVIEW

Well-child care can be one of the most rewarding things that a family physician does. Such care allows a clinician to deliver evidence based services to children to keep them healthy. It reassures parents about normal development and gives children the knowledge about their bodies to maintain their health as they mature into adults. It also gives the physician an often welcome opportunity to interact with a happy and healthy family. This chapter provides students with foundational materials to offer high quality well-child care. Infants, children, and adolescents require different areas of emphasis so this chapter focuses on each of these age groups in separate sections. Each section follows the RISE mnemonic presented in the overview chapter. Unless otherwise referenced, evidence presented in this chapter comes from the US Preventive Services Task Force (*www.ahrq.gov/clinic/uspstfix.htm*) (1) or the American Academy of Pediatrics "Bright Futures" publication (*brightfutures.aap.org*) (2).

Despite the potential rewards of well-child care, such care is often not adequately provided. The most common barriers to providing such care include: lack of time during the office visit, inadequate insurance reimbursement, patient refusal to discuss or comply with recommendations, and lack of physician expertise in counseling techniques (3). Providing effective well-child care thus requires more than a simple understanding of what risk factors to focus on, what immunizations to order, what screening tests to offer, and what educational topics to discuss. It also requires an understanding of how to redesign health systems to allow physicians to deliver such care more effectively.

The Patient Centered Medical Home concept, endorsed by the American Academy of Family Physicians, the American Academy of Pediatrics, American College of Physicians, and the American Osteopathic Society, provides such a system redesign (4). Key components include having a personal physician who knows the child well. Preventive services not offered during one visit can be provided during a subsequent visit. The personal physician leads a team of individuals at the practice level who collectively takes responsibility for the preventive care needed by the child. This team can effectively share the workload required to provide high-quality well-child care. A nurse, for example, can complete certain screening tests before the child is seen by the physician. A nurse educator can provide more in-depth educational counseling. Care is facilitated by registries and information technology that tracks care. Reminders pop up in the electronic health record when immunizations are due. Letters are generated to remind patients when it is time to schedule a preventive care visit. Payment systems appropriately reimburse clinicians because of the added value provided to patients who have a patient-centered medical home. Additional payments are available for ancillary services such as health educators. Pay-for-performance services reimburse practices who achieve defined quality goals such as target immunization rates. Practices have not yet adopted the Patient Centered Medical Home model universally but regional efforts such as Community Care of North Carolina have demonstrated feasibility as well as associated improved outcomes (5).

WELL-CHILD CARE FOR EARLY CHILDHOOD (AGES 0 TO 2 YEARS)

Parents who bring infants for well-child care are often happy but also anxious, with first-time parents still adjusting to their new roles. An important goal of these visits therefore is to establish trust and allay anxiety. Clinicians can do this by spending a short time interacting with the infant at the beginning of the visit, taking time to elicit any concerns or questions from the parent early in the visit, and remaining aware of nonverbal cues.

Risk Assessment

PERINATAL PERIOD

It is important to review the mother's pregnancy, delivery, and postpartum notes to identify important risk factors. For example, breech position during pregnancy, especially in young girls, may require a follow-up ultrasound at 6 to 8 weeks to evaluate for developmental dysplasia of the hip. A shoulder dystocia during delivery will require a more detailed physical exam to evaluate for a brachial plexus injury. Failure to pass the screening hearing exam in the newborn nursery will require further evaluation. If not done during prenatal care, clinicians should obtain a detailed family history to identify increased risks for genetically linked conditions such as sickle cell disease/trait, thalassemia, cystic fibrosis, muscular dystrophy, fragile X syndrome, and Down syndrome. Many of these conditions are also screened for on routine state-mandated newborn screens at birth.

Finally, an in-depth social history can provide important information to guide care for the infant and the family. Clinicians should explore social, environmental, and financial stressors to identify families in need of additional community resources, ask mothers about postpartum depressive symptoms and inquire about contraceptive intentions.

GROWTH AND DEVELOPMENT

Inadequate growth may be the presenting feature of a variety of disorders, such as endocrinopathies, cardiac diseases, and renal dysfunction but is more commonly a result of social stressors, poor bonding, and inadequate nutrition. Height, weight, and head circumference should be measured during all routine office visits during the first 2 years of life and plotted on a standardized growth chart. The growth *rate* may be more meaningful than individual measurements alone. After age 2, only height and weight need to be plotted and expressed as a BMI centile.

Development can be monitored by documenting achievement of age-appropriate milestones for intellectual, motor, and social skills. Early identification of developmental delays allows timely implementation of appropriate interventions and identification of available community resources. Unfortunately, clinical assessment alone detects <30% of children with developmental disabilities. Standardized developmental screening instruments such as Denver II screening test, Battelle Developmental Inventory, and others, are more sensitive. Parent report instruments, such as the Parents' Evaluation of Developmental Status and Child Development Inventories, can be similarly effective and require much less physician time. Clinicians generally begin using standardized developmental screening around 6 months of age (6).

Immunizations and Chemoprophylaxis

Immunization has probably saved more children's lives than any other public health intervention, with the possible exception of providing clean water (7). Although US childhood immunization rates have risen over the past two decades, disparities continue, with lower rates among children living in poverty, urban settings, and among black and Hispanic children (8). Clinicians should withhold immunizations only for true contraindications, which are rare (Table 5.1), and implement office systems to effectively track immunization status of patients, obtain appropriate informed consent from the patient and the family and use every visit to provide indicated immunizations.

RECOMMENDED VACCINES

The immunization schedule recommended by the Centers of Disease Control and Prevention (CDC) can be viewed online at (*www.cdc.gov/nip/recs/child-schedule.htm*). Clinicians should be aware that this schedule changes regularly and is likely to continue to change as new and more effective vaccines are introduced. In addition, the Society of Teachers of Family Medicine (STFM) has a very helpful and updated website: *http://www.immunizationed.org/*. Most vaccines are started in the first 2 years of life and the primary series is completed by the time children enter school. For children who fall behind the recommended schedule, the CDC offers detailed

TABLE 5.1 Contraindications and Precautions for Childhood Immunizations

True Contraindications and Precautions	Not True Contraindications (Vaccines May Be Given)
Anaphylactic reaction to vaccine	Mild to moderate local reactions (soreness, redness, swelling) after a dose of injectable vaccine
Moderate or severe acute illness following a dose of an injectable vaccine	Mild acute illness with or without low-grade fever
Known hypersensitivity to component of vaccine	Current antimicrobial therapy
Moderate or severe acute illness as it may be difficult to identify subsequent reactions from immunization	Convalescent phase of illness Prematurity (same schedule and indications as full-term infants)
Pregnancy in vaccine recipient (certain live vaccines only)	Recent exposure to an infectious agent History of penicillin or other nonspecific allergies in child or any allergy in a relative

Adapted from American Academy of Pediatrics. Guide to Contraindications and Precautions to Immunizations, Red Book 2009.

guidelines to catch up these children with accelerated schedules (*http://www.cdc.gov/vaccines/recs/scheduler/catchup.htm*). Current inactivated vaccines include vaccines against diphtheria, tetanus, pertussis, polio, hepatitis A and B, Haemophilus influenza type B, seasonal and H1N1 influenza, and rotavirus. Live vaccines include vaccines against measles, mumps, rubella, and varicella. These live vaccines are delayed until children reach 12 months of age and should in general be avoided in immune-compromised children. The intranasal influenza vaccine is also a live attenuated vaccine and should be delayed until children are 2 years of age.

VACCINE SAFETY

In recent years, an increasing number of articles in parent magazines and web site postings have questioned the safety of the vaccine programs. Do vaccines cause autism, sudden infant death syndrome (SIDS), seizures, encephalitis, and other neurologic problems? The evidence-based answer is consistently no. Although large and systematic analysis of the data have consistently found no links to such adverse effects, clinicians must take the time to address these questions and use available scientific knowledge to help parents make informed decisions.

The Institute of Medicine has released a comprehensive series of reports that examine adverse effects of the major vaccines and may be used as an evidence-based reference when discussing this topic with concerned parents (9) (the full text can be found online at *http://www.iom.edu*). Two other websites, one maintained by Johns Hopkins School of Public Health (*http://www.vaccinesafety.edu*) and one maintained by the Immunization Action Coalition (*http://www.immunize.org*), provide regularly updated advice and the latter provides subscribers with regularly e-mailed newsletters.

Thiomersal in particular has received much attention. This preservative has been used in vaccines since the 1930s and contains traces of mercury. In a review of all available data, the Institute of Medicine found that there are inadequate data to make a conclusion for or against any adverse side effects of thiomersal. Nevertheless, a thiomersal-free version of all vaccines given to children younger than 6 years of age is now available.

VITAMIN D CHEMOPROPHYLAXIS

Increasing evidence of vitamin D deficiency in the population has also prompted recent revisions of guidelines for supplementation with vitamin D (10). Vitamin D supplementation of 400 IU/day is now recommended for all infants and young children, both breast and formula fed. Because this would require consuming more than 1 L of formula per day, clinicians should recommend supplementation in the form of multivitamin drops.

Screening

Recommended screening tests are listed in Table 5.2. A clinician should also remain alert for conditions listed in Table 5.3, but realize that evidence of screening effectiveness is lacking.

RARE GENETIC DISEASES

Recent advances in technology have created a significant increase in screening tests available to newborns. States for many years have required a screening blood test for hypothyroidism and phenylketonuria because of the profound and irreversible effects if these conditions remain unrecognized. Today most states require screening for at least eight core conditions and many states have added further conditions. State by state requirements can be viewed at *http://genes-r-us.uthscsa.edu/resources/consumer/statemap.htm*. Most states do not require parental consent prior to screening, but do allow exemption for religious and other reasons. In addition, many states require that if the infant was screened before 24 hours of age, the screening should be repeated before 2 weeks of age, because of the greater possibility of false-negative results in the immediate postpartum period.

HEARING

Most states now require universal newborn hearing screening and 2 to 3 of 1,000 babies are born with some degree of hearing loss. Using auditory brainstem response (ABR) or otoacoustic emissions (OAE), congenital hearing loss can be identified in the newborn period. Early identification can prevent abnormal language and learning development. Parents should be reassured that both ABRs and OAEs have high false-positive rates and that repeat testing or referral to audiologist is required to further assess the child.

CONGENITAL HEART DISEASE

Congenital heart disease has an incidence of approximately 1% of births and accounts for half of all deaths from congenital abnormalities. Most cases can be detected in the first 6 months of life. Although not specifically evaluated by the USPSTF as a screening test, most clinicians advise auscultation of the heart and palpation of pulses (including femoral pulses) to detect asymptomatic septal defects and aortic coarctation, respectively.

ANEMIA (HIGH-RISK ONLY)

Iron deficiency anemia in infancy and early childhood has been associated with delayed growth and development and is reversible with adequate supplementation (note that the criteria for anemia in children are age dependent). In children with significant iron deficiency anemia, the effects of treatment are dramatic. Screening for and treating milder iron deficiency anemia remains more controversial. Hemoglobin as a screening tool for detecting iron deficiency in toddlers in the United States seems to lack sensitivity and specificity, and treating anemia found with such screening may not be beneficial (11). Universal supplementation with multivitamins and iron for high-risk infants (e.g., low-income populations, immigrants from developing countries, premature and low-birth-weight infants), may be a more effective strategy (12).

LEAD (HIGH-RISK ONLY)

Low-level lead toxicity (serum levels of 10 to 25 mg/dL) can lead to subtle effects on behavior, cognition, sleep patterns, and growth rate and eliminating such elevations is considered a national health objective (13). Over the past two decades, blood levels have decreased dramatically but it is still estimated that more than 300,000 children ages 1 to 5 years remain at risk for exposure to harmful lead levels (14). Elevated levels remain more common in children living: 1) in communities where prevalence of elevated lead levels is high, 2) in houses built before 1950 with dilapidated paint or

TABLE 5.2 US Preventive Services Task Force Screening Recommendations for Children and Adolescents

Age	Screening Test	Comments	Strength of Recommendation*
All children	Growth (including head circumference) and development younger than age 2, BMI centiles after age 6	The optimal frequency has not been defined	B
	Blood pressure, auscultation of heart (in children), and palpation of femoral pulses (in newborns)	The optimal frequency has not been defined; accurate blood pressure measurements are particularly difficult in children<3 years of age	B
Newborn	Newborn screen—content varies by state	Repeat TSH, PKU at 2 weeks of age if tested before 24 hours of life	A
	Hearing screen	Otoacoustic emissions (OAE) followed by Auditory Brain Response (ABR) for OAE failures	B
6–12 months	Blood-lead concentration	Screen only high-risk groups*	B
1–5 years	Vision screening for amblyopia and strabismus	Use cover-uncover test or Random Dot E; screening before age 5	B
	Mantoux test (using PPD) for TB	Screen only high-risk groups†; start screening at 12–15 months of age	B
Adolescents	Pap smear, chlamydia (female only)	Screen if sexually active*	A
	HIV	All adolescents >13 years old if sexually active	B
	Gonorrhea, syphilis	Screen high-risk group*	B
	Depression	When systems are in place to assure appropriate management	B

Data from US Preventive Services Task Force. Guide to Clinical Preventive Services. *http://www.ahrq.gov/clinic/uspstf/uspstopics.htm*
BMI = body mass index; PKU = phenylketonuria; TSH = thyroid-stimulating hormone; PPD = purified protein derivative; HIV = human immunodeficiency virus
*Level of evidence for effectiveness: A, strong or moderate research-based evidence (consistent across several studies, including at least two randomized controlled trials); B, limited research-based evidence (less consistent or extensive evidence, but preponderance of evidence supports use of treatment); C, common practice with little or no research-based evidence; X, moderate or strong evidence suggesting that this intervention is not effective
†High risk for anemia: low income populations, immigrants from developing countries, premature and low birth-weight infants
High risk for lead: persons living in communities where prevalence of elevated lead levels is high, living in houses built before 1950 with dilapidated paint or undergoing recent renovation, or living with someone whose hobby involves lead exposure such as stained glass work or metal sculpture
High risk for TB: persons infected with HIV, close contacts of persons with known or suspected tuberculosis, immigrants from countries with high tuberculosis prevalence, and medically underserved populations including the homeless
High Risk for STD: men who have had sex with men; men and women having unprotected sex with multiple partners; past or present injection drug users; men and women who exchange sex for money or drugs or have sex partners who do; individuals whose past or present sex partners were HIV-infected, bisexual, or injection drug users; persons being treated for sexually transmitted infections and persons requesting an HIV test

undergoing recent renovation, or 3) with someone whose hobby involves lead exposure such as stained glass work or metal sculpture. Children given food supplements contaminated by lead or eating from pottery containing lead are also at risk. This is seen more commonly in recent immigrants, especially from Latin American countries. It remains controversial whether reduction in blood lead levels leads to clinical improvement (behavior, cognition) in children with low to moderate levels of lead intoxication. Environmental lead abatement programs are effective at reducing risk of exposure for other children. Although the USPSTF found that the evidence is insufficient to support screening, many states still require that high-risk subgroups be screened between 1 and 2 years of age.

TUBERCULOSIS (HIGH-RISK ONLY)

The annual incidence of tuberculosis in children declined by nearly 50% in the United States between 1993 and 2001, to 1.5 cases/100,000. Certain subgroups, however, remain at much higher risk and should be screened as discussed in the following section. Screening is performed with the Mantoux test in which purified protein derivative is injected intradermally. When administered properly, the sensitivity of the test is 90 to 95%. Induration of 10 mm or more constitutes a positive test

TABLE 5.3 Important Conditions for Which Universal Screening Is Not Recommended by USPSTF but Clinical Vigilance Needed

Age	Condition	Additional Comments
All children	Early childhood caries Dental crowding or misalignment	
Newborn	Symptoms and signs of hip instability or dislocation Cataract	Consider screening ultrasound if breech position during pregnancy Assessment of red reflex with ophthalmoscope in newborn period remains standard practice in most settings
Children younger than 3 years of age	Congenital heart disease Undescended testes Anemia	Cardiac auscultation for murmurs remains standard practice in most settings Consider iron supplementation for at-risk children age 6–12 mo
Children and adolescents	Family violence Hyperlipidemia Exercise-induced asthma	Consider non fasting lipid panel for at-risk children age 2–20
Adolescents	Large spinal curvatures	

for high-risk individuals and children younger than 4 years of age. Induration of 15 mm for low-risk individuals is assumed to be specific for tuberculous infection (note that it is important to measure induration and not just erythema). If the test is positive, chemoprophylaxis is recommended to prevent subsequent development of active tuberculosis in an asymptomatic child. The true specificity of the test, however, remains poorly defined because there is no reliable gold standard for latent infection. Please see the chapter on tuberculosis for further details.

Because of false-positive results, cost, potential toxicity, and the inconvenience of Isoniazid treatment, screening is recommended only in high-risk groups. This includes people infected with HIV, close contacts of persons with known or suspected tuberculosis, immigrants from countries with high tuberculosis prevalence, and medically underserved populations including the homeless. Screening should begin at 12 to 15 months of age and be repeated annually or biannually if the child or adolescent remains in a high-risk group. Any child or adolescent found to have active tuberculosis should also be tested for HIV infection.

Education/Counseling

During well-child care for young children, education should focus on topics for which good evidence exists that counseling by physicians can change behavior. Based on the most current evidence, a summary of recommended counseling topics is presented in Table 5.4. But given the developmental stage of many young families, it may be even more important to spend time educating parents about normal development and thereby reducing anxiety and worry. Topics for which less supporting evidence exists but which are nonetheless an important part of well-child care visits in the first 2 years of the life are presented at the end of this section (bowel habits, stimulation, sleeping, crying, skin care).

SIDS

Although the pathophysiology of SIDS remains largely unknown, several studies have helped clinicians provide advice on how to reduce the chance of this devastating event. A modifiable association between SIDS and the child's sleeping position has been found in repeated studies (15). Children who slept on their stomachs had roughly twice the incidence of SIDS, an association that has prompted multiple organizations to recommend that healthy infants sleep only on their backs (Back to Sleep Campaign). The validity of this recommendation is supported by a decline in the incidence of SIDS since this new sleep position was first advocated (15).

CAR SEATS

Clinicians should use well-child care opportunities to remind parents that the child must remain in a car seat at all times while the car is moving. Motor vehicle crashes account for the highest number of deaths among children older than 1 year. A systematic review of randomized controlled trials showed that counseling about seat restraints for young children was more likely to be heeded by parents than guidance on other issues (16).

TABLE 5.4 Counseling Messages for Children and Adolescents

Age Group	Counseling Message*
Newborns	Place infant on back to sleep Breastfeed
Children	Install smoke detectors Use flame-retardant sleepwear Set hot water heaters below 125°F Use childproof containers for medication Use approved bicycle helmets Store firearms safely Supplement fluoride if inadequate in water Visit dentist regularly Brush teeth and floss regularly Eliminate exposure to passive smoking Use child safety seats, lap/shoulder belts Limit intake of dietary fat and portion size Limit television time Engage in regular physical exercise
Adolescents	Avoid tobacco Avoid alcohol Avoid drugs Maintain abstinence Use condoms regularly if sexually active Use contraception regularly if sexually active Develop strategies to avoid violence

Data from US Preventive Services Task Force (*http://www.ahrq.gov/clinic/uspstf/uspstopics.htm*) and from Bright Futures (*http://brightfutures.aap.org/pdfs/Guidelines_PDF/13-Rationale_and_Evidence.pdf*).
Topics were included in this table if there is level A, B, or C evidence that counseling in office changes behavior and there is clear evidence that behavior change leads to improved health outcomes. Levels of evidence are defined as follows: (A) strong or moderate research-based evidence (consistent across several studies, including at least two randomized controlled trials); (B) limited research-based evidence (less consistent or extensive evidence, but preponderance of evidence supports use of treatment); (C) common practice with insufficient evidence for or against.

OTHER INJURIES

Although suffocation and motor vehicle crashes are the most common causes of unintentional injury and death during early childhood, falls, fires and burns, poisoning, choking, and drowning also pose significant risks. Appropriate education can provide parents with the knowledge and confidence needed to reduce the likelihood of such injuries.

DENTAL HEALTH

Dental caries and periodontal disease are significant health problems for children. Daily brushing and flossing and frequent exposure to small amounts of fluoride have been proven to be effective. Brushing should start soon after the child has teeth, but toothpaste should not be added until the child is old enough to *not* swallow the toothpaste. Children living in an area with inadequate water fluoridation and exclusively breastfed children older than 6 months of age should be supplemented with daily fluoride drops (see CDC recommendations for dosage) (*http://www.cdc.gov/mmwr/preview/mmwrhtml/rr5014a1.htm#tab1*). Fluoride varnish may prove to be an equally effective alternative option. Routine visits to a dentist have also been shown to improve dental health, although the optimal frequency remains unknown. Many dentists like to see children first between the ages of 18 months and 3 years.

BREASTFEEDING AND NUTRITION

Clinicians should encourage exclusive breastfeeding in the first 6 months of life. Breastfeeding can be continued after introduction of foods. Breastfeeding is associated with a reduced risk of otitis media, gastroenteritis, respiratory illness, SIDS, necrotizing enterocolitis, obesity, and hypertension. Breastfeeding is also associated with improved maternal outcomes, including a reduced risk of breast and ovarian cancer, type 2 diabetes, and postpartum depression (17). Solid foods should be delayed until 4 to 6 months of age. Cow's milk should not be introduced until 12 months of age. Although routine screening for iron deficiency anemia is not recommended, evidence shows that iron-enriched foods should be included in the diet of infants and young children. No restriction of fat and cholesterol is currently recommended for children younger than age 2.

BOWEL HABITS

The most common concern regarding bowel habits relates to frequency and consistency. Frequencies in normal children can vary from one bowel movement every few days to several bowel movements per day. Consistency can vary from very loose and yellow in breastfed babies to more well formed in bottle-fed infants. Further exploration may be warranted if the stool has a very foul odor or is very voluminous. In otherwise healthy children, who are not volume depleted, reassurance is usually all that is needed.

STIMULATION

Parents will agree intuitively that stimulation is important to develop an alert and curious infant. Clinicians can play a pivotal role in providing ideas and encouragement. Parents and caregivers can stimulate the infant by talking, reading, and singing. Other ideas include creating a brightly colored environment, periodically changing the location of the bed, rearranging the toys in the crib, hanging attractive mobiles over the crib, dancing, and taking frequent walks with the baby. As the infant grows, early introduction of books in the child's life may improve literacy. Reach Out and Read is one nationwide program that provides doctors' offices low-cost books to be given out during well-child visits (*http://www.reachoutandread.org/*).

SLEEP ISSUES

Infant sleeping patterns vary, with the amount of sleep time generally decreasing from birth through the preschool years. To prevent dental caries, a baby should never be put to bed with a bottle of milk or juice. Sleep location (a crib versus the parents' bed, a separate room versus the parents' room) is controversial, with arguments in favor of all arrangements. Although cultural and personal preferences must be considered, there is evidence from observational studies that sleeping in the parent's bed in rare cases leads to inadvertent smothering when the parent rolls onto the child. The importance of putting children to sleep on their backs was discussed previously.

WELL-CHILD CARE FOR MIDDLE CHILDHOOD (AGES 2 TO 11 YEARS)

As children grow older, clinicians should spend a larger part of the visit interacting with the child. A 2-year-old may still be shy, and remember with anxiety the last set of immunizations. During the physical exam, clinicians should not approach the child too quickly. To build confidence and allay fears, the least invasive and least painful parts of the examination should be done first. A 6 year old should be encouraged to ask questions and be provided answers to their questions during the interview. By the time a child is 10 years old, it may be appropriate to offer the child the opportunity to spend part of the visit alone with the clinician.

Risk Assessment

SEXUAL DEVELOPMENT

The age range of pubertal development is quite wide and appears to be occurring earlier with successive generations for unknown reasons. In girls, it is now not uncommon for thelarche (breast bud development) and/or pubarche (pubic hair growth) to start at age 8, and this is no longer considered to represent precocious puberty. Menarche tends to follow 2 to 3 years later. Puberty generally starts earlier in African-Americans (18). The first physical manifestation for boys is gonadarche (enlargement of testes). A pronounced growth spurt is also associated with onset of puberty (about 1 year after onset of breast bud development in girls, and 2 years after onset of genital enlargement in boys). Significant deviations in development should prompt consideration of an endocrinologic workup, including assessment of bone age.

Immunizations

Children should continue to be immunized according to recommended schedules (*www.cdc.gov/nip/recs/child-schedule.htm* and *http://www.immunizationed.org.*) The primary series of all immunizations is completed by the time the child enters kindergarten and is usually required at school entry, although exceptions can be made for conscientious objection, health, or religious reasons. Catch-up schedules should be used for children who have fallen behind on immunizations or for children newly immigrated who are not adequately immunized (*http://www.cdc.gov/vaccines/recs/scheduler/catchup.htm*).

Screening

WEIGHT

Childhood obesity is rapidly becoming a major public health problem. Based on definitions by the CDC, 15% of children are overweight, a number more than three times as high as in 1980. These children are more likely to suffer socially, and have increased morbidity and mortality as adults. Unlike adult body mass index (BMI), normal BMI varies with age and thus should be plotted on norm referenced charts at each visit. Children whose BMI is between the 85th and 95th centile for that age and gender are considered "overweight" and those greater than the 95th centile are considered obese. Appropriate charts are available at *http://www.cdc.gov/growthcharts/*. Even experienced clinicians may have a hard time visually identifying children who are clinically overweight and therefore we should screen for obesity in children (particularly older than age 6; USPSTF Grade B) by plotting BMI as it prompts greater recognition of a weight problem than plotting height and weight separately (19).

VISION

In children younger than age 5 years, the primary aim of vision screening is to identify children with strabismus and decreased visual acuity. Between ages 3 and 5 years, stereograms such as Random Dot E can be used (sensitivity of 54% to 64% and specificity of 87% to 90%). The cover-uncover test (Fig. 5.1) can be more easily performed because no special equipment is needed, but its test characteristics remain unknown. Using these screening tools for children younger than 3 years has generally been unsuccessful. Although USPSTF could find no direct evidence that screening for visual impairment, compared with no screening, leads to improved visual acuity, there is fair evidence that early treatment of strabismus and refractive error prevents amblyopia. For this reason, vision screening is generally recommended.

BLOOD PRESSURE

Although hypertension is rare in children, prevalence has increased with increased prevalence of childhood obesity. Thus, there is a general consensus that blood pressure should be measured periodically in children and adolescents. No good evidence exists for when measurement should first occur and at what intervals it should be repeated. Guided by how well

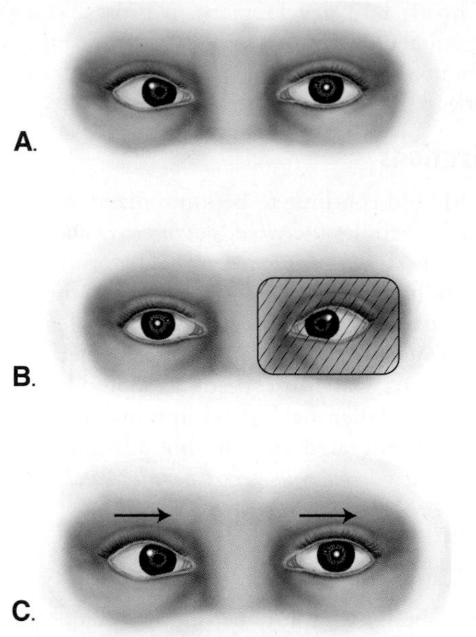

Figure 5.1 • Demonstration of cover-uncover test on child with nonparalytic right monocular esotropia. **A.** Examiner shines light in child's eyes, asking child to focus on light. *Corneal reflections not symmetrical*. **B.** Examiner covers left eye while still asking child to focus on light. *Right eye (weaker eye) moves to fix on light*. **C.** Examiner uncovers left eye while still asking child to focus on light. *The left eye (good eye) is uncovered and "takes over" and fixes on light. Right eye moves inward again*. From Bickley LS, Szilagyi P. Bates' Guide to Physical Examination and History Taking, 8th ed. Philadelphia: Lippincott Williams & Wilkins, 2003.

children can cooperate and the well-child check frequency, many clinicians first check blood pressures when a child is 3 years old and repeat these measurements periodically. Blood pressure measurements should be taken bilaterally using a cuff of correct width (two-thirds of upper arm length). An undersized cuff may give a falsely elevated reading. Criteria for childhood hypertension vary with age, but in general a blood pressure greater than the 95th percentile for that age group is diagnostic (reference ranges are available at: *http://www.nhlbi.nih.gov/guidelines/hypertension/child_tbl.htm*. As in adults, elevated blood pressure should be confirmed on at least two separate occasions before hypertension should be diagnosed.

SCREENING TESTS OF UNCERTAIN BENEFIT

There is disagreement whether we should screen for lipid disorders in children older than 2 years. Much of the controversy is due to the uncertainty whether early treatment will result in better outcomes. The USPSTF concluded in 2007 that evidence is insufficient to screen children for lipid disorders before age 20. By contrast, the American Academy of Pediatrics (AAP) recommended in 2008 to screen children and adolescents with a positive family history of dyslipidemia or premature coronary vascular disease once with a non-fasting lipid panel. The AAP also recommends that pediatric patients for whom family history is not known or those with other personal coronary vascular disease risks such as BMI greater than 85th percentile, blood pressure greater than 95th percentile, cigarette smoking, or diabetes mellitus be screened.

Routine urine dipstick testing of school-age children is also of uncertain benefit. This test is not supported by evidence because of the low prevalence of asymptomatic disease and the high proportion of false-positive tests.

Education/Counseling

WEIGHT

Despite the alarming trends in obesity, effective interventions continue to elude us. Nonetheless, as noted previously, the USPSTF recommends screening for obesity and then offering or referring obese children for intensive behavioral interventions based on some evidence (USPSTF Grade B). A recent Cochrane Review had found insufficient evidence for the effectiveness of behavioral counseling (or other preventive interventions with overweight children) that can be conducted in primary care settings (20). The issue of childhood obesity may require broader societal changes to affect a significant change in incidence.

In children older than age 2 and in adolescents, counseling should focus on limiting dietary intake of fat (<30% of total calories) and increasing the intake of fruits, vegetables (>5 servings), and grain products containing fiber (>6 servings). Children and adolescents should also be strongly encouraged to participate in regular physical exercise.

INJURY PREVENTION

Unintentional injury continues to be the leading cause of death and morbidity among children older than 1 year and adolescents. Motor vehicle crashes are responsible for the highest number of injuries but other causes such as falls, burns, firearms, bike, and other sport injuries contribute substantially. The well-child visit gives the clinician an opportunity to assess the family's strategies to avoid unintentional injuries and give guidance on avoiding risk. An acute visit for an injury provides another opportunity to educate as the family may be particularly receptive to changing behavior at that moment.

WELL-CHILD CARE FOR ADOLESCENTS (AGES 12 TO 18 YEARS)

Care for adolescents begins to resemble care for adults. Clinicians should make efforts to allow adolescents to be alone during the majority of the visit. Emancipated minors may receive all their care without adult consent. Emancipation is a legal definition that may be prompted by an adolescent marrying or living independently. In most states, even minors who are not legally emancipated may receive services related to mental health, evaluation and treatment of sexually transmitted diseases, and contraceptive management without adult consent.

Risk Assessment

RISKY SEXUAL BEHAVIOR

Clinicians frequently neglect inquiring about sexual activity in young adolescents, but by ninth grade 37% of males and 29% of females are sexually active (21). These youths are disproportionately affected by chlamydia, *Neisseria gonorrhea*, and other sexually transmitted infections. Asymptomatic carrier states are common and associated morbidity is high. Infection may also be a cofactor in the heterosexual transmission of HIV.

SUBSTANCE ABUSE

Three-quarters of young adolescents have tried alcohol at least once. Furthermore, 19% of 9th graders and 37% of 12th graders reported binge drinking (five or more drinks on one occasion) in the past month (21). Alcohol is also involved in half of all adolescent deaths from motor vehicle crashes, other unintentional injuries, suicides, and homicides. The burden of suffering of alcohol abuse, and the availability of alcohol abuse treatment resources makes this an important topic to address with all adolescents.

DEPRESSION AND SUICIDE

Seventeen percent of adolescents report having made a plan to commit suicide and it is the third leading cause of death in people 15- to 24 years old. Youth violence is also increasingly recognized as a major health problem. Clinicians should remain keenly alert for signs and symptoms of depression, problems with drugs or alcohol, a history of violent or criminal behavior, and the availability of weapons in the home. Prevalence rates for these risk behaviors come in large part from the Youth Risk Behavior Survey; updated results can be found at *www.cdc.gov/nccdphp/dash/yrbs/.*

EATING DISORDERS

Body image is a serious problem for many adolescents. The 2005 Youth Risk Behavior Survey found 61% of adolescent girls were attempting to lose weight. The prevalence of eating disorders is estimated to be between 1 to 3% among adolescents. Although some adolescents use unsafe means to be thin, others turn to supplements and steroids to gain muscle mass. Clinicians can assess whether a patient is at risk for an eating disorder by asking questions about goal weight and what the adolescent is doing to obtain/maintain that goal.

Immunizations

Although the majority of children in this age group will have completed the primary series of childhood immunizations, booster immunizations are recommended for children ages 10 to 12. In addition to boosters of the primary series, a vaccine against neisseria meningitis is recommended, as risk for n. meningitis is increased in the close quarters of college. For adolescent girls, the vaccine against the human papilloma virus is recommended, because it can reduce infection with strains of human papilloma virus responsible for the majority of cases of cervical cancer and some genital warts. Recommendations for vaccination against strains of influenza virus are rapidly changing and clinicians need to remain aware of current guidelines. Updated recommendations for all vaccines can be found on the CDC website (*http://www.cdc.gov/vaccines/recs/schedules/child-schedule.htm#printable*) or at *http://www.immunizationed.org/*.

Screening

SEXUALLY TRANSMITTED INFECTIONS

In 2006, the CDC revised its policy on HIV screening, now recommending universal HIV testing for adolescents and adults ages 13 to 64. Although the USPSTF agrees that evidence supports screening of high-risk populations, it gives a C recommendation for universal screening, given the issues of screening low prevalence populations.

All sexually active female adolescents should be routinely screened for chlamydia and gonorrhea. There is insufficient evidence to recommend for or against screening asymptomatic males. A number of tests exist to screen for chlamydia and gonorrhea, including cultures, direct fluorescent antibody testing, unamplified nucleic acid hybridization, and enzyme immunoassay performed on an endocervical, rectal, or urethral sample. Urine can also be used as a more convenient but more expensive test using nucleic acid amplification.

High-risk adolescents of both sexes should also be screened for syphilis. High risk is defined using epidemiologic data and includes: men who have had sex with men, men and women having unprotected sex with multiple partners, past or present injection drug users, men and women who exchange sex for money or drugs or have sex partners who do, individuals whose past or present sex partners were HIV-infected, bisexual, or injection drug users, persons being treated for sexually transmitted infections, and persons requesting an HIV test.

PAPANICOLAOU (PAP) SMEARS

Routine cervical cancer screening has traditionally been recommended within 3 years of initiating sexual activity for adolescents and young women. However, this recommendation was revised in December 2009 because many abnormal Pap smears in young women will revert to normal without treatment (22). At the time of this publication, it is recommended that adolescents and all women under age 21 not be screened for cervical cancer, irrespective of whether or not they are sexually active (22).

SUBSTANCE ABUSE

Although screening tools such as the CAGE questionnaire can be used with adolescents, the performance of such tools has not been well-validated in this age group. The USPSTF finds insufficient evidence to formally screen asymptomatic adolescents.

DEPRESSION

Depression screening tools have been adapted to the care of adolescents (PHQ-Adolescent) and the USPSTF recommends screening for depression when systems are in place for appropriate referral and treatment.

SPORTS PHYSICALS

Family physicians are often asked to do screening physicals for sport participation. The American Heart Association released revised guidelines in 2007 that recommend that such an exam include a detailed history including inquiries about chest pain, syncope or near syncope, and excessive shortness of breath. Clinicians should assess whether an adolescent has a personal history of heart murmurs or elevated blood pressure and a family history of premature sudden death or know cardiac conditions such as cardiomyopathies or arrhythmias. The physical exam should check blood pressure, assess for hear murmurs, palpations of the femoral pulses, and identification of stigmata of Marfan syndrome. Although European guidelines suggest that screening electrocardiograms based on population studies lead to decreases in sudden cardiac death, the American Heart Association has not endorsed this recommendation (23).

Education/Counseling

RISKY SEXUAL BEHAVIOR

Discussions should be based on a careful sexual history and tailored to the needs of individuals. As noted earlier, these conversations should take into account the early initiation of sexual activity by many teens. It is not unreasonable to begin these conversations between ages 10 and 12. Clinicians should discuss measures that can reduce risk, including abstaining from sex, maintaining a mutually faithful relationship with an uninfected partner, consistently using latex condoms, and avoiding sexual contact with casual partners. Other forms of contraception should also be discussed, but clinicians must emphasize that only latex condoms have been shown to effectively prevent transmission of most forms of sexually transmitted infections. Whereas these behavior changes are clearly effective, it remains less clear whether counseling adolescents in the office by clinicians can bring about such changes.

SUBSTANCE ABUSE

Strong evidence shows that brief counseling messages by clinicians can reduce tobacco use. Parents should be urged to stop smoking because of the documented ill effects on health of secondhand smoke. Clinicians should also give anti-tobacco messages to adolescents who smoke. Although the evidence is less strong for alcohol and other drugs, most guidelines urge clinicians to discuss these topics with adolescents. Although a discussion around drugs and alcohol may not change the adolescent's behavior on that visit, it encourages the adolescent to ask questions or raise concerns on that topic on future visits.

KEY POINTS

- Health care providers need to improve their rates of providing well child and adolescent care
- Systems developed within the health care medical home model can help improve the rates of children who are up to date with preventive interventions
- Immunizations remain our most effective method of primary prevention in children
- We should discontinue recommending interventions not supported by evidence
- US preventive services task force is the best non-partisan, evidence-based resource to guide preventive services recommendations for children

CHAPTER 6

Well-adult Care

Marguerite Duane and Ranit Mishori

CLINICAL OBJECTIVES

1. Identify which components of well-adult care are most evidence-based
2. Identify methods to implement well-adult care in a busy practice
3. Describe how to customize population-based guidelines to individual adult patients

SPECIFIC ISSUES IN PREVENTION AND SCREENING FOR AN ADULT POPULATION

Successful implementation of preventive services requires using every teachable moment with adult patients and documenting when preventive health topics have been addressed. Consider what, when, how, and to whom the range of preventive services should be provided. Use evidence of benefit to patients as the guiding principle in offering services. As when making a clinical diagnosis, history-taking is essential to ascertain an individual's risk factors: this is necessary to decide to whom which services should be offered. Concentrate efforts on delivering the most valuable services: specifically services with the greatest health impact or cost effectiveness (1). Employ a system that will automatically provide you with guideline updates and allow access to or reminders of these guidelines at the point of care. The overview chapter at the start of this section provides a list of useful web resources for preventive services. In this chapter, we will continue to implement the ***RISE*** mnemonic, using history and education as its cornerstone.

As outlined in the overview chapter, specific recommendations in this chapter continue to rely heavily on guidelines from the US Preventive Services Task Force (USPSTF), accessible at *http://www.ahrq.gov/clinic/USpstfix.htm*. Nearly 90% of family physicians surveyed agreed with all of the USPSTF recommendations (2). As noted previously, the USPSTF has developed a clear and rigorous grading system based upon the level of evidence that supports a recommendation *http://www.uspreventiveservicestaskforce.org/uspstf/gradespost.htm*. Individual patient preference becomes an important consideration particularly when discussing services with a "C" or "I" rating or when recommendations from other organizations differ significantly from those of the USPSTF, it is then critical for the clinician to engage in shared decision-making with the patient as they both consider the risks and benefits of an intervention for that individual. It has been shown that patients who are more actively involved in their care are more likely to follow through with health advice and to be satisfied with their health care (3). Weighing benefit to harm often depends on the value that an individual patient assigns to a service and will differ from person to person (e.g., one patient will be willing to risk erectile dysfunction or incontinence as a possible outcome of finding and treating prostate cancer, whereas to another patient these are unacceptable risks), especially when mortality reduction from prostate-specific antigen (PSA) screening has yet to be demonstrated (4).

ORGANIZING YOUR THINKING ABOUT PREVENTIVE HEALTH SERVICES

The Periodic Health Evaluation

With adult patients, the periodic health evaluation (PHE) is an ideal time to provide evidence-based preventive health services as outlined in Table 6.1. A systemic review of studies assessing the evidence of the benefits and harms of the PHE suggests patients benefit from a PHE through its role in improved delivery of some clinical preventive services and in reduction of patient worry (5). Although there is no clear consensus on the ideal frequency and content of the PHE, family physicians spend an average of 35% of their office time performing adult PHEs (6).

Unfortunately, clinicians still spend a disproportionate amount of time during a PHE performing a thorough physical exam: most of whose individual components perform poorly as screening tests. Worse yet, they may also perform screening laboratory or radiology tests of unknown usefulness or that may even be harmful, creating unnecessary discomfort, cost, waste, and potential harm (Table 6.2). Several examples of ineffective tests include screening tumor markers, screening whole body or coronary computed tomographic (CT) scans, routine cardiac stress tests, and Pap smears in women without a cervix. It is estimated that approximately 10 million women had unnecessary Pap smears performed between 1992 and 2002 in the United States (7). The money saved from these unnecessary Pap smears could help pay for the 17 million women not currently screened for cervical cancer, often because of lack of access to health care (8). There is a significant cost also associated with ordering inexpensive tests for a large number of people that are poor screening tests. Here, there are additional hidden costs that can add up, such as the cost of follow-up

(*text continues on page 65*)

TABLE 6.1 Well Adult—Recommended Preventive Services

Screen/Chemoprophylaxis	When to Begin/ When to End	Interval	Tools/Special Concerns	Strength of Recommendation
Alcohol misuse screening and counseling interventions	Adulthood	Unknown	May use CAGE or AUDIT to screen. May use 5 As—assess, advise, agree, assist, arrange—for behavioral counseling	B
Aspirin for primary prevention of cardiovascular events	Men older than 45 Postmenopausal women Younger people at risk for CHD; Stop at age 79		Address potential benefits and harms of aspirin therapy	A
Blood pressure	First visit	Every 1–2 years, optimum not been determined. If on medication then 2–3×/year	Chart record, flow sheet	A
Colon cancer screening:	Age 50 average risk Age 40 increased risk End when age >75 or comorbid conditions limit life expectancy	Depends on test; see next	All agree screening should be done, but how and how often varies	A
Fecal occult blood test (FOBT)	As above	Annually	High false positive rate; Lowest cost and risk	A
Flexible sigmoidoscopy (FS)	As above	Every 3–5 years	Some recommend use together with FOBT. Evidence for combined unclear. USPSTF recommends either FS or FOBT	A
Colonoscopy	As above	Every 10 years if no abnormality detected	Highest cost, highest risk, most accurate.	A
Depression	Adulthood No established age to stop screening	Unknown	Should have systems in place to ensure accurate diagnosis effective treatment and follow-up	B
Diabetes, type 2	Adults with sustained BP 135/80	1–3 years	ADA recommends fasting plasma glucose (>126) or A1C (>6.5) for screening; Insufficient evidence to recommend for or against screening asymptomatic adults	B

TABLE 6.1 (*Continued*)

Screen/Chemoprophylaxis	When to Begin/ When to End	Interval	Tools/Special Concerns	Strength of Recommendation
HIV	High-risk patients Pregnant women Universal screening	Periodic	High-risk: All pregnant women, men who have had sex with men, hx prior STD, new or multiple partners, IV drug users; men and women who exchange sex for money or drugs or partners who do; individuals whose past or present partners were HIV-infected, bisexual, or injection drug users	A C
Hyperlipidemia	Men 35 and older Women 45 and older 20 and older if risk factors for coronary heart disease No established age to stop screening	Every 5 years More often if lipid levels close to needing therapy Less often if lipid levels low	Risk factors: diabetes FH of heart disease in male <50 or female <60; multiple risks for CHD (e.g., HTN, smoking)	A
Obesity	First visit	Periodically	Use height/weight to calculate body mass index May use waist circumference as measure of central adiposity	B
Syphilis	High-risk adults All pregnant women	Unknown	High-risk adults include men who have sex with men, people who exchange sex for drugs, commercial sex workers, adults in a correctional facility	A
Tobacco use and counseling to prevent tobacco-caused disease	All adults	Unknown	Brief interventions–screening, counseling and/or pharmacotherapy have increased tobacco abstinence rates	A

(*continued*)

TABLE 6.1 *(Continued)*

Screen/Chemoprophylaxis	When to Begin/ When to End	Interval	Tools/Special Concerns	Strength of Recommendation
Women Only				
Breast cancer screening	Age 50–74 years	Every 2 years Women with limited life expectancy unlikely to benefit	Screening mammography with or without clinical breast exam	**B**
Cervical cancer	Beginning at age 21, irrespective of sexual activity. May discontinue at age 65 if three consecutive negatives	At least every 3 years (USPSTF, AAFP, ACPM, CTF); Annual (ACS, ACOG)	No need for routine Pap after hysterectomy for benign reasons	**A**
Chlamydia	All sexually active women <25; Asymptomatic women at increased risk for infection	Routine with pelvic exam until 25; also women older than 25 at increased risk; Pregnancy	Increase risk if prior STD, new or multiple partners, inconsistent use of condoms, African-American, or unmarried	**A** **C** (>25 and low risk)
Gonorrhea	All sexually active women <25; Asymptomatic women at increased risk for infection; High risk pregnant patients	Nonpregnant women interval uncertain In pregnancy–first prenatal visit, then may repeat in third trimester	Increase risk if prior STD, new or multiple partners, inconsistent use of condoms, sex work, drug use or African-American	**B** **D** (if low risk)
Osteoporosis	Age 65 Age 60 high risk	Minimum 2 years to measure change in BMD; Longer intervals okay for screening	DEXA scan of femoral neck best predictor of hip fx. High risk: Low body weight (<70 kg) best predictor of low BMD, then not using estrogen. Other risks: white/Asian, hx of fracture, hx of osteoporotic fx, hx of falls, smoking, alcohol or caffeine use, limited physical activity	**B**
Men Only				
Abdominal aortic aneurysm (AAA)	Age 65–75 with history of ever smoking	One time if initial screen negative; If intermediate size AAA (4–5.4 cm), periodic screening	Abdominal US has 95% sensitivity and 100% specificity in setting with adequate quality assurance	**B**

TABLE 6.1 *(Continued)*

Screen/Chemoprophylaxis	When to Begin/ When to End	Interval	Tools/Special Concerns	Strength of Recommendation
Prostate cancer (includes PSA testing and DRE)	Discontinue when Age ≥75; May consider to begin at Age 50; Age 45 high risk	Unknown	Most authorities do not recommend screening; High risk: African-American or first degree relative with prostate cancer	D I
Chlamydia	Uncertain	Uncertain	Urethral swab, urine tests being studied	I

Data are from The Guide to Clinical Preventive Services May consider to begin at Age 50. Recommendations of the U.S. Preventive Services Task Force. A = consistent, good-quality patient-oriented evidence; AAFP = American Academy of Family Physicians; ACOG =American Congress of Obstetricians & Gynecologists; ACPM = American College of Preventive Medicine; ACS = American College of Surgeons; ADA = American Diabetes Association; A1C = glycosylated hemoglobin A1C; AUDIT = Alcohol Use Disorders Identification Test; B = inconsistent or limited-quality patient-oriented evidence; BMD = bone mineral density; BP = blood pressure; C = consensus, disease-oriented evidence, usual practice, expert opinion, or case series; CAGE = Cut down, Annoyed, Guilt, Eye opener; CHD = coronary heart disease; CTF = Children's Tumor Foundation; DEXA = Dual Energy X-ray Absorptiometry; FH = family history; FOBT = fecal occult blood test; fx = fracture; HTN = hypertension; hx = history; IV = intravenous; STD = sexually transmitted disease; US = ultrasound; USPSTF = US Preventive Services Task Force.
For information about the evidence rating system, see *http://www.uspreventiveservicestaskforce.org/uspstf/gradespost.htm*

testing and the cost of the physician's time to explain the results of the unnecessary tests which could have been better spent discussing preventive health measures that are proven to be effective (9). One study estimated that screening with routine complete blood counts and urinalyses (both D recommendations not to use as screening tests) cost the US health care system as much as $80 million each year (10). Finally, it may be confusing to patients when clinicians in the same office have very different recommendations and practices regarding screening—for example, when one performs Pap smears in women who have had a hysterectomy and another does not. When developing your clinical office system, be sure to educate your patients, your colleagues, and your staff to encourage the use of effective services and discourage the use of ineffective ones.

Risk Assessment (R)

As part of risk assessment in adult patients, one must be aware of the leading causes of morbidity and mortality in the target population. Table 6.3 shows the leading causes of death by age in the US adult population. Many of the leading diseases causing mortality can be attributed to patient behaviors which are summarized in Table 6.4 (11, 12). Prevention of premature death is not our only goal, though; preventing unnecessary morbidity and disability is important as well. Table 6.5 lists the leading chronic health conditions associated with disability or limited ability in the US adult population.

The history should be used to assess the individual's risk factors and in conjunction with the patient's age, sex, and family history, this information can be used to tailor the screening, counseling, and preventive medication services that are offered to the patient. The USPSTF has developed an electronic tool, the Electronic Preventive Services Selector (*http://epss.ahrq.gov/PDA/index.jsp*) that allows you to determine preventive health services recommendations for an individual patient based on age, gender, and selective behavioral risk factors.

The USPSTF recognizes certain "high-risk" populations that may benefit from additional interventions beyond those recommended for the general population. Some of these risk groups include individuals with high-risk sexual behavior, intravenous drug use, the presence of certain chronic medical conditions, and several subpopulations who might benefit from additional vaccines or screening for tuberculosis. With the completion of the mapping of the human genome, the practicing clinician will soon have to start considering specific genetic risks for disease as well.

Immunizations and Chemoprophylaxis (I)

IMMUNIZATIONS

As previously noted, immunizations are among the most effective of all primary preventive interventions (13). Adults are less likely than children to be up-to-date with most recommended vaccinations (*http://www.cdc.gov/vaccines/recs/schedules/adult-schedule.htm*). For example, most adults do not know their tetanus immunization status, and most cases of tetanus now occur in inadequately immunized older adults. A survey conducted in 2009 revealed low immunization rates among American adults, and decreased knowledge and awareness of recommended vaccinations among young adults (*http://www.adultvaccination.com/doc/Survey_Fact_Sheet.pdf*). The up-to-date recommended adult immunization schedule can be found at: *http://www.cdc.gov/vaccines/recs/schedules/adult-schedule.htm#print*. Given the frequent changes in immunization recommendations it is important to **only** use current and regularly updated information sources and not rely on dated information. Table 6.6 summarizes the present vaccine information available at the time of writing but this information should be verified before use. An invaluable tool for point-of-care information on immunization in adults and children is "Shots" from the Group on Immunization Education of the Society of Teachers of Family Medicine.

TABLE 6.2 Well Adult Preventive Services NOT Recommended in Low-risk Asymptomatic Patients

Screen	Test	Potential Harms	Special Considerations	Strength of Recommendation*
Bacteriuria	Urinalysis (UA), microscopy	Overuse of antibiotics	Note: this is a Level A recommendation in pregnant women between 12 and 16 weeks' gestation	D
Bladder cancer	UA, microscopy or urine cytology	Many UA false positives lead to unnecessary invasive procedures	Smokers at increased risk Counsel on quitting smoking	D
CHD in low-risk adults	Electrocardiogram, exercise treadmill test, electron beam computed tomography	Unnecessary invasive testing, radiation exposure, over treatment and labeling		D
Hepatitis B	Blood test		Note: this is a Level A recommendation in pregnant women	D
Hepatitis C	Blood test	False positives; unnecessary biopsies	Insufficient evidence to recommend for patients at high risk for hepatitis C virus—intravenous drug use, dialysis, transfusion before 1990	D
Genital herpes–HSV	Serologic tests for HSV antibodies	False-positive test results, labeling, and anxiety	In symptomatic patients, antiretroviral therapy does improve outcomes	D
Hormone replacement therapy for prevention of chronic conditions in postmenopausal women	Combined estrogen and progesterone or unopposed estrogen if patient had hysterectomy	Breast cancer, deep vein thrombosis, CHD, stroke, cholecystitis, dementia	Does reduce risk for fracture, but harms outweigh benefits	D
Ovarian cancer	CA-125 or transvaginal ultrasound	Unnecessary surgery, anxiety	No evidence that early detection will reduce mortality	D
Pancreatic cancer	Abdominal palpation, ultrasound, serologic markers	Invasive diagnostic tests, poor treatment outcomes		D
Peripheral arterial disease	Ankle brachial index	False-positive results, unnecessary workups		D
Testicular cancer	Clinical or self-exam		No evidence that early detection will reduce mortality	D

The USPSTF recommends against routinely providing the service to asymptomatic patients. The USPSTF found at least fair evidence that [the service] is ineffective or that the harms outweigh benefits.
For information about the evidence rating system, see *http://www.uspreventiveservicestaskforce.org/uspstf/gradespost.htm*

TABLE 6.3 Leading Causes of Death, United States, 2007

Rank	Ages 25–44 (All Races)	Number
	All causes of death	108,658
1	Unintentional injuries	26,722
2	Malignant neoplasms	17,551
3	Diseases of heart	14,513
4	Suicide	10,983
5	Homicide	9,855
6	Human immunodeficiency virus (HIV) disease	4,782
7	Chronic liver disease and cirrhosis	3,154
8	Cerebrovascular diseases	1,472
9	Diabetes mellitus	1,467
10	Septicemia	817
Rank	**Ages 45–64 (All Races)**	**Number**
	All causes of death	425,338
1	Malignant neoplasms	148,322
2	Diseases of heart	135,675
3	Unintentional injuries	19,909
4	Diabetes mellitus	18,140
5	Chronic lower respiratory diseases	16,089
6	Cerebrovascular diseases	11,514
7	Chronic liver disease and cirrhosis	7,977
8	Suicide	7,079
9	Nephritis, nephrotic syndrome and nephrosis	5,804
10	Septicemia	4,019
Rank	**Over Age 65 (All Races)**	**Number**
	All causes of death	1,341,848
1	Diseases of heart	595,406
2	Malignant neoplasms	258,389
3	Cerebrovascular diseases	146,417
4	Chronic lower respiratory diseases	45,512
5	Alzheimer's disease	43,587
6	Diabetes mellitus	28,081
7	Influenza and pneumonia	25,216
8	Nephritis, nephrotic syndrome and nephrosis	24,844
9	Unintentional injuries	12,968
10	Septicemia	9,519

Source: Deaths: Final data for 2007. National vital statistics reports; vol 58 no 19. Hyattsville, MD: NCHS; 2010.
Available from: http://www.cdc.gov/nchs/data/hus/hus2009tables/Table029.pdf. (accessed Jan 6, 2011)

Updated each year, this free application for handheld devices is downloadable from *http://www.immunizationed.org/default.aspx*. In addition, a monthly newsletter called 'Needletips' produced by the Immunization Action Coalition can be obtained by registering at their website: *www.immunize.org*.

Travel Immunizations

International travel poses additional risks and unique preventive care needs. Travelers should be aware of local health risks. The most common risk with any travel is accidental injury, such as motor vehicle accidents, but there are other preventable causes of morbidity as well. Know where to access information about communicable disease risk, immunization recommendations, food and water precautions, advice on the prevention and treatment of traveler's diarrhea, and other health information. Local health departments have immunization clinics that usually include overseas travel information. You can also access pertinent travel information from travel guidebooks and obtain the most current information from the Centers for Disease Control and Prevention at *http://www.cdc.gov/travel/* (14). The main prevention targets for travelers include water and foodborne illnesses, such as traveler's diarrhea, hepatitis A, cholera, typhoid fever, and insect-borne illness, (primarily malaria, dengue, and yellow fever). Most countries expect travelers to have received basic childhood immunizations, and a current Td or TdaP. Some countries or authorities recommend or require the following: hepatitis A vaccine or γ-globulin, hepatitis B vaccine, malaria chemoprophylaxis, cholera vaccine, yellow fever, or typhoid vaccine.

Patient education about prevention of food, water- and insect-borne illness is very important. Additionally, advise travelers to be extra cautious about new sexual contacts. With safe sex education, they may avoid acquiring sexually transmitted diseases (STDs) and HIV. Recommend taking along extra supplies of regular prescription medication, needles, and over-the-counter medications, because these may be unavailable at their destination. Consider prescribing medications for travelers' diarrhea or malaria prophylaxis if travel will be to endemic areas.

CHEMOPROPHYLAXIS

The USPSTF recommends aspirin chemoprophylaxis in adults at increased risk for coronary heart disease. Physicians should discuss the potential benefits and harms of aspirin therapy in men 45 years or older, postmenopausal women, and younger people with risk factors for coronary heart disease (e.g., diabetes, hypertension, smoking). Given that there is good evidence that aspirin therapy decreases the incidence of coronary heart disease in patients at increased risk but increases the incidence of gastrointestinal bleeding, the USPSTF concluded that the balance of benefits and harms is most favorable in patients at high risk for coronary heart disease (5-year risk ≥3%). The USPSTF recommends against the use of aspirin for prevention of colorectal cancer in patients at average risk.

Approximately one-third of US adults take a multivitamin or mineral supplement on a regular basis (15). However, there is limited evidence to support vitamin supplementation for chemoprevention purposes. The USPSTF found there is not enough evidence to recommend for or against the use of

TABLE 6.4 Behaviors Linked with Actual Deaths in the United States 1990–2000

Behavior Linked to Death	No. (%) in 1990*	No. (%) in 2000†
Tobacco	400,000 (19)	435,000 (18.1)
Poor diet and physical inactivity	300,000 (14)	400,000 (16.6)
Alcohol consumption	100,000 (5)	85,000 (3.5)
Microbial agents	90,000 (4)	75,000 (3.1)
Toxic agents, unspecified	60,000 (3)	55,000 (2.3)
Motor vehicle	25,000 (1)	43,000 (1.8)
Firearms	35,000 (2)	29,000 (1.2)
Sexual behavior	30,000 (1)	20,000 (0.8)
Illicit drug use	20,000 (<1)	17,000 (0.7)
Total	1,060,000 (50%)	1,159,000 (48.2)

*Data from McGinnis and Foege, 1993.
†From Mokdad AH, Marks JS, Stroup DF, Gerberding JL, 2004 and 2005.
The percentages are for all deaths.

vitamins A, C, or E or multivitamins to reduce the risk of cancer or cardiovascular disease. Given the potential harm associated with the use of β-carotene, the USPSTF recommends against the use of β-carotene to prevent cancer or cardiovascular disease. The USPSTF does strongly recommend folic acid supplementation to prevent neural tube defects in women of child-bearing age. Although there is considerable interest in recommending routine vitamin D supplementation, at this time, the patient-oriented evidence of benefit is lacking.

The USPSTF no longer recommends routine hormone replacement therapy for chemoprophylaxis. Although the USPSTF found evidence that the use of combined estrogen and progestin results in both benefits and harms, they concluded that the harmful effects likely outweigh the chronic disease prevention benefits. The USPSTF also recommends against the routine use of unopposed estrogen for prevention of chronic conditions in women who have previously had a hysterectomy.

TABLE 6.5 Selected Chronic Health Conditions Causing Limitation of Activity

	18–44 Years	45–54 Years	55–64 Years
	Rate (SE)	Rate (SE)	Rate (SE)
Type of chronic health condition	**Number of people with limitation of activity caused by selected chronic health conditions per 1,000 population**		
Mental illness	12.9 (0.5)	23.1 (1.1)	24.1 (1.4)
Fractures or joint injury	7.0 (0.4)	15.5 (0.9)	20.6 (1.2)
Lung	5.0 (0.3)	12.6 (0.8)	25.6 (1.3)
Diabetes	2.5 (0.2)	13.4 (0.8)	33.4 (1.5)
Heart or other circulatory	5.9 (0.3)	28.4 (1.2)	74.3 (2.4)
Arthritis or other musculoskeletal	22.2 (0.7)	61.9 (1.8)	100.7 (2.6)

SE = standard error.
Notes: Data are for the civilian noninstitutionalized population. Conditions refer to response categories in the National Health Interview Survey; some conditions include several response categories. "Mental illness" includes depression, anxiety or emotional problems, and other mental conditions. "Heart or other circulatory" includes heart problem, stroke problem, hypertension or high blood pressure, and other circulatory system conditions. "Arthritis or other musculoskeletal" includes arthritis or rheumatism, back or neck problem, and other musculoskeletal system conditions. People may report more than one chronic health condition as the cause of their activity limitation. Starting with *Health, United States, 2005,* estimates for 2000 and later years use weights derived from the 2000 census. See related *Health, United States, 2005,* table 58. See Appendix II, Condition; Limitation of Activity.
Source: Centers for Disease Control and Prevention, National Center for Health Statistics, National Health Interview Survey.

TABLE 6.6 Well-Adult Care Recommendations—Immunization Recommendations 2010

Immunization	Indication	Schedule	Contraindications/Special Concerns
Tetanus, diphtheria acellular pertussis (TdaP/Td)	All adults 18 age 65 (TdaP) 65 and older (Td)	Two doses at least 4 weeks apart, 3rd dose 6–12 months after second dose Booster every 10 years	Give if wound present and >5 years since last dose Avoid if severe hypersensitivity
Measles, mumps, rubella vaccine	• Born after 1956, if no documentation • Health care personnel • Travelers to foreign countries • HIV without severe immunosuppression • Entering college	At least one dose A second dose is recommended for health care workers, international travelers, and college students	Measles and rubella considered for separate indications, but given as MMR unless contraindicated Measles: recent exposure Rubella: women of childbearing age who lack laboratory evidence of immunity Do not give to pregnant women
Varicella vaccine	• Absence of reliable history of disease or evidence of immunity • US born since 1980 • High-risk susceptible individuals*	Two doses at least 4–8 weeks apart	Avoid in active tuberculosis, immunosuppressed, immunodeficiency, pregnancy, recent immune globulin
Polio vaccine IPV—inactivated vaccine OPV—oral (live) vaccine	• Routine adult vaccine not necessary • Travelers to endemic areas • Community members if outbreak • Lab workers handling virus • Health care workers at risk of exposure	Primary series is three doses	OPV not recommended in the United States Complete primary or incomplete series with IPV Select travelers should consider a booster even if primary series complete
Influenza vaccine (including H1N1)	All patients greater than 6 months of age (CDC recommendation). In particular, high risk groups include: • Nursing home/institutional residents • Chronic disease† • Pregnancy, second and third trimester • Health care employees including those in long-term care or assisted-living facilities • Close contacts of high-risk people	Annually each fall	Avoid if: Anaphylactic allergy to eggs Acute febrile illness
Pneumococcal polysaccharide vaccine (PPV)	• 65 years and older • Cigarette smokers • Chronic disease† • Alaskan Natives/American Indian • Residents of nursing homes/long-term care	One dose needed if given after age 65 Consider 5-year booster if highest risk	Give 2 weeks before elective splenectomy Give to patients with unknown vaccine status if indicated. Track long-term care residents' status

(continued)

TABLE 6.6 *(Continued)*

Immunization	Indication	Schedule	Contraindications/Special Concerns
Hepatitis A vaccine	• Travelers to endemic areas • Chronic liver disease • Clotting factor disorder • Men who have sex with men • Illegal drug use • Lab exposure • Consider food handlers	Two doses given 6–12 months apart	Avoid if hypersensitivity to alum or 2-phenoxyethanol Pregnancy class C
Hepatitis B vaccine	• Occupational risk of blood exposure • Clients/staff at institutions for Development disabled • Hemodialysis • Clotting factor recipient • Household/sex contacts of HBV patients • Certain international travel • IVDU • Men who have sex with men • Multiple sex partners or recent STD • Prison inmates • Unvaccinated adolescents	Three doses: second dose 1–2 months after first; third dose 4–6 months after first Alternate two-dose schedule available for adolescent	Special dosing needed in certain subgroups
Meningococcal vaccine (MCV4, MPSV4)	• Asplenic adults • College students • Military recruits • International travel to hyperendemic countries	One dose A second dose may be indicated after 5 years for adults still at high risk previously vaccinated with MPSV4	Meningococcal conjugate vaccine (MCV4) is generally preferred as part of routine childhood vaccine series MCV4 does not require booster dose
Zoster vaccine	• Adults 60 and older	Once as a single dose	• History of anaphylaxis to gelatin, neomycin • Immunodeficiency including leukemia; lymphomas, AIDS • On immunosuppressive therapy • Active untreated tuberculosis • May be pregnant
Human papilloma virus (HPV) vaccine	• Females 11–16 (may start at 9) • Prior abnormal Pap, genital warts, and positive HPV okay to give	Three doses: second dose 2 months after first, third dose 6 months after first	Pregnancy

Adapted from the recommendations of the ACIP of the CDC, available at http://www.cdc.gov/vaccines/recs/ACIP/, accessed June 23, 2010.
Foreign travel and less commonly used vaccines such as typhoid, rabies, and meningococcal are not included.
*Chronic disease includes cardiovascular, pulmonary including asthma, metabolic including diabetes, renal dysfunction, hemoglobinopathies, immunosuppressive, or immunodeficiency disorders.
†Same as above plus asplenic, CHF, chronic liver dysfunction, alcoholism, CSF leaks, hematologic malignancies, organ transplant.

Screening (S)

The recommended screening tests for well adults based on the USPSTF guidelines are included in Table 6.1. For level A and B recommendations, there is sufficient evidence to support these recommendations; therefore, these should be recommended and provided to patients. Level C recommendations should not be offered routinely as the net benefit is small. In individual patients, clinicians can consider offering these services if there are other considerations, such as strong family history or personal concern, that support providing these services. Clinicians should not offer preventive health services that receive a D recommendation because there is moderate to high certainty that the harms outweigh the benefits or that there are no benefits at all. With level I recommendations, there is insufficient evidence to weigh the benefits versus the harms, so clinicians should review the clinical considerations and engage in shared decision making to ensure patients understand the uncertainty about the balance of the benefits and harms (16).

The USPSTF recommendations include a discussion of the clinical considerations and rationale that can further guide the clinician in offering preventive services. For example, colorectal cancer (CRC) screening is a Level A recommendation, but there are three different tests that can be used to screen for colon cancer. The fecal occult blood test is the least expensive, least invasive, and presents the lowest risk. Although it has the highest false-positive rate, the fecal occult blood test has been shown to reduce mortality in randomized controlled trials. Flexible sigmoidoscopy and colonoscopy are both operator dependent and comparable in terms of specificity. Colonoscopy is the most sensitive intervention and remains the "gold standard" for detecting colon cancer, but it is also the most expensive and is associated with the highest risk. The risks of this test include bleeding, intestinal perforation, irritation, and adverse effects from sedatives. The most serious risk of colonoscopy, perforation of the colon, occurs in 0.2% to 1% of procedures (17). Depending on the availability of testing in the area, all three options could be offered to patients with a discussion of the benefits and harms associated with each test, so the patient can be engaged in the decision making process.

Screening for type 2 diabetes in adults with sustained blood pressure greater than 135/80 (high normal) is a level B recommendation in that there is moderate certainty that screening for diabetes is beneficial in these patients by reducing cardiovascular mortality. The USPSTF found insufficient evidence to recommend screening for diabetes in all asymptomatic adults. In contrast, the American Diabetes Association (ADA) recommends screening all overweight or obese adults age 45 or older for diabetes and younger overweight or obese adults (<45 years old) if they also have one of the following risk factors: physical inactivity, first-degree relative with diabetes, member of high-risk ethnic group, hypertension, high-density lipoprotein cholesterol level <35 mg/dL or triglyceride level >250 mg/dL, history of cardiovascular disease, women with history of gestational diabetes or delivering a baby weighing >9 lb, women with polycystic ovarian syndrome, impaired glucose tolerance on previous testing, or other clinical conditions associated with insulin resistance, for example acanthosis nigricans (18). Although the USPSTF does not provide a recommendation for the frequency of screening, the ADA, based on expert opinion, recommends screening at 3-year intervals or less depending on initial results and risk status.

The breast cancer screening recommendation for women ages 40 to 49 revised in 2009 generated a significant amount of controversy when first released. The level C recommendation indicated that mammography should no longer be routinely recommended in this age range, but rather the decision to start screening before the age of 50 should be individualized based on the patient's values regarding specific benefits and harms. There is sufficient evidence to show there is moderate harm associated with mammography screening for every age group considered, with more false-positive results in women ages 40 to 49. Given the increase in harms and the higher number needed to invite to screening (NNI) to prevent one breast cancer death in women ages 40 to 49 (NNI = 1904 versus NNI = 1339 in women ages 50 to 59), there is moderate certainty that there is only a small net benefit for women in this age group. The potential harms of breast cancer screening include psychological harms and unnecessary imaging tests and biopsies in women with false-positive results. In fact, more than one-third of women ages 40 to 50 years undergoing annual mammography will experience a "cancer scare" (19).

Cancer scares that can lead to long-term worry are not limited to breast cancer. For example, men who receive a false-positive PSA test result report more worry about cancer and belief that their cancer risk is increased, despite negative biopsy (20). In addition to the psychological harm associated with false-positive test results, studies show significant harms associated with treatment for prostate cancer: including urinary incontinence, erectile dysfunction, bowel dysfunction, and death (20). Given that the treatment benefits for prostate cancer detected by screening are small to none in men 75 age years and older, the USPSTF made a D recommendation for prostate cancer screening in men 75 and older. For men younger than age 75 years, the benefits of screening for prostate cancer are uncertain, a level I recommendation. Given the documented harms associated with screening and treatment of prostate cancer, it is critical that clinicians accurately inform men of the limited evidence for the benefits and encourage them to consider their personal preferences before offering PSA testing. Despite the lack of evidence for its benefit, there is widespread disagreement on the role of PSA testing to screen for prostate cancer.

USPSTF has assigned a B rating to screening for depression in the general population in which systems are in place to effectively manage patients newly diagnosed with depression. The first 2 questions of the PHQ-9 (see Figure 6.1) serve as a brief 2 question initial survey tool (the PHQ-2) which has proven reliability as a screening instrument. Those who respond positively to the PHQ-2 should then complete the longer PHQ-9 which can reliably assist in the diagnosis of a major depressive disorder (Fig. 6.1).

Preventive care can be expensive. A major issue in screening is "who pays the bill?" Medicare, for example, covers mammography every 2 years, but pays for only a single preventive health exam on enrollment at 65. Some traditional third-party payers (insurance companies) do not pay for preventive care. One advantage of some prepaid (HMO, PPOs) health insurance plans is that preventive care may be a higher priority, and the patient might not be directly billed for these services. Several managed care plans also use performance of screening tests as a measure of physician quality.

Figure 6.1 • Patient Health Questionnaires (PHQ-2).

PATIENT HEALTH QUESTIONNAIRE (PHQ-9)

NAME: ______________________ **DATE:** ____________

Over the *last 2 weeks,* how often have you been bothered by any of the following problems? *(use "✓" to indicate your answer)*	Not at all	Several days	More than half the days	Nearly every day
1. Little interest or pleasure in doing things	0	1	2	3
2. Feeling down, depressed, or hopeless	0	1	2	3
3. Trouble falling or staying asleep, or sleeping too much	0	1	2	3
4. Feeling tired or having little energy	0	1	2	3
5. Poor appetite or overeating	0	1	2	3
6. Feeling bad about yourself — or that you are a failure or have let yourself or your family down	0	1	2	3
7. Trouble concentrating on things, such as reading the newspaper or watching television	0	1	2	3
8. Moving or speaking so slowly that other people could have noticed. Or the opposite — being so fidgety or restless that you have been moving around a lot more than usual	0	1	2	3
9. Thoughts that you would be better off dead, or of hurting yourself in some way	0	1	2	3
add columns:			+	+
(Healthcare professional: For interpretation of TOTAL, please refer to accompanying scoring card.) **TOTAL:**				

10. If you checked off *any* problems, how *difficult* have these problems made it for you to do your work, take care of things at home, or get along with other people?	
	Not difficult at all ______
	Somewhat difficult ______
	Very difficult ______
	Extremely difficult ______

PHQ-9 is adapted from PRIME MD TODAY, developed by Drs Robert L. Spitzer, Janet B.W. Williams, Kurt Kroenke, and colleagues, with an educational grant from Pfizer Inc. For research information, contact Dr Spitzer at rls8@columbia.edu. Use of the PHQ-9 may only be made in accordance with the Terms of Use available at *http://www.pfizer.com*.

ZT242043

Educating Patients (E)

The last element of the RISE mnemonic is patient education. This aspect of prevention emphasizes risk factor identification to tailor educational messages about lifestyle change. Patient education or counseling can be in the form of brief advice or as more comprehensive counseling. For patients resistant or ambivalent to change, using techniques of motivational interviewing may be effective to move patients along the path to change (21). The continuity of care that is provided in family medicine and other primary care specialties provides the opportunity to reinforce a message, such as the importance of smoking cessation over time and multiple visits. Group and one-to-one behavioral change programs have also both been shown to be effective (22). For example, recent reductions in coronary artery disease mortality have at least in part resulted from public education and individual counseling about diet and exercise as well as from better control of hypertension (23). Likewise, declining HIV infection rates among gay men can be attributed to education and behavior change.

When educating patients, provide written materials, because the average patient retains only about 50% of what is said during the physician visit. A good source for patient information is *http://www.familydoctor.org* sponsored by the American Academy of Family Physicians and MedlinePlus (*http://medlineplus.gov/*) sponsored by the National Institutes of Health. The Agency for Health Care Research and Quality, the parent agency for the USPSTF program, has a personal health guide for patients, available at *http://www.ahrq.gov/ppip/adguide/*. This guide provides patients brief information about various preventive services, and allows for self-tracking. The Department of Health and Human Services also has a website, *http://healthfinder.gov/*, which provides information in English and Spanish on hundreds of health topics, and also includes links to more than 6,000 government and nonprofit health groups.

The USPSTF makes specific recommendations regarding counseling and patient education. The most relevant for the family physician are summarized here.

SMOKING CESSATION

Physicians should systematically identify smokers and provide strong, clear, and personalized advice to quit. The first step is to assess readiness to quit. For patients who are ready, clinicians should provide smoking cessation counseling, consider drug therapy with nicotine products and/or medications, and offer referral to in-person or telephone-based smoking cessation programs, such as 1-800-QUIT-NOW. Counseling should be done on a regular basis to smokers, as multiple messages are often needed; the harmful effect of smoking on children's health should be emphasized to smoking parents.

EDUCATION ON ABUSE OF ALCOHOL AND OTHER DRUGS

The USPSTF recommends screening and behavioral counseling interventions to reduce alcohol misuse by adults, including pregnant women (see Table 6.1). There is insufficient evidence to recommend for or against routine screening for drug abuse. Screening tools for harmful drinking and alcohol abuse include CAGE and AUDIT. CAGE (representing key words Cut down, Annoyed, Guilt, Eye opener in a 4-question screening tool) and the Alcohol Use Disorders Identification Test (AUDIT), a 10-question tool are validated measures to detect patients at risk for problem drinking. All people who use alcohol should be counseled about the dangers of operating a motor vehicle or performing other potentially dangerous activities after drinking alcohol. Pregnant women should be advised to limit or cease drinking. Even minimal interventions by primary care clinicians, such as advice to modify current use patterns and warnings about adverse health consequences, can have beneficial effects, especially for patients in the early stages of addiction (24). Patients identified as drug abusers require appropriate treatment or referral.

PROMOTING DENTAL AND ORAL HEALTH

Patients should be advised to see a dentist regularly. They should also be encouraged to avoid unhealthy snacks and to brush regularly with toothpaste that has fluoride.

UNINTENTIONAL INJURY PREVENTION

Advise patients to use seatbelts. The American Academy of Family Physicians additionally advises counseling on the use of child safety seats, bicycle safety, motorcycle helmet use, smoke detectors, poison control center numbers, and driving while intoxicated. The USPSTF recommends counseling elderly patients on specific measures to reduce the risk of falling.

DOMESTIC VIOLENCE PREVENTION

The American College of Obstetrics and Gynecology (ACOG) recommends counseling on abuse and neglect to young women, teens, and the elderly. However, the USPSTF found insufficient evidence to recommend for or against routine screening of women for intimate partner violence, or of older adults or their caregivers for elder abuse.

Family violence is at times a difficult and avoided issue. The victims are generally women and children, but men and the elderly are also at risk in some settings. People encountering violence rarely reveal this to the physician as a part of their chief complaint. Often, they present, instead, with symptoms of chronic pain, anxiety, insomnia, drug use, or depression (25, 26). The patient may not be willing to bring up the issue, but may be relieved to discuss it when asked. ACOG, American Medical Association, and American Academy of Family Physicians all have published statements stressing the importance of screening patents (women in particular) about violence (25–27). A set of questions known as the SAFE screen (28) has been advocated by some, even though its validity as a screen has not yet been proven. SAFE is a simple pneumonic representing a screening tool with eight questions in four areas.

1. **S**tress and **S**afety: do you feel safe in your relationship?
2. **A**fraid or **A**bused: Has your partner ever threatened you or your children? Has your partner ever abused you or your children?
3. **F**riends and **F**amily: If you were hurt, would your friends or family know? Would they be able to help you?
4. **E**mergency **P**lan: Do you have a safe place to go in an emergency? Do you need help in locating a shelter? Would you like to talk to a counselor about this?

NUTRITION EDUCATION

The USPSTF recommends that clinicians screen all adult patients for obesity using body mass index measurements and offer intensive counseling and behavioral interventions to promote sustained weight loss for obese adults (body mass index >30). Most major authorities recommend counseling patients on nutrition though a clinician or a dietician. Counseling should provide patients with basic information about managing a healthy diet. Use the food pyramid (*http://www.mypyramid. gov/*). The US Department of Agriculture and the US Department of Health and Human Services recommend the following in their publication, *Dietary Guidelines for Americans:*

- Eat a variety of foods.
- Balance the food you eat with physical activity; maintain or improve your weight.
- Choose a diet with plenty of grain products, vegetables, and fruits.
- Choose a diet low in fat (less than 30% of calories), saturated fat (less than 10% of calories), and cholesterol (300 mg or less per day).
- Choose a diet moderate in sugars.
- Choose a diet moderate in salt and sodium (less than 2,400 mg per day).

- If you drink alcoholic beverages, do so only in moderation (no more than one drink daily for women or 2 drinks daily for men). (One drink is 12 oz of regular beer, 5 oz of wine, or 1.5 oz of 80-proof distilled spirits).

Obese patients should be counseled to limit their calorie intake and increase activity to achieve a weight loss goal of 1/2 to 1 lb per week. Women of all ages should getting adequate amounts of calcium and women of childbearing age should be counseled to have adequate folate intake to prevent neural tube defects.

PHYSICAL ACTIVITY EDUCATION

Although the USPSTF found insufficient evidence to support the promotion of physical activity in primary care settings, the benefits of physical activity are seen at even modest levels of activity. Experts agree that physical activity that is at least of moderate intensity, for 30 minutes or longer, and performed on most days of the week is sufficient to confer health benefits. Patients who are not willing or able to reach these goals should be encouraged to increase the amount of physical activity in their daily lives, such as taking stairs or walking when available. Exercise programs should be medically safe, gradual, enjoyable, convenient, realistic, and structured. For those at higher risk and all women, adequate calcium intake should be coupled with weight-bearing exercise for adequate bone development and prevention of bone loss (an effective online resource on Osteoporosis Prevention and Treatment is available at: *http://www.nof.org/professionals/clinical-guidelines*). Providers can and should be role models for physical fitness. Studies show that providers who exercise regularly are significantly better at providing exercise counseling to their patients than those who do not (21).

STDS, HIV, AND UNINTENDED PREGNANCY PREVENTION

All adults at increased risk should be counseled about STDs and HIV. Counseling should be tailored to each patient based on his or her risk factors, needs, and abilities. Unintended pregnancy is the responsibility of both partners and can be avoided with proper planning. The periodic health exam, a visit for an STD, or an acute ill visit may provide an opportunity to assess a patient's risk and provide information to encourage patients to reduce their own risk. Specific education materials or advice about abstinence, avoidance of high-risk behaviors and high-risk partners, barrier methods including latex and condom use, may reduce the risk of STDs. The clinician should also advise the patient that the use of drugs or alcohol increase the risk of acquiring STDs or becoming pregnant unintentionally.

SKIN CANCER PREVENTION

Although the USPSTF found insufficient evidence to recommend that primary care clinicians provide counseling to prevent skin cancer, the use of sunscreen has been shown to prevent squamous cell skin cancer. Therefore, clinicians should consider advising patients to avoid excessive sun exposure and to recommend appropriate use of clothing and sunscreen, especially to parents of young children and in patients with a personal history of sunburn.

DON'T GIVE UP!

Some students and health care providers develop a certain fatalism about the ineffectiveness of patient education. This attitude can develop after seeing patients repeatedly over time who, despite compelling advice, will not make lifestyle changes that would obviously benefit their health. When this happens, remember that education is only one element in the process needed to produce change. Another crucial element is motivation, which comes largely from the individual, the family, and their social support network. From this perspective, as a provider, it is often better to be content with partial results and to be encouraged by the few patients who do follow your recommendations.

CHALLENGES IN PROVIDING PREVENTIVE CARE

Though the value of prenatal, well-baby, and well-child care may be fairly well-established in both the physicians' and patients' minds, well-adult care is not. Neither the patient nor the physician may have a good understanding of what services should be offered, or what services are likely to be beneficial. Evidence supporting the usefulness of some common preventive health services may be lacking, or may not apply to an individual patient. Significant customization is required in well-adult care.

As with most of medicine, preventive care cannot be learned from one article, one chapter, or one chart; it takes practice. There is a growing body of evidence to support or refute a variety of traditional preventive clinical practices. Evidence-based guidelines are growing in number and are now readily available via the internet at the point of care for both patients and physicians. These are becoming integrated within electronic health records. These resources can support a good doctor–patient relationship and a well-organized office system to deliver preventive services. In addition to resources listed in the overview chapter, further links to electronic preventive health services to further adult preventive care are presented here.

- National Guidelines clearing house—*http://www.guideline.gov/*
- American Academy of Family Physicians Recommendations for Clinical Preventive Services—*http://www.aafp.org/online/en/home/clinical/exam.html*
- Pocket Guide to Good Health for Americans—*http://www.ahrq.gov/ppip/adguide/*
- Putting Prevention Into Practice—*http://www.ahrq.gov/clinic/ppipix.htm*

Handheld/PDA Applications

- USPSTF selector download—select appropriate services by age gender service type and level of evidence *http://epss.ahrq.gov/PDA/index.jsp*
- Shots—Updated each year includes adult and pediatric immunization schedules and information on each vaccine *http://www.immunizationed.org/default.aspx*

- American Cancer Society (ACS) C-Tools 2.0—ACS recommendations for cancer screening as well as tools to assist with smoking cessation and PSA decision making *http://labs.cancer.org/ctools.asp*

KEY POINTS

- Not all preventive interventions benefit our patients.
- It is important to recommend interventions supported by evidence of benefit.
- The costs of performing ineffective interventions are significant.
- There are considerable resources available to guide clinicians and patients in the most recommended interventions.
- It is important to empower the patient and involve her or his preferences and values in shared decision-making particularly when making decisions about interventions lacking conclusive benefit.

CHAPTER

7

Promoting Quality of Life in Chronically Ill and Older People

James T. Pacala

CLINICAL OBJECTIVES

1. Describe the varying needs for preventing both mortality and morbidity of a heterogeneous elderly population.
2. List primary, secondary, and tertiary disease preventive strategies in chronically ill people and older adults.
3. Identify strategies for preventing geriatric syndromes and iatrogenic problems in chronically ill and older adults.
4. Apply preventive services appropriately to different health and functional strata of older adults.

SPECIAL CONSIDERATIONS FOR ADDRESSING PREVENTIVE CARE IN CHRONICALLY ILL AND OLDER ADULTS

There is a demographic shift toward aging populations in many regions of the world. Many countries are faced with formidable challenges of caring for an ever-increasing segment of older adults. For example, the population of the United States older than age 65 is expected to double in the next 30 years (1). Life expectancy is at an all-time high. The fastest growing segment of the US population is centenarians (2). Care of the aging population has become dominated by management of chronic disease, which now accounts for approximately 80% of health care spending in this population (3).

Despite the growing number and disease burden of older adults, they remain the most heterogeneous age segment of the population in terms of health and functional status. Whereas children, young adults, and middle-aged adults are characterized by relatively small numbers with chronic disease and functional deficits, the older adult population exhibits a broad scope of health and functionality, ranging from significant numbers who are free of disease and fully functional to a considerable portion who carry high disease burden and disability. Addressing preventive care in the chronically ill and older adult populations warrants classification of this heterogeneity in health status, recognition of the types of conditions that affect these patients, careful consideration of the overall goals of medical care for chronically ill and older individuals, incorporation of life expectancy into decision making, and a broadened definition of the activities typically included under the umbrella of "prevention."

Heterogeneity of the Older Adult Population

In general, populations of patients can be divided into four categories of health and functional status (see Table 7.1):

1. *Healthy* individuals who have no, or isolated, early chronic illnesses and are functionally independent. Significant health problems are usually acute in nature.
2. *Chronically ill* people have one or more advanced chronic illnesses that significantly impact their lives, and these illnesses dominate their medical status. Chronically ill individuals see health care providers more often, are periodically hospitalized for exacerbations of their conditions, spend significantly more of their financial resources on medical care, and often need assistance with instrumental activities of daily living.
3. *Frail* patients have multiple advanced chronic illnesses across organ systems, frequently combined with non-medical stressors (financial hardship, social isolation, etc.), resulting in disability and dependence in activities of daily living. Older frail patients frequently present with the so-called geriatric syndromes—problems such as falls, incontinence, confusion, and so on that will be addressed later in this chapter—that are the result of complex, multifactorial medical and non-medical etiologies.
4. *Dying* patients have a terminal condition that will result in death within a period of days to months.

These four health status categories have differing frequencies among middle-aged and older adults, the most significant of which is the dramatic increase of the chronically ill and frail segments observed in the geriatric population (Figs. 7.1 and 7.2; *activities of daily living dependency* being used in Figure 7.2 as a proxy for frailty). Table 7.1 presents profiles of each health status population segment and their approximate frequencies in younger and older adults. The marked heterogeneity of health and functional status in the older adult population warrants a more heterogeneous approach to preventive care.

Life Expectancy

Preventive medicine represents a tradeoff between the short-term morbidity (for example, the discomfort, inconvenience,

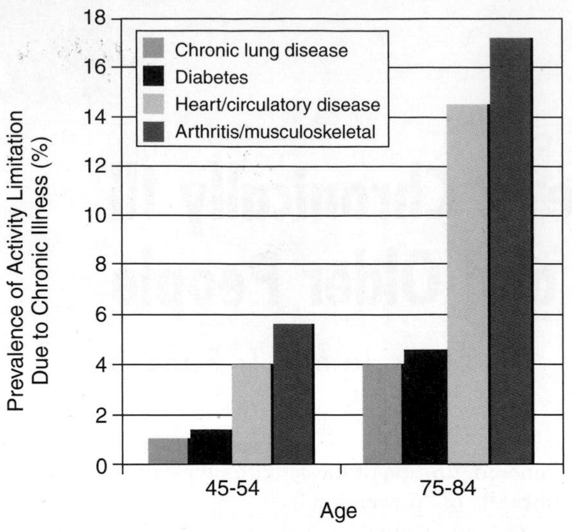

Figure 7.1 • Chronic Illness in Middle-aged and Older Adults

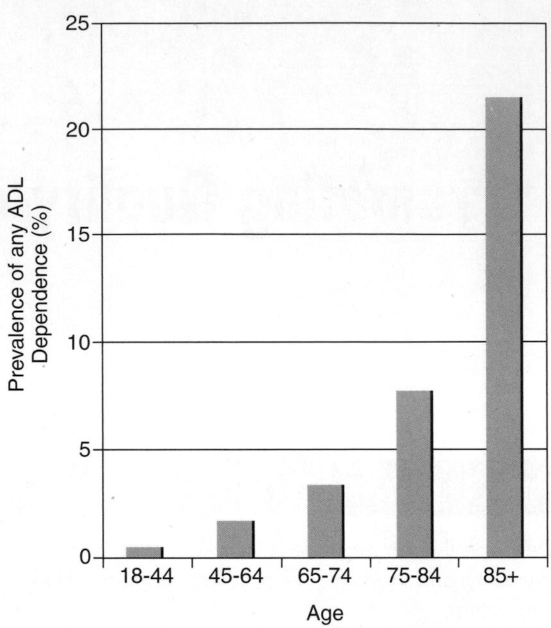

Figure 7.2 • Activities of Daily Living (ADL) Dependency by Age

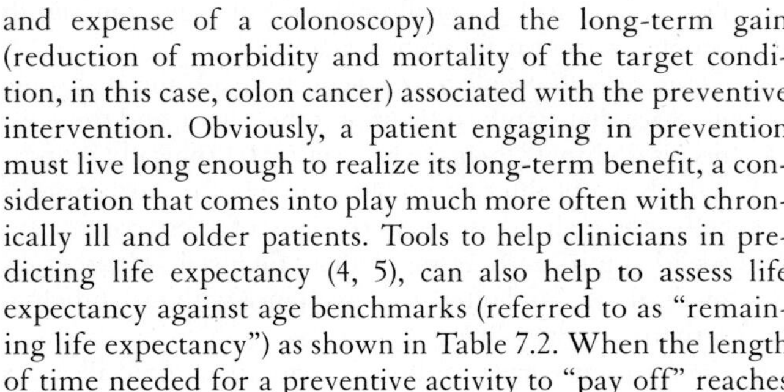
and expense of a colonoscopy) and the long-term gain (reduction of morbidity and mortality of the target condition, in this case, colon cancer) associated with the preventive intervention. Obviously, a patient engaging in prevention must live long enough to realize its long-term benefit, a consideration that comes into play much more often with chronically ill and older patients. Tools to help clinicians in predicting life expectancy (4, 5), can also help to assess life expectancy against age benchmarks (referred to as "remaining life expectancy") as shown in Table 7.2. When the length of time needed for a preventive activity to "pay off" reaches or exceeds remaining life expectancy, it becomes unlikely that an individual patient will benefit from the intervention and *more* likely it will create harm. A related, and perhaps more relevant concept, is that of "active life expectancy" (ALE; i.e., the number of years of disability-free existence). At age 65, ALE is approximately 80% of remaining life expectancy, but this percentage gradually decreases with advancing age to about 60% in 85-year-old adults.

TABLE 7.1 Health Status Population Segments

	Health Status Population Segments			
Feature	**Healthy**	**Chronically Ill**	**Frail**	**Dying**
Types of conditions	Acute illness; early chronic disease	Advanced chronic disease	Multiple chronic diseases; geriatric syndromes	Terminal illness
Degree to which conditions significantly impact quality of life	Little	Some	Profound	Profound
IADL functional status	Independent	Partially dependent	Dependent	Dependent
ADL functional status	Independent	Independent	Dependent	Dependent
Approximate frequency of segment in middle-aged population	85–90%	8–12%	2–3%	<1%
Approximate frequency of segment in geriatric population	50–65%	25–40%	5–10%	1–2%

TABLE 7.2 Remaining Life Expectancy, United States, by Age

Age	Remaining Life Expectancy in Years	
	Male	**Female**
65		
25th percentile	10	13
50th percentile	17	20
75th percentile	24	27
70		
25th percentile	8	10
50th percentile	14	16
75th percentile	19	22
75		
25th percentile	5	7
50th percentile	11	13
75th percentile	15	18
80		
25th percentile	4	5
50th percentile	8	10
75th percentile	12	14
85		
25th percentile	2	3
50th percentile	6	7
75th percentile	9	10
90		
25th percentile	2	2
50th percentile	4	5
75th percentile	6	8

Source: Reuben DB, Herr KA, Pacala JT, et al. *Geriatrics At Your Fingertips: 2010, 12th ed.* New York: The American Geriatrics Society; 2010:7. Reprinted with permission.

TABLE 7.3 Top 10 Causes of Mortality and Morbidity for People Age 65 and Older

Rank	Mortality*	Morbidity†
1	Heart disease	Arthritis
2	Cancer	Hypertension
3	Cerebrovascular disease	Hearing impairment
4	Chronic lung disease	Heart disease
5	Alzheimer disease	Orthopedic problems
6	Diabetes mellitus	Chronic sinusitis
7	Influenza and pneumonia	Cataracts
8	Kidney disease	Diabetes
9	Accidents	Tinnitus
10	Septicemia	Allergic rhinitis

*Centers for Disease Control and Prevention. Deaths, Percent of Total Deaths, and Death Rates for the 15 Leading Causes of Death in Selected Age Groups, by Race and Sex: United States, 1999–2006. *http://www.cdc.gov/nchs/nvss/mortality/lcwk3.htm*

†Centers for Disease Control and Prevention. Prevalence of Selected Chronic Conditions: United States, 1990–1992. *http://www.cdc.gov/nchs/data/series/sr_10/sr10_194.pdf*

Common Conditions in Chronically Ill and Older Adult Populations

The clinician should know the common causes of morbidity and mortality in each age group. As shown in Table 7.3, the diseases primarily responsible for killing older adults (mortality) are not congruent with those responsible for making them feel poorly (morbidity). Diseases causing mortality tend to have a shorter period of morbidity before causing death such as that seen in cancer, stroke, and pneumonia. Diseases causing morbidity often have long periods (from years to decades) of increasing morbidity until a catastrophic or fatal endpoint, such as diabetes leading to limb loss or osteoporosis resulting in a hip fracture.

Goals of Care

Medical management of these populations is predicated on the goals of care as agreed upon in shared decision making by patient and doctor. Although extension of life can tacitly be understood as an ultimate care priority in young and middle-aged patients, one cannot make this assumption in older and debilitated adults, in whom symptom management may take preference over survival. Elucidation of the patient's care goals will inform care planning as to the conditions that are prioritized for management.

CONDITIONS TO BE PREVENTED

Besides primary and secondary disease prevention, tertiary prevention—namely, avoiding adverse sequelae of existing conditions—becomes quite important in patients with chronic disease. Strategies to prevent geriatric syndromes and iatrogenic illness have particular applicability to the older adult population.

Primary and Secondary Disease Prevention

As in younger adults, primary preventive activities in older adults include risk factor assessment, immunizations, patient education of various types, and health-promoting behaviors such as exercise. The RISE mnemonic can still be usefully followed for primary prevention during health care maintenance encounters. The US Preventive Services Task Force (USPSTF) issues guidelines for many of these activities, but does not always provide age or functional status parameters for their appropriate use (6).

The USPSTF also provides guidance for secondary preventive activities achieved through screening. One type of secondary preventive strategy, cancer screening for detection of subclinical malignancy, deserves special consideration in older adults. Because most cancers become more prevalent and the accuracy of some screening tests (such as mammography) increases with age (7, 8), cancer screening can result in fewer false positives and less expense per year of life saved in older adults compared with younger patients. However, the mortality benefit of cancer screening is generally not realized until 5 or more years after a true-positive case is detected by screening (9), implying that in patients with 5 or fewer years of remaining life expectancy (or ALE), cancer screening would likely result in harm (i.e., morbidity associated with detection and treatment of the cancer) without the benefit of extended life.

Tertiary Prevention

Very often, the presence of a chronic disease or the occurrence of an adverse outcome from a chronic condition dominates a patient's overall risk profile for morbidity and mortality. In other words, after a patient has acquired a serious chronic disease, adverse manifestations of that disease often become the patient's greatest risk of future morbidity and mortality. Myocardial infarction, kidney failure, vision loss, and loss of a limb become the principal threats to the overall health of someone with diabetes. Therefore, in people with established or advanced chronic disease, tertiary prevention—preventing further complications of the disease—becomes a clinical priority.

Tertiary prevention is generally accomplished by optimal treatment, including control of risk factors, of the chronic disease in question. Chronic disease management models such as that described by Wagner have been developed for optimal tertiary prevention (10). The Wagner Chronic Care model is built on creating a productive interaction between what is described as an informed activated patient and a prepared proactive practice team. Several features of the model foster this type of productive interaction. *Self-management support* extensively involves the patient in actively managing his or her own illness, including participation in learning about the illness, care planning, goal setting, and monitoring of the target condition. A team-oriented *delivery system design*, in which all personnel taking part in care of the patient have well-defined roles, includes planned proactive patient visits, care coordination, and regular follow-up. *Decision support* is another critical feature, with point-of-care guidelines and prompts to assist providers in practicing evidence-based care. This proactive, team-care model is also supported by *clinical information systems* capable of establishing patient registries to facilitate standardization of care processes and efficient measurement of outcomes.

Successful chronic disease management programs use case managers for coordination of all care associated with the target condition. Patients are proactively and periodically assessed for unmet needs, both medical and non-medical, and the care manager is usually responsible for arranging services for addressing those unmet needs. Group visits of patients with the same target condition have been shown to be successful for improving outcomes (11). During these sessions, patients participate in educational activities designed to promote better self-care of their illness.

Chronic disease management models have demonstrated better health outcomes, including fewer readmissions to the hospital for the target condition and improved patient satisfaction at the same or less overall cost than standard care. Target conditions for which chronic disease management models have achieved these outcomes include heart failure (12), dementia (13), chronic obstructive pulmonary disease (14), and depression (15).

Prevention of Geriatric Syndromes

People who have transitioned into the frail functional state as outlined in Table 7.1 often present with geriatric syndromes. *Frailty* generally refers to a state of diminished physiologic reserve rendering the patient more likely to decompensate from minor stressors, to suffer from geriatric syndromes, and to be more vulnerable to disability. However, the term frailty has varying definitions in research and clinical care. A traditional and less specific definition refers to frailty as the result of unrelated chronic disease conditions acquired by an individual, who then crosses a functional tipping point into disability. More recently, frailty has been described as a specific syndrome (sometimes referred to as the *frailty syndrome*) characterized by sarcopenia (muscle wasting), poor exercise tolerance, slowed motor performance, decreased physical activity, and undernutrition (16). At the organ system level, the frailty syndrome is characterized by age-associated disregulation of physiologic systems that help to maintain homeostasis, such as pathologic inflammation, impaired immune function, and hormonal imbalances.

Whatever the cause of frailty, patients in this functional state will often develop and present with geriatric syndromes that pose serious risk of further functional decline and death. As such, a strategy of preventing these syndromes or their sequelae is warranted in frail older adults. Table 7.4 outlines suggested preventive services related to geriatric syndromes. The etiology of these syndromes is not confined to a single organ system or pathophysiologic process, but rather to multiple causes arising from both medical and non-medical conditions and stressors. Preventive efforts for geriatric syndromes can be primary, as in counseling older adults about accident prevention in the home; secondary, as in screening older adults for gait disorders; or tertiary, as in enrolling a patient with an injurious fall in a comprehensive falls prevention program.

Prevention of Iatrogenic Illness

The age-associated disregulation of homeostatic processes described in the previous section render the older adult more vulnerable to adverse affects related to medical care itself. In general, the older a person becomes, the more he or she is likely to experience an adverse affect associated with medical care. Iatrogenic illness becomes particularly prominent in older adults who have multiple chronic illnesses or have become frail. These older adults not only possess the physiologic predisposition to decompensate under the stress of medical care, but also invariably require more complex care involving greater numbers of providers across different care settings, leading to further problems arising from uncoordinated care. Frequently the treatment prescribed by one provider for a single problem makes another problem worse. It is essential for the family physician to recognize instances in

TABLE 7.4 Geriatric Syndrome Preventive Services

Syndrome	Preventive Assessment Instruments/Methods
Confusion/cognitive decline	Mini-Cog (27), Mini-mental status exam (28), Confusion Assessment Method (29)
Falls	Screening: inquiry about falls in the previous year; in those who have fallen: falls prevention program (30)
Functional decline	Activities of daily living and instrumental activities of daily living
Gait and balance disorders	Semitandem stand, Get-Up-And-Go test (31)
Incontinence	Inquiry if patient has lost urine >5 times/previous year
Sarcopenia/weight loss	Measurement of height and weight, calculation of BMI
Social withdrawal	Depression screening instrument (PHQ-2) (32), (PHQ-9) (33), Geriatric Depression Scale (34); inquiry about possible mistreatment such as the screening question, "Is there any difficult behavior in your family you would like to tell me about?"; caregiver burden assessment

which treatments directed by multiple consultants clash, and to appropriately reconcile these treatments to minimize iatrogenic illness.

There are several well-recognized risk factors for iatrogenic problems. Perhaps foremost is hospitalization, which is associated with numerous risks such as nosocomial infection, complications from hospital procedures, and adverse drug affects. Adverse drug affects are also quite common in the outpatient setting and have been associated with the following clinical features: older age, six or more chronic diagnoses, reduced creatinine clearance, having multiple prescribers for an individual patient, and taking nine or more total medications (17). Another well-described risk factor is transitioning care from one setting to another, most commonly on discharge from the acute hospital to another care facility or to home. Transitions are often marred by a lack of communication between providers at each end of the transition, resulting in errors of overuse, underuse, and inappropriate use of medications and treatments.

Several interventions have been shown to minimize or prevent iatrogenic problems. Acute care for the elderly units are modified hospital wards that are specifically designed for older inpatients (18). Architectural modifications include grab bars for safer mobility, indirect lighting for better vision, raised toilet seats for improved transfers, clocks and calendars with large font for better orientation, and low beds for preventing injurious falls. Acute care for the elderly wards are staffed by nursing and social work personnel that have been specially trained in geriatrics and use protocols for independent self-care, optimal skin integrity, proper nutrition, and facilitation of a smooth discharge from the hospital.

Pharmacy consultation provides regular review of medications to minimize adverse drug events on acute care for the elderly units. Pharmacist consultation, targeted at complicated hospitalized older adults and outpatients who are at high risk for functional decline, has been demonstrated to minimize adverse drug affects in both inpatient and outpatient settings (19). Geriatric Evaluation and Management, when properly targeted to frail older inpatients or outpatients with multidisciplinary needs, has been effective at reducing iatrogenic problems such as adverse drug events or readmission to the hospital for relapses of chronic illnesses (20). Problems with care transitions can be ameliorated by timely transfer of information between sites, education and preparation of the family and patient about the transition, a plan for self-management by the patient after the transfer, and a way for the patient and/or caregiver to be empowered to assert preferences for care (21). Systems for ensuring that these provisions are carried out can be accomplished through rigorous and proactive discharge planning, enhanced care coordination, and the use of "transitions coaches" who help guide patients through a transition of care (22).

One other type of iatrogenic problem bears mention: end-of-life care that does not match a patient's preferences. Advance directives, which should include designation of a proxy for health care decision-making, can help to avoid mismatches in patient preferences and the actual care that is rendered (SOR = C). Completion of a Physician Orders for Life-Sustaining Treatment form, endorsed by some states and being developed in many others, can potentially enhance patient-centered care at the end of life (23).

MATCHING PREVENTIVE STRATEGIES TO PATIENTS' HEALTH AND FUNCTIONAL STATUS

Table 7.5 summarizes preventive service recommendations for older adults using the RISE (Risk factor identification, Immunizations [and Chemoprophylaxis], Screening, and Education) classification scheme. These services correspond to the categories of prevention outlined in the previous section—those of primary, secondary, and tertiary disease prevention along with prevention of geriatrics syndromes and iatrogenic problems. In some instances, a preventive service may represent more than one of these categories. For example, detection and treatment of hypertension to prevent cardiovascular illness may represent primary (in people with no vascular disease), secondary (in people with asymptomatic vascular disease), or tertiary prevention (in those who have prior myocardial infarction or stroke). Table 7.6 lists preventive

TABLE 7.5 Preventive Recommendations for Older Adults

Preventive Service	Condition to be Detected/Prevented	Frequency	Strength of Recommendation*
Risk Factor Identification (R)			
Blood pressure screening	Hypertension	Yearly	A
Blood glucose	Diabetes mellitus	Every 3 years in patients with blood pressure >135/80	B
Blood lipids	Dyslipidemia	Every 5 years if low risk; more often in those with cardiac risk factors or history of CAD, stroke, or PAD; Uncertain age to discontinue	C for low-risk people, A for high-risk people
Bone mineral density (DEXA scan)	Osteopenia	At least once after age 65 in women	A
Delirium risk assessment	Delirium	On admission to hospital	B
Fall risk assessment	Injurious falls	Yearly	C
Height/weight	Malnutrition	Yearly	B
Immunizations and Chemoprophylaxis (I)			
Herpes zoster vaccine	Zoster	Once after age 60	A
Influenza vaccine	Influenza	Yearly	A
Pneumococcal vaccine	Pneumococcal pneumonia	Once after age 65; consider repeating after 7 years	A
Tetanus vaccine	Tetany	Every 10 years	B
Aspirin therapy	Cardiovascular events	Up to age 80 when benefit is assessed to outweigh risk; uncertain for age >80	A
Calcium and vitamin D supplementation	Falls, osteoporotic fractures	Assess at initial visit and at least yearly	A
Screening (S)			
Abdominal aortic ultrasound	AAA	Once between age 65–75 in men who have ever smoked	A
Alcohol misuse	Alcoholism	Perform initially and consider periodic rescreening	A
Fecal occult blood testing (FOBT) and/or colonoscopy	Colon cancer	Age 50–75: FOBT yearly; colonoscopy every 10 years. Stop after age 75	A
Delirium screening instrument	Inpatient complications	On the second postoperative day	C
Depression screening instrument	Depression	Yearly	B
Elder mistreatment Screening	Mistreatment	At least once, particularly in frail elderly	C
Falls screening	Injurious falls	Yearly	B
Gait and balance assessment	Gait disorders; injurious falls	Yearly	B
Hearing assessment	Hearing loss	Yearly	B
Mammography	Breast cancer	Every 1–2 years in women 50–74; consider continuing screening if life expectancy is >5 years	A (age 50–74); C otherwise
Pap smear	Cervical cancer	Every 3 years in women with a cervix up to age 65; can be stopped in most women after age 65 if previous 3 are negative	B

TABLE 7.5 (*Continued*)

Preventive Service	Condition to be Detected/Prevented	Frequency	Strength of Recommendation*
Thyrotropin (TSH)	Hypothyroidism	Every 2–5 years	C
Urinary incontinence screening instrument	Urinary incontinence	Every 2 years	B
Vision assessment	Visual impairment including Glaucoma assessment	Yearly after age 50	B
Education (E)			
Advance directive completion	Iatrogenic problems at the end of life	At initial visit and updated periodically, especially with change in condition or function	B
Accident prevention counseling	Falls, burns, motor vehicle accidents	At least once; periodic reassessment after significant change in functional status	C
Exercise counseling	Falls, frailty, cardiovascular events	Yearly	B

*A = consistent, good-quality patient-oriented evidence; B = inconsistent or limited-quality patient-oriented evidence; C = consensus, disease-oriented evidence, usual practice, expert opinion, or case series.
For information about the Strength of Recommendation Taxonomy evidence rating system, see *http://www.aafp.org/afpsort.xml*.

services that have been shown to create harm without significant added benefit and are thus not recommended. Table 7.7 summarizes the relative importance of the main preventive services in each of the four categories of older adults already defined. A rational approach to prevention in chronically ill and older adults involves prioritizing the services in Table 7.5 according to the patients' health and functional status described in Table 7.1, and is discussed in the following sections.

Healthy Older Adults

Healthy older adults have a relatively long life expectancy (e.g., on average 20 years for women and 17 years for men at age 65) and they receive many of the same preventive services applicable to younger adult populations (see Chapter 6). The most applicable preventive services for these patients center on primary and secondary disease prevention.

Any health promotive activities designed to stave off the development of chronic illness and frailty are also prioritized in healthy older adults. Long-term observational studies show that frailty can be primarily prevented through regular physical activity and proper nutrition (24). Young and middle-aged adults who regularly exercise (i.e., aerobic, weight training, and balance-related activities) are less likely to become frail when they are old. Similarly, diets that include low saturated fats, low sodium, adequate calcium and vitamin D, high fiber, and moderate alcohol intake are also associated with robust health in older adults. Even among older adults who lack a life-long pattern of exercise and good dietary habits, adoption of these behaviors is associated with less functional decline.

TABLE 7.6 Screening Tests Not Recommended By the USPSTF in Asymptomatic Older Adults*

Condition	Screening Tests Not Recommended
Bacteriuria	Urinalysis, urine culture
Bladder cancer	Urinalysis for hematuria, bladder tumor antigen measurement, NMP22 urinary enzyme immunoassay, urine cytology
Coronary artery disease in low risk patients	Electrocardiogram, exercise treadmill test, electron beam computed tomography
Colon cancer in people >75 years old	Fecal occult blood testing, colonoscopy
Chronic obstructive pulmonary disease	Spirometry
Ovarian cancer	Transvaginal ultrasonography, CA 125 measurement
Pancreatic cancer	Ultrasonography
Prostate cancer in men >74 years old	Prostate-specific antigen measurement, digital rectal exam

*Strength of Recommendation = D.

TABLE 7.7 Prevention Priorities

Target Condition for Prevention	Health Status Population Segments			
	Healthy	Chronically Ill	Frail	Dying
Primary and secondary disease prevention	++	+	+	−
Tertiary prevention of chronic disease	+	++	++	−
Geriatric syndromes	−	+	++	+
Iatrogenic illness	−	+	++	++

++ = high priority; + = moderate priority; − = low priority or inappropriate.

Chronically Ill Adults

People with serious chronic diseases are likely to have complications related to those diseases. Although someone with osteoporosis and diabetes could still die of an unrelated cancer, it is more likely that she will become disabled or die from a hip fracture or a complication of diabetes. For chronically ill older adults, tertiary prevention becomes a higher clinical priority.

As chronic illnesses accumulate and worsen over time, the greater the likelihood that the chronically ill older adult will become frail and develop geriatric syndromes; thus, screening for these syndromes (see Table 7.4) becomes important in this population. Multiple chronic illnesses also result in higher numbers of care providers, more prescription medications, and periodic hospitalizations, prompting attention to possible increased threat of iatrogenic problems and their prevention.

Frail Older Adults

The clinician should be able to recognize when an older adult is transitioning from a healthy or chronically ill state into a frail one. Signs of frailty can be identified through clinical vigilance or regular screening of adults for conditions such as decreasing body mass index, worsening exercise tolerance, bradykinesia (for both fine and gross motor activity), and especially immobility. Once identified as being frail, efforts focus more on prevention of geriatric syndromes (see Table 7.4) and iatrogenic illness, with primary and secondary prevention becoming deemphasized. The risks and benefits of aggressively managing individual chronic diseases need to be scrutinized and appropriate treatment goals for tertiary prevention established. For example, in a frail older woman with atrial fibrillation who is also at high risk of falls and hip fracture, one might highly prioritize aggressive treatment of osteoporosis while foregoing or relaxing treatment international normalized ratio (INR) goals for anticoagulation.

Several newer care model interventions have been demonstrated to prevent further functional decline and poor outcomes in frail older adults that are often cost-neutral or cost-saving compared with usual care (25). A small sample of these models is described in Table 7.8. A common feature of these effective models is comprehensive, physician-directed primary care with care coordination provided by co-located nurse-physician teams, supplemented by:

TABLE 7.8 Care Models for Frail Older Adults

Model Name	Description	Features	Outcomes	Strength of Recommendation*
Program of All-Inclusive Care for the Elderly (PACE) (35)	Combines funding from acute and long-term insurance sources (Medicare and Medicaid) for nursing home eligible patients	Extensive use of adult day care, through which all care is primarily coordinated; primary medical care provided by a geriatrician-led interdisciplinary team; regular assessment of clients' medical, functional, cognitive, and social needs; and use of a single hospital and nursing home for acute and long-term care if necessary	Cost neutral or cost saving, improved quality in process of care measures, and increased patient satisfaction when compared to non-PACE controls (36)	B

TABLE 7.8 *(Continued)*

Model Name	Description	Features	Outcomes	Strength of Recommendation*
Social Health Maintenance Organization (SHMO)	Bundled acute and long-term sources of payment, designed for all older adults	Annual screening of all program members to identify those at highest risk of adverse outcomes, use of case managers to assess and coordinate care for those at highest risk, extended home and community-based services, and linkage to providers with expertise in geriatrics, while having the patient retain his or her own primary care practitioner	Lower hospitalization among patients at highest risk of adverse outcomes (37)	B
Geriatric Evaluation and Management (GEM)	Proactive interdisciplinary team approach to the care of frail elders in both inpatient and outpatient settings	Teams usually consist of geriatricians, nurses, and social workers as a core team, with the addition of physical therapists, occupational therapists, pharmacists, dieticians, and other health care personnel in some programs; GEM teams assume primary care of patient for extended period or permanently	Improvement in functional outcomes, decreased nursing home use, increased satisfaction, and increased recognition and management of previously undetected conditions; mostly a cost neutral intervention compared with usual care (20, 38, 39)	A
Geriatric Resources for Assessment in Care of Elders (GRACE)	Proactive care management focused on low-income older adults	Home-based care management by a specially trained nurse practitioner and social worker who assess patients, coordinate care, and serve as a liaison between geriatrics practitioners acting as consultants and the patients' primary care physicians	Improved process of care quality measures and decreased acute care hospitalization among study subjects who were at highest risk of future adverse events (40, 41)	A
Guided care	Nurse-directed enhancement of primary care	Specially trained nurse works with two to five primary care physicians to enhance care of older adults through improved disease management, self-management, case management, lifestyle modification, transitional care, caregiver education and support, and GEM	Less use of expensive services and cost savings (42, 43)	B

*A = consistent, good-quality patient-oriented evidence; B = inconsistent or limited-quality patient-oriented evidence; C = consensus, disease-oriented evidence, usual practice, expert opinion, or case series.
For information about the Strength of Recommendation Taxonomy evidence rating system, see *http://www.aafp.org/afpsort.xml*.

- Periodic preventive home visits by nurses
- Medication counseling by pharmacists
- Ambulatory rehabilitative services
- Coordination and coaching at the time of transitions between sites of care
- Intensive care management for people with one predominant chronic condition
- Community-based training in self-management and informal caregiving

One might note that this list corresponds closely to the characteristics of a successful primary care medical home (26).

Dying Adults

The paramount priority in the care of the dying is to alleviate suffering while respecting the patient's preferences for care. Clinical priorities should focus on high quality end-of-life care (see Chapter 24) and on iatrogenic illness prevention, with prevention becoming irrelevant.

KEY POINTS

- Older adults are medically heterogeneous and thus have varying preventive needs based on their health and functional status.
- Remaining life expectancy and active life expectancy must be factored into decision making about preventive activities, because there is often a time lag between the preventive activity and when its health benefit becomes realized.
- In healthy older adults, primary and secondary disease prevention should be prioritized. The US Preventive Service Task Force recommendations are an evidence-based guide to these activities.
- In chronically ill older adults, tertiary prevention of sequelae of their most prominent chronic conditions should be prioritized.
- Frail older adults often develop geriatric syndromes such as falls, incontinence, immobility, and confusion. Preventive activities for these patients should focus on preventing geriatric syndromes, manifestations of chronic illness leading to disability, and iatrogenic illnesses.
- In terminally ill older adults, prevention should focus on minimizing iatrogenic illness particularly that brought on when patients' preferences for end-of-life care are not followed.

III

Common Problems

CHAPTER

8

Approach to Common Problems

Philip D. Sloane and Mark H. Ebell

CLINICAL OBJECTIVES

1. List the most common symptoms and diagnoses seen in family medicine.
2. Describe common decision-making approaches used by family physicians and give an example of when each is appropriate.
3. Apply the threshold model of decision-making to a common problem such as sore throat or deep vein thrombosis.
4. Explain how a family physician should approach the following issues: dealing with clinical uncertainty, identifying hidden agendas, and deciding how far to pursue rare diagnoses.

The "bread and butter" of family medicine is the outpatient management of medical problems. These problems come in all shapes, sizes, and presentations. Not surprisingly, different problems are approached quite differently. Basic principles discussed earlier in this book, such as understanding the patient in the context of their family and community, and considering whether they are up to date with health care maintenance, are incorporated to varying extents into all patient visits.

The remaining chapters of this book discuss the most common problems seen in family medicine. This chapter provides a brief overview of these problems and a general approach to their management. We will begin by discussing what we mean by common problems.

THE PROCESS OF PRIMARY CARE

Every patient who comes into a physician's office does so for a purpose. We usually refer to this purpose as the reason for visit (or chief complaint) Table 8.1 lists the most common reasons patients visit family physicians, according to the National Ambulatory Medical Care Survey (1). As you review Table 8.1, note the following.

- Family medicine is broad and complex, and involves knowledge of a wide array of different problems. In contrast, physicians in many medical or surgical specialties spend the majority of their time regularly treating only a handful of diseases.
- Preventive care is a key element of office practice; however, the majority of patients want help with specific medical problems.
- Many of the common reasons for visiting a family physician are symptoms (noted in boldface in Table 8.1). Symptoms can be thought of as mysteries that need to be solved before the family physician can come up with a treatment plan.
- Another common reason for visiting is chronic illness. For these patients, the challenge is not making a diagnosis but rather effective management over time.
- Types of visits that have increased between 1993 and 2007 include preventive visits, chronic illnesses such as diabetes and arthritis, and return visits for management of medications and review of test results. These trends reflect the increasing emphasis in family medicine on prevention and chronic disease management over the past two decades.

Note that no psychological conditions are listed among the 20 most common reasons for visiting, although as many as half of family physician visits involve issues such as stress, adjustment problems, depression, and anxiety. The explanation for this apparent contradiction is that the stated reason for a visit is often not the patient's actual reason for coming to see their family physician. Often, people who are in psychological distress either consciously or unconsciously use symptoms as their "admission ticket" to a medical office. At other times, the patient's psychological distress is interwoven with medical and often social issues. Thus, the family physician must not only address the patient's presenting complaint, but also be vigilant for less obvious issues that may constitute the patient's underlying reason for coming.

The broad training of family physicians allows multiple problems to be addressed during a single visit. In fact, a study that directly observed a large group of family physicians found that they addressed an average of 2.8 problems during each visit and took an average of eight clinical actions (i.e., one action is "ordering a test" or "prescribing a drug") (2). Juggling diverse problems and making good decisions during a 15- to 20-minute visit is part of the challenge of being a good family physician.

For patients who present with symptoms, the physician's first task is to arrive at a diagnosis. After the diagnosis is established, a management plan can be developed. Thus, the process that occurs in the examining room could be diagrammed like this:

Symptom ➔ Clinical diagnosis ➔ Diagnostic testing (optional) ➔ Management

Often, the family physician's initial diagnosis is provisional, and the management plan is designed to both treat the symptoms and confirm the diagnosis. Providing an estimate of prognosis (i.e., what the patient should expect in the coming days or weeks) is also an important of the care process.

TABLE 8.1 Primary Reason for Visit Making Up at Least 1% of a Typical Family Physician's Practice in Either 1993 or 2007*

	1993 N = 120,723,258 visits		2007 N = 214,675,650 visits	
Reason for Visit	**% of Visits**	**Rank**	**% of Visits**	**Rank**
General medical examination	4.0	2	9.2	1
Cough	5.6	1	4.5	2
To review test results†	1.7	16	4.3	3
Progress visit, reason not otherwise specified (NOS)	1.2	21	4.2	4
Medication, other and unspecified kinds	1.1	22	4.0	5
Back and low back pain, ache, soreness, discomfort†	3.0	4	3.7	6
Hypertension	2.6	8	3.0	7
Throat soreness	3.2	3	2.6	8
Diabetes mellitus	1.0	23	2.0	9
Abdominal or stomach pain, cramps, spasms, NOS†	2.0	11	1.5	10
Earache, pain	2.3	9	1.5	11
Headache, pain in head	1.6	18	1.4	12
Blood pressure test	2.8	5	1.4	13
Physical examination required for employment or school†	1.9	12	1.4	14
Skin rash	1.6	17	1.4	15
Nasal congestion	1.8	14	1.2	16
Knee pain, ache, soreness, discomfort	0.6	39	1.2	17
Medical counseling, NOS	0.5	47	1.1	18
Fever	1.9	13	1.1	19
Prophylactic inoculations	0.8	25	1.0	20
Head cold, upper respiratory infection	2.7	6	1.0	21
Well baby examination	2.6	7	0.8	29
Prenatal examination, routine	2.2	10	0.7	33
Pap smear	1.7	15	0.7	35
Vertigo, dizziness	1.2	19	0.8	26
Chest pain	1.2	20	0.9	24

Data source: National Ambulatory Medical Care Survey (NAMCS), 1993, 2007: *http://www.cdc.gov/nchs/ahcd.htm;* totals are estimated from a national probability sample.
*Symptoms are noted in boldface type.
†Combines multiple categories used in the NAMCS survey.

Table 8.2 lists the most common diagnoses coded by family physicians in 2007.

- The most common diagnoses are chronic diseases (e.g., hypertension, diabetes, chronic sinusitis, asthma) and acute respiratory problems (e.g., upper respiratory infections, bronchitis, pharyngitis).
- Several of the common diagnoses are outside of the traditional realm of internal medicine—for example, well-child care, strains/sprains, depression, and contact dermatitis. These exemplify why family medicine training extends into a variety of specialty fields.

Clinical Decision Making

Medical students often feel quite confused as they begin to observe a busy private medical practice. Many patients have problems that seem to defy classification, and the causes of illness are often multifactorial. Patient management proceeds often at an unfamiliarly fast pace, often without detailed histories or comprehensive examinations. The physician seems to be cutting corners much of the time. Decisions are made that often have a social rather than a medical context. Yet outcomes of care are mostly good and the patients seem satisfied. Why and how is this done?

TABLE 8.2 The 30 Most Common Diagnoses Recorded for Family Physician Visits in 2007*

Diagnosis	ICD9†	% of Visits
1. Essential hypertension	401.9	7.6
2. Diabetes mellitus, type II, without complications	250.0	3.9
3. Acute upper respiratory infection	465.9	3.3
4. Routine infant or child health check	V20.2	3.0
5. Routine general medical examination at a health care facility	V70.0	2.8
6. Chronic sinusitis	473.9	2.0
7. Hyperlipidemia	272.4	1.6
8. Depressive disorder	311	1.5
9. Bronchitis, not specified as acute or chronic	490	1.4
10. Acute pharyngitis	462	1.4
11. Urinary tract infection	599.0	1.3
12. Otitis media	382.9	1.1
13. Low back pain	724.2	1.1
14. Asthma	493.9	1.1
15. Other specified aftercare	V58.8	1.1
16. Routine gynecologic examination	V72.31	1.1
17. Sprains and strains of shoulder and upper arm	840.9	0.9
18. Osteoarthritis	715.9	0.9
19. Contact dermatitis and other eczema unspecified cause	692.9	0.9
20. Chronic obstructive pulmonary disease	496	0.8
21. Obesity	278.00	0.8
22. Allergic rhinitis	477.9	0.8
23. Anxiety	300.00	0.8
24. Other specified counseling	V65.49	0.8
25. Backache, unspecified	724.5	0.7
26. Supervision of other normal pregnancy	V22.1	0.7
27. Depressive symptoms	300.4	0.6
28. Encounter for therapeutic drug monitoring	V58.83	0.6
29. Hypothyroidism	244.9	0.6
30. Abdominal pain	789.00	0.6

*Primary diagnosis only; many patients had additional, secondary diagnoses. Total estimated number of visits = 214,675,650 visits. Data source: National Ambulatory Medical Care Survey (NAMCS), 2007: *http://www.cdc.gov/nchs/ahcd.htm;* totals are estimated from a national probability sample.
†International Classification of Diseases, Ninth Edition.

The answer is, partly, because the physician is experienced and well-trained and often knows his or her patients well. However, just as important is that decision making in primary care differs in certain respects from what students are taught in hospital settings. Traditional medical education, which focuses on mechanisms of disease, teaches that symptoms result from disease and that treatment of the disease heals the symptoms. In primary care, this concept is often reversed. Symptoms are often quite likely to get better on their own so that making a specific diagnosis may be neither necessary nor beneficial to the patient. Thus, the clinical reasoning and decision-making styles learned in traditional inpatient care often are not appropriate in the outpatient primary care setting.

Decision making develops from three main activities: gathering information (the history, physical examination findings, and test results), analyzing the information (the reasoning process), and making judgments about the data. It is

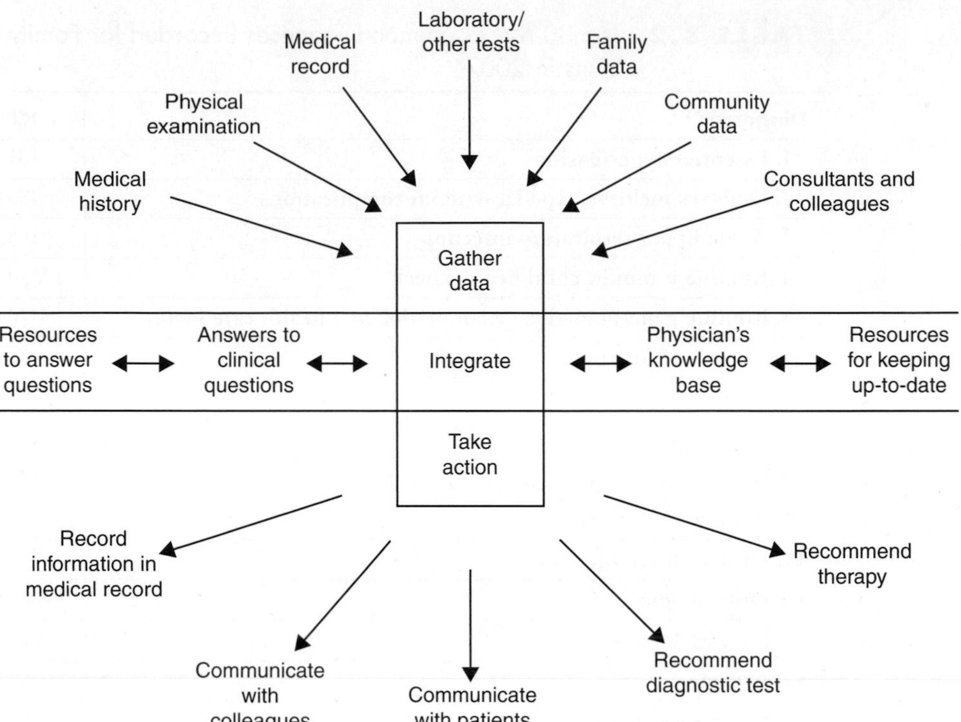

Figure 8.1 • The flow of information in primary care practice. (Reprinted from Ebell MH, Frame P. What can technology do to, and for, family medicine? Fam Med 2001;33:311–319. Used with permission.)

enriched by previous knowledge of the patient and the patient's environment—the context of the decision. Throughout the process, the family physician directs the encounter to efficiently obtain specific information. The result is a working diagnosis and management strategy. This is communicated to the patient, and the decision is confirmed or rethought, with the patient generally being a partner in management decisions.

This flow of information is shown in Figure 8.1. Considerable time and effort goes into managing this flow of information, and family physicians are increasingly using sophisticated electronic health records (EHRs) and clinical decision support tools to assist them with this process.

Primary care physicians use four distinct clinical reasoning styles to develop working diagnoses: hypothesis generation and testing, pattern recognition, algorithmic reasoning, and exhaustive methods. Each has its place in primary care. Furthermore, they are not mutually exclusive; a particular patient encounter may involve more than one of the styles. The four methods are briefly discussed in the following section.

HYPOTHESIS GENERATION AND TESTING

Hypothesis generation and testing is commonly used in primary care. The physician begins generating diagnostic hypotheses within seconds of reviewing the rooming note and scanning the record, even before meeting the patient. The initial hypothesis is often quite general, such as "this child may have something serious." The physician directs the interview to obtain information that will test and refine this hypothesis (in the case of a sick child, asking about fever, vomiting, fluid intake, activity, etc.). While testing and refining hypotheses, the physician remains open to information that would suggest other hypotheses, because the biggest danger in using this diagnostic method is making too hasty a decision and missing or ignoring key information. In a typical clinical encounter, expert clinicians generate a short list of likely diagnoses within 30 seconds and correct hypotheses within 6 minutes. This is an efficient and low-cost reasoning process, widely applied in office practice. Examples of problems effectively addressed with this reasoning style are abdominal pain, chest pain, and dizziness.

PATTERN RECOGNITION

In pattern recognition, the physician rapidly arrives at a diagnosis (or a very limited differential diagnosis) because the clinical picture looks like something he or she has seen before. The pattern itself could be any combination of data from the history and examination. This method is quick, efficient, and inexpensive, but it requires considerable clinical experience to be successful. It is used extensively by office-based clinicians, but one drawback is that some diagnostic evaluations may be closed prematurely, missing important problems or cues. Conditions that are often diagnosed using this method include those whose diagnosis relies largely on physical findings, such as rashes, arthritis, or bursitis, and common diseases with distinctive clinical patterns, such as otitis media, depression, and cystitis.

ALGORITHMIC REASONING

Algorithmic reasoning involves following a consistent, logical method that does not vary from patient to patient. The physician's decision-making process can be diagrammed as a flowchart with branching decision points, in which objective data from the history, examination, or laboratory allow the physician to choose one pathway or another. This method is most useful when the data required are relatively discrete (i.e., black-and-white choices), the diagnostic possibilities are few, and the data required are modest. Because so many primary care problems are vague or have many diagnostic possibilities, algorithmic decision making is used for a minority of visits. Problems often approached algorithmically include anemia, hyperlipidemia, vaginal discharge, and dysuria. Practice guidelines often use algorithms, and the best ones are flexible enough to allow for the possibility of missing or inaccurate data.

EXHAUSTIVE METHODS

Exhaustive methods involve gathering comprehensive history and physical examination data and pursuing intensive laboratory testing to cover all possibilities. The data are then sifted for abnormal findings. This reasoning style was the model traditionally taught in medical schools for inpatient care. However, it is too inefficient, time-consuming, and expensive for management of most problems seen in the office. More importantly, this method may be hazardous for patients because it poses real risks of laboratory errors and adverse effects of invasive tests such as radiation exposure. Therefore, this method is reserved for unusual and complex medical problems, such as an elderly patient with a persistent fever of unknown origin, or a patient with chronic fatigue.

Pitfalls in the Diagnostic Process

In making a diagnosis, the language we use moves from the words of the patient to those of the doctor. This reflects the significant responsibility that rests with the physician—to interpret the patient's problem in medical terms. The diagnostic label we supply will help us communicate with other health professionals and plan treatment. It also helps the patient understand his or her problems in the broader context of health care and health information. Not surprisingly, however, many patients are less interested in diagnosis than they are in the prognosis and the treatment plan.

Among the many pitfalls to accurate diagnosis are premature closure, hidden agendas, zebras, "I got burned once" (IGBOs), and the rare disease rule. Each of these is discussed briefly below; your goal as a clinician is to be aware of them and to keep them from steering you off course as you evaluate patients in the office.

PREMATURE CLOSURE

Premature closure occurs when the physician settles on a diagnosis before all of the information is in or sticks with a diagnosis despite compelling information to the contrary. In studies of diagnostic reasoning, this was the most common reason for misdiagnosis (3). It is related to our general tendency as human beings to ignore nonconfirmatory data—for example, the man who complains about a "typical woman driver" but ignores all of the excellent women drivers that he encounters every day as he drives around town (not to mention some dangerous male drivers!) Because primary care always involves a certain element of uncertainty—even as the patient walks out the door—the important thing is to remain receptive to unexpected information and be willing to alter or amend your diagnosis. This is particularly true when initial tests or the response to empiric therapy do not support the diagnosis—always be prepared to question your original diagnosis.

HIDDEN AGENDA

Hidden agendas exist when the actual reason for coming to the doctor is not initially stated. This is very common, particularly when a psychosocial concern underlies the patient's complaint. For example, why does one patient with a "common cold" schedule an appointment when another does not? Usually, there is a hidden agenda. Perhaps the patient is concerned that it might develop into pneumonia, because this happened in the past. Or perhaps it is because he is a smoker and wants reassurance that he does not have cancer or because she will be going to an important job interview in a few days and believes that an antibiotic will help her get better quicker. Or perhaps his son was killed in an auto accident 1 year ago, and he is feeling depressed and wants to talk.

Thus, it is the family physician's job to discover the underlying issues behind the visit so the patient can receive the treatment, education, or reassurance that he or she needs. Useful strategies include asking the patient "Is there any reason you are especially concerned about this symptom?" and asking early in the interview: "Is there anything else you want to discuss today?" It is better to identify hidden agendas early in the visit than to discover the true reason as you leave the room when your hand is on the doorknob.

ZEBRAS

"Think horses, not zebras" is familiar advice. In practical terms, this means that you should first consider the diseases that are most common in a given clinical situation. Within the United States, certain diseases, although rare in many areas, are relatively common in others. Examples include Rocky Mountain spotted fever in North Carolina (fever and headache); lead poisoning in the inner cities (exhaustion, muscle cramps); and Lyme disease in New England (fever, rash, arthritis). You must, therefore, be aware of the incidence and prevalence of illness in your community when making diagnostic and treatment decisions. Remembering the frequency of a disease is also important when interpreting diagnostic tests, since the diagnostic accuracy of a test relates to the prevalence of the condition being sought: a positive test result for a rare disease is likely to represent a false positive, while a positive test for a common disease is probably a true positive. For further information on test interpretation, see Chapter 2.

IGBO

"I got burned once" is a kind of personal zebra. It occurs when a physician's practice style is too heavily influenced by an unusual, often recent, patient outcome. Although we all need to learn from experience, IGBOs can steer the unwary physician into inappropriate tests, referrals, or therapies. For example, the physician who misses a pulmonary embolism may subsequently order too many helical computed tomography scans on future patients. The best antidote to an IGBO is for physicians to discuss problem cases with colleagues and process the implications of the experience. Formal groups, such as morbidity and mortality conferences, are excellent settings for working through an IGBO.

RARE DISEASE RULE

The rare disease rule reminds us that zebras do, in fact, exist. It states that "if you don't think of it, you won't make the

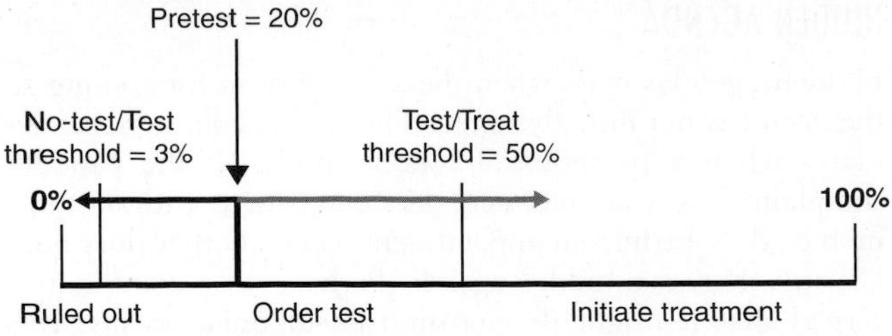

Figure 8.2 • The starting point is a 20% estimate of the overall risk of strep throat among patients in your practice presenting with a complaint of sore throat. Your "no test/test" threshold is 3% (e.g., if the probability is less than 3%, you consider that strep is effectively ruled out, remembering that you can never achieve perfect diagnostic certainty), and the "test/treat" threshold is 50% (e.g., if probability of strep is greater than 50%, you would initiate antibiotics) (5).

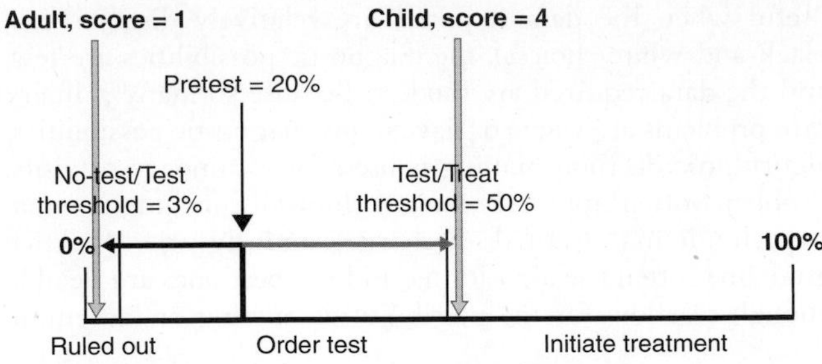

Figure 8.3 • Using the validated clinical decision rule for strep pharyngitis (Chapter 18, Sore Throat), a 50-year-old patient with sore throat and fever, but no tonsillar findings, no adenopathy, and with a cough, would get 1 point (1% probability of strep). A 10-year-old patient with sore throat, fever, adenopathy, no exudates, and no cough would get 4 points (51% probability of strep). Their probability of strep, revised after using the clinical decision rule, is shown above. Note that for these patients the probability of strep either dropped below the no test/test threshold (adult) or exceeded the test/treat threshold (child) using the clinical examination alone (5).

diagnosis." It acknowledges that, although common things occur commonly, rare diagnoses cannot be forgotten. It reminds you that when the pieces do not fit together, you may have to do some rethinking or research. Strategies include leaving the patient's room to reflect on the case (long hallways in group practices are great for this!), consulting an electronic reference or textbook, or presenting a problem case to a colleague or consultant (in person, by phone, or even online). Good physicians use these strategies daily.

Diagnostic Tests and Clinical Decision Rules

Although you may think of a diagnostic test as something done in a laboratory or radiology department, it is useful to think of tests more broadly. Indeed, the most commonly used diagnostic tests are the questions we ask and the examination maneuvers we carry out. In recent years, all of these aspects of diagnostic testing have been increasingly evaluated for their accuracy.

As an example from the clinical history, the following single question was developed by a family medicine researcher as a diagnostic test: "When was the last time you had more than five drinks in 1 day (more than four drinks for women)?" If the patient responds that they have done so in the past 3 months, this positive response is 86% sensitive and specific for alcohol dependence (4). In the original study, 77% responding in the affirmative were problem drinkers compared with 7% who responded "more than 3 months ago" and 1% who responded "never." (See Chapter 2, Information Mastery: Basing Care on the Best Available Evidence, for more on use of diagnostic tests.)

Physical examination maneuvers are also diagnostic tests. Some widely used maneuvers are actually very inaccurate (e.g., Homan sign for deep vein thrombosis [DVT], epigastric tenderness for peptic ulcer disease, and Tinel sign for carpal tunnel syndrome). Conversely, some little-used maneuvers are actually quite accurate (e.g., square wrist sign for carpal tunnel and spider angiomas for serious hepatic disease).

However, individual elements of the history and physical examination are rarely accurate enough on their own to rule in or rule out a diagnosis. Instead, it is better to use combinations of findings. An increasing area of research, much of it by primary care physicians, seeks to identify the best individual predictors of a disease from the history and physical examination, combine them into a simple score and then test or "validate" that score in a separate group of patients. These scores are often called clinical decision rules or clinical decision guides. Well-known examples include the Ottawa ankle rules for determining the need for an x-ray and the Wells score for DVT.

A clinical decision rule is often used to place the patient in a low-, intermediate-, or high-risk group. This information then informs the decision to order (or not order) further diagnostic tests, and even the interpretation of their results. It is useful to think in terms of two thresholds, the "no test/test" threshold and the "test/treat" threshold. When the probability of disease goes below the "no test/test" threshold, the physician has at least provisionally ruled out the diagnosis in question. When the probability exceeds the "test/treat" threshold, the physician is comfortable enough with the diagnosis to initiate treatment (although further confirmatory diagnostic testing may still be considered). When the probability of a disease lies between these thresholds, further diagnostic evaluation (i.e., questions, examination, or testing) is required.

Although there are formal methods for setting these thresholds, physicians generally establish them implicitly based on their values and those of their patient. When tests are inexpensive and noninvasive, the "no test/test" threshold tends to move lower; when they are noxious, costly, or dangerous, it moves higher or may even merge with the "test/treat" threshold (e.g., brain biopsy for Alzheimer disease). Similarly, the "test/treat" threshold is lower when treatment is benign, cheap and effective and higher when there are significant dangers to treatment (e.g., prescribing anticoagulants for DVT). A fully worked out example of using a validated clinical decision rule is shown in Figures 8.2 through 8.4. (See Chapter 18, Sore Throat, for the full clinical decision rule.)

The "no test/test" threshold is also influenced by the potential seriousness of the differential diagnoses. So, in

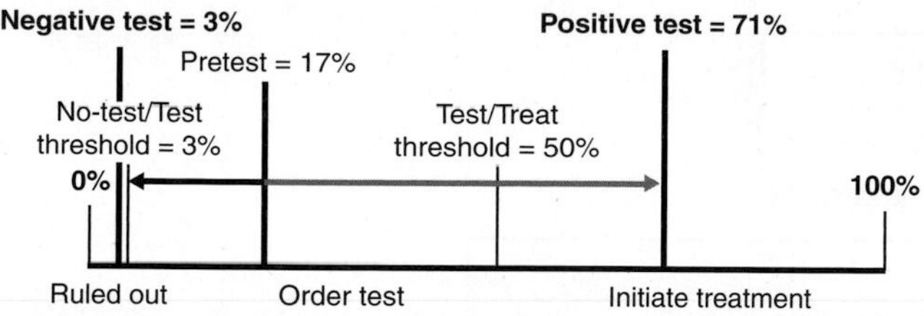

Figure 8.4 • A 20-year-old patient with sore throat, fever, adenopathy, no exudates, and who is coughing, would receive 2 points and have an intermediate risk of strep. This becomes the starting point when interpreting the result of a rapid strep test. Further testing with the rapid strep test moves the probability above or below the two thresholds (to 71% if positive or 3% if negative) (5).

patients with atypical chest pain, for example, even though the pretest probability of significant coronary artery disease may be low we are more likely to pursue testing to rule out cardiac disease because this diagnosis is potentially fatal. After we are satisfied that life-threatening causes are highly unlikely to be present, our test/treat threshold may be lowered so that we may prescribe antacids even thought acid reflux may not be a likely cause of the symptom.

Figure 8.5 provides a general framework for linking clinical decision rules (that use the history and physical exam to stratify risk) with subsequent diagnostic tests. For example, DVT can be ruled out on the basis of a low risk on the Wells score and a normal D-dimer or venous ultrasound. On the other hand, patients with moderate or high DVT risk based on the Wells score who have a negative D-dimer or ultrasound require further testing or close follow-up because they still have a moderately high "posttest" probability of DVT, as their "pretest" probability was so high.

This approach to clinical decision making is widely used for important conditions such as DVT, heart disease, pulmonary embolism, and pneumonia. It makes the best possible use of the physician's history and physical examination skills and customizes the diagnostic evaluation to the patient rather than using a wasteful and potentially inaccurate "one-size-fits-all" approach.

CHRONIC DISEASE MANAGEMENT

There are two types of patient visits in family medicine in which the doctor does not have to make a diagnosis during the encounter. The first—preventive care—is discussed in Part II of this book. The other is the care of people with chronic conditions for which a diagnosis has already been established before the office visit. Examples include hypertension, congestive heart failure, asthma, and arthritis. As you can see from Table 8.2, this type of office visit is very common in family medicine.

Effective chronic disease management is an important and growing element of family medicine. It often requires the patient to make and maintain lifestyle changes, such as dietary modification, exercise, administration of medication, and self-monitoring. These lifestyle modifications affect the patient's personal and family life; therefore, addressing psychosocial issues is an important element of chronic disease visits.

In addition to helping the patient make and maintain the necessary lifestyle changes, chronic disease care involves periodically assessing the patient's wellbeing through history-taking, examination, and selected laboratory tests. These periodic evaluations require considerable skill and organization on the part of the physician. Often, optimal chronic disease management involves a team approach in which other professionals, such as nurses, pharmacists, podiatrists, psychologists, physical therapists, and other medical specialists (e.g., ophthalmology for patients with diabetes), regularly participate in patient management.

In chronic disease management visits, the primary care process can be diagrammed like this:

Established diagnosis → Review of progress since last visit → Management

The visit involves addressing the patient's concerns, reviewing certain subjective and objective indicators of disease status, and revisiting behavioral goals, especially those agreed on by the doctor and patient at previous visits (e.g., weight loss, physical activity).

For patients with one or more chronic diseases, it is imperative that the medical record be well-organized and that communication with other health care professionals be clear and frequent. This is facilitated by use of an EHR, ideally one that includes evidence-based guideline recommendations and flowcharts for monitoring chronic diseases. For example, physicians can be reminded by an EHR if a diabetic patient has not seen the ophthalmologist in more than a year or is overdue for a foot exam.

Deciding on a Management Plan

After analyzing the data and developing a working diagnosis, you often need to make a judgment about whether to order a test, initiate a treatment, or refer the patient. This decision should be based on recommendations from evidence-based guidelines (see Chapter 2, Information Mastery, for more on choosing a good guideline). Good guidelines provide flexibility for patients and physicians and recognize that patients may have different degrees of tolerance for risk and different financial resources. For example, some patients may choose not to have their first mammogram until age 50, because the evidence is much less compelling for its use between the ages of 40 and 50 years.

Thus, cost, time, convenience for the patient, and potential adverse effects of testing or therapy may all impact clinical decisions. Finally, and most important, the patient's personality, anxieties, and social situation may all influence your clinical decision. Does the patient have insurance, or will he or she need to pay out of pocket if you order an expensive test? How high is the patient's need for reassurance that he or she is not seriously ill? How far does he or she trust the doctor (unaided by laboratory tests) to provide this reassurance?

Knowledge of the patient represents relevant data accumulated from experience. Long-term continuity with an individual and family helps the physician learn about their beliefs regarding illness and health, how they deal with stress, how they take their medications, and how responsible they are in managing their own problems. All of these factors enter the melting pot of clinical decision making.

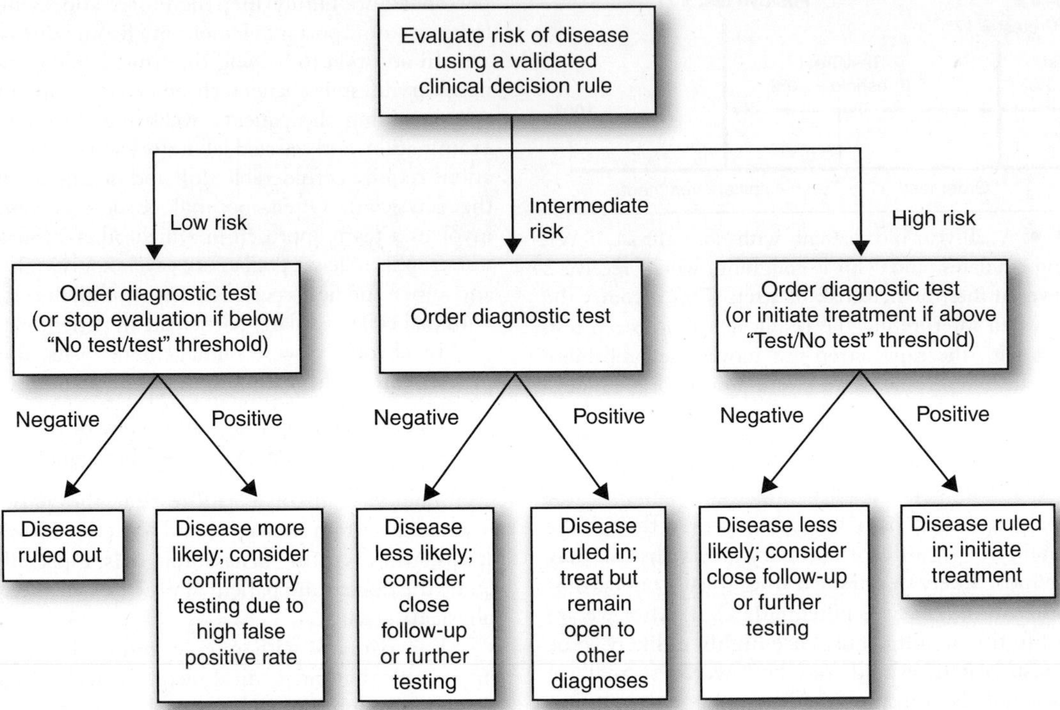

Figure 8.5 • A general approach to diagnostic test interpretation that makes use of the history and physical examination.

Clinical Uncertainty

In primary care practice, uncertainty goes with the territory (6). The degree of uncertainty faced by primary care clinicians is greater than that faced by other physicians because of the larger numbers of undifferentiated problems, the self-limited nature of many complaints, and the relative lack of research data about many primary care conditions. As a result, good communication and follow-up between doctor and patient are essential. Management of clinical uncertainty is one of the keys to practicing good primary care.

Diagnostic uncertainty comes from four sources:

- Cognitive uncertainty, which is related to the physician's perception or knowledge (or lack thereof) of the clinical problem
- Accuracy of the test—many commonly used tests only have modest predictive value, especially when the disease is rare
- Emotional state (anxiety, usually) of the physician
- Variability of the patient's response to communication and therapy

In resolving uncertainty, time is a very powerful diagnostic tool. In many cases, you will need to wait some time before the diagnosis becomes clear or the patient gets better. It is not uncommon for physicians to identify and treat symptoms, realizing that they may resolve spontaneously before a diagnosis is made; examples include diarrhea and abdominal pain, both of which typically resolve without a specific laboratory confirmed diagnosis.

The effective use of time as a diagnostic and therapeutic strategy requires considerable skill, however. The physician who is too anxious to await the evolution of a symptom may order unnecessary tests and have the patient return too frequently, at considerable cost. Take for example computed tomography (CT), which has mushroomed in usage in the United States from 3 million scans per year in 1980 to an estimated 62 million in 2007 (7). It was recently estimated that 1 solid cancer resulting from radiation exposure will occur for every 1,000 abdominal or pelvic CTs ordered in a middle-aged man, and 1 in approximately every 500 scans performed on 20-year-old women (i.e., the number needed to harm is 500) (8). So, for many types of abdominal pain, watchful waiting is more prudent than obtaining a CT scan. On the other hand, the physician who fails to consider alternative diagnostic hypotheses or who does not ask the patient to return may miss an important diagnosis. Methods of managing uncertainty include sharing your uncertainty with colleagues and patients, educating patients about possible outcomes, and reassuring patients that you will continue to observe them for diagnostic clues.

Some physicians worry a great deal about medical malpractice, and they use that as an excuse to order unnecessary tests or questionable treatments. The risk of malpractice can be reduced by documenting visits carefully and clearly, by communicating well with the patient (including what to do if not improving), and by maintaining a good relationship with the patient.

Shared Decision Making

There is an increasing emphasis among primary care physicians on shared decision making, a process by which the clinician and patient work as partners to review data, share treatment preferences, and agree on a treatment plan. This sharing of decision making with the patient has been demonstrated to improve patient satisfaction, enhance treatment adherence, and reduce the overall cost of medical care (9, 10). However, although this approach is gaining increasing acceptance in practice, its actual application requires considerable individualization, because patients vary in how much they want to know in order to participate actively in decision making, how well they can process medical information (especially statistics on such things as likelihood ratios and complication rates), and how much they desire the physician to make recommendations versus offer choices. It appears especially relevant and useful in chronic disease management, where behavior change is an especially important part of the treatment process, and where patient involvement in decision making is especially critical.

USING THE REMAINDER OF THIS BOOK

The rest of this book consists of chapters devoted to common problems. Many are organized around a symptom, such as abdominal pain, back pain, or dizziness. Others are devoted to a specific chronic disease, such as hypertension, obesity, and asthma. A few discuss clusters of diseases whose presentation, pathophysiology, and approach overlap (e.g., upper respiratory infections, sexually transmitted diseases).

In choosing what to put in each chapter, we have tried to focus on the issues that are most important to good patient management. Thus, some chapters focus on diagnosis, others on treatment, and others on both. When appropriate, we have tried to include easy-to-use tables and algorithms, detailed information about the accuracy of diagnostic tests, evidence-based treatment recommendations, dosages for commonly used drugs, and the general approach to management.

KEY POINTS

- Family medicine practice addresses a diverse array of clinical issues and often addresses multiple problems in a single clinic encounter.
- Several different diagnostic reasoning approaches are used in primary care, depending on the type and complexity of the problem being evaluated.
- The test/treat threshold model is suitable to assist clinical decision making in primary care.
- Some level of clinical uncertainty cannot be avoided in primary care decision making.

Acknowledgment

Special thanks to David Reed, PhD, of the Cecil G. Sheps Center for Health Services Research at the University of North Carolina at Chapel Hill for conducting the analyses for Tables 8.1 and 8.2.

CHAPTER

9

Chest Pain

Phillip E. Rodgers and Lee A. Green

CLINICAL OBJECTIVES

1. Evaluate chest pain in a primary care setting using a structured, evidence-based approach
2. Readily identify uncommon but life-threatening causes of chest pain in the primary treatment
3. Manage non-life threatening but important causes of chest pain

Chest pain is a common reason for a patient to visit his or her family physician. It is also one of the most challenging problems to treat; the differential diagnosis covers the entire spectrum of family medicine, from acute life-threatening conditions to somatoform sensations and worries. The possibility of an acute coronary syndrome (ACS)—ST-elevation myocardial infarction (STEMI), non-ST-elevation myocardial infarction (NSTEMI), or unstable angina (UA)—weighs most heavily in the evaluation of chest pain. Much in the chest aside from the heart can hurt, however, and heart disease is actually one of the less common causes of chest pain in the primary care setting.

The general approach to the patient with chest pain is rapid assessment and treatment of possible life-threatening conditions if present, followed by a careful biopychosocial evaluation and management of underlying causes. Simply "ruling out MI" is not an adequate stopping point for the family physician's evaluation.

PATHOPHYSIOLOGY

Pain in the chest may emanate from the heart, great vessels, lungs, pleura, ribs, shoulders, muscles, esophagus, or upper abdomen. Pain can also be felt in the chest as part of systemic processes such as panic attacks, thyrotoxicosis, or stimulant use. Although a full discussion of chest pain pathophysiology is beyond the scope of this chapter, familiarity with basic mechanisms of the most common and important sources of chest pain is essential to understanding their clinical management.

Acute Coronary Syndrome

The pain of ACS is caused by hypoperfusion of the myocardium, usually from occlusion of a coronary artery by thrombus formed on the disrupted endothelium of a ruptured atherosclerotic plaque. If perfusion is not restored within 3 to 6 hours, cells begin losing integrity and leaking contents such as cardiac troponins, myoglobin, and creatine kinase. If ischemia persists, cell death occurs and acute ischemia becomes myocardial infarction.

UA is defined as rest pain for 20 minutes or more that is likely to be associated with an unstable coronary artery occlusion and hypoperfusion. However, unstable angina also includes new-onset, effort-dependent angina and a recent (within 2 months) clinically significant increase in chronic angina symptoms. Such accelerations of angina may represent rupture or other acute changes in a plaque, formation of a thrombus not fully occluding an artery, or simple progression of atheroma. Although the long-term mortality of unstable angina is substantial and not much less than that of myocardial infarction (1, 2), it is important to distinguish UA from MI as their acute management strategies differ. Unfortunately, such a distinction can often be made only in retrospect, well after critical initial treatment decisions have been made.

Variant angina, also known as vasospastic or Prinzmetal angina, is caused by spastic narrowing of otherwise normal coronary arteries. Although frequently considered in the differential diagnosis, true coronary vasospasm is quite uncommon (3). Other important but rare sources of ACS include nonatherosclerotic coronary artery inflammation or dissection, as well as systemic conditions that either severely limit oxygen delivery to the heart (severe anemia, hypotension) or dramatically increase consumption (sepsis, thyrotoxicosis). Preexisting coronary artery disease (CAD) increases the risk for ischemia in the setting of these and other extraordinary physiologic stressors.

Stable Angina

Stable angina, also known as chronic effort-dependent angina, is caused by lack of sufficient oxygen delivery to myocardium during exertion, most often because of impaired blood flow past the hallmark atherosclerotic plaques of CAD. This imbalance produces the characteristic squeezing or dull "pain" of stable angina, as well as characteristic electrical changes on electrocardiogram (ECG) (ischemic muscle conducts electricity differently) and wall motion abnormalities on echocardiography (ischemic muscle does not contract normally).

Panic Disorder

Panic-associated chest pain can be severe and lead to extensive and invasive intervention, though its mechanism remains unknown (4). Panic attacks may occur in isolation, as part of panic disorder, or as part of other anxiety disorders. Even in referral settings, panic disorder is present in more than 30% of chest pain patients, and may coexist with CAD (5).

Gastroesophageal Reflux Disease and Esophageal Spasm

Approximately 10% of the adult population experience regular gastroesophageal reflux disease (GERD) symptoms, though fewer than 1% seek medical attention for it (6, 7). GERD-related chest pain can result from both irritation of the esophageal mucosa and esophageal spasm, the latter of which can mimic angina. Reflux can be exacerbated by triggers that relax the lower esophageal sphincter, most notably caffeine, alcohol, and fatty foods.

Other Causes

Musculoskeletal chest pains commonly arise from ribs or thoracic soft tissue, though most people who have them do not present for medical evaluation. Mitral valve prolapse is often blamed for chest pain among young people (especially women), though there is evidence that reflux may be the actual cause of most pain attributed to mitral valve prolapse (8). Pulmonary embolism may produce pain, usually pleuritic in nature, though its symptoms are notoriously variable and entirely absent in at least half of cases. Pleuritic pain can also be produced by inflammation from an infectious process or by neoplasm. Spontaneous pneumothorax is uncommon and is associated with vigorous exercise, primarily (by a ratio of 5:1) in men in their 20s.

Chest pain can rarely result from dissection of the thoracic aorta (almost exclusively found among hypertensive patients; Marfan syndrome and syphilis are very rare causes), vertebral or rib metastases from any of several different malignancies (and enlarged mediastinal nodes resulting from lymphoma), sarcoidosis, and collagen-vascular diseases.

DIFFERENTIAL DIAGNOSIS

Perhaps nowhere in medicine is the clinical epidemiology of a problem as varied—or as important—as in the evaluation of chest pain. The four most common and important causes of chest pain in primary care are ischemic heart disease, panic, reflux, and musculoskeletal pain. Musculoskeletal pain is the most common, followed by reflux and other gastrointestinal sources. Heart disease is the most life-threatening, although panic causes substantial morbidity that is often inadequately recognized. Pulmonary embolism and aortic dissection are also associated with substantial morbidity and mortality, although both are rare in the primary care setting.

The probabilities of the various causes differ sharply across the clinical settings in which chest pain is commonly encountered. Table 9.1 presents the final diagnoses of cases of chest pain from a network of family physicians' offices (9). GERD alone accounts for at least 13% of all patients. "Psychosocial" sources mainly represent panic attacks, either isolated or in the setting of panic disorder. Pulmonary causes are pleuritic for the most part. Causes such as aortic dissection and pneumothorax are very rare in outpatient family medicine, and were not observed at all in the 399 cases used to construct Table 9.1. By contrast, about 30% of patients seen in the emergency department with chest pain will have an acute coronary syndrome, and 15% or more will actually suffer MI (10). Thus, decisions appropriate in the emergency department may not be valid in the office.

TABLE 9.1 Differential Diagnosis in Patients with Chest Pain

Diagnostic Category	% of Episodes in Family Practice Settings
Musculoskeletal pain	36
Gastrointestinal pain	19
Nonspecific chest pain	16
Stable angina	11
Psychosocial pain	7
Pulmonary pain	5
Nonischemic cardiac pain	4
Acute cardiac ischemia	2

Reprinted with permission from Klinkman MS, Stevens D, Gorenflo DW. Episodes of care for chest pain. J Fam Pract 1994;38:344–352.

CLINICAL EVALUATION

Proper evaluation of chest pain involves a complete medical history and physical examination, which is time consuming. However, time can be critical to managing potentially life-threatening conditions. Therefore, the evaluation of the chest pain patient proceeds in two steps: 1) rapid evaluation using a few key predictors of ACS, followed by immediate initiation of treatment if indicated (within 10 to 20 minutes of initial presentation); and 2) a complete evaluation after an ACS has either been excluded or properly triaged. Treatment for ACS or other life-threatening conditions should never be delayed while the complete evaluation phase is being performed, unless the diagnosis is in doubt and information from the complete evaluation is crucial to resolving it.

Studies have identified a small set of factors that are of genuine predictive utility for the diagnosis of ACS in the primary care setting (9, 11). Table 9.2 presents these validated diagnostic cues in approximate order of importance for both rapid and detailed evaluation.

The Acute Cardiac Ischemia Time-Insensitive Predictive Instrument (ACI-TIPI) is a well-validated clinical prediction rule for estimating the likelihood of an ACS in patients with chest pain in the emergency department. The ACI-TIPI can be used in primary care settings, although its positive predictive value is lower because of the lower incidence of an ACS in that setting. A second well-validated tool has been developed for patients with acute chest pain and a normal or nonspecific ECG (see Table 9.3).

TABLE 9.2 Key Elements of the History and Physical Examination of the Patient with Chest Pain

Rapid Evaluation for Potential Acute Coronary Syndromes

History
- Onset and character of pain
- Prior history of coronary artery disease

ECG within 10 minutes of presentation (findings in descending order of importance)
- ST segment elevation or depression of ≥1 mm in at least two consecutive leads
- Q waves in at least two leads, not including aV_R, not known to be old
- T-wave hyperacuity or inversion in at least two leads, not including aV_R
- New bundle-branch block

Complete evaluation

History
- Anxiety symptoms (choking feeling, fear, light-headedness, paresthesias)
- Nighttime symptoms
- Previous episodes; age at onset
- Tachycardia
- Acid regurgitation, heartburn
- Relationship to activity
- Relationship to respiration
- Cardiac risk factors (hypertension, diabetes, smoking, family history, hyperlipidemia)
- Claudication
- Use of cocaine
- Thromboembolic risk factors (recent fracture or immobilization, hypercoagulable states, history of DVT or PE)

Physical examination
- Blood pressure
- Oxygenation assessment (respiratory effort, color, pulse oximetry or arterial sampling if indicated)
- Heart murmurs
- Third, fourth heart sounds
- Pulmonary edema (dyspnea, bilateral rales)
- Stigmata of vascular disease (bruits, diminished pulses, arterial changes or A-V nicking on retinal examination, skin changes, or ulceration of lower extremities)
- Xanthelasma
- Edema
- Obesity

A-V = atrioventricular; DVT = deep vein thrombosis; ECG = electrocardiogram; PE = pulmonary embolism.

History and Physical Examination

RAPID EVALUATION

The initial chest pain history seeks to identify any likely symptoms of acute, life-threatening conditions. Although not always a simple task, it should be obtained concurrently with other elements of the rapid evaluation (physical exam, ECG) for efficiency.

The pain of an ACS is typically dull, aching, pressing, squeezing, or heavy and steady. It is seldom sharp or burning. Pain or pressure may be located in the chest (angina pectoris) with radiation elsewhere, or it may be located entirely outside the chest in the upper epigastrium, shoulder, upper arm (left or right), jaw, or neck. Pain is often severe, but some patients describe their discomfort as pressure or heaviness rather than pain. Asking only about pain will fail to identify many of these patients. Chest symptoms are often accompanied by palpitations, diaphoresis, pallor, dyspnea, and a feeling of impending doom (*angor animi*). Less severe and less persistent pain of the same type, triggered by activity and relieved by rest, is characteristic of chronic stable angina.

Women are more likely to report their ischemic cardiac pain in the neck, back, or epigastrium (12). Diabetic patients may have little or no pain, and elderly patients often present with shortness of breath rather than chest pain (13). Atypical angina (anginal-type pain appearing in patterns other than exertional angina) suggests a lower probability of an ACS, but does not rule it out. Such atypical pain may be right-sided or midepigastric. Inferior MI may present with only a profound sense of unease, accompanied by nausea and vomiting. Well-localized sharp or pleuritic pain suggests noncardiac causes. Similarly, very brief pains lasting a few seconds each or pain present continuously for days are unlikely to represent an ACS.

TABLE 9.3 Clinical Prediction Rule for Patients with Normal ECG or Nonspecific ECG Changes

1. Read the ECG, and decide whether it is normal or has nonspecific changes (note: this clinical rule does not apply to clearly abnormal ECGs):
   Normal: ECG is completely within normal limits without any ST- or T-wave abnormalities
   Nonspecific changes: ECG has nonspecific ST- or T-wave changes, including minor ST- or T-wave abnormalities not suggestive of ischemia or strain
2. Count the number of risk factors that your patient has:

Risk Factor	Points
Age >60 years	1
Male sex	1
Pain described as pressure	1
Pain radiating to arm, shoulder, neck, or jaw	1
Total:	

3. Find your patient's risk of AMI below for his or her number of points and type of ECG:

	Normal ECG		Nonspecific ECG	
Number of Points	Number in Group	% with AMI	Number in Group	% with AMI
0	177	0	114	0
1	374	1.1	309	2.6
2	354	2.5	333	4.8
3	137	9	149	11
4	19	26	26	23

AMI = acute myocardial infarction; ECG = electrocardiogram.
Modified and reprinted with permission from Rouan GW, Lee TH, Cook EF, Brand DA, Weisberg MC, Goldman L. Clinical characteristics and outcome of acute myocardial infarction in patients with initially normal or nonspecific electrocardiograms. Am J Cardiol 1989;64:1087–1092.

Not all heart pain is ischemic. The pain of pericarditis is typically worse when recumbent, and relieved by sitting forward. ECG changes are often diffuse and can involve both precordial and limb leads. Diagnosis may be difficult at first, only confirmed once enzymes have excluded MI while extensive ECG changes persist. Aortic dissection may cause a tearing or cutting pain, perhaps felt posteriorly in the chest or midback.

A history of established CAD is a key risk for ACS, but is not always easily elicited. Ask the patient about a history of previous MI, abnormal noninvasive test results, the results of previous catheterizations, and nitroglycerin use for pain relief. The best-studied element of history to predict CAD is the type of chest pain. Typical anginal symptoms (substernal dull, heavy, or squeezing chest pain/pressure appearing with exertion and relieved by rest) are highly predictive of CAD (LR+ >100). Atypical angina (anginal-type pain that occurs without exertion) is moderately predictive, whereas pain that is nonanginal in character is rarely caused by CAD.

Figure 9.1 presents the likelihood of CAD for men and women of varying ages and symptom descriptions (14); the practical importance of these symptom distinctions is readily apparent. It is important to note that while the likelihood of ACS increases with age for both men and women, age is not a powerful predictor. Premenopausal women can be regarded as having roughly the same risk as a man with the same history and examination findings but 10 years younger. Postmenopausally, women's risks for ACS converge over time to become similar to those of men.

Although epidemiologic risk factors such as smoking, family history, hyperlipidemias, diabetes, and hypertension are good predictors of the long-term risk of developing CAD, they are only minimally useful in discriminating between an ACS and noncardiac chest pain in the acute setting (15, 16). These traditional risk factors are important to assess when counseling patients both in primary prevention and after the diagnosis of CAD is established, but they should not color the evaluation of a patient who has acute chest pain.

The rapid history of chest pain must be obtained without delay, but care should be taken to notice clues to nonemergent causes whose symptoms may initially appear quite similar to angina. Specifically, the chest pain of a panic attack can mimic an ACS, with substernal chest pressure accompanied by a fear of imminent death, choking sensations, shortness of breath, palpitations, sweating, lightheadedness, tremulousness, or nausea. On the other hand, the paresthesias that can occur with panic are uncommon with ACS, as are a fear of "going crazy," derealization (feelings of unreality), and depersonalization (feelings of being outside of or detached from oneself). Although panic attacks may occur at any age, they usually begin in the patient's teens or 20s. Age of onset of symptoms

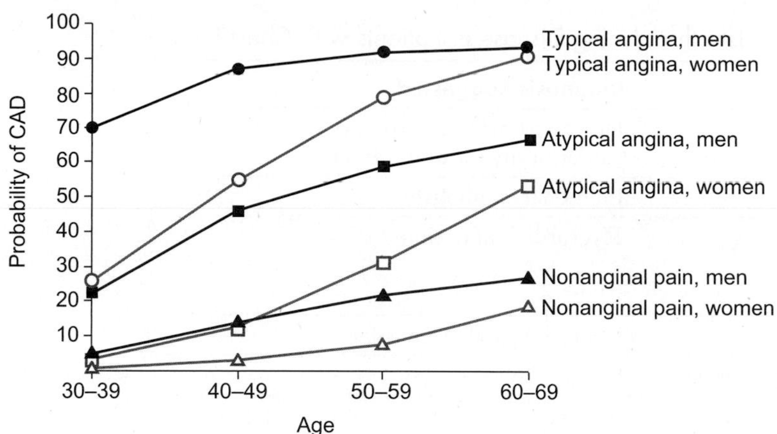

Figure 9.1 • Likelihood of coronary artery disease (CAD) by patient and symptom characteristics. Definitions: typical angina, substernal dull, heavy or squeezing chest pain or pressure appearing with exertion and relieved by rest; atypical angina, anginal-type pain appearing in patterns other than on exertion; nonanginal pain (atypical chest pain), pain with a character that is not that of typical angina (e.g., chest wall pain, epigastric burning).

can be helpful: ACS is rare before age 35 in men or 45 in women and uncommon until 10 years later than that.

GERD can mimic angina when associated with severe, prolonged spasm of the esophageal smooth muscle ("nutcracker esophagus"). Esophageal spasm can be partially relieved by nitroglycerin, furthering its mimicry of an ACS. Relief with antacids or histamine 2 antagonists also suggests GERD, although its absence does not exclude the diagnosis. See Chapter 21, Dyspepsia, for a more detailed discussion of the diagnosis of GERD.

Musculoskeletal pain can be sharp or dull, whereas the pain of ACS is not sharp. Musculoskeletal pain that is reproducible with palpation of the chest wall is a strong negative predictor of MI (LR 0.3), particularly with the suspicion of ACS is low (17). Pulmonary causes of pain may behave like musculoskeletal pain, but are more often pleuritic (sharp pain worsened by breathing). Tachycardia and tachypnea associated with pleuritic chest pain are red flags for pulmonary embolism or pneumonitis. See Table 9.4 for other red flags and Chapter 12 for a more detailed discussion of the diagnosis of pulmonary embolism.

The most important part of the physical examination is the patient's overall appearance. If pain is present at the time of examination, is the patient simply describing a pain that is annoying, or is he or she pale and sweaty? The patient presenting with chest pain should have vital signs assessed promptly and monitored closely for changes during the evaluation. Tachycardia in particular is characteristic of panic and pulmonary embolism (the latter especially when accompanied by tachypnea). Bradycardia, especially if new or symptomatic, may be associated with inferior myocardial ischemia. Hypertension can occur as a result of acute pain of any source, but can also be associated with acute MI or, more rarely, aortic dissection. Although a very uncommon outpatient presentation, acutely symptomatic hypotension may indicate inferior ischemia or, more ominously, left ventricular (LV) failure caused by large anterior wall MI or massive pulmonary embolus.

The examination of the rapid evaluation phase should be brief, directed specifically toward the red flags of immediate danger (see Table 9.4). The sensitivity and specificity of these findings are generally not defined. However, the finding of sudden or "flash" pulmonary edema, a new mitral regurgitant murmur, hypoxia, bradycardia, hypotension, or a new S3 sound is ominous.

COMPLETE EVALUATION

As in any thorough outpatient evaluation, a complete chest pain history should document the pattern of discomfort, what makes it better or worse, and any associated symptoms. The temporal pattern—whether the pain is constant or intermittent, brief or long-lasting, or associated with particular times of day—may help differentiate causes. Fleeting pains or pain continuously present for days are unlikely to be caused by coronary disease, although the latter may be seen in patients with pericarditis.

Ask the patient about the frequency of recurrence and any changes in frequency, such as acceleration of angina or increasingly frequent panic attacks. If the pain is exertional in nature, you should ask how much exertion is required to bring it on and how much rest is needed to relieve it. Angina that occurs after less-strenuous exertion than before suggests progression of the disease and compels further investigation.

Exacerbating and relieving factors also help differentiate causes. Pain occurring with specific movements suggests pulmonary or musculoskeletal etiologies (as well as pericarditis), and pain with respiration suggests pulmonary etiologies. Reflux is commonly worse after fatty or large meals and while bending at the waist or lying supine; it usually improves with antacids (see Chapter 21, Dyspepsia, for more information on reflux).

Other symptoms occurring with chest pain should be noted because they can be associated with specific diagnoses: paresthesias and palpitations (panic); cough or hemoptysis (pulmonary embolism, pneumonia); shortness of breath (pulmonary embolism, pneumothorax). For a more detailed discussion of the diagnosis of pulmonary embolism, see Chapter 12, Venous Thromboembolism. Absence of subjective fear does not exclude panic, because up to one-third of patients have the subtype of nonfear panic disorder (3). Diminution of chest pain with sitting up and leaning forward is typical of pericarditis. Regurgitation of acid and even food into the pharynx is highly specific for GERD.

The patient's medical history also includes clues to the differentiation of chest pain. A history of hypertension, diabetes, claudication, or cerebrovascular disease increases the likelihood of vascular disease. A recent viral illness or prodrome suggests either pleuritis or pericarditis. A history of multiple complaints across organ systems should prompt inquiry for primary somatization disorder or somatization as a manifestation of depression.

TABLE 9.4 Red Flags Suggesting Life-threatening Disease in Patients with Chest Pain

Finding	Diagnosis Suggested
Hypotension, poor tissue perfusion, pulmonary edema, or oliguria	Decreased cardiac output, possible large anterior myocardial infarction
Tachycardia, tachypnea, hypoxia	Pulmonary embolism
Electrocardiogram changes, especially ST segment elevation or new left bundle-branch block	Myocardial infarction
New systolic mitral murmur	Ruptured papillary muscle
Arrhythmia and/or chest pain in younger patient	Cocaine abuse
Mediastinal widening on chest radiograph	Aortic dissection with severe tearing or ripping pain

Coronary risk factor assessment is useful when addressing your patient's long-term risk of developing CAD. Risk factors include family history, hyperlipidemia, and smoking in addition to the medical history described above. Cocaine abuse should also be noted because it can cause cardiac death in young patients. Caffeine intake predisposes to GERD, but does not increase the risk of CAD.

During the physical examination, palpate pulses in all four extremities, and listen for bruits over the carotids, abdominal aorta, and renal vessels. Diminished or absent pedal pulses or an audible bruit suggests vascular disease. In patients with leg complaints (not chest pain), absence of a femoral pulse or presence of a femoral artery bruit are useful for ruling in peripheral vascular disease (LR+, 5 to 7), but do not rule it out when absent. Although young patients with scaphoid abdomens often have bruits on auscultation, essentially all have normal vessels. Reduction or disappearance (perhaps intermittent) of the brachial and carotid pulses is associated with aortic dissection, as is inequality of blood pressure in the two arms in patients with chest pain. Extremities should also be examined for clinical evidence of deep venous thrombosis (erythema, tenderness, unilaterally increased limb diameter, palpable cord, Homan sign), the presence of which should raise suspicion of pulmonary embolism.

Cardiac auscultation is ordinarily normal or nonspecific in the chest pain patient (8). A new murmur, although uncommon, is a red flag for adverse outcome, and a rub may aid in the diagnosis of pericarditis. Pulmonary auscultation is typically normal as well, but rubs, rales, and consolidation should be sought. Percussion of the chest can reveal the rare spontaneous pneumothorax.

Diagnostic Testing

RAPID EVALUATION

The sole laboratory investigation in the rapid evaluation phase is a 12 lead ECG. If there is no reason to doubt a diagnosis of ACS, therapy should be started without delay. An ECG should be performed on any patient in whom ACS is suspected, and should be completed and read within 10 minutes of the patient's arrival.

Three features of the presenting ECG are established predictors of ACS (Table 9.5). Of these, ST segment changes (or new left bundle-branch block [LBBB]), either ≥0.5-mm elevation or ≥1 mm depression in at least two leads, is the most important. T-wave hyperacuity (at least 50% of QRS amplitude) or inversion in at least two leads (excluding aV_R, in which the T wave is normally inverted) is also important. A finding of new Q waves of ≥1 mm in at least two leads is strongly associated with acute injury, but may not be present in the first 24 to 36 hours after infarction. ST segment elevation during chest pain is useful for ruling in acute MI (LR+, 5.1; LR−, 0.59) (24); ST segment depression is associated with ischemia but less specifically with infarction.

The ECG changes associated with pulmonary embolism are far less specific. In the approximate order of positive predictive value (none have substantial negative predictive value) they are sinus tachycardia, $S_1Q_3T_3$ pattern, rightward axis deviation, right bundle-branch block, ST depression in the right precordial leads, p pulmonale, and ST elevation in lead III (18). None of these findings is very good at ruling out PE when absent.

COMPLETE EVALUATION

A chest radiograph is recommended for patients with chest pain who do not have a clearly identifiable source on history and physical. Chest films will show widening of the mediastinum in half of the patients with aortic dissection (19). Other useful findings include consolidation in patients with pneumonia; the boot-shaped shadow of a fluid-filled pericardium; a tumor producing pleural irritation; a pneumothorax; or rarely, the wedge-shaped shadows of pulmonary infarcts from emboli.

Cardiac troponins T or I have become the laboratory test of choice because of their high sensitivity and particularly high specificity for cardiac injury. Normal serial troponin measurements at 10 hours after symptom onset can essentially exclude myocardial infarction. Furthermore, normal troponins can help to inform short term prognosis: only 1 in 300 patients with a normal ECG and a normal troponin I level 6 hours after chest pain onset will have an adverse cardiac outcome in the next 30 days (20). This can be particularly helpful when deciding where and how quickly to proceed with a diagnostic workup.

Significant troponin elevation in patients with characteristic chest pain—even with a normal ECG and normal or

TABLE 9.5 Characteristics of Diagnostic Tests Useful in Patients with Chest Pain

Test	LR+	LR−
Coronary Artery Disease		
Nonsloping ECG ST segment depression during ECG stress (21)		
>2.5 mm	39	
2–2.5 mm	11	
1.5–1.99 mm	4.2	
1–1.49 mm	2.1	
0.05–0.99 mm	0.9	
Reversible perfusion defect on thallium scintigraphy (19)	11.8	0.31
Reversible wall motion abnormality on stress echocardiography (20)	7.4	0.21
Acute Coronary Ischemia		
ECG findings for ruling in ACI (21)		
New ST segment elevation >1 mm	6–54	
New left bundle-branch block	6.3	
Q wave	3.9	
T wave hyperacuity	3.1	
Serum Markers for Ruling out ACI (22)		
Myoglobin in normal range and not doubling over 2 hours within 6 hours of presentation	17	0.1
CK-MB normal, single test	2.8	0.75
CK-MB normal, serial measurements		0.04
Total CK normal, single test		0.85
Total CK normal, serial measurements		0.11
Serial troponin T <0.18 ng/mL with normal ECG (23)		0.003
Serial troponin T <0.18 ng/mL with ST-depression or T-wave inversion		0.013

ACI = acute cardiac ischemia; CK-MB = creatinine kinase myocardial bands; ECG = electrocardiogram; LR = likelihood ratio.

borderline creatinine kinase myocardial bands—yields a diagnosis of myocardial infarction. Troponin elevation also has prognostic significance, carrying a 2% to 6% risk for further cardiac injury (MI or sudden cardiac death) within 6 months. These patients are candidates for intensive medical therapy or percutaneous coronary intervention (PCI) (21, 22). Troponins T and I are similar in accuracy and either may be used; individual laboratories should be consulted for their preference and reference ranges.

When working with a patient who has more chronic symptoms, testing for CAD may be done by exercise ECG, exercise echocardiography, or gated blood pool scanning. For any of these tests, pharmacologic stress testing can be substituted for exercise. The addition of radionuclide imaging improves the specificity of these tests. Graded exercise ECG using the Bruce or equivalent graduated protocols is the usual test of choice for men with suspected CAD (23). Pharmacologic stress testing should be reserved for patients who are physically unable to exert themselves, because it yields less prognostic information than physiologic stress.

Simultaneous nuclear perfusion imaging can reveal areas of reversible ischemic myocardium and is recommended for patients with baseline ECG abnormalities such as bundle-branch block, preexcitation syndrome (i.e., Wolff-Parkinson-White) baseline ST depression >1 mm, mechanical pacing, or digoxin therapy. The American College of Cardiology/American Heart Association Guidelines for Exercise Testing (24) also suggests adding radionuclide imaging for symptomatic women and elders, two groups in whom ECG stress alone is often less reliable. Stress echocardiography also reveals areas of wall motion abnormality induced by ischemia, and has seen increased use in centers staffed by experienced interpreters, on whom much of its utility rests. The accuracy of stress ECG, stress radionuclide, and ECG testing is summarized in Table 9.5.

Five-year mortality prognosis can also be estimated for outpatients from exercise ECG data (25). Angina is scored 0 for none, 1 for angina induced by but not limiting the treadmill test, and 2 for angina that limits the test. The score is (exercise in minutes) − (5 × maximal ST deviation) − (4 × angina score). Patients with scores of 5 or greater have a 5-year survival rate of 99%; those with scores of −10 to +4 have a 5-year survival rate of 95%; and those with scores of −11 or lower have a 5-year survival rate of only 79%.

Coronary artery calcium scoring by computed tomography is in increasingly widespread clinical use, though enthusiasm for it exceeds the evidence base at this time. There is evidence for its use to estimate prognosis for patients with uncertain causes of chest pain, negative initial troponin, and non-ischemic ECG findings (26). Patients with coronary artery calcium scoring of 0 are at extremely low near-term risk for coronary events.

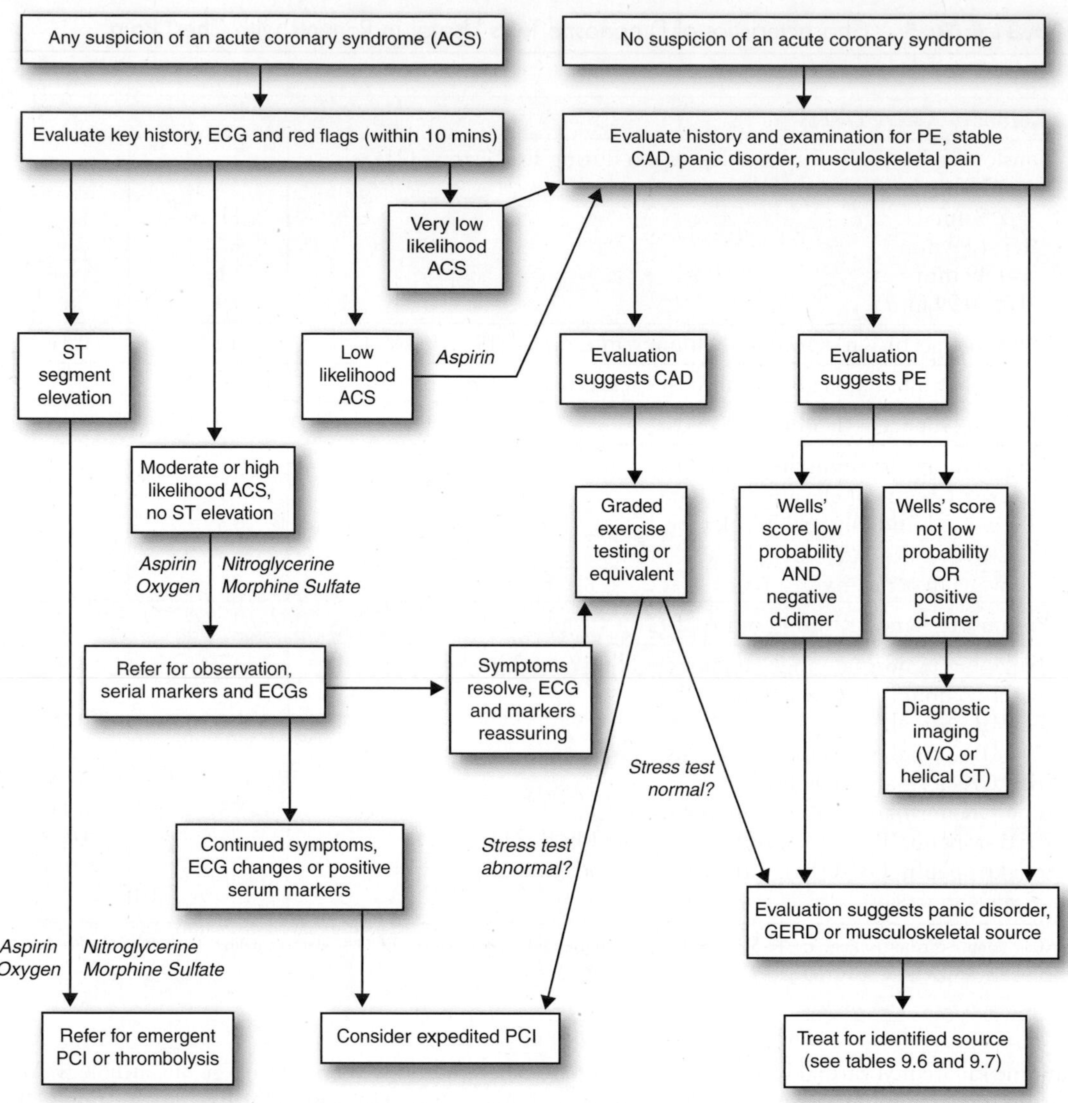

Figure 9.2 • Approach to the patient with chest pain. CAD = coronary artery disease; ECG = electrocardiogram, GERD = gastroesophageal reflux disease; PCI = percutaneous coronary intervention.

Suspected dissection of the aorta can be evaluated with angiography, transesophageal echocardiography, helical computed tomography, or magnetic resonance imaging. Although all perform well in high-risk groups and effectively rule out the diagnosis when normal (27), angiography performs surprisingly poorly as the likelihood of disease decreases. Only magnetic resonance imaging appears to offer better than a 50% positive predictive value when the risk of aortic dissection is low (<1%) (28).

It is important to evaluate the possibility of pulmonary embolism in patients with chest pain. The recommended diagnostic strategy is described in detail in Chapter 12, Venous Thromboembolism.

MANAGEMENT

Management of the patient with chest pain is very different for each of the many causes previously discussed. Key elements in managing chest pain are listed in Table 9.6. Figure 9.2 illustrates the approach to the patient. The basic principles of therapy for the most important causes of chest pain in primary care are summarized in the following section. Table 9.7 summarizes the pharmacotherapy for chest pain. Management of GERD (Chapter 21) and pulmonary embolism (Chapter 12) are discussed elsewhere in this text.

Acute Coronary Syndromes

ANTI-PLATELET THERAPY

All patients with suspected ACS should receive aspirin, 325 mg swallowed or chewed, immediately and then continued daily indefinitely. Aspirin therapy prevents three to 10 deaths or MIs per 100 ACS patients, making it the most effective medical intervention available (29–32). It should only be withheld for true absolute contraindications, such as anaphylaxis, other major allergic reaction, or current active gastrointestinal bleed

TABLE 9.6 Key Elements in Management of Chest Pain, by Cause

Target Disorder	Intervention	Strength of Recommendation*	Comments
ACS, CAD	Aspirin	A	Withhold only for absolute contraindications
	β-blockers	A	Withhold only for absolute contraindications; oral administration only
	Nitroglycerin	B	Pain relief and improvement of hemodynamic indices; unclear if improves survival
CAD	Coronary revascularization (bypass or angioplasty)	A	For patients meeting very specific selection criteria
	Lipid lowering	A	Reduce LDL cholesterol to <100 mg/dL; <70 mg/dL for patients with history of ACS
	Smoking cessation	B	Largest absolute risk reduction of any treatment if patient successfully quits
ACS	Clopidogrel	A	For ASA contraindicated patients suspected of UA/NSTEMI; duration of therapy depends on diagnosis
	Unfractionated or low-molecular-weight heparin	A	Usually reserved for ongoing symptoms of pain or instability
	Morphine sulfate	C	Clearly effective for pain and anxiety relief, although not formally studied; inadequate dosing is common and inexcusable
MI	ACE inhibitors	A	Improve survival post-MI in anterior infarcts with ejection fraction <40%
	Emergent reperfusion (thrombolysis or PCI) for STEMI patients	A	Target time to thrombolysis: <30 minutes Target time to PCI: <60 minutes
PE	Unfractionated or low-molecular-weight heparin	A	Treatment should not be delayed while confirming a strong clinical suspicion of PE
GERD	H_2 receptor antagonists	A	
	Proton pump inhibitors	A	
	Elevation of head of bed	B	
	Decreased fat intake	B	
	Avoidance of chocolate, onions, peppermint, and garlic	B	
Panic	Benzodiazepines	A	High rate of placebo response, and much better short-term than long-term efficacy
	Tricyclic antidepressants	A	
	Cognitive therapy	A	
	Combined drug and cognitive therapy	A	
Musculoskeletal pain	NSAIDs	C	

ACS = acute coronary syndromes; CAD = coronary artery disease; GERD = gastroesophageal reflux disease; LDL = low-density lipoprotein; MI = myocardial infarction; NSAIDs = nonsteroidal anti-inflammatory drugs; PE = pulmonary embolism.
*Strength of Recommendation Taxonomy (SORT): A, Consistent, good quality patient-oriented evidence; B, Inconsistent or limited-quality patient-oriented evidence; C, Consensus, disease-oriented evidence, usually practice, expert opinion or case series for studies of diagnosis, treatment prevention, or screening; X, moderate or strong evidence suggesting that this treatment is not effective.

TABLE 9.7 Pharmacotherapy of Chest Pain, by Cause

Drug	Dose Range	Comments	Cost*
Acute Coronary Syndrome			
Metoprolol	Acute: 5 mg IV every 2 minutes for three doses, then 50 mg orally BID starting 15–60 minutes after last IV dose Chronic: 50–100 mg orally every day	Monitor as for atenolol	$$
Aspirin	325 mg immediately, 81–325 mg daily	Effect disappears at doses >325 mg/day	$
Clopidogrel	300 mg at diagnosis, 75 mg daily	For aspirin contraindicated patients	$$$
Nitroglycerin	IV: 5–10 mg/minute, titrate up by 10 mg/minute every 10 minute until relief is achieved or until baseline in hypertensive patients, headache, or hypotension occurs Oral: 0.4 mg sublingual; may repeat every 5 minutes, with 3 doses being the usual maximum	Monitor for SBP <90, or 30% below normal	$
Lisinopril	5 mg orally every day, titrate to max 20 mg/day		$
Enalapril	2.5–5 mg daily, to max of 40 mg/day in single or divided dose		$
Benazepril	2 mg daily, titrated to max of 20 mg/day		$$
Fosinopril, quinapril	5 mg daily, titrated to max of 30 mg/day		$$
Morphine sulfate	2–4 mg IV every 10–20 minutes as needed	Underdosing common; 10–30 mg may be required	$
Panic Disorder SSRIs			
Paroxetine	20–50 mg orally every day	May cause increased agitation in the short run; consider starting at 10 mg	$$
Sertraline	50–200 mg every day	May start at 25 mg for elders or complexly ill patients	$$
Citalopram	10–60 mg every day		$$
Desipramine	25–300 mg every day (usually at HS)	Side effects may limit titration to effective doses. Start low, increase slowly once weekly	$$
Nortriptyline	10–150 mg	May be more well tolerated than other tricyclics	$
Diazepam	2.5–5 mg TID	Many other benzodiazepines are available and probably equally effective	$$
Alprazolam	0.25 mg TID, titrated to max of 4 mg/day	Some antidepressant effect; may require careful dose adjustment for panic	$
Clonazepam	0.5 mg TID, titrated to maximum of 20 mg/day		$$
Buspirone	Start with 7.5 mg BID; increase by 5 mg every day for 3 days to a max dose of 15–30 mg/day divided BID-TID	See text	$$$

BID = twice daily; GERD = gastroesophageal reflux disease; HR = heart rate; IV = intravenously; SBP = systolic blood pressure; SSRI = selective serotonin reuptake inhibitor; TID = three times per day.
*Relative cost: $ = <$33.00; $$ = $34.00–$66.00; $$$ = >$67.00.

(not merely positive occult blood or a history of bleed). Patients with true contraindications should receive clopidogrel 300 mg as a loading dose as soon as an ACS is diagnosed and 75 mg daily thereafter. Clopidogrel should also be considered in addition to aspirin ("dual antiplatelet therapy") for patients with UA or NSTEMI, as the combination lowers risk of death or urgent revascularization versus aspirin alone (33, 34). The duration of therapy is guided by subsequent evaluation and intervention.

REPERFUSION THERAPY

The patient with chest pain and ST segment elevation greater than 1 mm in two or more contiguous leads or new LBBB is experiencing STEMI, and should be considered for immediate reperfusion. Restoring coronary blood flow limits infarct size, preserves LV function, and enables myocardial remodeling, all of which contribute to substantial decreases in short- and long-term mortality. Both thrombolytic therapy and emergent PCI provide these benefits: treatment choice depends on characteristics of both the patient and the treating institution.

Indications for thrombolytic administration for STEMI are very narrow: characteristic pain onset within 6 hours of presentation (perhaps up to 12 hours, but with lesser benefit) plus either ST segment elevation in more than two contiguous leads or new LBBB. Thrombolysis is contraindicated for patients who do not meet these criteria (23, 27). Other contraindications include active gastrointestinal and genitourinary bleeding (not menses), abdominal or thoracic surgery within 1 month, head trauma, recent stroke, hypertensive crisis, aortic dissection, and pancreatitis. Although age is not an absolute contraindication to thrombolytic therapy, patients older than age 75 are at greater risk for bleeding complications from thrombolysis, and may be better served by emergent PCI (35).

Evaluation and administration of thrombolysis should occur within 30 minutes of presentation to an equipped facility (usually an emergency department). For properly screened patients, thrombolysis reduces in hospital and 1-year mortality by approximately 6 per 100 patients treated, although it probably does not improve 3-year outcomes (36). Hospitals typically administer thrombolytic agents (usually streptokinase or recombinant tissue plasminogen activator—rtPA) under specific protocols; see your institution's policy for details.

PCI refers primarily to percutaneous transluminal coronary angioplasty with or without intracoronary stenting. Emergent PCI yields better short- and long-term outcomes than thrombolysis for patients with STEMI in centers suitably staffed, equipped, and experienced to provide it without delay (37, 38). PCI is not superior in hospitals with lower volumes, and if a "door-to-balloon" time of 90 minutes cannot be achieved, delaying thrombolysis to seek PCI can worsen outcomes (39).

For patients with NSTEMI, early PCI (within 24 hours) has also demonstrated improved survival and rehospitalization rates compared with conservative medical therapy (40). Additionally, platelet inhibition with intravenous glycoprotein IIb/IIIa receptor antagonists (abciximab, eptifibatide, or tirofiban) can improve early survival, primarily for patients with NSTEMI and UA who are at high risk for complications and will undergo PCI (41).

MEDICAL THERAPY

In addition to immediate anti-platelet therapy, patients with a suspected ACS should receive oxygen, nitroglycerine and morphine, if necessary. Oxygen via nasal cannula has no proven outcomes benefit in the absence of significant hypoxia, though it carries low risk and can improve comfort. Nitroglycerin can provide preload and afterload reduction and significant relief of chest pain, but should not be given if the patient is hypotensive (systolic blood pressure <90 mm Hg), bradycardic, or has suspected right ventricular infarction. Nitroglycerin can be given sublingually every 5 minutes for three doses before consideration of intravenous or transdermal administration. Morphine can provide important analgesia and anxiety relief, but is frequently underdosed—start at 2 to 4 mg intravenously, and repeat every 20 to 30 minutes until effective.

β-blockers can improve both short- and long-term mortality in patients with ACS, and should be administered *orally* within the first 24 hours of onset, in the absence of contraindications such as uncompensated heart failure, symptomatic hypotension or bradycardia. Intravenous β-blockade is now relatively contraindicated due to an increase in risk of cardiogenic shock, and should be reserved for specific and urgent indications such as tachyarrhythmias and hypertensive crises (42). Oral metoprolol has been studied at 200 mg daily in either BID regular- or QD long-acting dose preparations. Atenolol is disfavored based on metaanalysis that show it to be substantially less effective than other agents in its class (43).

Anticoagulant therapy has become standard for higher risk UA/NSTEMI patients because it decreases infarction and PCI rates (44). Recently, low-molecular-weight heparin has gained a small but definite advantage over unfractionated heparin both in efficacy and safety (45). Angiotensin-converting enzyme (ACE) inhibitors are indicated within 24 hours of onset for patients who sustain MI, but not for ACS patients in general. For patients with large anterior infarcts, ejection fractions below 40%, or transient LV dysfunction, ACE inhibitors provide an approximately 0.5% absolute risk reduction for mortality (1 fewer death for every 200 patients treated) (46, 47). Benefit for other MI patients is unclear, and ACE inhibitors should not be given to patients with hypotension, hyperkalemia, or rising creatinine.

Calcium channel blockers do not generally improve outcomes and may increase mortality among patients with LV dysfunction or pulmonary edema (27). They should generally not be used in acute treatment of ACS, except for specific indications such as atrial arrhythmias and genuine variant angina, which is rare. Antiarrhythmic therapy can increase mortality and should be reserved for sustained, symptomatic ventricular arrhythmias (48, 23).

Coronary Artery Disease

Therapy for CAD is aimed at controlling symptoms that interfere with the patient's function and reducing the risk of death or infarction. Aspirin should be given to all patients who do not have absolute contraindications (see those listed previously) (49). Likewise, β-blockers are standard of care because of their long-term mortality benefit, and they are also effective antianginal drugs.

Smoking cessation, although challenging to accomplish, is essential. Smokers with CAD who quit reduce their absolute risk of death over the ensuing decade by 11% to 16%, making smoking cessation the single most important intervention in this group (50, 51). Smoking cessation also reduces the risk of disability and hospitalization.

In patients with known CAD and baseline low-density lipoprotein levels ≥130 mg/dL on diet alone, reduction in low-density lipoprotein cholesterol to below 100 mg/dL can prevent 4 deaths in 100 patients treated for 5 years (52). HMG-CoA reductase inhibitors (statins) used in combination with diet are the preferred agents because they are the only agents shown to achieve this level of benefit. Very aggressive lipid lowering with statins, to target low-density lipoproteins <70, can further reduce subsequent events among patients with a recent ACS (53).

Nitrates are used for additional symptomatic relief. Sublingual or spray forms are used for acute symptoms, and long-acting oral agents or transdermal patches are used for daily prevention. If patches are used, they should be removed at night to prevent disappearance of effect due to tachyphylaxis. Calcium channel blockers are also useful for symptomatic relief, and long-acting agents seem to be safe, but the short-acting agents should be avoided because case-control studies suggest a nearly four fold increase in odds ratio for cardiovascular mortality among hypertensive patients (54). Calcium channel blockers can supplement, but should not replace, survival enhancing β-blockers in patients' antianginal regimens.

Revascularization reduces mortality for patients with 50% or greater left main coronary artery stenosis, three-vessel disease and diminished LV function, or two-vessel disease involving the left anterior descending artery (23, 27). Revascularization does not reduce mortality or major coronary events compared with optimal medical therapy outside of these indications (55); angioplasty or stenting should not be considered a "given" for all or even most stenoses. Symptom improvement may be achieved for patients with any degree of CAD who suffer lifestyle-limiting anginal symptoms not adequately controlled by medical therapy. In general, the debate between coronary artery bypass graft and angioplasty is beyond the scope of this chapter, but it should be noted that diabetic patients requiring insulin or oral agents seem to have a lower mortality rate with coronary artery bypass graft (56).

Nonsteroidal Anti-inflammatory Drugs and CAD Risk

Chronic use of a nonsteroidal anti inflammatory drug (NSAID) increases risk for MI and cardiac death for patients with CAD, in direct proportion to the agent's degree of COX-2 inhibition (57). Higher risk NSAIDs include not only those marketed as "COX-2 selective inhibitors" such as rofecoxib, celecoxib, and valdecoxib, but also relatively COX-2 selective drugs such as diclofenac and nabumetone—all should be avoided in patients with CAD.

First-line analgesic medications for CAD patients should include acetaminophen, non-acetylated salicylates (e.g., salsalate) and aspirin. Should these be insufficient or not well-tolerated, a trial of NSAIDs with lower COX-2 selectivity (e.g., naproxen, piroxicam) could be considered. Patient with CAD needing high, daily doses of even these NSAIDs for pain management may be good candidates for a trial of low-dose opioids or adjuvant medications.

Panic Disorder

The two primary approaches to treatment of panic disorder are cognitive therapy (also called cognitive behavioral therapy) and pharmacotherapy. The best results are obtained by combining the two modalities because they have been shown to be mutually potentiating in the few trials in which they were combined (58).

Cognitive therapy teaches the patient to interpret the somatic sensations that accompany an attack as something other than evidence of serious illness. Panic patients have been shown to interpret such sensations in much more alarming ways than nonpanic patients. Cognitive therapy has been shown both to change those interpretations successfully and to provide improvement similar to that from pharmacotherapy (59).

Pharmacotherapeutic management with either antidepressants or anxiolytics is often necessary for more than 6 months. Treatment with either class of agent is more effective than placebo among patients in blinded trials willing to maintain treatment (60).

Due to their tolerability and safety profile, selective serotonin reuptake inhibitors (SSRIs) have become first-line pharmacologic treatment for panic disorder. SSRIs have been shown to be better than placebo in a meta-analysis of randomized controlled trials (61) and are equivalent in effect to tricyclics and benzodiazepines. Patients should be warned that they can cause increased agitation in the first few weeks of use; a short-term prescription for benzodiazepines is often prescribed during these initial weeks to counter this adverse effect. Tricyclic antidepressants are the most thoroughly studied antidepressants for panic disorder. If chosen, therapy should be initiated at low doses, and physicians should be careful to explain the expected adverse effects as normal so that panic patients do not interpret them as serious.

Benzodiazepines are the primary anxiolytic class; buspirone may be useful but is not well studied yet. Alprazolam and lorazepam are often used for panic disorder, but it is likely that all members of the class are effective. Although tolerance is common with long-term use and tapering may be necessary to prevent withdrawal, addiction (e.g., increasing dose requirements, behavioral "drug seeking," concealment of multiple sources) is generally uncommon. Care should be taken, however, in prescribing these medications for patients with a significant history of addiction, personality disorder or complex chronic pain, as rates of overuse rise in these groups. Benzodiazepines should be used on a fixed schedule, never as needed, for panic disorder treatment.

Relaxation therapy has been shown to improve patients' ability to tolerate anxiety, but has not been shown to reduce the frequency or severity of panic attacks. It is therefore not a primary treatment recommendation for panic disorder, although it may be for other anxiety disorders.

Musculoskeletal Pain

Musculoskeletal chest pain is traditionally treated with NSAIDs or acetaminophen. It is unclear what fraction of patients derives symptomatic improvement from this therapy. Considerable attention to the patient's worry about heart disease, with appropriate reassurance, is an important part of management.

KEY POINTS

- Chest pain is a common symptom in outpatient primary care practice, though much more likely to be caused by musculoskeletal, anxiety or gastrointestinal disorders than an acute coronary syndrome (ACS) (9).
- Patients presenting to the office with chest pain should immediately be assessed for potentially life-threatening conditions with a focused history, targeted physical examination, 12-lead electrocardiogram (ECG), and emergency interventions if indicated.
- After life-threatening diagnoses are excluded, a complete evaluation should proceed to determine the underlying source of chest pain: simply "ruling out ACS" is insufficient.
- Evidence-based therapy should be initiated to address likely diagnoses, which may include gastroesophageal reflux disease (GERD) (62), panic disorder (63), musculoskeletal dysfunction, stable angina (64), and others.

CHAPTER

10

Common Chronic Cardiac Conditions

Philip M. Diller and Douglas R. Smucker

CLINICAL OBJECTIVES

1. List the diagnostic criteria
2. Assess and detect signs and symptoms indicating functional capacity, and acute exacerbation or worsening status at each encounter
3. Offer specific treatment interventions for patients whose clinical status has worsened
4. Describe the evidence-based interventions that prevent further disability or death
5. Describe how a continuity relationship between a family physician and a patient with a common cardiac condition leads to high-quality care and better clinical outcomes

Chronic heart disease has a tremendous impact on clinical care, public health, and national resources. Heart disease is the leading cause of mortality in the United States. On average, 2,300 Americans die each day from cardiovascular disease (1). This chapter will review three of the most common chronic cardiac conditions encountered in family practice: coronary artery disease (CAD), heart failure (HF), and atrial fibrillation (AF).

Patients with known CAD are routinely cared for by family physicians (2). Angina affects more than 6 million Americans, and CAD is responsible for 1 in every 6 deaths (1). Heart failure, one of the common complications of CAD, is the most common cause of hospitalization for individuals older than age 65. Each year 670,000 new cases develop and 280,000 deaths occur from HF (1, 3). The family physician will also encounter many patients with cardiac arrhythmias in clinical practice, of which AF is the most common arrhythmia (4). For each of these three conditions, we will review evidence regarding diagnosis, treatment, and long-term monitoring.

The general approach to patients with any chronic cardiac condition includes two overarching goals: 1) to prevent further disability or death from chronic cardiac disease and 2) to help patients cope with their condition by treating symptoms and improving physical capacity. These goals can best be achieved in the context of a continuity doctor–patient partnership using a combination of evidence-based approaches including lifestyle changes, modification of cardiac risk factors, disease monitoring with diagnostic testing, medications, and specialty consultation or referral when appropriate.

CORONARY ARTERY DISEASE

CAD is a metabolic/inflammatory disease of the coronary arteries that leads to build up of an atherosclerotic plaque and narrowing of the arterial lumen. Atherosclerotic plaques can rupture and the body's response to repair the rupture (thrombosis) can lead to symptoms of angina, myocardial infarction (MI), and/or sudden death. Patients who are discharged after an episode of angina or have survived an MI have known CAD, and family physicians are often closely involved in managing and preventing further complications (3). CAD is one of the top 20 diagnoses seen by family physicians. The primary tasks in the management of patients with known CAD during ambulatory visits include (5–8):

- Identifying the type of angina and detecting changes in the pattern and severity of angina symptoms
- Treating angina symptoms when they occur
- Reducing and controlling risk factors to prevent progression of coronary artery disease and in turn, decrease the likelihood of MI and death

The ambulatory management of a patient with known CAD who presents to the office is shown in Figure 10.1 and discussed in more detail below.

DIAGNOSIS

Differential Diagnosis

When a patient with known CAD presents to the office, the following symptoms should suggest CAD: chest pain with or without exertion, pain radiating from chest to jaw or left shoulder, dyspnea with exertion, or sudden "indigestion" poorly responsive to antacids. These symptoms can also be caused by common other conditions such as those coming from: *the heart*, myocarditis, heart failure, mitral valve prolapse; *the major arteries*, dissecting aneurysm; *the lungs*, pulmonary embolus, pneumothorax; *the esophagus*, spasm, esophagitis, ulceration; *the stomach*, hiatal hernia, peptic ulcer disease; *the skin and musculoskeletal structures*, herpes zoster, trauma, costochondritis; and *psychological conditions*, panic attack. A thorough history and physical examination and familiarity with these common conditions are necessary to diagnose CAD as the underlying cause. Patients with known CAD may have experienced angina before and often recognize when angina recurs.

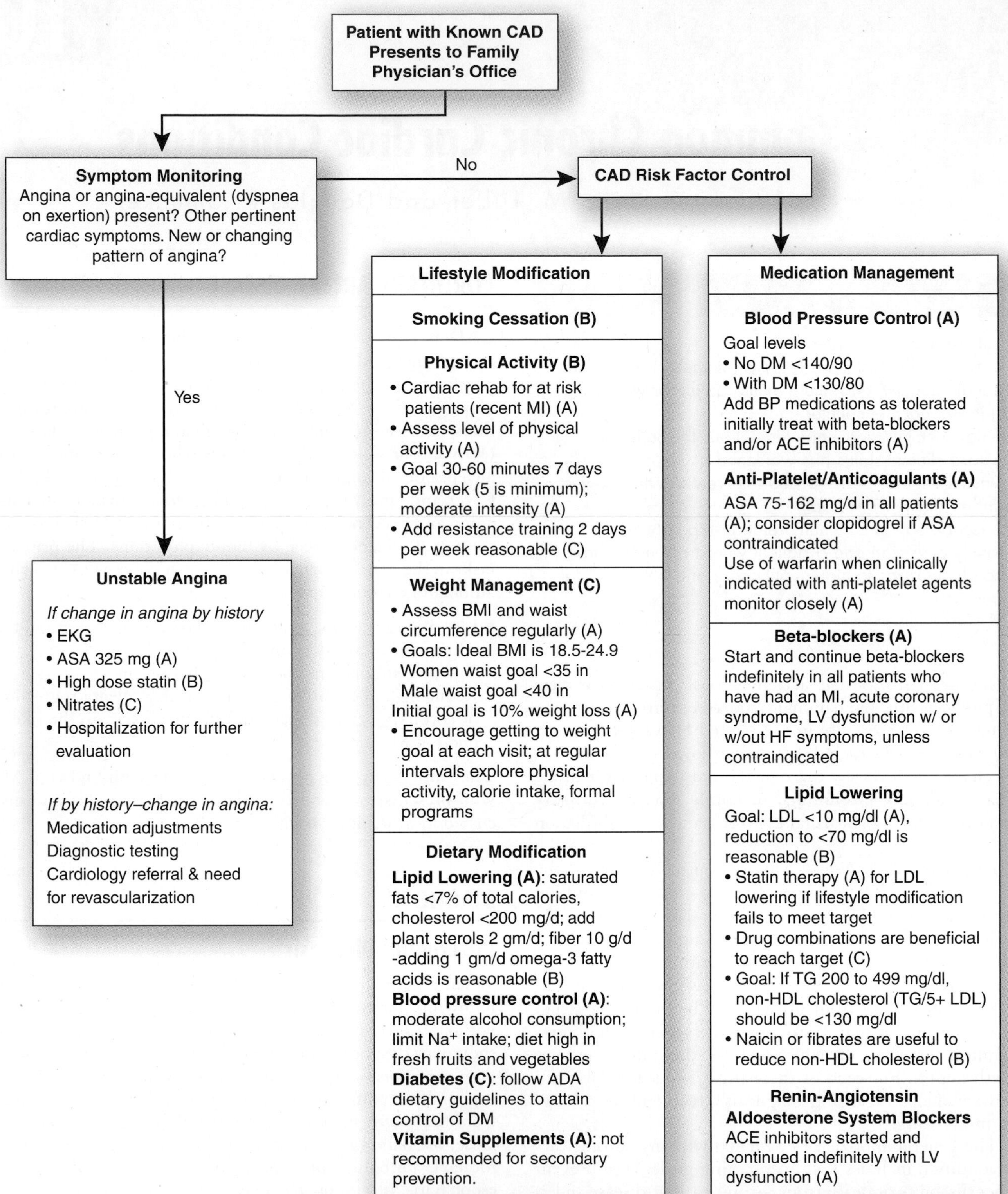

Figure 10.1 • Office management of patients with known coronary artery disease. A = consistent, good-quality patient-oriented evidence; B = inconsistent or limited-quality patient-oriented evidence; C = consensus, disease-oriented evidence, usual practice, expert opinion, or case series. For information about the Strength of Recommendation Taxonomy evidence rating system, see *http://www.aafp.org/afpsort.xml*.

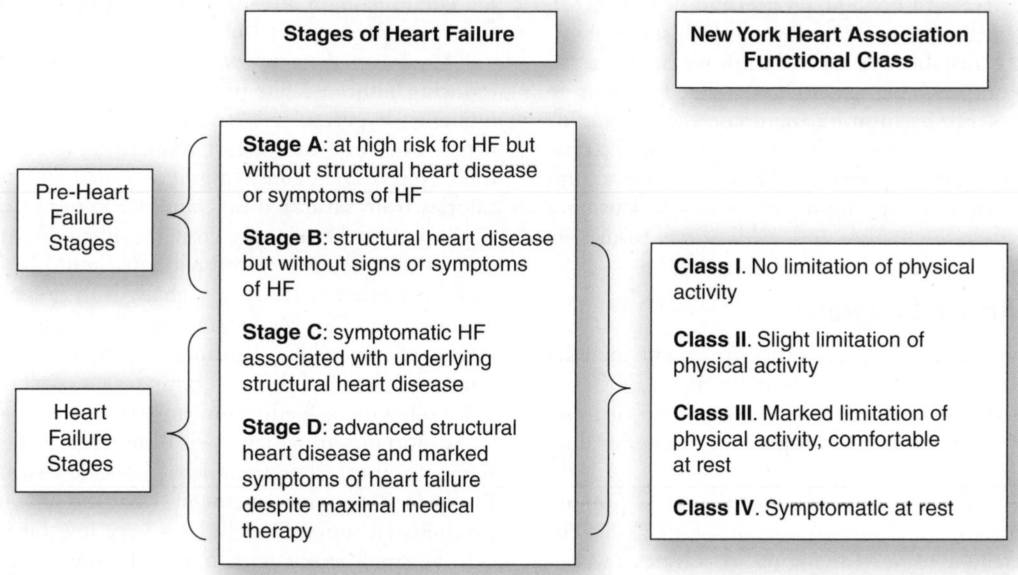

Figure 10.2 • How the stages of heart failure related to the New York Heart Association functional classification.

History and Physical Examination

When a patient with known CAD presents to the office, ask about the patient's experience of angina since the last visit. If angina is present, identify the type of angina. Characterizing the quality, pattern, and frequency of chest pain is a crucial task in evaluating patients with known CAD (2). Chest pain can be categorized as typical angina, atypical angina, or noncardiac chest pain. Typical angina is defined as having all three of the following characteristics: 1) substernal chest discomfort or pressure, 2) discomfort/pressure that is provoked by exertion or emotional stress, and 3) discomfort/pressure that is relieved by rest or by taking nitroglycerin. If only two of those three characteristics are present, the patient is said to have atypical angina. For example, a patient with substernal pain or pressure that occurs at rest, but is relieved by nitroglycerin has atypical angina. The third category is noncardiac chest pain in which a patient has only one of the three characteristics listed (2, 6).

You should ask patients about the quality, location, and duration of the pain, and about associated symptoms such as diaphoresis, shortness of breath, nausea, and palpitations. It is also important to identify factors that worsen or relieve pain. Patients with a fairly predictable pattern of chest pain with exertion are categorized as having stable angina. Patients who have new onset angina or a worsening pattern of pain have unstable angina. Unstable angina is associated with a much higher short-term risk for an acute myocardial infarction or other cardiac event, and calls for prompt evaluation and often requires immediate hospitalization (5, 6).

ASSESSING THE FUNCTIONAL STATUS

The family physician should regularly assess the impact of CAD on the patient's physical functioning. The New York Heart Association (NYHA) classification scale is widely used for this purpose (see Figure 10.2).

MONITORING FOR PHYSICAL SIGNS OF VASCULAR DISEASE

During an initial physical examination, the physician should also search for signs of vascular disease (abnormal fundi, decreased peripheral pulses, bruits), end-organ damage caused by hypertension (abnormal fundi, carotid bruit), aortic valve stenosis (systolic murmur, abnormal pulses), left heart failure (third heart sound, displaced apical pulse, basilar rales), and right heart failure (jugular venous distension, ascites, pedal edema).

Diagnostic Testing

In a patient with known CAD, exercise testing with thallium or technetium imaging is a valuable clinical tool (2, 5, 6). Stress imaging can be used to evaluate changes in anginal patterns, to assess exercise capacity, or to detect disease in patients being considered for cardiac rehabilitation programs. For CAD patients who are unable to exercise, who have left bundle branch block, or who have an electronically paced ventricular rhythm on baseline electrocardiogram (ECG), stress imaging using a pharmacologic agent is recommended (2). Dobutamine, dipyridamole, and adenosine can be used to stress the cardiac muscle while the patient is at rest, causing differences in perfusion and wall motion in the areas with coronary artery obstruction.

Coronary angiography remains the "gold standard" for evaluation of CAD. Patients with known CAD are first diagnosed and evaluated by this procedure. Patients with known CAD who experience unstable angina are reevaluated with coronary angiography for both diagnostic and therapeutic indications and require the family physician to consult a cardiologist.

TREATMENT OF PATIENTS WITH KNOWN CAD

There are two primary goals in the management of patients with known CAD, particularly those with angina. The first, and highest priority, is to prevent progression of CAD, MI, and death from cardiac events. To accomplish this, the physician must identify unstable angina and improve cardiovascular risk factor control. The second and related goal is to improve quality of life by limiting the occurrence of angina and other symptoms of cardiac ischemia that can be distressing and impair functional capacity (5). These goals are accomplished primarily by treating angina symptoms and using a combination of lifestyle changes and medications to modify cardiac risk factors and, as outlined in Figure 10.1.

Treatment of Angina Symptoms

For patients with unstable angina, office treatment includes immediate evaluation with history and physical, an ECG and initiation of treatment with nitrates, oxygen, aspirin, and high-dose statin before transfer to hospital for further evaluation and treatment.

For patients with symptoms of stable angina, a primary goal is to limit symptoms and improve quality of life (5–8). The two agents primarily used to treat angina are nitrates and calcium antagonists. Neither of these agents has been shown to reduce mortality in patients with known CAD, but their use can reduce the frequency and distress caused by angina. Nitrates decrease venous return, reduce left ventricular wall stress, and dilate stenotic coronary arteries. They exist in several forms of administration (sublingual, oral, spray, transdermal, and intravenous) that are similarly effective in relieving ischemic episodes. All patients with CAD should have a rapid-acting nitroglycerin for rescue from acute anginal episodes. A long-acting nitrate, such as isosorbide dinitrate or isosorbide mononitrate, can be used for individuals with frequent angina. Hypotension and headache are common side effects of nitrates.

Calcium channel blockers are often added or substituted for long-acting nitrates to control angina symptoms (5, 6). They function by blocking movement of calcium into myocardial and smooth muscle cells, resulting in muscular and vascular relaxation. Two classes of calcium channel blockers exist: nondihydropyridines (i.e., verapamil, diltiazem) and dihydropyridines (i.e., nifedipine, amlodipine). The dihydropyridines produce significant peripheral vasodilatation and may produce a reflex tachycardia. Verapamil and diltiazem modestly reduce peripheral resistance, decrease heart rate, reduce contractility, and slow electrical conduction. The physician must be cautious with certain drug combinations in patients with known CAD. Dihydropyridine calcium channel blockers and a nitrate can produce profound hypotension while diltiazem or verapamil combined with a β-blocker can cause significant bradycardia or conduction defects.

LIFESTYLE CHANGES

The modification and control of CAD risk factors is an important goal in the management of patients with known CAD. The classical risk factors for CAD include: age, male sex, being postmenopausal for women, family history of early CAD, smoking, hypertension, hyperlipidemia, and diabetes mellitus (9). Other related risk factors include obesity and a sedentary lifestyle. Lifestyle interventions for CAD include smoking cessation, diet modification, weight loss, and exercise (5–7). The family physician should encourage the patient and family to stop smoking and should provide counseling, nicotine replacement, and suggest cessation programs. It is never too late to gain an advantage over chronic cardiac disease by cessation of smoking (10).

Common dietary goals in patients with CAD include reducing saturated fats (if hyperlipidemic), reducing sodium intake (if hypertensive), and controlling blood sugar (if diabetic). The American Heart Association (AHA) recommends their Step II Diet, consisting of less than 30% total fat, 7% of calories from saturated fats, and <200 mg of cholesterol/day (9). However, there is only limited evidence to support the efficacy of this diet. Motivated patients should be encouraged to go even further with dietary changes to prevent further cardiac disease. The Mediterranean diet emphasizes increased intake of vegetables, legumes, fruits, cereal, fish, reduced intake of meat and dairy, and moderate consumption of alcohol. Following a Mediterranean-style diet reduced cardiovascular mortality in patients with known CAD (11). An intensive program to change multiple lifestyle risk factors (Ornish Program: stress management, smoking cessation, exercise, psychosocial support) includes a very low-fat vegetarian diet (12). A small study with 5 year follow up showed that in patients who could adhere to the Ornish program stabilized or even reversed coronary artery obstruction and reduced the number of subsequent cardiovascular events (12).

Medications that Improve Risk Factor Control and Decrease CAD Mortality

Interventions that have the greatest evidence for preventing infarction or death remain underused in appropriate patients with known CAD (5, 6). Medications with evidence for CAD mortality reduction in patients with known CAD include: 1) antiplatelet medications, 2) β-blockers, 3) lipid-lowering agents, and 4) angiotensin-converting enzyme inhibitors (ACE) (see Figure 10.1) (5).

ANTIPLATELET AGENTS

Aspirin should be taken routinely by all patients with known CAD, particularly higher risk patients with chronic stable angina. For patients who do not tolerate aspirin, who have experienced worsening CAD while taking aspirin, or for patients who have had recent angioplasty with stenting, clopidogrel (Plavix) is another option (2). Apart from these circumstances, there is no evidence to routinely prescribe clopidogrel for all patients with CAD (13).

β-BLOCKERS

β-blockers have been repeatedly shown to reduce the risk of MI and other adverse cardiac events in patients with CAD, particularly in patients who have had a previous MI. β-blockers reduce heart rate, decrease myocardial contractile force, and block deleterious sympathetic tone on coronary arteries (5, 6). No one β-blocker has shown superiority over others in reducing angina or adverse outcomes. Some β-blockers are cardioselective (atenolol, metoprolol) and affect primarily β1 receptors. Propranolol is a common nonselective β-blocker that demonstrates β2 (pulmonary smooth muscle) and β1 effects. Nonselective β-blockers may induce bronchospasm in patients with asthma or chronic obstructive pulmonary disease. Other potential side effects of β-blockers are bradycardia, impaired glucose control in diabetes, exercise intolerance, depression, and impotence (although depression and impotence are much less common than previously supposed) (14). Physicians should ensure that all eligible patients with known CAD, particularly those who have had an MI, are taking a β-blocker. Although diabetes mellitus has traditionally been considered a relative contraindication to β-blocker therapy, several randomized trials have shown that β-blockers improve morbidity and mortality in hypertensive patients with diabetes mellitus (15).

LIPID-LOWERING AGENTS

Patients with known CAD should have close attention paid to their lipids and an aggressive approach to lowering levels of low-density lipoproteins (LDL). For patients with CAD, the National Cholesterol Education Program recommends that LDL cholesterol be maintained at less than 100 mg/dL, high-density lipoproteins at greater than 40 mg/dL, and non-high-density lipoproteins cholesterol (serum triglycerides/5 + LDL) at less than 130 mg/dL (9). Extrapolating from randomized trials suggest that an even lower goal for LDL to <70 mg/dL may be beneficial for patients with CAD and multiple other risk factors for an acute cardiac event, most importantly diabetes mellitus (16). If diet and exercise do not achieve these goals, drugs that lower cholesterol should be prescribed, beginning for most patients with a statin (9). Statins consistently have shown a mortality benefit in patients with known CAD (17).

ACE INHIBITORS

In addition to aspirin, a β-blocker, and close attention to lipids, the addition of ACE inhibitors should be considered for every patient who has known CAD. Several studies have shown that ACE inhibitors reduce the risk of cardiovascular death, MI, and stroke in patients who have vascular disease (18). Even small doses of ACE inhibitors with only a small change in blood pressure may have a vasoprotective effect in preventing adverse events among patients with CAD.

LONG-TERM MONITORING

The American College of Cardiology/AHA guidelines suggest five questions that should be answered regularly during the follow up of a patient with chronic stable angina (Table 10.1). In addition to a follow up history, a brief focused physical exam covering the cardiovascular and pulmonary systems should be performed at each visit. Laboratory assessments should be directed by the history, physical exam, and clinical course of the patient with particular attention to meeting recommended goals for blood lipids. An ECG is indicated when there is a change in the patient's anginal pattern, symptoms of dysrhythmia, or syncope. Cardiac stress imaging or angiography should be considered for any CAD patient with a change in the pattern of angina symptoms (5–8).

Deciding on Need for Revascularization

A challenge for the clinician caring for patients with known CAD is recognizing when revascularization is indicated as opposed to attempting to further maximize medical management (5, 19). Decisions regarding revascularization should generally be made in consultation with a cardiologist or cardiovascular surgeon. Percutaneous transcutaneous coronary stenting should be considered instead of coronary artery bypass graft in patients with one-, two-, or three-vessel disease who have anatomy suitable for stent therapy and who have normal left ventricular function. The presence of significant left main coronary disease, multivessel disease not amenable to stenting, or significant CAD in the presence of left ventricular dysfunction (ejection fraction <50%) indicates that revascularization with coronary artery bypass grafts may be beneficial (20).

TABLE 10.1 History Questions to Monitor Symptoms in Patients with Chronic Stable Angina

- Has your level of physical activity decreased since the last visit?
- Have your anginal symptoms increased in frequency or become more severe since the last visit?
- How well are you tolerating therapy?
- How successful have you been at modifying risk factors and improving knowledge about ischemic heart disease?
- Have you developed any knew comorbid illness or has the severity of treatment of known comorbid illnesses worsened your angina?

Adapted from Snow V, Barry P, Fihn S, et al. Primary care management of chronic stable angina and asymptomatic suspected or known coronary artery disease: a clinical practice guideline from the American College of Physicians. Ann Intern Med 2004;141:562–567. Used with permission.

HEART FAILURE

HF is a heterogeneous condition caused by impaired function of the left ventricle either during systole, diastole, or both (3, 18). Subsequent signs and symptoms are due to the body's maladaptive response to impaired left ventricular (LV) function. In the United States, CAD is the most common etiology of HF. CAD leads to myocardial injury and infarction, with the eventual development of systolic HF, in which the LV ejection fraction (LVEF) is reduced (LVEF <40%). Other etiologies of systolic HF include hypertension, valvular heart disease, alcohol abuse, congenital abnormalities, viral infections, and idiopathic cardiomyopathy.

Not all HF is systolic, however; an estimated 40% of HF arises in patients with normal LV systolic function (20). These patients have diastolic HF, in which the left ventricle is stiff, fails to relax, and does not fill adequately at normal diastolic pressures. Aging, hypertension, and CAD are the most common causes of diastolic HF.

The pathophysiology of HF is a complex interplay of hemodynamic and neurohormonal mechanisms as the body attempts to compensate for ventricular dysfunction. Reduced renal perfusion stimulates the renin-angiotensin-aldosterone system and the sympathetic nervous system. Heightened activity of these two neurohormonal systems leads to myocardial toxicity, peripheral vasoconstriction, and renal salt and water retention. In systolic failure, the left ventricle dilates and loses contractility. In diastolic dysfunction, the neurohormonal systems are also activated but to a lesser degree.

Five tasks are important in the clinical evaluation of HF patients (3, 20–22): 1) establish HF as the patient's diagnosis, 2) determine the type of HF (systolic or diastolic), 3) manage HF symptoms and determine the severity of a patient's functional limitation, 4) optimize medication interventions to slow disease progression and delay mortality, and 5) identify patients who are at risk for developing HF or who have structural heart disease but without signs and symptoms of HF.

DIAGNOSIS

Differential Diagnosis

HF is a symptom complex that may includes fatigue, dyspnea, orthopnea, peripheral edema, and tachycardia. Causes of this symptom complex or some of these symptoms other than HF include cirrhosis, anemia, nephrotic syndrome, myxedema (hypothyroidism), obesity, medications (vasodilators, estrogens, nonsteroidal anti-inflammatory drugs), obstructive sleep apnea, pregnancy, varicose veins, pulmonary hypertension, and the precursors of HF if poorly controlled such as hypertension, ischemic heart disease, atrial fibrillation, and valvular heart disease.

History And Physical Examination

ESTABLISH HEART FAILURE AS THE DIAGNOSIS

To assist with the management of HF, recent guidelines categorize HF in four stages (3). Stages A and B are pre-HF stages when a person is at risk for HF, whereas Stages C and D are when a person experiences symptoms of HF. Figure 10.2 shows how the stages of HF relate to the NYHA classification. Asking about previous chest pain or MI is important in determining the cause of and planning treatment of HF. Attention to risk factors (hypertension, diabetes mellitus, dyslipidemia, smoking) and symptoms that suggest underlying CAD is also important in the initial evaluation of heart failure. Other risk factors for HF include obesity, alcoholism, viral infections, valvular heart disease, and congenital heart disease.

A complete history is important in order to elicit symptoms of HF (Stage C) and search for clues regarding its etiology (3). The classic symptoms are fatigue, dyspnea, and edema. In HF, dyspnea on exertion often progresses to paroxysmal nocturnal dyspnea, orthopnea, and dyspnea at rest. Peripheral edema, typically of the feet and legs, is the result of fluid overload and poor cardiac function. Other symptoms of HF include nocturia, anorexia, abdominal bloating, cachexia, and mental confusion.

The physical examination helps establish the diagnosis of HF, assess for fluid retention, and provides clues to the etiology and type of the HF (23). The physical findings that best rule in systolic HF are gallop rhythm (positive likelihood ratio [LR+] = 24), displaced point of maximum impulse or PMI (LR+ 16), and jugular venous distention (LR+ 9). All of these signs are very specific but not very sensitive, meaning that when present they are strong evidence in favor of HF but when absent do not rule it out. Other useful signs and symptoms include dyspnea on exertion or at night when recumbent (paroxysmal nocturnal dyspnea), unexpected weight gain, wheezing or rales, and presacral or leg edema (3). Tachycardia may be a compensatory response for a low cardiac output, and a reduction in heart rate in response to medical treatment is an indicator of treatment efficacy. Low blood pressure (systolic <90 mm Hg) indicates poor cardiac output and is a predictor of poor outcome. A weight gain of 1 to 2 kg over 1 to 3 days suggests fluid retention, although some patients may initially present with much greater weight gains (5 to 10 kg or more). Pulmonary congestion is suggested by wheezes on auscultation, whereas rales suggest frank pulmonary edema.

Diagnostic Testing

Patients should undergo diagnostic testing to confirm the diagnosis and determine whether the HF is systolic or diastolic (3, 22). A transthoracic two-dimensional echocardiogram with Doppler flow studies is the most important initial diagnostic study because it defines the type(s) and severity of LV impairment. It allows measurement of the EF, ventricular mass, chamber dimensions, and wall motion in addition to evaluation of valvular, pericardial, and vascular structures. It also allows measurement of flow across the mitral valve, categorizing patients into normal (E > A), delayed relaxation (E < A), and restrictive (E >> A) filling patterns. An abnormal E:A ratio is associated with diastolic HF (24). Radionuclide angiography or cardiac catheterization with LV angiography also provides reliable measurement of LVEF and regional wall motion. The latter also permits confirmation of diastolic HF by the measurement of ventricular filling pressures and indices of LV diastolic relaxation. However, because it is more invasive than other studies, it is not part of the routine evaluation of all patients with suspected HF.

In the acutely dyspneic patients, the B-natriuretic peptide level can be helpful in ruling out HF in a dyspneic patient. A B-natriuretic peptide level >100 pcg/dL is moderately accurate for the diagnosis of systolic HF in acutely dyspneic patients presenting to the emergency department (LR+ 3.8, LR- 0.13) (25). Routine studies for all patients with suspected HF include complete blood count, urinalysis, comprehensive metabolic profile (including serum magnesium, phosphorus, and calcium), thyroid-stimulating hormone, chest radiograph, and ECG.

Ongoing assessment of functional status also plays an important role in the management of HF patients (3). Functional status is an indicator of disease severity and treatment success and is strongly associated with prognosis. Evaluation of functional status includes measurement of physical capacity, emotional status, social function, and cognitive abilities. Just as with chronic stable angina, the NYHA classification of heart disease is a useful functional assessment tool (Figure 10.2). A validated prediction model is also available online *(www.ccort.ca/CHFRiskModel.asp)* (26).

TREATMENT OF HEART FAILURE

The management of a HF patient when the follow-up in the office includes the goals of enhancing quality of life, preventing hospitalizations due to worsening status, and preventing disease progression and avoidable death (Fig. 10.3).

To enhance quality of life, you should routinely assess the patient's functional capacity (NYHA class), monitor HF signs and symptoms, and review self-care strategies with the patient or family. Changes in NYHA class indicate disease progression and need for more intensive therapy or possible conversations about end-of-life and prognosis. The patient's weight

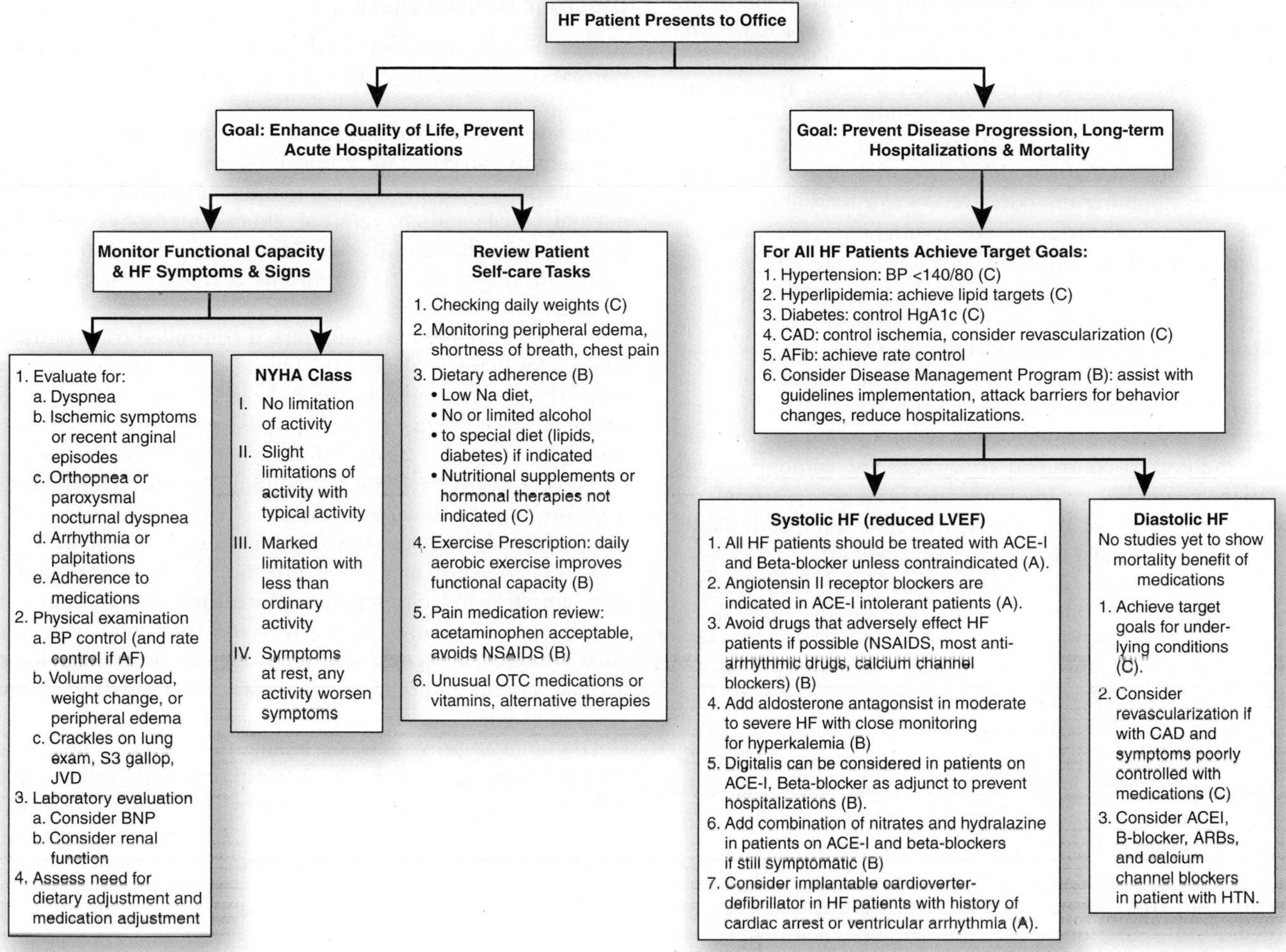

Figure 10.3 • Patient with heart failure symptoms. A = consistent, good-quality patient-oriented evidence; B = inconsistent or limited-quality patient-oriented evidence; C = consensus, disease-oriented evidence, usual practice, expert opinion, or case series. For information about the Strength of Recommendation Taxonomy evidence rating system, see *http://www.aafp.org/afpsort.xml.*

and volume status with its corresponding signs (peripheral edema, crackles on lung exam) may prompt discussion of diet and medication adherence, medication adjustments (diuretics). Changes in dyspnea may direct the conversation to exercise prescription or further evaluation of ischemic heart disease, or rate control if atrial fibrillation is present.

Management of HF requires a partnership between the physician and patient. At each encounter, inquire about specific self-care tasks such as monitoring daily weights, symptom monitoring (understanding symptoms), dietary and medication adherence, following exercise prescription, and avoiding medications that worsen symptoms. Many hospitalizations can be avoided if patients follow these simple self-care tasks and understand how to intervene when signs of early volume overload appear.

To prevent disease progression and its attendant consequences such as hospitalizations, decline in functional status, and premature death requires close attention to control the upstream contributing causes of HF and medication regimens with demonstrated benefit. Achieving optimal control of the conditions that have caused or contribute to HF applies to both systolic and diastolic HF (Figure 10.2). Thus, you should help the patient keep his or her blood pressure under 140/90, achieve lipid target goals, keep the hemoglobin A1c between 7.0 and 7.5%, manage ischemia to prevent ongoing cardiac damage, and keep the heart rate in patients with atrial fibrillation between 60 and 80 beats per minute (bpm). Case management is another care option that can help HF patients follow treatment guidelines, attack barriers to behavior changes, and reduce hospitalizations (27).

In addition to these interventions, it is also important to prescribe therapies that have been shown to reduce disease progression and confer mortality benefit. Although several drugs have been shown to improve mortality for patients with systolic HF, for diastolic HF, the data for a mortality benefit are lacking.

Systolic Heart Failure

ACE inhibitors (ACEIs) such as enalapril, captopril, and lisinopril are the cornerstone of treatment for chronic systolic HF (3, 28) (see Figure 10.2). Many large clinical trials have shown that ACEIs improve symptoms, reduce mortality, decrease hospitalizations, and improve quality of life in all NYHA classes of HF. All HF patients who do not have contraindications should receive an ACEI. Contraindications include pregnancy, bilateral renal artery stenosis, hypotension (systolic blood pressure <90), worsening renal, potassium retention (K+ >5.5), angioedema, and chronic cough. Treatment with ACEIs should be initiated at low doses and increased by doubling the dose every 3 to 7 days until recommended target doses are achieved. Serum blood urea nitrogen, creatinine, potassium, and blood pressure should be measured before initiating therapy, again at 2 weeks, and with any change in dose. Angiotensin receptor blockers (ARBs such as losartan, valsartan, and candesartan) are alternatives for those who are intolerant of ACEIs (29). ARBs have been shown to be equivalent to ACEIs in reducing mortality; but adding an ARB to an ACEI was associated with worse outcomes in one large randomized controlled trial (30). The combination of hydralazine and isosorbide dinitrate may be a particularly effective treatment for black patients, either as an addition or an alternative to ACEI to decrease afterload (31).

All patients with stable NYHA class II and III HF should receive a β-blocker unless there is a contraindication (3). β-blockers (i.e., carvedilol, bisoprolol, and extended-release metoprolol) are usually taken together with ACEIs. Studies have shown that they delay clinical progression of HF and reduce mortality. They also should be initiated at low levels and titrated to target heart rates of approximately 70 bpm (a decrease from a mean heart rate of 85 in one large trial) (32). Contraindications include hypotension, fluid retention, worsening HF, bradycardia, and heart block.

Diuretics are an important component of successful HF therapy, primarily to improve symptoms. They act rapidly to reduce fluid retention, and complement treatment with ACEIs and β-blockers (3, 28). Measuring daily body weight is helpful in assessing the response to diuretic therapy and for defining when increased dosing is needed. Diuretic resistance, often seen in severe failure, can be overcome by using a combination of two diuretics (i.e., furosemide and metizoline). Spironolactone or eplerenone, potassium-sparing diuretics that block aldosterone receptors, reduce the risk of morbidity and mortality in NYHA class III and IV HF patients. In conjunction with ACEIs and a loop diuretic, one of the potassium-sparing diuretics should be considered for use in all advanced HF patients (3, 33). The risks of treatment with diuretics include electrolyte depletion, activation of the renin-angiotensin-aldosterone system, hypotension, and azotemia. It is important to monitor closely for hyperkalemia if potassium-sparing diuretics are used; research trials measured potassium as often as once each month after the initiation phase (3).

Digitalis glycosides have long been used for HF and are also used to control the ventricular response rate in patients with atrial fibrillation (AF) (3, 28). Their benefit for selected patients includes the alleviation of symptoms and reduction in hospitalizations. Digitalis has no effect on mortality, and may even increase mortality in women (34). Treatment is initiated with a dose of 0.125 to 0.25 mg daily with an optimal serum digoxin range of 0.5 to 0.8 ng/mL (35). It is important to monitor serum levels of digoxin to detect toxicity, but serum levels do not correlate with therapeutic effects. Risks of digoxin include arrhythmias, gastrointestinal symptoms, and neurologic complaints.

Diastolic Heart Failure

Approximately one-third of HF patients have normal or near-normal systolic function. They have diastolic HF, in which the ventricles are stiff, cannot fill without high end-diastolic pressures, and have impaired capacity to change filling with varying activity levels. The clinical diagnosis is made when patients have typical symptoms of HF, only mildly reduced or normal LVEF, and changes on echocardiography suggesting poor diastolic filling of the left ventricle. Distinguishing diastolic and systolic HF is important because their treatment strategies are different.

There have been no randomized controlled trials of intervention for diastolic HF (3, 20). Thus, the management of diastolic HF must be guided by limited clinical trials, clinical experience, and knowledge of pathophysiology. Initially, treatment should be directed at treating underlying causes of diastolic HF such as CAD, hypertension, arrhythmias, severe anemia, thyrotoxicosis, hemochromatosis, and constrictive pericarditis. The next management goal is to reduce symptoms of fluid overload and elevated ventricular filling pressure (3, 20). Careful use of loop diuretics and nitrates can reduce fluid volume and pulmonary artery pressure. However, even small reductions in vascular volume may significantly reduce ventricular filling, lower cardiac output, and worsen symptoms. Nondihydropyridines calcium channel blockers, β-blockers, and ACEIs have properties that may improve diastolic failure. Calcium channel blockers have been shown to improve symptoms and exercise tolerance in clinical trials. β-blockers act by slowing heart rate and thereby enhancing ventricular filling. ACEIs, over time, may reverse LV hypertrophy (LVH) in diastolic failure.

LONG-TERM MONITORING

Figure 10.3 includes the approach to long-term monitoring of HF.

Atrial Fibrillation

AF is the most common chronic cardiac rhythm disturbance that causes significant morbidity and mortality in the general population (1, 4). The prevalence of AF increases with age, from 2% in the general population to 8% to 10% of individuals older than age 80 years (4). AF is characterized by chaotic atrial activity caused by simultaneous discharge of multiple atrial foci that produces an irregularly, irregular cardiac rhythm with varying ventricular rate. AF is the most common cardiac condition that predisposes individuals to thromboembolic stroke (relative risk = 7 for patients with AF) (1, 4).

Atrial fibrillation can be classified as paroxysmal (self-terminating), persistent (not self-terminating, lasting >7 days), or chronic (failed cardioversion, lasting >1 year). Figure 10.4 outlines a general approach to the evaluation and management of patients with atrial fibrillation. Key tasks for the physician include (4):

- Detecting underlying causes for AF and coexisting cardiovascular disease
- Treating patients who are acutely symptomatic
- Determining whether to attempt cardioversion to sinus rhythm

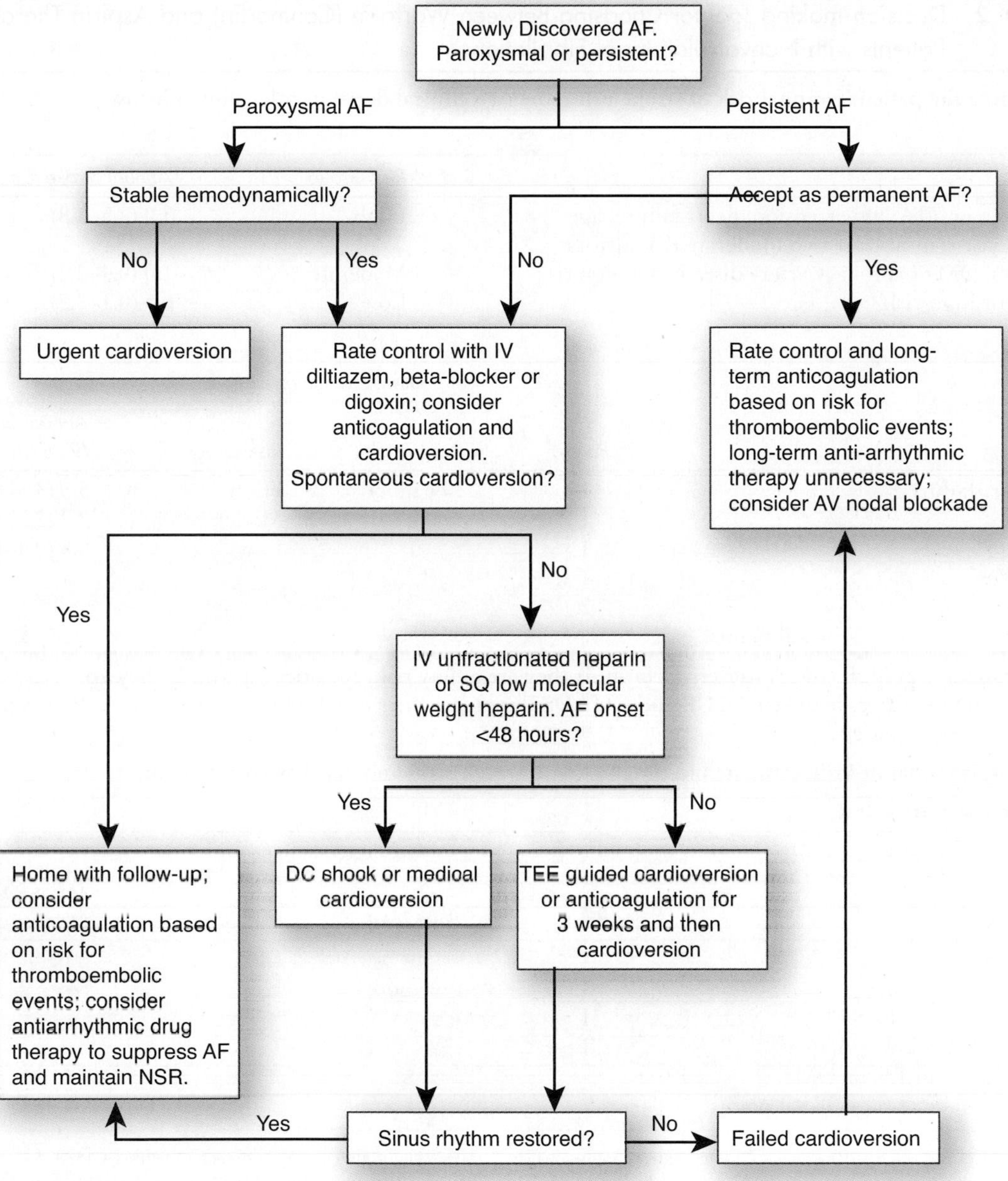

Figure 10.4 • Management of atrial fibrillation.

- Controlling ventricular rate for patients with chronic atrial fibrillation
- Determining a plan for anticoagulation to prevent thromboembolic events (e.g., stroke)

DIAGNOSIS

Differential Diagnosis

Patients with AF can present with no symptoms, or with palpitations, dyspnea, lightheadedness, chest pain, or even significant respiratory distress (36). The differential diagnosis of palpitations with or without dyspnea include anxiety disorder, electrolyte abnormalities, hyperthyroidism, ischemic heart disease, HF, chronic obstructive pulmonary disease, pulmonary embolus, stimulants (caffeine, cocaine), alcohol, medication toxicity, sepsis, pneumonia, mitral valve prolapse, and cardiac arrhythmias.

History and Physical Examination

A complete history and physical examination is directed toward identifying the possible causes, establishing the onset and duration of symptoms because the timing of new onset AF determines appropriate therapy, and determining if the patient is hemodynamically stable. Patients with asymptomatic AF may be detected when routine cardiac auscultation uncovers an irregular rhythm. Physical examination can also reveal an anxious patient with significant respiratory distress,

TABLE 10.2 Decision-making Tool for Choosing Between Warfarin (Coumadin) and Aspirin Therapy in Patients with Nonvalvular Atrial Fibrillation

Step 1. Determine the patient's annual risk of stroke using the two clinical decision rules shown below:

ACCP Rule

Definition	*Risk Group*	*Annual Stroke Rate, % (95% CI)*
History of stroke or TIA; hypertension; heart failure; age older than 75 years; or at least two moderate risk factors	High	3.0 (2.5–3.8)
Age 65–75 years, DM or coronary artery disease; not high risk	Moderate	1.0 (0.4–2.2)
Not moderate or high risk	Low	0.5 (0.1–2.2)

CHADS$_2$ Rule

		Risk Score Interpretation		
Risk Factor	*Points*	*Point Totals*	*Risk Group*	*Annual Stroke Rate, % (95% CI)*
Congestive heart failure	1	3 or more	High	5.3 (3.3–8.4)
Hypertension	1	1 or 2	Moderate	2.7 (2.2–3.4)
Age older than 75 years	1	0	Low	0.8 (0.4–1.7)
Diabetes mellitus	1			
Stroke or TIA	2			
Total points:				

Step 2. If the patient is at high risk, consider warfarin. If they are at low risk, consider aspirin. If they are at moderate risk or if the risk estimate differs between ACCP and CHADS2, evaluate their bleeding risk in step 3 and discuss pros and cons of treatment with patient.

Step 3. If patient is moderate risk, estimate bleeding risk and weigh risks and benefits with patient.

Outpatient Bleeding Risk Index

		Risk Score Information		
Risk Factor	*Points*	*Point Total*	*Risk Group*	*Major Bleeds per Total Number of Patients*
Age at least 65 years	1	0	Low	0 per 128
History of GI tract bleeding	1	1 or more	High	5 per 92
History of stroke	1			
Recent MI, hematocrit lower than 30%, creatinine higher than 1.5, or DM	1			
Total points:				

ACCP = American College of Chest Physicians; CI = confidence interval; TIA = transischemic attack; DM = diabetes mellitus; CHADS = congestive heart failure, hypertension, age greater than 75 years, diabetes and history of stroke or TIA; GI = gastrointestinal; MI = myocardial infarction; TIA = transient ischemic accident.

(Adapted from Ebell M. Choosing between warfarin (Coumadin) and aspirin therapy for patients with atrial fibrillation. Am Fam Phys 2005;71:2348–2351. Used with permission.)

hypotension, tachycardia with heart rates ranging from 80 to 150 bpm, tachypnea, and crackles on pulmonary exam.

Diagnostic Testing

Atrial fibrillation is confirmed by ECG (absence of P waves, irregular chaotic QRS complexes). Laboratory tests for the initial workup of AF include a complete blood count, thyroid-stimulating hormone, renal, hepatic function, and consideration of drug screen. If the patient has significant respiratory distress, a chest x-ray can be helpful with identifying pulmonary processes. An ECG should be ordered to detect underlying valvular or cardiac disease and to evaluate the size of the left atrium, which is an indicator of reversibility. If cardioversion is likely within the next 48 hours for rhythm control then a transesophageal echo (TEE) is indicated to identify a possible mural thrombus.

TREATMENT OF ATRIAL FIBRILLATION

Treatment of patients with AF considers the type, the presence of hemodynamic instability, contributing conditions, deciding on rate or rhythm control, and the plan for anticoagulation therapy (Figure 10.4). The decision for anticoagulation therapy includes balancing the risk for thromboembolic events without anticoagulation with the risks of bleeding with anticoagulation, and is part of the care of every patient with AF. The decision for long-term anticoagulation of patients with AF to prevent a future event is separate from deciding on rate or rhythm control to treat symptoms. Fortunately, treatment with antiplatelet agents or warfarin significantly reduces the risk of stroke (4). Table 10.2 outlines a practical decision rule to identify low-risk AF patients who can be treated with aspirin rather than warfarin, and identifies the intermediate and high-risk AF patients when warfarin is indicated (37).

New-onset AF

If the patient is hemodynamically unstable (ventricular rate >140 bpm and with acute MI, chest pain, dyspnea, or HF), the treatment is urgent synchronized cardioversion. If a hemodynamically stable patient has early onset AF (identified within <48 hours of onset), start heparin, perform TEE to rule out atrial thrombus, and cardioversion. If new AF is identified more than 48 hours after onset, TEE can be performed to rule out atrial thrombus and cardioversion can be done, but if thrombus is present, anticoagulation with warfarin is begun and cardioversion delayed for 3 weeks. The heart rate should be controlled with IV diltiazem or a β-blocker to maintain the ventricular rate between 60 and 80.

Paroxysmal AF

Paroxysmal AF is self limiting; two-thirds of patients convert, often within 24 hours, and if the patient is hemodynamically stable they require no further rhythm management. Appropriate treatment of correctable causes is the primary intervention, and the need for anticoagulation should be determined.

For patients successfully converted to sinus rhythm from atrial fibrillation, some will benefit from short-term use of medications. However, most should not be placed on long-term rhythm maintenance therapy because the risks appear to outweigh the benefits (36, 38). The choice of medication depends upon the presence of comorbid conditions (4). If a pattern of recurrent paroxysmal episodes occurs, for the patient with minimal heart disease the first line suppressive antiarrhythmic therapy is flecainide propafanone, or sotalol. If these drugs fail to prevent AF episodes, then amiodarone is second-line therapy. For patients with AF and heart failure, safety data support the use of amiodarone as first line therapy (39, 40). For patients with AF and coronary artery disease, sotalol is the drug of choice because of its antiarrhythmic and β-blocking properties (41, 42). For AF and hypertension, the initial drug choice is based on the presence or absence of LVH (4). If LVH is absent, flecainide and propafenone are first-line and amiodarone or sotalol second-line therapies. If LVH is present, then amiodarone is first line.

Persistent AF

When AF does not terminate spontaneously or with initial medications and persists, then the physician and patient are faced with the decision to accept progression to permanent AF or to attempt cardioversion to normal sinus rhythm. The decision to choose either rate or rhythm control depends on individual patient factors such as age, symptoms, and risk for thromboembolic events. Cardioversion does not confer better survival or improved quality of life when compared to rate control (42–44). Successful cardioversion does not reduce the need for long-term anticoagulation in those patients who are at increased risk of thromboembolic events (i.e., congestive heart failure, hypertension, age greater than 75 years, diabetes and history of stroke or transient ischemic accident 2 score >1, Table 10.2 [37]).

Permanent AF

Management of permanent AF focuses on rate control. Target heart rate is 60 to 80 bpm and is accomplished with drugs that block the AV node: β-blockers, nondihydropyridine calcium channel blockers, and digoxin. β-blockers are considered first line, but if bronchospastic disease is present, verapamil and diltiazem are effective alternatives. Digoxin is not as effective as these two classes for rate control, but is synergistic when added to them.

KEY POINTS

- Regularly screen patients with known coronary artery disease (CAD) for new or increasing chest pain episodes, and intervene aggressively if an unstable angina pattern is suspected.
- Consider prescribing an antiplatelet medication, β-blocker, lipid-lowering agent, and angiotensin-converting enzyme inhibitor (ACEI) for all patients with CAD to decrease mortality from progressive coronary heart disease.
- Complete an echocardiogram with Doppler flow for all patients with a clinical diagnosis of heart failure to define the type(s) and severity of left ventricular impairment.
- All patients with systolic heart failure who do not have contraindications should receive either an ACEI or angiotensin receptor blocker to improve symptoms, reduce mortality, decrease hospitalizations, and improve quality of life.
- For patient with atrial fibrillation, the family physician's key tasks are to detect underlying causes, treat acute symptoms, control ventricular rate, and understand the evidence, timing, and mechanisms for cardioversion and anticoagulation.

CHAPTER 11

Hypertension

Brian R. Forrest and Anthony J. Viera

CLINICAL OBJECTIVES

1. Define hypertension and discuss its epidemiology and clinical importance.
2. Describe the initial approach to evaluating and managing a patient with elevated blood pressure.
3. Name the major classes of medications used to reduce blood pressure and describe the approach to choosing antihypertensive therapies.

Hypertension—defined as a sustained systolic blood pressure (SBP) greater than 140 mm Hg, a sustained diastolic BP (DBP) greater than 90 mm Hg, or being on antihypertensive treatment—is a chronic condition that affects more than 72 million Americans (1, 2). Its prevalence greatly increases with age, affecting more than three-quarters of those age 75 years or older (1). The estimated lifetime risk of developing hypertension in the United States is 90% (3). Hypertension is one of the major contributors to death from cardiovascular disease, responsible for 35% of all myocardial infarctions (MIs) and strokes as well as half of all episodes of congestive heart failure (CHF) (4). Hypertension is also a major contributor to peripheral vascular disease, end-stage renal disease, aortic aneurysm, and retinopathy (5–8). Nearly 1 of 4 premature deaths is caused by hypertension, making it the single most important cause of premature death in developed countries (7, 9). It is the most common diagnosis in the United States, and annual costs attributable to hypertension are estimated to be nearly $77 billion (1).

Nationally, the death rate from stroke has dropped by 60% in the last 3 decades, and mortality from coronary heart disease has declined by 53%. Both changes are in part attributable to better detection and control of hypertension (10). Yet, despite what is known about the benefits of treatment, 35% of patients with hypertension are not being treated and 63% do not have their hypertension under control (2, 11). More than 30% of people with hypertension are not even aware of their problem (12). Although lack of access to medical care might explain some of this quality gap, much of the undiagnosed and uncontrolled hypertension occurs in patients who have health insurance and access to a physician (13).

The bulk of detection and treatment of hypertension is done by family physicians and other primary care clinicians. This chapter focuses on what you should know about adult hypertension, such as making the diagnosis, the initial evaluation, recommending lifestyle modification and drug therapy, and planning long-term management.

SCREENING

The first step in treating hypertension is finding it. Every family physician should have a strategy for detecting hypertension in his or her patient population. The US Preventive Services Task Force strongly recommends that clinicians screen adults 18 years and older for hypertension, but makes no recommendation regarding the interval at which screening should take place (7). Most screening for hypertension occurs opportunistically, in that patients presenting to a clinic for any reason will have their BP measured. This approach works well for those patients who come to the physician several times per year. Some groups, however, such as younger to middle-aged men and underserved populations do not regularly seek medical care and may require special contact via mailings, health fairs, or worksite screening. Within practices, quality improvement efforts for hypertension care might include electronic health records, patient registries, and reminder systems to identify people with elevated BP who remain undiagnosed or undertreated (14).

ACCURATE MEASUREMENT OF BLOOD PRESSURE

Although measurement of BP is one of the most commonly performed tasks in clinical medicine, it is also fraught with error. The gold standard for noninvasive measurement of BP is the auscultatory method using a mercury sphygmomanometer with an appropriately sized cuff. However, concerns over potential environmental hazards posed by mercury have led to phasing out of mercury instruments (15). Aneroid sphygmomanometers use a column of air rather than a column of mercury and can easily lose calibration (16). With either type of sphygmomanometry, several sources of error are introduced by the person obtaining the measurement. These include errors of technique, and terminal digit bias (the tendency to record 5 or 0 as the last digit). Further, different observers may use different Korotkoff sounds in their interpretation of BP. Increasingly, clinical settings are relying on automatic devices to obtain BP measurements. These devices obviously eliminate some of the observer factors (e.g., digit bias), but they cannot accurately assess BP in people with arrhythmias (e.g., atrial fibrillation) or severe atherosclerosis (because of poor compliance of arteries). Palpation of the radial pulse on the measured arm (to ensure that the cuff occludes the brachial artery) can help prevent measurement error from arrhythmia or less than full compression. Some devices have a digital display that demonstrates the measured pulse wave as well. Finally, automatic devices should be periodically calibrated against a gold standard (i.e., a mercury manometer).

Because BP may be elevated by acute stressors or recent activity, patients should be relaxed and seated for at least 5 minutes before the measurement is taken. A distended bladder or the recent use of tobacco or caffeine may give spuriously high readings. The patient should be seated, with the arm bare and supported. The cuff should be centered with the air bladder portion of the cuff encircling 80% of the arm. A wider cuff should be used on obese or thick arms. A small cuff or the presence of thick or restrictive clothing under the cuff will falsely elevate the readings by as much as 10 to 15 mm Hg. With the auscultatory method, the ipsilateral radial pulse should be palpated during inflation to be certain that systolic pressure has been exceeded. The pulse should disappear when the cuff is adequately pressurized; otherwise, the presence of an auscultatory gap will confuse the systolic reading. Listen with the bell of the stethoscope (or with light pressure in stethoscopes with a tunable diaphragm) to hear the low-frequency Korotkoff sounds. The first repetitive sound corresponds to the systolic pressure. Diastolic pressure should be noted at the disappearance of the sounds, not muffling, because disappearance is a more reliable criterion for diagnosis, and most studies of treatment have used it. Finally, on the initial measurement, BP should be checked in both arms (16, 17). Significant variations between pressures in each arm should prompt further evaluation for underlying causes such as coarctation or stenosis.

Some patients have BP that is elevated when measured in the office setting but not when measured out of the office setting using either self-BP monitoring or 24-hour ambulatory BP monitoring. Sometimes, this "white-coat hypertension" will be suspected because the patient will tell you that his or her BP is always "normal" when checked elsewhere. The incidence of white-coat hypertension is less than 25% of measured hypertension, and therefore should be confirmed with structured home measurements or ambulatory BP monitoring (18). Automatic BP devices stationed in grocery stores and pharmacies are likely to be inaccurate and should not be relied on (19). Home (or self) BP monitoring may be extremely useful as an adjunct to diagnosis or management (20). A website listing automatic devices that have been validated is maintained at *www.dableducational.com* (21). In patients who have an elevated BP in the office setting, but in whom you suspect white-coat hypertension based on no evidence of target organ damage, a 24-hour ambulatory BP monitor measurement may be useful (8, 22). Keep in mind, however, that white-coat hypertension, while conferring less risk than sustained hypertension, may not be entirely benign (23–25). Also, masked hypertension, defined as BP that is not elevated in the office but elevated elsewhere, carries nearly the risk of sustained hypertension (25). How best to detect masked hypertension is a subject of ongoing research. The different cutoffs for what is considered an elevated BP are shown in Table 11.1. Note that "normal" out-of-office BP is about 5 mm Hg lower than "normal" office BP (20).

CLINICAL ASSESSMENT

Making the Diagnosis

After you have identified a patient with an elevated BP, remember that the final diagnosis of hypertension is a clinical one—a function of the actual BP, risk factors, and the effect of the diagnosis on the patient. A single, greatly elevated BP reading in the office setting (SBP >200 mm Hg and/or DBP >120) is adequate to make the diagnosis of hypertension in the absence of a recognized cause of secondary elevation, and treatment should be immediately initiated. For most patients with somewhat elevated blood pressure (SBP 140 to 200 mm Hg or DBP 90 to 120 mm Hg), an average of three readings over at least 6 weeks should be used. If the average SBP is higher than 140 mm Hg or the average DBP is higher than 90 mm Hg, the diagnosis is confirmed. If uncertainty remains, base your assessment on additional readings.

The term "isolated systolic hypertension" refers to a SBP >140 mm Hg when the DBP is <90 mm Hg. Isolated systolic hypertension is common in the elderly partially because of decreased vascular compliance. Historically, DBP was used to

TABLE 11.1 Cutoffs for Diagnosis of Hypertension based on Type of BP Measurements

Setting	Systolic BP	Diastolic BP	Comment
Office measurements	140 mm Hg	90 mm Hg	Two readings, 5 minutes apart, sitting in chair. Confirm reading in other arm.
Home or self-BP measurements	135 mm Hg	85 mm Hg	Average of measurements taken on 4 consecutive days, three measurements taken in the morning and three measurements taken in the evening (20).
Awake average of 24-hour ambulatory BP measurements	135 mm Hg	85 mm Hg	There is normally a 10% to 20% decrease of BP during sleep. Patients that do not have this decrease ("nondippers") may be at increased cardiovascular disease risk (22).
Entire average of 24-hour ambulatory BP measurements	130 mm Hg	80 mm Hg	

classify the severity of hypertension. However, longitudinal studies have demonstrated that SBP is a better predictor of future morbidity and mortality, especially for middle-aged and older individuals (8, 26). Patients are thus classified based on whichever level of BP (systolic or diastolic) is in the higher range (8). Those in whom the SBP is between 140 and 159 or the DBP is between 90 and 99 mm Hg are said to have stage 1 hypertension, whereas those in whom SBP is greater than 159 mm Hg or DBP is greater than 99 mm Hg are said to have stage 2 hypertension (8).

Initial Evaluation

Table 11.2 lists the key elements of history, physical examination, and laboratory tests that should be considered in all patients with a new diagnosis of hypertension. The initial evaluation should screen for end-organ damage and other cardiovascular risk factors, address the possibility of secondary causes of hypertension, and begin educating the patient and family. The rationale for including each component is based primarily on an understanding of the natural history of cardiovascular disease, not necessarily on outcome-proven evidence.

HISTORY

As a first step, make note of symptoms suggesting end-organ disease, such as chest pain, orthopnea, paroxysmal nocturnal dyspnea, lower extremity edema, or claudication. Then address the possibility of secondary or treatable causes of hypertension. The most common secondary causes in primary care settings are significant alcohol use, chronic renal disease, and drugs (including over-the-counter agents such as decongestants and illicit drugs); also consider renovascular hypertension, hyperaldosteronism, pheochromocytoma, and obstructive sleep apnea (OSA). More than 50% of patients with OSA have hypertension, and treatment of OSA reduces BP in these patients (27). A useful mnemonic to help think about the secondary causes of hypertension is shown in Table 11.3 (27). Ask about specific symptoms that suggest secondary causes, such as sweating, palpitations, or flushing.

Keep in mind that in primary care settings at least 90% to 95% of newly diagnosed hypertensive patients will not have a secondary cause. More extensive workup is indicated only for patients younger than age 25, and for those in whom a secondary disease is suspected on clinical grounds, such as severity of hypertension, malignant course, a lack of response to therapy, or physical findings of secondary disease, such as a renal bruit or a Cushingoid appearance.

ASSESS GLOBAL CARDIOVASCULAR RISK

It is important to identify other cardiac risk factors that interact with hypertension to increase risk such as smoking, diabetes, dyslipidemia, or a family history of early cardiac disease. Cardiovascular disease risk calculators can provide an estimate of a person's risk over a specified time frame (e.g., next 10 years) (28, 29). For example, using the free web-based or personal digital assistant calculator available from *http://www.med-decisions.com/cvtool/*, a 56 year old male nonsmoker, nondiabetic with a SBP of 175 mm Hg, a total cholesterol of 243 mg/dL with high-density lipoprotein of 30 mg/dL, and no evidence of left ventricular hypertrophy on electrocardiogram has a 10 year risk of having a cardiovascular event of approximately 29%. Such information may be useful in helping patients understand the importance of controlling blood pressure and other risk factors.

PHYSICAL EXAMINATION

Start by making note of the patient's body mass index (BMI). To assess end-organ damage, cardiovascular examination should note cardiac size and rhythm, the presence of a third heart sound (S3), peripheral edema or other signs of cardiac failure; decreased pulses; or carotid bruits. Focal weakness, abnormal gait, or other abnormalities on neurologic testing may suggest a prior cerebrovascular accident. Ophthalmoscopic examination may disclose hypertensive retinopathy. Physical features that suggest a secondary cause of hypertension include Cushingoid features such as moon facies and central adiposity, a diastolic abdominal bruit suggestive of renovascular hypertension, or the diminished femoral pulses with hypertension in the arms that suggest coarctation of the aorta.

INITIAL LABORATORY OR OTHER DIAGNOSTIC TESTS

Laboratory tests should include urinalysis to identify proteinuria and hematuria, as well as serum blood urea nitrogen (BUN) and creatinine to assess renal function. In those in whom the urinalysis shows no protein, consider a urinary microalbumin to screen for early nephropathy. Obtain an electrocardiogram to check for left ventricular hypertrophy (Table 11.4), arrhythmia, and baseline ST segment changes or signs of previous MI. An echocardiogram is indicated if left ventricular hypertrophy is suspected based on the electrocardiogram or physical examination. Obtain a fasting blood glucose level and a full cholesterol panel (including low-density lipoprotein, high-density lipoprotein, and triglycerides) to detect diabetes mellitus and hyperlipidemia. A complete blood count revealing mild anemia may be a sign of chronic renal insufficiency. Hyperaldosteronism is suggested by a low serum potassium level.

PATIENT EDUCATION

Patients may find it difficult to understand hypertension (30). There are no symptoms, and for most patients, the major issue is a risk of stroke or heart attack 15 to 20 years later, far removed from their current experience. They may also have fears and negative images about BP medications (30). By taking time for a thorough history and physical examination, you underscore the importance of hypertension and begin to teach the patient how lifestyle influences the problem. Over the long term, your effectiveness in managing the hypertensive patient depends on your ability to educate your patient. Ultimately, it is the patient who decides what recommendations to follow, including whether or not to take a medication for the rest of his or her life.

TREATMENT

General Approach

After the initial evaluation, take time to develop an individualized treatment plan that contains elements of lifestyle modifications and, if appropriate, pharmacotherapy. Figure 11.1 provides an algorithm describing initial management. In patients who have stage 1 hypertension and no signs of target organ damage, a 3-month period of lifestyle modifications

TABLE 11.2 Recommendations for Initial Evaluation of Hypertension (Based on Expert Opinion)

History	
Look for features suggesting secondary disease	
Age <25	
Malignant course	
Lack of response to therapy	
Ask about symptoms of end-organ disease	
Chest pain	
Orthopnea	
Paroxysmal nocturnal dyspnea	
Lower extremity edema	
Claudication	
Left ventricular hypertrophy	
Identify other cardiovascular risk factors	
Diabetes	
Smoking	
Family history of early coronary artery disease	
History of elevated cholesterol level	
Physical examination	**Evaluating For**
Pulse	Arrhythmia
Body mass index	Obesity
Cardiac: size, rhythm, S3, JVD, edema	Left ventricular hypertrophy, heart failure
Vascular: carotids, peripheral pulses	Carotid artery disease, peripheral artery disease
Back: renal bruits	Renovascular hypertension
Fundus	Hypertensive retinopathy
Neurologic	Prior cerebrovascular event
Laboratory tests	
Urinalysis	Hypertensive nephropathy
Urine microalbumin	Microalbuminuria (early hypertensive nephropathy)
BUN/creatinine	Renal dysfunction
Potassium and sodium	Aldosteronism
Glucose	Diabetes
Fasting lipid panel (HDL, LDL, triglycerides)	Hyperlipidemia
Electrocardiogram	Left ventricular hypertrophy, prior myocardial infarction

BUN = blood urea nitrogen; HDL = high-density lipoprotein; JVD = jugular venous distention.

without pharmacotherapy may be sufficient to bring a patient's BP to goal. Left unaddressed, however, approximately 20% of patients with stage 1 hypertension will progress to stage 2 over a 4 year period (31). In patients at high risk of cardiovascular events, delaying treatment may result in poorer long-term outcomes (32).

In patients between 40 and 69 years of age, observational studies have found that for every 20/10 mm Hg increase in blood pressure, the risk of stroke and cardiovascular events is doubled (33). Treating hypertension dramatically lowers the incidence of end-organ complications such as stroke and heart disease (34). Patients with greater BP elevations and those with

TABLE 11.3 "ABCDE" Mnemonic for Secondary Causes of Hypertension

Mnemonic	Think About	Comment
A	Accuracy Alcohol Apnea Aldosteronism	Are the blood pressure readings accurate? Could chronic alcohol use be playing a role? Does the patient have obstructive sleep apnea? Does the patient have hypokalemia or other suggestions of primary hyperaldosteronism?
B	Bruits Bad kidneys	Is there an abdominal bruit suggestive of renovascular hypertension? Does the patient have renal parenchymal disease (which can be cause or a consequence of hypertension)?
C	Catecholamines Coarctation Cushing	Is the patient having palpitations, tachycardia, diaphoresis, headaches, and/or paroxysmal hypertension suggestive of pheochromocytoma? Are there decreased or delayed femoral pulses, or rib notching on chest x-ray suggestive of coarctation of the aorta? Any weight gain, hirsutism, amenorrhea, striae, or moon facies suggestive of Cushing syndrome?
D	Drugs Diet	Any use of sympathomimetics, corticosteroids, NSAIDs, oral contraceptive pills, MAOIs, or other drugs that can elevate BP? Are excess dietary sodium or obesity contributing?
E	Endocrine Erythropoietin	Is there untreated thyroid disease or hyperparathyroidism? Is there another disorder (COPD) leading to increased erythropoietin levels?

NSAID = nonsteroidal anti-inflammatory drug; MAOI = monoamine oxidase inhibitor; COPD = chronic obstructive pulmonary disease.
Adapted from Onusko E. Diagnosing secondary hypertension. Am Fam Phys 2003;67(1):67–74.

higher overall cardiovascular disease risk derive the greatest benefit from treatment (35–38). Using data from the Hypertension Detection and Follow up Program, only three patients with DBP between 115 and 129 mm Hg would have to be treated for 5 years to prevent one death, stroke, or MI (number needed to treat $[NNT]_{5y} = 3$) (39). In a stage 1 hypertensive patient with additional cardiac risk factors, a reduction of 12 mm Hg in SBP over 10 years will prevent one death for every 11 patients treated ($NNT_{10y} = 11$). For those with preexisting cardiovascular disease or target organ damage treating only nine patients for 10 years will prevent one death (40).

The extent to which BP should be lowered has been the subject of several studies. In the Hypertension Optimal Treatment trial, 18,790 participants 50 to 80 years of age were randomly assigned to a DBP goal of ≤90 mm Hg ≤85 mm Hg, or ≤80 mm Hg (41). Rates of overall cardiovascular events were similar among the groups. In a subgroup analysis of the 1,501 participants with diabetes, those randomized to a goal DBP of ≤80 mm Hg had 12.5 fewer major cardiovascular events per 1,000 patient-years ($p < 0.01$) compared with the participants randomized to a goal DBP ≤90 mm Hg (41). In a United Kingdom Prospective Diabetes Study Group (UKPDS) trial, 1,148 patients with type 2 diabetes were randomized to tight control (goal BP <150/85 mm Hg) or less tight control (goal BP <180/105 mm Hg) (42). Achieved mean BP levels were 144/82 mm Hg in the tight control group and 154/87 mm Hg in the less tight control group. At follow-up after a mean of 8.4 years, the tight control group had approximately 7 fewer diabetes-related deaths ($p = 0.02$) and 5 fewer strokes ($p = 0.01$) per 1,000 patient-years (42). In a trial to investigate the effects of different levels of BP control among nondiabetics, the Cardio-Sis investigators randomized 1,111 patients (open-label) to goal SBP of <140 mm Hg (usual control) or goal SBP of <130 mm Hg (tight control) (43). Approximately 6% fewer patients in the tight control group had left ventricular hypertrophy at 2 years for an NNT of 18 over 2 years.

TABLE 11.4 Simplified Criteria for Left Ventricular Hypertrophy (LVH) on Electrocardiogram

The presence of ALL three of the following criteria suggests LVH:

- Deepest S wave in lead V_1 or V_2 plus tallest R wave in lead V_5 or $V_6 \geq 35$ mm, OR R wave in lead a VL ≥ 12 mm
- Age ≥ 35 years
- Left ventricular "strain" pattern (asymmetric ST segment depression and T wave inversion, usually seen in leads I, aVL, V_4–V_6)

Adapted from Goldberger AL. Clinical electrocardiography: a simplified approach, 6th ed., Mosby, St. Louis, 1999; Grauer K. 12-lead ECGs: a "pocket brain" for easy interpretation, 2nd ed., KG/EKG Press, Gainesville, FL, 2001.

The 7th report of the Joint National Committee on Prevention, Detection, Evaluation, and Treatment of High Blood Pressure (JNC 7) guidelines recommend that the target BP should be less than 140/90 mm Hg for most patients and less than 130/80 mm Hg for patients with diabetes mellitus or renal disease (8). Although lowering BP to these goals is beneficial, keep in mind that excessive lowering can be harmful. Lowering DBP to a level below 70 mm Hg diastolic has been associated with increased mortality, stroke, and MI in patients with coronary artery disease, which may be a particular concern for older patients (44). Also, although adverse effects of

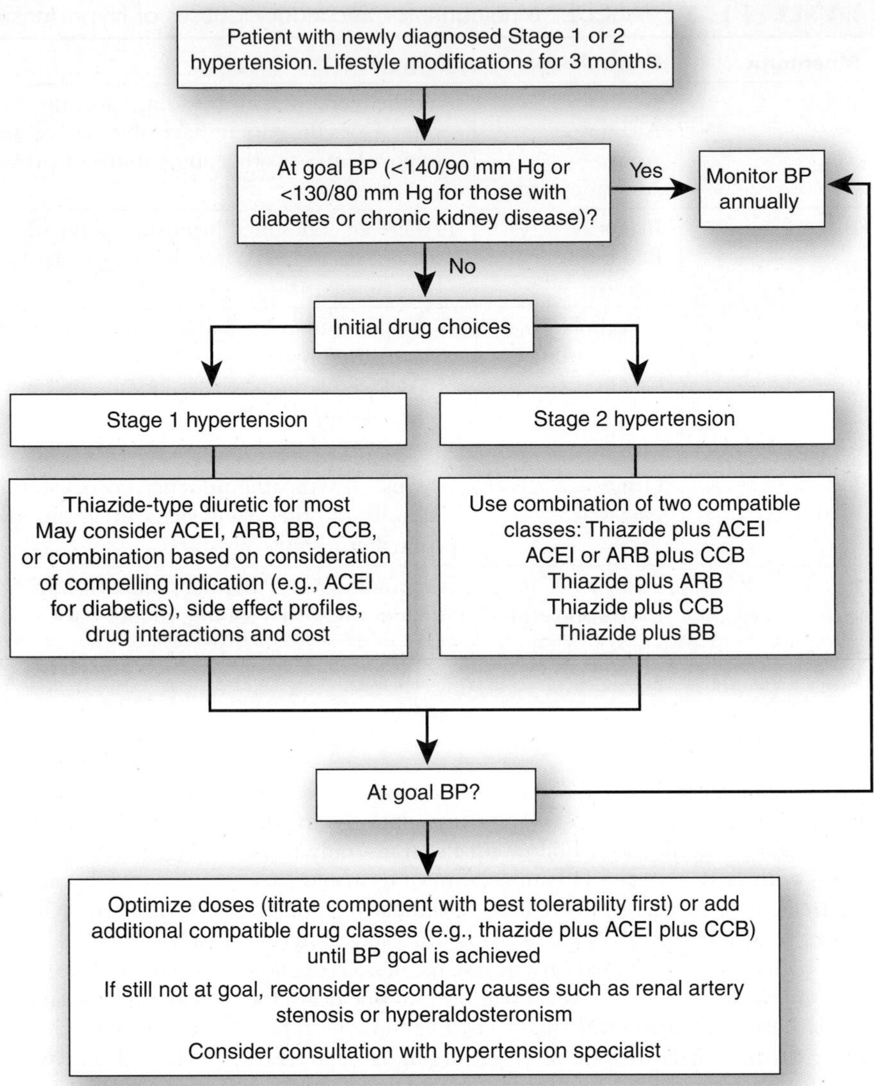

Figure 11.1 • Suggested management of Stage 1 or 2 hypertension. BP = blood pressure; ACEI = angiotensin-converting enzyme inhibitor; ARB = angiotensin receptor blocker; BB = β-blocker; CCB = calcium channel blocker.

some medications may be greater in the elderly, antihypertensive medications should not be withheld from a patient based solely on older age (45, 46).

Lifestyle Modifications

Consider lifestyle modifications for every patient. Table 11.5 lists individual strategies, with an approximation of their BP-lowering efficacy. A multicenter, randomized trial demonstrated that patients with hypertension can sustain multiple lifestyle changes over 18 months, and such changes improve control of their blood pressure (47). Multiple lifestyle modifications (e.g., weight loss, exercise, and Dietary Approaches to Stop Hypertension [DASH] diet) are more effective than a single modification (e.g., diet alone). In fact, a low-sodium (1,600 mg) DASH diet can be as effective as single drug therapy (48, 49). The challenge with any of the lifestyle modification recommendations is to actually get the patient to adopt them.

Lifestyle modifications offer additional health benefits, fewer adverse effects, and are generally inexpensive. In most cases, the proper use of lifestyle modifications, such as an exercise prescription or a weight loss program, requires a great deal of commitment by both physician and patient. Furthermore, some therapies, such as biofeedback, may be very expensive and offer relatively little in terms of efficacy (50).

EXERCISE

Several different trials have found that an exercise regimen lowers BP in patients with both normal and high initial BPs and may decrease the number and dosage of medications needed to control BP (51, 52). The effect of exercise on lowering BP is even more pronounced in those with hypertension (51). Exercise is an appropriate first step for most hypertensive patients. An example of an initial, minimal exercise regimen would be walking briskly for 30 minutes three to five times per week.

WEIGHT LOSS

For overweight (BMI $\geq$25 kg/m^2) and obese (BMI $\geq$30 kg/m^2) patients—who currently constitute over 65% of the US adult population (53)—weight reduction should be an essential part of the management plan. There is a strong correlation between obesity and hypertension, especially in people with centrally distributed body fat. Clinical trials of weight loss, often

TABLE 11.5 Lifestyle Modifications: Least to Most Effective

Recommendation	Average SBP Reduction (mm Hg)
Two or fewer alcoholic drinks* per day for men; 1 or fewer drinks per day-women	2–4 mm Hg
<2.4 g sodium/day	2–8 mm Hg
30 minutes aerobic activity/day	4–9 mm Hg
DASH diet	8–14 mm Hg
Losing weight	5–20 mm Hg/10 lb lost

*A drink is defined as one 12 oz beer, 5 oz of wine, or 1.5 oz of liquor.

combined with exercise, have resulted in lowered BP and increased the impact of pharmacotherapy (54, 55). If a weight loss program is prescribed, a simple instruction such as "you should try to lose some weight" is insufficient. The physician should specify a target weight, coordinate a dietary intervention (such as a calorie-restricted diet), give an exercise prescription, and use frequent follow-up office visits (such as every 4 to 6 weeks) or local community groups, such as Weight Watchers, to help the patient lose weight. Patients do not need to attain ideal body weight to benefit. Weight loss of as little as 10 lb may result in substantial reductions in BP, perhaps eliminating the need for medication (or a second medication). Further, weight loss has numerous additional health benefits.

DIET

The DASH diet is an eating plan rich in potassium, magnesium, and calcium obtained from fruits, vegetables, and low-fat dairy products (56, 57). An example of a DASH eating plan based on a 2,000-calorie diet is shown in Table 11.6. Randomized trials have demonstrated a significant decrease in both SBP and DBP for as long as 18 months in patients adhering to the DASH diet (47). Even though patients may not completely adhere to a DASH eating plan, partial dietary changes may give a graduated response.

Population studies show a consistent correlation between salt intake and hypertension. Recent clinical trials have demonstrated that reducing sodium intake can lower BP (58, 59). However, sodium restriction is probably best thought of as a population approach rather than a clinical approach. Whereas not all patients are "salt-sensitive," it is recommended that all patients with hypertension reduce their sodium intake to less than 2.4 g/day (8). On a population level, such a reduction can lower BP and could reduce strokes, MIs, and CHF (59). Today's salt substitutes offer improved palatability and can help your patients reduce their sodium intake. Caution should be exercised in patients on medications that can elevate potassium levels as most of the salt substitutes are high in potassium.

ALCOHOL REDUCTION

Alcohol acts as a vasopressor, and meta analysis of randomized controlled trials has shown that reduction of heavy alcohol use can lower BP (60). Intake of alcohol should be limited to no more than 1 oz of ethanol per day for men and 0.5 oz per day for women (8). This amounts to no more than 24 oz beer, 10 oz wine, or 3 oz of 80-proof whiskey per day for men (two drinks) and half that amount (one drink) for women. Keep in mind that patients who have recently started abstaining from alcohol may have transiently elevated BP associated with alcohol withdrawal.

ANTIHYPERTENSIVE MEDICATIONS

There are more than 125 agents in the United States approved to treat hypertension, each belonging to one of several drug classes (Table 11.7). Reducing BP with any BP-lowering medication will improve cardiovascular and stroke outcomes in both the young and the elderly (61). The ideal medication is one that improves patient oriented outcomes, is well-tolerated, and is affordable. Keep in mind that generic formulations are as effective as brand name pharmaceuticals (62). A single antihypertensive medication typically reduces SBP by approximately 9 to 10 mm Hg. To reach goal BP, many patients will require a combination of BP-lowering medicines from different classes. Particular evidence for using a medicine for a compelling indication is an important factor to consider when prescribing antihypertensives (Table 11.9). For example, in patients who have had a myocardial infarction, β-blockers, and angiotensin-converting enzyme (ACE) inhibitors have been shown to reduce morbidity and mortality independently of their BP-lowering effects (8, 63).

In the absence of a compelling indication, the preferred initial medication is usually a low-dose thiazide or thiazide-like diuretic (64). An ACE inhibitor is also a good first choice. The regimen should be kept as simple as possible; patients are more likely to adhere to once-daily medications (65). You should also consider the side effect profile of the various antihypertensive agents. Most side effects tend to be dose related. Using antihypertensive medications in combination (e.g., thiazide diuretic with an ACE inhibitor) often allows lower doses of agents to be prescribed, thereby reducing the potential for adverse reactions or bothersome side effects (66). Another component of tolerability is the potential for drug interactions. If no other compelling reason exists to choose one medication over another, the one with the fewest potential drug interactions is optimal.

Affordability is another important consideration for many patients. Uninsured or underinsured patients may not take their medication regularly if they cannot afford it. Some insured patients will not be able to afford the copays on multiple medications. Fortunately, there are generic formulations available for nearly every class of antihypertensive medications. Even certain combination pills are available in a generic form. It is thus important to consider costs to the patient when considering antihypertensive medications, but cost does not need to be a barrier to attaining good BP control.

Diabetic Patients with Hypertension

Patients who have diabetes warrant special consideration when it comes to hypertension. At least four trials provide evidence for the benefit of aggressive BP control in patients who have diabetes (41, 42, 67, 68). For diabetic patients, a goal BP less than 130/80 mm Hg is desirable. Setting a target of 155/85, the UKPDS showed a reduction of diabetic complications ($NNT_{8y} = 6$) and deaths from diabetes ($NNT_{8y} = 15$) (42). In fact, in the UKPDS study, "tight" glucose control did not

TABLE 11.6 Sample Dietary Approaches to Stop Hypertension (DASH) Diet

Food Group	Daily Servings	Serving Sizes	Examples and Notes	Significance
Grains and grain products	7–8	1 slice bread, ½ cup dry cereal, ½ cup cooked rice, pasta, or cereal	Whole wheat bread, English muffin, pita bread, bagel, cereals, grits, oatmeal	Major sources of energy and fiber
Vegetables	4–5	1 cup raw, leafy vegetable, ½ cup cooked vegetable, 6 oz vegetable juice	Tomatoes, potatoes, carrots, peas, squash, broccoli, turnip greens, collards, kale, spinach, artichokes, sweet potatoes, beans	Rich sources of potassium, magnesium, and fiber
Fruits	4–5	6 oz fruit juice, 1 medium fruit, ¼ cup dried fruit, ½ cup fresh, frozen, or canned fruit	Apricots, bananas, dates, oranges, orange juice, grapefruit, mangoes, melons, peaches, pineapples, prunes, raisins, strawberries, tangerines	Important sources of potassium, magnesium, and fiber
Low fat or nonfat dairy foods	2–3	8 oz milk, 1 cup yogurt, 1.5 oz cheese	Skim or 1% milk, skim or low-fat buttermilk, nonfat or low-fat yogurt, part skim mozzarella cheese, nonfat cheese	Major sources of calcium and protein
Meats, poultry, and fish	2 or less	3 oz cooked meats, poultry, or fish	Select only lean; trim away fat; broil, roast, or boil, instead of frying; remove skin from poultry	Rich sources of protein and magnesium
Nuts, seeds, and legumes	4–5/week	1 ½ oz or 1/3 cup nuts, ½ oz or 2 Tbs seeds, ½ cup cooked legumes	Almonds, filberts, mixed nuts, peanuts, walnuts, sunflower seeds, kidney beans, lentils	Rich sources of energy, magnesium, potassium, protein, and fiber

Table is based on a 2,000-calorie diet; oz = ounces; Tbs = tablespoon.
From National Heart, Lung, and Blood Institute, "Your Guide to Lowering Your Blood Pressure with DASH," *http://www.nhlbi.nih.gov/health/public/heart/hbp/dash/*, accessed December 1, 2009.

reduce mortality, whereas "tight" BP control with a β-blocker or ACE inhibitor reduced both diabetes-related complications and mortality (42). Based largely on such evidence, hypertensive patients are the only group for which the USPSTF currently gives a grade A recommendation for screening for diabetes (69). Many patients who have type 2 diabetes are also overweight, and obesity and diabetes both make BP more difficult to control. Because of their renal protective effects and their favorable metabolic profile, renin-angiotensin system agents (ACE inhibitors or angiotensin receptor blockers) are the preferred initial agent for BP control in patients with diabetes. Starting a two-drug combination (e.g., ACE inhibitor plus low-dose thiazide diuretic) should be a strong consideration in any diabetic patient whose SBP is 150 mm Hg or greater because it will usually take two medications to reduce SBP by 20 mm Hg (41).

LONG-TERM MANAGEMENT

Initially, the patient should be seen every 1 to 2 weeks until the BP is stabilized. Then, gradually decrease the frequency of visits to every 3 to 6 months with follow-up evaluations of electrolytes, BUN, and creatinine. A trial considering whether a 3- or 6-month interval was preferred found similar rates of BP control and patient satisfaction with either follow-up interval (70). Patients should be told to bring their medications with them to each visit. Ideally, patients should have their BPs checked occasionally between visits, either at work or at home. Reliable home BP monitoring devices are readily available, but even when a patient obtains a monitor that has been independently validated and recommended for use, you should make sure the cuff size is appropriate and check that the device is measuring BP accurately (e.g., against your calibrated office sphygmomanometer) for that particular patient. Finger monitors and wrist monitors should be avoided (21). Home monitoring has been shown to increase BP control and the proportion of people who get to goal BP, perhaps by improving medication adherence and self-efficacy in hypertension management (71). Patients who perform BP monitoring on their own should be told to bring a record of their BP readings to each visit.

In addition to a review of all medications and possible adverse effects, each visit should include an assessment for cardiac symptoms, BP, heart rate, rhythm, new murmurs, S3, jugular venous distention, edema, and rales. A more detailed examination should be performed annually to detect evidence of end-organ damage, such as left ventricular hypertrophy, stroke, or vascular disease. Urinalysis, BUN, and creatinine

TABLE 11.7 Characteristics of Antihypertensive Medication Classes

Drug Class	Drug Subclass	Examples	Most Common or Concerning Side Effect(s)	Comment
Thiazide diuretics*	Thiazide and thiazide-like	Chlorthalidone, hydrochlorothiazide	Hypokalemia, hyperuricemia, hyponatremia, erectile dysfunction	Chlorthalidone is longer-acting and more potent than hydrochlorothiazide
ACE inhibitors*		Benazepril, enalapril, lisinopril, ramipril	Hyperkalemia, cough, angioedema, rise in creatinine	A rise in creatinine of <30% from baseline is acceptable and not a reason to stop these medications
Calcium channel blockers*	Dihydropyridines	Amlodipine, felodipine, nifedipine	Peripheral edema	
	Nondihydropyridines	Diltiazem, verapamil	Dizziness	
Angiotensin receptor blockers		Candesartan, irbesartan, losartan	Hyperkalemia, angioedema (less than with ACE inhibitors)	Useful when cough limits the use of an ACE inhibitor; no generics available
β-blockers	Noncardioselective	Nadolol, pindolol, propranolol	Bradycardia bronchoconstriction (mostly a concern with noncardioselective), erectile dysfunction, hypertriglyceridemia, hyperglycemia	Limited data regarding cardiovascular or all-cause mortality benefit
	Combined α-β blockers	Labetalol, carvedilol		
	Cardioselective	Atenolol, bisoprolol, metoprolol		Indicated in the patient who is post-MI
	Vasodilating	Carvedilol, nebivolol		
Loop diuretics	Loop	Bumetanide, furosemide, torsemide	Hypokalemia, ototoxicity	Use instead of thiazide when glomerular filtration rate is severely reduced
Aldosterone antagonists		Spironolactone, eplerenone	Hyperkalemia, gynecomastia (spironolactone), erectile dysfunction	These are also known as "potassium-sparing diuretics"
Alpha1-blockers		Doxazosin, prazosin, terazosin	Dizziness, orthostasis	Should not be used as monotherapy for hypertension
Centrally acting agents		Clonidine, guanfacine, methyldopa	Constipation, dry mouth, rebound hypertension, erectile dysfunction	Clonidine available in a transdermal preparation
Direct vasodilators		Hydralazine, minoxidil	Orthostasis, lupus-like syndrome (hydralazine), hair growth (minoxidil)	Minoxidil causes fluid retention and is reserved for severe resistant hypertension; hydralazine can be used with nitrates for heart failure when renin-angiotensin system blockers are unable to be used
Postganglionic neuronal inhibitors		Reserpine	Bradycardia, depression	Rarely used today
Direct renin inhibitors		Aliskiren		

ACE = angiotensin-converting enzyme; ARB = angiotensin receptor blocker; MI = myocardial infarction.
*Best initial choices for patients without special indications (Table 11.9).

TABLE 11.8 Key Recommendations

Recommendation	Strength of Recommendation (SOR)*
Adults age 18 years and older should be screened for hypertension (7).	A
In patients with newly diagnosed hypertension, perform a urinalysis, BUN/creatinine, potassium, sodium, glucose, fasting lipid panel, and an electrocardiogram (8).	C
Recommend lifestyle modifications for all patients with hypertension (8).	B
For patients with uncomplicated hypertension in whom pharmacotherapy is needed, prescribe a low-dose thiazide diuretic as first-line (8).	A
For hypertensive patients who have a compelling indication, prescribe antihypertensive medication(s) based on the compelling indication(s) (8).	B
Because ACE inhibitors and ARBs are associated with favorable effects on renal function and can improve insulin sensitivity, they are good first choices in treating diabetic hypertensive patients (8).	C

ACE = angiotensin-converting enzyme; ARB = angiotensin receptor blocker; BUN = blood urea nitrogen.
*A = consistent, good-quality patient-oriented evidence; B = inconsistent or limited-quality patient-oriented evidence; C = consensus, disease-oriented evidence, usual practice, expert opinion, or case series. For information about the Strength of Recommendation Taxonomy evidence rating system, see *http://www.aafp.org/afpsort.xml*.

levels should be checked at regular intervals, along with serum potassium if the patient is taking a diuretic, an angiotensin receptor blocker or an ACE inhibitor. A flowsheet in the patient's chart or the electronic health record will allow you to easily follow the patient's BP, physical findings, laboratory study results, and prescribed treatments over time.

Keeping up to date with advances in hypertension can be a challenge for the physician. Because of the scope of the problem, there are thousands of studies and scores of clinical guidelines from a variety of different perspectives published yearly. Clinicians should look for practice guidelines that have explicit descriptions of how the literature was reviewed and summarized, and that emphasize long-term, patient-oriented outcomes. The best source of summary information is the report of the Joint National Committee on Prevention, Detection, Evaluation, and Treatment of High Blood Pressure (the most recent, the seventh report, can be found at *http://www.nhlbi.nih.gov/guidelines/hypertension/*). Key recommendations are summarized in Table 11.8.

TABLE 11.9 Compelling Indications for Antihypertensive Medication Selection

Compelling Indication	Antihypertensive Medication Options
Chronic kidney disease	ACEI, ARB
Diabetes	THIAZ, BB, ACEI, ARB, CCB
Heart failure	THIAZ, BB, ACEI, ARB, ALDO ANT
High cardiovascular disease risk	THIAZ, BB, ACEI, CCB
Post-myocardial infarction	BB, ACEI, ALDO ANT
Recurrent stroke prevention	THIAZ, ACEI

ALDO ANT = aldosterone antagonist; ACEI= angiotensin converting enzyme inhibitor; ARB = angiotensin receptor blocker; BB = β-blocker; CCB = calcium channel blocker; THIAZ = thiazide diuretic.

KEY POINTS

- Hypertension affects 1 of every 3 American adults and is a major contributor to deaths from cardiovascular disease.
- Although screening for elevated blood pressure is common, hypertension still remains underdiagnosed and undertreated.
- Accurate assessment of a person's blood pressure status relies on proper technique using calibrated equipment and repeated measurements.
- Initial evaluation of a person with hypertension has three underlying goals: (1) assess for other cardiovascular comorbidities, (2) assess for target organ damage, and (3) evaluate for common secondary causes of hypertension.
- Treatment of hypertension reduces the risk of developing major cardiovascular events such as myocardial infarction, stroke, and congestive heart failure.
- Lifestyle modifications for patients with hypertension include weight loss (if overweight), exercise, moderation of alcohol intake, and a low sodium DASH eating plan.
- Initial pharmacologic treatment of hypertension is usually with a thiazide diuretic or angiotensin converting enzyme (ACE) inhibitor, and may be influenced by a compelling indication (such as comorbid diabetes). Many hypertensive patients will require at least two agents from different classes to attain blood pressure control.

CHAPTER

12

Venous Thromboembolism

David Weismantel

CLINICAL OBJECTIVES

1. Estimate the probability of deep vein thrombosis and pulmonary embolism based on the clinical signs and symptoms
2. Appropriately use imaging studies to confirm or rule out venous thromboemboism
3. Recommend the appropriate duration of anticoagulant therapy
4. Identify patients who might require long-term anticoagulation

Venous thromboembolism (VTE) describes related clinical diagnoses that include deep venous thrombosis (DVT) and pulmonary embolism (PE). DVT is defined as a partial or complete occlusion of a deep vein by thrombus; PE is the blocking of a pulmonary artery or one of its branches by a thrombus or foreign material. Most pulmonary emboli originate from thrombi within the deep vessels of the lower extremities and pelvis—the popliteal, femoral, or iliac veins (1). Upper extremity DVT is less common but may also lead to PE, especially in the presence of a venous catheter.

The age- and sex-adjusted annual incidence of VT is 117 cases per 100,000 persons (DVT is 48 per 100,000; PE is 69 per 100,000). The incidence increases steadily with advancing age and reaches 900 episodes per 100,000 by the age of 85 years (2, 3). PE is diagnosed in more than 500,000 patients in the United States each year and results in approximately 200,000 deaths (4–6). These numbers certainly underestimate the true incidence of PE as it is thought that half of all patients remain undiagnosed. In addition to age, other risk factors for the development of VTE include previous thromboembolism, obesity, pregnancy, the postpartum period, malignancy, inherited thrombophilias, oral contraceptive use, and exogenous estrogen therapy. Environmental risk factors include immobility, trauma, and surgery. More than half of all VTE events are associated with antecedent trauma, surgery, immobilization, or diagnosis of cancer (7). The classic Virchow triad of stasis, vascular damage, and hypercoagulability describes the basic pathophysiologic factors that alone, or more commonly in combination, promote the development of thrombosis.

Leg pain and swelling are relatively common presenting complaints in primary care practice. In the 1995 National Ambulatory Medical Care Survey, 1.3% of patients presenting to family physicians had a complaint of leg pain or leg swelling (8). Although these symptoms may be caused by a number of vascular, musculoskeletal, infectious, or dermatologic causes, DVT must always be a primary consideration. Yet when evaluating a patient with suspected DVT, it is important to appreciate that only a minority of patients will actually have the disease. For this reason, noninvasive testing is required to minimize the likelihood of inappropriate invasive testing or anticoagulation. Considering the risks of postphlebitic syndrome, PE, and death associated with a delayed or missed diagnosis of DVT, and the potential risk of chronic anticoagulation in a patient who does not have a DVT, accurate diagnosis is essential. Likewise, because the most common symptoms (dyspnea, pleuritic pain, cough) and signs (tachypnea, rales, tachycardia) of PE are also extremely common among patients without PE, additional testing is needed to confirm or exclude the diagnosis of PE (9, 10).

This chapter describes an effective diagnostic approach to patients with suspected DVT or PE, making the best possible use of the history and physical examination in validated clinical decision rules. Subsequently, an evidence-based and efficient approach to the treatment of VTE will be outlined.

DIAGNOSIS OF DEEP VEIN THROMBOSIS

Pathophysiology and Differential Diagnosis

Leg pain and swelling are typically caused by an imbalance of the oncotic and fluid pressures between the intravascular and extravascular spaces. Acute causes of leg pain and swelling include superficial thrombophlebitis, trauma, cellulitis, and dermatitis. Superficial thrombophlebitis often presents with erythema, induration, and tenderness of a superficial vein caused by thrombus and inflammation; the long saphenous vein is most commonly involved. Twenty-three percent of all patients with superficial thrombophlebitis have simultaneous DVT by duplex ultrasound evaluation (11). Trauma from fractures, muscle tears, and hematomas may also cause pain or swelling in a lower extremity. Symptoms will typically be unilateral with a specific time of injury noted; however, trivial or occult injuries may at times present as a painful and swollen extremity. Cellulitis is a bacterial infection of the dermis and subcutaneous tissues most often caused by group A β-hemolytic *Streptococcus* or *Staphylococcus aureus*; chronic lower extremity edema, minor trauma, or a dermatosis may predispose the patient to this problem by damaging the skin. Dermatitis can also cause diffuse tenderness and swelling of a leg; local histamine action causes pruritus and discomfort, with secondary edema of the dermis and subcutaneous tissues.

Chronic causes of leg pain and swelling include chronic venous insufficiency, postphlebitic syndrome, congestive heart failure, pretibial myxedema, and hypoalbuminemia. Often bilateral in nature, chronic venous insufficiency is a result of incompetent valves in the greater or lesser saphenous veins. There is a hereditary predisposition, and women are more commonly affected. DVT and venous hypertension can cause valvular damage and incompetence resulting in postphlebitic syndrome, which in turn can cause chronic lower extremity discomfort, edema, and ulceration. Decreased cardiac output from congestive heart failure may result in systemic venous congestion and lower extremity edema. Nonpitting pretibial myxedema is a characteristic finding among patients with hypothyroidism; other accompanying symptoms often include weakness, fatigue, weight gain, and cold intolerance. Decreased intravenous oncotic pressure secondary to hypoalbuminemia may cause a chronic, bilateral, lower extremity pitting edema. Primary etiologies include malnutrition, hepatocellular failure, or excess renal or gastrointestinal loss of albumin. The decrease in intravascular volume stimulates salt retention and leads to further edema formation because the underlying oncotic deficit remains.

A concise differential diagnosis of the painful and swollen lower extremity is shown in Table 12.1. Specific historical and physical examination findings that would suggest a progressive or life-threatening illness are listed in Table 12.2.

TABLE 12.1 Differential Diagnosis of Leg Pain and Swelling

Diagnosis	Frequency in Primary Care Practice
Vascular	
Superficial thrombophlebitis	Very common
Chronic venous insufficiency	Very common
Congestive heart failure	Common
Deep venous thrombosis	Uncommon
Postphlebitic syndrome	Uncommon
Lymphedema	Uncommon
Dermatologic	
Cellulitis	Very common
Dermatitis	Very common
Endocrine and metabolic	
Lymphedema	Uncommon
Hypoalbuminemia	Rare
Traumatic	
Fracture, muscle tear, hematoma	Very common

History and Physical Examination

The patient presenting with an acutely painful and swollen leg is at risk for DVT and requires rapid assessment through a focused history and physical examination. Individual historical elements and physical examination findings are of limited value in the diagnosis of DVT. Larger and better designed studies (12, 13) generally find lower sensitivities and specificities for physical examination findings than poorly designed studies (14). The historical elements with the greatest positive predictive values for DVT are recent surgery and immobilization for more than 3 days in the past 4 weeks (15). The test characteristics of individual historical elements and physical examination findings from the highest quality studies are outlined in Table 12.3. Note that Homan's sign is of no value in the diagnosis of DVT and should be omitted from the examination.

Clinical Decision Rule

Although the individual elements of the history and physical examination have limited value, groups of these signs and symptoms can be very useful. A clinical decision rule combining the results of nine carefully defined signs and symptoms was developed by Wells et al (15). Later validation of this rule in different groups of patients found that it effectively stratified patients into groups according to their risk of having

TABLE 12.2 Red Flags Suggesting Progressive or Life-Threatening Disease in the Patient Suspected of DVT

History and Physical Examination Finding	Diagnoses Suggested
Dyspnea, tachypnea	Pulmonary embolism, congestive heart failure, dysrhythmia
Chest pain	Pulmonary embolism, congestive heart failure, dysrhythmia
Syncope	Pulmonary embolism, dysrhythmia
Hypotension, pulmonary edema, cyanosis	Pulmonary embolism, congestive heart failure, dysrhythmia
Fever	Pulmonary embolism, systemic infection
DVT = deep venous thrombosis.	

TABLE 12.3 Key Elements of the History and Physical Examination for Leg Pain and Swelling

Element of History and Physical	Sensitivity (%)	Specificity (%)	LR+	LR−
Immobilization (>3 days in past 4 weeks) (14)	24	90	2.4[a]	0.8
Venous dilatation (13)	25	89	2.3	0.8
Recent surgery (14)	9	94	1.5	1.0
Swelling (12)	84	44	1.5	0.4
Temperature difference (11)	72	48	1.4	0.6
Edema (11)	97	33	1.4	0.1*
Calf pain (11)	86	19	1.1	0.7
Homan sign (12)	56	39	0.9	1.1
Local tenderness (12)	76	11	0.9	2.2
Erythema (12)	24	62	0.6	1.2

*Best individual signs and symptoms for ruling in (immobilization) and ruling out (no edema) deep vein thrombosis in symptomatic patients.

DVT (16, 17). Patients stratified to the low-, moderate-, and high-risk groups based on this rule had a 3%, 17%, and 75% risk of DVT, respectively. The ability to sort these patients by risk with a clinical decision rule will significantly influence the interpretation of subsequent noninvasive tests. The decision rule is found in Table 12.4.

Laboratory Testing

Diagnostic tests for DVT include duplex venous ultrasound, magnetic resonance imaging (MRI), helical computed tomography, D-dimer, and contrast venography. The latter is an invasive test and is considered to be the reference standard. The accuracy of noninvasive tests varies with the study population (symptomatic versus asymptomatic), and the type of DVT being diagnosed (proximal, distal, or both). The tests are generally less accurate in asymptomatic patients, and less accurate for diagnosis of distal DVT than for proximal DVT. Table 12.5 summarizes the risk stratified performance of the various tests for the diagnosis of DVT in symptomatic patients (18–22). Impedance plethysmography and duplex venous ultrasound have excellent positive predictive values to rule in DVT in the high-risk patient, whereas D-dimer testing has an excellent negative predictive value to rule out the diagnosis in the low-risk patient.

Duplex venous ultrasound is the most widely used modality for evaluating patients with suspected DVT. Ultrasound assessment is operator-dependent, unable to distinguish between acute and chronic thrombus, inaccurate in detection of pelvic and calf DVT, and less reliable in the presence of significant edema or obesity. False-positive examinations may be caused by superficial phlebitis, popliteal cysts, and abscess.

Yet when used in combination with a clinical prediction rule, ultrasound examination is accurate in predicting the need for anticoagulation. However, a normal ultrasound study in a moderate- to high-probability patient requires additional investigation (D-dimer or repeat ultrasound) before DVT can be ruled out. If suspicion for DVT persists despite an initial negative duplex ultrasound result, one should repeat the test 4–7 days later and educate the patient about warning signs of pulmonary embolism or worsening DVT. Two studies with a total of 2,107 patients repeated the ultrasound 5–7 days later if the first ultrasound result was normal and did not anticoagulate patients with two normal ultrasound results (23, 24). Only 0.6% of these patients had a thromboembolic complication (DVT or PE) during the next 3 months, and only one of these occurred during the week between ultrasounds. A third study repeated the ultrasound 1 day and again 6 days later in patients with a normal initial ultrasound result (25). Of 390 patients with three normal ultrasound results, only 6 had a thromboembolic complication during the next 3 months. Thus, in patients with two normal ultrasound results a week apart, the risk of a thromboembolic complication during the next 3 months is only about 1%.

Although there is considerable interest in MRI for the diagnosis of DVT, the studies to date have been small (26–28) or methodologically flawed, with limitations ranging from a failure to blind, to a retrospective design, to a poor-quality reference standard (29–31). When compared with contrast venography, MRI sensitivity ranges from 80% to 100%, and specificity from 93% to 100%. Use of MRI to diagnose DVT should currently be limited to cases in which there is considerable local experience with the technique and in which contrast venography may be indicated but there are relative contraindications to the use of intravenous contrast agents (32, 33). Likewise, there is insufficient evidence to support the routine use of helical computed tomographic (CT) venography for the diagnosis of DVT (34). Both MRI and CT venography remain relatively expensive compared to duplex venous ultrasound.

Elevated levels of D-dimer, a fibrin degradation product, are associated with an increased risk of DVT. Different D-dimer assays vary considerably in their performance. Latex agglutination assays are quick and inexpensive but are not

TABLE 12.4 Wells Clinical Decision Rule to Evaluate the Probability of DVT Using the History and Physical Examination

1. Count the number of risk factors for your patient and calculate the risk score:

Risk Factor	Points
Active cancer (treatment ongoing or within previous 6 months or palliative)	1
Paralysis, paresis, or recent plaster immobilization of the lower extremities	1
Recently bedridden for >3 days or major surgery within 4 weeks	1
Localized tenderness along the distribution of the deep venous system	1
Entire leg swelling	1
Calf swelling by >3 cm when compared with the asymptomatic leg (measured 10 cm below the tibial tuberosity)	1
Pitting edema (greater in the symptomatic leg)	1
Collateral superficial veins (nonvaricose)	1
Alternative diagnosis as likely or greater than that of deep vein thrombosis	−2
Total (range, −2 to 8)	

2. Determine the pretest likelihood of DVT:

Risk Score	Risk Category	Probability of DVT
≤0	Low	3% (95% CI, 2%–6%)
1–2	Moderate	17% (95% CI, 12%–23%)
>2	High	75% (95% CI, 63%–84%)

CI = confidence interval; DVT = deep venous thrombosis.
(Adapted from Wells PS, Anderson DR, Bormanis J, et al. Value of assessment of pretest probability of deep-vein thrombosis in clinical management. Lancet. 1997;350:1795–1798.)

recommended because they are less accurate. Microplate enzyme-linked immunosorbent assays (ELISAs) are accurate but expensive; membrane ELISAs are less expensive and almost as accurate. Note that a negative D-dimer test alone does not rule out DVT; 2–5% of patients with suspected DVT and a negative D-dimer test result actually have a DVT. This is similar to the performance of ultrasound alone in unselected patients with suspected DVT. The D-dimer test is most useful in patients with a moderate risk of DVT, and a normal duplex venous ultrasound result. In one study, only 1 of 598 patients with a normal duplex ultrasound and a normal D-dimer test result developed a DVT during the next 3 months. Of 88 patients with a normal duplex ultrasound result but an elevated D-dimer test result, 5 had a DVT detected 1 week later with a repeat ultrasound, and an additional 2 patients had a venous thromboembolic complication during the next 3 months (35).

Another recent study found that the combination of a low-risk assessment by a validated clinical prediction rule and a negative D-dimer test effectively ruled out DVT (36). Finally it has been demonstrated that patients with a Wells clinical prediction rule score of less than 2 points and a negative D-dimer test were less likely to have VTE during follow-up than were patients with a negative ultrasound examination (0.4% vs 1.4%) (37). It is important to note that a positive D-dimer test does not raise the likelihood of DVT appreciably and is therefore of limited diagnostic value.

Approach to the Patient

The indiscriminate application of diagnostic testing to all patients with suspected DVT would risk the overtreatment of low-risk patients and the undertreatment of high-risk patients. Initial use of the Wells DVT Clinical Decision Rule will stratify patients into low-, moderate-, or high-risk groups. The rule was developed and validated in nonpregnant patients with a first episode of DVT; pregnant patients and those with a history of previous DVT should be evaluated more aggressively, as they have an increased risk of DVT.

After a patient has been placed in the low-, moderate-, or high-risk group, the algorithm in Figure 12.1 should guide further evaluation. This algorithm was developed by the Institute for Clinical Systems Improvement (ICSI) and incorporates evidence-based recommendations for the use of pretest clinical probability with prediction rules, D-dimer testing, and imaging in the diagnosis of DVT (38). The diagnosis may be considered ruled out in low-risk patients with a negative duplex venous ultrasound and in moderate-risk patients with a normal D-dimer and negative ultrasound. Moderate- and high-risk patients with a normal initial ultrasound but an abnormal D-dimer should undergo a repeat ultrasound in 1 week or

TABLE 12.5 Risk-Stratified Characteristics of Diagnostic Tests for Venous Thromboembolism in Symptomatic Patients

Deep Venous Thrombosis			Pretest Probability by Wells Clinical Decision Rule (%)					
			High Risk: 75%		Moderate: 17%		Low Risk: 3%	
Test	Sensitivity (%)	Specificity (%)	PPV	NPV	PPV	NPV	PPV	NPV
Duplex ultrasonography (17)	88–97	80–96	93–99	69–91	47–83	97–99	12–42	99–100
Helical computed tomography (18)	71	93	97	52	68	94	24	99
Magnetic resonance imaging (19)	56–100	88–100	93	40	49	91	13	99
D-dimer (20)	89	77	39	89	—	—	14	99
	Pulmonary Embolism		High Risk: 78.4%		Moderate: 27.8%		Low Risk: 3.4%	
Helical computed tomography (42)	77	89	96	52	73	91	20	99
Magnetic resonance imaging (42)	77	87	96	51	70	91	17	99
Transthoracic echocardiography (42)	68	89	96	43	70	88	18	99
Transesophageal echocardiography (42)	70	81	93	43	59	88	12	99
D-dimer erythrocyte agglutination (SimpliRED) (42)	89	59	89	60	46	93	7	99
Ventilation perfusion scanning (43)	98	10	80	58	30	93	3	99

DVT = deep vein thrombosis; NPV = negative predictive value; PPV = positive predictive value.
(Adapted from Ramzi DW, Leeper KV. DVT and pulmonary embolism: Part I. Diagnosis. Am Fam Physician. 2004;69:2829–36.)

proceed to contrast venography. Moderate- and high-risk patients with an abnormal ultrasound should be treated for DVT. It is important that this algorithm not be used inflexibly. Patients with new or progressive symptoms, such as a patient with suspected DVT who then develops signs and symptoms of PE, should be evaluated immediately.

DIAGNOSIS OF PULMONARY EMBOLISM

Although acute PE is an important diagnostic possibility in the patient presenting with chest pain and shortness of breath, many other cardiac, pulmonary, gastroenterologic, and musculoskeletal etiologies are possible and should always be considered in the evaluation. Table 12.6 presents a concise differential diagnosis of chest pain.

History and Physical Examination

The patient presenting with chest pain and shortness of breath is at risk for PE and requires rapid assessment through a focused history and physical examination. Individual historical elements and physical examination findings are of limited value in the diagnosis of PE. The classic triad of signs and symptoms (chest pain, dyspnea, hemoptysis) are neither sensitive nor specific. They occur in fewer than 20% of patients in whom the diagnosis of PE is made, and most patients with these symptoms are found to have another diagnosis to account for them. The most common symptoms and signs are summarized in Table 12.7 (9, 10).

Clinical Decision Rule

A clinical decision rule combining the results of seven carefully defined signs and symptoms was developed and validated by Wells and colleagues (39). Patients stratified to the low-, moderate-, and high-risk groups based on this rule had a 3%, 28%, and 78% risk of PE, respectively. The ability to sort these patients by risk with a clinical decision rule will again significantly influence the interpretation of subsequent noninvasive tests. The decision rule is found in Table 12.8.

Laboratory Testing

Diagnostic tests for PE include ventilation-perfusion (V/Q) scanning, helical CT, D-dimer testing, and pulmonary angiography. The latter is an invasive test and is considered

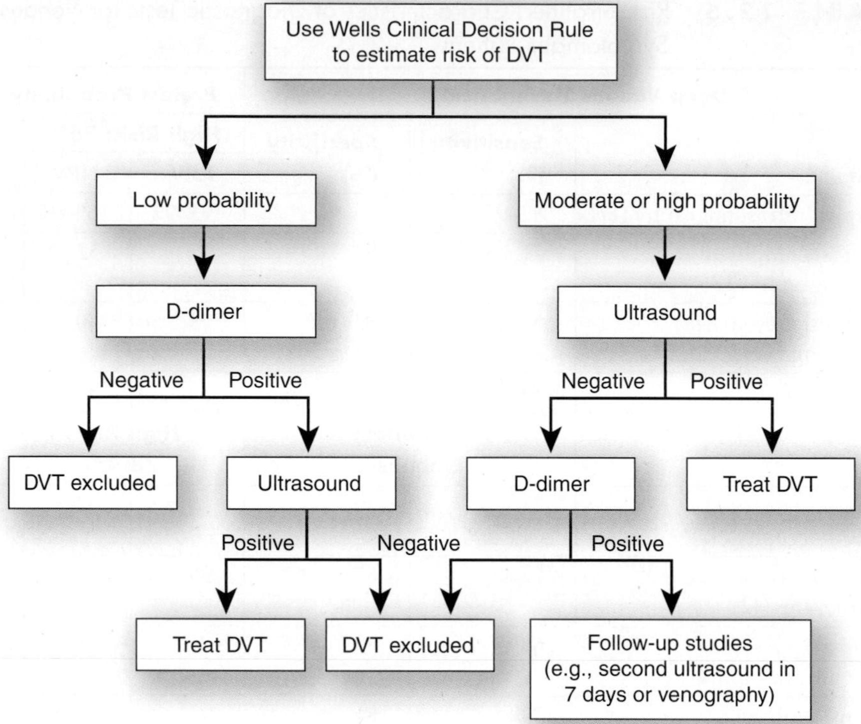

Figure 12.1 • Algorithm for evaluation of DVT using a combination of the Wells Clinical Decision Rule and diagnostic testing. DVT = deep venous thrombosis. (Adapted from Institute for Clinical Systems Improvement. Healthcare guidelines. Venous thromboembolism diagnosis and treatment. *http://www.icsi.org/venous_thromboembolism/venous_thromboembolism_4.html*. Accessed August 1, 2010.)

to be the reference standard. Table 12.5 summarizes the risk-stratified performance of the various tests for the diagnosis of PE in symptomatic patients (40, 41). Helical CT has an excellent positive predictive value to rule in PE in the high-risk patient, whereas D-dimer testing has an excellent negative predictive value to rule out the diagnosis in the low-risk patient.

The V/Q scan has historically been the standard diagnostic study in patients with suspected PE. Defects in radioactive tracer uptake from ventilated and perfused areas of the lungs are reported as normal, nearly normal, or indicating a low, intermediate, or high probability of embolus. A high-probability V/Q scan provides sufficient evidence and specificity for the initiation of treatment for PE. Likewise, a normal or near-normal

TABLE 12.6 Differential Diagnosis of Chest Pain and Shortness of Breath

Diagnosis	Frequency in Primary Care Practice
Cardiac	
Coronary artery disease	Common
Aortic dissection	Uncommon
Pericarditis	Uncommon
Pulmonary	
Pneumonia	Very common
Pulmonary embolism	Uncommon
Pneumothorax	Uncommon
Gastroenterologic	
Gastroesophageal reflux disease	Very common
Esophageal spasm	Uncommon
Musculoskeletal	
Trauma	Very common
Costochondritis	Very common

TABLE 12.7 Symptoms and Signs in Acute Pulmonary Embolism

Symptom	Frequency (%)
Dyspnea	73
Pleuritic chest pain	66
Cough	37
Hemoptysis	13
Sign	
Tachypnea	70
Rales	51
Tachycardia	30
Fourth heart sound	24
Accentuated pulmonic component of second heart sound	23
Circulatory collapse	8

TABLE 12.8 Wells Clinical Decision Rule to Evaluate the Probability of PE Using the History and Physical Examination

1. Count the number of risk factors for your patient and calculate the risk score:

Risk Factor	Points
Clinical signs or symptoms of DVT (leg swelling, pain with palpation of deep veins)	3
Alternative diagnosis less likely than PE	3
Heart rate greater than 100 beats per minute	1.5
Immobilization or surgery within past 4 weeks	1.5
Previous DVT or PE	1.5
Hemoptysis	1
Malignancy	1
Total (range, 0–12.5)	

2. Determine the pretest likelihood of DVT:

Risk Score	Risk Category	Probability of DVT
<2	Low	3.3% (95% CI, 1.7%–4.8%)
2–6	Moderate	20.2% (95% CI, 17.1%–23.3%)
>6	High	62.9% (95% CI, 52.9%–73.0%)

CI = confidence interval; DVT = deep venous thrombosis; PE = pulmonary embolism.
(Adapted from Wells PS, Anderson DR, Rodger M, et al. Derivation of a simple clinical model to categorize patients' probability of pulmonary embolism: increasing the model utility with the SimpliRED D-dimer. Thromb Haemost. 2000;83:418.)

scan should be considered sufficiently sensitive to rule out the diagnosis. Unfortunately, at least half of scans are indeterminate (low or intermediate probability). In the Prospective Investigation of Pulmonary Embolism Diagnosis study, 40% of patients with confirmed PE had a high-probability V/Q scan, 40% had an intermediate-probability scan, and 14% had a low-probability scan (41).

Helical CT scanning has a sensitivity and specificity of nearly 90% to detect large main and lobar emboli, yet is less able to detect smaller subsegmental involvement (42). Helical CT scanning is increasingly the standard imaging study for patients with suspected PE (43, 44). However, it is important to remember that it exposes patients to a large radiation dose and is likely to miss smaller or subsegmental PE's. In addition, the diagnostic accuracy of helical CT scanning appears to vary widely from institution to institution because of differences in image quality and interpreter experience (45, 46).

D-dimer testing in combination with the Wells Clinical Prediction Rule has been shown to be effective in ruling out PE in patients presenting to the emergency department (47). Use of D-dimer for the diagnosis of PE has been extensively studied and is best characterized as having good sensitivity and negative predictive value, but poor specificity. It is helpful at ruling out VTE when negative, especially in low-risk patients, but is not helpful when positive.

Approach to the Patient

As with DVT, the indiscriminate application of diagnostic testing to all patients with suspected PE would risk the overtreatment of low-risk patients and the undertreatment of high-risk patients. Initial use of the Wells PE Clinical Decision Rule will again stratify patients into risk groups. After a patient has been placed in the low-, moderate-, or high-risk group, the algorithm in Figure 12.2 guides further evaluation with helical CT scanning. This algorithm was also developed by the ICSI and incorporates evidence-based recommendations for the use of pretest clinical probability with prediction rules, D-dimer testing, and imaging in the diagnosis of PE (38). The diagnosis may be considered ruled out in low-risk patients with a normal D-dimer. Moderate- and high-risk patients require imaging by helical CT. It should again be stressed that this algorithm not be used inflexibly.

MANAGEMENT OF VENOUS THROMBOEMBOLISM

The algorithm in Figure 12.3 outlines a basic, evidence-based approach to the treatment of VTE, including initial heparin anticoagulation, oral warfarin therapy, and other supportive measures. It emphasizes interventions that have been shown to minimize the likelihood of acute or long-term complications. Because DVT and PE are clinical manifestations of the same pathophysiologic process, the standard anticoagulation protocols are identical.

Initial Management of VTE

Prompt anticoagulation with heparin is the first priority in treating the patient with VTE; this prevents the local extension,

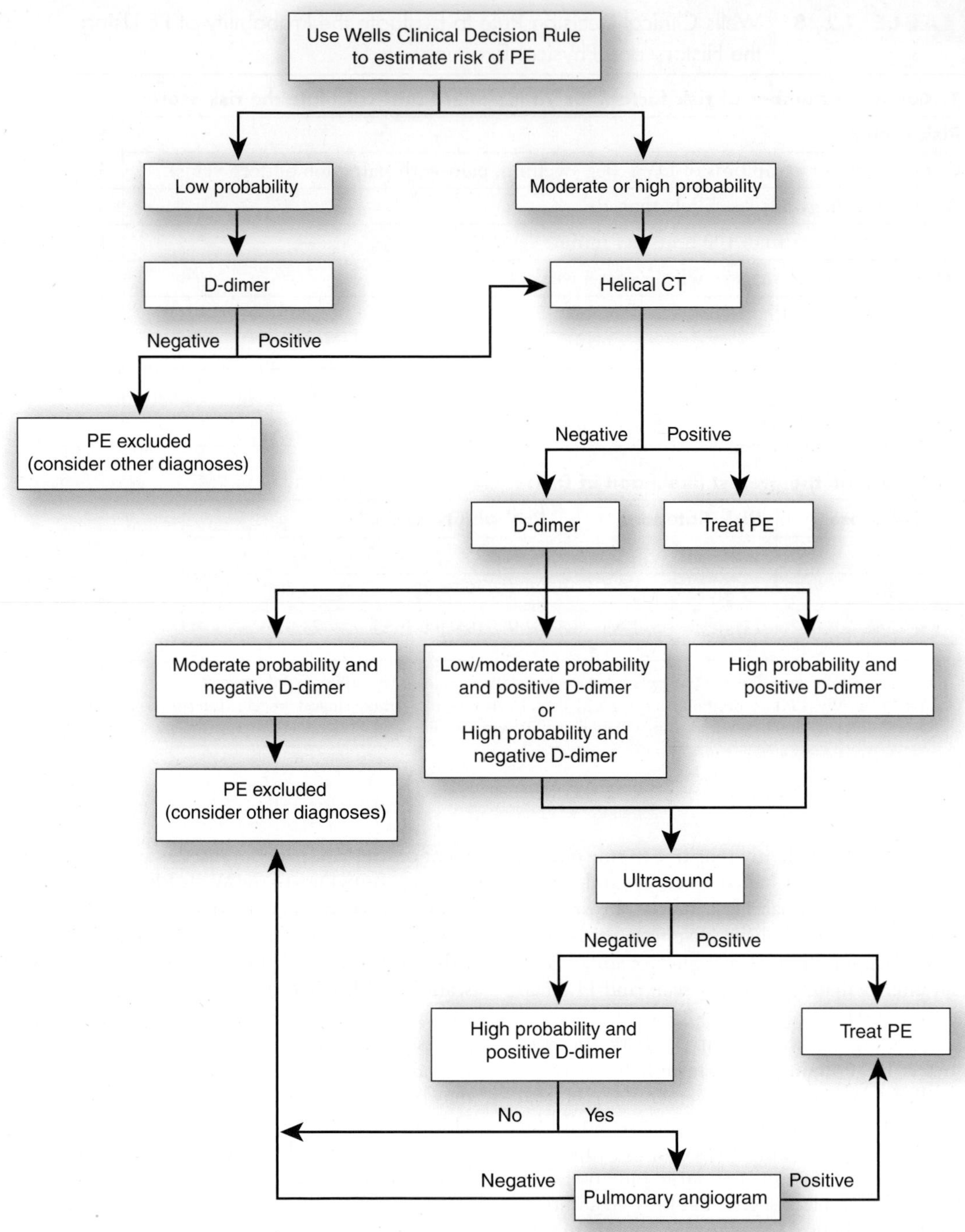

Figure 12.2 • Algorithm for evaluation of PE using a combination of the Wells Clinical Decision Rule and helical CT scan. CT = computed tomography; PE = pulmonary embolism. (Adapted from Institute for Clinical Systems Improvement. Healthcare guidelines. Venous thromboembolism diagnosis and treatment. *http://www.icsi.org/venous_thromboembolism/venous_thromboembolism_4.html*. Accessed August 1, 2010.)

embolization, and recurrence of venous thromboembolic disease. Oral warfarin is started simultaneously. Heparin acts immediately to catalyze the inhibition of several activated coagulation factors and leads to the stabilization of the intravascular thrombus. Heparinization is typically continued for 5 days and until a stable and therapeutic international normalized ratio (INR) is established with oral warfarin therapy. There are three approved approaches to the initial anticoagulant treatment of a patient with acute VTE: intravenous unfractionated heparin (UH), subcutaneous low-molecular-weight heparin (LMWH), and subcutaneous fondaparinux, a synthetic factor Xa inhibitor.

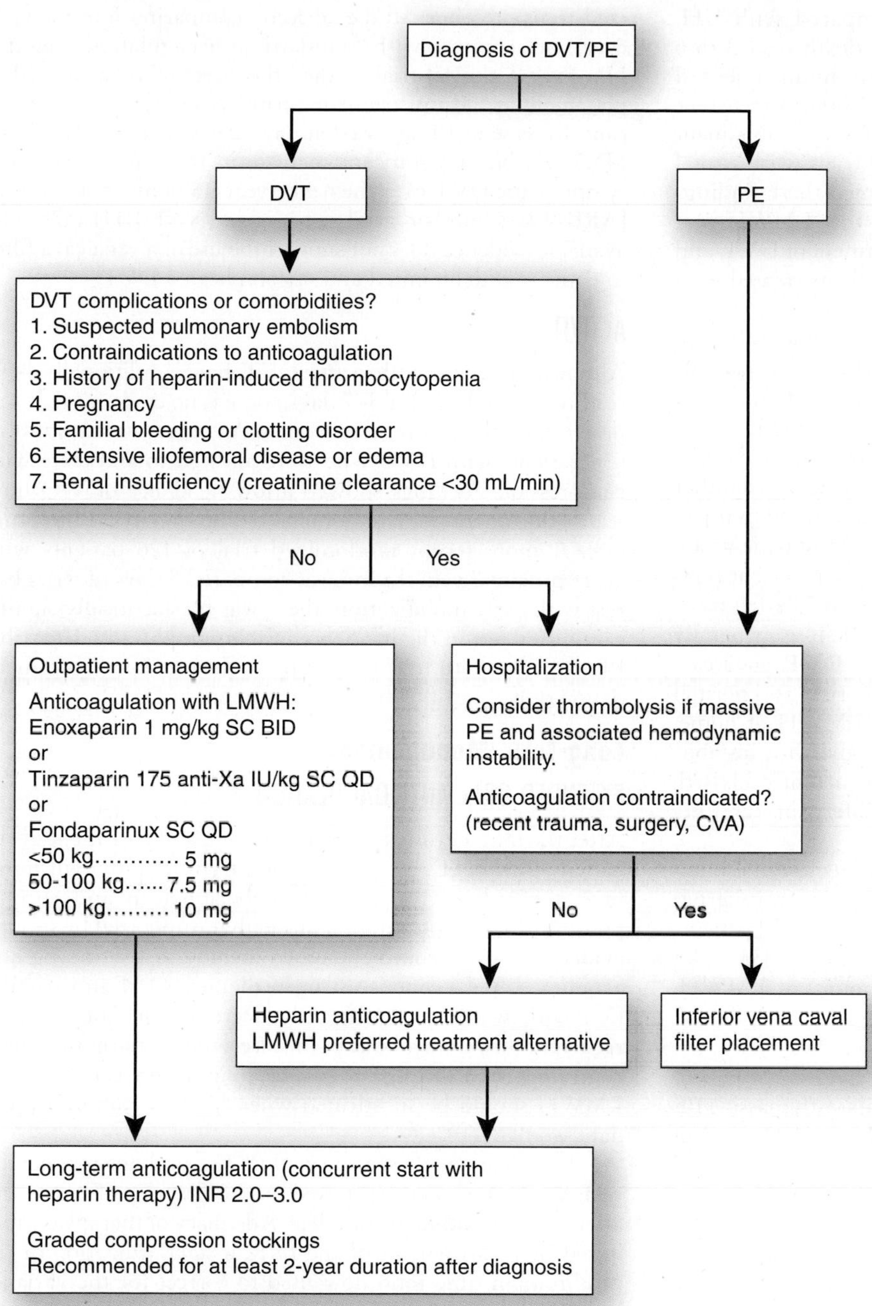

Figure 12.3 • Algorithm for treatment of VTE. BID = twice daily; DVT = deep venous thrombosis; LMWH = low-molecular-weight heparin; PE = pulmonary embolism; QD = every day; SC = subcutaneously; VTE = venous thromboembolism.

HEPARIN AND FONDAPARINUX

The traditional treatment of VTE has been anticoagulation with intravenous UH; the goal of this therapy is the prompt establishment of an activated partial thromboplastin time of 1.5 to 2.5 times the control (48). More recently, LMWHs have been introduced that have the advantage of fixed dosing, a subcutaneous route of administration (making outpatient treatment possible), and a more predictable anticoagulant response. Laboratory monitoring is typically unnecessary as a result of better bioavailability, a longer half-life, and dose-independent clearance. If monitoring of LMWH is necessary, an anti-Xa level of 0.4–0.7 U/mL is the goal of therapy (49). The only LMWHs currently approved and labeled by the US Food and Drug Administration for the treatment of acute VTE are enoxaparin at a dosage of 1 mg/kg administered subcutaneously twice daily (outpatient or inpatient therapy) or 1.5 mg/kg once daily (inpatient therapy only), or tinzaparin at a dosage of 175 anti-Xa IU/kg administered subcutaneously once daily. Fondaparinux (<50 kg, 5 mg; 50–100 kg, 7.5 mg; >100 kg, 10 mg) administered subcutaneously once daily is another option; it is a synthetic inhibitor of activated factor X (Xa).

A meta-analysis of 11 randomized controlled trials with a total of 3,674 patients demonstrated the safety and effectiveness of LMWH therapy for acute DVT. Compared with UH, LMWH significantly reduced the risk of death over 3 to 6 months (absolute risk reduction [ARR] 1.65%; number needed to treat [NNT] 61). A trend toward a reduction in recurrent thromboembolic events was also observed (50). A subsequent meta-analysis of 13 randomized controlled trials, with a total of 4,447 patients with DVT or PE, confirmed these findings (51). From this information, it is apparent that LMWH is at least as safe and effective as UH for the treatment of DVT, and that one death is prevented for every 60 patients treated with LMWH instead of UH.

Several studies have shown the efficacy and safety of administering LMWH at home. One study of 400 patients with DVT compared home therapy with LMWH to inpatient UH and failed to show any significant difference in the risk of recurrent thromboembolism or major bleeding (52). No difference in these clinical outcomes was found in another prospective study comparing patient self-injection with injection administered by a home care nurse (53). Most patients are both capable and willing to participate in this treatment regimen; 91% were pleased with home therapy and 70% felt comfortable with self-injection of LMWH (54). It is generally agreed that patients with an uncomplicated DVT, good cardiopulmonary reserve, no excessive bleeding risk, and normal renal function can be safely treated with LMWH at home. Because of the risks of hypoxemia and hemodynamic instability, initial outpatient treatment of PE is not currently advised, although clinical trial evidence for its safety in carefully selected patients is building.

There is emerging evidence that subcutaneous unfractionated heparin given in a relatively high fixed dose is an alternative to LMWH or intravenous UFH. In a study of 708 patients with VTE randomized to subcutaneous UFH (333 U/kg initially followed by 250 U/kg every 12 hours) or LMWH, outcomes were similar (55).

THROMBOLYSIS

Thrombolytic therapy is indicated in patients with massive PE and associated hemodynamic instability. However, the role of thrombolysis in the treatment of patients with submassive PE remains controversial. In the largest study to date, improved survival was observed in patients treated with alteplase plus heparin compared with heparin alone. Using death and major complications as the end point, the number needed to treat was 7.3 for patients with PE and pulmonary hypertension or right ventricular dysfunction but without arterial hypotension or shock. One fewer death was observed for every 82 patients treated with this combination therapy (56). In patients with PE, the usual dose of 100 mg of alteplase is given by intravenous infusion over a period of 2 hours. Streptokinase is given in a 250,000 IU loading dose, followed by 100,000 IU per hour for 24 hours. Delivery of thrombolytics directly into the thrombus by catheter has not been shown to be superior to peripheral infusion.

VENA CAVA FILTER PLACEMENT

Placement of an inferior vena cava filter is reserved for patients with a contraindication to anticoagulation, a serious complication of anticoagulation, or recurrent thromboembolism despite adequate anticoagulation. To date there have been no randomized trials or cohort studies directly comparing inferior vena cava interruption with standard anticoagulation therapy. However, a clinical trial studied the effect of vena cava filter placement in 400 anticoagulated patients and showed a significant decrease in PE assessed at day 12 of therapy (ARR 3.7%; NNT 27) but a significant increase in the rate of recurrent symptomatic DVT over the next 2 years (absolute risk increase [ARI] 9.2%; number needed to harm [NNH] 11) (57). The available evidence does not support the use of a vena cava filter in patients with an initial and uncomplicated DVT.

ACTIVITY

Although patients with acute DVT have traditionally been confined to bed rest for 3–7 days, there is no evidence that this practice improves clinical outcomes. An observational study of 638 patients with DVT who were allowed to ambulate with compression stockings showed a low incidence of V/Q lung scan—documented PE as compared with that in the literature (58). A more recent randomized trial of 126 patients with acute proximal vein thrombosis compared 8 days of strict bed rest with early mobilization; there was no statistically significant difference in the incidence of scintigraphically detectable PE (59). These studies do not support the previous recommendation of bed rest for the acute treatment of DVT.

Long-term Management

EXTENDED ORAL ANTICOAGULATION

After the initial evaluation, stabilization, and treatment of the patient with VTE, subsequent long-term therapy will minimize the risk of recurrent thromboembolism and chronic postphlebitic complications. Although unsupported by specific evidence, most recommendations include discontinuing and avoiding any exogenous estrogen therapy. Oral anticoagulation with warfarin significantly decreases the incidence of recurrent thromboembolic events. Because warfarin therapy is contraindicated during pregnancy, long-term treatment with LMWH should be substituted when VTE occurs in a pregnant woman (60).

For a patient presenting with VTE, oral anticoagulation with warfarin should be started on the first day of treatment, after heparin loading is complete. Adequacy of therapy is monitored by measurement of the INR, a standardization of the prothrombin time ratio now used to correct for the variance between laboratories resulting from the use of different thromboplastin reagents. The full antithrombotic effect of warfarin requires 3–5 days to establish; therefore, heparin is overlapped with warfarin for at least the first 5 days of therapy.

Both 5- and 10-mg algorithms have been proposed and validated for initiation of warfarin. Two studies in hospitalized patients receiving heparin found that the 5-mg algorithm was preferable (61, 62), whereas a larger, more recent study in outpatients receiving LMWH supports a 10-mg algorithm (63). Unless new data demonstrate that one or the other of these algorithms is definitely better, both should be considered reasonable options for the initiation of warfarin (64); the algorithms are shown in Tables 12.9 and 12.10. For older patients, an initial 2.5-mg dose is sometimes used. The heparin may be discontinued after 5 days if the INR is within the therapeutic range of 2.0–3.0 (60).

The optimal duration of oral anticoagulant therapy for a first episode of VTE varies and depends on whether risk factors are transient or persistent. In general, patients with a clear reversible risk factor for an initial DVT or PE, such as a long plane flight or being postoperative, only require 3 months of treatment. A comparison of 3 months anticoagulation with extended oral anticoagulation of approximately 10 months for patients with DVT or PE found a reduction in the risk of recurrent VTE (ARR 26%; NNT 4), but an increased risk of major bleeding (ARI 3.8%; NNH 26) in the extended therapy group over a period of 2 years (65). In general, longer durations of oral anticoagulant therapy are associated with a decreased risk of venous thromboembolic recurrence, yet an increased risk of bleeding complications. A Cochrane review of 2,994 patients with DVT or PE in eight studies similarly found a decreased risk of recurrent VTE with prolonged warfarin therapy (0.9% vs 7.8%; ARR 6.9%; NNT 14), but an increased incidence of major bleeding (2.0% vs 0.2%; ARR 1.8%; NNH 56) (66). Therefore, some recent recommendations promote long-term anticoagulant therapy in those patients with a first unprovoked VTE in whom risk factors for bleeding are absent and for whom good anticoagulant monitoring is possible (60).

There has been some recent investigation of the utility of D-dimer measurement after completion of anticoagulation therapy. A large randomized controlle trial showed that a normal D-dimer 1 month after anticoagulation suspension for unprovoked VTE was associated with a low risk of late recurrences (4.4% patient-years) (67). Another prospective multicenter study, assessed the D-dimer time course and its relation

TABLE 12.9 Algorithm for Initiation of Warfarin Using 5 mg Initial Dose

Day	INR	Dosage
1		5.0 mg
2	<1.5 1.5–1.9 2.0–2.5 >2.5	5.0 mg 2.5 mg 1.0–2.5 mg 0.0 mg
3	<1.5 1.5–1.9 2.0–3.0 >3.0	5–10 mg 2.5–5.0 mg 0.0–2.5 mg 0.0 mg
4	<1.5 1.5–1.9 2.0–3.0 >3.0	10 mg 5.0–7.5 mg 0.0–5.0 mg 0.0 mg
5	<1.5 1.5–1.9 2.0–3.0 >3.0	10 mg 7.5–10.0 mg 0.0–5.0 mg 0.0 mg
6	<1.5 1.5–1.9 2.0–3.0 >3.0	7.5–12.5 mg 7.5–10.0 mg 0.0–7.5 mg 0.0 mg

TABLE 12.10 Algorithm for the Initiation of Warfarin Using 10 mg Initial Dose

Patients are given 10 mg of warfarin on days 1 and 2.

Day 3 INR	*Warfarin Dose in mg on Days 3 and 4*		*Day 5 INR*	*Warfarin Dose in mg on Days 5, 6, and 7*
<1.3 1.3 to 1.4	15.0, 15.0 10.0, 10.0	→	<2.0 2.0–3.0 3.1–3.5 >3.5 <2.0	15.0, 15.0, 15.0 7.5, 5.0, 7.5 0.0, 5.0, 5.0 0.0, 0.0, 2.5 7.5, 7.5, 7.5
1.5 to 1.6 1.7 to 1.9	10.0, 5.0 5.0, 5.0	→	2.0–3.0 3.1–3.5 >3.5	5.0, 5.0, 5.0 2.5, 2.5, 2.5 0.0, 2.5, 2.5
2.0 to 2.2 2.3 to 3.0	2.5, 2.5 0.0, 2.5	→	<2.0 2.0–3.0 3.1–3.5 >3.5 <2.0	5.0, 5.0, 5.0 2.5, 5.0, 2.5 0.0, 2.5, 0.0 0.0, 0.0, 2.5 2.5, 2.5, 2.5
>3.0	0.0, 0.0	→	2.0–3.0 3.1–4.0 >4.0	2.5, 0.0, 2.5 0.0, 2.5, 0.0 0.0, 0.0, 2.5

INR = international normalized ratio.
(Adapted from Kovacs MJ, Rodger M, Anderson DR, et al. Comparison of 10-mg and 5-mg warfarin initiation nomograms together with low-molecular-weight heparin for outpatient treatment of acute venous thromboembolism. A randomized, double-blind, controlled trial. Ann Intern Med. 2003;138:716.)

TABLE 12.11 ACCP Recommendations for Long-term Anticoagulation in Patients with DVT or PE (INR goal: 2.0–3.0)

Thromboembolism	Anticoagulation	Duration	SOR
First episode of VTE with a reversible or time-limited risk factor (e.g., trauma, surgery)	Warfarin	3 months	A
First episode symptomatic thrombosis confined to deep veins of calf	Warfarin	3 months	A
First episode of idiopathic or unprovoked VTE	Warfarin	At least 3 months, consider indefinite therapy	A
Recurrent VTE	Warfarin	Indefinitely	A
Any episode VTE with cancer	LMWH	Indefinitely, or until cancer is resolved	A

ACCP = American College of Chest Physicians; DVT = deep venous thrombosis; PE = pulmonary embolism; VTE = venous thromboembolism.
(Adapted from Kearon C, Kahn SR, Agnelli G, et al. Antithrombotic therapy for venous thromboembolic disease: American College of Chest Physicians Evidence-Based Clinical Practice Guidelines (8th ed.). Chest. 2008 Jun;133(6 Suppl):454S–545S.)

with late recurrences in patients with normal D-dimer 1 month after anticoagulation suspension for a first episode of unprovoked VTE. Patients with a normal D-dimer 1 month after stopping anticoagulation repeated D-dimer testing every 2 months for 1 year. The D-dimer was normal in 68% (243/355) of patients 1 month after anticoagulation suspension. Patients in whom D-dimer became abnormal at the third month and remained abnormal afterward had a significantly higher risk of recurrence (7/31; 27% patient-years) than patients in whom D-dimer remained normal at the third month and afterward (4/149; 2.9% patient-years; adjusted hazard ratio 7.9) (68). It has been suggested that repeated D-dimer testing after anticoagulation suspension for a first episode of unprovoked VTE may be used to further tailor the duration of treatment.

In the case of recurrent VTE, lifetime anticoagulant therapy should be encouraged in the absence of risk factors for bleeding. The specific recommendations for duration of oral anticoagulation have been adapted from the American College of Chest Physicians and are included in Table 12.11 (60).

The incidence of recurrent VTE is increased in patients with cancer, and these patients also are more likely to have complications from long-term warfarin therapy. A large multicenter trial in patients with cancer and VTE found that the likelihood of recurrent thrombosis was lower in the patients who received long-term treatment with LMWH than in those who received warfarin. In this trial, 13 patients needed to be treated with LMWH instead of warfarin to avoid one episode of recurrent DVT (69). However, 6 months of treatment costs more than $10,000, making the cost of preventing one recurrent DVT in excess of $100,000.

COMPRESSION STOCKINGS

The addition of compression stockings to standard oral anticoagulant therapy is supported by a study of 194 patients. Those using knee-high 30- to 40-mm Hg custom-fitted graded compression stockings for 2 years had a lower risk of developing mild-moderate postphlebitic syndrome (ARR 27.1%; NNT 4), and the incidence of severe postphlebitic syndrome was also decreased (ARR 12%; NNT 8) (70). Another study confirmed that although there was no reduction in the rate of recurrent VTE, extended use of compression stockings improved the long-term clinical course and should be considered a valuable addition in the management of DVT (71).

INVESTIGATION FOR POSSIBLE MALIGNANCY OR INHERITED THROMBOPHILIA

Although there is an increased incidence of cancer at the time of presentation in patients with idiopathic VTE (i.e., no clear predisposing cause such as bed rest), a complete medical evaluation including history, physical examination, and basic laboratory studies, and further evaluation as indicated based on these findings, has been shown to adequately detect malignancy in this setting. A retrospective study with 986 consecutive patients (142 with DVT and 844 with DVT ruled out) found no difference in the incidence of cancer over the next 34 months (72). A study of 260 patients with DVT followed for 2 years of regular visits found that all subsequent cancers were diagnosed because the patient became symptomatic and sought care from a family physician (73). Beyond initial and age-appropriate cancer screening, there is no evidence that an aggressive search for an underlying malignancy is warranted.

The inherited thrombophilias are associated with an increased risk for VTE, yet the diagnosis of one of these defects does not substantially change the clinical management of initial or recurrent VTE. Likewise, counseling regarding the increased risk associated with prolonged immobilization, surgery, pregnancy, and exogenous estrogen therapy would be unchanged. A sensible approach may be to screen for hereditary thrombophilias (factor V Leiden, prothrombin G20210A mutation, protein C deficiency, protein S deficiency, antithrombin III deficiency, anti-phospholipid antibodies, and hyperhomocysteinemia) in the case of recurrent VTE, a younger patient, or a patient with a family history of thromboembolic disease. If an inherited thrombophilia is diagnosed, further screening and possible identification of other family members could lead to avoidance of known secondary risk factors. The typical patient with an initial episode of VTE will not benefit from the investigation for an inherited coagulation defect.

PATIENT EDUCATION

Patients with VTE should be instructed about the importance of an extended course of oral anticoagulation in decreasing the likelihood of recurrent thromboembolism. Oral anticoagulation therapy requires regular evaluation of the INR and adjustment of the warfarin dosage. The patient should also avoid periods of prolonged immobilization and exogenous estrogen therapy in the future. Most importantly, each patient should learn to recognize the symptoms of a recurrent VTE so that therapy may be started in a timely fashion.

KEY POINTS

- Use the Wells rule or another validated clinical decision rule to determine the probability of VTE.
- D-dimer is useful when used as part of an algorithmic approach, especially for ruling out VTE in low-risk patients.
- High resolution CT is accurate for diagnosis of larger pulmonary emboli but may miss smaller or subsegmental lesions.
- Anticoagulation with low molecular weight heparin followed by at least 3 months of warfarin (Coumadin) is the standard of care for patients with uncomplicated VTE with a clear provoking factor.
- Selected patients with idiopathic or recurrent VTE should be anticoagulated for a longer period.

CHAPTER

13

Diabetes

Katrina Donahue, Sam Weir, Mary Roederer, and Evie Sigmon

CLINICAL OBJECTIVES

1. Describe clinical situations that should prompt evaluation for possible diabetes.
2. List the diagnostic criteria for diabetes.
3. Discuss how to convey the diagnosis of diabetes to a patient.
4. Describe the initial evaluation and management of a patient with diabetes.
5. List the necessary components to manage diabetes over time.

Diabetes mellitus (DM) is a chronic disease characterized by hyperglycemia resulting from defects in insulin secretion, insulin action, or both. It is one of the five most common diagnoses in primary care (1). An estimated 23.6 million people in the United States have DM, more than 5 million of whom are undiagnosed (2). Estimated costs attributed to DM in the United States are $174 billion, including direct medical costs and indirect costs of disability, work loss, and premature mortality (2). Type 1 DM results from autoimmune β-cell destruction, which leads to absolute insulin deficiency. Type 2 DM involves insulin resistance, which leads to relative insulin deficiency. Type 2 DM is much more common. Only 5–10% of patients diagnosed with diabetes have type 1 DM (3). Throughout this chapter, we will use the term "diabetes" to refer to both types of DM.

Diabetes causes multiple micro- and macrovascular complications and often leads to premature death (2). Microvascular complications include neuropathy, nephropathy, and vision changes. Macrovascular complications include heart disease, stroke, and peripheral vascular disease. Adults with diabetes are two to four times more likely to die from heart disease or have a stroke. Diabetes is the leading cause of blindness among adults and the leading cause of kidney failure. More than 60% of people with diabetes have neuropathy, and more than 60% of nontraumatic limb amputations are for complications of diabetes (2). Periodontal (gum) disease is more common among patients with DM. Poorly controlled diabetes in pregnant women can also cause major birth defects and excessively large infants.

Diabetes is a lifelong disease that requires a multifaceted approach to prevent complications. This approach must include lifestyle change, self-management, and negotiation of behavior goals, in addition to the treatment of hyperglycemia and addressing micro- and macrovascular risks.

DIAGNOSIS

Clinical Presentation and Differential Diagnosis

A person with diabetes can present with obvious symptoms or can be completely asymptomatic. Classically, severe hyperglycemia generates symptoms of fatigue, weight loss, polydipsia (excessive thirst), polyphagia (frequent eating), and polyuria (excessive urination). More subtle presentations of diabetes require the physician to consider combinations of signs and symptoms consistent with the disease and deserving of further evaluation. Such signs and symptoms include:

- obesity
- recurrent infections (especially yeast vaginitis, skin infections, and periodontal infections)
- slow healing wounds
- neurological syndromes (especially focal limb neuropathies presenting with paresthesias, burning, and tingling in the extremities)
- visual changes and blurry vision
- abdominal pain from nonalcoholic fatty liver or chronic pancreatitis (often from chronic excessive alcohol consumption)
- heart disease or stroke, especially among people who have not had consistent medical care
- in women, menstrual irregularity and obesity, polycystic ovarian syndrome, history of gestational diabetes or giving birth to an infant weighing more than 9 lb (4)

Red Flags: Hyperglycemic Crises

Diabetes can also present acutely as either diabetic ketoacidosis (DKA), which is common in patients with type 1 diabetes, or hyperosmolar hyperglycemic state (HHS), which is more likely to occur in type 2 diabetes. These conditions are jointly referred to as hyperglycemic crises to emphasize their seriousness and the need for rapid and intensive management. Table 13.1 lists the common presenting signs and symptoms that constitute "red flags" suggesting these states (5).

The hallmark of DKA is the triad of hyperglycemia, ketosis, and acidosis. Common clinical settings for DKA include previously undiagnosed type 1 diabetes or precipitating conditions in patients with known diabetes. Precipitating conditions include omission of previously prescribed insulin dose as well as problems such as pneumonia, urinary tract infection, alcohol abuse, trauma, pulmonary embolus, or myocardial infarction (MI). Symptoms suggestive of DKA include a fairly rapid course (<24 hours) of, nausea, vomiting, and abdominal pain. Signs of DKA include rapid, deep respirations

TABLE 13.1 Clinical Red Flags Suggesting a Hyperglycemic Crisis

Red Flags		
Symptoms	**Signs**	**Suggesting a Diagnosis of**
Rapid onset (<24 hours) Nausea and vomiting Abdominal pain Malaise	Mild dehydration Rapid, deep breathing Fruity smelling breath	Diabetic ketoacidosis (DKA)
Gradual onset (days to a week or more) Nausea and vomiting Abdominal pain Headache Thirst Polydipsia Polyuria Weight loss Lethargy Dizziness Headaches	More severe dehydration Mental status changes Obtundation Coma Focal neurologic signs (hemiparesis, visual field deficits) Seizures	Hyperglycemic hyperosmolar state

(Kussmaul breathing), fruity smell to the breath, signs of dehydration, and mental status changes.

HHS can present with more extreme levels of hyperglycemia (more than 1,000 mg/dL) than seen with DKA, but without ketosis or acidosis. The hyperglycemia causes profound dehydration that leads to hyperosmolality. The typical presentation is an insidious onset over days to weeks, with increasing thirst, polydipsia, polyuria, weight loss, and mental status changes. Physical examination reveals signs of dehydration and often includes mental status changes, obtundation, or coma. HHS may also present as seizures or with focal neurologic signs, such as hemiparesis or visual loss. Although HHS is more common in older adults, it can present in adolescents with previously undiagnosed type 2 diabetes.

History and Physical Examination

The initial evaluation should include a history, physical exam, laboratory evaluation, and referrals for specialized evaluation. The evaluation should classify the patient into diabetes type, identify any current diabetes complications, and help develop the patient's diabetes continuity care plan (4).

The patient's medical history, social history, health habits, and family history can provide information regarding current status and future risk of complications. Given the increased risk of heart disease, a high priority is to identify other cardiovascular risk factors, especially hypertension, dyslipidemia, and smoking. Symptoms to ask about include visual problems, periodontal irritations, skin rashes, fatigue, sexual dysfunction, and paresthesias (4). Within the family history, you should also ask about diabetes and premature cardiovascular disease. If there is a family history of diabetes, inquire about any complications of diabetes in family members. For women who have had children, a history of gestational diabetes or having a baby weighing more than 9 lb are important evidence of prior insulin resistance. In addition to current and past use of alcohol and tobacco, the social history should include current dietary habits (especially sweets, snacks, and regular soft drinks) and current physical activity.

The physical examination (Table 13.2) should pay close attention to organ systems and findings that indicate possible complications. Body mass index (BMI) should be calculated from height and weight. Blood pressure is critical and will guide treatment. A funduscopic examination will assess for cataracts and retinopathy. The oral cavity should be thoroughly examined for periodontal disease. Palpation of the thyroid and examination of the skin can give clues about possible coexisting hypothyroidism. Because they are a common site of neurological, vascular, and cutaneous manifestations of diabetes, the lower extremities should be a major focus of the physical examination. The skin should be inspected and palpated for skin color, temperature, dryness, nail thickness, and hair distribution on the lower extremities and feet. Corns, calluses, and any bony deformities deserve a thorough description. Neurologic examination includes vibratory sensation, light touch, and proprioception of the feet; light touch can best be assessed with the use of a monofilament. The dorsalis pedis and posterior tibial pulse should be palpated and described.

Referrals

An initial referral for dilated eye exam is indicated for all patients with type 2 diabetes shortly after diagnosis and for patients with type 1 diabetes within 5 years of diagnosis (Strength of Recommendation Taxonomy = B). Podiatry referral may also be indicated depending on the findings on the foot exam. Diabetes education and medical nutrition referrals are also indicated to help support self-management.

Diagnostic testing

Table 13.3 lists the diagnostic criteria for diabetes. The best test to obtain depends on the clinical presentation. In the presence of classic symptoms (polyuria, polydipsia, weight loss) or if there is a concern of hyperglycemic crises, a random plasma

TABLE 13.2 Components of Physical Exam of a Newly Diagnosed Patient with Diabetes

Exam Component	Rationale	Strength of Recommendation
Height, weight for calculating BMI	Comparison to norms, identify/document obesity	C
Blood pressure	Comparison to norms, identify hypertension	A
Funduscopic exam	Screen for retinopathy, cataracts	B (for ophthalmologist/ optometry referral)
Oral exam	Screen for periodontal disease	C (for dental referral)
Thyroid palpation	Increased risk of concomitant thyroid disease in diabetics	C
Cardiac exam	Screen for cardiovascular disease (e.g., CHF, murmurs)	C
Abdominal exam	Screen for hepatomegaly	C
Evaluation of pulses	Screen for peripheral vascular disease	C
Skin	Screen for infections, signs of glucose intolerance (acanthosis nigricans), evaluate sites for blood glucose monitoring	C
Foot and neurologic	Screen for lesions and infections, evaluate for peripheral neuropathy	B

A = consistent, good-quality patient-oriented evidence; B = inconsistent or limited-quality patient-oriented evidence; BMI = body mass index; C = consensus, disease-oriented evidence, usual practice, expert opinion, or case series; CHF = congestive heart failure.
For information about the Strength of Recommendation Taxonomy evidence rating system, see *http://www.aafp.org/afpsort.xml*.

glucose is the appropriate test. Values greater than or equal to 200 mg/dL are diagnostic of diabetes. In the absence of these classic symptoms, any one of three possible tests (glycosylated hemoglobin [A1C], fasting plasma glucose, or the 2-hour oral glucose tolerance test [OGTT]) can be used depending on availability (3). In the absence of significant hyperglycemia, these three tests require repeat testing for confirmation. An A1C level of 6.5% or higher has recently been recommended (6) and added as an option by the American Diabetes Association (ADA) (4). However, the A1C assay must be one that is certified by the National Glycohemoglobin Standardization Program; point-of-care A1C assays are not accurate enough at this time to be used for diagnosis (3). Patients may also be asked to return for a fasting plasma glucose (i.e., after at least 8 hours without any calories). Any fasting glucose result greater than 125 mg/dL is strongly suggestive of diabetes and should be repeated; two results above 125 mg/dL from different days are needed to make the diagnosis. The 2-hour OGTT is rarely used for routine clinical use given the cumbersome nature of the test.

TABLE 13.3 Diagnostic Criteria for Diabetes and Categories of Increased Risk*

Diagnosis	Criteria
Diabetes	Symptomatic and a random plasma glucose ≥200 mg/dL. OR A1C ≥6.5%+ OR Fasting plasma glucoses ≥126† mg/dL. OR 2-hour (75 g) glucose tolerance test ≥200 mg/dL.†
Increased risk for diabetes	Fasting plasma glucose 100–125 mg/dL (impaired fasting glucose/ prediabetes) 2-hour (75g) glucose tolerance test 140–199 mg/dL (impaired glucose tolerance/prediabetes) A1C 5.7–6.4%

*Based on the 2010 American Diabetes Association recommendations (3).
†Should be confirmed with repeat testing.

All three tests include ranges that place patients at increased risk for diabetes (3). If fasting plasma glucose is greater than 100 but less than 126 mg/dL, the patient is said to have impaired fasting glucose or prediabetes (4). Additionally, OGTT values between 140 and 200 mg/dL define impaired glucose tolerance or prediabetes. Patients with an A1C of 5.7–6.4% are also considered at increased risk for developing diabetes. Patients found to be in these increased risk categories should be counseled on ways to lower their risk, such as diet and physical activity (3).

In addition to confirming the diagnosis of diabetes, the laboratory evaluation is used to obtain several baseline measures. Obtain hemoglobin A1C to examine blood glucose control over the previous 3 months. A fasting lipid profile is obtained for cardiovascular risk stratification. Also, obtain a serum creatinine and calculated GFR to assess for the presence of kidney disease. Screen all type 2 diabetics with a microalbumin/creatinine test to determine future risk of renal disease (type 1 patients begin after having had diabetes for at least 5 years) (7). Finally, order a thyroid-stimulating hormone in all patients with type 1 and if clinically indicated, in those with type 2 diabetes.

Conveying the Diagnosis

The first task of the clinician who has made a diagnosis of diabetes is to convey this news to the patient. Patients with a recent diagnosis of diabetes need additional time and attention. Diabetes is a condition that requires patient participation in its management. Patients face the prospect of a lifelong medical condition with the potential for serious complications. If they are supported and well informed it encourages their involvement in self-management of diabetes at an early stage.

When delivering a new diagnosis of diabetes it is useful to present the information quickly and clearly and then use open-ended questions and reflective listening to explore the patient's reaction to the diagnosis. One technique that fosters open discussion is: deliver information (inform), allow for patient response (listen), and reflect response back to patient (ask guiding questions) (8). For example, "It sounds like you have had many family members who have had diabetes. Tell me more about that." Exploring the meaning of diabetes for your patient can provide valuable clues that can help you identify his or her individual motivation. Often patients will have erroneous information about diabetes, and this can be an opportunity to dispel those myths. If your patient relates that a grandmother had kidney failure from diabetes, this can open a conversation. For example, you might say, "It sounds like your grandmother had many of the problems that are related to diabetes including kidney failure, dialysis, and other complications." This statement can lay the groundwork for a discussion about managing diabetes. You could say something like, "The good news is we know so much more about the treatment of diabetes now than we did even a few years ago. I want to work with you to reduce your chances of developing the problems your grandmother had."

At this point you are ready to introduce the basic concepts of managing diabetes. Being able to convey the importance of making lifestyle changes in a nonjudgmental way is important and critical to getting the patient "on board" with self-management (9). Developing the skill of discussing the consequences of unhealthy choices without passing a moral judgment of the behavior takes practice. For example, if the patient relates that he developed diabetes because of laziness or lack of exercise, acknowledge the response and follow it with a possible solution or open ended question, such as, "Yes, lack of exercise might have contributed, but it's not too late to start exercising now, and you can really make a difference in your blood sugar." Exploring practical strategies with the patient can be helpful. Asking the patient if he can take walks in the neighborhood may be more practical than asking him to join a gym, for example.

Although having a patient go from accepting the diagnosis to making a solid commitment to longstanding behavior change will often take more than one visit, you will want to touch on the key issues of behavior change as part of this initial visit. Closure of the visit acknowledges that it takes time to learn to live well with diabetes. A key message the patient should hear is that he or she can make a difference in his diabetes care and that you will work with the patient to keep him or her healthy. It is a good idea to provide the patient with some reading materials that will reinforce these initial concepts. The ADA website (*www.diabetes.org*) has good and reliable information for patients.

MANAGEMENT

Comprehensive management of diabetes must deal with both the metabolic problems and the increased risk of cardiovascular disease. It requires ongoing attention to cardiovascular risk factors, education, and support in self-management of the disease, and a focus on metabolic goals of therapy. To meet these goals, patients and their physicians need to combine behavioral strategies with pharmacologic interventions. Table 13.4 summarizes the components of comprehensive management of diabetes. Within the table and in the subsequent discussion, different management strategies are prioritized by the evidence.

Blood Pressure Control

Evidence from well done clinical trials demonstrates the importance of blood pressure (BP) control in the comprehensive care of people with diabetes (10–13). Tight management of BP to goals of a systolic BP <130 mm Hg and a diastolic BP <80 mm Hg lowers the risk of both macrovascular and microvascular complications. In one large randomized trial, control of BP to a goal of <130/85 mm Hg reduced diabetes-related endpoints by 24%, compared with a BP goal of <150/105 mm Hg (10). In contrast, tight blood glucose control reduced the same endpoints by only 12% (10). In another randomized trial, the number needed to treat (NNT) for 10 years to a diastolic BP goal of 80 mm Hg (compared with a diastolic BP goal of 90 mm Hg) to prevent 1 cardiovascular death was 14 (11).

In addition to diet and activity, many patients will require medications to reach BP targets. Antihypertensives that have been shown to reduce cardiovascular events in diabetic patients include angiotensin-converting enzyme (ACE) inhibitors, angiotensin receptor blockers (ARBs), β-blockers, diuretics, and calcium channel blockers. Although all of these drug classes have proven efficacy against macrovascular complications in patients with diabetes, the ACE inhibitors (e.g., enalapril) and ARBs (e.g., losartan) have particular benefit in reducing the risk of microalbuminuria and the progression to nephropathy. With ACE inhibitors and ARBs, renal function and serum potassium require monitoring (14).

Drug therapy for hypertension in diabetes mellitus should include an ACE inhibitor or ARB with the addition of a thiazide diuretic to achieve BP targets. The ADVANCE trial (12) examined the combination of an ACE inhibitor with a diuretic and showed a reduction in the risk of major macrovascular and microvascular events (NNT of 77 over 4.3 years). In patients with any degree of albuminuria or nephropathy who are unable to tolerate ACE inhibitors or ARBs, BP management with β-blockers, diuretics, or nondihydropyridine calcium channel blockers is indicated (15). See Chapter 11 for further information on treatment of hypertension.

Tobacco Cessation

One of the most important things that a smoker with diabetes can do to improve his or her health is to quit smoking (16). Smoking cessation counseling from a provider is particularly effective (17). The number needed to counsel for one smoker to quit varies between 8 and 13 depending on the length of the counseling and the number of counseling sessions (16). Quit lines (e.g., 1–800-QUIT-NOW) can assist busy physicians by providing follow-up phone counseling to smokers who are

TABLE 13.4 Management of Diabetes: Key Recommendations for Practice

Area/Topic	Recommendation	NNT	Strength of Recommendation*
Treatment of hypertension	Maintain BP below 130/80 mm Hg	NNT for 10 years to prevent 1 diabetes-related endpoint: 6	A
	Advise patients to follow DASH diet		C
	If microalbuminuria is present, treat with ACE inhibitors or ARBs		A
Smoking cessation	Counseling on smoking cessation	NNT for 10 years to save 1 life: 11	A
Aspirin therapy to prevent stroke	For women with increased 10-year risk of stroke: take 81 mg aspirin daily to reduce risk of stroke For men with increased 10-year risk of CHD: take 81 mg aspirin daily to reduce risk of heart attack	NNT for 10 years to prevent 1 stroke: 16 NNT for 10 years to prevent 1 MI: 46	A
Management of dyslipidemia	Use statins to treat to LDL goal <100 mg/dL	NNT for 10 years to prevent 1 major CHD event: 15	A
Management of hyperglycemia	A team approach to care (e.g., provider, nurse, pharmacist, diabetes educator) improves outcomes and patient satisfaction		A
	Long-term A1C below or around 7.0% lowers risk of microvascular and possibly macrovascular complications	NNT for 10 years to prevent 1 diabetes related endpoint 17; NNT for 10 years to prevent 1 CVD event: 47	A
	Metformin is the initial drug of choice for patients who can take it		A
	When insulin is started, oral agents should be continued, to reduce total insulin needs and weight gain		A
	Glucose self monitoring improves overall management of hyperglycemia in patients treated with insulin		C
	Monitor A1C every 6 months and more frequently if target levels have not been reached		C
Screening for and management of complications	In patients with retinopathy, control of blood pressure and glucose, laser photocoagulation, vitrectomy, and other interventions can help preserve sight		A
	Screen for nephropathy annually using the spot microalbumin/creatinine ratio (<30 mg/g is normal)		C
	Screen annually for peripheral neuropathy		B
	Perform foot exam annually		C

A = consistent, good-quality patient-oriented evidence; B = inconsistent or limited-quality patient-oriented evidence; BP = blood pressure; CVD = cardiovascular disease; C = consensus, disease-oriented evidence, usual practice, expert opinion, or case series; CHD = coronary heart disease; DASH = Dietary Approaches to Stop Hypertension; NNT = number needed to treat; MI = myocardial infarction.
*For information about the Strength of Recommendation Taxonomy evidence rating system, see *http://www.aafp.org/afpsort.xml*.

ready to quit. See Chapter 47 (Addiction) for further information on smoking cessation.

Aspirin Prophylaxis

Any patient with diabetes and any form of cardiovascular disease (coronary heart disease [CHD], cerebrovascular disease [CRVD], or peripheral arterial disease) will benefit from aspirin as a secondary preventive intervention. Doses of 81 mg to 325 mg daily have been tested in many trials. The most recent update of the Antiplatelet Trialists Collaborative meta-analysis reported that in patients with CHD, risk of death from any cause is reduced by 20% (OR = 0.80, 95% CI 0.75–0.86) with aspirin. For patients with a history of CRVD, aspirin reduced the risk of all-cause mortality by 9% (OR= 0.91, 95% CI 0.85–0.98) (18).

For patients with diabetes who do not have cardiovascular disease, the use of aspirin for primary prevention is less well established. Multiple primary preventive trials have found modest benefits for aspirin in the primary prevention of CHD for men and CRVD for women. These benefits of aspirin have to be weighed against the risks of gastrointestinal (GI) bleeding and hemorrhagic stroke. The US Preventive Services Task Force (USPSTF) has recently reviewed the available evidence and updated their recommendations (19). The benefit of aspirin, stated as numbers of MIs prevented, varies based on the 10-year risk of heart disease. On the other hand, the risk of aspirin from GI bleeding varies with age. Evidence-based recommendations need to take both of these factors into account.

In practice, the 10-year risk of CHD or CRVD is easy to calculate using internet-based tools. A tool that is specific for patients with diabetes is based on the UKPDS study and can be downloaded from *http://www.dtu.ox.ac.uk/index.php?maindoc=/riskengine/*. The majority of men with diabetes older than age 45 and women with diabetes older than age 55 will have risks of CHD or stroke that are above the thresholds where benefits of aspirin outweigh the risks.

Two recent randomized controlled trials of aspirin as a primary preventive strategy in patients with diabetes have been reported (20, 21). Ogawa and colleagues randomized 2,539 patients with type 2 diabetes from more than 160 institutions throughout Japan. After a median follow up of 4.37 years, there were no statistically significant differences in atherosclerotic events (hazard ratio of 0.80, favoring aspirin, but 95% CI 0.58–1.10). In terms of cardiovascular mortality, there was 1 death in the aspirin group (stroke) and 10 deaths in the nonaspirin group (5 strokes and 5 fatal MIs). This difference was statistically significant (HR = 0.10, 95% CI 0.01–0.79). There was a 10% reduction in all cause mortality in the aspirin group, but this did not achieve statistical significance (21). Despite these data, many other trials have found benefit in specific populations and based on cardiovascular risk, aspirin should still be considered.

A meta-analysis of aspirin for primary prevention of CVD events in patients with diabetes included seven trials with a total of 11,618 patients (22). Aspirin therapy reduced risk of cardiovascular events by 8% (RR = 0.92, 95% CI 0.71–1.27), which was not statistically significant. The authors did find that trials with a higher percentage of male participants showed a 29% nearly significant reduction in MI risk from aspirin (RR = 0.71, 95% CI 0.5–1.0, $p = 0.05$). In a hypothetical cohort that was 55% male, one would need to treat 95 people for 4.5 years to prevent one MI. Trials with more women showed a 33% reduction in risk of stroke (RR = 0.67, 95% CI 0.48–0.92). Similarly, in a hypothetical cohort that is 86% women, one would need to treat 56 women for 3 years to prevent one stroke. The rationale for recommending aspirin as a primary preventive strategy for patients with diabetes may vary based on gender, but the end result is in keeping with the USPSTF recommendation. The number of GI bleeds with aspirin overall is low (0.4 to 6.0 per 1,000 person/years depending on age/gender in patients with no GI bleeding risk factors, and the cost is very low) (23, 24).

Even in those with a history of GI bleeding or prior peptic ulcer, the benefit of aspirin is still possible. Such patients should be tested for *Helicobacter pylori* and treated if infected. If the patient is on a second antiplatelet agent, on concomitant anticoagulant therapy, or has GI symptoms of dyspepsia or reflux, coadministration of a proton pump inhibitor with aspirin is appropriate (25). For patients with an absolute contraindication to aspirin therapy, other antiplatelet therapy may be an option, but the evidence is scant (19).

Lipid Lowering

Diabetes is associated with multiple lipid abnormalities, including increased total cholesterol, triglycerides, and low-density lipoprotein (LDL) cholesterol, and a decreased high density lipoprotein (HDL) cholesterol. These abnormalities often cluster with obesity, insulin resistance, and hypertension to form the metabolic syndrome or, more recently, the construct of global cardiometabolic risk (26). Behavioral management with the DASH diet and exercise improves all of these abnormalities (27). Use of statins to lower LDL-cholesterol to levels as low as 70 mg/dL (non HDL-cholesterol <100 mg/dL) has been proven to reduce CVD events in diabetics with a 10 year CVD risk of 12 percent or greater (28,29). In this group of patients with diabetes and no CHD, the number needed to treat for 1 year to prevent 1 CHD event is 150. Now with generic statins available at low cost and given their low incidence of side effects, statins are a reasonable and advocated measure to decrease overall cardiovascular risk in people with diabetes.

The most recent guidelines from the ADA advocate an LDL target of less than 100 mg/dL for all adults with diabetes, with less than 70 mg/dL deemed an 'option' for those with known cardiovascular disease (4). Achieving these lipid targets requires a combined approach with statin therapy and lifestyle modification in most patients. If the target LDL goal <100 mg/dL cannot be reached with maximal doses of statin therapy, reduction in LDL of 30–40% is an acceptable alternative goal (4). In patients unable to take a statin, consider fibrates over other antihyperlipidemics as they have been shown to decrease cardiovascular events (30).

In addition to lowering LDL, the ADA has identified triglyceride levels less than 150 mg/dL and high density lipoproteins (HDL) greater than 40 mg/dL in men and greater than 50 mg/dL in women as desirable, although these goals are secondary to the LDL targets mentioned previously (4). Patients with combined hyperlipidemia and very high triglyceride levels (>400 mg/dL) may need to have the triglyceride abnormalities addressed primarily, usually with either a fibric acid derivative or niacin. Non-statin drugs might also be considered for patients whose HDL cholesterol is lower than target and whose LDL cholesterol is less than 140 mg/dL. Niacin has been found to be effective in a secondary prevention trial in such patients

(31). Although historically there have been concerns of worsening glucose levels in people treated with niacin to improve HDL, other evidence has shown that the negative effect on blood glucose is minimal (32). Overall, the level of evidence for combining statins with other agents is not as strong as high-dose statins alone, and combination therapy increases the risk of liver abnormalities, myalgias, and rhabdomyolysis (33).

Glucose Control

Long-term successful management of blood glucose to a goal of A1C below 7.0 % clearly lowers the risk of microvascular complications. This has been shown for both type 1 (34) and type 2 (35) diabetes. The relationship between management of hyperglycemia and risk of macrovascular complications has historically been less clear. The Action to Control Cardiovascular Risk in Diabetes study halted the glycemic control trial because of increased mortality in the intensive control arm (A1C <6%) versus the standard control arm (A1C 7–7.9%) (5% vs 4%; HR 1.22, 95% CI 1.01–1.46, number needed to harm = 100) (36). For patients with type 1 diabetes, a 17-year follow-up from the Diabetes Care and Complications Trial demonstrated that successful management of blood glucose to a goal A1C of 7.0% early in the course of disease is associated with a 3.6% statistically significant reduction in absolute risk of CHD events. Thus, the NNT for an A1C target of 7.0% to prevent one patient from developing CHD over 17 years (heart disease death, nonfatal MI, angina, coronary revascularization) is 28 (37). The relationship between glycemic control and subsequent complications is more logarithmic than linear. Clinically, this means that there is a greater reduction in subsequent risk of complications from lowering an A1C from 10% to 8% than there is from lowering the A1C from 8% to 6%. As one might expect, the risk of hypoglycemic complications goes up as the A1C value gets closer to 6%. Management of hyperglycemia begins with behavioral management. For women of reproductive age, contraception until excellent glycemic control has been achieved is important to minimize risk of fetal abnormalities.

BEHAVIORAL MANAGEMENT

The initial behavioral changes that are required with diabetes include dietary changes and physical activity. Carbohydrates (CHO) are the nutrients that have the largest effect on blood sugar levels and remain the initial focus in a patient with diabetes. A major nutrition goal therefore is limitation of CHO intake. Patients should learn the sources of CHO in their diet and how to balance CHO intake with oral medication or insulin. Most patients will have to eliminate high CHO items (e.g., regular sodas, syrup, fruit juices, sweeteners) to be able to regulate their blood sugar. Helping the patient identify the CHO sources in his or her diet can provide ideas for clear practical changes. For example, if a patient tells you he is having sugar-sweetened tea each night with dinner, you might ask if he would be willing to switch to unsweetened tea or tea with an artificial sweetener. Open discussion of changes patients are willing to make empowers them in mastering the dietary changes that diabetes often requires (38). Non-nutritive or artificial sweeteners are considered safe when used in recommended amounts. Reducing overall calorie intake is recommended for weight loss but popular low CHO diets (<130 g/day) are not recommended. Patients on such diets may demonstrate greater weight loss and blood sugar lowering effect in early months of the diet, but both weight and blood sugar levels are similar at 1 year (39). Further, low-CHO diets are difficult to maintain and can raise LDL cholesterol levels. Other general dietary recommendations include increasing fiber intake, whole grains, fruits and vegetables, and reducing saturated fats and trans fats. Some patients may benefit from a visit with a registered dietician who can provide an individualized nutrition assessment and plan.

Patients with diabetes should be encouraged to exercise. Exercise is an essential component of management of diabetes. The ADA exercise recommendation is 150 minutes per week or 20 minutes per day of moderate intensity aerobic physical activity, and in the absence of comorbid contraindications, strength training 2 days per week. In one trial, an endurance and strength training program of 24 months' duration reduced participants'A1C levels, insulin levels, and blood pressure. Of note, A1C values decreased from an average of 8.2 to 7.6% (40). Exercise, whether moderate or vigorous has been shown to increase insulin sensitivity in patients with diabetes (41). Another study found that exercise lowered abdominal visceral fat, increased insulin sensitivity, and improved lipid profiles (42).

Many patients may be resistant to exercise. Emphasis should be on "starting low and going slow" if they have not been exercising on a regular basis. Often patients need help identifying barriers to exercise. Open ended nonjudgmental questions will help patients come up with their own ideas. For example, you might ask, "If you were going to exercise, what would you do?" This may lead to, "What keeps you from exercising?" Asking questions that prompt patients' own solutions will help overcome the barriers to making behavior changes.

PHARMACOLOGIC MANAGEMENT

For patients who do not reach their A1C goal with behavioral management, drug therapy is recommended. There are three major classes of oral agents available for treatment of type 2 DM: metformin, the sulfonylureas, and the thiazolidinediones. Table 13.5 summarizes the common medications and their use.

The United Kingdom Preventive Diabetes Study (UKPDS) provides the best evidence to guide the initial choice of medication to control hyperglycemia. The major findings of this 10-year study can be summarized as follows:

- Sulfonylureas, metformin, and insulin were equally effective as initial therapy at reaching the intensive goal of an A1C of 7.0%.
- Over the 10 years of follow-up, glycemic control deteriorated equally in all groups, requiring dosage increases and/or additional agents to reach glycemic goals.
- The risk of major hypoglycemic episodes was lower for metformin (0.6% per year) than for sulfonylureas (1% per year) or insulin (2% per year).
- Patients randomized to metformin had fewer deaths than patients randomized to other forms of intensive therapy or to conventional therapy (NNT for 1 year to prevent one death = 141).

Given the UKPDS findings along with its low cost and lack of associated weight gain, metformin is recommended as initial pharmacologic therapy for people with type 2 DM when behavioral management is unsuccessful in meeting

TABLE 13.5 Medications Commonly Used for the Treatment of Diabetes Mellitus

Medication	Medication Brand Name	Dosing Forms	Dosing Pearls	Comments
Biguanides				
Metformin	Glucophage, Glucophage XR	Tablets Oral solution XR tablets	Renal excretion (avoid in men with SCr >1.5 mg/dL or women with SCr >1.4 mg/dL) Start at a low dose to avoid GI side effects	Watch for signs and symptoms of lactic acidosis
Sulfonylureas				
Glimepiride	Amaryl	Tablets	Titrate dose to effect	Renal excretion
Glipizide, Glipizide extended release (ER)	Glucotrol, Glucotrol XL	Tablets ER tablets	Titrate dose to effect	Renal excretion May be best for use in elderly or decreased renal function because of shorter half-life
Glyburide	DiaBeta, Micronase, Glynase	Tablets	Titrate dose to effect	Renal excretion
Micronized Glyburide	Glynase PresTab	Tablets	Titrate dose to effect	Renal excretion
Thiazolidinediones				
Pioglitazone	Actos	Tablets	Titrate dose to effect	Hepatic elimination Risk of CHF Expensive
Rosiglitazone	Avandia	Tablets	Titrate dose to effect	Hepatic elimination Risk of CHF Expensive
Newer Agents				
Sitagliptin	Januvia	Tablets	Renal elimination Dose for renal function	Expensive Risk of pancreatitis
Exenatide	Byetta	Injection Solution Injection pens	Administer 60 minutes before food or drugs that require threshold	Very expensive Risk of pancreatitis

CHF = congestive heart failure; CrCl = creatinine clearance; CV = cardiovascular; GI = gastrointestinal; LFTs = liver function tests; OCPs = oral contraceptives; SCr = serum creatinine; TZD = thiazolidinediones; XR/ER = extended release.

glycemic management goals (43). It was the only glycemic therapy in the UKPDS trial to show a positive impact on mortality and was associated with the lowest risk of hypoglycemia.

Metformin

As discussed previously, metformin is recommended as initial pharmacologic therapy for type 2 DM. It acts primarily by reducing hepatic glucose production and increasing peripheral glucose utilization. It lowers A1C by an average of 1.5–2.0%. In addition to its beneficial effects on blood glucose, metformin also positively affects other important physiologic processes in patients with diabetes, including blood lipids, blood pressure, and clotting activity. Metformin also consistently causes weight loss of 1–5 kg when compared with thiazolidinediones, second-generation sulfonylureas, or combination therapy with metformin and a second-generation sulfonylurea, all of which tend to increase weight (44). Metformin is eliminated by the kidneys; therefore, it is to be avoided when the serum creatinine is 1.5 mg/dL or greater in men or 1.4 mg/dL or greater in women.

The most common side effects of metformin are gastrointestinal; they include nausea, vomiting, anorexia, and diarrhea. These effects tend to be transient for 2–4 weeks after initiation or dosage increases, and are dose-related. To minimize these effects, start at 500 mg once per day (with the evening meal) and increase the dose slowly, titrating upward on a weekly basis. The maximum dose is 2,550 mg daily given in divided doses with meals. If side effects occur, the dose can be reduced for a period of time or the drug can be stopped temporarily. Metformin alone rarely causes hypoglycemia; however, hypoglycemia can occur with strenuous exercise without caloric intake or with concomitant intake of alcohol or other hypoglycemic medications.

Metformin inhibits lactate metabolism, and the greatest risk of metformin is lactic acidosis, occurring at a rate of 3–5 cases per 100,000 patient-years (45). Risk factors include age older than 80 years, concurrent diuretic therapy, recent radiographic contrast, and dehydration (e.g., from acute diarrhea or vomiting, septicemia, impaired hepatic function, acute renal failure, hypoxemia, or alcohol abuse). To minimize the risk of lactic acidosis, metformin should not be used in people with renal insufficiency (creatinine level ≥1.5 mg/dL in men, 1.4 mg/dL in women). Also, the drug should be discontinued before and for 48 hours after radiographic studies with intravenous contrast that may transiently affect renal function.

Caution should be used in patients who are pregnant or lactating, have active liver disease, chronic obstructive pulmonary disease, or active alcoholism. Education for patients prescribed metformin should include temporarily stopping its use when undergoing any radiographic procedure involving intravenous contrast and during any acute GI illness with vomiting or diarrhea.

The monthly cost of generic metformin is approximately $13.00–32.00 depending on dose. The only advantage of the more expensive extended release form is that the maximum dose can be taken once a day (46, 47).

Sulfonylureas

Sulfonylureas lower blood glucose by stimulating pancreatic insulin secretion and increasing tissue sensitivity to insulin. Sulfonylureas lower A1C an average of 1.5–2.0%. Although there are seven sulfonylureas, only the three second-generation drugs (glipizide, glyburide, and glimepiride) are commonly used. Several general principles guide the use of these agents:

- Choose an agent with a relatively short half-life to minimize the risk of hypoglycemia (glipizide has the lowest rate).
- Start with a low dose given with the morning meal.
- Increase the dose every 5–7 days, as needed to reach glycemic goal.
- Divide doses above 50% of the maximum—the second dose given with the evening meal.
- Do not switch back and forth between agents. There are no major differences in their efficacy, and switching from one to another is rarely helpful.

The biggest risk of sulfonylureas is hypoglycemia, occurring in about 1% of patients per year. This risk is higher when using drugs that have a longer half-life and in patients with impaired renal function. For this reason, education for patients prescribed sulfonylureas should include reducing the dose if they are going to skip a meal or are not eating because of an acute GI illness. All of the sulfonylureas are now available generically; the monthly cost is approximately $12.00–20.00 depending on dose. There is no advantage to the long-acting forms except that they can be given once per day (46, 47).

Thiazolidinediones

The two thiazolidinediones (TZDs), pioglitazone and rosiglitazone, act primarily by decreasing peripheral insulin resistance in skeletal muscle and adipose tissue. These drugs lower A1C by an average of 1.0% to 1.5%. In addition to lowering glucose values, they also lower triglycerides slightly and increase both LDL and HDL cholesterol. They can be used alone or in combination therapy with metformin, sulfonylureas, or insulin.

TZDs are extensively metabolized in the liver; therefore, they are contraindicated in patients with active liver disease or liver enzymes greater than 2.5 times normal. Elevations in liver enzymes and liver failure can occur due to these agents, so liver transaminases (aspartate aminotransferase or alanine aminotransferase) should be monitored before beginning these drugs and every 2 months during the first year of therapy. Signs and symptoms of liver disease at any time require immediate testing of liver function, and the development of jaundice should prompt immediate drug discontinuation while further evaluation is pending.

TZDs can cause fluid retention, which can lead to weight gain, edema, and new or worsening congestive heart failure (CHF). Therefore, preexisting New York Heart Association Class III or Class IV CHF is a contraindication to their use. A meta-analysis of published and unpublished trials evaluating rosiglitazone and the effects on cardiovascular outcomes revealed an increased risk of MI (RR 1.43; 95% CI, 1.03 to 1.98; $p = 0.03$) (48). Subsequent studies have neither confirmed nor refuted these findings for rosiglitazone. The current black box warning on the Food and Drug Administration (FDA) package insert for rosiglitazone states that its effects on myocardial ischemia are inconclusive.

The TZDs have not been evaluated in pregnant or lactating women and therefore should not be used during pregnancy or breastfeeding. They can occasionally induce ovulation in premenopausal women who are anovulatory; therefore, women of childbearing age taking these drugs need to use effective contraception.

Given the possible risks of cardiovascular events with rosiglitazone and lack of a similar association with pioglitazone, pioglitazone is the TZD of choice (49). Certainly, education for patients taking one of these drugs should include the need to seek prompt medical attention for any unexplained anorexia, fatigue, nausea, vomiting, abdominal pain, or dark urine, which might represent liver toxicity. Patients should also be encouraged to report potential symptoms of CHF, such as rapid weight gain, orthopnea, paroxysmal nocturnal dyspnea, or worsening dyspnea on exertion. The average monthly cost of these medications varies from $80 to $160 depending on the dosage (47).

Newer Agents

Sitagliptin exerts its glucose lowering effect by inhibiting dipeptidyl peptidase-4, a protease that degrades glucagon-like peptide 1 (GLP-1). GLP-1 is a glucose-dependent stimulator of insulin secretion and an inhibitor of glucagon release. Therefore, sitagliptin indirectly increases insulin secretion and decreases circulating glucagons. Sitagliptin has been studied alone and in combination with metformin, glimepiride, and pioglitazone in patients with Type 2 DM. In monotherapy trials, sitagliptin decreases A1C by an average of 0.4% to 1%, and in combination with metformin, glimepiride, or pioglitazone, it decreases A1C by an average of 0.7–1% (50). One trial examined triple therapy with sitagliptin, metformin, and glimepiride with an additional A1C decrease of 0.9% versus glimepiride and metformin alone (51). As with other antidiabetic agents, sitagliptin decreases A1C to a greater extent in those with diabetes for a shorter time and those with higher A1Cs at baseline.

The FDA changed the prescribing information for sitagliptin (marketed as Januvia or the combination product Janumet) to highlight the risk of acute pancreatitis with use. In less than 3 years of postmarketing use, 88 cases of acute pancreatitis were reported to the FDA as associated with sitagliptin. When prescribing sitagliptin, prescribers should consider the patients risk of pancreatitis and discuss the warning signs of pancreatitis with patients. In clinical trials, the most common side effects in treated patients versus placebo were nasopharyngitis, back pain, osteoarthritis and pain in extremities (50). The effect of sitagliptin on serum lipids is likely unchanged, but the trials have had inconsistent results (50). Sitagliptin does not appear to increase weight in patients with diabetes (50). A concern for drugs that affect GLP-1 is the potential for increased blood pressure based on animal models, but a study of nondiabetic patients with hypertension did not show a significant effect on BP (52).

Exenatide, another newer agent, is a GLP-1 receptor agonist that directly stimulates glucose-dependent release of insulin and depresses glucagon levels. Exenatide is indicated for the treatment of type 2 DM and decreases A1C by about 0.9%. Potential side effects include GI effects such as nausea, vomiting, and diarrhea, and when combined with a sulfonylurea there is an increased risk of hypoglycemia. Reports of pancreatitis, although not causally proven, have occurred with exenatide. Use caution in patients with a history of pancreatitis (53).

The major deterrents to exenatide use are the need for twice-daily injections and the high cost. Although it is available as a pen for injection, easing the preparation of the injection for the dose, most patients prefer an oral tablet to an injectable product.

Insulin

Rational therapy with exogenous insulin is based on knowledge of the physiology of endogenous insulin secretion. The pancreatic β-cell constantly secretes insulin even in a fasting state. This *basal* insulin secretion is supplemented with *bolus* insulin secretion after a meal, in response to rising levels of glucose. In type 2 DM, insulin therapy is usually begun as a basal insulin strategy with once a day long-acting insulin injections. The pancreas, assisted by oral agents, continues to deal with postprandial bolus insulin secretion. Pancreatic failure is progressive in type 2 DM; however, many patients end up requiring a twice-a-day or more intensive insulin regimen. These regimens are designed to meet both basal and bolus insulin requirements. Basal insulin for type 2 DM can be given at nighttime or as a twice-daily regimen.

When adding basal insulin for management of type 2 DM, oral agents are generally continued as well. The continuation of metformin, alone or in combination with other agents, results in slightly better glucose control and reduced weight gain when initiating basal insulin therapy (54). If a patient taking a sulfonylurea is begun on basal insulin and develops hypoglycemia, it is appropriate to reduce the dose of the sulfonylurea by 50%. Dosage adjustment after initial dosing of insulin is crucial for success of any insulin regimen. A commonly used algorithm is to ask patients to adjust their insulin dose every 3 days, as follows: If the mean fasting plasma glucose is greater than 100 mg/dL for the preceding 3 days, the patient is asked to increase the bedtime insulin dose by 2 units. Table 13.6 summarizes these recommendations.

There are three insulin preparations available for nighttime insulin therapy (Table 13.7). Neutral protamine hagedorn (NPH) insulin is the older, now generic, preparation. Glargine and detemir insulins are the newer insulin analogs. All are equally effective at lowering A1C and fasting plasma glucose when added to oral therapy in patients with type 2 DM. However, there is a significantly lower rate of hypoglycemia with glargine insulin than with NPH insulin; the NNT with glargine insulin compared with NPH insulin for 1 year to prevent one severe hypoglycemic event is 71 (54). Hypoglycemic events with NPH were more likely to occur during the night; hypoglycemic events from glargine were more likely to occur between 9:00 a.m. and 1:00 p.m. A 26-week noninferiority trial comparing insulin detemir and insulin glargine found comparable efficacy and safety outcomes in patients with type 2 DM (55). Patients randomized to detemir experienced significantly less weight gain than with glargine (1.2 ± 3.96 kg vs 2.7 ± 3.94 kg, $p = 0.001$) (55). Choice among the insulin preparations will depend on provider and patient preference, risk of hypoglycemia, and ability to pay for the different preparations.

As type 2 DM progresses, bedtime insulin and oral agents may not be adequate, and patients may once again exceed their A1C goal. In this situation, twice-daily insulin injections are indicated. A logical next step is to initiate a combined form of insulin, usually a 70/30 mix of a rapid and intermediate duration form of insulin—either 70/30 regular/NPH or 70/30 aspart/protamine aspart.

Insulin Therapy in Type 1 Diabetes

All patients with type 1 diabetes require insulin therapy to avoid hyperglycemia and diabetic ketoacidosis. Given the insulin deficiency that accompanies type 1 diabetes, all of these regimens will need to replace both basal and bolus insulin requirements. More recent regimens include three or four injections per day or continuous infusion insulin pumps. A common regimen would be the use of glargine insulin to replace basal needs (either once a day or equal injections twice a day) and multiple injections of lispro or aspart insulin solution 15 minutes before meals. The short-acting insulin analogues have shown to have a modest 0.1% greater reduction in A1C when compared with regular insulin in patients with type 1 diabetes (56). They also have a lower rate of hypoglycemia than traditional insulin therapy. These insulin analogues seem to offer more of an advantage when used with an insulin pump in continuous subcutaneous insulin infusion. For patients using basal bolus regimens with injections (as opposed to an infusion pump), basal insulin adjustments are made every 3 to 5 days in the same way as in the nighttime regimen for type 2 DM described previously.

Strategy for Use of Hypoglycemic Medications in Type 2 DM

Figure 13.1 illustrates an overall strategy for the management of hyperglycemia in patients with type 2 DM. Initial evaluation includes the development of an individualized A1C goal. For most patients this will be <7.0%; it may be higher in

TABLE 13.6 Insulin Therapy Guidelines (55,69)

Visit	Goals of Visit	Details
I. Starting a Patient on Nighttime Basal Insulin		
Before initiating insulin	Review behavioral management Teach or review self monitoring blood glucose monitoring (SMBG) Teach adjustment of insulin dose based on SMBG results Teach injection technique Review signs, symptoms, and treatment of hypoglycemia	Best done by a certified diabetes educator (CDE) Follow-up in 1 week
Visit at which insulin is initiated	Calculate initial insulin dose Review patient's injection technique Review SBGM, adjustment algorithm and hypoglycemia instructions	Initial dose = FPG (mg/dL)/18 Dosage adjustment: If mean of previous 3 FPG measurements is >100 mg/dL and no PG measurement is less than 70 mg/dL, increase bedtime insulin dose by 2 units Rx for daytime hypoglycemia: • Mild hypoglycemia (can be managed by patient) during the day, reduce sulfonylurea dose by 25% • Severe (requires assistance from someone else) hypoglycemia during the day, reduce sulfonylurea dose by 50% • Rx for nighttime hypoglycemia: • For any documented hypoglycemic episode at night, reduce insulin dose by 2 units, wait 1 week before any dose increases • Follow-up (phone or visit) in 1 week
Subsequent visits	Consider nonvisit review of SBGM (fax, e-mail, electronic transmission from glucose meter)	Initial monitoring is daily, can become less frequent once patient has reached goals
II. Initiating and Adjusting BID Insulin		
Before starting BID regimen	Discontinue sulfonylurea; continue metformin, TZD agent Review SBGM, new insulin adjustment algorithm, diet and exercise plans; if not already SBGM BID, begin BID monitoring (fasting, before evening meal)	
Starting dose	AM: 50% of previous nighttime insulin dose	PM: 50% of previous nighttime insulin dose
Dose adjustment	AM dose adjustments based on before-evening-meal SBGM readings	PM dose adjustments based on fasting before-breakfast SBGM readings
Dose adjustment frequency	Make dose *reductions* based on a reading <70 mg/dL the very next day	Make dose *increases* based on the average glucose reading from the previous 3 days every 3 days
Dose decrease details	If any before supper PG measurement is <70 mg/dL, reduce the before-breakfast insulin dose by 2 units beginning the next morning	If any FPG measurements is <70 mg/dL, reduce the before-supper insulin dose by 2 units beginning that afternoon

AM = morning; CDE = certified diabetes educator; BID = twice per day; FPG = fasting plasma glucose; F/U = follow-up; PG = plasma glucose; PM = evening; SBGM = self blood glucose monitoring; TZD = thiazolidinedione.

TABLE 13.7 Pharmacology and Use of Insulin Preparations

	Insulin	Onset (hours)	Peak (hours)	Duration (hours)	Compatibilities*	Practical Use
Rapid-acting	Lispro insulin solution (analog); *Brand: Humalog*	0.25	0.5–1.5	2–5	NPH, ultralente	Rapid-acting insulin analogs are used with meals to decrease post-prandial rise in BG
	Insulin aspart solution (analog); *Brand: NovoLog*	0.25	1–3	3–5	NPH	
	Insulin glulisine solution; *Brand: Apidra*	0.25	1–1.5	3–5	NPH	
Short-acting	Insulin (regular); *Brand: Humulin R; Novolin R*	0.5–1	2–5	8–12	All except glargine	Regular human insulin used with meals to decrease postprandial rise in BG Less expensive than rapid-acting insulin analogues
Intermediate-acting	Isophane insulin suspension (NPH); *Brand: Humulin N; Novolin N*	1–1.5	4–12	24	Regular, aspart, lispro	Used with regular insulin to manage total daily insulin requirements Usually administered twice daily Infrequent use
	Insulin zinc suspension (lente); *Brand: Humulin L*	1–2.5	7–15	24	Regular, semilente, ultralente	
Long-acting	Extended insulin zinc suspension (ultralente); *Brand: Humulin U*	4.8	10–30	20–36	Regular, lente, semilente, lispro	Infrequent use Used as once daily long-acting insulin Can be used once or twice daily
	Insulin glargine solution (analog); *Brand: Lantus*	1.1	No real peak	24	None	
	Insulin detemir solution; *Brand: Levemir*	Data not available	6–8	Dose-dependent	None	

BG = blood glucose.
*Compatibilities are important for mixing insulins to minimize the total number of subcutaneous injections daily.

patients who are diagnosed after 60 years of age or in whom some other disease is likely to shorten their life expectancy (4). It is important to remember that behavioral management is the cornerstone of hyperglycemic management of diabetes and deserves to be reemphasized at every visit. Many patients will require the addition of drug therapy, and metformin is the initial choice for patients who can take it (35). On the basis of their safety, efficacy, and relatively low cost, sulfonylureas are an appropriate choice for a second agent if one is needed. Pioglitazone or sitagliptin may be considered if a third agent is needed (choice based on hypothesized reason for hyperglycemia—insulin resistance versus insulin deficiency), although in patients who pay for their own prescriptions, cost issues may favor the addition of bedtime insulin at this point. If A1C goals have not been met with multiple oral agents, bedtime basal insulin therapy is indicated. Failure of bedtime basal insulin therapy justifies the change to a bid insulin regimen and the discontinuation of sulfonylureas.

A primary care-based team approach improves outcomes and patient satisfaction (57). Comprehensive management of diabetes may require several visits with different members of a diabetes care team, including a family physician and a diabetes case manager (dietician, nurse practitioner, pharmacist, etc).

Complementary and Alternative Medicines in Diabetes

According to the National Institutes of Health National Center for Complimentary and Alternative Medicines (58), there is a

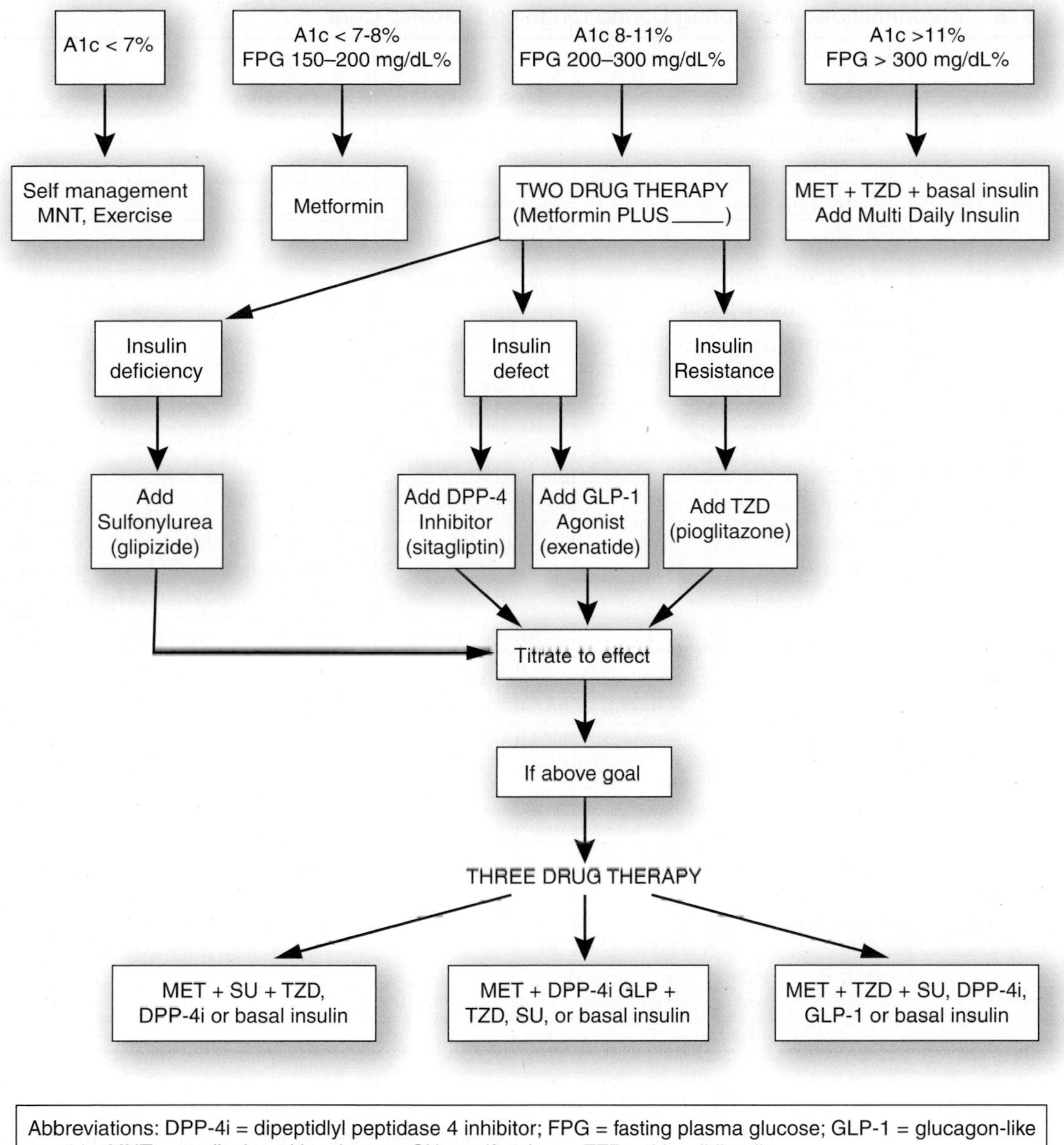

Figure 13.1 • Hypoglycemic agents for treatment of type 2 diabetes.

lack of scientific evidence to support the use of complementary and alternative medicines (CAM) in the treatment of diabetes. The most important point to convey to patients is to avoid replacing a proven conventional medication therapy with an unproven CAM. However, patients should be encouraged to report the use of CAM to prescribers to assure no drug interactions and to give a full picture to manage a patient's overall health.

One systematic review from 2003 found the best evidence for efficacy with Coccinia indica and American ginseng. The trials of Coccinia indica showed a decrease in fasting glucose and postprandial glucose over short durations of 6–12 weeks. Similarly, the review found small trials of short duration (8 weeks) with American ginseng that revealed a decrease in A1C and fasting glucose. None of the trials with Coccinia indica or American ginseng found pervasive side effects. The other herbs and supplements did not have rigorous trial designs or compelling evidence of efficacy (59).

Subsequent reviews and meta-analyses with commonly considered CAM supplements for diabetes have failed to show a benefit in the treatment outcomes of type 2 DM through well-designed, randomized controlled trials. In fact, an evidence-based review of chromium picolinate intake and insulin resistance, like that seen in type 2 DM, conducted by the FDA found a lack of data and highly uncertain relationship (60). Another systematic review of cinnamon on glucose control in type 1 and type 2 DM found a lack of evidence to support an improvement in A1C or fasting glucose (61). Alternatively, a meta-analysis evaluating magnesium intake and the risk of type 2 diabetes found that increasing the dietary intake of magnesium through magnesium-rich foods like beans, whole

TABLE 13.8 Recommended Monitoring During Ongoing Diabetes Care

Category of Monitoring	What to Monitor	Frequency	Comments
Health behaviors and self-care	Confidence in self-management	At each visit	
	Eating habits	At each visit	
	Activity level	At each visit	
	Medication adherence (including aspirin)	At each visit	
	Home glucose monitoring	At each visit	
	Tobacco use	At each visit	
	Readiness to change	At each visit	
Physical examination	Height, weight, BMI	At each visit	
	Blood pressure	At each visit	
	Foot exam and foot care instruction	Annually	If high risk (history of ulcer, foot deformity, loss of protective sensation), exams should be every 3 months.
Laboratory	Hemoglobin A1C	At least every 6 months	More frequently if ≥7.0%
	Fasting Lipids	Annually	More frequently if hypercholesterolemia
	Retinal exams	Annually	Begin within months of diagnosis of type 2, within 5 years of diagnosis for type 1. If low risk, eye professional may recommend 2-year interval.
	Microalbumin/creatinine	Annually	Begin within months of diagnosis of type 2, within 5 years of diagnosis for type 1. Two positive screens within 6 months required to diagnose nephropathy

BMI = body mass index.

grains, nuts and green leafy vegetables (as in the DASH diet) may reduce the risk of type 2 diabetes (62).

LONG-TERM MONITORING

Monitoring of diabetes begins with monitoring the behavioral management of the disease. Providers can explore in a nonjudgmental, caring way the issues their patients face living with the disease. They can support their patient's efforts at self management through assessment of current behaviors, assessment of readiness to change, and appropriate self-management counseling to adjust behavioral management.

The question, "On a scale of 1 (not at all confident) to 10 (totally confident), how confident are you that you can do the different tasks and activities needed to manage most of your health condition(s) so as to reduce your need to see a doctor?" is a good way to begin the conversation. Low self-management confidence is correlated with decreased self management behaviors (63).

In addition to a global inquiry about confidence, more detailed information is usually needed. One broadly studied inventory of diabetes self management is the Summary of Diabetes Self-Care Activities questionnaire which has now been validated in both English and Spanish versions (Figure 13.2) (64, 65). The last question about readiness to change was added to the summary to help busy practitioners know how to approach the discussion of self-management. An answer of 7 or greater indicates readiness to make additional behavioral changes. Less than 7 indicates that a patient is either ambivalent about making any changes (score of 3–6) or is not even considering lifestyle change at this time (score of 1–2). In either case, brief encouragement to continue considering behavioral changes is indicated.

Other aspects of periodic monitoring involve specific components of physical examination as well as laboratory measures (Table 13.8). BMI monitoring is an important aspect of longitudinal diabetes care. Insulin resistance increases as BMI rises, and weight loss improves blood glucose, lipids, and BP. Blood pressure should also be monitored at each office visit. In patients with labile BP or in those with "white coat" hypertension, home BP monitoring may be appropriate. Other key parts of the interval physical exam for patients with diabetes are the foot exam and the retinal exam (66).

Diabetes Self-Care Questionnaire

The questions below ask you about your diabetes self-care activities during the past 7 days. If you were sick during the past 7 days, please think back to the last 7 days that you were not sick. For each item, circle the number that best represents what actually happened.

Eating Habits

1. On how many of the last SEVEN DAYS have you followed a healthful eating plan?

   0 1 2 3 4 5 6 7

2. On how many of the last SEVEN DAYS did you eat five or more serving of fruits and vegetables?

   0 1 2 3 4 5 6 7

3. On how many of the last SEVEN DAYS did you eat high-fat foods such as red meat or full-fat dairy products?

   0 1 2 3 4 5 6 7

Exercise Habits

4. On how many of the last SEVEN DAYS did you participate in at least 30 minutes of physical activity?

   0 1 2 3 4 5 6 7

5. On how many of the last SEVEN DAYS did you participate in a specific exercise session (such as swimming, walking, biking) other than what you do around the house or as part of your work?

   0 1 2 3 4 5 6 7

Blood Sugar Testing

6. On how many of the last SEVEN DAYS did you test your blood sugar the number of times recommended by your health care practitioner?

   0 1 2 3 4 5 6 7

Medications

7. If you take aspirin, on how many of the last SEVEN DAYS did you take your recommended aspirin pills?

   0 1 2 3 4 5 6 7 Not applicable

8. If you take diabetes pills, on how many of the last SEVEN DAYS did you take your recommended diabetes pills?

   0 1 2 3 4 5 6 7 Not applicable

9. If you take insulin, on how many of the last SEVEN DAYS did you take your recommended insulin injections?

   0 1 2 3 4 5 6 7 Not applicable

Foot Care

10. On how many of the last SEVEN DAYS did you check your feet?

    0 1 2 3 4 5 6 7

11. On how many of the last SEVEN DAYS did you inspect the inside of your shoes?

    0 1 2 3 4 5 6 7

Smoking

12. Have you smoked a cigarette–even one puff–during the past SEVEN DAYS?

    0 No

    1 Yes. *If* yes, how many cigarettes did you smoke on an average day?

    Number of cigarettes: ____________

Readiness to Change

13. On a scale of 1 to 10, how ready are you to make changes in your lifestyle to improve your diabetes care?

    Not ready Very ready

    0 1 2 3 4 5 6 7 8 9 10

Thank you for completing this survey.

Figure 13.2 • A version of the summary of diabetes s self-care activities adapted for primary care practice.

Review of glucose monitoring data is another element of periodic visits. For patients taking insulin, the results of self blood glucose monitoring are used to adjust subsequent insulin doses, and this does lead to improved levels of A1C (4). For patients with type 2 diabetes who are not taking insulin, there is not enough scientific evidence to know whether review of glucose values improves management or not. A1C monitoring definitely improves glycemic control in patients with type 1 diabetes (67) and is recommended for patients with type 2 DM (3). Fasting lipid monitoring is also recommended. ADA guidelines call for glucose monitoring every three (in patients with recent changes to therapy) to 6 (for patients at target on stable regimens) months and lipid monitoring annually (4).

Screening for Early Signs of Complications

Retinopathy screening with either retinal photography or a retinal exam by an eye professional is an essential strategy to reducing the burden of blindness caused by diabetes. Improved BP and glucose control, laser photocoagulation, vitrectomy and other interventions can help preserve sight if retinopathy is identified in a timely fashion (4). The ADA recommends annual retinal exams soon after the discovery of type 2 diabetes and within 5 years of the diagnosis of type 1 diabetes.

The earliest sign of what may become diabetic kidney disease is microalbuminuria. The gold standard test is a 24-hour urine specimen analyzed for albumin. Although there are false positives and occasional false negatives, the spot albumin/creatinine ratio on a random urine specimen is much more practical and is now the preferred test (4). To minimize the false positives, two positive results within 6 months are needed before a patient is diagnosed as having microalbuminuria. If the second specimen is negative after an initial positive, a third test is recommended. Microalbuminuria is defined as an albumin: creatinine ratio of between 30 and 300 mg/g; values greater than 300 represent frank proteinuria, and values of less than 30 are normal. False positives can occur in the setting of a urinary tract infection, CHF, gross hematuria or fever. The ADA recommends annual screening (4).

Screening to prevent foot ulcers and amputation is done by annual physical examination. The foot exam for patients with diabetes includes inspection, palpation, monofilament testing, and vibratory sensation testing. The feet are inspected for corns, calluses, ulcers, deformities, and nail abnormalities. Monofilament testing identifies patients who have lost protective sensation and will not be aware of the tissue damage that precedes foot ulcers (69). Perception to light touch is assessed with the monofilament at five sites on each foot. Loss of protective sensation at 8 or more sites is a strong predictor of subsequent foot ulcer and increased risk of limb loss (68). The exam should be accompanied by patient education and encouragement for patients to care for their feet at home (4).

KEY POINTS

Table 13.4 summarizes the key points presented in this chapter, and the level of evidence supporting each recommendation. Diabetes management is challenging because of the need to provide ongoing support and encouragement for difficult behavior changes; the stringent standards for control of blood pressure, blood sugar, and serum lipids; the multiple organ systems that need to be monitored; the complexity of many medication regimens; and the relentless, longstanding demands that the disease places on patients. For these reasons, ongoing, regular care by a provider team, working in partnership with a motivated patient, leads to the best results.

CHAPTER 14

Thyroid Disorders

Jeri R. Reid

Thyroid problems are commonly encountered in family medicine and can lead to significant clinical consequences if undiagnosed. The initial presentation is often subtle, making clinical diagnosis challenging. Fortunately, when diagnosed, most thyroid disorders can be satisfactorily treated but will require long-term monitoring. In this chapter, the current evidence and consensus recommendations on the evaluation and management of the most common thyroid disorders will be reviewed.

HYPOTHYROIDISM

CLINICAL OBJECTIVES

1. List the common causes and classification schemes of hypothyroidism.
2. Outline the steps in the evaluation of hypothyroidism and describe the role that antithyroid antibodies play in the diagnostic workup.
3. Outline the recommended treatment strategy for hypothyroidism and how management differs in certain high-risk groups.

Hypothyroidism is one of the most commonly encountered endocrine problems in primary care. The syndrome we recognize as hypothyroidism results from decreased action of thyroid hormone at the tissue level. In most cases, this results from decreased production and secretion of thyroid hormone by the thyroid gland. Chronic autoimmune (Hashimoto's) thyroiditis is the most common cause of hypothyroidism in iodine-sufficient areas. The diagnosis and management of this disease has been simplified by the availability of sensitive biochemical testing and effective pharmacotherapy (1).

The prevalence of hypothyroidism in the United States is between 0.3% and 2.0%. It is approximately 3 times more common in African-Americans than whites, 5 times more common in people age 65 and older than in younger populations, and 10 times as frequent in women as in men (1, 2). Other risk factors include a personal or family history of thyroid or autoimmune disease, Turner syndrome, Down syndrome, multiple sclerosis, and primary pulmonary hypertension (3).

Diagnosis

Hypothyroidism can be classified as congenital or acquired based on the time of onset. Congenital hypothyroidism is most commonly caused by endemic iodine deficiency. In countries with sufficient iodine intake, this disorder is usually caused by thyroid gland dysgenesis or defective hormone synthesis. Acquired hypothyroidism occurs later in life and is usually the result of autoimmune thyroiditis (Hashimoto's). Other causes of acquired hypothyroidism include surgical removal of thyroid tissue or destruction of the thyroid by radioactive iodine, other external radiation, or toxin exposure. Certain drugs such as amiodarone and lithium interfere with glandular hormone release and can also cause hypothyroidism. A transient hypothyroidism can also be caused by subacute or lymphocytic thyroiditis (e.g., postpartum thyroiditis) with most patients returning to a euthyroid state after 2–8 months (3).

Hypothyroidism can be further classified as primary and secondary. Primary hypothyroidism relates to disease that directly affects the thyroid gland. Secondary hypothyroidism refers to a central cause, such as an adenoma impinging on the hypothalamus or pituitary. Central causes are very rare.

The last classification scheme for hypothyroidism is based on severity. Clinical (overt) is distinguished from subclinical (mild) on the basis of the serum free thyroxine (FT4) level in a patient with an elevated thyroid stimulating hormone (TSH) (3). Clinical hypothyroidism will be reviewed in this section, and subclinical disease will be reserved for later discussion. Table 14.1 lists the differential diagnosis of hypothyroidism.

History and Physical Examination

The most common signs and symptoms of hypothyroidism are listed in Table 14.2. Other symptoms include weight gain, hoarseness, hair loss, muscle cramping and weakness, arthralgias, paresthesias, menstrual irregularity (usually menorrhagia), and infertility (4). However, the clinical manifestations of hypothyroidism can be subtle, especially in the elderly. The detection of hypothyroidism is complicated by its insidious onset and the fact that the symptoms overlap with those of many other health problems. Occasionally, in very advanced disease, the presentation is dominated by hypothermia, congestive heart failure, pleural effusion, intestinal ileus, coagulopathy, ataxia, seizures, psychosis, severe depression, dementia, or coma (3).

The physical exam may reveal a diffuse or nodular goiter, sluggish movements, bradycardia, pretibial edema, facial puffiness, coarse skin, brittle nails, carpel tunnel syndrome and prolongation of ankle reflex. Congenital hypothyroidism may present with hypothermia, poor feeding, bradycardia, jaundice, enlarged posterior fontanelle, and umbilical hernia. Most infants are asymptomatic, warranting the routine screening of all newborns (1, 3).

Laboratory abnormalities that may be associated with hypothyroidism include increased total and low-density

TABLE 14.1 Causes of Hypothyroidism*

Primary—resulting from underfunction of the thyroid gland (95% of cases)
Idiopathic (most commonly "burned out" Hashimoto's thyroiditis)
Hashimoto's thyroiditis
Irradiation of the thyroid to treat Graves' disease
Surgical removal of the thyroid
End-stage invasive fibrous thyroiditis
Severe iodine deficiency
Drug therapy (e.g., lithium, interferon)
Infiltrative systemic disease: Sarcoidosis Amyloidosis Scleroderma Hemochromatosis
Secondary—resulting from undersecretion of thyroid-stimulating hormone (5% of cases)
Neoplasms of the pituitary gland or hypothalamus
Congenital hypopituitarism
Pituitary necrosis (Sheehan syndrome)

*Excludes congenital hypothyroidism

TABLE 14.2 Common Signs and Symptoms of Hypothyroidism

Symptom	**Percent of Patients Affected***
Weakness	99
Lethargy	91
Cold intolerance	89
Decreased sweating	89
Forgetfulness	66
Constipation	61
Physical Findings	
Coarse or dry skin	97
Slow speech	91
Eyelid edema	90
Skin cold to touch	83
Thick tongue	82
Facial edema	79
Coarse hair	76
Skin pallor	67

These statistics are adapted from a textbook of endocrinology. Findings may be more subtle in the primary care setting. (Adapted from Wilson JD, et al, eds. Williams Textbook of Endocrinology, 9th ed. Philadelphia, PA: Saunders, 1998. [In Hueston WJ. Treatment of hypothyroidism. Am Fam Physician. 2001;64:1717–1724.] Used with permission from Elsevier.)

lipoprotein (LDL) cholesterol, elevated homocysteine levels, anemia, and hyponatremia (1).

Diagnostic Testing

Making the definitive diagnosis begins with the measurement of highly sensitive TSH in a reliable laboratory. An elevated level suggests hypothyroidism and should be followed by a FT4 level. If this value is below the normal range, the diagnosis of hypothyroidism is confirmed.

A normal TSH level does not rule out secondary (central) hypothyroidism. This should be suspected in a patient with a normal TSH who exhibits clinical features of hypothyroidism and should prompt further testing with FT4. A normal TSH and T4 usually do not require further evaluation; however, severe nonthyroid illness and some drugs (e.g., glucocorticoids, dopamine, dobutamine) can falsely lower the TSH level and mask mild hypothyroidism. If the T4 level is low, clinical findings suggesting pituitary dysfunction or an intracranial mass should be sought, especially in patients with sarcoidosis, cranial injury, radiotherapy, or cancers known to metastasize to the pituitary (3). Imaging of the pituitary gland and hypothalamus would be indicated in these patients. If a mass or other central cause is found, appropriate referrals (e.g., to neurosurgery, endocrinology) would be indicated. Secondary causes are rare, but many practitioners routinely order both TSH and FT4 in all patients suspected of hypothyroidism to rule out this possibility. Triiodothyronine testing (T3) is not useful in making the diagnosis of hypothyroidism (4).

The measurement of thyroid autoantibodies (specifically antithyroperoxidase antibodies) confirms autoimmune thyroiditis as the cause of sustained primary hypothyroidism, because they are present in high titers in 95% of these patients (5). This diagnosis should already be clinically suspected in patients who do not have other risk factors for hypothyroidism (3). The measurement of antibodies is still useful because it alerts the clinician to the possibility of other autoimmune diseases in the patient or their family (6). Thyroid ultrasound or radionuclide scanning is only necessary if structural abnormalities are suspected.

Treatment

The treatment for primary hypothyroidism is hormone supplementation with levo-thyroxine (L-thyroxine). When used properly, this medication is highly effective with few side effects. The L-thyroxine dose needs to be individualized, and controversy exists regarding the starting dose, the titration method, and the final goal of treatment. The generally accepted replacement dose is 1.6 mcg/kg (5), which equates to 100 mcg/day for the average woman and 125 mcg/day for the average man. In young, healthy adults with no significant comorbidities, starting with the full replacement dose is safe, convenient and cost-effective (7). Dosages of 12.5–25 mcg (or 25% of the calculated replacement dose) are recommended for patients aged 60 and older or with heart disease (3, 5, 8). These precautions are taken because of the concern that an abrupt increase in metabolic rate could precipitate angina, myocardial infarction, congestive heart failure, or arrhythmia in such patients (8). Dosages are titrated by 25–50 mcg every 6 weeks until a euthyroid state (normal TSH level) is achieved. Smaller titration doses of 12.5 mcg are sometimes advocated in people with severe ischemic heart disease (3).

Most authorities recommend that the TSH be maintained in the lower half of the reference range (0.4–2.5 mcU/mL). If the patient is doing well with the TSH in the upper half of the reference range (2.5–4.5 mcU/mL), then no dosage increase is recommended. Low TSH levels (below 0.4 mcU/mL) should be avoided especially in patients older than age 60 because of an increased risk of osteoporosis and atrial fibrillation (9).

L-thyroxine has a narrow therapeutic range, as well as potential interactions with several common medications. Malabsorptive states and medications such as cholestyramine, ferrous sulfate, sucralfate, calcium, and aluminum hydroxide can interfere with L-thyroxine absorption. Rifampin and sertraline accelerate L-thyroxine metabolism. Nephrotic syndrome and the anticonvulsant medications phenobarbital, phenytoin, and carbamazepine can decrease thyroid hormone binding. Warfarin doses need to be monitored closely during titration since the metabolism of clotting factors increases as thyroid function improves. Pregnancy increases thyroid hormone requirements by as much as 75% (3). Most thyroidologists recommend the use of brand-name LT4 (5) despite a recent study suggesting that generic products are bioequivalent (10). The LT4 product chosen should remain the same throughout treatment to ensure as much stability as possible. The use of triiodothyronine in combination with LT4 for patients who remain symptomatic on LT4 alone is not currently recommended (11). Table 14.3 summarizes treatment recommendations for thyroid disease.

Long-term Monitoring

Because the half-life of thyroid hormone is nearly a week, it takes 3–6 weeks after initiating a dosage change for a steady state to be achieved. For this reason, the patient should be assessed every 6 weeks during the titration process. At such assessments, serum TSH should be measured and the patient questioned about thyroid symptoms and medication side effects. When the TSH becomes normal, follow-up visits should be scheduled at 6 months and 1 year. If the TSH and LT4 dosage remain stable, annual visits should continue indefinitely (5). Any changes in dosage should be followed by a repeat TSH level in 6 weeks. The importance of compliance should be emphasized at each visit, because as many as 40% of patients on L-thyroxine do not receive enough medication to achieve a TSH in the normal range (12). This can have significant health consequences, because undertreated hypothyroidism can lead to cardiac dysfunction, depression, elevated cholesterol levels, and persistent symptoms (6).

HYPERTHYROIDISM

CLINICAL OBJECTIVES

1. List the common causes of hyperthyroidism.
2. Outline the most efficient workup of hyperthyroidism.
3. Describe the treatment options for hyperthyroidism and discuss the indications and adverse effects of each treatment.

Technically, thyrotoxicosis is the clinical state caused by increased circulating levels of thyroid hormone in the body and hyperthyroidism refers exclusively to the condition caused by excess production and release of thyroid hormone from the thyroid gland. This section will use the term *hyperthyroidism* to refer to all conditions caused by thyroid hormone excess. The prevalence of hyperthyroidism is 2% in women and 0.2% in men (13).

Diagnosis

The most common causes, in approximate order of frequency are:

- Graves' disease. An autoimmune disease that leads to increased thyroid hormone secretion. Graves' disease accounts for 60–80% of all cases with 15% of these cases occurring in patients older than 60 years of age.
- Toxic nodular goiter and solitary hyperfunctioning nodules. Toxic nodular goiter causes 5% of cases in the United States but may be more common in iodine deficient areas. This condition typically occurs in patients older than 40 years with longstanding multinodular goiter. Autonomously functioning solitary nodules are found in younger patients and are associated with iodine deficiency. Both cause symptoms because of autonomous thyroid hormone production.
- Thyroiditis. A series of diseases that cause transient leakage of thyroid hormone from a damaged gland. They include subacute thyroiditis after a viral illness and lymphocytic and postpartum thyroiditis.
- Excess iodine ingestion, either from diet, radiographic contrast, or medication. Amiodarone can produce hyperthyroidism either as a result of its high iodine content or by inducing thyroiditis.
- Factitious hyperthyroidism. This occurs from intentional or accidental ingestion of excess thyroid hormone.

Rare causes include metastatic thyroid cancer, ovarian tumors that produce thyroid hormone (struma ovarii), trophoblastic tumors, or TSH-secreting pituitary tumors (13).

History and Physical Examination

The clinical manifestations of hyperthyroidism (Table 14.4) vary depending on the duration of the illness, the age of the patient, and comorbid conditions. Elderly patients often present with decreased appetite or atrial fibrillation; however, they occasionally present with only fatigue and lethargy (apathetic hyperthyroidism). Thyroid storm is a rare complication of hyperthyroidism, usually resulting from a stressful illness in a patient with inadequately treated hyperthyroidism. It presents with fever, delirium, vomiting, diarrhea, and dehydration (14).

The physical examination may demonstrate weight loss, elevated systolic blood pressure, tachycardia, pretibial edema, tremor, or proximal muscle weakness. A tender diffuse goiter suggests subacute thyroiditis. Painless goiter is present in other forms of thyroiditis and in Graves' disease. Single or multiple nodules may be present with or without tenderness. In up to 40% of patients with Graves' disease, there are distinctive eye findings that include proptosis, lid retraction, extraocular muscle dysfunction, and keratitis (14).

TABLE 14.3 Summary of Treatment Recommendations for Thyroid Disorders

Problem and Intervention	Strength of Recommendation*	Comment
Hypothyroidism		
Thyroid hormone replacement at full starting dose	B	As effective as other regimens in patients under age 60 without cardiac disease
Thyroid hormone replacement with gradual titration to replacement dose	C	This is recommended by most experts with lower starting doses and more careful titration in elderly or cardiac patients
Titration to TSH goal of 0.5–2.5	C	
Thyroid hormone replacement with generic L-thyroxine	B	Combining triiodothyronine with L-thyroxine is not supported by scientific evidence. Patient should minimize changing formulations.
Hyperthyroidism		
Antithyroid drugs	A	Effective in 40–50% of patients. Less effective in smokers and larger goiters.
Radioactive iodine therapy	A	Effective in 80% of cases; can be redosed. Treatment of choice for Graves' disease in the United States.
Total thyroidectomy	A	100% effective, but carries 100% risk of permanent hypothyroidism. Preferred over subtotal for most patients.
Subtotal thyroidectomy	A	92% effective; 25% risk of permanent hypothyroidism but significant risk of recurrence. Recommended only for toxic nodules.
Thyroid Enlargement		
Observation without treatment	C	Treatment of choice with no compressive symptoms or thyroid dysfunction. Hormone suppression to reduce goiter size has been demonstrated to be ineffective and is not recommended.
Surgery to reduce size of goiter	C	100% success with total thyroidectomy; 40% success with subtotal thyroidectomy. Postoperative L-thyroxine does not prevent recurrences.
RAI for toxic goiter	A	80% effective
RAI for nontoxic goiter	B	Typically decreases goiter size by 40–90%. Recombinant TSH increases RAI uptake and reduces doses needed.
Thyroid Nodules		
Observation if nontoxic nodules and <1 cm in diameter	C	If no abnormal US characteristics and no risk factors for thyroid cancer
Near-total thyroidectomy for cancers other than medullary	C	
Total thyroidectomy with lymph node resection for medullary cancer	C	
Lobectomy for indeterminate or suspicious nodules	C	
Subclinical Thyroid Dysfunction		
L-thyroxine therapy -Symptomatic patient with TSH < 10 -Asymptomatic patient with TSH > 10	 C C	Risks outweigh benefits in asymptomatic patients with TSH < 10
Treatment of subclinical hyperthyroidism when TSH < 0.1	C	Risks outweigh benefits in patients with TSH above 0.1 except in elderly, heart disease or osteoporosis

A = consistent, good-quality patient-oriented evidence; B = inconsistent or limited-quality patient-oriented evidence; C = consensus, disease-oriented evidence, usual practice, expert opinion, or case series; RAI = radioactive iodine; TSH = thyroid-stimulating hormone; US = ultrasound.
For information about the SORT evidence rating system, see *http://www.aafp.org/afpsort.xml*.

TABLE 14.4 Common Signs and Symptoms of Hyperthyroidism

Signs and Symptoms	Patients Older than 70 Years (%)	Patients Younger than 50 Years (%)
Tachycardia	71	96
Fatigue	56	84
Weight loss	50	51
Goiter	50	94
Tremor	44	84
Apathy	41	25
Atrial fibrillation	35	2
Anorexia	32	4
Nervousness	31	84
Hyperactive reflexes	28	96
Depression	24	22
Increased sweating	24	95
Polydipsia	21	67
Heat intolerance	15	92
Increased appetite	0	57

Adapted from Trivalle C, Doucet J, Chassagne P, et al. Differences in signs and symptoms of hyperthyroidism in older and younger patients. J Am Geriatr Soc. 1996;44:51. Used with permission.

Diagnostic Testing

The diagnostic approach to hyperthyroidism is outlined in Figure 14.1. It is important to identify the cause of the hyperthyroidism so that appropriate treatment can be offered. This is best accomplished by ordering a radionuclide uptake and scan. Increased uptake occurs in Graves' disease, toxic multinodular goiter and solitary hyperfunctioning nodules. However, Graves' disease is easily distinguished from the nodular causes because there will be a diffuse uptake in the gland instead of a nodular or focal pattern. Thyroiditis is also easy to distinguish from Graves' because there will be a decreased uptake on the scan with thyroiditis rather than an increase (13).

Thyroid autoantibody measurement is not routinely recommended, because it offers little assistance in differentiating between Graves' disease and thyroiditis. Antithyrotropin antibodies can help predict the success of certain treatment regimens that will be discussed in the following sections (15).

Treatment

The management goal is to correct the hypermetabolic state with the fewest complications. β-blockers can resolve many of the adrenergic symptoms, such as tremor, tachycardia, heat intolerance, and nervousness. Propranolol titrated to doses between 80 and 320 mg per day is most commonly used. Calcium channel blockers can resolve some of the symptoms if β-blockers cannot be tolerated. These drugs are usually the only treatment needed for thyroiditis-induced hyperthyroidism, because it is usually self-limited. β-blockers (except atenolol) are safe for short-term use in pregnancy (13). Persistent hyperthyroidism is treated with antithyroid drugs, radioactive iodine, or surgery. Each of these has been shown to be effective and well tolerated if used as recommended (16).

PHARMACOTHERAPY

Antithyroid drugs (ATDs) interfere with the organification of iodine and are the preferred treatment for Graves' disease in many parts of the world outside the United States. In this country, ATDs are generally reserved for pregnant patients, children, and those who refuse radioactive iodine (RAI) therapy. They can also be used in cardiac and elderly patients to normalize thyroid function before surgery or RAI, because thyrotoxicosis can be temporarily exacerbated by these treatments (16).

Methimazole is the agent used most often in nonpregnant patients because it can be given less frequently at maintenance doses and has a lower incidence of side effects. The starting dose is 15–30 mg in a single daily dose. β-blockers can be given in conjunction with ATDs and tapered as the patient becomes euthyroid. After 4–12 weeks, the patient is usually euthyroid, as evidence by symptoms and T4 levels. The methimazole dose can usually be tapered to a maintenance dose of 5–10 mg as a single daily dose and should be continued for 12–18 months (14). Symptoms, rather than TSH levels, should be used to monitor early response to treatment, because TSH levels can take months to normalize.

Propothiouracil (PTU) is the alternative medication. However, it has to be dosed more frequently and has more side effects. Its main use is in pregnancy because methimazole has been linked to a rare fetal scalp abnormality. Both drugs are compatible with breastfeeding.

Remission rates are estimated at 40–50% and do not seem to be affected by the dosage or the duration of therapy beyond

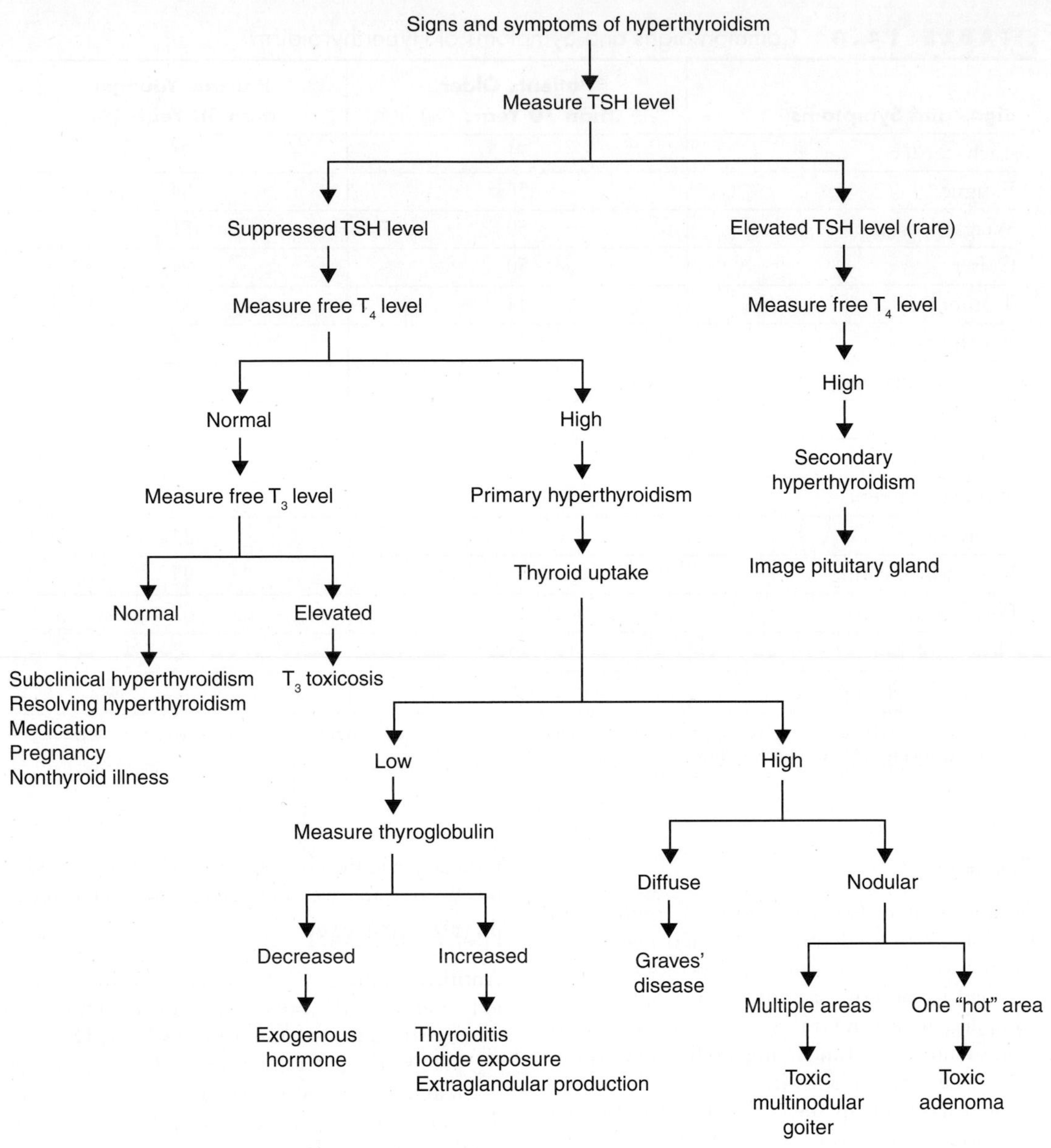

Figure 14.1 • Management algorithm for hyperthyroidism. (From Reid JR, Wheeler SF. Hyperthyroidism: diagnosis and treatment. Am Fam Physician. 2005;72:623–630. Used with permission.)

12–18 months. Treatment success decreases as the severity of the hyperthyroidism and thyroid gland size (goiter) increase. Smokers and those with elevated antithyrotropin receptor antibody titers have lower remission rates. Relapse usually occurs in the first 3–6 months after ATDs are discontinued. There is no current evidence to support using T4 in combination with ATDs to improve remission rates (16).

Major side effects of ATDs include polyarthritis (1–2%) and agranulocytosis (0.1–0.5%). Agranulocytosis usually occurs within 3 months of starting therapy. PTU has a higher dose-related risk of this reaction, and it is very rare with methimazole doses less than 30 mg. Patients should be warned to discontinue the drug if they experience a sudden fever or sore throat. Routine monitoring of white cell counts is controversial (16) but may be beneficial in the early detection of agranulocytosis (17). PTU causes elevated liver function tests in 30% of patients, and immunoallergic hepatitis in 0.1–0.2%. Methimazole can cause cholestasis, but this is rare. Minor side effects occur in less than 5% of patients and include rash, fever, gastrointestinal symptoms, and arthralgias. Most of the minor side effects do not require cessation of therapy except for arthralgias, because they could be the first sign of a more serious polyarthritis syndrome (16).

Iodides block the conversion of T4 to T3 and inhibit hormone release from the gland. They can cause paradoxical hormone release and interfere with radioactive iodine or antithyroid drug treatment, so they are not routinely used. They can, however, be used preoperatively with β-blockers for rapid control of symptoms before emergency nonthyroid surgery or to reduce the vascularity of the gland before Graves' disease surgery (16).

RAI

RAI concentrates in the thyroid gland and destroys thyroid tissue. It is the treatment of choice for Graves' disease in the United States and the preferred treatment for multinodular goiter and toxic nodules in patients older than 40 years. When relapse occurs after ATD therapy, RAI is generally recommended. The cure rate with single-dose treatment is 80–90%, with thyroid function returning to normal within 2–6 months (16). The treatment is safe and cost-effective but causes permanent hypothyroidism in 82% of patients with Graves' disease at 25 years. There is a lower incidence of hypothyroidism (32%) in patients with toxic nodules or toxic multinodular goiter because the rest of the gland may start to function normally when the hyperthyroidism is treated (18).

RAI treatment is contraindicated in pregnancy, and conception should be delayed for 4–6 months after treatment. If these guidelines are followed, RAI poses no increased risk of future birth defects or infertility in women of childbearing age (16). RAI is also being used more often in patients younger than 20 years old but is still controversial (19). Women who are breastfeeding should avoid RAI because it appears in breast milk.

Achieving remission and earlier onset of the hypothyroidism allows for better long-term outcome for the patient (18). If relapse does occur, RAI can be repeated as soon as 3 months (20). Potential complications of RAI include radiation thyroiditis (1% of patients), exacerbation of Graves' ophthalmopathy, transient neck soreness, facial flushing, and decreased taste. Radiation thyroiditis occurs in 1% of patients and can cause a transient, reversible thyrotoxicosis. Pretreatment with ATDs, preferably methimazole, can be used for cardiac and elderly patients to prevent this possibility. The drugs need to be stopped 4 days before RAI and can be restarted 1 week after the treatment because they can reduce the effectiveness of RAI treatment (16). Exacerbation of Graves' ophthalmopathy occurs in15% of patients, especially smokers, and can be prevented by starting prednisone before RAI and continuing it for 2–3 months. Consultation with an experienced ophthalmologist is recommended. Because of this complication, many endocrinologists prefer not to treat patients with severe Graves' ophthalmolopathy with RAI (14).

Patients should avoid children and pregnant women for 24–72 hours after RAI and use frequent hand washing and flushing to minimize the exposure of others to contaminated urine, saliva, and feces during this time (13).

SURGERY

Toxic nodules in healthy patients younger than 40 years old are usually removed surgically. Surgery could also be considered a treatment option for pregnant women or children who cannot tolerate ATDs, in patients experiencing compressive symptoms from their goiters, in noncompliant patients, in those who have failed ATDs but do not want RAI, or patients with such severe disease that a recurrence would not be tolerated (13). Total (or nearly total) thyroidectomy is preferred over subtotal thyroidectomy in all cases except for the toxic nodule because of the significantly lower risk of recurrence (16). Hypothyroidism occurs in most patients after surgery, and this should be anticipated and treated appropriately.

A recent meta-analysis of thyroidectomy revealed a low morbidity rate (3%) and no mortalities (21). Complications include hypoparathyroidism or recurrent laryngeal nerve damage (1–2% of patients regardless of the type of surgery performed). Patients should be rendered euthyroid with antithyroid drugs preoperatively. Iodinated contrast agents, β-blockers, and corticosteroids may also be needed if surgery needs to be done urgently (22).

Long-term Monitoring

Patients should be monitored closely after any treatment for hyperthyroidism. After ATD treatment, the patient should be monitored every 4–12 weeks until the thyroid status stabilizes, then every 3–4 months for the 12- to 18-month duration of therapy. When the medication is withdrawn, visits should continue at 3- to 4-month intervals for the first year, when relapse is more likely to occur.

Recommended follow-up after RAI includes frequent visits every 4–6 weeks for the first 3 months as the thyroid status normalizes and, in most cases, hypothyroidism develops. After the patient's condition has stabilized, 3- and 6-month follow-up visits should be planned. Regardless of the treatment, annual visits should continue indefinitely because relapse can occur years later and because thyroid replacement may need to be adjusted (13).

Despite appropriate treatment, some patients with hyperthyroidism continue to experience ocular, cardiac, and psychological complications of the disease. There seems to be no significant increase in the risk of cancer mortality in these patients (23), but there may be an increased risk of mortality related to cerebrovascular disease, cardiac disease, and hip fractures in those treated with RAI (24). Interestingly, a recent study on bone mineral density in hyperthyroid patients showed a return to baseline bone density in women 3 years after treatment (25). It seems prudent, however, to monitor hyperthyroid patients carefully for osteoporosis and atherosclerotic risk factors.

THYROID ENLARGEMENT

CLINICAL OBJECTIVES

1. Describe the causes of thyroid enlargement.
2. List the diagnostic testing indicated in the workup of thyroid enlargement.
3. Discuss the evidence related to the treatment of thyroid enlargement with surgery, L-thyroxine, or RAI.
4. Outline the long-term management of thyroid enlargement regardless of treatment.

Thyroid enlargement, or goiter, is the most common thyroid disorder in clinical practice. The prevalence in the United States is variable depending on the regional iodine intake but is estimated at 4–7% (26). Goiter is 5–10 times more common in women (27). The development of goiter is influenced by autoimmune, genetic, and extrinsic factors.

Diagnosis

There are three general ways of describing goiter:

- Endemic versus sporadic. Goiter is termed endemic if it occurs in 10% or more of the population; otherwise, it is sporadic. Endemic goiter is the result of iodine deficiency and is very rare in the United States.
- Simple or multinodular. Goiter is described as simple when the gland is diffusely enlarged. Multinodular goiters have multiple nodules within the gland.
- Nontoxic or toxic. Nontoxic goiter exhibits normal thyroid function, whereas toxic goiter refers to an enlarged gland associated with either hypo- or hyperthyroidism.

Certain drugs (including lithium, iodides, and amiodarone) and certain foods (including rutabagas, cabbage, turnips, soybeans, and kelp) can act as goitrogens by disrupting normal thyroid hormone synthesis and release. Cigarette smoking is also associated with goiter; this occurs because thiocyanate, a degradation product of cyanide in tobacco smoke, competes with iodine for uptake in the thyroid gland. Pregnancy can induce goiter by exacerbating an existing iodine deficiency (28).

Goiter occurs in 50% of patients with Hashimoto's thyroiditis (29) as a result of defective hormone synthesis, lymphocytic infiltration, and increased growth factor secretion. Typically there is a goiter present with Graves' disease that is caused by the effects of TSH (30). Multinodular goiter results from the disordered growth of thyroid cells and the gradual replacement of the gland by fibrosis. A painful goiter is usually (in 90% of cases) caused by subacute thyroiditis or acute hemorrhage into a thyroid cyst or adenoma. Rare causes are acute suppurative thyroiditis or a rapidly enlarging carcinoma (29).

History and Physical Examination

Most patients with goiter are asymptomatic. History should be directed toward eliciting symptoms of hypo- or hyperthyroidism (discussed previously) and determining the presence of risk factors for thyroid disease or malignancy. The patient should be questioned about the ingestion of goitrogens, pregnancy, and smoking. Risk factors for malignancy include a family history of thyroid pathology, personal history of neck radiation therapy, previous thyroid surgery, and cervical adenopathy (31). Rarely, there could be worrisome symptoms of mechanical pressure if the goiter is very large or extends into the thorax. These could include dyspnea, dysphagia, hoarseness, cough, or symptoms of thoracic outlet syndrome (32). Physical exam should include a thorough palpation of the thyroid gland to determine the size, tenderness, and presence of nodules. The patient should be examined for signs of hypo- or hyperthyroidism.

Diagnostic Testing

Laboratory investigation should begin with TSH measurement. If abnormal, the appropriate workup for hypo- or hyperthyroidism should follow. Elevated levels of antithyroid antibodies occur in 15–20% of patients with multinodular goiter and help predict the development of Graves' thyrotoxicosis and Hashimoto's-induced hypothyroidism (33). Basal serum calcitonin has been associated with thyroid cancer; it has been recommended in evaluating goiter in people with a family history of thyroid cancer or multiple endocrine neoplasia. Because of a high incidence of false positives and a lack of standardization of measured values, routine calcitonin measurement is not recommended (34).

Thyroid ultrasound should be considered in multinodular goiter to rule out the presence of a dominant nodule that would need further workup. Some authors recommend ultrasound for all patients with goiter, because it has been estimated that up to 50% of nodules are not palpable on physical exam (35). A dominant nodule is investigated in the same way as a solitary nodule, with fine-needle biopsy (FNB).

Pulmonary function testing or a barium swallow may be needed if compressive symptoms are present. Screening for suspected tracheal compression or intrathoracic extension of goiter is indicated in all patients with large multinodular goiters having compressive symptoms or in whom the lower margin of the goiter cannot be palpated. Chest radiographs may sometimes reveal these goiters, but computed tomography scanning or magnetic resonance imaging are much more sensitive tests for this purpose. Because computed tomography scanning involves the use of iodinated contrast agents, pretreatment with ATDs may need to be considered to prevent iodine-induced thyrotoxicosis (33).

Treatment

The management of goiter includes monitoring without treatment, thyroidectomy, L-thyroxine suppression, or RAI. The choice of treatment is dependent on the whether the goiter is toxic or nontoxic, simple or multinodular, or associated with compressive symptomatology.

Monitoring without treatment can be considered in patients with nontoxic goiter who have no compressive symptoms. These patients should be followed with clinical exam, thyroid laboratory testing, and, possibly ultrasound to detect growth of the thyroid, thyroid dysfunction, or the presence of dominant nodules (35).

Surgery is the treatment of choice for patients with large symptomatic goiters or those with risk factors for thyroid cancer. Total thyroidectomy is becoming preferred over subtotal thyroidectomy because it results in no risk of recurrence and, in the hands of an experienced surgeon, carries the same rate of complications. The recurrence rate of goiter after a subtotal thyroidectomy is as high as 60% (36). Permanent hypoparathyroidism or damage to the recurrent laryngeal nerve occurs in 1% of patients. These complications become 3–10 times more likely in recurrent goiter operations. The postoperative use of L-thyroxine to prevent goiter recurrence in patients undergoing partial thyroidectomy is used by many clinicians but is not supported by the current evidence (35).

Long-term suppression of TSH with the use of L-thyroxine has been extensively studied as a treatment for nontoxic goiter. In general, this therapy is not recommended because there is not a significant reduction in the size of the goiter with therapy and long-term treatment could result in subclinical hyperthyroidism (see the following section) (32).

In the treatment of toxic goiter associated with hyperthyroidism, RAI is considered the treatment of choice. In nontoxic goiter, treatment with RAI can result in a decrease in goiter volume by 40–60% and a reduction in compressive symptoms with a low incidence of complications. The use of recombinant human TSH has been found to increase the uptake of RAI in multinodular goiter, allowing for lower dosages to be used. The incidence of hypothyroidism is 22–58% over 5–8 years, and there is a rare chance of radiation thyroiditis or induction of Graves' disease (35). There is still reluctance among clinicians to use RAI treatment in patients without hyperthyroidism despite studies supporting its safety. Perhaps this results from the lack of evidence regarding the long-term risk of thyroid and nonthyroid cancers after treatment of these patients. When used, it tends to be restricted to patients older than 40 years of age and those with contraindications for surgery (37).

Long-term Monitoring

The natural history of nontoxic goiter is characterized by gradual growth (averaging 4.5% per year), nodule formation, and development of functional autonomy. Here are a few key issues to consider in following patients with goiter:

- Progression to clinical hyperthyroidism occurred in 10% of patients with goiter within a 5-year follow-up period (32). Therefore, patients with goiter who do not receive treatment need to be educated about these complications and followed clinically at least annually.
- Patients who have been treated for goiter require the same diligent follow-up. Those treated with subtotal thyroidectomy need to be monitored for goiter recurrence (15–40% of patients) and hypothyroidism (10–20%). Of course, patients undergoing total thyroidectomy need lifelong monitoring of their iatrogenic hypothyroidism. Eight percent of patients who have received RAI will experience recurrent goiter; Graves' disease associated with ophthalmopathy can occur in up to 5% of these patients (32).
- Even though L-thyroxine suppression is no longer recommended in most cases of goiter, a clinician may still encounter patients treated in this manner. It is important to monitor these patients for the development of subclinical and overt hyperthyroidism, which become more likely the longer the therapy is continued. It might be beneficial to counsel these patients about these risks so they can consider other treatment options.
- Regardless of the treatment, monitoring for the development of thyroid cancer must always be one of the goals of follow-up. Although simple goiter is not a risk factor for thyroid cancer, the tendency to form nodules over time increases the risk. The incidence of malignancy in both solitary nodules and multinodular goiter is approximately 5% (38).

SOLITARY THYROID NODULE

CLINICAL OBJECTIVES

1. List the common types of thyroid nodules.
2. Outline the steps in the diagnostic evaluation of thyroid nodules.
3. Discuss the malignant potential of thyroid nodules and risk factors associated with the development of malignancy.
4. Describe the management of thyroid nodules based on cytology.

Solitary thyroid nodules are frequently found incidentally during a physical examination or on non-thyroid neck imaging. Their prevalence increases with age, so that as many as half of patients older than age 60 years will have a thyroid nodule (38). Many nodules are quite small, but palpable nodules are present in 4–7% of the adult population. Thyroid nodules are 4–5 times more common in women than men (39).

As in the development of goiter, the formation of a solitary nodule depends on environmental, genetic, and autoimmune factors. Exposure to ionizing radiation or external beam radiation increases the risk of nodule, both benign and malignant (38). Thyroid nodules are also more likely to occur in areas of low iodine intake (40). Thirty-five percent of patients with Graves' disease have nodules and approximately 10% of these may be malignant (39).

Diagnosis

The most common type of nodule is a colloid nodule, which has no malignant potential. Cysts and thyroiditis are also common and, with colloid nodules, account for 80% of all nodules. Of the remainder, 10–15% are benign follicular adenomas, and about 5% are cancerous (41). Nonmedullary carcinomas account for 90% of thyroid malignancies. Of these, 85% are papillary, 11% follicular, 3% Hürthle, and 1% anaplastic. Medullary carcinoma represents 5% of thyroid malignancies (38).

History and Physical Examination

In a euthyroid patient, history and physical should be directed toward identifying risk factors for malignancy. Table 14.5 lists

TABLE 14.5 Red Flags Raising Concern for Thyroid Cancer in a Patient with a Thyroid Nodule

Data Source	Factors Raising Strong Concern	Factors Raising Moderate Concern
Clinical history	• Family history of medullary thyroid cancer or multiple endocrine neoplasia • Rapid growth of nodule	• Male sex • Patient age younger than 20 or older than 65 years • Previous radiation to the head or neck
Physical examination	• Firm or hard nodule • Nodule fixed to adjacent structures • Paralysis of vocal cords • Regional lymphadenopathy	• Nodule greater than 4 cm or partially cystic • Symptoms suggesting compression (dysphagia, hoarseness, dyspnea)

Adapted from Hegedus L, Bonnema SJ, Bonneddback FN. Management of simple nodular goiter: current status and future perspectives. Endocr Rev. 2003;24:102–132.

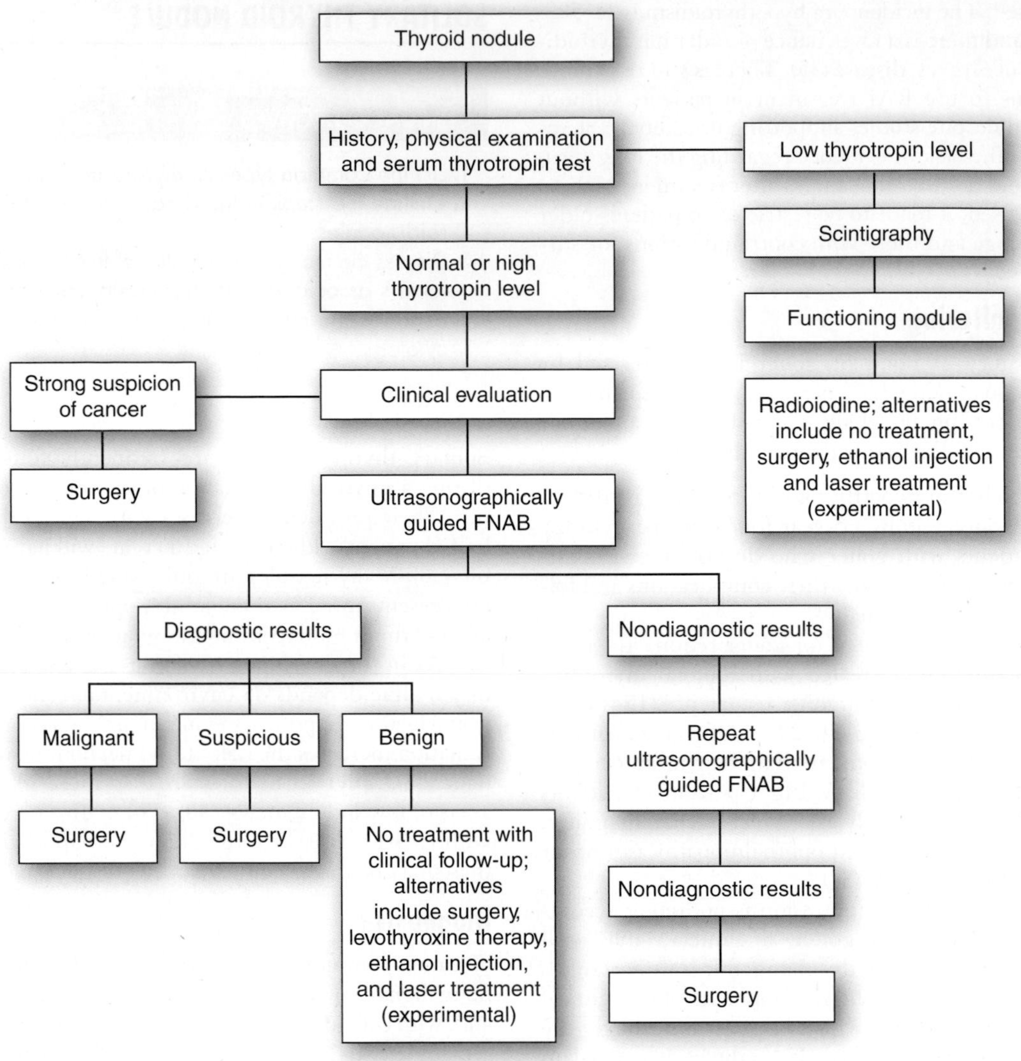

Figure 14.2 • Management algorithm for thyroid nodule. (From Hegedus L. The thyroid nodule. N Engl J Med. 2004;351:1764–1771. Copyright 2007 Massachusetts Medical Society. All rights reserved. Used with permission.)

the clinical findings that may suggest thyroid carcinoma according to the degree of suspicion. Additionally, papillary carcinoma occurs in 4–8% of patients with a family history of the same tumor. Patients with familial adenomatous polyposis and multiple hamartoma syndrome also have an increased risk of thyroid carcinoma (34).

The physical examination should include a thorough examination of the thyroid and surrounding lymph node beds, noting the size, tenderness, and consistency of any nodule or lymph node.

Diagnostic Testing

TSH and, if indicated, FT4 should be obtained in all patients; however, only 1% of solitary nodules cause hyper- or hypothyroidism (42). The presence of hyperthyroidism or hypothyroidism lowers the suspicion of cancer but does not exclude it. Serum calcitonin levels should be measured in patients with family history of medullary carcinoma or multiple endocrine neoplasia II, as described earlier under thyroid enlargement (39).

Ultrasonography is a relatively inexpensive, noninvasive examination that is becoming a routine part of the evaluation of thyroid nodules. It is estimated that half of all nodules cannot be detected on physical exam but are easily identified by ultrasound. In addition, ultrasound can distinguish cystic from solid nodules and improve the yield of FNB. Ultrasound and color-flow Doppler criteria that may indicate an increased risk of malignancy include irregular margins, intranodular vascular spots, and microcalcifications. Computed tomography, magnetic resonance imaging, and positron emission tomography have no established role in the evaluation of thyroid nodules. However, thyroid nodules found incidentally on positron emission tomography scans have been found to have a higher malignant potential and should always be biopsied (38). Radionuclide scanning is indicated only if hyperthyroidism is diagnosed by laboratory testing. The toxic nodule is easily identified on the scan, and the uptake in the rest of the gland will be reduced. The cancer risk in a toxic nodule is less than 1% (34).

FNB of a thyroid nodule is the most accurate and cost-effective way to differentiate benign from malignant nodules. The sensitivity is estimated at 93% and the specificity at 96%. The use of FNB has reduced the number of nodules for which surgery is recommended from nearly 50% to less than 20% (43). Ultrasound-guided FNB decreases the rate of unsatisfactory specimens from 15% to 3% and is especially helpful in nodules less than 1.5 cm and in all nonpalpable nodules (44).

Treatment

The algorithm in Figure 14.2 depicts the current recommendations for the evaluation and treatment of a clinically detected solitary thyroid nodule. Euthyroid patients with no risk factors for malignancy and a nodule less than 1 cm that shows no suspicious ultrasound findings have a very low risk of malignancy and need no further follow-up (45). However, the American Thyroid Association suggests that these patients should be followed by periodic ultrasonography (46). All nodules 1 cm or greater, any nodule in a patient with risk factors, or any nodule with suspicious ultrasound characteristics should be biopsied by an experienced clinician (39).

If the specimen is found to be adequate and reveals benign follicular cells, no further treatment is needed. Because false negative results occur in 5% of biopsies, the patient should be reevaluated at 6 and 18 months and have a repeat biopsy if the nodule enlarges. The presence of malignant cells is always an indication for surgery; this is usually a near-total thyroidectomy, except in the case of medullary carcinoma, which requires total thyroidectomy and bilateral regional lymph node resection (39).

Approximately 10% of biopsy specimens will be read as "suspicious follicular lesions" or "indeterminate." Surgical excision is recommended for this diagnostic dilemma. The surgery performed is usually a lobectomy with a total thyroidectomy to follow if malignancy is confirmed (38).

The use of L-thyroxine in the suppression of benign solitary nodules is controversial. It is recommended by many clinicians as an alternative to surgery or to prevent recurrence postoperatively. However, the results of numerous studies on this issue have failed to provide conclusive evidence that the benefit of L-thyroxine for solitary nodules outweighs the risks of this therapy, and observation without L-thyroxine treatment is the current evidence-based choice (39). RAI treatment of thyroid nodules is restricted to hyperfunctioning nodules (13) and those with locally invasive or metastatic thyroid cancer (39). Percutaneous ethanol injection and laser photocoagulation are new techniques being investigated in the treatment of solitary nodules. The safety and long-term efficacy of either technique has yet to be established through controlled clinical trials (47).

Long-term Monitoring

The natural history of benign thyroid nodules is to grow slowly over time (48). The patient should be followed at least annually with palpation and ultrasound. Interval history should be elicited especially regarding the development of risk factors for cancer. Serum TSH should be monitored during these visits because autonomous functioning may occur within the nodule. Although nodule size alone does not predict malignancy, all benign nodules that increase in size by more than 20% at annual follow-up should be rebiopsied (3). The primary care physician may encounter patients taking long-term L-thyroxine therapy for thyroid nodule suppression and should monitor them for thyrotoxic side effects as well as discuss the risks and benefits of continuing this therapy.

SUBCLINICAL THYROID DYSFUNCTION

CLINICAL OBJECTIVES

1. Define subclinical thyroid dysfunction.
2. Describe the recommendations for thyroid screening in the general population and identify high-risk groups targeted for screening.
3. Discuss the evidence that links subclinical thyroid dysfunction to adverse health outcomes.
4. Outline the treatment and/or long-term monitoring recommended for each type of subclinical thyroid dysfunction.

Subclinical thyroid dysfunction is a subject of considerable concern and debate among professional societies. Untreated subclinical thyroid dysfunction may have significant clinical consequences. Subclinical thyroid dysfunction is a laboratory diagnosis made when the TSH level is outside the reference range, and the freeT4 (and T3, if measured) are normal. There is some debate over the reference range used for TSH, but a recent consensus panel, with representatives from the major endocrinological societies, concluded that the range of normal TSH is between 0.45 and 4.5 mIU/L (49).

Diagnosis

Subclinical hypothyroidism is estimated to be present in 4–8% of the general population and in as many as 20% of women age 60 or older (50). It has been linked to increased cardiac risk factors, including elevations in cholesterol and LDL levels, diastolic hypertension, and elevated C-reactive protein and homocysteine levels (51). It has also been associated with the development of other systemic and neuropsychiatric symptoms. However, the consensus panel found little or no evidence that it caused any of these effects, except for significantly elevated cholesterol and LDL levels in patients with TSH greater than 10 mIU/L (49).

Subclinical hyperthyroidism occurs in about 2% of the population. It has been associated with atrial fibrillation and other cardiac events and with increased cardiac mortality in patients 60 years and older. There is about a threefold increase in the incidence of atrial fibrillation, but only in patients with TSH levels below 0.1 mIU/L. Bone mineral density decreases in prolonged subclinical hyperthyroidism if TSH is below 0.1 mIU/L but there is insufficient evidence to link fractures to this condition (49).

Important subsets of patients to consider in subclinical thyroid dysfunction are those who have known thyroid disease and are being treated with L-thyroxine medication. It is estimated that 20% of these patients have subclinical hypothyroidism due to inadequate thyroid replacement, and 14–20% have subclinical hyperthyroidism from overtreatment with L-thyroxine (49).

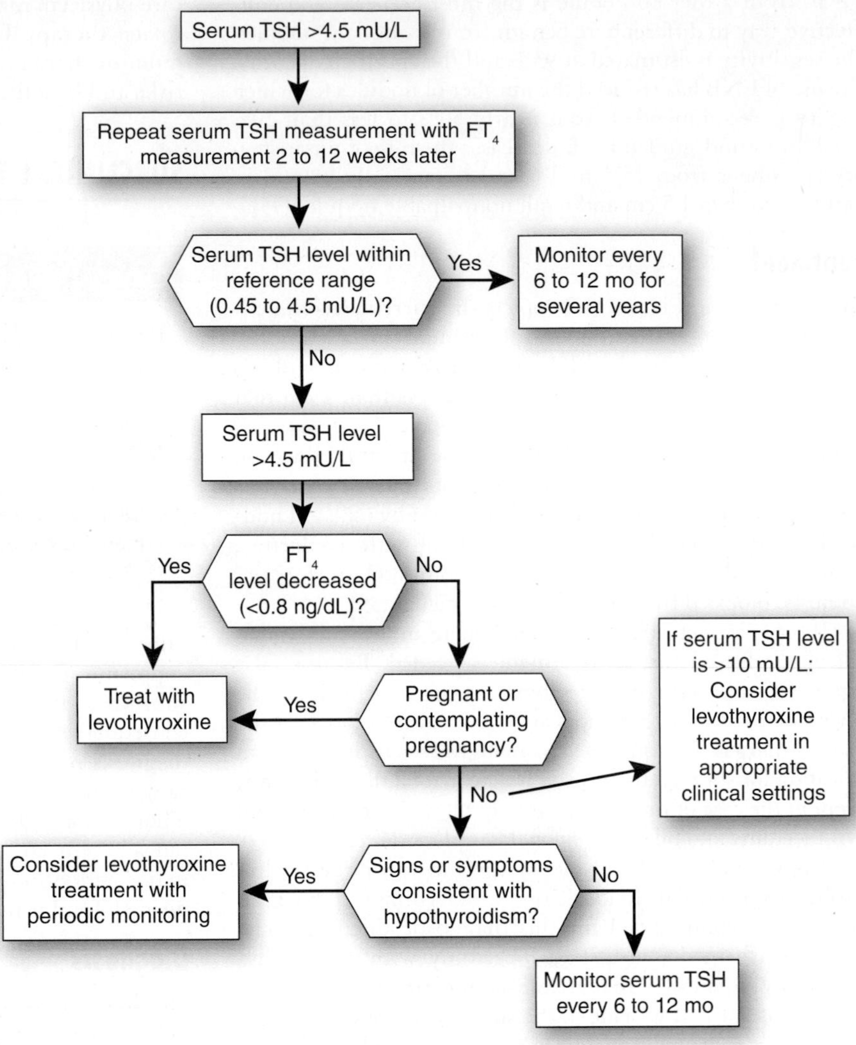

Figure 14.3 • Management algorithm for subclinical hypothyroidism. (Adapted from Col NF, Surks MI, Daniels GH. Subclinical thyroid disease: clinical applications. JAMA. 2004; 291:239–243.)

Screening and Diagnostic Testing

There has been considerable debate over who should be screened for thyroid disease. The United States Preventive Services Task Force found insufficient evidence to recommend for or against routine screening for thyroid dysfunction in the general population (52). All people with previous thyroid radiation, surgery or dysfunction; type 1 diabetes or other autoimmune disease; atrial fibrillation; or a family history of thyroid disease should be tested for thyroid dysfunction. Patients with any signs or symptoms of thyroid dysfunction, including any thyroid enlargement or nodule, should undergo diagnostic testing (49).

Subclinical hypothyroidism is diagnosed when the TSH is above the normal range and the free T4 is normal. It is important to exclude other causes of elevated TSH, such as undertreated clinical hypothyroidism, early pituitary or hypothalamic disorders, and recovery from severe illness or thyroiditis. Before treatment decisions are made, the TSH should be repeated along with the free T4 measurement within 2–12 weeks, and the patient should be evaluated for signs and symptoms of hypothyroidism. Lipid profiles should be considered. Measurement of antithyroid antibodies are not needed to diagnose subclinical hypothyroidism, but their presence predicts about twice the likelihood of developing clinical hypothyroidism (49).

Subclinical hyperthyroidism is diagnosed when the TSH is below the normal range and the free T4 and free T3 are normal. Other causes that need to be excluded include overtreatment or inappropriate treatment with L-thyroxine, delayed recovery from treatment for hyperthyroidism, pregnancy, euthyroid sick syndrome, or treatment with certain medications (e.g., dopamine and glucocorticoids). An asymptomatic patient with a low TSH should have repeat testing with free T4 and T3 in 3–12 weeks. Patients with atrial fibrillation or any cardiac signs or symptoms need follow-up within 2 weeks. A radioiodine scan is useful to determine the etiology of the subclinical hyperthyroidism, as described in the hyperthyroidism section. This test is recommended in the workup of a patient with subclinical hyperthyroidism whose TSH is <0.1 mIU/L, or in patients with heart disease, osteoporosis, or hyperthyroid symptoms. Bone mineral density testing may also be considered (53).

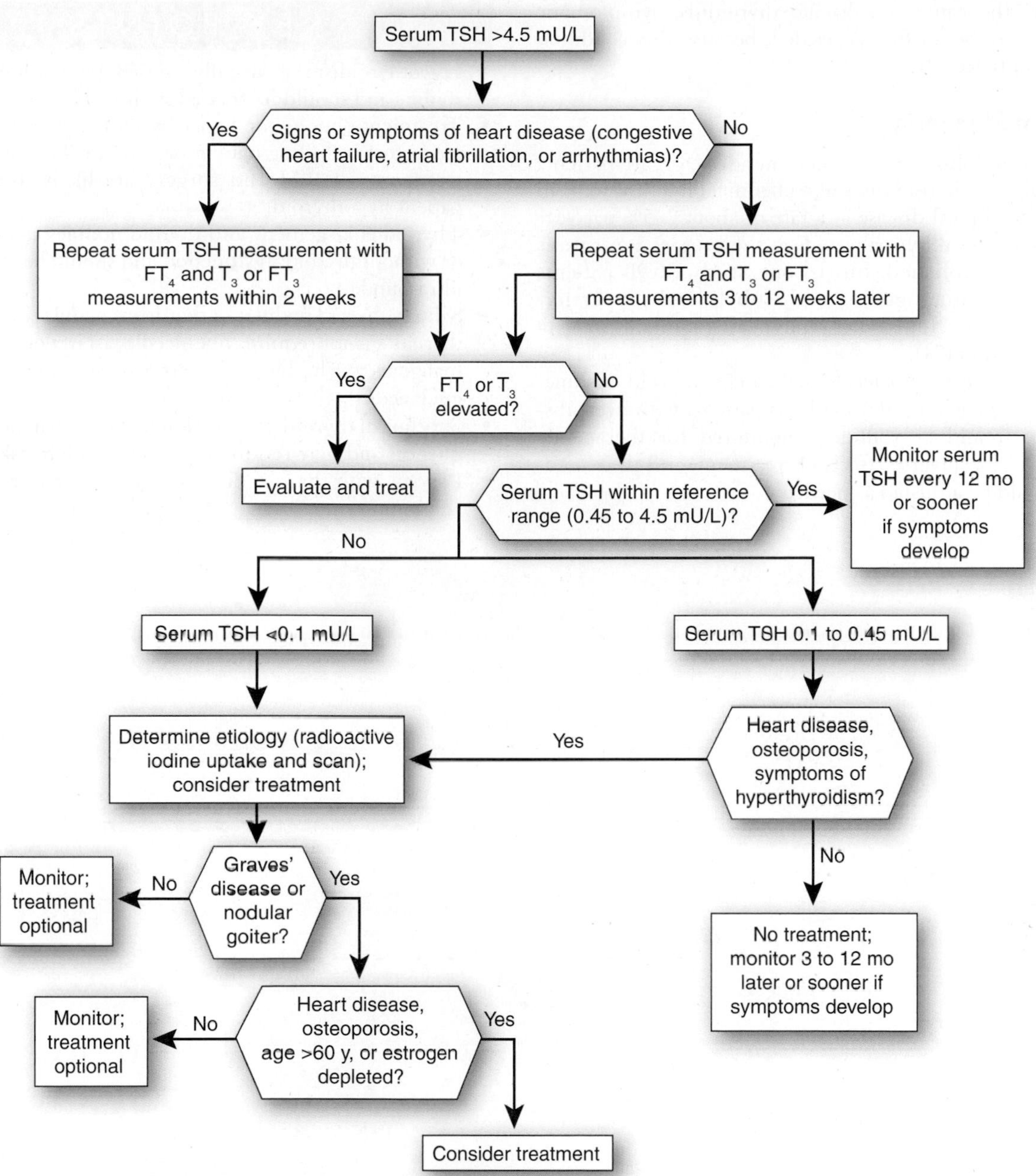

Figure 14.4 • Management algorithm for subclinical hyperthyroidism. (Adapted from Col NF, Surks MI, Daniels GH. Subclinical thyroid disease: clinical applications. JAMA. 2004;291:239–243.)

Treatment

The decision to treat subclinical hypothyroidism with L-thyroxine must be an individualized one, since the benefits of treatment based on the current literature are limited to a possible improvement in symptoms, a lowering of LDL cholesterol and improved left ventricular function. There has been no evidence to support improved survival, decreased cardiac morbidity, or improved quality of life (50). The consensus panel did not recommend treatment of TSH levels less than 10 mIU/L. However, if the patient has significant hypothyroid symptoms, a trial of L-thyroxine therapy could be considered. In patients with TSH higher than 10 mIU/L, L-thyroxine therapy is considered reasonable (49). These recommendations are depicted in Figure 14.3.

Figure 14.4 outlines a detailed approach to the evaluation and management of patients with subclinical hyperthyroidism. Treatment for subclinical hyperthyroidism is recommended for any patient with a TSH persistently less than 0.1 mIU/L. Patients who are elderly, have heart disease or osteoporosis may benefit from treatment of TSH between 0.1 and 0.45 mIU/L (49). These treatments are described in detail in previous sections. If the cause is subacute thyroiditis, symptomatic treatment may be all that is needed, because this condition resolves spontaneously.

Long-term Monitoring

Close clinical follow-up is recommended for all patients with subclinical thyroid disease. Subclinical hypothyroidism progresses to clinical disease at a rate of about 2–5% per year (49). For subclinical hyperthyroidism the progression rate is not as well established, but in one study of 90 patients with multinodular goiter and subclinical hyperthyroidism, 8% developed overt hyperthyroidism over a period of 7 years (54).

Patients who are treated for subclinical thyroid dysfunction have the same long-term risks as patients with overt disease. They should be routinely monitored for therapeutic response and for adverse effects of treatment, and their medication should be adjusted as needed.

KEY POINTS

- Hypothyroidism is usually caused by Hashimoto's thyroiditis and should be treated with L-thyroxine.
- Treatment options for hyperthyroidism depend on multiple factors including patient preference. The most effective treatments of RAI and surgery are likely to render the patient hypothyroid.
- Thyroid enlargement and thyroid nodules can occur with or without thyroid dysfunction and should be imaged with ultrasound.
- Solitary thyroid nodules or dominant nodules in an enlarged thyroid gland require fine-needle aspiration to rule out malignancy. The biopsy is best achieved under ultrasound guidance.
- Subclinical thyroid dysfunction has long term health consequences and may require treatment in high-risk groups.
- Patients with thyroid disorders need long-term follow-up and monitoring.

CHAPTER

15

Nutrition and Weight Management

Margaret E. Thompson and Mary Barth Noel

CLINICAL OBJECTIVES

1. Describe how obesity and overweight are defined.
2. List factors that influence the nutritional status of people throughout the life-cycle.
3. Be able to perform a nutritional assessment on patients.
4. List factors contributing to overweight and obesity in children.
5. Describe different strategies for managing underweight, overweight, and obese patients.

In trying to educate patients about nutrition, it is useful to think of diet, genetics, and environment. It is important to consider the role of each component in relation to the others. It is also important to consider potential disease states and their influence on nutritional needs.

The Recommended Dietary Allowances and the newer Adequate Intakes acknowledge the human variation in dietary requirements. These guidelines set ranges of two standard deviations around the mean requirement, thus taking into account genetic, age, and health status differences. Models such as the United States Department of Agriculture food pyramid are practical illustrations of the nutrient needs for the US population based on the current medical evidence and cultural trends regarding issues such as obesity, diabetes, cancer, and heart disease. Models such as the food pyramid may be helpful for some, but the recommendations need to vary with age, health status, and genetic makeup. The 2005 iteration of the food pyramid allows customization depending on these factors (see *www.mypyramid.gov*).

The most prevalent nutritional disorders in the United States are overweight and obesity. In considering these problems, it is important to consider the defining parameters for these two classifications, as well as the prevalence of these conditions and the importance of nutrition, overweight, and obesity with regard to overall health of the individual. Current standards define overweight and obesity based on the body mass index (BMI), which can be determined from tables, or calculated using the formula:

$$\text{BMI} = \text{Weight (kg)}/(\text{height in meters})^2.$$

In 1999, a National Institutes of Health (NIH) consensus panel lowered the threshold for overweight from a BMI of 27 kg/m^2 to a BMI of 25 kg/m^2 (1). Likewise, the cutoff for obesity has been lowered from a BMI of 32 kg/m^2 to a BMI of 30 kg/m^2 (Table 15.1). This new classification has nearly doubled the number of people who qualify as overweight. These definitions are not without controversy, primarily because we do not know whether the risk comes from the excess weight, the genetic makeup, or the lifestyle and behaviors of the overweight population (2, 3). The weight guidelines also do not take into consideration the location of the fat and health risk. Weight carried in the abdominal region of the body seems to confer greater risk for heart disease and diabetes. Additionally, there may be differences between racial groups; for example, the increased risk associated with obesity may occur at higher BMIs for populations of African-American descent than for Asian populations.

The prevalence of obesity in the United Sates was approximately one third of adults in 2007–2008 (4). Obesity is common in all races, ages, and both genders. The prevalence of obesity in African-Americans is 51% higher than in whites, and the prevalence in Hispanics is 21% greater than in whites (4). The question of whether these weight differences are attributable to gender, cultural, genetic, or racial differences is still under consideration, as are the health risks associated with these differences.

Scientific knowledge and advice vary about the health significance of increased weight. Some studies indicate that a 10-lb weight gain for a woman over her lifetime significantly increases her risk of cancer (5). One study found that for people whose BMI was greater than 40 kg/m^2, the death rate for cancer was 52% higher for men and 62% higher for women than in people of normal weight (6). Table 15.2 summarizes the current consensus on the health implications of overweight and obesity (7).

DIAGNOSIS

A nutritional assessment is the process of determining whether an individual is consuming and using appropriate amounts of the nutrients that are required for vital life processes. All patients deserve some level of nutritional assessment. It is important to note that weight alone is not a good indicator of nutritional status. In a relatively healthy person, the assessment may take the form of a simple screen, whereas a patient with risk factors for malnutrition requires a more thorough evaluation. The latter category includes overweight and obese patients, those who are underweight, or have chronic or severe acute illness, children, the elderly, and those living in poverty or who have other factors that may make access to nutrients difficult.

TABLE 15.1 Classification of Overweight and Obesity in Adults by Body Mass Index (BMI), Waist Circumference, and Associated Disease Risks

Category	Definition Based on BMI	Obesity Class	Disease Risk* Relative to Normal Weight and Waist Circumference	
Waist circumference			Normal	Increased men >102 cm, women >88 cm
Underweight	<18.5			
Normal	18.5–24.9			
Overweight	25.0–29.9		Increased	High
Obesity	30.0–34.9	I	High	Very high
Obesity	35.0–39.9	II	Very high	Very high
Extreme obesity	≥40	III	Extremely high	Extremely high

*Risk of developing type 2 diabetes, hypertension, and/or cardiovascular disease.
(From National Heart, Lung, and Blood Institute. Clinical guidelines on the identification, evaluation, and treatment of overweight and obesity in adults. Executive summary. Bethesda, MD: National Institutes of Health; 1998.)

History

All patients should undergo a brief screening history that inquires about changes in weight and appetite, eating habits (e.g., the number of meals per day and the variety of foods consumed), and symptoms of chronic disease (e.g., fever, chronic pain, fatigue). A significant weight loss is defined as a 5% weight loss in 1 month, 7.5% in 3 months, or a 10% loss in 6 months. A severe weight loss is defined as anything greater than those parameters. Acute weight loss or weight gain (over a day or two) is usually because of a change in fluid status rather than an indication of nutritional change.

In patients with known or newly identified chronic illness, a more thorough history is appropriate. In addition to a complete review of gastrointestinal symptoms, the physician should ask about supplemental vitamins and other products, alcohol and illicit drug use, appetite suppressants or stimulants, glucocorticoids, and laxatives. Chronic disease frequently increases nutritional requirements. For example, inflammation causes an increase in basal metabolic rate (BMR), which raises the daily caloric requirement.

In considering which patients might be at risk for poor nutrition, consider the various steps involved in nutritional intake, from acquiring food to absorbing nutrients (Table 15.3). Poverty and other access issues impair the ability to acquire food. Age or disability may preclude preparation of proper foods. Problems with dentition or coordination may impair ingestion of nutrients. Various gastrointestinal diseases, enzyme deficiencies, or medications may interfere with the taste, digestion, absorption, or metabolism of nutrients. Table 15.4 lists "red flags" that suggest the need to look especially hard for nutritional disease.

Dietary History

The dietary history should relate to both usual and recent food intake patterns. Reasonable questions include number of meals per day and examples of what is consumed at each meal.

TABLE 15.2 Risks of Overweight and Obesity

Overweight and obesity are known risk factors for	Obesity is associated with
• Diabetes	• High blood cholesterol
• Heart disease	• Complications of pregnancy
• Stroke	• Menstrual irregularities
• Hypertension	• Hirsutism
• Gallbladder disease	• Stress incontinence
• Osteoarthritis	• Depression
• Sleep apnea	• Increased surgical risk
• Uterine, breast, colorectal, kidney, and gallbladder cancer	• Increased risk of stillbirth (8) • Increased risk of neural tube defects (9)

Source unless noted: National Institute on Diabetes and Digestive and Kidney Disease. Statistics related to overweight and obesity. Bethesda, MD: National Institutes of Health; 2000.

TABLE 15.3 Areas to Consider in Identifying Patients at Risk for Poor Nutrition

Aspect of Nutrition	Examples
Acquiring food	• Poverty • Transportation needs • Infirmity • Language barriers • Inability to prepare food • Substance abuse • Depression
Ingestion of nutrients	• Poor dentition • Pain with chewing or swallowing • Lack of taste • Depression • Anxiety • Dementia • Medications • Substance abuse
Digestion	• Complete or partial gastrectomy • Pancreatic disease
Absorption	• Lack of absorptive surface due to surgery, Crohn's disease
Metabolism and excretion	• Inborn errors of metabolism • Nonabsorbable fat substitutes, leading to steatorrhea

A more thorough investigation includes cultural practices, personal preferences, and the use of a food pyramid to help patients identify the numbers of servings in each food group that they consume. Clinicians may use either retrospective methods (i.e., recall) or prospective food diaries to evaluate nutrient intake. The retrospective analysis has less validity than a prospective food diary, in which the patient is assigned the task of tracking all intake over the course of 1–2 days (10).

Physical Examination

A systematic physical examination is important in evaluating nutritional status. General inspection may readily reveal overweight or underweight status. Temporal wasting, decreased muscle mass, proximal muscle weakness, scaling skin, poor wound healing, and excessive bruising are signs suggesting malnutrition. Dietitians often use anthropometric measurements, including height, weight, skin fold thickness, head circumference (especially in infants and children), and waist to hip ratio. Clinicians tend to use the BMI is, which is a standardized and reliable measurement of body fat in adults (11, 12).

BMI tables and a downloadable tool for calculating BMI with personal digital assistants are readily available at *http://www.nhlbi.nih.gov*. When using BMI, be aware that it may overestimate body fat in trained athletes and underestimate body fat in older patients and others who have low lean body mass, including some obese individuals.

Circumference measurements are also useful in determining nutritional status. The waist circumference assesses abdominal fat content. Waist measurements of greater than 40 inches in men and 35 inches in women are independent risk factors for disease (13). In individuals with BMI >35 kg/m^2, measurement of waist circumference does not add to assessment of risk of disease (strength of recommendation [SOR]=C) (13). A high waist circumference is associated with an increased risk for type 2 diabetes, dyslipidemia, hypertension, and cardiovascular disease (CVD) in patients with a BMI in a range between 25 and 34.9 kg/m^2 (14).

TABLE 15.4 Red Flags Suggesting High Risk of Serious Nutritional Problems

- Weight loss of >5% in 1 month, 7.5% in 3 months, or 10% in 6 months
- Weight loss or gain associated with other systemic symptoms
- History of upper gastrointestinal surgery or disease

Laboratory Evaluation

No single laboratory test can diagnose malnutrition. Protein status is one of the oldest and most important measures of nutritional health. Commonly used measures include serum albumin, serum transferrin, and other serum proteins, such as transthyretin (also known as prealbumin). It is important to remember that the serum albumin level lags behind actual protein nutrition, because serum albumin has a half-life of 2–3 weeks. Serum proteins such as albumin and transferrin also are acute phase reactants and may actually increase under conditions of inflammation. Transferrin has a serum half-life of 8 days, and thus may be a more accurate parameter than albumin for measuring recent nutritional changes. However, the transferrin concentration is related to the overall iron status of the patient.

Micronutrients may be assessed directly via vitamin and mineral assays, or indirectly using tests such as the complete blood count and peripheral blood smear. Common patterns of vitamin and mineral deficiency include:

- Low levels of vitamin A, zinc, and magnesium in protein-calorie malnutrition;
- Deficiencies of fat-soluble vitamins (A, D, K, and E) in syndromes involving fat malabsorption. (Vitamin D production and metabolism is dependent on activation and adequate sunlight exposure.)
- Folic acid and iron deficiency in celiac disease. Changes in red blood cell production may result from insufficient levels of iron, vitamin B_{12}, folic acid, and other vitamins.

Patients with poor nutritional status may also demonstrate weak immune status in the form of poor T-lymphocyte responses. Evaluating the total lymphocyte count can be helpful in assessing T cells. Using a skin test for anergy is another way of assessing T-cell function.

EVALUATION OF OVERWEIGHT AND OBESITY

Overweight patients generally present to the family physician's office with a concern other than that of losing weight. Common presenting problems include type 2 diabetes mellitus, hypertension, musculoskeletal complaints (particularly back, knee, hip, or foot pain), and breathing difficulties. It is important to identify the excess weight or obesity as a problem, even if that is not the presenting complaint.

Questions should focus on the history of the weight problem and identification of risk factors for overweight as well as for co-morbid conditions. Patients with established coronary heart disease, other atherosclerotic diseases, type 2 diabetes, and sleep apnea are classified as being at very high risk for disease complications and mortality (13). Other obesity-associated conditions include polycystic ovarian disease, osteoarthritis, gallstones, and stress urinary incontinence. Smokers present a particular challenge. Epidemiologically, smokers are leaner than nonsmokers, and past smokers are heavier than those who have never smoked. This can be an issue when encouraging smoking cessation. Table 15.5 outlines the assessment of the overweight or obese patient.

It is important to determine the patient's readiness to lose weight. Gather information on previous attempts at losing weight, and whether those were successful. Ascertain the number of meals consumed each day, and how the patient's family life may affect the eating pattern. Many overweight patients admit to skipping meals in an attempt to lose weight. This practice should be discouraged because it may actually result in lowered BMR as well as an increase in caloric intake during the less frequent meals, both of which retard weight loss. Some overweight patients may give a history of using medications such as laxatives and diuretics in an attempt to lose weight.

The usual daily activity level of an individual plays a role in weight. Many patients think that they are very active during their jobs, and that exercise is therefore unnecessary for them. Social and emotional histories may reveal obstacles to losing weight, or even a history of emotional or physical abuse.

TABLE 15.5 Evaluation of the Overweight or Obese Patient

Evaluation	Element
History	• Dietary history • Activity history • Presence of heart disease; hypertension; diabetes; sleep apnea; polycystic ovaries; hypothyroidism; osteoarthritis; gallbladder disease; gout • Medications or nutritional supplements • Number of previous pregnancies • Family history of overweight • Social and emotional histories • Employment history
Physical examination	• Blood pressure • Calculated body mass index • Waist circumference • Thyroid examination • Striae, centripetal fat distribution (Cushing syndrome) • Leg edema • Cellulitis • Acanthosis nigricans (coarse hyperpigmentation seen with hyperinsulinemia) • Intertriginous rashes
Laboratory evaluations to consider	• Electrolytes • Liver function tests • Complete blood counts • Lipid profile • Thyroid-stimulating hormone • Fasting or random serum glucose

Focus patients on lifestyle changes and weight loss attempts that have been successful in the past.

Physical Examination

Obese patients deserve a complete physical examination to rule out signs of secondary causes of obesity, such as Cushing syndrome, hypothyroidism, or other pituitary abnormalities. Measurement of the waist circumference is also important as noted above.

Laboratory Evaluation

Obesity is a known risk factor for CVD and diabetes mellitus; therefore, other risk factors should be evaluated. Consider serum testing for hyperlipidemia and hyperglycemia.

THE UNDERWEIGHT PATIENT

A person is defined as underweight if the BMI is below 18.5 kg/m^2. The underweight patient presents unique considerations in a culture that is not sympathetic to this problem. As with the overweight person, careful assessment is needed because there are multiple causes of being underweight. One should not assume that underweight individuals are healthier than overweight patients. One problem of underweight is that there is little caloric reserve as a margin of safety if there are major health problems. Another concern is that people with restricted diets frequently have inadequate intake of vitamins and trace minerals. Additionally, the insulating function of body fat is not present, and the person may feel cold and is, therefore, at risk for hypothermia.

Causes of underweight status include dieting and eating disorders, genetically low normal body weight, wasting diseases, and high activity levels. Also, movement disorders (e.g., Parkinson disease) can cause extra energy expenditure, leading to decreased weight. Assessment of the underweight individual should consist of a good nutritional assessment, as outlined earlier in the chapter.

GENERAL RECOMMENDATIONS FOR NUTRITION GUIDANCE

A good source of evidence-based advice is the "USA Nutrition and Your Health: Dietary Guidelines for Americans," available at *www.nutrition.gov* (15). Its key recommendations for healthy people older than age 2 include:

- Consume a variety of nutrient-rich foods and beverages from among the various food groups.
- Limit the intake of saturated and trans fats, cholesterol, added sugars, salt, and alcohol.
- Obtain recommended intakes within caloric needs by adopting a balanced eating pattern, such as the US Department of Agriculture Food Guide or the Dietary Approaches to Stop Hypertension (DASH) eating plan.

This web site also makes recommendations for specific population groups, such as women of childbearing age and the elderly.

TREATMENT OF OVERWEIGHT AND OBESITY

Many treatment modalities are available to foster weight loss. In prescribing a weight loss regimen, it is crucial to remember to set goals with the patient, to negotiate a customized plan for weight loss, and to let the patient know that you will be there with him or her over the long haul, regardless of weight loss success. Assistance from experts such as nutritionists is often helpful. The best practice is to prevent overweight and obesity from occurring by instilling in patients the healthy habits of good nutrition and avoiding a sedentary lifestyle. There are critical periods in life when weight gain is more likely. These include after childbirth and menopause (16). If patients can learn to anticipate these changes, it is possible that they can institute appropriate lifestyle changes to prevent weight gain.

Once overweight or obesity is identified, it is important to set appropriate goals with the patient. The National Heart, Lung, and Blood Institute (NHLBI) practice guideline suggests an initial weight loss of 10% of body weight; however, this may not always be practical or achievable (13). Remind patients that even a 10-lb weight loss may ameliorate related conditions, such as hypertension and elevated blood glucose. A general timeline for a 10-lb weight loss is 6 months. Additional goals should include the maintenance of weight loss over time, and prevention of further weight gain. Modification of other cardiovascular risk factors, such as smoking, hypertension, elevated cholesterol, and physical inactivity, and recognition and treatment of diabetes deserve equal emphasis in the management of overweight or obese patients. Note that as patients quit smoking, they are likely to gain weight, so anticipatory guidance about this is essential. Patients should not expect to be able to quit smoking and lose weight at the same time.

Table 15.6 outlines the evidence regarding recognition and management of obesity in adults. Table 15.7 shows expected outcomes for the various treatments of obesity in adults. Modification of the diet affects the "energy input" side of the weight loss equation. Research continues in determining appropriate diets for weight loss. Any macronutrient—carbohydrate, protein, or fat—causes weight gain when overconsumed. Conversely, diets that decrease calories, whether as carbohydrate, protein, or fat, will be effective in helping adults lose weight, and reduce cardiovascular risk (17, 18). A large, randomized controlled trial comparing high or low fat, high or low protein, and high or low carbohydrate diets demonstrated that the type of caloric restriction had no bearing on eventual success at weight loss, but that sticking to the diet and showing up at group therapy sessions were the most important factors in weight loss success [SOR=A] (19).

Current evidence supports the use of calorie restriction for weight loss. An excess intake of 3500 kcal results in the gain of one pound, so in order to lose a pound, there must be a deficit of 3500 kcal. In an individual with a BMI $\geq$35 kg/m^2, reducing the kcal consumed by 500–1,000 kcal/d would result in weight loss of 1–2 lb per week, and thus a 10% weight loss in 6 months. A combination of reducing calories and increasing physical activity could be used to get the 500-kcal deficit. The caloric content of the macronutrients and alcohol is

TABLE 15.6 A Summary of Evidence-based Clinical Guidelines on the Identification, Evaluation, and Treatment of Overweight and Obesity in Adults

Recommendation	Strength of Recommendation*
Advantages of weight loss	
Lower elevated blood pressure	B
Improve hyperlipidemia	A
Lower blood glucose in obese patients with type 2 diabetes mellitus	A
Reduced osteoarthritis-related disability	A
Measurement of degree of overweight and obesity	
Body mass index to assess obesity and estimate relative risk	B
Waist circumference	C
Waist circumference cutoffs for patients with body mass index of 25–34.9 kg/m^2	C
Goals of weight loss	
Initial goal = 10% from baseline	A
Loss of 1–2 lb/week for 6 months	B
Methods of weight loss	
Dietary therapy	
Low-calorie diet	A
Reduced fat as part of a low-calorie diet	A
Diet with deficit of 500–1,000 kcal/d (will achieve weight loss of 1–2 lb/week)	A
Physical activity	
Weight loss	A
Decreased abdominal fat	B
Increased cardiorespiratory fitness	A
Maintenance of weight loss	C
30 minutes or more of moderate-intensity physical activity on most and preferably all days of the week as an integral part of weight loss therapy and weight maintenance	B
Behavior therapy	
As adjunct to diet in promoting weight loss and weight maintenance	B
Assessment of patient's motivation and readiness to implement a plan	C
Combined low-calorie diet, increased physical activity, and behavior therapy	A
Pharmacotherapy with lifestyle modification	B
Weight loss surgery—see text for indications	B
Maintenance	
After successful weight loss, maintenance program consisting of low calorie diet, physical activity, and behavior therapy, which should be continued indefinitely	B

*A, consistent, good-quality patient-oriented evidence; B, inconsistent or limited-quality patient-oriented evidence; C, consensus, disease-oriented evidence, usual practice, expert opinion, or case series. For information about the SORT (Strength of Recommendation Taxonomy) evidence rating system, see *http://www.aafp.org/afpsort.xml*

shown in Table 15.8. Reducing the amount of fat in the diet is helpful as long as the excess calories are not added back through increased consumption of carbohydrates. Many patients do not realize that sweetened and alcoholic drinks are loaded with calories which certainly contribute to the daily energy balance.

Physicians should work to individualize goals with patients. The balance between increased activity and decreased caloric consumption should be determined jointly by the patient and the physician. For example, the overall goal of 1–2 lb per week (with a 500–1,000 kcal/d difference between intake and output) may be more of a change than many

TABLE 15.7 Comparison of Obesity Treatment Strategies in Adults

Treatment	Outcome	Level of Evidence	Reference
Low calorie diet (1,000–1,200 kcal/day)	8% weight loss over 3–12 months	A	13
Very low calorie diet (400–500 kcal/day)	Greater weight loss than low calorie diets, but the difference disappears after 1 year	A	13
Aerobic activity	Aerobic exercise independent of dietary change results in modest weight loss (3–6 lb)	A	13
Surgery	Substantial weight loss in patients with BMI >40 or BMI >35 with comorbidities	B	13
Orlistat	5% reduction in body weight	B	52
Behavioral therapy	Up to 9 lb over 4 years when used in combination with other therapies	B	52
Group-based behavioral interventions	Greater loss in BMI than individual therapy	A	53

individuals can manage. More moderate goals (such as 1 lb/month or developing/improving health habits), with moderate changes (the difference of about 100 kcal/day), might be more realistic. In developing the plan for weight loss, the physician needs to investigate what the individual has done in the past that has been successful or unsuccessful. The individual who determines how she or he will change is far more likely to implement that change. For example, a patient who is reluctant to change his or her diet may be counseled to increase activity by an amount equivalent to the required caloric deficit. A weight loss prescription should be written with specific numbers, such as number of calories and number of minutes of specific exercises. Figure 15.1 contains helpful tips to discuss with your patients.

When counseling a patient in techniques for losing weight, an exercise prescription is essential, unless there is a medical contraindication to exercise. Promoting an increase in "physical activity" might be a more acceptable term to patients who think that exercise is too difficult for them. Lifestyle activities, such as walking, parking farther away from destinations, and using the stairs, are appropriate suggestions. The patient needs to decide what type and amount of exercise is achievable. Note that the use of pedometers to guide physical activity has been shown to promote modest weight loss among sedentary overweight individuals [SOR=A] (20). Though the actual number of kilocalories consumed per session of exercise is small, increased activity is crucial to overall energy balance. Calorie counters as part of the display on commercially available exercise machines are notoriously inaccurate because they do not take into account variables such as lean body mass and level of fitness. Table 15.9 lists types of activities and the time needed to consume a given number of calories. Exercise is especially important in maintaining weight loss, and has the added benefits of decreasing insulin resistance and reducing cardiovascular risk. Exercise may also convey an increased sense of well-being.

Some experts suggest that 1 hour per day of physical activity is necessary to lose weight. This does not have to be over a continuous period, in contrast to the 20–30 minutes, three times per week needed to reduce CVD risk. Another difference between exercises for CVD and physical activity for weight loss is that physical activity for weight loss does not require a specific heart rate elevation. The goal of increased physical activity is that when combined with dietary changes, it should result in a caloric deficit of 250–500 kcal/day.

TABLE 15.8 Macronutrient and Alcohol Caloric Content

Nutrient	Kilocalories/gram
Protein	4
Carbohydrate	4
Fat	9
Ethanol	7

Behavioral Therapy

Self-monitoring of eating habits may help patients lose weight. Food diaries are a simple form of this monitoring. The risk is that some patients may become obsessed with excessive dieting behaviors; therefore, this type of monitoring is best used to gain a short-term understanding of problem areas in eating. Patients may also benefit by recognizing and avoiding food triggers and enlisting the social support of friends, relatives, or others attempting to lose weight. A system of rewards for reaching certain goals is also effective in many patients. Table 15.10 lists web-based resources for both patients and clinicians.

Medications

Patients desiring weight loss should complete a trial of diet, exercise, and behavioral modification before pharmacotherapy is considered. According to the NHLBI and the US Food and Drug Administration (FDA), medications are indicated in patients who have a BMI greater than 30 kg/m^2 with no cardiac risk factors, or a BMI greater than or equal to 27 kg/m^2 with

Cookbooks

Here are some good reliable sources of advice and recipes:
- The *Cooking Light* magazine or series for each year
- The *American Heart Association Cookbook*
- The *Better Homes and Gardens* Cookbooks

Eating Out

Many Americans eat out frequently. Here are some tips that may be helpful:
- It is usually easier to control what you eat if you eat at home. However, if you plan ahead you can choose lower calorie options, such as baked or broiled foods; no added butter/margarine/sour cream/cream sauces to foods.
- Beware that American restaurants generally serve very large portions; share the meal, take part home, or leave part of the meal to make the portions represent portion sizes that should be consumed by most people. Children's meals are actually the portion size that most children need—don't buy an extra meal for a child; adults consume more than a child needs so we often don't understand the smaller portions that the child needs and then encourage over-consumption.
- Never super-size any meal or beverage; super-sizing adds more than 600 calories and sometimes as much as 1000 calories to the meal/beverage.
- Be aware that many chain restaurants publish lists of nutritional information for each of their selections, usually at that location where the food is paid for.
- Here are two websites you can use in planning healthy meals out:
  www.restaurant.org/nutrition/index.cfm
  www.healthy-dining.com

How to Feel Full While Eating Less

- Drink water instead of caloric drinks to quench thirst. If you have to flavor the water, use lemons or limes. Also, remember that you can sometimes feel hungry when you are thirsty instead.
- Small snacks can add up to big calories. Small candies range from 20 to 60 calories a piece. If you eat 10 pieces, that could as much as 600 calories.
- Changing from one food item (such as small candy that is 20 calories to one that is 60 calories, or 1 glass of wine to 1 bottle of wine cooler) can add significant calories without any change in what the body feels is consumed. The example of the eating 10 pieces of 20 calorie candy (200 calories) to eating 10 pieces of 60 calorie candy (600 calories) is an added consumption of 400 calories or 1 pound weight gain in less than 10 days!

Make Changes that You Can Stick With, and Then Be Patient

- Most overweight individuals have become that way by eating only about 50 calories too many a day. So most people don't have to make big changes to start losing weight—they just have to make and keep the changes, and then be patient.
- A combination of healthy eating with moderate diet and exercise is the best way to lose weight, or at the very least, improve one's health.
- Changes for weight loss in a person's diet need to be individualized. Everyone does not gain weight in the same way nor are they going to be able to lose weight and not regain it in the same way. The above suggestions are based on some areas that research has shown to be problematic, but these suggestions need to be tailored to each person's problematic areas of eating and physical activity.

Figure 15.1 • Helpful tips to losing weight.

two or more risk factors (e.g., hypertension, dyslipidemia, CVD, type 2 diabetes mellitus, sleep apnea). Medications should not be used in isolation; diet, exercise, and behavior modification are also necessary. There are currently three FDA-approved medications for weight loss; in October 2010, the manufacturer of sibutramine voluntarily withdrew it from the market due to adverse effects. Table 15.11 lists medications for weight loss. A recent meta-analysis demonstrated that such medications can lead to a weight loss of about 5 kg after 1 year, with little evidence for long-term sustained weight loss (21).

TABLE 15.9 Examples of Moderate Activities

Moderate physical activity uses approximately 150 calories of energy per day, or 1,000 calories/wk. Everyday chores and sports are moderate activities.
Examples are listed below.

Common Chores	Sporting Activities
Washing and waxing a car for 45–60 minutes	Playing volleyball for 45–60 minutes
Washing windows or floors for 45–60 minutes	Walking 1.75 miles in 35 min (20 minutes/mile)
Gardening for 30–45 minutes	Basketball (shooting baskets) for 30 minutes
Wheeling self in wheelchair for 30–40 minutes	Bicycling 5 miles in 30 minutes
Pushing a stroller 1.5 miles in 30 minutes	Dancing fast (social) for 30 minutes
Raking leaves for 30 minutes	Water aerobics for 30 minutes
Walking 2 miles in 30 min (15 minutes/mile)	Swimming laps for 20 minutes
Stair walking for 15 minutes	Basketball (playing a game) for 15–20 minutes
	Jumping rope for 15 minutes

More vigorous activities, such as running, bicycle racing, and stair climbing take less time to consume the same number of calories.

TABLE 15.10 Web-based Resources for Nutrition and Weight Management

Organization and/or Web Site	Web Address
The American Dietetic Association	*http://eatright.org*
The National Association of Anorexia Nervosa and Associated Disorders	*http://www.anad.org*
The National Academy of Sciences	*http://www.nas.edu*
Overeaters Anonymous	*http://www.overeatersanonymous.org*
National Heart, Lung, and Blood Institute	*http://www.nhlbi.gov/guidelines/obesity*
US Food and Drug Administration	*http://www.fda.gov*
National Health Information Council (a part of the Public Health Service—Office of Disease Prevention and Health Promotion)	*http://nhic-nt.health.org*
The National Institutes of Health information clearinghouse for diabetes, digestive diseases, and related areas such as obesity	*http://www.niddk.nih.gov*
US Department of Agriculture—Food and Nutrition Consumer Service (food pyramid and related materials)	*http://www.mypyramid.gov*
Nutrition site for all government information	*http://www.nutrition.gov*
Disease-specific nutrition information (Medline Plus)	*http://www.medlineplus.gov*

A general guideline is that if a patient taking a weight loss medication has not lost at least 2 kg after 4 weeks, the medication should be discontinued.

Complementary Therapies

Both ephedrine and ephedra have been used by patients for weight loss, though ephedra is no longer legally available in the United States. There is evidence that these drugs promote only a small amount of weight loss (2.5–10.5 lb in 6 months), with the tradeoff of a relatively large risk (1/1,000) of a serious adverse event (22). Hence, these drugs are not recommended for use in helping patients lose weight. Other complementary therapies, none of which has been shown over a six month period to cause lasting weight loss, include Garcinia (hydroxyacetic acid), chitosan, chromium picolinate, and glucomannate [SOR=A] (23).

Surgery

Surgical procedures for weight loss should be reserved for patients in whom medical weight loss treatment has failed, and who are suffering from complications of extreme obesity. Bariatric surgery can be considered an option for patients with a BMI greater than or equal to 40 kg/m^2, or greater than or equal to 35 kg/m^2, if cardiovascular risk factors are present [SOR=C]. Bariatric surgery has been shown to be highly effective in managing the comorbidities associated with obesity,

TABLE 15.11 Drugs Used for Weight Loss

Drug	Dose	FDA Approval	Action	Adverse Effects	Cost
Orlistat (Xenical)	120 mg 120 mg orally three times daily before fat-containing meals	Long-term use, over-the-counter	Inhibits pancreatic lipase, decreases fat absorption	Decrease in absorption of fat-soluble vitamins; soft stools and anal leakage	$$$
Phentermine (Adipex-P, Fastin, Oby-trim, Pro-fast, Zantryl)	8, 15, 18.75, 30, 37.5 mg 8 mg three times daily 30 minutes before meals, or 15–37.5 mg daily before breakfast	Short-term use (controlled substance C-IV)	Appetite suppressant	Abuse, hypertension, tachycardia, restlessness, insomnia	$
Diethylpropion (Tenuate, Tenuate Dospan, generic available)	25 mg, 75 mg SR 25 mg three times daily, 1 hour before meals, or 75 mg SR once daily in the midmorning	Short-term use (controlled substance C-IV)	Appetite suppressant	Pulmonary hypertension, arrhythmias, psychosis, dry mouth, restlessness	$

CNS = central nervous system; FDA = US Food and Drug Administration; MAOIs = monoamine oxidase inhibitors.

such as type 2 diabetes, hypertension, obstructive sleep apnea, and hyperlipidemia. [SOR=A] (24). Available procedures include placing a restrictive band around the stomach to reduce the capacity (gastric banding), ligating off part of the stomach (gastroplasty), or bypassing the stomach altogether (gastric bypass). Good illustrations of the procedures are available from the National Library of Medicine at *http://www.nlm.nih.gov/medlineplus/ency/article/007199.htm*.

Gastric bypass has been shown to be more effective than gastric banding for weight loss and requires fewer surgeries for revision, but has more side effects [SOR=A] (25). Some evidence suggests that gastric bypass produces more weight loss than gastric banding [SOR=B]) (26). It should be noted that bariatric surgery has a significant complication rate, depending largely on the experience of the surgeon who performs the operation (24).

MANAGEMENT OF THE UNDERWEIGHT PATIENT

The underweight person works with the same energy balance principles as the overweight person (kcal eaten vs energy expended). Food, exercise, and weight goals need to take these factors into consideration. Practical food considerations include the following:

- High-fat foods do not necessarily help an underweight person gain weight because they cause the person to feel full for long periods and therefore can act as an appetite suppressant.
- Snacks or small frequent meals may help and should be taken at least two hours before the next meal.
- Adding calories without adding volume to liquids consumed may be effective (e.g., adding powdered milk to regular milk to increase protein calories).

A physician who is concerned with an underweight patient should investigate the problem with the same clinical tools that are used for the overweight patient. Treatment should consist of measures appropriate to the diagnosis; for example, increased calories for increased energy expenditure or mental health treatment for eating disorders.

WEIGHT MANAGEMENT IN CHILDREN AND ADOLESCENTS

Through the last decades in the United States, the average weights of children have increased. There is some evidence that parental overweight or obesity is a risk factor for the development of overweight in children though this relationship is probably multifactorial, involving not only genetics, but also environment and culture, which affect diet (27).

Evaluation of Overweight and Obesity in Children

The United States Preventive Services Task Force (USPSTF) recommends that clinicians screen children age 6–18 years for overweight and obesity and offer them comprehensive behavioral intervention to improve weight status. Although these comprehensive interventions have been found to improve weight in the short term, there is only limited evidence that these patients maintain improved weight status beyond one year [SOR=B] (28). There is hope that early intervention also helps children and adolescents develop health eating and activity patterns, which should be the focus of the intervention (29).

The definition of overweight and obesity in children is based on comparison to children of the same age and sex as follows:

- Overweight: BMI at or above the 85 percentile and lower than 95 percentile.
- Obesity: BMI at or above the 95 percentile.
- Child BMI charts are available from: *http://www.cdc.gov/healthyweight/assessing/bmi/*.

History

Appropriate, weight specific questions include those about diet, activity level, and hours of television viewing, breast versus formula feeding as an infant, as well as presence of family history of obesity, and conditions frequently comorbid with obesity, such as type 2 diabetes, hypertension, and lipid disorders. There is a long-standing body of evidence supporting the theory that consumption of sweet drinks (fruit juices and soft drinks) is associated with overweight in children [SOR=B] (30). However, a recent publication on the study called Project Eating Among Teens (Project EAT) did not show any association between sugar-sweetened beverages, juice consumption, and weight gain among teenagers over a 5-year period (31).

Physical and Laboratory Examination

There are no set parameters for appropriate waist circumference in children so measurement of waist circumference is not helpful in screening or diagnosis [SOR=C] (27). Along with a general physical examination to look for secondary causes of obesity (for example, purple striae may suggest hypercortisolism), laboratory evaluation should include fasting lipid profiles in patients with a strong family history of lipid disorders or cardiovascular disease, as well as a fasting blood glucose in children with a family history of type 2 diabetes mellitus (32).

The medical concern for this weight increase in children has been focused on problems such as mature onset diabetes in youth, where type 2 diabetes mellitus occurs at young ages (33). However, it is unclear from the data that childhood overweight is carried into adult overweight or that it is associated with medical risk (34). It is important not to label children as overweight, as this may affect their body image well into the future. Because many children "fill out" before they "grow up," this may well be a misdiagnosis. In a child with normal growth in stature, it is unlikely that overweight or obesity is caused by an underlying metabolic or genetic form of overweight (29). Overweight children with the highest risk for adverse health outcome include those with current weight-related comorbidities, high risk of developing weight-related comorbidities in the future, or significant negative psychosocial ramifications of their overweight status [SOR=A] (32).

Management of Overweight and Obesity in Children

Several studies to date have directly linked increased hours of watching television to overweight (35, 36). Other investigators have explored school-based programs aimed at increasing

TABLE 15.12 Evidence-based Interventions in Children

Intervention	Strength of Recommendation and Source
Physical activity and diet better than diet alone	A (32)
No evidence that physical activity alone is effective	C (32)
Lifestyle exercise more effective than aerobic/calisthenics in maintaining weight loss	B (32)
Behavioral weight loss programs more effective if implemented by parents, rather than child	A (32)
Programs targeting sedentary behavior (such as television watching) equally effective to promoting physical activity	B (32)
Combined behavioral lifestyle interventions can produce a significant and meaningful reduction in overweight in children and adolescents	A (40)

*A = consistent, good-quality patient-oriented evidence; B = inconsistent or limited-quality patient-oriented evidence; C = consensus, disease-oriented evidence, usual practice, expert opinion, or case series.
For information about the Strength of Recommendation Taxonomy evidence rating system, see *http://www.aafp.org/afpsort.xml*.

physical activity and improving intake of fruits and vegetables (35, 37). The standard tools of a healthy diet and plenty of activity seem to be the standbys for physicians and dietitians at this point. There is evidence that moderately intense exercise for one half to one hour most days per week reduces total body and visceral fat in overweight children and adolescents [SOR=A] (38). However, not all treatments with diet and exercise have been shown to be beneficial (39). Tables 15.12 and 15.13 contain a summary of recommendations regarding management of overweight in children. Organizations that have published evidence-based guidelines on management of obesity and overweight in children include the American Heart Association, the Scottish Intercollegiate Guideline Network, and the USPSTF. Notably, the USPSTF states that there is insufficient available evidence on the effectiveness of interventions that can be offered in the primary care setting. The guideline committees agree that diet alone, without changing activity, is ineffective in treating overweight in children.

Recent studies show that parents (primarily mothers) who restrain the eating of their children actually cause the reverse of what might have been intended (41, 42). Instead of the child then moderating her food intake, the child no longer has the internal inhibition because it was replaced by the parent. In other words, dieting does not work in children, especially when enforced by a parent.

Two recent areas of interest in treatment interventions in diet have been the following: 1) reduction of sugar-sweetened beverages because the consumption of these beverages has increased steadily and 2) fast food/convenience food consumption. Studies demonstrate no apparent difference in consumption of high calorie fast foods between leaner and overweight youth (43).

TABLE 15.13 Comparison of Obesity Treatment Strategies in Children

Treatment	Outcome	Level of Evidence	Reference
Moderately intense exercise for 30–60 minutes per day	Reduction of visceral fat and total body fat	A	38
Orlistat	Reduction of weight over placebo	B	32, 45
Comprehensive behavioral intervention with medium to high intensity	Reduction in BMI of 1.9–3.3 kg/m^2	B	28
Orlistat combined with behavioral modification	Reduction in BMI of 0.85 kg/m^2	B	28
Parental involvement in comprehensive intervention with lifestyle change	Better than lifestyle changes alone	B	54

Psychosocial issues surrounding the diagnosis of overweight, or "fat" in a child should not be underestimated (44). Communication with the child and family must revolve around moderating health risks and making positive lifestyle changes rather than cosmetic issues.

There is evidence that drug treatment can be effective in treating obesity in children and adolescents. Studies demonstrate that in combination with general recommendations for diet, exercise, and behavior modification, orlistat can improve weight management in adolescents [SOR= B] (32, 45). Current guidelines suggest that surgery as a treatment for extreme obesity in children should be used rarely and as a last resort [SOR=C] (32).

WEIGHT MANAGEMENT IN THE ELDERLY PATIENT

Nutritional guidelines for older adults can be found at *http://www.nutrition.org/chi/content/full/129/3/751* (46). Note that, although generally similar to adult guidelines, these include information on water intake, increased calcium, and selected vitamin supplements. The DASH study found that consuming increased fruits, vegetables, and calcium-containing foods, combined with physical activity, decreased hypertension. The study also recommended weight loss, but within the context of the changes suggested, the improved dietary content and physical activity seemed as important as caloric reduction (47). It is important to note that when older adults lose weight, a relatively high percentage of the weight lost is lean body mass. In active older adults, at least 30% of the weight reduction is loss of lean body mass, and this percentage is even higher in nonactive older adults.

The BMR decreases with age, and this may lead to weight gain despite consistency in diet and exercise patterns. In spite of this, the trend is for weight to decrease in older age. Peak weights for men occur on average at 55 years of age and for women at 65 years (48, 49). Even without intervention, the weight will tend to decrease after these ages. Treatments of overweight in this age group have not been investigated for any conclusions regarding their efficacy. However, the mortality and morbidity data seem to show that the slightly overweight older adult fares better in longevity than the underweight older adult (50). In fact, when there are no obesity associated comorbidities such as hypertension and cardiovascular disease, longevity actually increases with increasing BMI [SOR=A] (51).

KEY POINTS

- All patients deserve some level of nutritional assessment. Those with chronic disease or evidence of a nutritional disorder deserve a detailed nutritional assessment.
- Nutritional status, including overweight and obesity, is affected by a combination of genetics, environment, and behavior.
- In assessing overweight and obese adults, BMI and waist circumference are key in assessing health risk.
- The most effective weight loss methods in adults and children include increased activity, decreased caloric intake, and behavior modification.
- Addressing a sedentary lifestyle may be the most important aspect of managing overweight in children.
- A higher BMI in otherwise healthy elderly patients is associated with longevity.

CHAPTER 16

Ear Pain

William J. Hueston and Arch G. Mainous III

CLINICAL OBJECTIVES

1. List the most common infectious and noninfectious causes of pain in the ear.
2. Discuss the reliability of the diagnostic tests for otitis media.
3. Describe the optimal management of acute suppurative otitis media.
4. Compare and contract strategies that are most effective for preventing recurrence of otitis media in children with frequent infections.

Ear pain is one of the most common reasons why parents seek care for their children from primary care physicians. Otitis media was the third most common reason for visiting a physician in a study of community practices (1) and ranked 11th in reasons for visits among the more than 500,000 patient problems recorded in a sentinel large cross-sectional study (2). In addition, ear wax, serous otitis media, and otitis externa also ranked in the top 50 most common diagnoses (1). Although these problems are infrequently life-threatening, they commonly cause a significant amount of anxiety and suffering in primary care patients as well as posing significant costs to the health care system (3).

APPLIED ANATOMY

The ear is innervated by three different neural pathways (4). Figure 16.1 presents an overview of ear anatomy. The external ear, conchae, and external auditory canal receive primary sensory innervation from somatic sensory fibers of the facial nerve (7th cranial nerve). Parts of the external auditory canal also receive sensory innervation from the auricular branch of the vagus (*Arnold nerve*), which contains nerve fibers from the 7th cranial nerve as well as the 9th and 10th nerves. The stimulation of the Arnold nerve in the external auditory canal sometimes produces cough through vagal stimulation. The Arnold nerve also is involved in herpes zoster infections of the external ear canal. On the other hand, the middle ear receives its neural innervation through branches of the glossopharyngeal nerve (9th cranial nerve) only. Because this nerve innervates the throat and tongue, it is common for throat pain to be referred to the middle ear.

The separate innervation of the middle and external ears can be useful in differentiating the source of pain. Retraction of the conchae or pressure on the tragus (the *tragus sign*) in the case of external otitis or trauma to the external auditory canal will cause pain because of local inflammation of the 7th cranial nerve. However, stimulation of the external ear typically will not produce pain with otitis media.

The inner ear, on the other hand, is innervated by the 8th cranial nerve, the vestibulocochlear nerve. The nerve is made up of two large divisions (the vestibular and cochlear nerves) that transmit information relating to balance and sound to the medulla. Dysfunction in the vestibulocochlear nerve results in symptoms such as hearing loss, vertigo, or tinnitus.

The function and integrity of the Eustachian tube is a major factor influencing the likelihood of a child developing middle ear infections. The role of the eustachian tube is to ventilate the middle ear and provide mucociliary clearance for bacteria and other materials that migrate from the nasopharynx. Ventilation is controlled by the tensor veli palatini muscle, which opens and closes the eustachian canal to normalize pressures in the middle ear. Mucociliary clearance is performed primarily in the lower half of the eustachian tube that is provided with many mucous glands.

Dysfunction of the eustachian tube disrupts proper ventilation of the middle ear and can result in a negative pressure that pulls fluid into the middle ear space. Stasis of this fluid (middle ear effusion) combined with colonization with nasopharyngeal organisms can result in otitis media. Conditions that are associated with poor eustachian tube function or occlusion of the lower eustachian tube such as allergic rhinitis or upper respiratory tract infections increase the risk of otitis media. Additionally, poor function of the tensor veli palatini muscle which is seen in some families as well as in patients with Trisomy 21 (Down syndrome) also increase the risk of otitis media. Finally, patients with craniofacial abnormalities that may involve the eustachian tube also have higher incidences of otitis media.

DIFFERENTIAL DIAGNOSIS

Table 16.1 summarizes the usual differential diagnoses for ear pain. The most common cause of inflammation in the middle or external ears is infection. Additionally, some pain may accompany the impaction of the external ear by foreign bodies or with excessive cerumen due to excessive pressure in the auditory canal causing mucosal irritation. Generally, cerumen impaction or foreign body presence does not produce pain, but rather results in hearing loss.

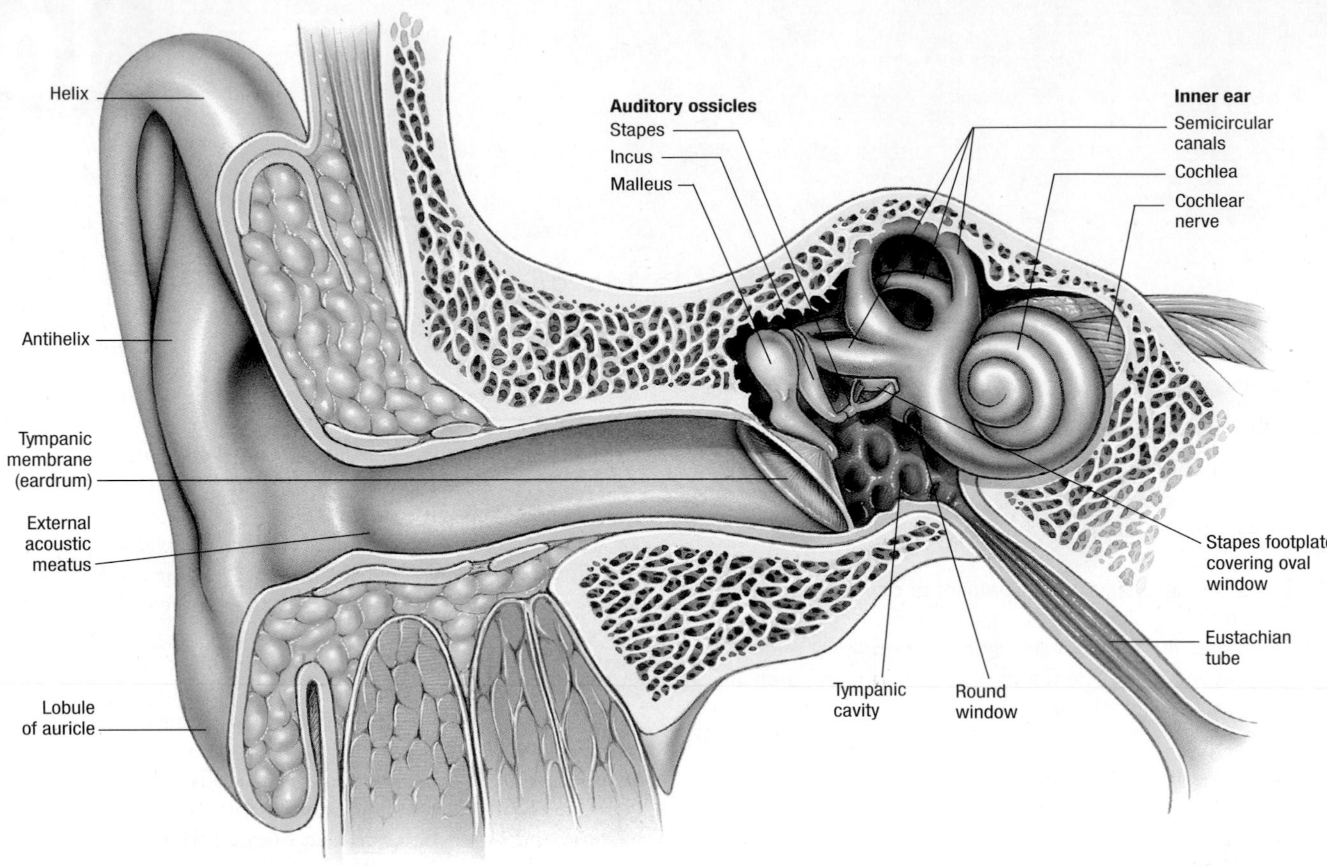

Figure 16.1 • Anatomy of the ear.

Infections of the external ear and auditory canal are defined primarily by their location:

- Perichondritis is used to describe infection of the pinna. These infections usually produce a red painful, swollen external ear.
- Furunculosis refers to infection of the hair follicles in the outer third of the auditory canal. Both perichondritis and furunculosis are usually caused by staphylococcal species or, occasionally, streptococcal species.

TABLE 16.1 Differential Diagnosis of Ear Pain

Diagnosis	Frequency in Primary Care
Acute otitis media	Very common
Cerumen impaction	Very common
Otitis externa	Common
Referred pain from throat or temporal bone	Common
Acoustic trauma	Less common
External ear dermatitis	Less common
Perichondritis	Less common
Foreign body in the canal	Less common
Furunculosis	Rare
Mastoiditis	Rare
Ear tumors (eosinophilic granulomas, rhabdosarcomas)	Rare

- Otitis externa refers to infection of the fibrocartilaginous inner two-thirds of the auditory canal, which is devoid of hair follicles and glands and has a very friable, thin skin layer. The most common organism cultured from the auditory canal in otitis externa is *Pseudomonas*, which can be found in association with other bacteria such as *Staphylococcus* and *Proteus* (5). Infection causes edema of the ear canal and disrupts the normal squamous cell shedding that occurs on a regular basis. This leads to the accumulation of a keratin layer in the canal along with exudate and necrotic debris.

Patients with repetitive trauma to any of these areas are at highest risk for the development of an infection.

CLINICAL EVALUATION

History

Table 16.2 summarizes the most common risk factors for the development of acute otitis media (AOM).

Decreased hearing, pain, and associated systemic signs of infections such as fever or malaise characterize middle ear infections. The peak onset of middle ear infections is in the first 6 years of life. About one-third of children have their first episode of otitis media in the first year of life and often have repetitive episodes throughout their childhood. Another third of children have only a small number of ear infections (<3) in their childhood. The remaining third of children do not have any ear infections.

TABLE 16.2 Risk Factors for Development of Acute Otitis Media

Age <2 years
Male
Genetic predisposition
Previous episode(s) of otitis media
Cigarette smoking in household
Attendance at day care
Recent upper respiratory infection

From *Rosenfeld R, Bluestone C, Evidence based Otitis Media St Louis, MO, BC Decker Inc. 1999.*

In general, the most useful elements of the history in a patient with ear pain are: the location of the pain, type of pain, and actions that make the pain worse. Outer ear infections are sensitive to touch of the ear as described above. Otitis media is a deeper pain that is unaffected by movement of the outer ear. The most predictive symptoms for otitis media are ear pain (LR + of 3.0–7.4) and rubbing of the ear (LR + 3.4) (6).

The degree of accompanying hearing loss also can be a useful historical sign. Complete hearing loss can occur with foreign bodies or complete canal occlusion with cerumen. Severe otitis externa may totally obstruct the auditory canal as well. Middle ear infections generally cause a dulling of sound, but hearing is still present.

Finally, it is important to ask about dental problems, pain with chewing, throat pain, or other problems that are affecting the throat and jaw. Referred pain to the ear is common and other sources of the problem should be sought. Temporomandibular disorders are particularly prone to ear pain (7). In patients with temporomandibular disorders, the prevalence of otalgia without infection varies between 12 and 16% (8). Patients with suspected temporomandibular disorders should generally be referred to a dentist for further assessment.

Physical Examination

The first step in evaluating ear pain is differentiating middle ear pain, external ear pain, and referred pain. Again, manipulation of the external ear will exacerbate most pain located in the external ear or the auditory canal. However, referred pain and middle ear pain will be unaffected by this maneuver. Inspection of the outer ear and auditory canal will confirm the presence of foreign bodies or inflammation.

If manipulation of the outer ear fails to reproduce or worsen the pain, the source is more likely to be the middle ear or referred pain. The presence of an earache along with night restlessness and a fever increase the likelihood of an otitis media (9). The next step in the evaluation is visualization of the tympanic membrane (TM) plus possible ancillary testing such as pneumatic otoscopy and tympanometry to determine if the membrane is mobile. A mobile TM suggests that no fluid is present in the middle ear and that the diagnosis of otitis media cannot be made.

When examining the TM when AOM is suspected, the most useful positive findings for otitis media include a bulging (positive likelihood ratio [LR] of 51) or cloudy (LR of 34) TM. These findings are caused by effusion which is a necessary component to diagnose AOM and a much better predictor than observing redness of the TM (9). A TM that is only slightly red (LR 1.4) is not useful (6). The combination of a cloudy effusion, bulging membrane, and loss of mobility has a predictive value for AOM in the mid-90th percentile (10). Note if the tympanic membrane is perforated as this will allow purulent material to exude into the auditory canal.

Classic presentation of AOM is rare. In a study of practicing primary care doctors, in only 58% of cases could clinicians could state with confidence that the person they diagnosed with AOM really had an infected-looking ear (11). Other investigations have shown significant disagreement between expert examiners for the presence of effusion (12). When clinical otoscopy to diagnose effusion was compared to myringotomy as the gold standard in a study of 226 children, the sensitivity of clinical examination was only 74% and the specificity was 60% (13).

To improve diagnostic accuracy, pneumatic otoscopy can be used as an adjunctive maneuver. In this test, air is introduced into the auditory canal while the TM is being visualized. Movement of the TM with increased air pressure is believed to indicate that no middle ear effusion is present. However, this test does not improve the positive predictive value of clinical otoscopy significantly (14). Other ancillary tests are described in the following section. Table 16.3 lists key elements of the history, physical examination and diagnostic testing.

Red Flags Signaling Problems

Table 16.4 summarizes important “red flags” to watch for. Most ear infections are localized to the ear canal and middle ear, but contiguous spread to adjoining structures can occur infrequently.

External ear infection (perichondritis) is generally located in the body of the auricle, but spares the noncartilaginous lobule.

TABLE 16.3 Key Elements in the History, Physical Examination, and Diagnostic Testing for Ear Pain

Diagnosis	Diagnostic Maneuvers	Reliability of Diagnostic Test
Otitis externa	Pain on manipulation of outer ear	Not tested
Acute otitis media	Pneumatic otoscopy	Sensitivity: 74–93%; specificity: 58–60%
	Tympanometry in cooperative children	Sensitivity: 78–95%; specificity: 79–93%
	Tympanometry in uncooperative children	Sensitivity: 71%; specificity: 38%
	Acoustic reflectometry	Sensitivity: 79–90%; specificity: 79–86%

TABLE 16.4 Red Flags Suggesting Progressive or Life-Threatening Disease in Patients with Ear Pain

Red Flag	Diagnosis Suggested
Ear lobule erythema	Erysipelas
Seventh cranial nerve palsy	Malignant otitis externa (*Pseudomonas* infection)
Ulceration in external ear canal	Auditory canal tumor or tumor eroding into the canal such as myosarcoma or lymphoma
Nonhealing lesion in the auditory canal	Auditory canal tumor or tumor eroding into the canal such as rhabdomyosarcoma or lymphoma
Tenderness over the mastoid	Mastoiditis

Involvement of the lobule of the auricle, which does not contain cartilage, is an ominous sign that suggests a more virulent infection such as erysipelas. If the lobule is involved in infection, rapid initiation of antistreptococcal antibiotics is imperative to keep the infection from rapidly progressing into the surround neck tissue.

In otitis externa, invasion into adjoining tissue occurs most frequently in infections caused by *Pseudomonas aeruginosa*. Infection with this organism, termed *malignant otitis externa*, can cause widespread local invasion and bacteremia with sepsis and death. The hallmark warning signs of *Pseudomonas* malignant otitis include a seventh nerve palsy on the affected side. Other infections, in particular, herpes zoster of the ear, also can produce a seventh nerve palsy and must be differentiated from malignant otitis externa.

Other warning signs in the auditory canal include an ulcerated or nonhealing lesion in the canal. Either of these signs can indicate erosion of an adjoining tumor into the canal. If these lesions are seen, biopsies of the ulcerated or nonhealing area are indicated.

A final red flag seen in otitis media is tenderness over the mastoid process of the temporal bone. This could signal mastoiditis, a chronic osseous infection that in the preantibiotic era was a significant cause of morbidity and usually will not resolve without surgical debridement of the mastoid.

Diagnostic Testing

Tympanometry improves the sensitivity and specificity of the diagnosis of middle ear effusion necessary to diagnose AOM. Tympanometry measures the amount of a test sound that transverses the TM at given positive and negative auditory canal pressures. The tympanometer forms an airtight seal around the auditory canal, and a sound wave is introduced by pushing a button on the instrument. The machine monitors the amount of the sound reflected back from the TM. This procedure is repeated as various positive and negative pressures and the results are plotted based on the amount of sound transmitted: usually a bell-shaped curve reflects normal TM movement. Figure 16.2 is an example of a normal tympanogram result. In a series of studies evaluating this test, the sensitivity of tympanometry to diagnose effusion compared to myringotomy as the gold standard ranged from 79% to 95% with a corresponding specificity of 57–93% (10). However, the reliability of the test is influenced by the level of cooperation by the patient. In poorly cooperative children, the predictive value drops substantially (15).

Acoustic reflectometry, another adjunctive test, measures reflected sound off the TM. The amount of sound reflected is measured in decibels. The most appropriate cutoff value for a positive test is still controversial. Studies of acoustic reflectometry have used either tympanometry or clinical examination as the gold standard, which limits their interpretation. Even given these weak gold standards, positive and negative predictive values are in the 80% range (10).

Recommended Diagnostic Strategy

A combination of history, physical examination, and diagnostic testing to diagnose otitis media is recommended by the Agency for Healthcare Research and Quality (16). A 2004 American Academy of Pediatrics and American Academy of Family Physicians (AAP/AAFP) guideline defined AOM as: 1) the presence of middle ear effusion (based on either diagnostic tests or physical examination findings of opacification or a full or bulging tympanic membrane or otorrhea) **plus** 2) an acute onset of signs and symptoms, together with 3) signs and symptoms of middle ear inflammation such as erythema, otalgia, and systemic unwellness such as fever or irritability in an infant or toddler. All three elements should be present before AOM is diagnosed. Figure 16.3 illustrates a useful approach to the evaluation and treatment of ear pain.

MANAGEMENT

Table 16.5 summarizes management approaches for the following common ear conditions.

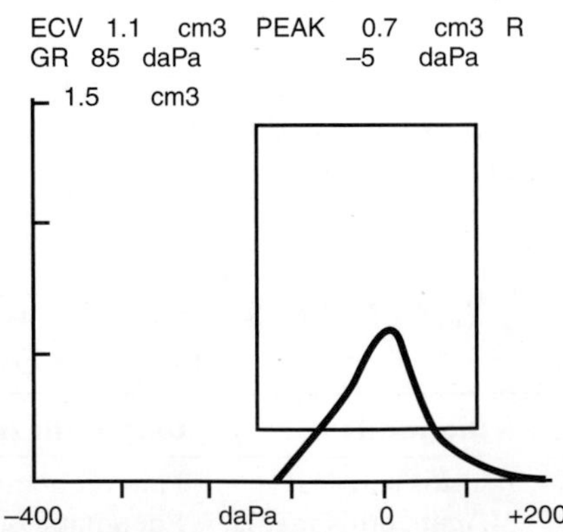

Figure 16.2 • Normal tympanogram.
Key: ECV = external canal volume. The other variables describe the characteristics of the curve which with a normally functioning TM, should be bell-shaped and peak in the outlined rectangle. Generally, ECV > 2 cm3 and a flat curve suggests a TM perforation.

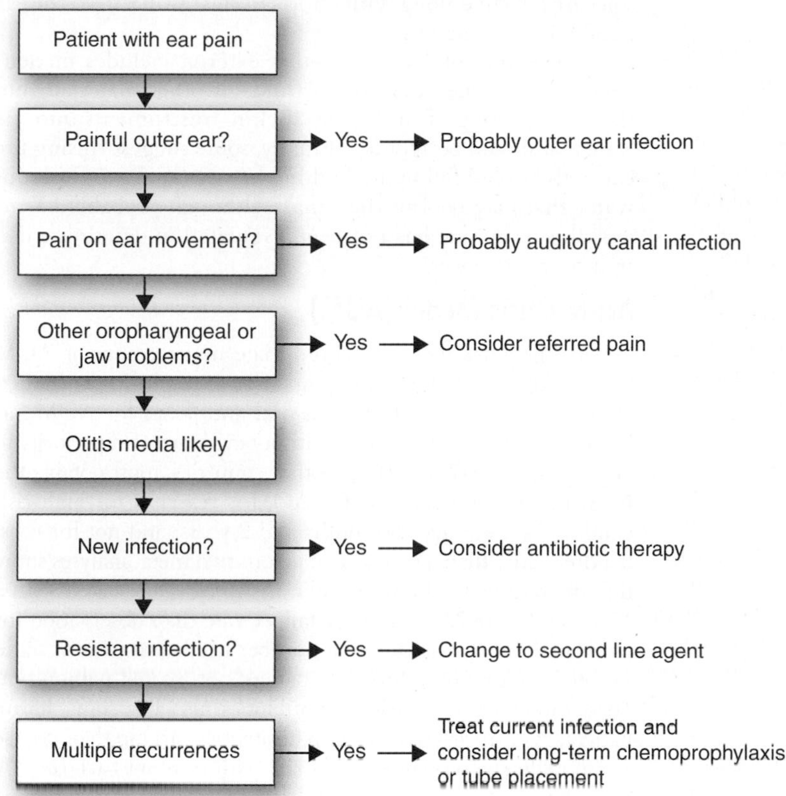

Figure 16.3 • General approach to the patient with ear pain.

TABLE 16.5 Management of Common Causes of Ear Pain

Treatment Strategy	Strength of Recommendation*	Recommendations/Conclusions
Antibiotic for AOM Media		
Routine antibiotics use in children <6 months of age	A	Antibiotics associated with 12.3% reduction in failure rate (NNT = 6)
Observation acceptable in healthy children >6 months of age with uncertain diagnosis, mild/moderate severity of illness, and reliable follow-up available	B	Patients have to meet all criteria for observation and those who return with continuing symptoms in 48–72 hours should receive antibiotics
Comparison of amoxicillin, penicillin, cefaclor, cefixime	A	No differences in effectiveness
Trimethoprim-sulfamethoxazole versus cefaclor	A	No difference in effectiveness
Single dose ceftriaxone versus amoxicillin-clavulanate	A	No differences in effectiveness
High dose versus regular dose amoxicillin-clavulanate dose	A	No differences in effectiveness
Duration of antibiotic therapy for AOM		
Multiple studies of 3–5 days of therapy versus 10 days of therapy	A	No difference in effectiveness; greater incidence of antibiotic side effects in patients treated for longer duration
Dosing frequency of amoxicillin		
Twice-a-day dosing versus three-times-a-day dosing	A	No difference in effectiveness

*A, consistent, good-quality patient-oriented evidence; B, inconsistent or limited-quality patient-oriented evidence; C, consensus, disease-oriented evidence, usual practice, expert opinion, or case series; NNT = number needed to treat.
For information about the SORT evidence rating system, see *http://www.aafp.org/afpsort.xml*.

Cerumen Impaction

Disimpaction of cerumen is usually achieved by irrigation of the auditory canal with either water or a 50:50 water-peroxide solution. Water temperature should be tepid and as close to body temperature as possible. This is important both for the comfort of the patient and because the use of water that is either too cold or too hot can precipitate a strong vestibular nerve reaction with nystagmus and dizziness. Topical cerumen softening agents can be used either before irrigation (to first soften the wax) or for cerumen that persists after irrigation, but prolonged use may cause irritation of the canal with subsequent edema, which worsens the cerumen entrapment. As a last resort, cerumen can be removed with direct suction under direct microscopic visualization, which is usually performed by an otolaryngologist.

Cerumen impaction that does not impair hearing probably does not require removal and efforts should generally be directed at avoiding total canal occlusion rather than a patient becoming reliant on frequent irrigations. In addition, patients should be advised not to insert foreign objects such as cotton-tipped swabs or other paraphernalia into the ear canal because this is likely to push cerumen further into the canal and result in an impaction.

Perichondritis and Furunculosis

Broad spectrum antibiotics effective against staphylococcal and streptococcal species, such as cephalosporins, are necessary. Because blood flow to the outer ear cartilage is scanty, cartilage necrosis with long-term ear deformity (cauliflower ear) can occur if treatment is delayed or inadequate.

Infection of the outer ear also is common after trauma, especially injuries such as frostbite. Close attention to tissue healing and protection against infection is an important aspect of managing outer ear frostbite or other traumas such as bites or scratches.

Otitis Externa

Treatment includes debridement of necrotic tissue through gentle rinsing followed by the application of a broad-spectrum antibiotic topical solution that will cover the most common organisms in what is usually a polymicrobial infection. For patients whose canal is obliterated by edema, the insertion of a gauze wick may be necessary to draw antibiotics into the infected canal.

The choice of topical antibiotic for otitis externa has not been studied extensively (Table 16.6). Neomycin/polymyxin B ear drops and ofloxacin ear drops are both popular because of their ability to eradicate *Pseudomonas*. Because of ototoxicity associated with aminoglycosides, neomycin should be avoided when the tympanic membranes is ruptured or cannot be visualized well. The addition of corticosteroids is popular in some ear drops, although there is little evidence that this speeds healing or prevents recurrences. Based on a clinical practice guideline (5), oral antibiotics such as ciprofloxacin should be added to topical therapy for severe or recurrent cases along with aggressive aural toileting usually performed under direct microscopic observation by an otolaryngologist.

"Swimmers ear" is a form of recurrent or chronic otitis externa caused by chronic irritant fluid accumulation in the acoustic canal, such as can occur in competitive swimmers. Often, this is more of an inflammatory etiology than infective and the use of topical astringent drops, such as acetic acid, sometimes combined with topical steroids such as hydrocortisone are effective along with efforts to clear water from the ear canal when drying off.

Prevention of recurrent otitis externa includes maneuvers to reduce the intrusion of fluids or other materials into the ear. Cleaning of the ear by sticking instruments into the ear canal should be avoided. Finally, some suggest rinsing the ear with alcohol following bathing or swimming to flush out water that may pool in the canal. Although probably harmless, this technique has not been evaluated to determine if it reduces recurrences.

Acute Otitis Media (AOM)

What constitutes the most appropriate management of AOM has sparked debate for many years. For example, in the United States, routine use of 10 days of oral antibiotics for AOM has been the traditional treatment without evidence of superiority to other strategies (17, 18). But in other countries, most notably the Netherlands, antibiotic use for AOM is reserved for high-risk children between ages 6 months and 2 years, and not for most children older than age of 2. Data from two meta-analyses show that the routine use of amoxicillin in AOM is associated with a 12.3% (17) to 13.7% (19) lower failure rate than observation (or placebo). This translates into a number needed to treat of six to prevent one case of failure in a patient not treated with antibiotics. However, early use of antibiotics also has some harm: patients with AOM treated with antibiotics early in their course are more likely to become colonized with resistant bacteria (20). It has been noted in a Dutch study that children initially treated with amoxicillin had more episodes of recurrent AOM than those not treated with antibiotic further emphasizing the need for judicious prescribing of antibiotics (21).

The value of antibiotics in otitis media was evaluated in two randomized placebo-controlled studies in children 6 to either 23 or 35 months treated with amoxicillin-clavulanic acid. Compared to placebo, children receiving antibiotics had fewer treatment failures at 3 or 4 days and less time to symptom resolution. However, children receiving amoxicillin-clavulanic acid had nearly twice the rate of side effects, principally diarrhea (22, 23).

To help guide clinicians, the AAP and the AAFP published an evidence-based guideline for treatment in 2004 that remains in effect. For children younger than 6 months of age diagnosed with AOM, the guideline recommends routine antibiotic administration starting with amoxicillin at a dose of 80–90 mg/kg per day (24). For children older than age 6 months, the AAP/AAFP recommendations include the option to observe selected children without antibiotic treatment. This option should be based on the certainty of diagnosis, the child's age, the severity of illness, and the assurance that the patient will be able to follow up if the symptoms do not improve in 48–72 hours. If the child is otherwise healthy, the diagnosis is uncertain, the illness not severe, and the child's caregiver can reliably follow-up if symptoms do not improve, then observation and symptom treatment alone is a reasonable strategy. If the child returns with a more definitive examination or worsening of symptoms within 72 hours, then antibiotic therapy should be started. Another useful strategy is a "wait and see" approach where an antibiotic is provided but parents are instructed not to fill the prescription unless the child has persistent pain and fever. In one study looking at this approach (25), only 1 in 5 parents filled the antibiotic prescription and there was no difference in outcomes.

TABLE 16.6 Antibiotics commonly used in Ear Infections

Drug	Dosage	Contraindications/Cautions/Adverse Effects
Otitis Externa		
Neomycin solutions	3–4 drops QID × 7 days	Rupture of tympanic membrane, potential ototoxicity with ruptured tympanic membrane
Ofloxacin solutions	Children 1–12 years: 5 drops BID × 10 days Patients ≥12 years: 10 drops BID × 10 days	Warm bottle in hands to avoid dizziness
Acute Otitis Media (AOM)		
First Line		
Amoxicillin	80 mg/kg split at least BID × at least 5 days	Penicillin allergy, diarrhea (~2%)
Sulfamethoxazole (SMX)-trimethoprim (TMP)	40 mg/kg SMX/8 mg/kg TMP divided BID × 10 days	Sulfa allergy; avoid in patients with glucose-6-phosphatase deficiency; avoid in folate deficiency; light sensitivity, skin reactions (2%) with severe reactions in (<0.1%); may cause bone marrow suppression possible with chronic use
Second Line		
Ceftriaxone	50 mg/kg up to 1 g	Cross-reactivity with penicillin allergy; pain at injection site, diarrhea (5–6%)
Amoxicillin-clavulanate	20–45 mg/day of amoxicillin component in 2 or 3 doses	Penicillin allergy; history of jaundice; select appropriate concentration; diarrhea (up to 40%)
Azithromycin	30 mg/kg as a single dose OR 10 mg/kg QD × 3 days OR 10 mg/kg × 1 day then 5 mg/kg on days 2 through 5	Macrolide allergy; diarrhea (~5%), nausea (~3%), abdominal pain (~3%)
Other second- or third-generation cephalosporins (e.g., cefaclor, cefuroxime, cefixime)	Varies with drug	Caution in penicillin allergy, diarrhea (3–5%), rash
Prophylaxis for recurrent AOM		
Amoxicillin	Half daily dosage at bedtime	Penicillin allergy, diarrhea (2%)
Sulfamethoxazole-Trimethoprim	40 mg/kg SMX/8 mg/kg TMP QHS	Sulfa allergy, skin reactions (2%) with severe reactions in (<0.1%)

When the effectiveness of multiple different antibiotics was compared in their ability to treat AOM, there appeared to be no benefit of any one drug over any other (see Table 16.6). Antibiotics used for 5 days or less showed equal effectiveness with longer durations of therapy (26). One study has suggested, though, that 2 days of therapy with oral antibiotics is not as effective as treatment for 7 days (18). In addition to a cost benefit of shorter durations of therapy, reports have noted fewer drug-related side effects in patients taking short courses of antibiotics. One study estimated that the number needed to treat with short-duration therapy to avoid one gastrointestinal adverse effect was eight children. In addition to short-duration therapy compared to long-duration therapy with oral antibiotics, a single intramuscular dose of ceftriaxone was just as effective as a longer duration of other antibiotics (27).

Because of the emergence of multiple drug resistant strains of *Streptococcus pneumoniae*, there has been some concern that standard doses of medications might not be sufficient to cover strains that are intermediately resistant. Higher dose regimens of beta-lactam resistant antibiotics, such as amoxicillin-clavulanate have been suggested to deal with this potential problem. However, two controlled studies of high-dose amoxicillin-clavulanate have shown no greater effectiveness than standard dosing regimens. It should be noted that whereas the higher doses of amoxicillin are not supported by these studies and remain theoretical, the AAP/AAFP guideline on treating AOM recommends doses of amoxicillin of 80–90 mg/kg to overcome intermediate resistance.

The treatment of recurrent otitis media after a previous resistant episode is another area of controversy. Some physicians treat a second episode of AOM with a second-line drug after a previous treatment failure. However, recurrences several weeks after an initial episode are usually produced by a new organism and do not necessarily have the same resistance pattern as previous infections. One nonrandomized study that investigated the effectiveness of a second-line drug versus a first-line agent (amoxicillin or trimethoprim-sulfamethoxazole) showed no benefit of the broader spectrum second-line agent in a recurrent infection after a previously resistant episode (28). To reduce the development of resistance, new episodes should be treated with narrower spectrum agents, such as amoxicillin or sulfamethoxazole/trimethoprim.

Non-antibiotic treatments for AOM include autoinflation, steroids, or antihistamines. Autoinflation refers to having children "pop" their ears by blowing out with a closed airway and nose. Modest improvements at short and longer intervals (more than a month) have been demonstrated with autoinflation although the number of studies is small. Based on the low risk from this activity, a Cochrane review stated that this maneuver is reasonable to consider (29). The use of oral or nasal steroids during AOM has also shown quicker clearing of effusion. Finally, antihistamine-decongestant combination medications were shown to result in no greater clearing of effusion than placebos but were associated with a greater incidence of side effects in a study of 553 children with otitis medica with effusion (30). Based on this, and a Cochrane review on the topic (31), Antihistamine-decongestants are not recommended for AOM.

Children who have ear perforations may experience persistent ear drainage with AOM. These conditions can be treated with oral antibiotics, but a Cochrane review found that fluoroquinolone-containing ear drops were superior at clearing discharge compared to oral antibiotics (32).

During episodes of AOM, management of ear pain can be accomplished with either an oral analgesic such as acetaminophen or ibuprofen or with topical ear drops containing mild anesthetics. A study evaluating pain control in older children (ages 5–18) also showed that naturopathic ear drops work equally as well as anesthetic ear drops to control pain (33).

Long-Term Monitoring and Prevention

In children with multiple, recurrent episodes of AOM, prevention of recurrent infections may be necessary. Recurrent otitis is defined as three or more episodes of AOM in a 6-month period or four episodes in a year with a normal examination documented between each infection (34). The first approach in preventing recurrences is to identify conditions that predispose children to Eustachian tube dysfunction. Most commonly, this is an upper respiratory infection that cannot be prevented. However, some children have chronic allergic rhinitis that results in eustachian tube dysfunction. Treatment of these children with antihistamines or nasal steroids may reduce their risk of a recurrent infection.

For children with no evidence of allergy, options include chronic antibiotic prophylaxis or surgical ventilation of the inner ear through the placement of tubes. Tympanostomy tubes and antibiotic prophylaxis have nearly equal effectiveness for the prevention of recurrence (35), but medication use is associated with fewer side effects. Antibiotic prophylaxis can be achieved with either amoxicillin or sulfamethoxazole given as a single dose at bedtime. The usual dose is half of the total daily treatment dose. Selected antibiotics are listed in Table 16.5.

If the clinician and family elect to try antibiotic prophylaxis and this approach fails, axis, the insertion of tympanostomy tubes is indicated. If antibiotic prophylaxis does fail, it is most likely to fail in the first 6 months, so a short trial of antibiotic suppression is probably indicated in most patients (36). An exception to this may be in children who already have language delay and recurrent infections complicated by persistent otitis media (otitis media with effusion), for whom tympanostomy tubes are indicated as initial therapy (37). Controlled trials have showed no benefit for early insertion of tubes either in the short term (3 years of age) (38) or long term (9–10 years of age) (39).

For patients with tubes in place, families often are told to limit children's exposure to water such as swimming. One study examining the validity of this restriction showed that children allowed to participate in surface swimming had no higher rate of ear pain or complications such as recurrent AOM than those who were not allowed to swim. The place where swimming occurred (lake, ocean, pool, etc.) did not appear to influence either pain or complication rates (40).

PATIENT EDUCATION

Ear pain is very common in childhood and may create a great deal of anxiety in parents in addition to causing sleepless nights and days off from work. When encountering the family with a young child who has ear pain, clinicians should recognize the stress that this illness places on the family as well as try to dispel myths that may have arisen regarding treatment of the problem. Some of the issues that physicians should be prepared to counsel families about include the following.

Antibiotic therapy may hasten resolution of symptoms and reduce treatment failures in children between 6 months and 3 years of age, but also is associated with more side effects. Parents are accustomed to receiving antibiotics but physicians should alert parents to the possibility of drug reactions. Prescribing decisions should weigh parent expectations and desires along with the acuity of illness in the child. For a mildly ill child, taking a watchful waiting approach may be suitable.

A treatment failure in one infection does not indicate that a second-line antibiotic must be used for all subsequent infections. Many parents assume that because amoxicillin did not work the last time, it is not going to work this time. This can lead to the unnecessary use of broader spectrum, more expensive agents, and speed the development of drug resistance. When treatment failures occur, physicians should emphasize at that time that the use of a different drug should not influence the treatment if the child should get another infection in the future.

Prevention of recurrent otitis media is indicated in few patients and nonsurgical options are effective.

Children with tympanostomy tubes can be allowed to participate in surface swimming without increasing their risk of ear pain or other complications.

A nice patient education handout is available from the members of the American Academy of Family Physicians at: *http://www.aafp.org/afp/2007/1201/p1659.html*

KEY POINTS

- AOM can only be diagnosed in the presence of a middle ear effusion.
- Tympanography is a useful test if clinical exam cannot confirm the presence of a middle ear effusion.
- AOM will resolve spontaneously in some children without antibiotics.
- High dose amoxicillin is indicated to treat intermediately resistant *S. pneumonia*.
- Otitis media with effusion can be treated with ventilation tubes but early insertion of tubes offers no advantage to speech development over watchful waiting.

CHAPTER 17

Common Eye Problems

Gary R. Gray and Rebecca Rosen

CLINICAL OBJECTIVES

1. List the differential diagnoses for a patient presenting with a red eye or eyelid disorder.
2. Describe the physical exam findings that are most useful for clarifying the diagnosis of specific eye disorders.
3. Define historical findings to aid the physician in evaluating a patient with an ocular complaint.
4. List the key physical exam or historical findings suggesting a possible serious or vision threatening eye disorder.

Red eye is the most common ophthalmic disorder encountered in the family physicians' office practice (1). Although most cases represent a relatively benign self-limited process, the physician must be able to accurately assess the patient and rule out potential vision-threatening disorders. Therefore, a thorough understanding of the potential etiologies coupled with a careful history and physical exam is essential.

Infectious and inflammatory disorders of the eyelids are frequently encountered in the family physician's office practice. Many conditions may be successfully treated by the family physician, though some require surgical intervention and referral to an ophthalmologist. Although it is not common in daily practices, most family physicians will occasionally face a patient with sudden visual loss. An accurate, quick assessment is the key to preserving vision.

There is considerable overlap in the symptomatology and differential diagnosis of ocular conditions. Patients' descriptions are often not precise, and they may focus only on the particular symptom that is most bothersome to them, overlooking other symptoms that a physician would find more alarming. A systematic approach is, therefore, needed in primary care practice.

DIFFERENTIAL DIAGNOSIS

The Red Eye

Conjunctivitis, inflammation of the thin transparent membrane covering the sclera and inner surfaces of the eyelids, is the most common cause of red eye (1,2). However, four additional diseases cause a painful red eye—corneal lesions, uveitis, acute glaucoma, and scleritis—all of which represent involvement of deeper eye structures (3). Subconjunctival hemorrhages are a common cause of a painless red eye.

Historical clues and clinical findings guide the physician to the appropriate diagnosis and plan of action. Table 17.1 summarizes the differential diagnosis of red eye. Although the frequency of more serious diseases is low in the family physicians' office, they must always be considered.

CONJUNCTIVITIS

Conjunctivitis has both infectious and noninfectious causes. Table 17.2 describes the most common etiologies of conjunctivitis. Although widely used, the actual diagnostic usefulness of specific signs and symptoms in conjunctivitis is poor. Conjunctival hyperemia (redness) is a common finding in all cases of conjunctivitis. Tearing, itching, foreign body sensation, and ocular discharge are all characteristic of conjunctivitis, although these findings vary according to underlying etiology.

Infectious conjunctivitis can be caused by a variety of viruses and bacteria. The most common infectious etiologies are listed in Table 17.2. Clinical findings and history serve as primary guidance for diagnosis. For example, a purulent ocular discharge is more likely to be associated with a bacterial etiology, whereas a serous discharge is more likely associated with a viral cause.

Allergic conjunctivitis is often seasonal and found in people with history of allergic rhinitis, asthma, or atopic dermatitis. Clinical clues include bilateral involvement, ocular itching, and watery or mucoid discharge.

Mechanical or irritative conjunctivitis may be associated with contact lens use, chemical exposure, and dry eyes (keratoconjunctivitis sicca). A detailed history is crucial. Patients should be asked specifically about contact lens wear, including the use of sterilizing and wetting solutions. Thimerosal, a mercury-based preservative in contact lens solutions, has been associated with irritation. Potential workplace irritants include ultraviolet light, dust, chemicals, and tobacco smoke. Patients who use topical capsaicin for musculoskeletal pain may complain of irritation if they touch their eyes while their fingers are contaminated with the medication.

ACUTE NARROW-ANGLE GLAUCOMA

Acute narrow-angle closure glaucoma is an ophthalmologic emergency. Its pathophysiology involves blockage of the aqueous humor flow through the canal of Schlemm, resulting in increased intraocular pressure. Most patients with acute narrow-angle glaucoma have preexisting shallow anterior chamber angles (between the iris and the cornea). The following are associated with an increased risk for acute angle closure (5): hyperopia, family history of angle closure glaucoma, advancing age, female gender, Asian or Inuit descent, and pupillary dilation from medication.

TABLE 17.1 Differential Diagnosis of the Patient with a Red Eye

Diagnosis	Frequency
Conjunctivitis	Very common
Keratitis	Uncommon
Uveitis	Uncommon
Corneal lesions/abrasions	Common
Scleritis	Uncommon
Acute glaucoma	Uncommon
Subconjunctival hemorrhage	Common

Patients with acute angle closure glaucoma have a dramatic presentation of pain and blurred vision. Patients may see halos around lights. Characteristic physical findings include conjunctival hyperemia, corneal cloudiness, and papillary dilation, with a sluggish or absent response to light.

SUBCONJUNCTIVAL HEMORRHAGE

A subconjunctival hemorrhage is an easily recognized condition in which blood accumulates between the conjunctiva and sclera. Usually a benign process, it may be caused by minor trauma, excessive coughing, pushing in labor and delivery, vomiting, or other conditions associated with a significant Valsalva maneuver (6). Patients with hypertension and diabetes are more susceptible, as well as those taking anticoagulant medications.

CORNEAL ABRASIONS

Corneal abrasions represent mechanical damage to the corneal epithelium. Symptoms include pain, photophobia, and a foreign body feeling associated with excess tearing (7). The history often includes a distinct precipitating event.

SCLERITIS, UVEITIS, AND KERATITIS

These inflammatory conditions of the deeper eye structures are significantly less common causes of red eye than conjunctivitis (8). The hallmark clinical finding in these conditions is pain in the eyeball rather than on the surface. Reduced visual acuity is common in both uveitis and keratitis and may accompany scleritis as well.

Keratitis represents the clinical manifestation of inflammation involving the corneal epithelium. Underlying causes include: dry eyes, severe viral conjunctivitis, ultraviolet light exposure (sunburn), and contact lens use (8).

Uveitis represents inflammation of the iris and ciliary body. This condition is also commonly termed iritis or iridocyclitis and is associated with several common autoimmune diseases including: juvenile rheumatoid arthritis, ankylosing spondylitis, systemic lupus erythematosus, and sarcoidosis (8).

Scleritis refers to inflammatory conditions involving the sclera and has been associated with systemic lupus erythematosus, rheumatoid arthritis, and polyarteritis nodosa (8).

Eyelid Disorders

BLEPHARITIS

Blepharitis, one of the most common ocular disorders (9), is a chronic bilateral inflammatory process affecting the eyelid margins. There are two types of blepharitis, defined by their anatomic location—anterior (affecting mainly the outside of the eyelid) or posterior (affecting mainly the inside of the eyelid). The two main causes of anterior blepharitis are seborrheic dermatitis and staphylococcal infection, or a combination of the two (10,11). Posterior blepharitis is caused by Meibomian gland dysfunction in which the openings of the Meibomian glands become clogged, resulting in thickening of the eyelids, chalazion, and eventual atrophy of the Meibomian glands (9). The Meibomian glands secrete oils that prevent the tear layer from evaporating too quickly, thus keeping the surface of the

TABLE 17.2 Common Causes of Conjunctivitis and Associated Symptoms and Clinical Findings

Etiology	Symptoms and Clinical Findings
Infectious Conjunctivitis	
1. Viral Conjunctivitis:	**Viral Conjunctivitis:**
Adenovirus: Pharyngoconjunctival fever types 3 and 7, epidemic keratoconjunctivitis types 8 and 19; enterovirus: hemorrhagic conjunctivitis; herpes simplex; varicella zoster	Unilateral involvement; minimal itching marked tearing, minimal exudative discharge; may be associated with upper respiratory infection symptoms (adenovirus); preauricular adenopathy common
2. Bacterial Conjunctivitis:	**Bacterial Conjunctivitis:**
Pneumococcus; Haemophilus influenzae; Staphylococcus aureus; Neisseria gonorrhoeae	Unilateral involvement; minimal itching, moderate tearing; profuse exudative (purulent) discharge; preauricular adenopathy uncommon
Chlamydia	
Allergic conjunctivitis	Bilateral involvement; marked ocular itching, moderate tearing; watery or mucoid discharge

eye moist and hydrated. If the glands atrophy and the oils dry up, dry eye and possible subsequent conjunctivitis and keratitis will result. Anterior and posterior blepharitis may exist simultaneously. Blepharitis can begin in childhood but occurs more commonly in the 6th and 7th decades (10,11) and in people who suffer from acne rosacea or seborrheic dermatitis of the face and scalp. Other more acute causes include contact dermatitis, head lice (pediculosis), and association with the use of isotretinoin (Accutane) (9).

Patients with blepharitis complain of a burning or gritty sensation in their eyes as well as itching, irritation, and redness of the eyelid margins. They also complain of their eyelids sticking together, especially on awakening. The history should include questions directed at systemic symptoms, exacerbating factors, duration, allergies, infected contacts, and previous and current medications (9). On physical exam, the lid margins are erythematous and swollen, and there are fine flakes or debris and scales or collarettes (a crust that encircles the base of an eyelash) clinging to the base of the lashes, which are themselves often small, thin, broken, or sometimes white (9,10). There may also be vesicles or ulcers along the eyelid margin, and a hordeolum or chalazion may also be present (see color plate Figures 17.2 and 17.3).

The differential diagnosis of blepharitis includes: atopic dermatitis, contact dermatitis mechanical irritation (allergic conjunctivitis → increased rubbing), sebaceous cell CA (asymmetric eyelash loss), ocular rosacea, contact lens complications, conjunctivitis, dry eye syndrome, and herpetic eye disease.

Hordeolum and Chalazion

A hordeolum or sty is an acute suppurative infection of either the Meibomian gland (internal hordeolum) or of the eyelash follicle or tear gland (external hordeolum). The main causative organism is usually *Staphylococcus aureus*.

The patient presents with the complaint of a swollen, painful, and often red mass along the lid margin. This mass may be indurated and may rupture (see color plate Figures 17.4 and 17.5). On examination, in addition to the above findings, there may also be preauricular lymphadenopathy (18).

A chalazion is a chronic, sterile, granulomatous lesion of the Meibomian glands (deep chalazion) or of the Zeis glands (superficial), which results from gland obstruction. An acute chalazion may appear and present similarly to a hordeolum, or may result from a persistent hordeolum. Chalazia, as discussed previously, are often associated with chronic blepharitis, acne rosacea, seborrhea, conjunctivitis, and hordeolum.

Although the initial presentation may involve a tender, erythematous swelling or nodule, a chalazion is usually a painless lump on the eyelid. If large enough, chalazia may cause discomfort and even compress the cornea causing astigmatism. Patients may complain of nothing other than the unpleasant appearance of the lump (see color plate Figures 17.6 and 17.7).

Visual Loss

Causes of painless loss of vision that the family physician may encounter include retinal detachment, vitreous hemorrhage, central or branch retinal vein occlusion, and central retinal artery occlusion.

RETINAL DETACHMENT

To understand retinal detachment, it is important to understand the physiology of the vitreous and retina. The vitreous is composed of a gel-like substance that makes up 80% of the ocular globe volume (12). Consisting mostly of water interwoven by collagen fibrils, this gel also contains salts, soluble proteins, glycoproteins, and glycosaminoglycans. Over time, the vitreous undergoes liquefaction, especially in people with high myopia (12). Retinal detachment occurs when the pigmented retina separates from the inner sensory retina, allowing the liquid vitreous to seep between the two layers. Retina becomes ischemic, and the photoreceptors degenerate resulting in vision loss.

The presenting symptoms are usually flashes of light (photopsia), which result from the retinal traction and not from direct retinal stimulation, and a sudden shower of black dots, which are red blood cells in the vitreous after rupture of a retinal vessel. The incidence of retinal detachment is approximately 10–15 per 100,000 people per year (13,14). It occurs more commonly in men, in the elderly, and in people with degenerative myopia (15). Risk factors include myopia, cataract surgery, trauma, history of retinal detachment in the other eye (13), and, to a lesser extent, family history (14). Early diagnosis and referral to an ophthalmologist for timely treatment are critical to preserve vision.

VITREOUS OR RETINAL HEMORRHAGE

Vitreous hemorrhage, caused by rupture of the retinal vessels, has multiple etiologies. The rupture of the blood vessel releases red blood cells into the avascular vitreous, which are seen by the patient as floaters or dark lines. A large hemorrhage can cause sudden, painless loss of vision. Among the most common causes are: 1) tearing of neovascularized blood vessels seen in diabetic retinopathy (most common etiology) or in the retinopathy that accompanies sickle cell disease; 2) retinal detachment; 3) posterior vitreous detachment; 4) central or branch retinal vein occlusion; and 5) trauma.

CENTRAL OR BRANCH RETINAL VEIN OCCLUSION AND CENTRAL RETINAL ARTERY OCCLUSION

These two conditions share a similar pathophysiology, with branch retinal vein occlusion being more common. Risk factors for these conditions are similar to those associated with other thrombotic conditions such as stroke and myocardial infarction; they include: hypertension, smoking, diabetes, and advanced age.

Central retinal artery occlusion (CRAO) is an ocular emergency, as permanent blindness can result from infarction of the retina. In CRAO, an embolic or thrombotic event results in sudden, painless vision loss (16). Embolic etiologies include cardiogenic or carotid emboli. Thrombosis may result from arteriosclerosis, which is the most common underlying systemic etiology (17), giant cell arteritis, collagen vascular diseases, or hypercoagulable states (16).

EVALUATION OF PATIENTS WITH EYE COMPLAINTS

History and Physical Examination

Important general elements of the history and physical examination are summarized in the following sections and in Tables 17.3 and 17.4. The history should focus on the duration

TABLE 17.3 Key Historical Elements to Ask About in Taking a History of an Eye Condition

1. Symptoms and signs: itching, discharge, irritation, pain, photophobia
2. Duration of symptoms
3. Unilateral or bilateral disease
4. Type of discharge: mucoid, watery, purulent
5. Exposure to infection
6. History of trauma
7. Contact lens wear
8. Use of eye cosmetics
9. Signs of systemic disease: urethritis, cervicitis, skin lesions
10. History of atopy
11. Decreased vision

of symptoms, unilateral versus bilateral involvement, and presence and characterization of any discharge. Inquire about systemic illnesses (e.g., connective tissue diseases, Marfan syndrome) that may have ocular manifestations. A medication history is useful to identify systemic and topical agents that may cause ocular symptoms, such as dryness or blurred vision. A sexual history may identify those patients at risk for *Chlamydia trachomatis* and *Neisseria gonorrhoeae* eye infection. Penetrating trauma is an ophthalmic emergency requiring immediate ophthalmic attention. One should always inquire regarding decreased visual acuity, photophobia, and globe pain, which signify involvement of the deeper structures of the eye, necessitating referral to an ophthalmologist (Table 17.5).

Ask additional questions to uncover exactly what the patient is experiencing. Blurred vision is a very nonspecific term, and may be used by patients to describe a variety of disparate complaints, including glare, diplopia, refractive errors, impaired accommodation, and photophobia. Accurate identification of the patient's true complaint is essential for the formulation of the differential diagnosis. This will help you focus the physical examination on the relevant findings.

TABLE 17.4 Key Elements of the Physical Examination of a Patient with an Eye Problem

1. Visual acuity
2. Slit-lamp examination (if available)
3. Fluorescein testing
4. External examination:
   a. Regional lymphadenopathy
   b. Conjunctiva: injection, hemorrhage, discharge
   c. Cornea exam facilitated by dye staining: abrasions, erosions, ulcerations, presence of dendritic lesions
   d. Eye lashes and lids: swelling, lesions, crusting
   e. Pupillary reflex

TABLE 17.5 Red Flags for Patients Presenting with a Red Eye, for Which Prompt Ophthalmologic Consultation is Indicated

Symptom or Sign	Significance
Globe pain	Suggests problem within the eye, such as iritis, uveitis, or glaucoma
Decreased visual acuity	Suggests a severe problem
Sluggish papillary reflex	Retinal or central nervous system involvement
Dendritic corneal lesions	Suggest herpes simplex infection
Vesicular lesions around the eye	Suggesting herpes zoster

The physical examination of the eye should begin with a visual acuity exam. If the patient wears eyeglasses, test acuity with and without glasses. The physical exam should be performed in a well-lit room. The patient's skin and scalp should be inspected for signs of seborrheic dermatitis, rosacea, atopic dermatitis, or head lice. In addition, check for:

- Regional lymphadenopathy, especially preauricular adenopathy, which would suggest adenoviral conjunctivitis.
- Vesicular skin lesions associated with ocular complaints; they suggest herpes simplex or varicella zoster.
- If available, fluorescein staining and a slit-lamp exam should be performed to evaluate for foreign bodies, corneal ulcerations, abrasions, or other lesions.
- Pupillary abnormalities suggest a serious process, such as acute glaucoma, uveitis, scleritis, or keratitis.
- Check for eyelid eversion (ectropion) or entropion, which may cause irritation.
- Assess the function of extraocular muscles and check for foreign bodies.
- Eversion of the upper eyelid, gently folding it over a soft swab stick, allows inspection of the inner surface for lesions or embedded foreign bodies.

An algorithm for evaluation of the red eye is provided in Figure 17.1.

Diagnostic Testing

Cultures and other laboratory evaluations are generally not useful or required. Specific instances in which culture is indicated include: neonatal conjunctivitis, recurrent or severe purulent conjunctivitis, and suspected *N. gonorrhoeae* or *Chlamydia* infections. Radiologic imaging is not helpful unless a foreign body is suspected. Magnetic resonance imaging may be contraindicated, if it causes movement of a metallic object.

The evaluation of a patient with suspected retinal detachment includes a fundus exam with the ophthalmoscope. In patients with a retinal detachment, the fundus appears gray and thin. A horseshoe-shaped tear may be visible (see color plate Figure 17.8).

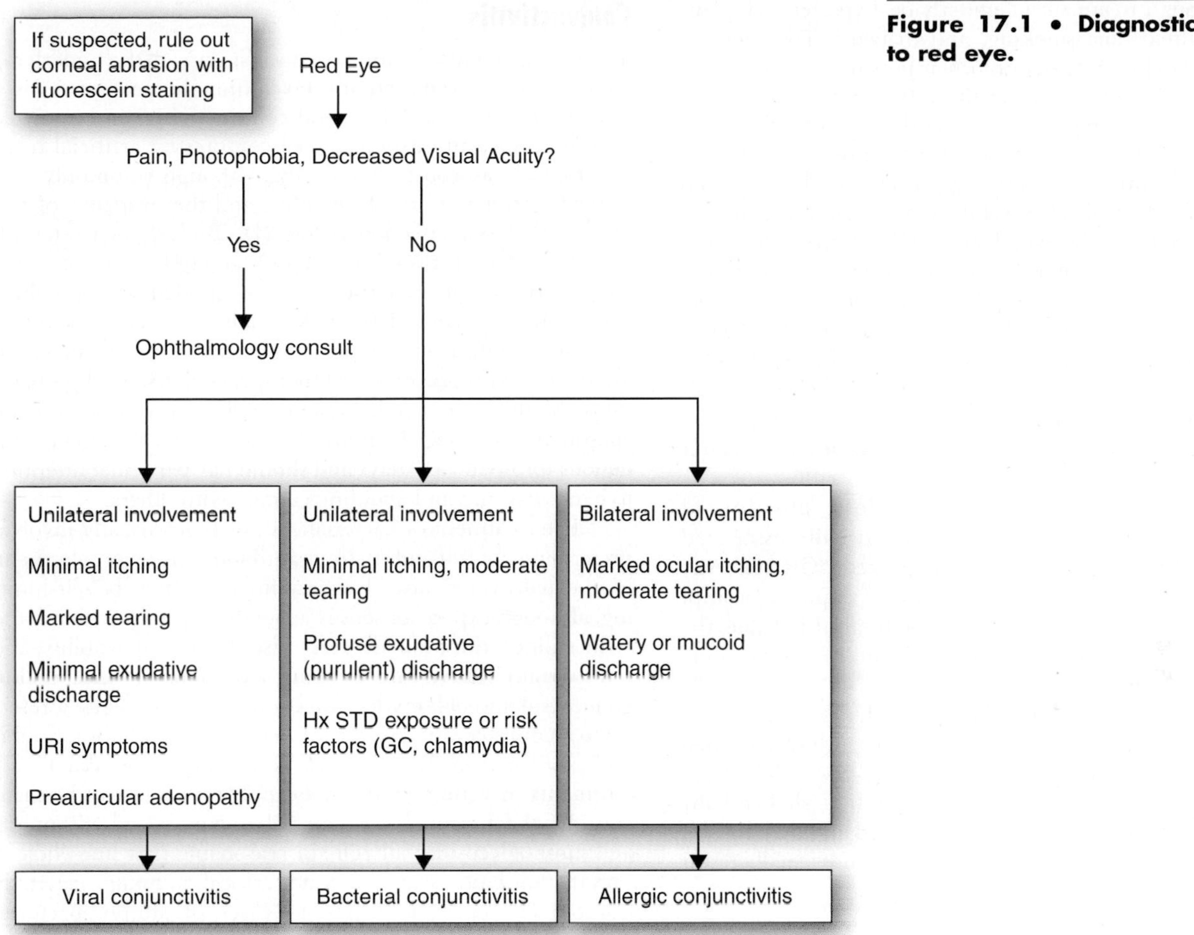

Figure 17.1 • Diagnostic approach to red eye.

Physical exam findings in patients with vitreous or retinal hemorrhage include a blood meniscus or collection of blood, which can be seen in the vitreous, or preretinal space. In the case of a retinal hemorrhage, areas of red or yellow punctuations, or streaks, or "flame-like" lesions can be appreciated on the retinal surface (see color plate Figure 17.9).

Patients with CRVO or branch retinal vein occlusion will present with painless unilateral vision loss or diminished visual acuity; they may also complain of floaters. Visual acuity may be 20/15 or decrease to 20/100–20/200, or be reduced to just light perception (19). The patient may also have visual field defects, especially if the occlusion is in a branch of the central retinal vein. On exam, it is common to see retinal hemorrhages, cotton wool spots (retinal ischemia), a swollen optic disc (because RVO inhibits venous return), and dilated and tortuous veins along the retinal surface (see color plate Figure 17.10).

The funduscopic exam in cases of CRAO may show diffuse whitening of the fundus because of ischemia as well as a pathognomonic cherry-red spot, which is the choroid showing through the ischemic macula. There may also be "box car" segmentation of the venous vessels, which represents occlusion of the circulation, and sometimes emboli can be visualized. The physical exam should include auscultation of the heart and carotids and, after the immediacy of the situation has passed, imaging of the heart and the carotids should be performed as well.

TREATMENT

Many common eye conditions can be managed at the primary care level; other, often less common, conditions require referral to an eye specialist.

Conditions That Should Generally Be Referred for Specialty Care

Many eye diagnoses should generally not be managed by primary care physicians. Scleritis, uveitis, and keratitis have the potential to cause permanent visual impairment. Acute narrow-angle glaucoma is an absolute ophthalmologic emergency requiring immediate specialty consultation. All patients with suspected retinal detachments should be immediately referred to an ophthalmologist, even if both visual acuity and fundus exam appear normal, as treatment is surgical and 95% can be repaired (13,15). Patients with vitreous or retinal hemorrhages should be referred for evaluation; however, the family doctor should work to control the underlying diabetes, hypertension, and hyperlipidemia.

Referral to an ophthalmologist is imperative for diagnosis of branch and CRVOs and for CRAOs. The contralateral eye may be affected in 12% of CRVO patients within 4 years (22). There is no established treatment except to prevent further damage through treatment of underlying hypertension, glaucoma, hyperlipidemia, smoking, and diabetes. Treatment of CRAO involves lowering of intraocular pressure and/or vasodilation to dislodge or move the thrombus distally into more peripheral arterioles, thereby reducing the area of infarct (17). Vasodilation can be attempted through compression and rapid decompression of the eye by putting pressure on the globe and then letting go suddenly for several attempts, with intermittent fundal exams to assess blood flow (17). Other treatment modalities include topical beta blockers, oral nitrates, paracentesis of aqueous humor, retrobulbar anesthetic block, hyperbaric oxygen, inhalation of carbogen (a mixture of 95% oxygen and 5% carbon dioxide), and direct infusion of thrombolytics into the ophthalmic artery (17,23). Despite these varied modalities, prognosis for vision recovery is poor; however, prompt diagnosis and initiation of treatment correlates with better prognosis (23).

A transient, painless monocular loss, blurring of vision, (amaurosis fugax) is a symptom usually associated with strokes. However, it may also precede CRAO. Any patient presenting with amaurosis fugax requires prompt attention and workup to assess and then treat, if possible, the underlying disease processes that could lead to further morbidity and mortality.

Vitreous or retinal hemorrhages in infants and children less than 3 years old (20), especially after 1 month of age when most birth trauma retinal hemorrhages have resolved (21), are considered pathognomonic for child abuse (i.e., shaken baby syndrome), and these cases must be addressed and investigated immediately. These types of hemorrhages do not usually result from falls off of diaper tables or beds (20).

Conjunctivitis

The management of conjunctivitis is specific to the underlying etiology. Viral conjunctivitis (excluding herpesviruses) is a self-limited process. Adenoviral conjunctivitis can be treated with local measures, such as cool compresses, artificial tears, and topical vasoconstrictor drops. Although commonly prescribed, antibiotics are of no value, and the incidence of secondary bacterial infection is low (1). Topical corticosteroids have been demonstrated to reduce scarring in cases of severe conjunctivitis, but their use should be guided by ophthalmic consultation because of the risk of adverse events, including herpesvirus infection. Herpes simplex and varicella infections are treated with oral antiviral therapy; ocular steroid preparations should be avoided. Patients with suspected adenoviral conjunctivitis should be reminded that they will remain contagious for up to 7–10 days and should pay particular attention to hand washing and avoiding contact with others.

The treatment of bacterial conjunctivitis usually involves prescribing topical ophthalmic antibiotic drops or ointment. Nonsexually transmitted bacterial infections may be self-limiting, although expert consensus generally supports treatment to reduce illness duration, decrease disease communicability, and reduce complication rate. Systemic antibiotics are indicated in gonococcal and chlamydial infections, and necessitate a referral to an ophthalmologist. Commonly used ophthalmic antibiotics are listed in Table 17.6. It is generally advisable to use ointments in young children, as applying drops can be difficult. Erythromycin, bacitracin-polymyxin B, sulfacetamide, and aminoglycosides all remain reasonable first-line choices. Specific antibiotic selection is not critical, although generally quinolones are unnecessary in cases of simple bacterial

TABLE 17.6 Common Ophthalmic Antibiotics

Drug	Cautions	Dosage
Bacitracin-polymyxin B (ointment)	History of allergy	Small ribbon of ointment to eye every 3–4 hours
Gramicidin-neomycin-polymyxin B (solution)	History of allergy	1–2 drops every 4 hours
Erythromycin (ointment)	History of allergy	Small ribbon of ointment to eye every 4 hours
Sulfacetamide (10% solution) (10% ointment)	History of allergy Contact lenses Age <2 months	1–2 drops every 4 hours, small ribbon of ointment to eye every 3–4 hours
Gentamicin (solution and ointment)	History of allergy	1–2 drops every 4–6 hours; small ribbon of ointment to eye every 8 hours
Tobramycin (solution and ointment)	History of allergy	1–2 drops every 4–6 hours, small ribbon of ointment to eye every 8 hours
Ciprofloxacin (solution and ointment)	History of allergy Age <1 year	1–2 drops every 4 hours, small ribbon of ointment to eye every 8 hours × 2 days then BID
Ofloxacin (solution)	History of allergy Age <1 year	1–2 drops every 4 hours

TABLE 17.7 Common Ophthalmic Allergy Drugs

Drug	Cautions	Dosage
Mast cell stabilizers		
Lodoxamide	Age <2 years	Age 1–2 drops QID
Cromolyn	Age <4 years	1–2 drops QID
Nedocromil	Age <3 years	1–2 drops BID
Pemirolast	Age <3 years	1–2 drops QID
Nonsteroidal anti-inflammatory steroids (NSAIDs): Ketorolac	Aspirin or NSAID-induced asthma or allergy Age <3 years	1 drop QID
Antihistamines		
Levocabastine	Age <12 years	1 drop QID
Olopatadine	Age <3 years	1 drop BID
Antihistamine/vasoconstrictor		
Naphazoline/pheniramine	Age <6 years Narrow-angle glaucoma MAO use	1–2 drops QD-QID as needed

conjunctivitis. Topical antibiotics should generally be continued until resolution is noted. Aminoglycosides such as neomycin and gentamicin have been associated with ocular allergic reactions, a consideration if the patient notes worsening symptoms with the use of these agents. Many providers recommend that antibiotics be stopped 24 hours after the initial resolution of redness and other symptoms. Follow-up is generally unnecessary, although patients should be told to return if their symptoms fail to improve over several days, or worsen.

Allergic conjunctivitis is treated symptomatically with topical antihistamine drops, either alone or in combination with a vasoconstrictor. Persistent symptoms may be treated with topical mast cell stabilizers. Ketorolac, a topical nonsteroidal anti-inflammatory drug, may help with allergic conjunctivitis, and oral antihistamines may provide symptomatic relief. Ophthalmic corticosteroids, although beneficial, should be used only with the recommendation of an ophthalmologist. Commonly used ophthalmic allergy preparations are listed in Table 17.7.

Most cases of conjunctivitis can be managed by the primary care physician. Herpes simplex and varicella zoster infections are indications for ophthalmologic evaluation, and require treatment with oral antiviral mediations. Patients with suspected glaucoma and inflammatory disorders of the deeper eye structures should also be urgently referred for specialty care.

Management of Corneal Abrasion

The recommended management of corneal abrasions has changed over the past decade. Historically, eye patching was commonly used in patients with corneal abrasions. This habit has proven hard to break despite evidence that it may increase pain and slow the healing process (7). Appropriate management of corneal abrasions should include (7):

- Analgesics, oral or topical nonsteroidal anti-inflammatory drugs
- Topical antibiotics (ointments are more lubricating) erythromycin and bacitracin are reasonable first choices. Antipseudomonal coverage with gentamicin or quinolones is indicated in contact lens wearers
- No contact lens worn in the affected eye until the abrasion has healed
- Follow-up within 24 hours
- Instructions regarding primary prevention of eye injuries with eye shields and safety glasses

Common pitfalls in management include the continued use of ophthalmic anesthetics, which may mask worsening symptoms.

Management of Subconjunctival Hemorrhage

Subconjunctival hemorrhages require no specific treatment. Patients should be reassured that resolution should occur within approximately 2 weeks. Failure to resolve warrants a referral to an ophthalmologist to evaluate for less common causes, such as Kaposi sarcoma (6).

Treatment of Blepharitis

This condition is chronic, with frequent relapses, so it is important to treat any underlying conditions, to maintain lid hygiene, and to avoid exacerbating triggers such as eye makeup. Treatment includes warm compresses, for about 3–5 minutes once or twice daily, to loosen and then remove the matted material and debris from the lids. The compresses can also be used to perform gentle massage of the Meibomian glands to express secretions and unclog the gland openings. It is important to avoid overmanipulation of the eyelids, as this can cause mechanical irritation. The compresses can be followed by cleansing of the lid margins with a cotton tip applicator soaked in a solution of diluted baby shampoo (3 oz water plus 3 drops of baby shampoo) (11) or with over-the-counter solutions (EyeScrub or OcuClenz), as needed (9). Patients should be advised to discard their current eye makeup (in case of staph infection), to never share eye makeup, to choose eyeliner and mascara that wash off easily (avoid waterproof), and to replace eye makeup every 6 months.

In more recalcitrant cases, topical antibiotic ointments like bacitracin, erythromycin, and sulfacetamide can be applied once to twice daily with a cotton swab (11). Bedtime is usually more convenient, as the ointment may lead to blurry vision and make daily activities more difficult. If eyelid hygiene and topical antibiotics do not relieve symptoms in patients with Meibomian gland dysfunction, a course of oral antibiotics may be warranted, either doxycycline 50 mg twice daily or tetracycline 250 mg four times daily with the antibiotics being tapered as symptoms regress. In patients who have rosacea or severe inflammation, systemic tetracycline can be added (erythromycin in children and pregnant women) (11). In some cases, topical corticosteroids applied sparingly may also help. Patients should be made aware that this is a chronic condition, and that lid hygiene may need to be continued indefinitely. They should avoid allergens and other exacerbating factors, and they should work with their doctor to treat underlying systemic diseases.

Patients should be referred to an ophthalmologist if there is vision loss, moderate to severe pain, corneal involvement, lack of response to therapy, or suspicion of cancer (unilateral involvement) (9).

Management of Hordeolum

Treatment includes warm compresses for 10–15 minutes three to five times a day (with a clean washcloth). Compresses alone are often sufficient intervention. However, because this is a bacterial infection and may spread to other glands or follicles, an erythromycin or sulfacetamide ophthalmic ointment applied four times a day for 7 days hastens recovery. Culture is seldom required unless initial treatments are unsuccessful (10).

If the patient also suffers from blepharitis, which may have been the inciting factor, the underlying blepharitis should be treated as well. If the lesion does not show improvement in 48 hours, referral to an ophthalmologist for incision and drainage is necessary.

Management of Chalazion

Chalazion is one of the most common eye diseases managed by nonophthalmologists (24). Approximately 25% resolve spontaneously. The treatment for chalazion is similar to that of hordeolum. Warm compresses are applied three to four times a day. This conservative treatment is often sufficient and, as this is a lipogranuloma, antibiotics are not indicated unless infection is suspected. If the chalazion persists or is causing visual changes, referral to an ophthalmologist is appropriate. The chalazion can be excised or injected with steroids, although steroid injections are not always successful (18,25). Treatment of any associated underlying condition is necessary.

KEY POINTS

- Conjunctivitis, corneal lesions, and subconjunctival hemorrhage are the most common causes of a red eye; however, primary care physicians must be on the lookout for more serious causes such as keratitis, uveitis, scleritis, and acute glaucoma.
- Clinical signs and symptoms suggesting a serious eye problem include loss of visual acuity, globe pain, sluggish pupillary reflex, dendritic corneal lesions, and vesicular lesions around the eye.
- Every patient with an eye complaint should have a careful examination, including visual acuity testing.

Many common eye conditions can be managed at the primary care level.

CHAPTER 18

Sore Throat

Mark H. Ebell

CLINICAL OBJECTIVES

1. Describe the differential diagnosis of sore throat for patients of different ages.
2. Describe an evidence-based approach to diagnosis of strep throat and infectious mononucleosis that integrates the history and physical with judicious use of the laboratory.
3. Choose appropriate treatment for various causes of sore throat.

Sore throat is one of the most common symptoms evaluated in primary care and has been well studied as a model for clinical decision-making. Approximately 4% of patients seeing a family physician report "sore throat" as the primary reason for the visit, making it the second-most common reason for an office visit (1). Patients often present to the physician with the preconceived notion that they have a "strep throat" and expect antibiotic therapy. However, streptococcal pharyngitis is responsible for only a minority of cases of sore throat, and you should thoroughly consider all possible infectious and noninfectious causes of the symptom.

Antibiotic therapy for streptococcal pharyngitis reduces the duration of symptoms by about 1 day, the incidence of complications such as abscess formation, the risk of spread to others, and the incidence of rheumatic fever (2–4). However, the incidence of rheumatic fever in particular has declined substantially over the past 40 years (since the widespread introduction of penicillin) from approximately 20 cases per million to 1.5 cases per million (5). Because complications are rare in the modern era and overtreatment increases the development of resistant strains of bacteria, an accurate diagnosis is important. This chapter presents an approach to therapy that builds on our knowledge of the differential diagnosis for different ages, a rational approach to the history and physical examination, and judicious use of the laboratory.

DIFFERENTIAL DIAGNOSIS

Infectious Causes

Sore throat can be caused by bacterial, viral, or fungal infection of the posterior pharynx and tonsillar tissue. Infection by group A β-hemolytic streptococcal (GABHS) bacteria is the most important cause of bacterial infection because of rare but serious possible complications such as peritonsillar abscess, rheumatic fever, and acute glomerulonephritis. Other serotypes (notably group B and group C) are relatively common in the posterior pharynx, but are not thought to cause sore throat. An exception may be large colony count group C strep, although there is no evidence that antibiotics reduce symptoms in these patients (6).

The role of other bacterial pathogens such as *Chlamydia pneumoniae, Branhamella* species, *Haemophilus* species, and *Mycoplasma pneumoniae* remains controversial. These diagnoses should be considered in patients with lingering infections who do not have evidence of GABHS pharyngitis. *M. pneumoniae* in particular is more common in patients who are older, are less ill, and have less evidence of pharyngeal inflammation (7). Although uncommon in most settings, gonococcal pharyngitis should be considered in patients who are otherwise at higher risk for sexually transmitted infection.

Most episodes of pharyngitis are caused by viruses, including adenoviruses, influenza viruses, parainfluenza virus, and respiratory syncytial virus (8). However, it is not usually necessary or important to determine the specific virus responsible for an episode of viral pharyngitis. An exception is pharyngitis caused by Epstein-Barr virus infection, also known as infectious mononucleosis, because of the protracted course and rare but potentially serious complications of this illness (such as splenic rupture and respiratory compromise because severe tonsillar hypertrophy and cervical adenopathy) (9).

The incidence of infectious mononucleosis peaks between the ages of 10 and 29 years and is rare in patients older than age 40 or younger than age 10. Although the infection is thought to occur relatively often in younger children, it generally results in a mild or subclinical infection, so blood tests for infectious mononucleosis are only rarely ordered. Few data are available on the precise likelihood of mononucleosis in patients presenting to a family physician with a complaint of sore throat; estimates by age and setting are shown in Table 18.1 (10–13). These estimates were derived by combining incidence data (in cases/100,000 population) with reports of the likelihood of infectious mononucleosis among specific age groups.

A gram negative rod, *Fusobacterium necrophorum*, has recently been reported as a cause of pharyngitis in 10% of adolescents and young adults. It cannot be identified by any presently available commercial tests. Most importantly, it is associated with Lemierre syndrome, a rare condition occurring in about 1 in 400 episodes of *F. necrophorum* pharyngitis that has a 5% mortality rate (14).

Acute cytomegalovirus infection is a rare cause of pharyngitis, and although it resembles infectious mononucleosis in some respects, it is associated with a greater degree of hepatic

TABLE 18.1 Likelihood of Group A β-hemolytic Streptococcal (GABHS) Pharyngitis and Infectious Mononucleosis in the Primary Care Setting by Age*

Infection	Age (Years)	%
GABHS pharyngitis	0–4	15
	5–9	30
	10–19	15
	Adult	5–10
Infectious mononucleosis	0–4	<1
	5–14	1–2
	15–24	5–10
	25–34	1–2
	>34	<1

*Data are from Ehrlich TP, Schwartz RH, Wientzen R, Thorne MM. Comparison of an immunochromatographic method for rapid identification of group A streptococcal antigen with culture method. Arch Fam Med 1993;2:866–869; Holmberg SD, Faich GA. Streptococcal pharyngitis and acute rheumatic fever in Rhode Island. JAMA. 1983;250:2307–2312; Wigton RS, Connor JL, Centor RM. Transportability of a decision rule for the diagnosis of streptococcal pharyngitis. Arch Intern Med. 1986;146:81–83; Komaroff AL, Pass TM, Aronson MD, et al. The prediction of streptococcal pharyngitis in adults. J Gen Intern Med. 1986;1:1–7; Hoffman S. An algorithm for a selective use of throat swabs in the diagnosis of group A streptococcal pharyngo tonsillitis in general practice. Scand J Prim Health Care. 1992;10:295–300; Fry J. Infectious mononucleosis: some new observations from a 15-year study. J Fam Pract. 1980;10: 1087–1089; Everett MT. The cause of tonsillitis. The Practitioner. 1979;223:253–259; Hanson CJ, Higbee JW, Lednar WM, Garrison MJ. The epidemiology of acute pharyngitis among soldiers at Ford Lewis, Washington. Mil Med. 1986;7:389–394.

involvement. Candidiasis is a rare cause of sore throat. It should be considered in immunosuppressed patients, especially those with AIDS, and in patients using nasal or inhaled steroid preparations.

Noninfectious Causes

Gastroesophageal reflux disease causes pain by direct irritation of the pharyngeal tissue by stomach acid. Allergic rhinitis or sinusitis, with chronic posterior drainage from the nasopharynx, can cause pharyngeal irritation through a combination of chemical irritation and repeated drying. Persistent coughing can cause sore throat without any direct infection of the pharynx. Acute thyroiditis causes anterior neck pain that may be mistaken for pharyngitis but is typically associated with more local tenderness to palpation. Other causes of throat pain include trauma (either external or internal, such as from a fish bone) and referred dental pain.

The differential diagnosis of sore throat in the primary care setting is summarized in Table 18.2. No reliable estimates are available for the likelihood of noninfectious causes of sore throat. Depending on the age of the patient and the setting in which they present, the prevalence of GABHS pharyngitis varies from 5% to 36%; estimates of the likelihood of streptococcal pharyngitis by age are shown in Table 18.1. GABHS pharyngitis is more common in children, in emergency departments, and in the fall and winter (15–18).

CLINICAL EVALUATION

In most cases, the history will help you determine whether the sore throat is because an infectious or noninfectious cause. Noninfectious causes should be suspected in patients who are afebrile or who have no other signs of upper respiratory infection, have had symptoms longer than 1–2 weeks, and have associated symptoms such as heartburn, postnasal drip, or itchy eyes. Current use of antacid medications or a history of peptic ulcer disease should alert you to the possibility of gastroesophageal reflux disease. Symptoms are typically worse late at night or early in the morning, and patients will often report a bitter or unpleasant taste in the back of the throat on awakening.

When evaluating a patient with sore throat, be alert for red flags (summarized in Table 18.3). These patients need more rapid assessment and may require urgent referral. Otherwise, the key clinical questions for the patient with infectious sore throat are whether it is caused by GABHS pharyngitis, infectious mononucleosis or in adolescents by infection with *F. necrophorum*. The remainder of this section focuses on the history, physical examination, and laboratory testing for these former two diagnoses.

HISTORY AND PHYSICAL EXAMINATION

GABHS Pharyngitis

The signs and symptoms most strongly associated with GABHS pharyngitis are a measured or reported (subjective) fever, absence of cough, tonsillar or pharyngeal exudate, cervical adenopathy, and tonsillar enlargement. Myalgias, recent strep exposure, a brief duration of illness before presentation, and headache also increase the likelihood of GABHS pharyngitis somewhat. Pharyngeal injection is commonly noted, but the sensitivity and specificity vary greatly, probably because physicians define it differently. The typical scarlatina rash (a fine sandpapery eruption)

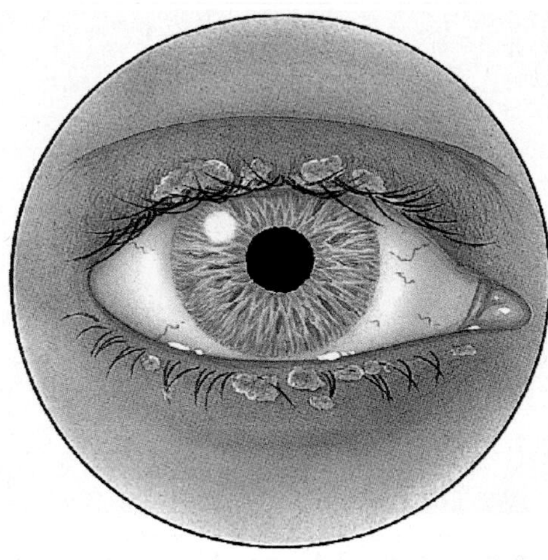

Figure 17.2 • Red-rimmed eyelids with scaling and debris at the eyelash base and broken lashes in blepharitis. (Provided by Anatomical Chart Company.)

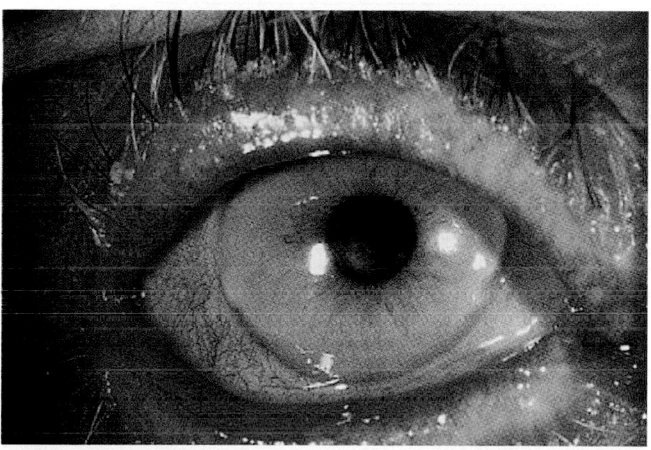

Figure 17.3 • Blepharitis. (From Weber J, Kelly J. Health Assessment in Nursing, 2nd ed. Philadelphia: Lippincott Williams & Wilkins; 2003.)

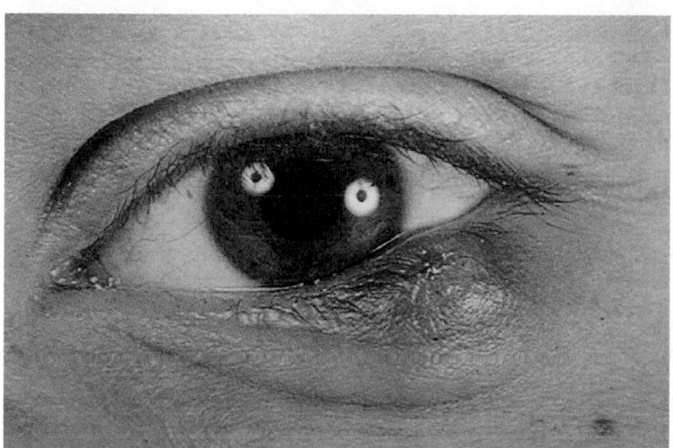

Figure 17.4 • Hordeolum: note the localized swelling and erythema with eyelash follicle involvement. (From Goodheart HP. Goodheart's Photoguide of Common Skin Disorders, 2nd ed. Philadelphia: Lippincott Williams & Wilkins; 2003.)

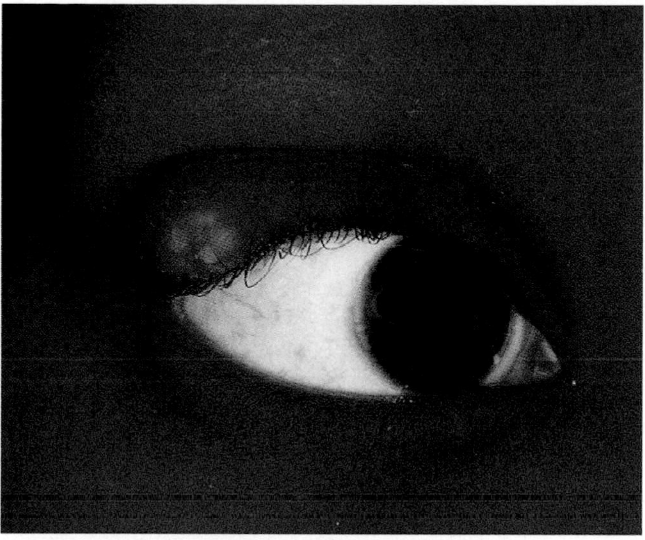

Figure 17.5 • Internal hordeolum. A 9-year-old female presented with a 3-day history of a painful, fast-growing lesion on her right upper eyelid. (From Fleisher GR, Ludwig W, Baskin MN. Atlas of Pediatric Emergency Medicine. Philadelphia: Lippincott Williams & Wilkins; 2004.)

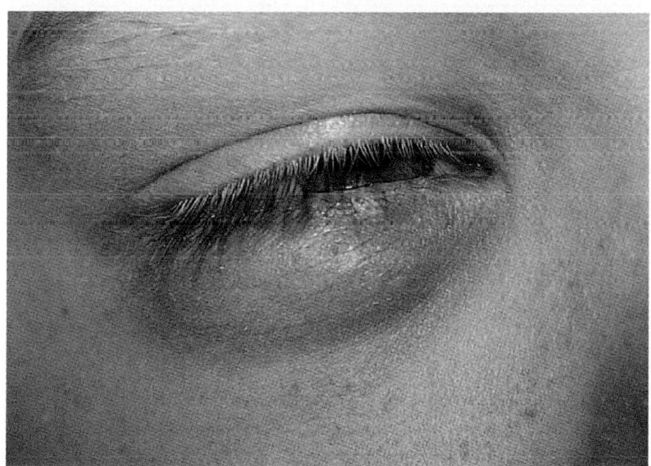

Figure 17.6 • Chalazion. A 7-year-old male presented with a large, slow growing, painless mass that developed on his lower lid over 4 months. (From Tasman W, Jaeger E. The Wills Eye Hospital Atlas of Clinical Ophthalmology, 2nd ed. Baltimore: Lippincott Williams & Wilkins; 2001.)

TABLE 18.4 Key Elements of the History and Physical Examination for Sore Throat

Symptoms and Signs	Sensitivity	Specificity	LR+	LR−
GABHS pharyngitis*				
Tonsillar or pharyngeal exudates	21%–58%	69%–92%	1.5–2.6	0.7–0.9
Fever (subjective)	30%–92%	23%–90%	1.0–2.6	0.3–1.0
Fever (measured temperature >37.8°C or 101°F)	11%–84%	43%–96%	1.1–3.0	0.3–0.9
Cervical adenopathy	55%–82%	34%–73%	0.5–2.9	0.6–0.9
Enlarged tonsils	56%–86%	56%–86%	1.4–3.1	0.6
No cough	51%–79%	36%–68%	1.1–1.7	0.5–0.9
No coryza	42%–84%	20%–70%	0.9–1.6	0.5–1.4
Myalgias	49%	52%–69%	1.4	0.9
Headache	48%	50%–80%	0.8–2.6	0.5–1.1
Pharynx injected	43%–99%	3%–62%	0.7–1.6	0.2–6.4
Duration <3 days	26%–93%	59%	0.7–3.5	0.2–2.2
Palatine petechiae	7%	95%	1.4	1.0
Strep exposure previous 2 weeks	19%	87%–94%	1.9	0.9
Scarlatina rash	4%	79%–99%	0.1–0.3	0.9–1.1
Infectious mononucleosis (adults)				
Any cervical adenopathy	87	58	2.1	0.2
Splenomegaly	7	99	7	0.9
Inguinal adenopathy	53	82	2.9	0.6
Palatine petechiae	27	95	5.4	0.8
Posterior cervical adenopathy	40	87	3.1	0.7
Axillary adenopathy	27	91	3	0.8
Fatigue	93	23	1.2	0.3
Anterior cervical adenopathy	70	43	1.2	0.9

Note: These data are from a meta analysis[†] of high-quality diagnostic studies. Signs and symptoms are organized from greatest accuracy (as measured by area under the receiver-operating characteristic curve) to least accuracy. A range is provided when the studies were heterogeneous, and a point estimate when they were homogeneous.
*Ebell MH, Smith MA, Barry HC, Ives K, Carey M. Does this patient have strep throat? JAMA. 2000;284:2912–2918.

with confirmed infectious mononucleosis, at least 98% had sore throat, lymph node enlargement, fever, and tonsillar enlargement. Other common physical signs included pharyngeal inflammation (85%) and transient palatal petechiae (50%). This presentation is typical in adolescents. Older adults are less likely to have sore throat and adenopathy but more likely to have hepatomegaly and jaundice (9, 10).

Although symptoms in general may be similar to those of streptococcal pharyngitis (sore throat, fever, chills, malaise, and headache) and the two coexist in 5–30% of patients, fatigue is a much more prominent symptom in infectious mononucleosis, and often interferes significantly with the patient's ability to function (9). Approximately 4% of patients have mild abdominal pain in the left upper quadrant; if this pain is severe, splenic rupture should be suspected and a surgical consultation obtained.

Cervical adenopathy and fever are present in over 99% of patients with infectious mononucleosis (9). In fact, if a patient does not have cervical adenopathy (either anterior or posterior) and fever (either by history or measured in the office), you can effectively rule out infectious mononucleosis. Because 90% of patients with mononucleosis have posterior cervical adenopathy, patients without this finding also have a very low probability of disease (5) unless they have other history or physical findings pointing strongly toward mononucleosis (e.g., recent exposure to someone with the disease, a protracted course, severe fatigue, or splenomegaly). Other signs found in patients with infectious mononucleosis include splenomegaly (present in 50%) (5), palatal petechiae (50%), jaundice (10%), and rash (3%) (9).

F. NECROPHORUM PHARYNGITIS

Relatively little is known about the clinical diagnosis of *F. necrophorum*. Lemierre syndrome, the rare complication of

TABLE 18.5 Clinical Prediction Rule for the Diagnosis of Group A β-hemolytic Streptococcal (GABHS) Pharyngitis*

1. Add up the points for your patient

Symptom or Sign	**Points**
History of fever or measured temperature >38°C	1
Absence of cough	1
Tender anterior cervical adenopathy	1
Tonsillar swelling or exudates	1
Age <15 years	1
Age ≥45 years	−1
Total:	

2. Find their risk of strep below

Points	**Likelihood Ratio**	**Percentage with Strep (Patients with Strep/Total)**
−1 or 0	0.05	1% (2/179)
−1	0.52	10% (13/134)
−2	0.95	17% (18/109)
−3	2.5	35% (28/81)
−4 or 5	4.9	51% (39/77)

Note: Baseline risk of strep = 17% in this population. This rule was validated in a group of 167 children over the age of 3 and 453 adults in Ontario, Canada.

*Data are from McIsaac WJ, Goel V, To T, Low DE. The validity of a sore throat score in family practice. CMAJ. 2000;163:811–815.

pharyngitis caused by *F. necrophorum*, is a disease of adolescents and young adults that typically begins 3–5 days after the onset of pharyngitis or tonsillitis. The patient develops rigors and suppurative thrombophlebitis of the internal jugular vein, followed by pulmonary abscesses. Unilateral neck swelling in a patient with symptoms of bacteremia several days after the onset of pharyngitis should trigger suspicion for Lemierre disease (14).

Diagnostic Testing

GABHS

A variety of rapid antigen tests and cultures are available to test for the presence of GABHS bacteria in the pharynx. Rapid antigen tests include enzyme immunoassays, latex agglutination tests, liposomal assays, and immunochromatographic assays. Their test characteristics vary considerably and are summarized in Table 18.6. You should know the type of test used in your office and its test characteristics in real clinical use. Relying on rapid antigen tests, even when strep is relatively common, will miss less than 5% of cases of strep throat (20), and can reduce the use of antibiotics (21).

Although the throat culture test is often considered a gold standard, a second throat culture taken simultaneously from a patient with an initial positive throat culture is only positive 90% of the time. Also, a small but significant percentage of sore throat patients with a positive throat culture for GABHS bacteria are actually carriers, in which a pathogen or mechanism other than GABHS bacteria is responsible for the sore throat.

INFECTIOUS MONONUCLEOSIS

Two types of laboratory tests are useful for confirming the diagnosis of infectious mononucleosis: the complete blood count with differential, and a variety of serologic tests. Most patients with infectious mononucleosis develop a lymphocytosis, which usually peaks 2 weeks after the onset of symptoms. Approximately 95% of patients have more than 60% lymphocytes; having less than that at 10–14 days after the onset of symptoms largely rules out the diagnosis. The total white blood cell count peaks above 10,000 cells/mm^3 in 77% of patients (9). Atypical lymphocytes are also common in patients with infectious mononucleosis. In fact, in one study all patients with more than 40% atypical lymphocytes and clinically suspected infectious mononucleosis had serologic evidence of acute Epstein-Barr virus infection. In the same study, 69% of patients with 20% to 40% atypical lymphocytes had evidence of Epstein-Barr virus infection (22). The likelihood ratios for different levels of atypical lymphocytosis are shown in Table 18.6. If the patient has more than 20% atypical lymphocytes, or more than 50% lymphocytes with 10% or more atypical lymphocytes, infectious mononucleosis is quite likely, and further confirmation of the diagnosis is not needed.

Serologic tests are often negative in the first week of infection because they rely on the body's immune response. The traditional test is based on the fact that heterophil antibodies produced in patients with infectious mononucleosis agglutinate sheep erythrocytes; the "Monospot" test that is still widely used is

TABLE 18.6 Characteristics of Tests Used to Detect Group A β-hemolytic Streptococcal (GABHS) Pharyngitis and Infectious Mononucleosis

Test	Sensitivity	Specificity	LR+	LR−
GABHS pharyngitis (all children with sore throat)				
Rapid test followed by culture if negative	96	96	25	0.04
Paired rapid antigen tests	91	95	18	0.1
Single rapid antigen test	88	96	23	0.13
GABHS pharyngitis (children at high risk for strep)				
Rapid test followed by culture if negative	97	98	46	0.03
Paired rapid antigen tests	94	97	29	0.07
Single rapid antigen test	91	97	28	0.1
Infectious mononucleosis				
>40% atypical lymphocytes*				39
36–40% atypical lymphocytes*				3.1
31–35% atypical lymphocytes*				1.2
20–30% atypical lymphocytes*				0.44
50% lymphocytes and >10% atypical cells†	39%	99%	39	0.61
Rapid slide agglutination				
(Monospot)†	86%	99%	86	0.14
1st week	69%	88%	5.7	0.35
2nd week	81%	88%	6.7	0.21
VCA-IgM‡				
1st week	0.80	0.99	80	0.20
2nd week	0.85	0.99	85	0.15
3rd week	0.97	0.99	97	0.03
Anti-EBV ELISA (Biotest anti-EBV recombinant)¶	0.99	0.99	99	0.01

EBV = Epstein-Barr virus; ELISA = enzyme-linked immunosorbent assay; Ig = immunoglobulin; VCA = viral capsid antigen.
*Ho-Yen DO, Martin KW. The relationship between atypical lymphocytosis and serological tests in infectious mononucleosis. J Infect. 1981;3:324–331.
†Fleischer GR, Collins M, Fager S. Limitations of available tests for diagnosis of infectious mononucleosis. J Clin Microbiol. 1983;17:619–624.
‡Evans AS, Niederman JC, Cenabre LC, et al. A prospective evaluation of heterophile and Epstein-Barr virus-specific IgM antibody tests in clinical and subclinical infectious mononucleosis: specificity and sensitivity of the tests and persistence of the antibody. J Infect Dis. 1975;132:546–554.
¶Farber I, Wutzler P, Wohlrabe P, et al. Serological diagnosis of infectious mononucleosis using three anti-Epstein Barr virus-recombinant ELISAs. J Virol Methods. 1993;42:301–308.

a rapid latex agglutination test based on the same principle. However, up to 20% of patients may not produce this antibody. Viral capsid antigen immunoglobulin M antibodies are produced relatively early in infection and do not persist once the acute infection is over. This test is quite sensitive and specific, although like the Monospot test, the sensitivity improves during the second week of the illness. Other laboratory tests that are sometimes abnormal in patients with infectious mononucleosis include aspartate aminotransferase (>40 μ/L in 76% of patients) and alkaline phosphatase (elevated in 71% of patients) (10). Characteristics of serologic tests are summarized in Table 18.6.

Recommended Diagnostic Strategy

The recommended approach to management of sore throat is summarized in Figure 18.1. If an infectious cause of sore throat seems likely, the physician should consider whether infectious mononucleosis is a possibility. If unlikely, the validated McIsaac clinical decision rule shown in Table 18.5 should be used to estimate the probability of strep (23, 24). The decision to order further testing, such as a rapid strep test, depends on this probability estimate. In adolescents, given emerging information about *F. necrophorum*, physicians should consider empiric antibiotic treatment for those with three or more points. Using this kind of a patient-centered, individualized, and evidence-based approach has even been shown to reduce cost and increase the quality of care (24).

MANAGEMENT

Viral pharyngitis is a self-limited condition, and only symptomatic treatment is indicated. Strategies for symptomatic

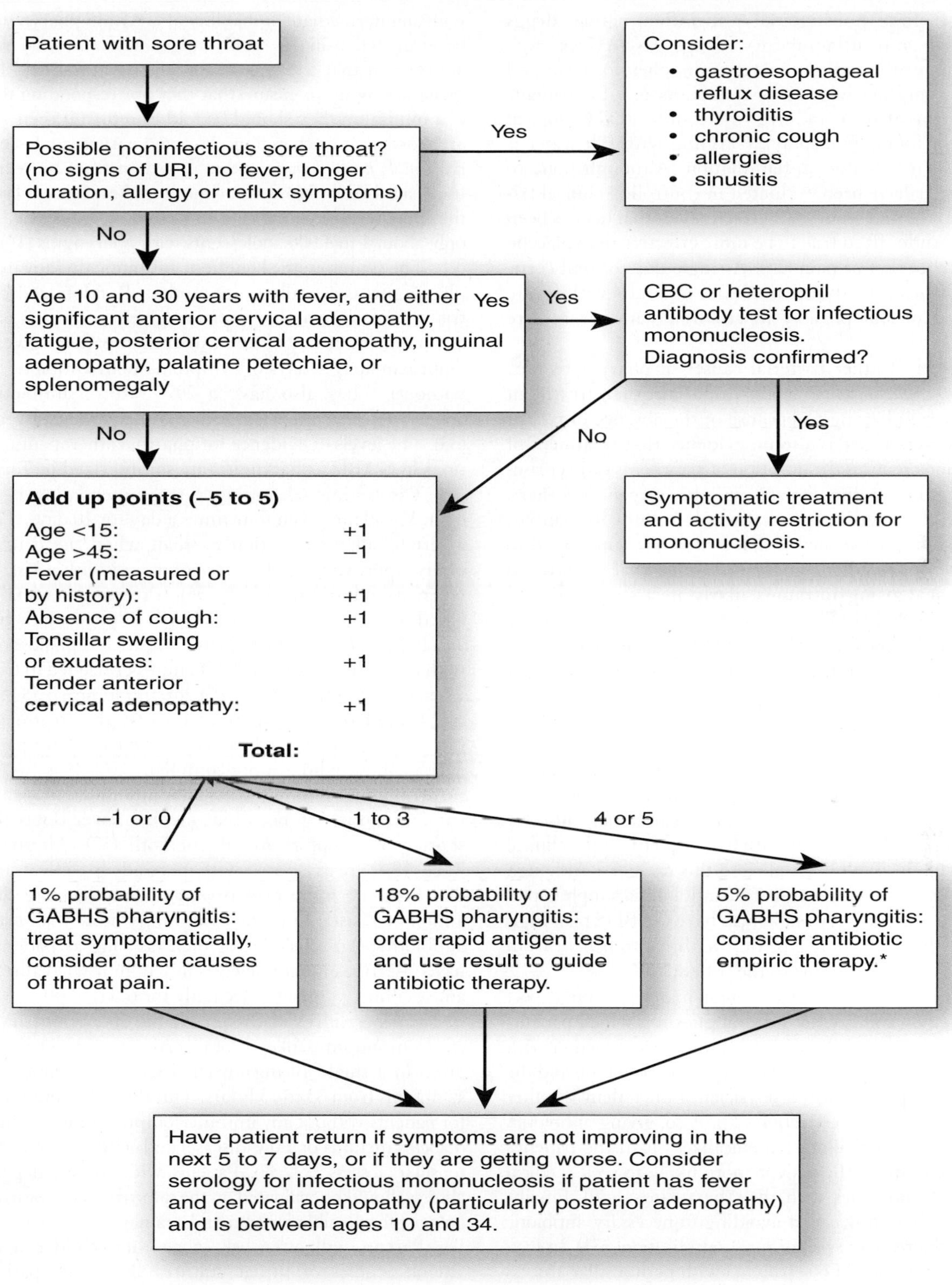

Figure 18.1 • General approach to the patient with sore throat.

treatment include nonsteroidal anti-inflammatory drugs (nonsteroidal anti-inflammatory drugs [NSAIDs]; e.g., ibuprofen, naproxen sodium) or acetaminophen for fever and throat pain, gargling with 2% viscous lidocaine for patients with severe throat pain, and over-the-counter (OTC) topical sprays (e.g., Chloraseptic spray). Gargling with salt water is soothing and may reduce inflammation. Although none of these strategies have been evaluated in controlled clinical trials, they are safe and seem to be effective. Herbal tea has been shown in a randomized trial to be more effective than placebo for short-term relief of pain (25). A single dose of oral corticosteroids reduces the duration of pain in adults with severe sore throat (26) and possibly in children with severe sore throat (27).

Treatment of other bacterial causes of pharyngitis (i.e., *Chlamydia, M. pneumoniae*) is less important than treatment of streptococcal pharyngitis because of the absence of risk of rheumatic fever. There is also no evidence that treatment of these infections reduces the duration of symptoms or decreases the likelihood that the disease will be spread to others. Gonococcal pharyngitis is generally only minimally symptomatic, but should be treated if detected to prevent spread to others. Recommended treatment for gonococcal pharyngitis is ceftriaxone 125 mg intramuscularly in a single dose or ciprofloxacin 500 mg orally in a single dose; azithromycin 1 g orally in a single dose (or doxycycline 100 mg orally twice daily for 7 days) should also be given if chlamydial infection is not ruled out (28).

GABHS Pharyngitis

Patients at very low risk for GABHS pharyngitis based on their demographics, history, and physical examination should be reassured that they do not seem to have a bacterial cause for their sore throat. Most patients with 0 or -1 points in the clinical prediction rule in Table 18.5 fall into this category. Although many patients have come to expect an antibiotic, a simple explanation of why they are very unlikely to have GABHS pharyngitis and why that is the only type of sore throat to benefit from antibiotics is usually satisfying to the patient.

Studies have shown that although many patients expect antibiotics, physicians are not good at guessing which patients want an antibiotic, and the patient's ultimate satisfaction with the encounter depends on the quality of the explanation and the length of time spent with the physician, rather than whether they got an antibiotic prescription (29). Also, giving antibiotics for a self-limited viral illness "medicalizes" it in the patient's mind, and may make the patient more likely to seek medical attention and antibiotics with their next illness (30). Finally, large studies have shown that avoiding unnecessary antibiotic use does not increase the risk of rare complications (31). In fact, an observational study of 606 patients with peritonsillar abscess found that antibiotic use did not prevent the condition in patients presenting initially with sore throat (32).

Patients with a very high probability of GABHS pharyngitis, based on the history and physical examination, can be considered for empiric treatment without further laboratory testing, because the likelihood of disease even in the presence of a negative rapid antigen test remains more than 5% because the number of false-negative results. Another (although more expensive) strategy is to use a rapid antigen test in these patients, and order a throat culture if the rapid test is negative. Patients with an intermediate probability of GABHS pharyngitis should be evaluated using a rapid antigen test and only receive an antibiotic if that test is positive. All patients should have adequate follow-up to ensure that they are responding to therapy; at a minimum they should be told to return if their symptoms are worsening or changing. As noted earlier, adolescents are at risk for *F. necrophorum* and may benefit from more aggressive use of antibiotics. However, clinical trial evidence is lacking and the most serious complication, Lemierre syndrome, occurs in only about 1 in 4,000 adolescents with pharyngitis (14).

The symptomatic benefit of antibiotic therapy in GABHS pharyngitis is actually quite modest. Randomized controlled trials have shown that patients given penicillin experience about one fewer day of sore throat than patients given placebo (approximately 4 days of symptoms with antibiotic vs 5 days without). They also have a 20% rate of antibiotic-related adverse effects compared with 5% for patients given placebo (33). The levels of evidence for pharmacotherapeutic interventions in GABHS pharyngitis are summarized in Table 18.7.

The traditional antibiotic recommendation is for penicillin V, 250 mg given four times a day for 10 days. The risk of a serious allergic reaction is small when the drug is given orally, approximately 0.025% compared with a risk of 0.64% when given intramuscularly (34). A recent meta-analysis combined data from 35 studies of GABHS pharyngitis treatment, and found a higher clinical cure rate with cephalosporins than with penicillin (93.6% vs 85.8%; number needed to treat = 13). The only exceptions were cefaclor and loracarbef (35).

Compliance is important because the treatment failure rate has been shown to be only 12% in compliant patients and 34% in those who are noncompliant (36). It is therefore not surprising that several studies have attempted to identify alternate antibiotic regimens that involve fewer doses per day, a shorter course of treatment, or both (37). Alternatives (see Table 18.8) are associated with more adverse effects (especially diarrhea), are more expensive, and may increase the risk of antibiotic resistance in the community more than use of older antibiotics. An effective regimen (as long as patients do not have infectious mononucleosis in whom it will cause a rash) is amoxicillin 1 g, given twice daily for 6 days (38).

Patients with exudative pharyngitis and severe pain may benefit from intramuscular or oral corticosteroids. Dexamethasone given in a single 10 mg injection halved the time to relief of symptoms from 33 to 15 hours. This therapy should be reserved for patients without any immunocompromising conditions (e.g., diabetes mellitus or HIV disease) and with no evidence of peritonsillar abscess (27, 39). Patients with suspected peritonsillar abscess should be evaluated on the same day by an otorhinolaryngologist for possible incision and drainage.

Parents will often ask when their child can return to school. Studies of throat cultures show that patients with GABHS pharyngitis become "culture-negative" within 24 hours of initiating antibiotic therapy. It is therefore reasonable to recommend that children spend the day following the office visit at home, but if feeling better and afebrile should be allowed to return to school on the second day after the office or emergency department visit (40).

Infectious Mononucleosis

Identification of patients with infectious mononucleosis is important because of the more protracted course of the disease

TABLE 18.7 Treatment of Sore Throat

Treatment	Strength of Recommendation	Comment
Antibiotics (cephalosporin for 7–10 days, penicillin VK 250 mg PO QID for 10 days, or amoxicillin 1 g PO BID for 6 days) for GABHS pharyngitis*	A	Reduces symptoms by about 1 day and reduces risk of rheumatic and suppurative complications
Dexamethasone 10 mg IM injection for severe pain and tonsillar enlargement†	B	Not in immunocompromised patients or those with peritonsillar abscess
2% viscous lidocaine gargle, salt water gargle, or throat lozenges	C	For relief of pharyngeal pain
Nonsteroidal anti-inflammatory drugs or acetaminophen	C	For relief of pain, fever, myalgias, headache. May also reduce pharyngeal pain.
Activity restriction for infectious mononucleosis	C	
Herbal tea	B	To relieve pain of sore throat

A = consistent, good-quality patient-oriented evidence; B = inconsistent or limited-quality patient-oriented evidence; C = consensus, disease-oriented evidence, usual practice, expert opinion, or case series.
For information about the SORT evidence rating system, see *http://www.aafp.org/afpsort.xml*.
*Peyramond D, Portier H, Geslin P, Cohen R. 6-day amoxicillin vs. 10-day penicillin V for group A β-hemolytic streptococcal acute tonsillitis in adults: a French Multicentre, open-label randomized study. Scand J Infect Dis. 1996;28:497–501.
†O'Brien JF, Meade JI, Falk JL. Dexamethasone as adjuvant therapy for severe acute pharyngitis. Ann Emerg Med. 1993;22:212–215.

(typically 1-2 months) and the possibility of serious complications in approximately 1% of patients. Complications include splenic rupture and respiratory compromise because pharyngeal edema and tonsillar swelling.

You should have a high index of suspicion for infectious mononucleosis in younger patients, particularly those ages 15–24 years, and in patients with posterior cervical adenopathy. Patients without anterior or posterior cervical adenopathy and fever are extremely unlikely to have the diagnosis, as are those older than age 35, which will help rule it out in many patients. Diagnostic tests are relatively insensitive during the first week of illness when many patients present.

Patients with infectious mononucleosis should be treated symptomatically with rest, oral fluids, and NSAIDs or acetaminophen for fever and myalgias. Aspirin should be avoided because Reye syndrome has been reported in association with infectious mononucleosis. Based on clinical experience and case reports, corticosteroids are recommended in patients with significant pharyngeal edema that causes or threatens respiratory compromise (41, 42).

Participation in contact sports (e.g., cheerleading, basketball, hockey, football, soccer) should be restricted during the acute phase of the illness and continue to be restricted for at least 4 weeks and as long as the spleen is palpable. One study followed 150 patients with newly diagnosed infectious mononucleosis for 6 months. The researchers found that sore throat, fever, headache, rash, cough, and nausea had largely resolved 1 month after the onset of symptoms. Fatigue resolved more slowly (77% initially, 28% at 1 month, 21% at 2 months, and 13% at 6 months), as did sleeping too much (45% initially, 18% at 1 month, 14% at 2 months, and 9% at 6 months) and sore joints (23% initially, 15% at 1 month, 6% at 2 months, and 9% at 6 months). Patients required about 2 months to achieve a stable level of recovery as measured by their functional status (43).

Patients with coexisting streptococcal pharyngitis or those at high risk for streptococcal pharyngitis based on their signs and symptoms (see Table 18.5) should be started on an antibiotic. Use an antibiotic other than amoxicillin, because it causes a rash in approximately 80% of patients with infectious mononucleosis. The mechanism of this reaction is not well understood. The level of evidence for treatment recommendations in infectious mononucleosis is shown in Table 18.7.

F. Necrophorum Pharyngitis

Because of the lack of a commercially available diagnostic test to identify this agent, consider empirically treating adolescents or young adults with 3 or more of the original Centor criteria (fever, anterior cervical adenopathy, tonsillar exudate, absence of cough). This bacterium is responsive to penicillin, clindamycin and cephalosporins but not to macrolide antibiotics.

PATIENT EDUCATION

Education of the patient with sore throat has several goals. First, patients should understand that only a minority of sore throats are caused by streptococcal pharyngitis or other bacteria, and that symptomatic treatment is usually sufficient. They should also be told how to relieve the symptoms of sore throat, using salt water gargles, NSAIDs, OTC throat sprays, and OTC lozenges (e.g., Chloraseptic). Finally, patients should know the symptoms of bacterial or complicated sore throat, such as fever, chills, sweats, swollen glands, and respiratory impairment, which require physician evaluation.

TABLE 18.8 Pharmacotherapy Recommended for the Treatment of Group A β-hemolytic Streptococcal (GABHS) Pharyngitis

Drug	Dosing Range	Adverse Effects	Comment
First-line drugs			
Penicillin VK	Children <12 years old: 25–50 mg/kg/day divided, Q 6–8 hours (max 3 g/day) Adults/children >12 yo: 250 mg PO QID for 7 to 10 days or 500 mg PO TID for 7 to 10 days	Mild diarrhea, vomiting, nausea	Compliance a problem, especially with QID dosing. Adjust dose for renal insufficiency. Available in suspension.
Amoxicillin*	Adults/children >12 years old: 500 mg PO TID for 7-10 days or 1 g PO BID for 6 days. Children <12 years old: 25–100 mg/kg/day divided Q 8 hours (maximum 2–3 g/day)	Rash in patients with infectious mononucleosis	Available as tablet, capsule, chewable tablet and oral suspension.
Alternate (second-line) drugs			
Azithromycin	Adults: 500 mg PO QD on day 1, 250 mg PO QD on days 2–5 Children >2 years old: 12 mg/kg (days 1–5)		Available as tablet or oral suspension. F. necrophorum does not respond to macrolides.
Cefixime	8 mg/kg (children) PO QD for 10 days. Children >50 kg or >12 years old and adults: 400 mg/day divided Q 12–24 hours		
Dexamethasone†	10 mg IM injection once for ages 12 and older		For severe sore throat only or pharyngeal edema

*Peyramond D, Portier H, Geslin P, Cohen R. 6-day amoxicillin vs. 10-day penicillin V for group A b-hemolytic streptococcal acute tonsillitis in adults: a French Multicentre, open-label randomized study. Scand J Infect Dis. 1996;28:497–501.
†O'Brien JF, Meade JI, Falk JL. Dexamethasone as adjuvant therapy for severe acute pharyngitis. Ann Emerg Med. 1993;22:212–215.

KEY POINTS

- Always remember that sore throat can be caused by noninfectious causes, and that infectious causes are usually viral (SORT=B).
- Use a clinical decision rule to estimate the probability of GABHS pharyngitis and guide testing and antibiotic therapy (SORT=A).
- In adolescents and young adults, consider infectious mononucleosis in those with persistent sore throat, fatigue, and posterior cervical adenopathy (SORT=B).
- Be aware of Lemierre syndrome, a rare complication of infection with *F. necrophorum* in adolescents and young adults that typically presents with rigors and unilateral neck swelling (SORT=C).

CHAPTER

19

Abdominal Pain

Steven Roskos, MD

CLINICAL OBJECTIVES

1. Use clues from the history and physical examination to establish a presumptive diagnosis on which to base diagnostic testing.
2. Determine when diagnostic testing is required and choose the most appropriate test to aid diagnosis of abdominal pain.
3. Determine when it is safe to forego further testing and begin empiric treatment for abdominal pain based on a presumptive diagnosis.

Abdominal pain, defined as any uncomfortable feeling in the abdominal region including the flank, is one of the most common presenting symptoms in primary care. Patients complaining of abdominal pain account for about 2% of all ambulatory patient visits, and the majority of these visits occur in primary care offices (1).

Although diagnostic technologies have advanced, a careful history and physical examination remain the keys to effective diagnosis and treatment. Evaluation of patients with abdominal pain begins with an assessment of whether the condition requires urgent treatment or surgery. If urgent treatment is not required, you can then develop a presumptive diagnosis based on clinical evaluation and choose either empiric treatment or diagnostic testing based on the best available evidence.

DIFFERENTIAL DIAGNOSIS

Conditions that cause abdominal pain range in severity from benign and self-limited to severe and life-threatening. Pathology causing abdominal pain may be within or outside the abdomen. A relatively limited number of conditions cause the great majority of episodes of abdominal pain in family medicine (Table 19.1 and 19.3). Less severe causes include gastroenteritis, dyspepsia, urinary tract infection, irritable bowel syndrome, ovarian cysts, and gastroesophageal reflux disease. More serious conditions that cause abdominal pain include appendicitis, pelvic inflammatory disease, diverticulitis, gallbladder disease, urinary stones, pyelonephritis, and intestinal obstruction. Myocardial infarction, pneumonia, muscle strain, and diabetic ketoacidosis are examples of pathology outside the abdomen that may also cause abdominal pain.

CLINICAL EVALUATION

When evaluating a patient with abdominal pain, first be certain the patient is stable. Arrange urgent hospital transport of patients with signs or symptoms of shock while the workup continues. Next determine the duration of pain. If pain is of less than 48 hours' duration, attempt to rule out an "acute abdomen" (a cause of abdominal pain that requires urgent surgery to prevent significant morbidity or death). Symptoms and signs that make an acute abdomen more likely include the red flags listed in Table 19.2. An acute abdomen is typically caused by either peritonitis or intestinal obstruction, which are discussed in more detail in the following sections. If you suspect the patient has an acute abdomen, urgently arrange hospital transport and surgical consultation. Of course, patients with a cause of acute abdomen such as appendicitis may rarely present with an atypical course; 48 hours is a general guideline, not a hard-and-fast rule.

If you do not suspect an acute abdomen or if the patient is in the emergency department already, use clues from the historical and physical examination to direct you toward a presumptive diagnosis (Figures 19.1 and 19.2). If your presumed diagnosis is ruled out, run through the appropriate algorithm again, broadening your differential diagnosis. The diagnostic clues apply in general, but may not describe all patients with a given diagnosis. Consider less serious diagnoses such as gastroenteritis, dysmenorrhea, simple pregnancy, diarrhea, constipation, or muscle strain. Consider less common diagnoses such as inflammatory bowel disease or cancer. If the etiology is still unclear, but immediately dangerous diagnoses are unlikely, consider providing symptomatic treatment, reassuring the patient, and arranging close follow-up.

History and Physical Examination

HISTORY

The duration, location, quality, and progression of pain are key historical data. The most likely diagnoses differ based on pain duration (see Figures 19.1 and 19.2). Patients with irritable bowel syndrome, dyspepsia, or gastroesophageal reflux disease typically do not seek care until the pain has been present for at least 48 hours, usually longer. Patients with a urinary stone, appendicitis, or cholecystitis usually seek care within the first 48 hours after the onset of pain.

Table 19.3 lists different causes of abdominal pain based on quality and location of pain. The quality of pain is usually either visceral or parietal. Visceral pain is typically deep, dull,

TABLE 19.1 Differential Diagnosis of the Patient with Abdominal Pain (23–25)

Diagnosis	Frequency in Family Physicians Office (%)	Frequency in Emergency Department (%)
Unknown or undocumented etiology	21–50	41
Gastroenteritis	9	7
Gastritis or dyspepsia	9	1
Urinary tract infection (not including pyelonephritis)	7	5
Irritable bowel syndrome	6–7	—
Ovarian cyst	6	—
Pelvic inflammatory disease	4	7
Gastroesophageal reflux disease (including hiatal hernia)	2–7	—
Diverticulitis	2	—
Diarrhea (undetermined or infectious)	2–6	—
Cholelithiasis/cholecystitis	2–3	2
Tumor, benign	1	—
Peptic ulcer	1–4	2
Urolithiasis	1	4
Appendicitis	1	4
Ulcerative colitis	1	—
Muscular strain	1–4	—
Intestinal obstruction	—	3
Constipation	—	2
Dysmenorrhea	—	2
Simple pregnancy	—	2
Pyelonephritis	—	2

and diffusely located in the midline. It results from spasm or stretching of the wall of a hollow viscus, distention of the capsule of a solid organ, or ischemia or inflammation of a visceral structure. Intestinal obstruction and early appendicitis usually cause visceral pain. Parietal pain results from irritation of the parietal peritoneum. This type of pain is sharper, more localized than visceral pain, and worsens with movement. An infection that has caused peritonitis, such as severe diverticulitis, will typically cause parietal pain. Some conditions characteristically progress from visceral to parietal pain. For example, appendicitis typically begins with epigastric visceral pain and progresses to right lower quadrant parietal pain.

TABLE 19.2 Red Flags for an Acute Abdomen (24,26,27)

Pain <48 hours
Pain followed by vomiting
Patient age ≥65 years
History of abdominal surgery
Abdominal guarding
Rebound tenderness

Many conditions commonly present with pain in a specific location (see Table 19.3, Figures 19.1 and 19.2). Urinary stones often begin with flank pain. Gallbladder disease usually causes right upper quadrant (RUQ) pain. Pain can also radiate or be referred from within the abdomen to outside the abdomen, such as in pancreatitis where pain radiates from the epigastrium to the middle of the back.

The timing of onset and progression of abdominal pain is also helpful information. Gradual onset of pain over a few hours to a few days is more likely to represent an inflammatory process or intestinal obstruction. The abrupt worsening of such pain may signal perforation of the inflamed or obstructed organ. Colicky pain that comes and goes may result from gastroenteritis, a partial bowel obstruction, obstructing urinary stone, or irritable bowel syndrome. Aspects of the history that are especially important in patients with abdominal pain are listed in Table 19.4.

TABLE 19.3 Causes of Abdominal Pain Based on Location and Quality

Intra-abdominal cause
Visceral pain
Epigastric: upper abdominal organs
Periumbilical: small intestine, cecum, appendix
Hypogastric: colon, rectum, pelvis
Parietal pain
Diffuse: generalized peritonitis from perforation or rupture of an organ
Right upper quadrant (RUQ): gallbladder
Right lower quadrant (RLQ): appendix
Left lower quadrant (LLQ): sigmoid colon
Visceral progressing to parietal pain
Periumbilical to RLQ: appendicitis
Hypogastric to LLQ: diverticulitis
Epigastric to RUQ: cholecystitis
Pain radiating to or referred to an extraabdominal location
Epigastric pain radiating to mid back: pancreatitis
RUQ pain radiating to right subscapular area: cholecystitis
Shoulder pain: ipsilateral subphrenic abscess
Extra-abdominal cause
Epigastric pain: myocardial infarction
Upper quadrant pain: ipsilateral pneumonia
Any location or diffuse abdominal pain: spinal nerve root irritation, stress, psychological illness, history of abuse
Abdominal wall pain: muscle strain, rectus sheath hematoma
Diffuse abdominal pain: sickle cell disease, diabetic ketoacidosis, uremia porphyria, lead poisoning, black widow spider bites

PHYSICAL EXAMINATION

Initially you should direct your physical examination toward the patient's general appearance and vital signs. Does the patient appear severely ill? Is the patient in distress because the pain? Is the patient's blood pressure low or is the pulse very fast? If the patient is in great distress or in shock, urgent action is required to restore normal vital signs or relieve pain. After you have addressed abnormal vital signs or severe pain, you should progress to examination of the abdomen, including inspection, auscultation, and palpation. Next, examine at least the flanks (checking for kidney tenderness) and any other areas of the body as indicated in Table 19.5. Pneumonia can cause abdominal pain so examination of the lungs is important. In men with pain below the umbilicus, perform a genital exam checking for an inguinal hernia or testicular pathology and a rectal examination, where one can sometimes detect appendicitis. Women with pain below the umbilicus should receive a pelvic and rectal examination, checking for uterine or ovarian pathology and cervical motion tenderness, a sign of pelvic inflammatory disease.

Based on findings from the history and examination, you can usually come up with a presumptive diagnosis, or perhaps several (Tables 19.3 and 19.6). For some diagnoses, such as gastroenteritis or irritable bowel syndrome, no further testing is required and you may begin empiric treatment (see Figure 19.2). For others, such as urinary tract infection or pelvic inflammatory disease, you may collect a test (urinalysis and culture or cervical DNA probe) and begin treatment while awaiting results (see Figure 19.1). Table 19.7 will help you determine whether historical or examination information is adequate to rule in or rule out a diagnosis, or whether additional testing is necessary. For example, a patient's self-diagnosis of urinary tract infection makes it 85.7% likely that the patient has a urinary tract infection. Because the treatment is relatively benign, you may initiate treatment without any further testing. On the other hand, presence of right lower quadrant pain makes it 73.7% likely that a patient has appendicitis, but the treatment (surgery) is invasive and risky, so further information would be helpful before making a treatment plan.

Diagnostic Testing

Because of the large number of conditions that can lead to abdominal pain, no diagnostic test is useful for all patients. You should base your diagnostic strategy on an assessment of the most likely diagnoses and the serious conditions that must be excluded (e.g., a pregnancy test should be performed in women of childbearing age to help exclude ectopic pregnancy; see Figure 19.1).

Exercise extra care in the elderly and for patients who are immunocompromised; for these patients, you should have a lower threshold for diagnostic testing or consultation. Use the algorithms in Figures 19.1 and 19.2 to choose a diagnostic strategy based on the presumptive diagnosis. The most helpful diagnostic tests for various diagnoses, as well as their accuracy, are listed in Table 19.8. Consider a patient with diffuse abdominal pain relieved somewhat by vomiting, a history of

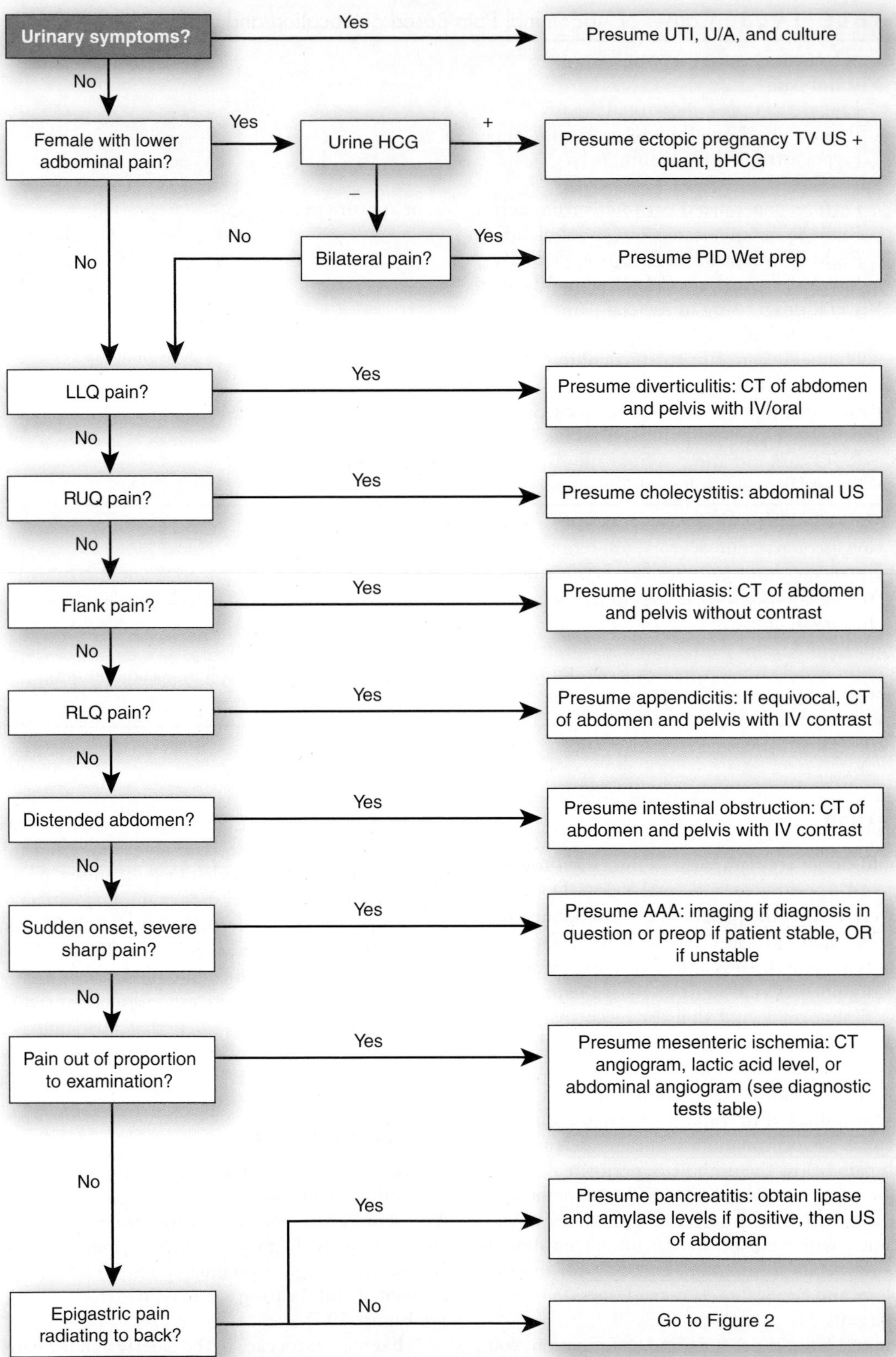

Figure 19.1 • Suggested approach to the initial evaluation of the adult with acute abdominal pain. Proceed to the next step if the diagnosis is not confirmed by suggested testing.

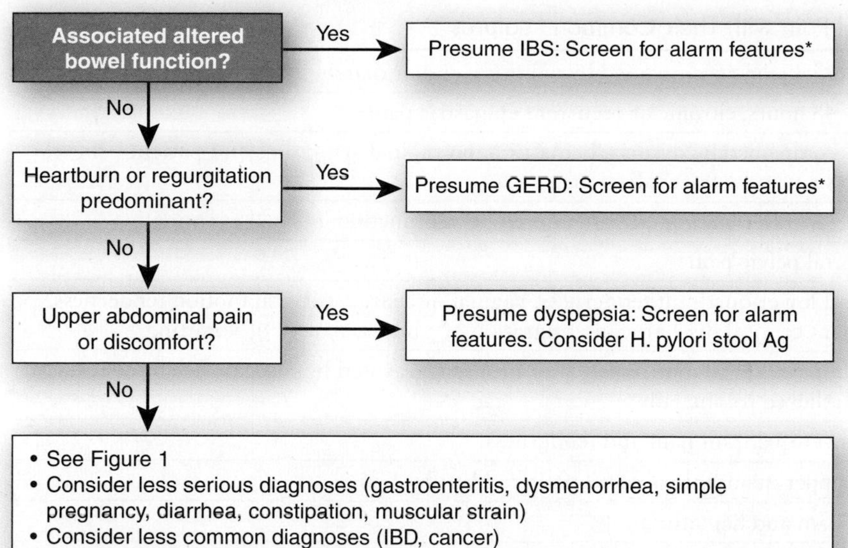

*Alarm Features: bleeding (melena, hematochezia, hematemesis) early satiety, progressive dysphagia, odynophagia, persistent vomiting, chronic severe diarrhea, recurring fever, previous GI malignancy, previous documented peptic ulcer, family history of GI cancer, unexplained weight loss >10% body weight or >10 lbs, lymphadenopathy, abdominal mass, anemia.

Abbreviations: IBS, Irritable bowel syndrome; GERD, gastroesophageal reflux disease, H. Pylori Stool Ag., Helicobacter pylori stool antigen; IBD, Irritable bowel disease; GI, gastrointestinal

Figure 19.2 • Suggested approach to the evaluation of the adult with chronic abdominal pain. Proceed to the next step if the diagnosis is not confirmed by suggested testing.

abdominal surgery, and constipation. If on examination the patient has abdominal distention, this patient is likely to have intestinal obstruction. Based on Figure 19.1 you should order a computed tomography (CT) scan of the abdomen and pelvis with intravenous contrast to confirm your diagnosis.

Recommended Diagnostic Strategy

The diagnostic strategy for abdominal pain depends on the presumptive diagnosis. The following presumptive diagnoses are discussed in detail in other chapters: dyspepsia and gastroesophageal reflux disease, Chapter 21; gastroenteritis and irritable bowel syndrome, Chapter 22; urinary tract infection, Chapters 27 and 30; pelvic inflammatory disease, Chapter 32; and ectopic pregnancy, Chapter 4. Other presumptive diagnoses are discussed in the following sections.

DIVERTICULITIS

Diverticulitis occurs when a diverticula in the colon becomes acutely inflamed. Typically, diverticulitis presents with gradual onset of continuous left lower quadrant pain (most inflamed diverticula are in the sigmoid colon). Patients may also develop fever, altered bowel habits, and vomiting. Urinary symptoms may be caused by inflamed bowel against

TABLE 19.4 Important Aspects of the History for Abdominal Pain

Duration of pain
Location of pain
Quality of pain
Severity of pain
Associated symptoms (nausea, vomiting, fever, diarrhea, etc.)
Precipitating or alleviating factors (e.g., food improving symptoms)
Underlying medical conditions (diabetes mellitus, cardiovascular disease, etc.)
Psychosocial factors (substance abuse, stress, travel, diet, etc.)
Menstrual and sexual history (to rule out pregnancy and sexually transmitted infection)

TABLE 19.5 Key Aspects of Physical Examination in Patients with Abdominal Pain

Abdomen, include inspection, auscultation, palpation, consider percussion
Flanks
Lungs
Male genital and inguinal (men with pain below the umbilicus or radiating to the groin)
Rectum (pain below the umbilicus)
Female pelvis (pain below the umbilicus)

TABLE 19.6 Causes of Abdominal Pain with Their Common Features

Gastroenteritis	Abdominal pain accompanied by vomiting and/or diarrhea
Dyspepsia (gastritis or ulcer)	Pain >48 hours, chronic or recurrent epigastric pain
Urinary tract infection (not including pyelonephritis)	Pain accompanied by dysuria, hematuria, no vaginal symptoms and patient believes she has a urinary tract infection
Irritable bowel syndrome	Pain >48 hours, associated with altered bowel function, normal examination
Ovarian cyst	Unilateral pelvic pain
Pelvic inflammatory disease	Bilateral lower quadrant tenderness, vaginal discharge, cervical motion tenderness, purulent cervical discharge, no migration of pain, no nausea or vomiting
Gastroesophageal reflux disease	Heartburn, regurgitation, often after meals, aggravated by recumbence or bending over, relieved by antacids
Diverticulitis	Left lower quadrant pain and tenderness
Cholecystitis	Right upper quadrant pain and positive Murphy sign
Urolithiasis	Flank pain and hematuria
Appendicitis	Right lower quadrant pain, migration from periumbilical to right lower quadrant area, fever, pain before vomiting, psoas sign
Intestinal obstruction	Constipation, vomiting relieves pain, history of abdominal surgery, abnormal bowel sounds, abdominal distention and rigidity
Dissecting abdominal aortic aneurysm	Sudden onset of severe, sharp pain, male gender, history of hypertension, new murmur, associated syncope, pulsatile abdominal mass, asymmetric pulses
Ectopic pregnancy	Women of childbearing age, lower quadrant pain, vaginal bleeding
Mesenteric ischemia	Pain out of proportion to examination, history of vascular or thrombotic disease
Pancreatitis	Epigastric pain radiating to back, vomiting, fever, history of alcoholism or gallbladder disease

the bladder. No symptoms or signs are particularly useful for distinguishing diverticulitis from other causes of abdominal pain. You may treat patients with mild symptoms empirically with broad spectrum antibiotics, clear liquid diet, and close follow up (2). Patients with more severe symptoms should have a CT scan (see Table 19.8); if it confirms diverticulitis, treat the patient with intravenous fluids, clear liquid diet, and intravenous broad spectrum antibiotics. Patients who do not improve or have signs of peritonitis require surgical consultation and possibly a sigmoid colectomy.

GALL BLADDER DISEASE

Causes of abdominal pain related to the gallbladder include biliary colic and acute cholecystitis (more common), as well as choledocholithiasis (common bile duct stones), cholangitis, pancreatitis, gallstone ileus, and gallbladder cancer (all less common). Biliary colic is caused by intermittent obstruction of the cystic or common bile duct by a gallstone. Patients typically have recurrent episodes of steady, severe pain in the epigastric region or RUQ that last for more than 15 minutes. Meals may precipitate pain, and the pain may radiate to the back or right scapula and be accompanied by nausea and vomiting. Cholecystitis is inflammation of the gallbladder caused by persistent obstruction of the bile duct, sometimes with bacterial infection. Patients with cholecystitis have persistent biliary pain as described above and may have fever and chills.

The best historical clues to acute cholecystitis include history of gallstones, characteristic unremitting RUQ pain lasting 3–5 hours, and associated fever and nausea (3). The best physical examination test for acute cholecystitis is Murphy sign, performed by palpating in the RUQ while the patient takes a deep breath (Table 19.7) (3, 4). The sign is positive if the patient suddenly stops the deep breath because of pain. However, it is not reliable in older patients.

Physical examination is not particularly helpful for biliary colic. If you suspect cholecystitis or biliary colic the best confirmatory test is an ultrasound of the abdomen. If findings from ultrasound are equivocal, and gallbladder disease is still strongly suspected, the next test to order would be a technetium 99 labeled dimethyl iminodiacetic acid scan (hepatobiliary scintigraphy, see Table 19.8). For this test, technetium 99 labeled dimethyl iminodiacetic acid is injected into the bloodstream, taken up by the liver and excreted in the bile, allowing visualization of the structure and function of the gallbladder and biliary tract. The best treatment for acute cholecystitis is early (within 72 hours) cholecystectomy, either laparoscopic or open (5).

UROLITHIASIS

Urinary stones form when the urine becomes supersaturated with soluble materials, most commonly calcium oxalate or calcium phosphate, although other materials such as uric acid or hydroxyapatite may also form stones. The stones form in the kidney and may cause severe pain when they block the flow of urine in the ureter. Pain from a urinary stone is typically colicky and radiates from the flank to the groin.

TABLE 19.7 Most Helpful Symptoms and Signs for Adults with Abdominal Pain

***Diagnosis*:** **Symptom or Sign**	**Pretest Probability**	**Probability of Diagnosis When Symptom or Sign is Present**	**Probability of Diagnosis When Symptom or Sign is Absent**
Urinary tract infection in women (28)			
Self-diagnosis (LR+4, LR− 0.1)	60%	85.7%	13%
Cholecystitis (4)			
Right upper quadrant (RUQ) pain (LR+2.5, LR−0.28)	10%	21.7%	3%
Murphy sign (LR+5.0, LR−0.4)		35.7%	4.3%
Appendicitis (29)			
Right lower quadrant (RLQ) pain (LR+8.4, LR−0.18)	25%	73.7%	5.7%
Pain before vomiting (LR+2.7, LR−0.02)		47.4%	0.7%
Intestinal obstruction (16)			
History of constipation (LR+8.80, LR−0.6)	8%	43.3%	5.0%
Visible peristalsis (LR+6.00, LR−0.9)		34.3%	7.3%
Distended abdomen (LR+5.70, LR− 0.4)		33.1%	3.4%
Ectopic pregnancy (30)			
History of tubal ligation (LR+16.7, LR−0.92)	15%	74.7%	14%
Uterine size <= 8 weeks (LR+17.5, LR−0.65)		75.5%	10.3%
Positive peritoneal signs (LR+6.2, LR−0.82)		52.2%	12.6%

LR+ = positive likelihood ratio, tests with higher values, especially >5, are good at ruling in disease; LR− = negative likelihood ratio, tests with lower values, especially <0.2, are good at ruling out disease; PP = pretest probability.

The most useful symptoms for diagnosing urolithiasis are acute onset (≤12 hours) and normal appetite (6). The most useful signs are groin or flank tenderness (6). Urinalysis may reveal red blood cells but a normal urinalysis does not exclude a urinary stone (7). The best test to rule in or rule out urolithiasis is a CT scan of the urinary tract without contrast (see Table 19.8) (8).

Urinary stones smaller than 5 mm will typically pass with conservative management, including alpha blockers, calcium channel blockers, or corticosteroids (9). Extracorporeal shock wave lithotripsy or ureteroscopy are both good treatments for patients with urinary stones greater than 10 mm or for stones that do not pass after 2–4 weeks of conservative management (10).

APPENDICITIS

Acute appendicitis is the most common condition leading to surgery for patients with abdominal pain. Distention of the appendix initially leads to poorly localized epigastric or periumbilical visceral pain, which may be accompanied by anorexia, nausea, or vomiting. With peritoneal involvement, the pain becomes localized to the right lower quadrant, often at McBurney point (5 cm from the anterior superior iliac spine on a line running to the umbilicus). Rupture of the appendix may lead to a temporary decrease in pain, followed by much more intense pain as well as higher fever and abdominal rigidity.

The most helpful symptoms for diagnosing appendicitis are right lower quadrant pain, and pain before vomiting (see Table 19.7). Vomiting before pain makes appendicitis very unlikely. The Alvarado score (11–13) combines several signs and symptoms (Table 19.9) and may be useful, particularly when the likelihood of appendicitis is in the intermediate range. You can use the mnemonic MANTRELL to remember the scoring categories. If you suspect appendicitis, obtain a complete blood count and use the Alvarado score to determine whether the patient is at low, intermediate, or high risk of appendicitis. Patients at low risk can be observed closely. Patients at intermediate risk should receive further diagnostic testing. A CT scan of the abdomen and pelvis with IV contrast is the most helpful test (see Table 19.8) although ultrasound is also useful (14). If a patient is at high risk or has appendicitis confirmed by diagnostic imaging, you should keep the patient from eating and drinking, start intravenous fluids, initiate antibiotics, provide adequate pain relief, and arrange surgical consultation.

INTESTINAL OBSTRUCTION

Adhesions from prior surgery may be responsible for 70% of cases of intestinal obstruction (15). Other causes of intestinal obstruction include tumors, gallstones, congenital bowel abnormalities, ingested materials, and incarcerated hernias. Pain from bowel obstruction is usually intermittent and generalized. It may be relieved by vomiting and worsened by eating. Strangulation (vascular compromise) becomes more likely with the passage of time and requires immediate surgery.

The most useful symptoms and signs for diagnosing bowel obstruction include history of constipation, visible peristalsis

TABLE 19.8 Most Helpful Diagnostic Tests for Adult Patients with Abdominal Pain

Diagnosis: Diagnostic Test	Pretest Probability	Probability of Diagnosis When Test is Positive	Probability of Diagnosis When Test is Negative
Diverticulitis (31)			
CT scan (LR+99, LR−0.01)	40%	98.5%	0.7%
Cholecystitis (32)			
Hepatobiliary scintigraphy (LR+4.2, LR−0.04)	30%	64.3%	1.7%
Ultrasound (LR+2.6, LR−0.52)		52.7%	18.2%
Urolithiasis (8)			
CT scan without contrast (LR+23, LR−0.05)	50%	95.8%	4.8%
Appendicitis in adults & adolescents (14)			
CT scan (LR+18.8, LR−0.06)	40%	92.6%	3.8%
Ultrasound (LR+4.5, LR−0.17)		75%	10.2%
Appendicitis in children (12, 13, 33)			
Alvarado score ≥7 (LR+4.0, LR−0.2)	20%	50%	5%
CT scan (LR+13.9, LR−0.03)	40%	90.3%	2%
Ultrasound (LR+17.2, LR−0.15)	40%	92%	9.1%
Intestinal obstruction (17)	8%		
CT scan (LR+93, LR−0.1)		89%	0.9%
Abdominal aortic aneurysm (AAA)			
Bedside ultrasound for AAA (34) (LR+97, LR−0.03)	50%	99%	2.9%
CT scan to detect rupture of AAA (35) (LR+3.4, LR−0.27)	40%	69.4%	15.3%
Pancreatitis (18)			
Serum amylase >360 U/L (LR+21, LR−0.05)	40%	93.3%	3.2%
Serum lipase >270 U/L (LR+14, LR−0.02)		90.3%	1.3%

LR+ = positive likelihood ratio, tests with higher values, especially >5, are good at ruling in disease; LR− = negative likelihood ratio, tests with lower values, especially <0.2, are good at ruling out disease; CT = computed tomography; PP = pretest probability.

TABLE 19.9 The Alvarado Score for Diagnosing Acute Appendicitis

Symptom, Sign, or Test	Points
Migratory pain	1
Anorexia	1
Nausea or vomiting	1
Tenderness of right lower quadrant	2
Rebound tenderness	1
Elevated temperature	1
Leukocytosis	2
Left shift	1
Total:	

Interpretation: Less than 4 points: low risk for appendicitis; 4–6 points: moderate risk of appendicitis; 7 or more points: high risk of appendicitis (11–13).

(seldom seen), and abdominal distention (see Table 19.7) (16). The most useful initial test for diagnosing bowel obstruction is a CT scan of the abdomen (see Table 19.8) (17).

Initial treatment for suspected bowel obstruction includes intravenous fluids, analgesics, and surgical consultation. Partial bowel obstruction may resolve with supportive treatment. The definitive treatment for complete bowel obstruction is surgery.

PANCREATITIS

Acute inflammation of the pancreas is most commonly caused by excessive alcohol use or gallstones. Other less common causes include hypertriglyceridemia, trauma, drugs, infections, and idiopathic. Patients with pancreatitis typically have epigastric pain radiating to the back, vomiting, fever, and may have a history of alcoholism or gallbladder disease. If you suspect pancreatitis you should initially order serum lipase and amylase. Amylase lower than 360 U/L effectively rules out acute pancreatitis; higher than 360 U/L rules it in. Lipase lower than 270 U/L rules out pancreatitis, and higher than

270 U/L rules it in (see Table 19.8) (18). You should order an ultrasound of the abdomen in all patients with pancreatitis to detect gallstones. Order a CT scan of the abdomen if the diagnosis is still unclear or if the patient's disease is severe according to Ranson's criteria (age >55, White Blood Cell >16,000, glucose >200 mg/dL, lactate dehydrogenase >350 IU/L, aspartate transaminase/serum glutamic-oxaloacetic transaminase >250 IU/L) (19,20). If three or more of Ranson's criteria are present the patient is likely to have severe pancreatitis. CT scan can detect pancreatic pseudocyst, necrosis, or abscess, as well as gallstone pancreatitis.

Treatment for pancreatitis is primarily supportive with enteral nutrition and pain control. Gallstone pancreatitis is best treated with endoscopic retrograde pancreatic cholecystogram and endoscopic sphincterotomy (21).

Abdominal Pain in Children

The differential diagnosis for abdominal pain in children is somewhat different than for adults. The most common causes are benign illnesses such as gastroenteritis, constipation, mesenteric lymphadenitis, and functional abdominal pain. Children may also have more serious illnesses that are unique to children such as Hirschsprung disease, intussusception, or pyloric stenosis. As they age, especially older than age 12 years, children are likely to have some of the same diagnoses as adults, such as appendicitis, which causes between 10% and 25% of cases of abdominal pain in children presenting to the emergency department (12). Extraabdominal causes of abdominal pain are especially prevalent in children, strep pharyngitis and right lower lobe pneumonia being most notorious. Keep in mind that for every 15 children with abdominal pain, 1 will have a serious condition (22).

Extraabdominal causes of abdominal pain in children can be rules out fairly easily. A chest x-ray will help exclude pneumonia and a rapid strep test will help exclude strep pharyngitis. For most school aged children, appendicitis is the major dangerous pathology that must be ruled out. If you suspect appendicitis, order a complete blood count and use the Alvarado score to risk stratify the patient (Table 19.9). Then if the patient is high risk for appendicitis, arrange surgical consultation. If the patient is moderate risk, order a CT scan of the abdomen to clarify the diagnosis. Low-risk patients can be observed closely, often in the hospital, to see if symptoms progress or improve.

KEY POINTS

- Use clues from the history and physical examination to establish a presumptive diagnosis on which to base diagnostic testing (C).
- History and physical examination alone are often adequate to begin initial treatment for urinary tract infection, as well as gastroesophageal reflux disease, dyspepsia, irritable bowel syndrome, and pelvic inflammatory disease (C).
- Lipase and amylase are the most useful tests for diagnosing pancreatitis; order CT if the patient has severe disease (C).
- Laboratory examinations are not very helpful in diagnosing cholecystitis, appendicitis, or urolithiasis (C).
- Ultrasound is the most helpful initial test if you suspect cholecystitis or ectopic pregnancy (C).
- CT scan is the most helpful test for diagnosing appendicitis, intestinal obstruction, urolithiasis, diverticulitis, and abdominal aortic aneurysm (C).

CHAPTER

20

Chronic Liver Disease

Thad Wilkins, Anila Jamal, Iryna Hepburn and Robert R. Schade

CLINICAL OBJECTIVES

1. List common causes of chronic liver disease.
2. Describe an efficient approach to evaluation of patients with abnormal liver tests.
3. Discuss the treatment of alcoholic and viral hepatitis
4. Use the Model of End Stage Liver Disease (MELD) score and METAVIR scoring system to determine the severity of liver injury.
5. Discuss the diagnostic criteria of non-alcoholic fatty liver disease.
6. Differentiate the various complications of cirrhosis.

The liver has several important roles, including digestive, immunologic, metabolic, excretory, and synthetic functions. The liver manufactures and secretes bile acids, such as chenodeoxycholic acid, which is secreted into the duodenum where it assists fat absorption. Liver sinusoids are lined with Kupffer cells, which serve as a first immune barrier between the gut and systemic circulation. The liver is rich in cytochromes and enzyme systems that oxidize and reduce exogenous substances such as alcohol, caffeine, drugs, vitamins, hormones, and toxins. Some drugs (i.e., clopidogrel) must be metabolized to their active form before they are effective. The liver excretes bilirubin, the final breakdown product of heme, as well as cholesterol and other fat soluble compounds. It synthesizes proteins such as albumin and clotting factors, and the urea cycle and gluconeogenesis take place in the liver as well.

Chronic liver disease is defined as the gradual destruction of normal liver tissue over time. This term encompasses many different etiologies including fibrosis and cirrhosis. In 2006, chronic liver disease and cirrhosis was the 12th leading cause of deaths in the United States, accounting for 27,555 deaths (9.2 per 100,000) (1). Common and preventable causes of chronic liver disease include excessive alcohol intake and chronic hepatitis B and C. This chapter will review the evaluation of patients with abnormal liver tests and includes a discussion of the most common causes of chronic liver disease.

EVALUATION OF ABNORMAL LIVER TESTS

Tests of Liver Function and Prognosis

Liver impairment may manifest as prolongation of prothrombin time (PT), hyperammonemia, hyperbilirubinemia, and hypoalbuminemia. PT or international normalized ratio (INR) is one of the most sensitive tests of liver synthetic function, because the liver is the site of synthesis of many blood clotting factors (factors II, V, VII, IX, X) and the PT reflects availability of the shortest lived compound of the coagulation cascade, factor VII. PT prolongation in the patient with known liver disease or with newly discovered liver tests abnormalities and no history of anticoagulants is a sign of impaired liver synthetic function and possible liver failure. Such patients should be evaluated promptly and monitored closely. The Model of End Stage Liver Disease (MELD) score is based on international normalized ratio (INR), creatinine, and total bilirubin, and is used to predict 90-day survival in individuals with liver impairment and to guide referral to specialized liver centers (2) (*http://www.unos.org/resources/meldpeldcalculator.asp*). Special quantitative liver function tests such as aminopyrine elimination tests are also available.

Tests of Liver Injury

Liver injury tests include serum aspartate aminotransferase (AST), alanine aminotransferase (ALT), alkaline phosphatase (AP), and gamma glutamyl transferase (GGT). Based on the pattern, liver abnormalities are often classified as either cholestatic or as hepatocellular injury.

CHOLESTATIC INJURY

Cholestasis refers to an arrest in the flow of bile. It can be categorized as intra- or extrahepatic in nature, and results in elevation of serum total bilirubin and bile acids (Figure 20.1). Cholestasis can occur at any level of the biliary system from biliary canaliculi to the common bile duct, and can be caused by mechanical obstruction (stones, tumors, infiltrative process) or by chemical substances (medications, hormones, herbal remedies). In cholestatic disease, elevation of AP and total bilirubin occurs with conjugated (direct) hyperbilirubinemia comprising greater than 50% of the total. Although AP also can come from bone and other sources, a concurrent increase in other cholestatic enzymes such as gamma glutamyl transpeptidase (GTP) and 5′-nucleotidase supports the diagnosis of a hepatic source of the increase. Similarly GTP, a microsomal enzyme, can be increased in response to drug metabolism because agents such as alcohol or phenytoin and can also increase in response to kidney injury.

Patients with cholestasis may have icterus, complain of colicky abdominal pain (gall stones), or pruritus. Extrinsic compression of the bile duct by a tumor may present with painless jaundice (Figure 20.2). AP and GTP may also

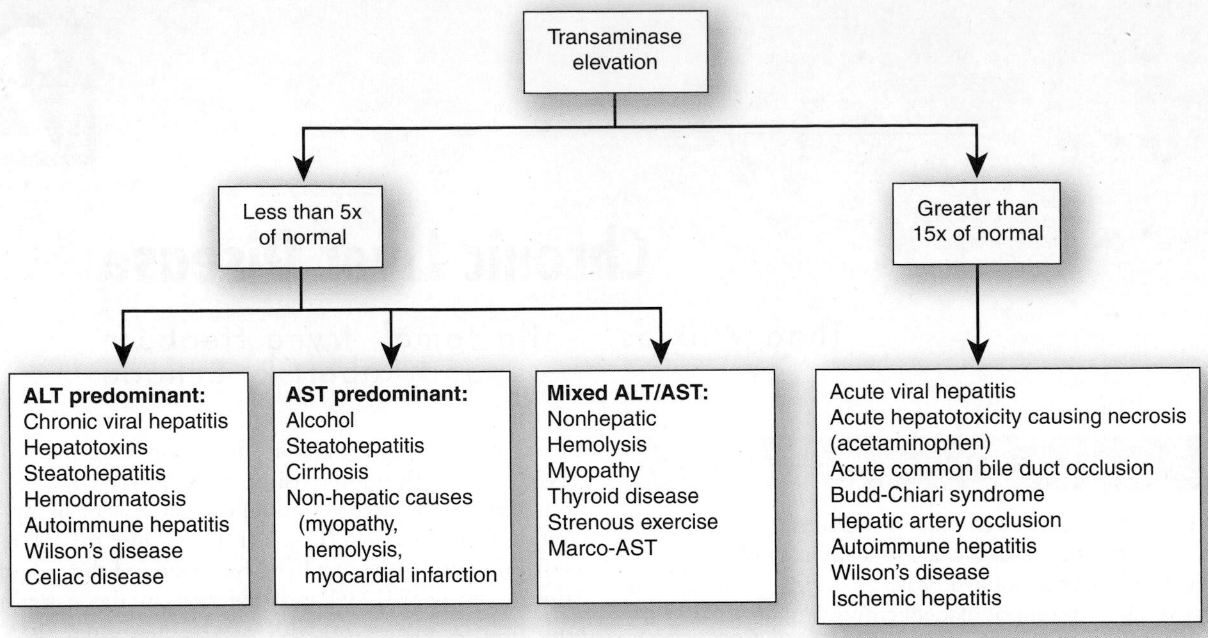

Figure 20.1 • Causes of elevated hepatic transaminases.

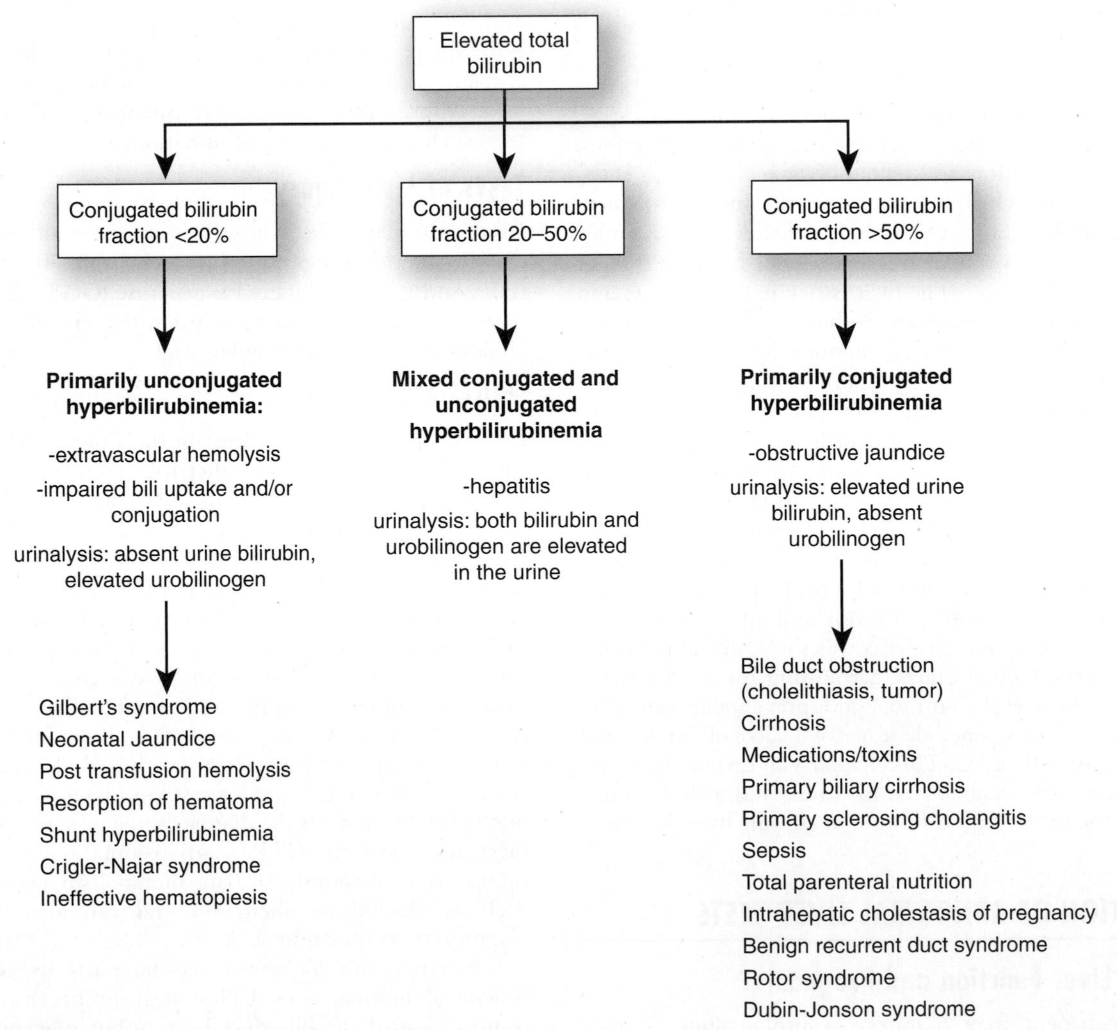

Figure 20.2 • Algorithm to evaluate elevated bilirubin.

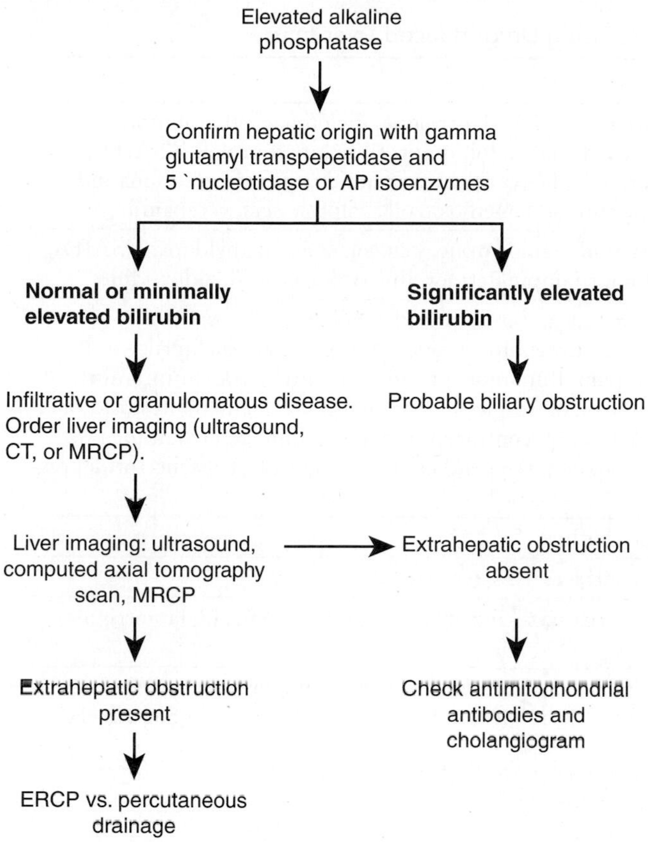

Figure 20.3 • Algorithm to evaluate elevated alkaline phosphatase.

increase in patients with space occupying or infiltrating liver lesions such as primary or metastatic tumors of the liver, amyloidosis, sarcoidosis, tuberculosis, or a liver abscess.

AP and GTP are characteristically increased in such cholestatic disorders as primary biliary cirrhosis (PBC) and primary sclerosing cholangitis (PSC). Indeed, an isolated elevation of the AP is often the first sign of these diseases. PBC occurs predominantly in women and is associated with antimitochondrial antibodies. PSC is found predominantly in men with inflammatory bowel diseases and may lead to development of cholangiocarcinoma.

Bilirubin, the break down product of heme from senescent red blood cells, is transported to the liver attached to albumin, where it is conjugated in hepatocytes and excreted. Serum bilirubin determination can measure total and direct bilirubin concentrations. Indirect bilirubin is calculated by subtracting the direct form from the total bilirubin, and in general reflects the unconjugated bilirubin level. Hyperbilirubinemia secondary to a hemolytic process results in elevation of unconjugated or indirect bilirubin. Another disorder of unconjugated bilirubin, Gilbert's syndrome, is a benign hereditary condition that occurs in approximately 5% of the population and causes a mild increase (<4 mg/dL) of unconjugated (indirect) bilirubin because impaired bilirubin conjugation. See Figure 20.3 for an algorithmic approach to hyperbilirubinemia.

HEPATOCELLULAR INJURY

ALT and AST are intracellular enzymes that are released from injured hepatocytes in response to cell damage. Overlap of cholestatic and hepatocellular injury pattern is common, and the patient's history and predominant abnormality should guide the investigation. Increases in AST can also occur as a result of muscle injury and in such cases measurement of creatine phosphokinase (CPK) can help determine its origin. Patients with acute hepatocellular injury are generally ill, have nausea, vague abdominal discomfort, and may have jaundice.

Since abnormal levels of liver tests are detected in 1–4% of an asymptomatic population, family physicians need a balanced approach for evaluation of such patients (3). Various factors may influence normal liver homeostasis and cause alteration in liver test patterns. These factors include age; gender; symptoms; medical, surgical, and family history; medications and supplements used history of substance abuse; and risk factors for liver disease. Additionally, the "normal value" may not be a reflective of normal values for a given patient: normal liver test values may vary with age, blood type, postprandial state, pregnancy, and gender (4). Also, normal liver tests do not exclude the presence of liver disease entirely. The significance of any test should be interpreted in the context of the clinical situation. If abnormal levels of liver tests are seen in an asymptomatic patient with low pretest probability of liver disease, the patient may be observed and laboratory workup should be repeated. Patients with signs and symptoms of chronic liver disease or clinically unstable patients with suspected liver disease require more prompt evaluation and possible referral to a specialized institution.

Many medications and their metabolites have been implicated in drug induced liver injury (DILI) (Table 20.1). Among those frequently implicated are nonsteroidal anti-inflammatory drugs, statins, antiretroviral agents, vitamin A, estrogens, and isoniazid. In addition to drug dose and total time of exposure to the drug, the patient's age, nutritional status, diet (toxigenic mushrooms), estrogen use, pregnancy, presence of chronic liver disease and genetic predisposition (cytochrome system variability) determine the probability of DILI in individual cases (5). DILI can present as hepatocellular injury, cholestasis, or a mixed pattern of liver test abnormalities. Elevation of bilirubin, PT, and ammonia are worrisome signs and correlate with increased mortality (5). Occasionally discontinuation of the hepatotoxic substance does not lead to complete resolution of liver test abnormalities and chronic liver disease develops (5–6% of patients) (5); therefore, a detailed past history of medications administered is important in ruling out iatrogenic causes of liver injury. History of alcohol use, injection drug use, and family history of liver disease should be obtained in every patient presenting with unexplained liver test abnormalities. Infectious etiologies should be excluded by appropriate testing (Table 20.2).

Hemochromatosis, a common genetic disorder of iron absorption that leads to iron overload, may initially present with isolated transaminase elevation and, if left untreated, may lead to end-stage liver disease. Presence of arthritis, erectile dysfunction, and heart failure in the patient with abnormal liver tests should prompt evaluation for hemochromatosis. The best initial test for detection of iron overload is elevated transferrin saturation. Demonstration of increased iron stores

TABLE 20.1 Common Medications and Supplements Causing Drug-induced Liver Injury

Type of the Liver Injury	Name of the Medication
Hepatic inflammation	Acetaminophen, allopurinol, carbamazepine, dantrolene, diclofenac, ethambutol, ethionamide, isoniazid, ketoconazole, labetalol, maprotiline, metoprolol, NSAIDs, penicillins, phenelzine, phenobarbital, phenytoin, pyrazinamide, quinidine, sulfonamides, tricyclic antidepressants, trimethoprim-sulfamethoxazole, valproic acid, verapamil.
Fatty liver	Acetaminophen, adrenocortical steroids, amiodarone, ketoconazole, methyldopa, NSAIDs, nifedipine, perhexiline, phenytoin, rifampin, tetracycline, valproic acid, zidovudine
Cholestasis	Amoxicillin/clavulanate, azathioprine, captopril, carbamazepine, cephalosporins, chlordiazepoxide, chlorpropamide, cloxacillin, cyclosporine, danazol, enalapril, erythromycin, flecainide, flurazepam, flutamide, griseofulvin, glyburide, imipramine, haloperidol, ketoconazole, megestrol, mercaptopurine, methimazole, methyltestosterone, nifedipine, nitrofurantoin, NSAIDs, oral contraceptives, phenytoin, penicillamine, propoxyphene, sulfonamides, tamoxifen, thiabendazole, tolbutamide, tricyclic antidepressants, verapamil.
Liver fibrosis or cirrhosis	Methotrexate, nitrofurantoin, terbinafine
Liver tumors	Anabolic steroids, danazol, oral contraceptives, testosterone
Fulminant hepatic failure	*Amanita phalloides* (mushroom), Carbamazepine, clarithromycin, isoniazid, lamotrigine, levetiracetam
Hepatotoxic herbs or supplements	Germander (Teucrium chamaedrys), chaparral (Larrea tridentata), kava kava, Ma huang; Heliotropium, Senecio, Crotalaria species, Valeriana officinalis and Scutellaria lateriflora mix, vitamin A.

NSAIDs = nonsteroidal anti-inflammatory drugs.
Source: (5).

and the presence of the characteristic genetic mutation (HFE) confirms this diagnosis (6). Lifetime reduction of body iron stores by removal of blood prevents disease progression.

Chronic autoimmune hepatitis (AIH) can cause elevation of liver enzymes. It is more common in women and is frequently associated with thyroid disease. Antinuclear antibodies, anti-smooth muscle antibodies, and liver-kidney microsomal antibodies should be measured when AIH is suspected. Liver biopsy helps confirm the diagnosis. The disease is managed with immunosuppressants such as prednisone and azathioprine.

Wilson disease (WD) is a rare genetic condition that impairs copper excretion and affects the liver and the central nervous system. Patients with WD usually present at a younger age or in childhood and may have psychiatric and neurologic abnormalities. Serum ceruloplasmin is decreased and serum and urine copper is increased in these patients. Slit-lamp examination of the eyes may demonstrate Kayser-Fleischer rings and liver biopsy can confirm elevated copper stores. Treatment is aimed at elimination of copper through enhanced urinary excretion by administration of d-penicillamine and by reduction of copper absorption.

Other less common causes of chronic liver injury include celiac disease and alpha-1-antitrypsin (A1TP) deficiency. Celiac disease occurs in patients with gluten hypersensitivity and presents with chronic diarrhea and failure to thrive, it may cause elevation of transaminases as well. Serum tissue transglutaminase antibodies and duodenal biopsy are diagnostic. Similarly, diagnosis of alpha-1-antitrypsin deficiency can be determined through measurement of A1TP serum levels and protease inhibitor (PI) phenotype. See Table 20.3 for a description of relatively uncommon causes of chronic liver disease. Most asymptomatic patients presenting with elevated transaminases and negative viral hepatitis serologies and normal iron studies will ultimately be diagnosed with either alcoholic injury or nonalcoholic steatohepatitis (NASH).

ALCOHOLIC HEPATITIS

Alcoholic hepatitis (AH) is a serious injury to the liver because alcohol ingestion that may occur in people who drink 60–100 g of alcohol daily for a prolonged period of time, or after an alcoholic binge in a chronic drinker (7–9). The type of alcoholic beverage is not important: a 12oz bottle of beer, a shot (1.5 ounces) of whiskey or vodka, and a 6 oz glass of wine all contain approximately 15 grams of alcohol. AH is associated with high morbidity and mortality: 30-day mortality is 20% in patients with mild to moderate AH and approaches 40% in patient with severe disease (7, 8). Women are at higher risk for development of AH and a lesser amount of alcohol is often required to cause severe hepatic inflammation. Additionally, AH may develop in the presence or absence of underlying cirrhosis.

Diagnosis

Patients with AH typically present with symptoms of weakness, anorexia, abdominal pain, mild fever, jaundice, nausea, and vomiting. In severe cases, signs of portal hypertension and its complications may be present, including ascites and bleeding. Patients may develop altered mental status because the presence of hepatic encephalopathy or because thiamine deficiency or

TABLE 20.2 Infections of the Liver

Viral
Hepatitis A, B, C, D, and E
Infectious mononucleosis
Cytomegalovirus
Bacterial
Tuberculosis
Atypical mycobacterial disease
Lepromatous leprosy
Brucellosis
Listeriosis
Bartonellosis
Secondary or tertiary syphilis
Tularemia
Rickettsial
Q fever
Fungal
Histoplasmosis
Coccidioidomycosis
Candidiasis
Cryptococcosis
Parasitic
Schistosomiasis
Visceral larva migrans
Fascioliasis
Toxoplasmosis

alcohol withdrawal. Clinical examination may reveal stigmata of chronic liver disease (spider angiomas, gynecomastia, proximal muscle loss, ascites, caput medusae), and tender hepatomegaly.

Patients with AH typically have a mild elevation of transaminases (less than five times the upper limit of normal), with a characteristic AST/ALT ratio >2, although this finding is neither specific nor sensitive. Elevated bilirubin and prolonged PT are indicative of severe hepatic disease and have prognostic value. The Maddrey discriminate function (DF) predicts prognosis and guides therapy: DF = 4.6 × (PT – control) + total bilirubin (mg/dL) (10). For example, a patient with PT 4 greater than control and total bilirubin of 8.0 has a DF = (4.6 × 4) + 8 = 26.4. A DF of 32 or higher indicates severe disease with a risk of death approaching 50% (10). Elevations of creatinine and blood urea nitrogen are ominous signs and may indicate the onset of hepatorenal syndrome and a very high probability of death. The MELD score may be used for determination of the severity of liver disease in AH: MELD ≥21 is associated with a 90-day mortality of 20% (11). Anemia and thrombocytopenia are frequently present from the effect of the alcohol on the bone marrow. Leukocytosis may occur as part of the hepatic inflammatory condition. Monitoring for signs of infection remains crucial since it is one of the major causes of death in patients with AH.

The differential diagnosis of AH includes acute viral hepatitis, fulminant Wilson disease, autoimmune hepatitis, ascending cholangitis, liver abscess, A1TP deficiency, decompensation of chronic liver disease from hepatocellular carcinoma, and ischemic hepatitis (7). Studies specific for each condition (see Table 20.2) and liver imaging (Doppler ultrasound, computed tomography [CT], or magnetic resonance imaging) are indicated, if the history of alcohol consumption is not clear. Ultrasound is usually the initial test because it is cost effective and there is no radiation exposure.

Treatment

Complete and permanent abstinence from alcohol is essential for treatment of AH. Depending on the severity of the disease, the patient may need to be admitted for supportive therapy with intravenous fluids and nutritional support which may include multivitamins, vitamin K, folate, and thiamine. Multiple medications have been studied in patients with AH, but only corticosteroids and pentoxifylline have demonstrated mortality benefit in patients with AH. Corticosteroids have been studied the most extensively and have demonstrated a 20% relative risk reduction and mortality in patients with AH and DF ≥32 (7). Initiation of prednisone 40 mg/day for 28 days is indicated in patients with DF ≥32 in the absence of contraindications (gastrointestinal bleeding, hepatorenal syndrome, sepsis, or chronic hepatitis B virus [HBV]) (12).

The Lille score (*www.lillemodel.com*) based on the laboratory response to treatment with steroids (serum bilirubin change on 7th day of corticosteroid therapy) has been used to determine whether steroids are effective in an individual patient (13). The Lille score >0.45 indicates no response to prednisone and allows its discontinuation. Pentoxifylline, a phosphodiesterase inhibitor with mild anti-tumor necrosis factor properties, has a demonstrated mortality benefit in AH and is associated with a decreased incidence of hepatorenal syndrome (14). Some authors suggest its superiority to steroids in treatment of AH (15), but more randomized trials are needed to confirm this. Currently pentoxifylline is indicated in patients who have not responded to or have contraindications to the use of corticosteroids (7).

NONALCOHOLIC FATTY LIVER DISEASE

Nonalcoholic fatty liver disease (NAFLD) may occur at any age and is characterized by large droplet fat deposition in hepatocytes. NAFLD is associated with the metabolic syndrome characterized by insulin resistance, central obesity, hypertension, and hyperlipidemia. It is the most common cause of elevated aminotransferases in adults in the United States and can rarely progress to cirrhosis (16–18). NAFLD refers to a spectrum of liver disorders ranging from steatosis to NASH; patients with the latter may progress to advanced fibrosis and cirrhosis. NASH is the most severe form of NAFLD and is histologically characterized by the presence of inflammation and fatty infiltration in individuals that do not consume alcohol (17). NAFLD does not include liver disorders caused by nutritional disorders, medications, toxins, and inborn errors of metabolism. Obesity and diabetes are risk

TABLE 20.3 Causes of Liver Tests Abnormalities with Common Clinical Findings and Treatments

Name of the Disease	Common Findings	Laboratory Evaluation	Treatment
Hereditary hemochromatosis	Family history, skin darkening, diabetes, arthritis, impotence, heart failure, conduction abnormalities	↑ALT and AST, serum transferrin, iron, ferritin, liver biopsy, genetic testing	Phlebotomy
Wilson disease	Family history, neuropsychiatric disease, cirrhosis	↑ALT and AST, occasionally ↑↑ALT and AST, serum ceruloplasmin, serum and urine cupper levels, slit-lamp eye examination, liver biopsy with quantitative copper measurement	Chelation
Alpha-1-antitripsine deficiency	Family history, lung disease	Alpha-1-antitripsine level, protease inhibitor phenotype analysis (Pi-type), liver biopsy	Supportive care, liver transplant
Autoimmune hepatitis	Female predominance, concomitant thyroid disease,	↑ALT and AST, occasionally ↑↑ALT and AST ANA, anti-smooth muscle Ab, anti-actin Ab, anti-liver- kidney microsomal Abs, IgG, liver biopsy	Steroids
Primary biliary cirrhosis	Female predominance, fatigue, pruritus, skin hyperpigmentation, jaundice, bone disease, xanthomas, arthropathy	↑AP, ↑bilirubin, anti-mitochondrial Ab, ANA, hyperlipidemia, IgM, bile acids, and hyaluronate	Ursodeoxycholic acid, liver transplant
Primary sclerosing cholangitis	Concomitant inflammatory bowel disease; often patient has no symptoms, but has liver tests abnormalities. Fatigue, fever, chills, night sweats, abdominal pain, pruritus	↑AP, ↑bilirubin, (fluctuating levels),↑IgM, ↑IgG, p-ANCA, cholangiogram demonstrating stricturing and dilatations of intra- and extrahepatic ducts, liver biopsy	Ursodeoxycholic acid, steroids, cyclosporine, methotrexate, azathioprine, tacrolimus, etanercept, endoscopic therapy for strictures, liver transplant
Acute Budd-Chiari syndrome	Ascites, jaundice	↑↑ALT&AST, hepatic vein thrombus present on imaging	Anticoagulation
Celiac disease	Failure to thrive, chronic diarrhea, anemia, nutritional deficiency	Antiendomysial Ab, antigliadin Ab	Gluten-free diet

ALT = alanine transaminase; AST = aspartate transaminase; ANA = antinuclear antibody; Ab = antibody; IgG = immunoglobulin G; AP = alkaline phosphatase; IgM = immunoglobulin M; p-ANCA = perinuclear antineutrophil cytoplasmic antibody.

factors for progressive fibrosis and diabetes is also a risk factor for death in patients with NAFLD (16).

Diagnosis

Most patients with NAFLD are asymptomatic; most initially present with an incidental laboratory abnormality or an abnormal imaging study. Approximately 50% will have hepatomegaly at the time of diagnosis (17,18). Although some patients may present with normal liver enzymes, most have an elevated ALT and AST, usually one to four times of upper limits of normal (18). Other lab abnormalities include an increase in alkaline phosphatase, increase in γ-glutamyltransferase, and less commonly hypoalbuminemia, prolonged prothrombin time, and hyperbilirubinemia (17,18). In the absence of other etiologies, liver imaging (initially ultrasound but could consider CT scan and magnetic resonance imaging) usually demonstrates increased fat deposition in the liver and liver biopsy is confirmatory.

Treatment

Treatment for NAFLD includes weight loss, exercise, and selective use of medications, as well as identifying and treating associated underlying metabolic conditions (i.e., diabetes, hyperlipidemia). Treatment may improve liver enzyme levels, steatosis, and histological findings, although good clinical trials are lacking. Among these, weight loss is the principal treatment in individuals that are obese. However, rapid weight loss especially after bariatric surgery can worsen NASH (16–18). Clinical trials have evaluated various medications and vitamins (ursodeoxycholic acid, vitamin E, vitamin C, and thiazolidinediones) but have found no evidence of effectiveness (16–19).

CHRONIC HEPATITIS B

In the United States, there are approximately 1.25 million hepatitis B carriers and hepatitis B virus (HBV) infection accounts for up to 5,500 deaths annually in the United States from cirrhosis, liver failure, and hepatocellular carcinoma (HCC) (20–22). Transmission of HBV is by perinatal, percutaneous, and sexual exposure. There are eight genotypes, A through H, and their prevalence depends on geographical location. All of these can be found in the U.S., with the prevalence of genotypes A, B, C, D, and E–G being 35%, 22%, 31%, 10%, and 2%, respectively (20).

Screening and Prevention

The US Preventive Services Task Force (USPSTF) strongly recommends screening for HBV in pregnant women at their first prenatal visit (strength of recommendation, SOR=A); but does not recommend routine screening of asymptomatic low risk individuals (SOR=D) (23). High-risk individuals who should be screened for HBV infection include patients with elevated liver tests and those at increased risk; these include homosexual men, intravenous drug users, patients on dialysis, individuals born in areas with high prevalence of HBV (i.e., Africa, South Asia, South America), individuals with HIV or hepatitis C infections, pregnant women, and close contacts, including sexual partners of HBV-infected individuals. Screening for HBV includes hepatitis B surface antigen (HBsAg) and hepatitis B surface antibody (HBsAb). Those who are seronegative for both HBsAg and HBsAb should be vaccinated (20). Newborns whose mothers are positive for HBV should receive hepatitis B immune globulin (HBIG) and begin the HBV vaccination series. Additionally, anyone younger than age 18 years who has not previously been vaccinated for HBV should be vaccinated (24).

Diagnosis

Clinical signs and symptoms of acute HBV infection include jaundice, dark urine, malaise, nausea, vomiting, abdominal pain, clay colored or pale stools, anorexia, and fever (24, 25). HBV is defined as chronic if an acute HBV infection persists more than 6 months. About 90% of infants infected with HBV during their first year of life will develop chronic HBV, whereas 90% of healthy adults infected with HBV will recover and have resolution of the disease within 6 months of infection (24). Chronic HBV increases the risk of cirrhosis and HCC.

Serologic tests of hepatitis B include HBsAg, HBsAb, hepatitis B core antibody (HBcAb), HBV DNA level, hepatitis E antigen (HBeAg), and hepatitis E antibody (HBeAb). Serum HBsAg is an indication for HBV infection, whereas HBsAb is a marker of immunity or vaccination to HBV (21,26). HBcAb is an indication of acute infection, although it may also appear in chronic hepatitis. HBV DNA levels may be obtained in chronic infection as part of an assessment of disease activity. The risk of advancing to cirrhosis and HCC is proportional to the level of HBV DNA and disease activity (21). Hepatitis B e-antigen positive infection is associated with high HBV DNA levels (>20,000 IU/mL) and seroconversion to HBeAb positive infection corresponds with a decrease in HBV DNA and clinical improvement (21) (Table 20.4).

Treatment

The goals of treatment are to suppress HBV replication and prevent cirrhosis, hepatic failure, and HCC. Parameters used to evaluate response to treatment include decrease in serum HBV DNA level, loss of HBeAg with or without detection of HBeAb, normalization of ALT levels, and improvement in liver histology (21,26). See Table 20.5 for phases of chronic HBV infection. There are seven drugs (interferon-alpha, pegylated interferon alpha, lamivudine, adefovir, entecavir, telbivudine, and tenofovir) available in the United States for the treatment of chronic HBV infection (21). Interferon-α is rarely used because of its frequent (three times a week) dosing, its route of administration (subcutaneous), and adverse reactions. Peginterferon-alpha given as a subcutaneous injection is expensive (~$350/week) and administered for 48 weeks. The other five medications are administered orally, are renally dosed, and must be given for a prolonged interval generally greater than 5 years. Viral resistance may occur during treatment with oral agents secondary to viral mutations.

CHRONIC HEPATITIS C

Hepatitis C virus (HCV) is a leading cause of chronic hepatitis and chronic liver disease, including cirrhosis and liver cancer. In the United States, the prevalence of hepatitis C antibody is 2% in adults 20 years of age and older, while about 150,000 new cases occur annually (27). HCV is the principal cause of death from liver disease and the primary indication for liver transplantation in the United States, accounting for 8,000–10,000 deaths annually (27–30). B 1980 when serologic testing became available, transmission of HCV is primarily by injection drug use or percutaneous exposure to contaminated blood. HCV may be transmitted sexually by individuals with high-risk behaviors, but this occurs much less frequently as compared to HBV (28,29). Perinatal transmission can occur, however it is uncommon (29). HCV is not transmitted via hugging, kissing, sharing of eating utensils, or breastfeeding, although breastfeeding should be avoided if the nipples are cracked or bleeding (28,29). There are six major genotypes of HCV with genotype 1 (1a and 1b) being the most common in the United States, followed by genotypes 2 and 3 (28).

Screening and Prevention

The USPSTF recommends against routine screening for HCV in asymptomatic adults who are not at increased risk for infection (grade of recommendation D) and found insufficient evidence to recommend screening in high risk individuals (31) The Centers for Disease Control and Prevention recommends

TABLE 20.4 Interpretation of HBV Immunologic Markers and Liver Enzyme Tests (22,26)

HBsAg	HBcAb	HBsAb	HBeAg	HBeAb	ALT/AST	HBV DNA	Interpretation
−	−	−	−	−	Normal	−	Susceptible (not immune) to HBV infection
−	+	+	−	−	Normal	−	Immune because of natural infection
−	−	+	−	−	Normal	−	Immune because of hepatitis B vaccination
+	+ (IgM HBcAb +)	−	+/−	+/−	Variable	+/−	Acute HBV infection
+	+ (IgM HBcAb −)	−	+/−	+/−	Variable	+/−	Chronic HBV infection
−	+	−	+/−	+/−	Variable	+/−	Four possible interpretations: 1. Resolved infection (most common) 2. False-positive HBcAb thus susceptible 3. "Low-level" chronic infection 4. Resolving acute infection
−	+	+/−	−	−	Normal	−	Resolved disease
+	+	−	+	↑	Variable	+++	Correlates with high level of viral replication; "marker of infectivity"
+	+	−	+	+	Variable	+	Correlates with low rates of viral replication
+ >6 months	+	−	+/−	+/−	Elevated	+++	Chronic disease
+ >6 months	+	−	−	+	Normal	++	Inactive carrier state

HBsAg = hepatitis B surface antigen (indicates that person is infectious); HBsAb = hepatitis B surface antibody (marker of immunity acquired through natural HBV infection, vaccination, or passive antibody [immune globulin]); HBcAb = hepatitis B core antibody (appears at the onset of acute hepatitis B infection; presence may also indicate chronic hepatitis B infection or false-positive test; HBeAg = hepatitis B early antigen (marker of infectivity); HBeAb = hepatitis B early antibody (correlates with low HBV DNA levels); HBV DNA = correlates with active replication; useful in monitoring response to treatment of HBV infection, especially in HBeAg-negative mutants.

TABLE 20.5 Phases of Chronic Hepatitis B Viral Infection

	Active	Inactive	Gray Zone	Immune Tolerant
ALT	Elevated	Normal	Elevated or Normal	Normal
HBeAg	+/−	−	+/−	+
HBeAb	+/−	+	+/−	−
HBV DNA (IU/mL)	>20,000	<20,000	Variable	>20,000
Histology:				
Inflammation	Active	None	Variable	Minimal
Fibrosis	Variable	Minimal	Variable	Minimal
Treatment	Indicated	Not Indicated	+/−	Not Indicated

Source: (26)

TABLE 20.6 Interpretation of HCV Markers

Anti-HCV	HCV RNA	Interpretation
+	+	Acute or chronic HCV depending on the clinical context.
+	−	Resolution of HCV; acute HCV during period of low-level viremia; false positive or negative result. Retest HCV RNA in 4–6 months to confirm resolution.
−	+	Early acute HCV infection; chronic HCV in setting of immunosuppressed state; false positive HCV RNA test. Retest anti-HCV and HCV RNA in 4–6 months.
−	−	Absence of HCV infection. Antibody testing in 4–6 months for confirmation.

Adapted from Source: (28)

that the following high-risk individuals should be tested for HCV infection: intravenous drug users, individuals who received blood transfusion or had organ transplant before 1992, people with HIV infection, hemophiliacs who received clotting factors before 1987, individuals on hemodialysis, individuals with unexplained abnormal liver function tests, children born to HCV-infected mothers, sexual partners of infected individuals, individuals with multiple sexual partners, spouses or household contacts of HCV-infected patients, and health care workers after a needle stick injury or mucosal exposure to HCV-positive blood (27, 28). HCV infected individuals should be advised against sharing toothbrushes or shaving equipment, donating blood, organs or semen, and drug users should avoid sharing or reusing syringes or needles (28). Currently, no prophylaxis, either with immunoglobulins or antiviral agents, or vaccine exists for pre- or postexposure to HCV (29,32)

Diagnosis

Symptoms of acute HCV include anorexia, abdominal discomfort, nausea, vomiting, fever, fatigue, and jaundice in about 20% of acutely infected patients. However, more than 80% of individuals who develop acute HCV have no symptoms. Twenty percent of the individuals exposed to HCV recover fully, but the rest develop chronic infection. Chronically infected patients may not have symptoms until liver failure becomes clinically evident (29,30).

Diagnosis of acute or chronic HCV consists of testing the serum for antibody to HCV (anti-HCV) and for HCV RNA (Table 20.6). HCV RNA may be discovered in the serum as early as 2 weeks after acute exposure, whereas anti-HCV is normally not detectable before 8–12 weeks after exposure to HCV-positive blood (28). ALT levels usually remain elevated throughout the course of the disease, but may fluctuate. Performing a liver biopsy provides information on the status of liver injury, helps identify features in order to decide whether to start therapy, and may show advanced fibrosis or cirrhosis that requires surveillance for HCC and screening for varices (28).

Treatment

The goal of treatment is to prevent complications, such as cirrhosis and HCC, and death from HCV infection (28). The combination of a pegylated interferon alpha and ribavirin is the recommended therapy for chronic HCV infection. Side effects of interferon include flulike illness, alopecia, depression, insomnia, irritability, weight loss, autoimmune disorder, and hematologic abnormalities. Side effects of ribavirin include hemolytic anemia, bone marrow suppression, and renal failure (29). Dosing and duration of treatment is based on viral genotype and body weight (Table 20.7).

Liver biopsy is not mandatory for deciding on treatment, although it is useful (28). Treatment responses are characterized by virological parameters rather than a clinical endpoint. Sustained virological response (SVR) is the most important parameter, which is defined as the absence of HCV RNA 24 weeks after discontinuation of therapy. End of treatment response is defined as undetectable virus at the end of either a 24- or 48-week course of therapy. Rapid virological response is defined as undetectable HCV RNA at week 4 of treatment; it is used to predict SVR. Early virological response is defined as complete absence of HCV RNA at week 12 of therapy compared with baseline level; this is the most accurate predictor of not achieving an SVR as discussed in Table 20.7 (28).

CIRRHOSIS

In patients with chronic liver injury and inflammation, the hepatic stellate cell can be stimulated to produce collagen leading to the development of intrahepatic fibrosis. This can culminate in cirrhosis, in which fibrous bands completely encircle groups of hepatocytes forming a nodule, altering hepatic architecture and resulting in portal hypertension. Physical findings in patients with cirrhosis can include scleral icterus, spider angiomata, palmer erythema, gynecomastia, Dupuytren's contracture, hepatomegaly, splenomegaly, presence of ascites,

TABLE 20.7 Treatment for Hepatitis C

Genotype	Treatment	Duration (weeks)	Rate of SVR (%)
1	Ribavirin 1,000 mg (≤75 kg) or 1,200 mg (>75 kg) PO daily + Peginterferon alpha-2a 180 μg SQ weekly *or* Peginterferon alpha-2b 1.5 μg/kg SQ weekly	48	45–50
2 and 3	Ribavirin 800 mg PO daily + Peginterferon alpha-2a 180 μg SQ weekly *or* Peginterferon alpha-2b 1.5 μg/kg SQ weekly	24	70–80
4	Ribavirin 1,000 mg (≤75 kg) or 1,200 mg (>75 kg) PO daily + Peginterferon alpha-2a 180 μg SQ weekly *or* Peginterferon alpha-2b 1.5 μg/kg SQ weekly	48	70

PO = by mouth; SQ = subcutaneously.
Source: (28,29,32)

asterixis, and fetor hepaticus. Table 20.8 lists the diagnostic accuracy of symptoms and physical exam findings for the diagnosis of hepatomegaly and ascites. The presence of cirrhosis can be determined either directly by observation of a nodular liver surface during surgery for example, or by liver biopsy.

Severity Assessment

Various histological scoring systems are utilized to measure the degree of hepatic inflammatory activity and fibrosis (33). The METAVIR scoring system grades fibrosis from 0 to 4 and activity from A0 to A3. See Table 20.8 for METAVIR scoring system. Indirect methods for evaluating the presence of cirrhosis include signs of portal hypertension such as splenomegaly and the presence of varices, an abnormal CT scan showing an irregular and nodular border to the liver, or newer ultrasonic techniques that indirectly score hepatic elasticity (33). Because cirrhosis is the 12th leading cause of death in the United States, scoring systems are often employed as prognostic indicators in patients with cirrhosis. The Child-Pugh (CP) system assigns points based on bilirubin level, prothrombin time, albumin level, presence or absence of ascites, and presence or absence of encephalopathy (34). Higher scores indicate a worse prognosis. In one study survival rates were: CP A-90% for 10 years, CP B- 95% 1-year and 75% 5-year survival rate, and CP C 85% and 50% 1- and 5-year survival rates, respectively (35). The MELD scoring system calculated using INR bilirubin level and serum creatinine is predictive of 90-day mortality for patients with advanced liver disease and is used as a basis for assigning priority to patients awaiting liver transplantation (2) (*http://www.unos.org/resources/MeldPeldCalculator.asp?index=98*).

TABLE 20.8 METAVIR Scoring System

Fibrosis score:
F0 = no fibrosis
F1 = portal fibrosis without septa
F2 = portal fibrosis with few septa
F3 = numerous septa without cirrhosis (bridging)
F4 = cirrhosis
Activity score:
A0 = no activity
A1 = mild activity
A2 = moderate activity
A3 = severe activity

Treatment

Complications of cirrhosis and portal hypertension include esophageal and gastric varices and the attendant risk of hemorrhage, ascites, spontaneous bacterial peritonitis, impairment of renal function, portal systemic encephalopathy, and the development of hepatocellular cancer. Primary goals for management of the patient with cirrhosis are to preserve existing hepatic function by prevention of further injury, and the management of complications. Preservation of hepatic function requires treatment of the underlying disease such as chronic hepatitis B or NASH, for example. Abstinence from alcohol is generally advised as is the avoidance of other hepatotoxic substances. Additionally, vaccination for hepatitis A and B in addition to routine vaccination for influenza annually and pneumococcal vaccination is recommended in patients with cirrhosis (36,37).

Management of Complications of Cirrhosis

VARICES

Normally the portal vein is a high flow (900 mL/minute), low pressure (4 mm Hg) vessel. In cirrhotic patients there is an alteration of hepatic architecture and an increase of hepatic vascular resistance from intrahepatic vasoconstriction resulting in portal venous hypertension and leading to shunting of blood and the development of collateral vessels and varices. In addition, there is reduced splanchnic and systemic vascular resistance which increases portal venous inflow. Portal vein pressure can be indirectly measured by determining the hepatic vein wedge pressure and subtracting vena caval pressure from this providing the hepatic vein pressure gradient. Varices do not form until this gradient is greater than 10 mm Hg.

Varices located in the gastric or esophageal lumen can rupture and hemorrhage. Screening endoscopy or a capsule study can identify those cirrhotic subjects at risk for bleeding by grading the size and number of varices and assessing them for stigmata of hemorrhage such as cherry-red spots or red wale lines on the veins. About 50% of patients with cirrhosis have varices on initial endoscopic evaluation. In those in whom no varices are seen, screening should be repeated every 2–3 years as about 8% of cirrhotic patients will develop varices each year. Therapy with nonselective β-blockers such as propranolol or nadolol used as primary prophylaxis to prevent bleeding can reduce the risk of hemorrhage; for every 10 patients with medium to large varices treated with β-blockers, one bleeding episode can be prevented (38). Patients may also be offered endoscopic band ligation (EBL). Hemorrhage from varices occurs in about 10% of patients per year and although 6-week mortality from hemorrhage is about 20%, those with the highest hepatic vein pressure gradient (>20 mm Hg) experience the greatest mortality, as high as 60%.

Patients with acute variceal hemorrhage should be resuscitated and have emergent upper endoscopy performed. Blood transfusion should be employed to maintain hemoglobin levels of 8 g/L. Antibiotic prophylaxis with either oral norfloxacin or oral ciprofloxacin or intravenous ceftriaxone should be administered to reduce the risk of pneumonia and other infections as this has been shown to reduce mortality (38). Management of acute variceal hemorrhage can include the use of pharmacologic agents such as octreotide or vasopressin, EBL, balloon tamponade, transhepatic variceal embolization, or performance of a Transjugular Intrahepatic Portosystemic Shunt (TIPS) or shunt surgery (38). The TIPS procedure entails percutaneously passing a catheter from the jugular vein into a hepatic vein. The guide catheter is then advanced through the hepatic parenchyma into the portal vein creating an artificial fistula and allowing placement of a stent between the portal vein and hepatic vein. The shunt then results in a lower hepatic venous pressure gradient. Bleeding varices can also be treated by embolization done either during a TIPS procedure or as a separate transhepatic catheterization. Patients who survive hemorrhage should be evaluated for liver transplant and should be treated with EBL until varices are obliterated.

ASCITES AND SPONTANEOUS BACTERIAL PERITONITIS

Cirrhosis and portal hypertension are associated with sodium retention and major changes in systemic vascular resistance, especially within the splanchnic circulation where there is reduced vascular resistance and an increase in blood flow. These conditions can lead to an accumulation of fluid within the peritoneal cavity: ascites, the most common of the three major complications of cirrhosis and one of the leading causes for hospital admission of cirrhotic patients. Development of ascites is a poor prognostic sign: as many as 15% of cirrhotic patients who develop ascites may expire within 1 year and 43.5% within 5 years (39). The patient who develops ascites notices weight gain and change in abdominal girth. On examination the flanks become bulging and shifting dullness is present (Table 20.9). The presence of ascites can be confirmed by ultrasound examination.

Cirrhosis is the cause for ascites development in the great majority (85%) of cases. Other etiologies such as heart failure, cancer, nephrotic syndrome, tuberculosis, and others account for approximately 15% of cases. Abdominal paracentesis, most commonly performed in the left lower quadrant, can permit analysis of ascitic fluid. Cell count and differential and measurement of ascitic fluid albumin and total protein concentration with determination of the serum-ascites albumin gradient (SAAG) should be obtained. A SAAG value ≥1.1 G/dL is 97% accurate for the diagnosis of cirrhotic ascites (40). Medical management of ascites generally consists of abstinence from alcohol, salt restriction to 2 g/day (88 mmol/day) and the use of diuretics: spironolactone in doses of 100–400 mg/day and furosemide 40–160 mg/day introduced in a stepwise manner targeting a daily weight-loss of 1 lb per day after peripheral edema has resolved (41). Urinary electrolytes can be used to monitor treatment: a "spot" urine sodium greater than the potassium value generally supports daily sodium loss of 78 mmol/day (40). Fluid restriction is generally not advised. In patients with tense or difficult to manage ascites large volume paracentesis can be employed, generally with concomitant administration of albumin intravenously 6–8 g/L of fluid removed (40). In all patients with cirrhotic ascites the MELD scores should be calculated and the patient evaluated for liver transplantation. Another therapeutic option is TIPS.

Some patients may develop the more serious complication of hepatorenal syndrome characterized by progressive reduction of renal function and low urinary sodium (42). Diuretics should be withdrawn from these patients and fluids administered. Therapy remains controversial but includes the use of octreotide, midodrine, TIPS, and transplantation.

Spontaneous bacterial peritonitis occurs when the ascitic fluid becomes infected. Diagnosis is made by paracentesis with fluid culture in blood culture bottles and cell count revealing >250 neutrophils/mL. Treatment is with a third-generation cephalosporin or with norfloxacin (43). In patients with low ascitic fluid protein or in those who previously had an episode of Spontaneous Bacterial Peritonitis (SBP) long-term prophylaxis with antibiotics is indicated (40,44).

HEPATIC ENCEPHALOPATHY

Hepatic encephalopathy has a spectrum ranging from mild impairment of cognitive function and motor skills to gross disorientation, to deep coma. It can be categorized into three types: hepatic encephalopathy from acute liver failure, that from portal systemic bypass in the absence of liver disease, and portal systemic encephalopathy (PSE) that occurs in patients with cirrhosis and portal systemic shunts. PSE is the most

TABLE 20.9 Accuracy of Clinical and Diagnostic Tests for Liver Disorders

Test Name	Sensitivity	Specificity	LR+	LR−
Clinical diagnosis of ascites (1)				
History of hepatitis	27	92	3.4	0.79
History of heart failure	47	73	1.7	0.73
History of carcinoma	13	85	0.9	1.02
History of alcoholism	60	58	1.4	0.69
Jaundice	33	90	3.3	0.74
Ankle swelling	93	66	2.7	0.21
Increased girth	**87**	**77**	**3.8**	**0.17**
Flank dullness	80	69	2.6	0.29
Bulging flanks	93	54	2.0	0.13
Recent weight gain	67	79	3.2	0.42
Shifting dullness	60	90	6	0.44
Telangiectasia	27	99	54	0.73
Flat or everted navel	33	88	2.7	0.76
Fluid wave	80	92	10	0.22
Edema	87	77	3.8	0.17
Hemochromatosis (2, 3, 11)				
Transferrin saturation >45%	98	99	98	0.01
Transferrin saturation >50%	82	88	6.8	0.2
Ferritin >200 ng/mL (men)	85	95	17	0.16
Ferritin >150 ng/mL (women)	85	95	17	0.16
Trans sat >50% or ferritin >150 ng/mL (women)	94	86	6.7	0.07
Trans sat >50% or ferritin >200 ng/mL (men)	94	86	6.7	0.07
Hepatic iron index ≥1.9	93	99.5	186	0.07
Serum iron >167 μg/dL	68	83	4	0.39
Hepatocellular carcinoma in patients with HCV or cirrhosis (4, 5)				
α-fetoprotein >200 mcg/L	27	99	27	0.27
Ultrasound	60	97	20	0.41
Helical computed tomography	67	92	8.4	0.36
Magnetic resonance imaging	81	85	5.4	0.22
Fatty infiltration of liver in patient with abnormal aminotransaminases (6)				
Ultrasound	83	93	11.8	0.18
Cirrhosis in patients with hepatitis C (7)				
Platelets <140 k AND AST/ALT >1	29	95	6.2	0.74
Platelets <140 k	85	87	6.4	0.16
AST/ALT ≥1	31	87	2.4	0.78
Clinical diagnosis of hepatomegaly (8)				
Palpation	67	73	2.5	0.45

TABLE 20.9 *(Continued)*

Test Name	Sensitivity	Specificity	LR+	LR−
Alcohol abuse or dependence (unselected population) (9)				
ALT ≥40 units/L (male)	11	96	2.8	0.93
AST ≥37 units/L (male)	11	93	1.6	0.96
MCV ≥96 (male)	39.4	75	1.6	0.81
MCV ≥96 (female)	41	79	2	0.75
GGT ≥50 units/L (male)	6.8	95.5	1.5	0.98
GGT ≥32 units/L (female)	6.5	91.8	0.8	1.02
Hepatobiliary disease (10)				
Alkaline phosphorus >170 units/L	65	83	3.8	0.42
Total bilirubin >1 mg/dL	56	91	6.2	0.48
GGT >28 U/L	75	85	5	0.29
ALT >25 units/L	56	90	5.6	0.49
AST >20 U/L	74	92	9.25	0.28

ALT = alanine aminotransferase; AST = aspartate aminotransferase; GGT = gamma glutamyl transferase; MCV = Mean cellular volume.

1. Simel DL, Halvorsen RA, Jr., Feussner JR. Quantitating bedside diagnosis: clinical evaluation of ascites. J Gen Intern Med 1988 Sep-Oct;3(5):423–428.
2. Bassett ML, Halliday JW, Ferris RA, Powell LW. Diagnosis of hemochromatosis in young subjects: predictive accuracy of biochemical screening tests. Gastroenterology. 1984 Sep;87(3):628–633.
3. McLaren CE, McLachlan GJ, Halliday JW, Webb SI, Leggett BA, Jazwinska EC, et al. Distribution of transferrin saturation in an Australian population: relevance to the early diagnosis of hemochromatosis. Gastroenterology. 1998 Mar;114(3):543–549.
4. Colli A, Fraquelli M, Casazza G, Massironi S, Colucci A, Conte D, et al. Accuracy of ultrasonography, spiral CT, magnetic resonance, and alpha-fetoprotein in diagnosing hepatocellular carcinoma: a systematic review. Am J Gastroenterol 2006 Mar;101(3):513–523.
5. Gupta S, Bent S, Kohlwes J. Test characteristics of alpha-fetoprotein for detecting hepatocellular carcinoma in patients with hepatitis C. A systematic review and critical analysis. Ann Intern Med 2003 Jul 1;139(1):46–50.
6. Hultcrantz R, Gabrielsson N. Patients with persistent elevation of aminotransferases: investigation with ultrasonography, radionuclide imaging and liver biopsy. J Gen Intern Med 1993 Jan;233(1):7–12.
7. Iacobellis A, Mangia A, Leandro G, Clemente R, Festa V, Attino V, et al. External validation of biochemical indices for noninvasive evaluation of liver fibrosis in HCV chronic hepatitis. Am J Gastroenterol 2005 Apr;100(4):868–873.
8. Naylor CD. The rational clinical examination. Physical examination of the liver. JAMA. 1994 Jun 15;271(23):1859–1865.
9. Aertgeerts B, Buntinx F, Ansoms S, Fevery J. Screening properties of questionnaires and laboratory tests for the detection of alcohol abuse or dependence in a general practice population. Br J Gen Pract. 2001 Mar;51(464):206–217.
10. Ferraris R, Colombatti G, Fiorentini MT, Carosso R, Arossa W, De La Pierre M. Diagnostic value of serum bile acids and routine liver function tests in hepatobiliary diseases. Sensitivity, specificity, and predictive value. Dig Dis Sci 1983 Feb;28(2):129–136.
11. Kowdley KV, Trainer TD, Saltzman JR, Pedrosa M, Krawitt EL, Knox TA, et al. Utility of hepatic iron index in American patients with hereditary hemochromatosis: a multicenter study. Gastroenterology. 1997 Oct;113(4):1270–1277.

common form and the subject of this section. PSE manifests as cognitive dysfunction that may progress to coma. On examination, asterixis (involuntary jerking movements especially in the outstretched hands) may be present and a fetor hepaticus (a strong, disagreeable, and peculiar odor to the breath) may be noted. PSE may present in a subclinical form, which can only be detected through sophisticated neurocognitive testing and may occur acutely or on a recurrent or persistent basis. It can be graded using the Glasgow coma scale or the West Haven criteria (45) (Table 20.10).

PSE occurs in 30–45% of patients with cirrhosis (46) and is related to abnormalities of ammonia metabolism with decreased urea synthesis associated with impaired hepatic function and with portal venous shunting resulting in hyperammonemia. Acutely, PSE may be precipitated by various conditions such as blood in the gut as may occur with variceal hemorrhage, infection such as SBP, constipation, dietary overload with proteins, or electrolyte abnormalities associated with the use of diuretics or from diarrhea. See Table 20.11 for a list of causes of hepatic encephalopathy in patients with cirrhosis. Because cirrhosis alters drug metabolism, standard doses of common medications such as sedatives and hypnotics may also lead to encephalopathy and coma. Standard treatment includes identification and elimination of any precipitating factors, and the use of nonabsorbable disaccharides such as sorbitol or lactulose. These agents are thought to inhibit bacterial ammonia formation in the colon and to trap ammonia as ammonium in

TABLE 20.10 West Haven Criteria to Evaluate Hepatic Encephalopathy

Grade 0, normal
Grade 1, mild lack of awareness
Grade 2, lethargic
Grade 3, somnolent but arousable
Grade 4, coma

TABLE 20.11 Causes of Hepatic Encephalopathy in Patients with Cirrhosis

Drugs: benzodiazepines, narcotics, alcohol
Increased ammonia production: excessive dietary protein, gastrointestinal bleeding, infection, electrolyte disturbances, constipation, metabolic alkalosis
Dehydration: vomiting, diarrhea, hemorrhage, diuretics, large volume paracentesis
Portosystemic shunting: radiographic or surgically placed shunts, spontaneous shunts
Vascular occlusion: portal vein thrombosis, hepatic vein thrombosis
Primary hepatocellular carcinoma

the bowel lumen (45). In addition, oral antibiotic treatment with neomycin, metronidazole, or rifaximin is sometimes used.

HCC

HCC is more common in patients with chronic viral hepatitis and cirrhosis. Although uncommon in the United States (incidence of 8,500–11,500 cases per year), the incidence has increased in the past 30 years; the prognosis is poor with a median survival of 8 months (47,48). Because of the skewed distribution of hepatitis C in the US population, the prevalence of HCC is likely to increase in the next 20 years (49). HCC surveillance by abdominal ultrasound has a high sensitivity and specificity and should be performed every 6–12 months in addition to monitoring α-fetoprotein levels (50,51). If a hepatic lesion is detected by ultrasound, a contrast-enhanced computed axial tomography scan, or magnetic resonance imaging should be performed to characterize the size and number of lesions. The decision to biopsy these lesions for confirmation of pathology is controversial and in many instances the finding of a hepatic mass with typical magnetic resonance imaging or CT appearance in patients with cirrhosis or chronic viral hepatitis and an elevated α-fetoprotein is sufficient for the diagnosis of HCC.

Treatment for HCC is determined by the size and number of lesions as well as the patient's overall condition as measured by CP classification. A variety of staging systems exist (52). For single small lesions, percutaneous ethanol injection is often used. For larger solitary lesions in patients with CP "A" status and good hepatic reserve hepatic resection may be possible. Other patients may be candidates for liver transplantation based on the size and number of lesions, their location, and whether there is evidence of vascular invasion or distant spread of the tumor. Liver transplantation has been shown to have the highest five-year survival rate of all options (50%). Patients who are not candidates for surgery may be eligible for radiofrequency ablation (49,53), transarterial chemoembolization, and chemotherapy.

Liver Transplantation

Liver transplantation is the critical salvage therapy for patients with end-stage liver disease. Candidates for transplant include any patient with signs of liver insufficiency as reflected in the MELD score, which is used as a guide for referring patients to a transplant center as well as for allocation of donor livers in the United States. Candidates should have a good social support network, and understand the lifetime risks associated with transplantation and the need to be compliant with immunosuppression.

Contraindications to transplant include extrahepatic malignancy, metastatic liver disease, unresolved infections, active alcohol or substance dependency and abuse, severe psychiatric disorders or mental retardation, extensive portal and mesenteric thrombosis, morbid obesity, and advanced age, among others. An adequate source of funding for the procedure is also required. One- and 5-year survival is about 85% and 75%, respectively, in adults. Most donor livers are obtained from brain dead donors, although living donor liver transplantation is becoming more common in which the donor contributes the right lobe of their liver.

KEY POINTS

- Common and preventable causes of chronic liver disease include excessive alcohol intake and chronic hepatitis B and C.
- The MELD score is based on INR, creatinine, and total bilirubin and helps to predict 90-day survival in individuals with liver impairment.
- Liver injury tests include AST and ALT, whereas AP and GGT and are classified as either cholestatic or as hepatocellular injury.
- Nonalcoholic fatty liver disease is the most common cause of elevated aminotransaminases in adults in the United States and is associated with the metabolic syndrome.
- The goal of treatment for chronic hepatitis B and C is to prevent cirrhosis, hepatic failure, and HCC.
- Complications of cirrhosis and portal hypertension include esophageal and gastric varices and their risk of hemorrhage, ascites, spontaneous bacterial peritonitis, impairment of renal function, portal systemic encephalopathy, and the development of HCC.

CHAPTER

21

Dyspepsia

William Y. Huang

CLINICAL OBJECTIVES

1. List common causes of dyspepsia
2. Discuss the pathophysiology of common causes of dyspepsia
3. Explain key diagnostic features of common causes of dyspepsia
4. Describe the evidence-based medicine approach to diagnosing and managing a patient with dyspepsia

Dyspepsia is defined as "chronic or recurrent pain or discomfort centered in the upper abdomen" (1). In addition to pain and discomfort, patients may note other symptoms including early satiety and fullness in the abdomen after meals (2). In the 2006 National Ambulatory Medical Survey, "stomach and abdominal pain, cramps, and spasms" was the eighth most frequent reason for patients to present to their physicians, estimated to account for more than 16 million visits per year (3). Family physicians most likely see patients with dyspepsia at least a few times each week.

If no alarm symptoms or signs are present, the family physician can effectively manage most patients through the use of simple diagnostic tests and medication. Patients who have alarm symptoms or fail to improve with standard treatment may require referral for further testing, including an upper endoscopy in most cases.

DIFFERENTIAL DIAGNOSIS AND PATHOPHYSIOLOGY

The most common causes of dyspepsia are functional dyspepsia (a diagnosis of exclusion), peptic ulcer disease (PUD), and gastroesophageal reflux disease (GERD). Esophageal or gastric cancers are rare causes. Other rare causes are mentioned in Table 21.1.

Gastroesophageal Reflux Disease

GERD is "a condition which develops when the reflux of stomach contents causes troublesome symptoms and/or complications" (6). Symptoms may include heartburn or the regurgitation of material from the stomach into the mouth. Complications may include esophagitis, erosions, ulcers, or other changes in the esophageal mucosa. There is a poor correlation between endoscopic findings and symptoms. Some patients may have signs of erosive esophagitis (erythema, friability, or an esophageal ulcer) whereas others may have no visible lesion (nonerosive reflux disease) (6). Our understanding of the underlying pathophysiology is evolving. One important causative factor is esophagogastric junction incompetence that can occur from transient lower esophageal sphincter relaxations, lower esophageal sphincter hypotension, or anatomic deformities of the esophagogastric junction such as a hiatal hernia. After the reflux occurs, another key factor is ineffective esophageal clearance of acid and reflux material that may result from impaired esophageal emptying, esophageal peristalsis dysfunction, or decreased salivary neutralizing capacity (7).

Peptic Ulcer Disease

The primary causes of PUD are *Helicobacter pylori* infection and nonsteroidal anti-inflammatory drug (NSAID) use. Although either of these alone is a significant cause, these two factors can act synergistically to further increase the risk of PUD (8). Cigarette smoking is an additional risk factor that may impair the healing of an ulcer and increase the likelihood of recurrence after successful treatment (9). Zollinger-Ellison syndrome is a rare cause of PUD.

Functional Dyspepsia

In up to 60% of patients with dyspepsia, there is no identifiable cause on endoscopy. In these cases, the patient is diagnosed as having functional dyspepsia. A number of potential mechanisms of functional dyspepsia have been proposed including impaired gastric accommodation to a meal, delay of gastric emptying of solid food, hypersensitivity to gastric distension, and others. Genetic factors, *H. pylori* infection, and psychosocial disorders may also contribute (10).

CLINICAL EVALUATION

History and Physical Examination

Ask about red flags or alarm symptoms that may indicate the possibility for serious disease such as a complicated peptic ulcer or malignancy (Table 21.2) (1,11,12). Although it is important to fully evaluate patients with any of these red flags, the sensitivity and specificity of these symptoms have been variable in previous studies (0% to 83%, 4% to 98%, respectively) and the positive predictive value is low (4% for cancer, 13% to 14% for ulcer disease or esophagitis) (13–15). Age is

TABLE 21.1 Differential Diagnosis of the Patient with Dyspepsia

Diagnosis	Typical Features	Frequency[†]
Functional dyspepsia	Epigastric pain or burning, postprandial fullness, early satiety	60%
Peptic ulcer disease	Postprandial epigastric burning pain	15%–25%
Reflux esophagitis	Heartburn, sour taste in the mouth	5%–15%
Gastric or esophageal cancer	Abdominal pain or heartburn, dysphagia, weight loss	<2%
Rare causes*		

*Rare causes include carbohydrate malabsorption, small intestinal mucosal disorders (e.g., sprue, intestinal parasites, chronic pancreatitis), infiltrative diseases of the stomach (e.g., Crohn disease), ischemic bowel disease, metabolic disorders (hypothyroidism, hypercalcemia), medications (e.g., erythromycin), cardiac conditions (e.g., inferior myocardial ischemia), and pulmonary conditions (e.g., lower lobe pneumonia).
[†]Frequency of diagnosis on endoscopy. The diagnosis of functional dyspepsia is made if there are no findings on endoscopy.
Compiled data from references 4 and 5.

another important factor; current guidelines recommend that all patients who are older than age 55 years with the new onset of dyspepsia should receive an endoscopy to evaluate for more serious disease (1,12).

TABLE 21.2 Red Flags for Patients with Dyspepsia Indicating More Serious or Life-threatening Disease*

Symptoms, Signs, or Laboratory Test	Disease
Unexplained weight loss	Cancer, obstruction
Anorexia	Cancer
Dysphagia	Cancer, obstruction
Hematemesis	Cancer, bleeding ulcer
Melena	Cancer, bleeding ulcer
Anemia	Cancer, bleeding ulcer
Heme-positive stool	Cancer, bleeding ulcer
Longstanding reflux symptoms	Cancer
Hematochezia	Bleeding ulcer
Orthostatic hypotension	Bleeding ulcer
Shock	Bleeding ulcer, perforated ulcer
Odynophagia	Obstruction
Early satiety	Obstruction
Recurrent vomiting	Obstruction
Sudden onset of severe abdominal pain	Perforated ulcer
Rigid board-like abdomen	Perforated ulcer
Other peritoneal signs	Perforated ulcer

*Compiled using data from 1,11,12.

Some patients may present with gastrointestinal bleeding. If the bleeding is severe, the patient may present with alarm symptoms and signs including hematemesis, melena, hematochezia, hypotension, tachycardia, anemia, syncope, and shock. In this situation or in other emergency situations such as a perforated ulcer, the physician must perform a quick history and physical examination, urgently stabilize the patient, and identify the cause the symptoms.

In nonemergent presentations typically seen in the office setting, the physician should perform a focused history and physical examination. In taking a focused history, the physician should ask about the location of discomfort, duration, quality, severity, associated symptoms, and both alleviating and exacerbating factors and use that information to refine the differential diagnosis of the patient's dyspepsia. Inquiring about a history of similar symptoms, use of medications, history of smoking, and the presence of any red flag symptoms also is important. In performing a focused examination, the patient's vital signs and appearance may give a clue on how urgent the patient's condition is. A careful examination of the abdomen is essential, although most patients with dyspepsia have a normal examination. A lung and cardiovascular examination may be useful in assessing whether an extra-abdominal cause of the patient's symptoms is present. If there are any alarm symptoms or concern about gastrointestinal bleeding, a rectal examination with stool heme testing is indicated. A discussion of additional items to look for during the history and physical examination follows in the next section.

GERD

Patients with GERD commonly present with heartburn, which is a sensation of a burning pain in the substernal area. This is frequently accompanied by acid regurgitation and a sour taste in the mouth (waterbrash). Symptoms may be aggravated by the foods discussed earlier, or by certain body positions such as bending forward or lying down. Food or antacids may alleviate the symptoms. The physical examination is usually normal. GERD may cause noncardiac chest pain or be associated with cough, asthma, laryngitis, and dental erosions (16).

A recent study reported the success of the GerdQ questionnaire in the primary care setting to diagnose a patient with

GERD. In using the GerdQ questionnaire, the physician documents the frequency of six key symptoms (heartburn, regurgitation, pain in the center of the stomach, nausea, difficulty sleeping due to heartburn or regurgitation, and use of medication) in the previous week and points are given for defined levels of frequency. The authors noted that patients with a point total between 11 and 18 points (18 = maximum number of points) had almost a 90% probability of GERD (17).

PUD

The classic presentation of PUD is epigastric abdominal pain that is burning or gnawing in character. Duodenal ulcers typically occur on an empty stomach or at least 2 hours after eating and are relieved by eating food or taking antacids. Gastric ulcers may occur sooner after eating and are less frequently relieved by food or antacids. A variety of other symptoms, including vomiting and loss of appetite may also be present (18). Epigastric tenderness may or may not be present on physical examination (19). The patient's stool may be heme-positive if bleeding has occurred.

FUNCTIONAL DYSPEPSIA

The Rome III committee defined functional dyspepsia as "the presence of symptoms thought to originate in the gastroduodenal region, in the absence of any organic, systemic, or metabolic disease that is likely to explain these symptoms" with a duration of symptoms at least 3 months and the onset of symptoms at 6 months before diagnosis. This committee categorized patients with functional dyspepsia into two subgroups: (i) epigastric pain syndrome (pain or burning in the epigastric area) and (ii) postprandial distress syndrome ("bothersome postprandial fullness" or "early satiation"), although the two syndromes can occur simultaneously in the same patient. A patient with functional dyspepsia must have at least one of these symptoms and no abnormality on endoscopy or other examination that explains the symptoms (2). The physical examination will mostly likely be normal.

Table 21.3 lists the accuracy of key elements of the history and physical examination of the dyspeptic patient. Although it is important to perform a history and physical examination to evaluate the patient's complaint of dyspepsia, studies have demonstrated that both generalist physicians and gastroenterologists have difficulty in making an accurate diagnosis of functional dyspepsia or organic conditions such as esophagitis or peptic ulcer disease based on their clinical assessment (20,21). Further diagnostic testing is needed.

Diagnostic Testing

GERD

There is no clear standard of diagnosis for GERD. In addition, generalists often make a presumptive diagnosis based on symptoms and empirically begin treatment, since in this setting serious disease is rare. They aim to "minimize danger" and identify those who may need more definitive diagnosis because of alarm symptoms or other urgent reasons. On the other hand, gastroenterologists may seek to "minimize uncertainty" by using invasive methods to establish a diagnosis (22). This is also appropriate given the referral nature of their population and the greater likelihood of serious disease.

The response to proton pump inhibitors (PPIs) has been evaluated as a diagnostic test for gastroesophageal reflux. Studies have investigated different dosages and drugs (mostly using higher than standard doses), varying lengths of time of medication use (from 1 to 4 weeks), and different reference standards (23,24) (Table 21.4). A meta-analysis using a 24-hour pH probe or endoscopy as the reference standard found that given a 50% pretest probability of GERD, a positive response to a trial of a PPI increases the likelihood of GERD to 75%, whereas a negative test reduces it to 21% (24). The PPI test can therefore be use as an initial diagnostic approach by primary care physicians when GERD is suspected.

Endoscopy has the advantage of allowing direct visualization of the esophageal mucosa and documentation and biopsy of any suspicious lesion. However, it is also important to understand that the endoscopic findings do not correlate with the severity of symptoms or the response to treatment. Patients with nonerosive reflux disease (no endoscopic findings) may still have significant symptoms and require strong medication for control of symptoms (11).

Patients who do not respond to usual treatment may be referred for other studies. Esophageal manometry is useful in determining the location of the lower esophageal sphincter for future pH monitoring, in diagnosing motor disorders and in evaluating peristaltic function before surgery. Esophageal pH monitoring may be useful in documenting persistent acid reflux events in patients with persistent symptoms or those with atypical symptoms (such as a cough) (11,16).

PUD

Diagnostic studies for peptic ulcer disease such as upper endoscopy or an upper gastrointestinal series (UGI) are needed to confirm the diagnosis of peptic ulcer disease. Upper endoscopy is very sensitive and specific (see Table 21.4) and has the added advantages of direct observation of the esophageal, gastric, and duodenal mucosa and the ability to perform biopsies of any lesions of concerns for cancer or for *H. pylori* infection. Patients who are noted to have a gastric ulcer on UGI should have an upper endoscopy and biopsy of the lesion, because as many as 3% of gastric ulcers may be malignant (4). The risk of complications from an upper endoscopy is extremely low (<0.3%) (4). Although an UGI is less sensitive and specific (see Table 21.4) and results in radiation exposure for the patient, it may still have a role in the diagnosis if the patient is not able to tolerate endoscopy or if a trained endoscopist is not available in the community.

H. Pylori INFECTION

H. pylori infection is the most common cause of peptic ulcer disease and its presence or absence should guide the management of a patient with dyspepsia and suspected PUD (see Management section). Available methods of diagnosing an *H. pylori* infection include ^{13}C and ^{14}C urea breath tests, serologic tests, and stool antigen tests. Breath tests are highly sensitive and specific (Table 21.4) (30). However, PPIs may increase the likelihood of false-negative results on breath tests for up to 2 to 4 weeks after stopping the PPI (31). Serologic tests include both serum antibody tests performed in a reference laboratory and whole blood tests performed at the point of care. The most commonly used serum antibody tests are enzyme-linked

(text continues on page 246)

TABLE 21.3 Diagnosis of Dyspepsia Using the History and Physical Examination

Diagnosis Suggested	Clinical Finding	Sensitivity	Specificity	LR+	LR−	Comments
GERD (20)	Overall clinical impression by GPs	62%	71%	2.14	0.54	Gold standard = endoscopic evidence of esophagitis
	Overall clinical impression by gastroenterologists	62%	81%	3.26	0.47	
GERD (21)	Systematic review of clinical impressions by primary care physicians, specialists and computer models			2.4	0.5	Gold standard = endoscopic evidence of esophagitis
GERD (17)	GerdQ questionnaire: Points given for frequency of six key symptoms and probability calculated from point total	65%	71%	2.24	0.49	Diagnosis of GERD confirmed by response to PPI, esophagitis on endoscopy or abnormal esophageal pH
Peptic ulcer disease (20)	Overall clinical impression by GPs	61%	73%	2.26	0.53	Gold standard = endoscopic evidence of peptic ulcer disease
	Overall clinical impression by gastroenterologists	55%	84%	3.44	0.54	
Peptic ulcer disease (21)	Systematic review of clinical impressions by primary care physicians, specialists and computer models			2.2	0.45	Gold standard = endoscopic evidence of peptic ulcer disease
Functional dyspepsia (20)	Overall clinical impression by GPs	37%	76%	1.54	0.83	Other diagnoses excluded by endoscopy
	Overall clinical impression by gastroenterologists	59%	72%	2.11	0.57	
Organic dyspepsia (21)	Systematic review of clinical impressions by primary care physicians, specialists and computer models			1.6	0.46	Gold standard = endoscopic evidence of esophagitis r peptic ulcer disease
Peptic ulcer disease (vs other condition such as gastritis, duodenitis, malignancy or esophagitis (18,19)	Male gender	61%	58%	1.45	0.67	Gold standard = confirmed peptic ulcer disease, method of diagnosis not specified Gold standard = endoscopic evidence of peptic ulcer disease
	Main symptom is pain	77%	45%	1.40	0.51	
	Duration <2 years	66%	65%	1.89	0.52	
	Episodic pain	80%	50%	1.60	0.40	
	Epigastric pain	68%	62%	1.79	0.52	
	Food reduces pain	39%	88%	3.25	0.69	
	Symptoms awaken patient at night and are relieved with food	48%	83%	2.82	0.63	
	Vomiting	33%	75%	1.32	0.89	
	Waterbrash	42%	77%	1.83	0.75	
	Heartburn	65%	45%	1.18	0.78	
	Flatulence	58%	52%	1.21	0.81	
	Loss of appetite	50%	63%	1.35	0.79	
	Family history of ulcer	47%	70%	1.57	0.76	
	Smoker	73%	50%	1.46	0.54	
	Epigastric tenderness to deep palpation	52%	27%	0.71	1.78	

GERD = gastroesophageal reflux disease; GP = general practitioner.

TABLE 21.4 Accuracy of Diagnostic Tests Useful in Patients with Dyspepsia

Test	Sensitivity	Specificity	LR+	LR−	Comment
Gastroesophageal Reflux Disease					
Proton pump inhibitor test* (23)	78% (meta-analysis of five studies)	54% (meta-analysis of five studies)	1.70	0.41	Gold standard = abnormal 24-hour esophageal pH
Proton pump inhibitor test* (23)	68% (meta-analysis of six studies)	46% (meta-analysis of six studies)	1.26	0.70	Gold standard = esophagitis on endoscopy
Proton pump inhibitor test in patients with noncardiac chest pain* (24)	80% (meta-analysis of six studies)	74% (meta-analysis of six studies)	3.08	0.27	Gold standard = esophagitis on endoscopy and/or abnormal esophageal pH
Endoscopy (25)					Gold standard = abnormal esophageal pH
Esophageal erythema	22%	74%	0.85	1.05	
Esophageal erosions or ulcerations	48%	64%	1.33	0.81	
24-hour pH monitoring (26)					
Clinical impression of a gastroenterologist as the gold standard	72%	60%	1.79	0.47	
Esophagitis on endoscopy as the gold standard	79%	44%	1.41	0.48	
Esophageal erosions as the gold standard	93%	41%	1.58	0.17	
Peptic Ulcer Disease					
Any peptic ulcer (27)					Final diagnosis jointly made by radiologists and endoscopists
Endoscopy	92%	100%†	92	0.08	
Upper GI barium study	54%	91%	6	0.51	
Gastric ulcer (28)					No gold standard. Method of Hui and Walter (29) used for calculations
Endoscopy	85%	98%	42.5	0.15	
Upper GI barium study	91%	99%	91	0.09	
Duodenal ulcer (28)					
Endoscopy	99%	100%†	99	0.01	
Upper GI barium study	50%	99%	50	0.51	
***H. Pylori* Infection**					
Urea breath test (30)	95% (mean of 6 studies)	96% (mean of 6 studies)	22.02	0.06	Most studies used an endoscopic based method of confirming *H. pylori* as the gold standard
Stool antigen test (33)	92% (systematic review of 43 studies)	92% (systematic review of 43 studies)	11.41	0.08	
Serum IgG antibody tests (32)	85% (meta-analysis of 21 studies)	79% (meta-analysis of 21 studies)	4.05	0.19	
Whole-blood antibody tests (30)	71% (mean of 8 studies)	88% (mean of 8 studies)	5.73	0.33	

GERD = gastroesophageal reflux; GI = gastrointestinal; Ig = immunoglobulin; PPI = proton pump inhibitor.

*In studies reporting the use of proton pump inhibitor tests, patients were given a PPI at a standard or high dose for a period of 1–4 weeks. Depending on the study, a positive test response was defined as a complete resolution of symptoms or a partial improvement of symptoms as measured by the use of a symptom questionnaire. All patients had an objective diagnosis of GERD confirmed by either an abnormal esophageal pH study or evidence of esophagitis or erosions on upper endoscopy.

†Specificities of 100% were changed to 99% to calculate positive likelihood ratios.

immunosorbent assays. There is no significant difference in the accuracy of commonly used serum antibody kits (32). Although whole blood tests used in the ambulatory setting may be more convenient for the physician and patient, they are less sensitive than serum antibody tests performed in a reference laboratory (71% vs. 85%) and are not recommended (30). Finally, stool antigen tests detect *H. pylori* antigen in the stool and are more accurate than whole blood or serologic tests, although somewhat less convenient (33). They can also be used to confirm eradication, but concurrent use of PPIs can cause false-negative stool antigen results (34).

Current guidelines recommend breath tests or stool antigen tests as the preferred initial test to detect *H. pylori* infection (35,36). Serologic tests at a reference laboratory are an alternative if breath tests or stool antigen tests are not available or if the patient has recently taken a PPI.

FUNCTIONAL DYSPEPSIA

Functional dyspepsia is a diagnosis of exclusion. To conclusively diagnose it, one would have to perform endoscopy to definitively exclude structural conditions such as peptic ulcer disease, GERD, and cancer (2). However, for patients younger than age 55 years with no alarm symptoms (especially if *H. pylori* negative and not an NSAID user), the likelihood of finding a serious condition is very rare and endoscopy is not needed (37). Extensive diagnostic testing is not recommended in patients with functional dyspepsia, unless the patient's symptoms and signs suggest an alternate diagnosis.

Recommended Diagnostic Strategy

The recommended strategy outlined here is based on evidence-based guidelines from the American Gastroenterological Association published in 2005 on the management of dyspepsia and in 2008 on the management of GERD (1,16,38). Figure 21.1 presents an algorithm for diagnosing and managing patients with dyspepsia. If the patient has any red flags (Table 21.2) or is older than age 55 with the onset of new symptoms, arrange endoscopy to look for malignancy or complicated peptic ulcer. Patients in acute distress or who are unstable require immediate, emergent stabilization, diagnosis, and management.

For patients with typical GERD symptoms of heartburn and acid regurgitation and without alarm symptoms, empirical treatment with a PPI is an option. If patients respond to the treatment, GERD is the likely diagnosis and one can continue the treatment. However, if the patient does not respond to initial treatment, further diagnostic evaluation such as an endoscopy may be considered.

Patients taking an NSAID or cyclooxygenase-2 inhibitor or other medications such as erythromycin or metformin should discontinue the drug if possible and use alternative medication. A PPI may be added if needed.

For patients with typical dyspeptic symptoms who are 55 years of age or younger and have no alarm symptoms, three possible strategies predominate: 1) a strategy of early endoscopy in which all patients with dyspepsia are referred for an endoscopy as part of the initial evaluation, 2) a strategy of empiric acid suppression in which all patients are given a PPI at the onset of symptoms, and 3) a "test and treat" strategy in which one tests the patient with dyspepsia for an *H. pylori* infection. Patients with a positive test result are treated with medication to eradicate *H. pylori*. Those with negative *H. pylori* test results are given acid suppression treatment with a PPI to control their symptoms.

In one study comparing the three strategies, the early endoscopy strategy resulted in fewer consultations for dyspepsia later on, whereas the empirical PPI strategy resulted in the lowest initial costs, though these were offset by the highest frequency of subsequent endoscopy. The "test and treat" strategy was the most cost effective strategy, although the authors were careful to remind readers to consider early endoscopy in older patients (39).

In comparing the "test and treat" strategy with early endoscopy, a long-term study following patients for a median of 6.7 years found that the "test and treat" strategy was more cost-effective than the immediate endoscopy strategy by resulting in fewer endoscopies and less antisecretory medication. Regarding the concern that the "test and treat" strategy would miss a case of cancer, this study found that in the "test and treat" group of 250 patients, only 2 were diagnosed with gastric cancer at the beginning of the study and only 1 was diagnosed with esophageal cancer 2.6 years into the study (40). Although other studies note a slight improvement in symptoms with an early endoscopy strategy (number needed to treat [NNT] = 25 to benefit one patient after 1 year), there is an increased cost of $255 per patient (1).

Previous studies confirm that an empiric PPI strategy is effective in relieving symptoms after 1 year (NNT = 5 compared with placebo and to a histamine$_2$ receptor antagonists [H_2RA]) (1). In comparing the "test and treat" strategy with the empiric PPI strategy, a recent study and a meta-analysis of recent trials concluded that there was no significant difference between the two strategies in terms of cost and improvement of symptoms (41,42). Current guidelines recommend using the prevalence of *H. pylori* infection in the community to determine which strategy to use. If the prevalence of *H. pylori* infection in the community is >5%, they recommend using the "test and treat" strategy, whereas if the prevalence of *H. pylori* infection is <5%, they recommend using the empiric PPI strategy (1). Because the prevalence of *H. pylori* is unknown in many communities, the most prudent strategy is to follow the "test and treat" strategy in most instances, and reserve the empiric PPI strategy for use in communities with a documented prevalence of *H. pylori* infection is <5%.

In further investigations of the "test and treat" strategy, additional studies confirm the effectiveness of the different management options that are used depending on the patient's *H. pylori* status. In patients found to have a *H. pylori* infection, a randomized trial confirms that giving eradication treatment and a PPI to *H. pylori*–infected patients is superior in relieving symptoms compared to giving a placebo antibiotics and a PPI for the *H. pylori* infection (43). In patients found not to have a *H. pylori* infection, another randomized trial confirmed that giving a PPI to *H. pylori* negative patients was more effective than a placebo and other medications in relieving symptoms (44).

Whether one uses the "test and treat" strategy or the empiric PPI strategy, one recent meta-analysis reports that many patients will still have some symptoms after 1 year (up to 83% using the "test and treat" strategy and up to 84.5% using the empiric PPI strategy) (42). Patients who have

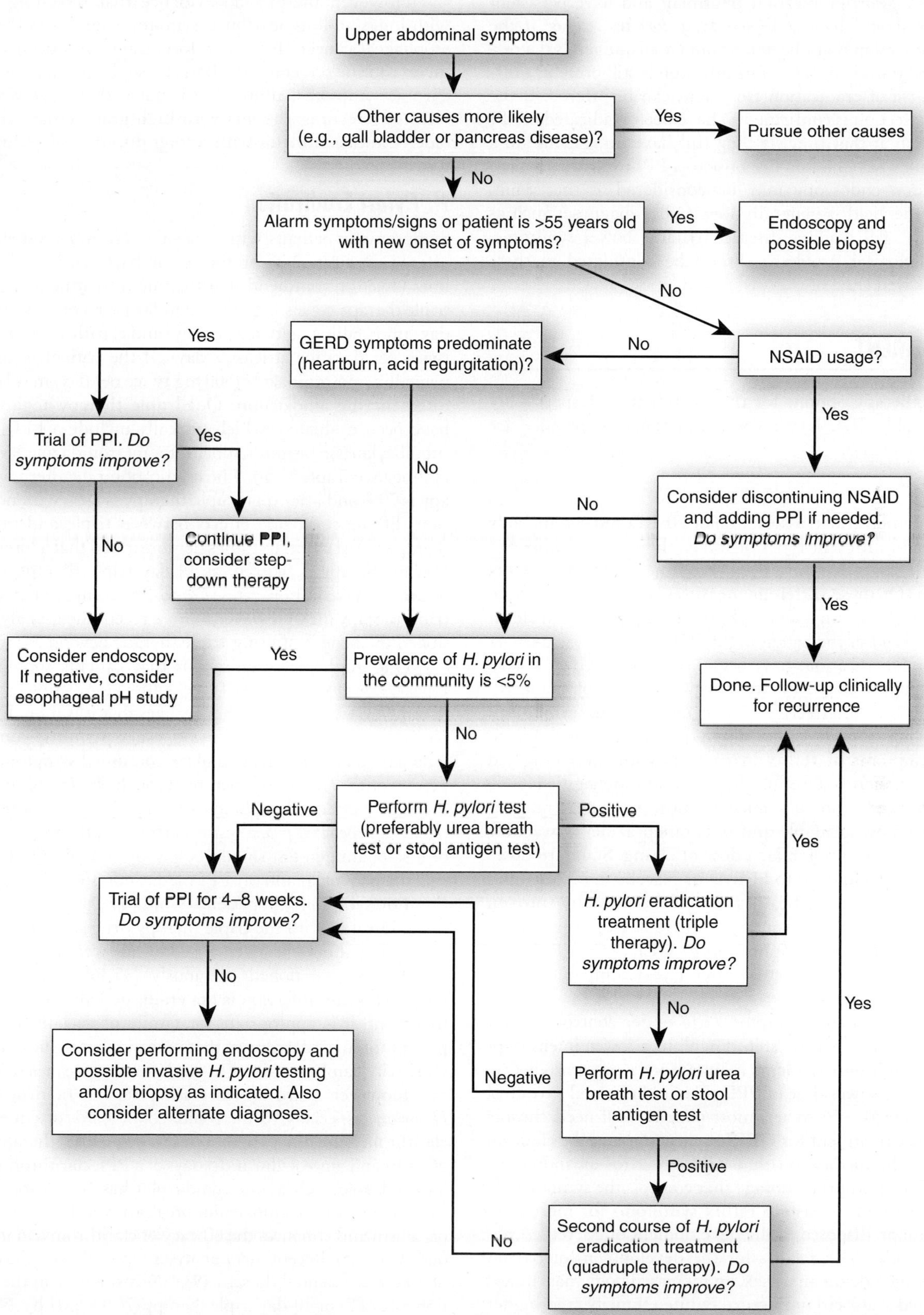

Figure 21.1 • Algorithm of diagnosis and management of patients with dyspepsia. (Compiled using data from 1,11,12,16,35,36,38.)

received *H. pylori* eradication treatment and have persistent symptoms should have a repeat *H. pylori* test to see if the *H. pylori* infection is eradicated or not (stool antigen is the recommended test). If the *H. pylori* infection is still present, a different course of eradication treatment can be offered. If the *H. pylori* infection is confirmed to have been eradicated, a PPI can be given at that time. If they still have no response to a PPI or if they have had no response to a PPI using the empiric PPI strategy, endoscopy may be considered at that point, although the yield is generally low. Other diagnoses such as pancreatitis, gall bladder disease, irritable bowel syndrome, and psychological problems should be considered in these patients as well (12,38).

MANAGEMENT

Pharmacotherapy options for the treatment of dyspepsia are listed in Table 21.5. Key recommendations for practice are listed in Table 21.6.

GERD

With the demonstrated association of GERD and certain body positions and different types of foods, there are a number of lifestyle measures that have been recommended to help reflux symptoms. Of these different measures, there is evidence to support weight loss in overweight or obese patients and elevation of the head of the bed at night (45).

Several medications have been used to treat GERD. Two types of medications, PPIs and histamine$_2$ receptor antagonists (H_2RAs), are effective in alleviating reflux symptoms. PPIs are more effective than H_2RAs as initial treatment to relieve symptoms of reflux in patients with uninvestigated heartburn, nonerosive reflux disease, and esophagitis (46,47) and are the medication of choice for most patients. A number of PPIs are now available and one, omeprazole, is available over the counter in a standard dose of 20 mg. Standard doses of PPIs are also superior to H_2RAs or placebo in maintaining symptom relief and healing of endoscopically proven esophagitis (48) and preventing recurrent esophageal strictures, an uncommon complication of GERD (NNT = 8 to prevent one recurrent stricture after 1 year compared with a H_2RA) (49).

After the patient's symptoms are under control, at least one-third of patients can "step down" to a lower intensity of treatment, with some patients maintaining symptom relief on H_2RAs or on a lower dose of PPIs than initially used to control symptoms (50,51). However, most patients will need chronic maintenance treatment for GERD symptoms and the clinician should use the medication that works best for an individual patient at an appropriate dosage that controls the symptoms.

Patients with persistent reflux symptoms for more than 10 years are predisposed to the development of Barrett esophagus (52). Other risk factors for the development of Barrett esophagus include the male sex, an increased body mass index, an increased waist circumference, white ethnicity, and higher socioeconomic status, although there is an inverse association with *H. pylori* infection (53–56). Long-standing reflux symptoms (57) as well as the development of high-grade dysplasia (58) in the Barrett epithelium are risk factors for esophageal adenocarcinoma.

However, there is no evidence that screening patients with longstanding heartburn symptoms decreases the risk of esophageal cancer (16). Therefore, guidelines do not recommend routine screening for Barrett esophagus in patients with chronic symptoms, although it is noted that there is a higher yield of screening patients with high-grade esophagitis or in older Caucasian males with a long duration of reflux symptoms (16,59).

H. Pylori Eradication

Symptomatic patients with a positive *H. pylori* test should be offered medication to eradicate the bacteria. Current guidelines (35,36) recommend that the initial treatment regimen be triple therapy consisting of the standard does of a PPI twice per day, amoxicillin (1 g twice per day) and clarithromycin (500 mg twice per day) for at least 7 days. If the patient is allergic to penicillin, metronidazole (500 mg twice per day) may be substituted for the amoxicillin. Quadruple therapy regimens also have been evaluated, which typically include a PPI, bismuth subsalicylate or bismuth subcitrate, metronidazole, and tetracycline (See Table 21.5.). The eradication rate after triple therapy is 79% and after quadruple therapy is 80% with no significant difference in side effects between triple and quadruple therapy (60,61). Initial studies demonstrated that a longer duration of therapy is helpful, as 14-day triple therapy regimens improved eradication rates 7% to 9% compared with 7-day triple therapy (62). However, a more recent meta-analysis questioned the benefit of using triple therapy beyond 7 days (63).

One guideline recommends that patients should have a repeat *H. pylori* test at least 4 weeks after completing eradication therapy (35), whereas another realizes that it is more feasible to recommend that a repeat *H. pylori* test be performed on patients who have a *H. pylori*-related ulcer, continued symptoms of dyspepsia after *H. pylori* treatment or have *H. pylori*–related mucosal associated lymphoid tissue lymphoma or gastric cancer (36). If a repeat *H. pylori* test is performed, the urea breath test or a stool antigen test should be performed (35,36). (For either test, the patient should off PPI medication for at least 2 weeks.)

For symptomatic patients whose *H. pylori* infection was not eradicated with the triple therapy drug regimen described above, they should be given a second-line treatment of quadruple therapy mentioned previously (35,36). For the patient whose *H. pylori* infection is not eradicated after two courses of treatment, it is appropriate for family physicians to refer the patient for an endoscopy at that point so that tissue culture and sensitivity can be obtained to guide further treatment (1).

However, there are increasing reports of drug-resistant *H. pylori*, especially to metronidazole (36.9% of patients) and clarithromycin (10.1%) (64). Ten-day sequential therapy (5 days of a PPI and amoxicillin and 5 days of a PPI, clarithromycin, and an imidazole such as metronidazole) has been proposed as a solution in that the amoxicillin breaks down the cell wall of the organism and enhances the efficacy of clarithromycin in the second stage (65). Recent meta-analyses report that eradication rate of 10-day sequential therapy (93.4%) is superior to the eradication rate of 7- or 10-day triple therapy (76.9%), with a NNT = 6 for one patient to benefit. However, limitations included some low-quality studies, publication bias, most studies occurring in Italy and no studies comparing sequential therapy to 14-day triple therapy or to quadruple therapy (66–68).

(text continues on page 252)

TABLE 21.5 Medications Options for the Treatment of Dyspepsia

Drug	Contraindications/Cautions/ Adverse Effects	Dosage	Relative Cost*
GERD, Peptic Ulcer Disease, and Functional Dyspepsia			
H_2 receptor antagonists	Headache, constipation, diarrhea, nausea/ vomiting, abdominal pain are rare adverse effects. Cimetidine interacts with some medications such as warfarin, theophylline and phenytoin; adjust for renal function.	Higher doses may be needed in GERD	$
Proton pump inhibitor	Diarrhea, abdominal pain and bloating are rare adverse effects Risk of community-acquired pneumonia, *Clostridium difficile* colitis, association with hip fractures	Standard dose every day	$$$ (trade) $ (generic)
***H. Pylori* Eradication Therapy**			
Triple therapy (35,36)			
PPI	See above	Standard dose 2 times/day	$$$
+Clarithromycin	Nausea, abnormal taste, headache or exacerbation of dyspepsia; diarrhea or antibiotic-associated colitis; not recommended for pregnant women; may interact with medication metabolized by the CYP3A system such as certain statin drugs	500 mg po 2 times/day	$$
+Amoxicillin (substitute metronidazole if allergic to penicillin)	Rash or drug allergy, diarrhea, antibiotic-associated colitis	1,000 mg po 2 times/ day for amoxicillin (500 mg po 2 times/ day for metronidazole)	$
Quadruple Therapy (Regimen reported in reference 36)			
PPI	See above	Standard dose 1 or 2 times/d	$$$
+Bismuth subsalicylate/ subcitrate	Bismuth subsalicylate cannot be used in aspirin-allergic patients. May cause a darkened tongue and dark stools.	525 po 4 times/day	$
+Metronidazole	May cause a metallic taste in the mouth. Causes a disulfiram-like reaction if the patient drinks alcohol while on this. Not recommended in the first trimester of pregnancy. Interacts with medications such as warfarin.	500 mg po 4 times/day	$
+Tetracycline	Not for use in pregnancy or children. Better absorbed on an empty stomach. Antacids may decrease its efficacy. Photosensitivity reactions are possible.	500 mg po 4 times/day	$

GERD = gastroesophageal reflux; H_2RA = histamine$_2$ receptor antagonists; Ig = immunoglobulin; PPI = proton pump inhibitor; po = by mouth.
*Relative cost: $, <$33.00; $$, $34.00–$66.00; $$$, >$67.00.

TABLE 21.6 Management Options and Efficacy

Intervention	Efficacy	Strength of Recommendation*
Initial Evaluation		
If alarm symptoms or patient is above the age of 55 years old with new symptoms, arrange endoscopy as the initial test (15)	Positive predictive value of alarm symptoms: • 4% for cancer • 13%–14% for ulcer disease or esophagitis	B
Gastroesophageal Reflux Disease		
Lifestyle measures: elevate head of bed and weight loss (45)	More randomized controlled studies needed for these and other lifestyle measures	B
Use of a PPI as a short-term medication to empirically relieve symptoms in patients with reflux symptoms (46)	PPIs more effective than placebo (RR = .37) and H_2RAs (RR = .66) in reducing heartburn	A
Use a PPI as short-term medication to relieve symptoms in patients with nonerosive reflux disease (46)	PPIs more effective than placebo (RR = .69) and H_2RAs (RR = .78) in reducing heartburn	A
Use of a PPI as maintenance medication for patients with nonerosive reflux disease (51)	At 6 months, 47% of patients taking placebo were more likely to discontinue medication due to inadequate relief of heartburn compared to 18.6% of patients taking omeprazole	B
Use of a PPI as short-term medication to relieve reflux symptoms and signs of esophagitis in patients with reflux esophagitis (47)	PPIs more effective than placebo (NNT = 1.7) and H_2RAs (NNT = 3) in healing esophagitis	A
Use of a PPI as maintenance medication for patients with reflux esophagitis (48)	PPIs at a standard dose more effective than placebo (NNT = 1.7) and H_2RAs (NNT = 2.5) in maintaining healed esophagitis.	A
Uninvestigated Dyspepsia without Alarm Symptoms and Age of 55 or Younger		
If the patient lives in a community with the prevalence of *H. pylori* infection >5%, test and treat for *H. pylori* infection as the initial diagnostic strategy in patients (1,40)	• No differences in symptoms, quality of life or satisfaction after a median of 6.7 years compared to a group that received early endoscopy. • Lower rates of anti-secretory therapy in the test and treat group (275 defined daily doses compared to 373 defined daily doses in the early endoscopy group) • Lower rates of endoscopy in the test and treat group (0.88 endoscopies per patient compared to 1.50 endoscopies per patient in the early endoscopy group) • In a meta-analysis of 5 studies, slightly greater likelihood of controlling symptoms at one year in early endoscopy group compared to a test and treat group (NNT = 25), but at the cost of $255 per patient	A
If *H. pylori*-positive, give *H. pylori* eradication treatment (1,43)	Eradication treatment more effective than placebo (NNT = 7–9) in relieving symptoms of dyspepsia at one year in *H. pylori* positive patients	A
If *H. pylori*-negative, use a PPI to control symptoms (44)	Omeprazole more effective than ranitidine (NNT = 7) and placebo (NNT = 4) in controlling symptoms of dyspepsia at 4 weeks in *H. pylori* negative patients	B

TABLE 21.6 *(Continued)*

Intervention	Efficacy	Strength of Recommendation*
If the patient lives in a community with the prevalence of *H. pylori* infection <5%, give a trial of PPI as initial therapy (1)	PPIs more effective than placebo and antacids (NNT = 5) and H_2RAs (NNT = 5) in relieving symptoms of dyspepsia	A
Documented Peptic Ulcer Disease		
If *H. pylori*-positive, give eradication treatment to heal duodenal ulcers, prevent recurrent ulcer, and prevent bleeding (69,70)	*H. pylori* eradication treatment + PPI vs PPI alone for healing duodenal ulcer. NNT is 2 to 3 for prevention of recurrent ulcer. NNT is 7 for prevention of recurrent bleeding.	A
If *H. pylori*-negative, but the ulcer is NSAID-related, give a PPI to heal ulcer and prevent recurrent ulcer (72,73)	PPI more effective than misoprostol or ranitidine. Recurrence also less likely with omeprazole than ranitidine (72% vs 59% for NSAID related ulcer).	B
If *H. pylori*-negative and the ulcer is not NSAID-related, give a PPI (74)		C
Perform an initial biopsy of gastric ulcers and repeat biopsy after appropriate treatment (76,77)	For 50 patients undergoing repeat endoscopy after treatment of a benign ulcer, 1 patient will be identified who will survive gastric cancer 5 years after a gastrectomy	B
Functional Dyspepsia (other conditions ruled out)		
If *H. pylori*-positive, give a triple therapy regimen to improve symptoms (78)	*H. pylori* eradication therapy has a small effect on relieving symptoms of functional dyspepsia at 1 year compared to placebo (NNT = 14)	B
If *H. pylori*-negative, give a PPI or H_2RA to relieve symptoms (80,81)	• PPIs more effective than placebo in relieving symptoms of functional dyspepsia (NNT = 10.0–14.6) • H_2RAs more effective than placebo in relieving symptoms of functional dyspepsia (NNT = 7) • PPIs more effective than H_2RAs in relieving symptoms of functional dyspepsia, but the difference is not significant (RRR = 7%)	B
***H. pylori* Eradication Regimens**		
Triple therapy (60,61)	Efficacy in eradicating *H. pylori* infection = 79%. See Table 5 for more detail. Conflicting evidence whether 14-day therapy more effective than 7-day therapy	A
Quadruple therapy (60,61)	Efficacy in eradicating *H. pylori* infection = 80%. See Table 5 for more detail	A
Sequential therapy (66,68)	93.4% efficacy for sequential therapy in eradicating *H. pylori* infection compared to 76.9% for triple therapy of 7–10 days (NNT = 6)	B

GERD = gastroesophageal reflux; H_2RA = histamine$_2$ receptor antagonists; Ig = immunoglobulin; NNT = number needed to treat; PPI = proton pump inhibitor; po = by mouth.
*A = consistent, good-quality patient-oriented evidence; B = inconsistent or limited-quality patient-oriented evidence; C = consensus, disease-oriented evidence, usual practice, expert opinion, or case series.
For information about the Strength of Recommendation Taxonomy evidence rating system, see *http://www.aafp.org/afpsort.xml*.

The patient whose infection is successfully eradicated but who has persistent dyspeptic symptoms likely does not have a peptic ulcer. A 4-week course of acid suppression treatment, usually with a PPI, is appropriate as a next step. If symptoms resolve at that point, the PPI can be discontinued. If symptoms do not resolve, the PPI can be continued with reevaluation for the need for the PPI every 6 to 12 months. Consideration can be given to performing an endoscopy at that point, although the diagnostic yield is low (1).

PUD

Patients with *H. pylori* positive PUD should have therapy to eradicate *H. pylori* and optionally a PPI for symptom control. The combination of *H. pylori* eradication and a PPI in patients with known peptic ulcer disease results in a slightly higher rate of duodenal ulcer healing compared with an ulcer-healing drug alone. In addition, *H. pylori* eradication prevents recurrent duodenal ulcers (69) and recurrent ulcer bleeding (70). Studies have confirmed the cost-effectiveness of eradicating an *H. pylori* infection in a patient with peptic ulcer disease (71).

For the patient who is *H. pylori*-negative but has an NSAID-related ulcer, PPIs are the most useful medication for both eradicating the ulcer and preventing its recurrence (72,73). If the patient with a peptic ulcer has no *H. pylori* infection and has not used NSAIDs, PPIs can be offered for symptomatic relief of the peptic ulcer, although a recent study cautioned that *H. pylori*-negative, NSAID-negative ulcers are rare and patients with this condition deserve further investigation to rule out *H. pylori* infection or NSAID use; *H. pylori*-negative ulcers may also be more difficult to treat (74). Empiric *H. pylori* eradication is also an option, especially if the patient is from a community with a high prevalence of *H. pylori* infection (75).

Special consideration should be given to patients with gastric ulcers. A biopsy of the ulcer should be performed on the initial endoscopy. *H. pylori* eradication treatment if indicated or a PPI can then be offered to heal the ulcer. Because there are reported cases of gastric cancer occurring despite a negative initial biopsy (76), a repeat endoscopy with biopsy should be performed after treatment, since a recent study reporting that for every 50 patients undergoing repeat endoscopy, 1 patient will be identified who will survive gastric cancer 5 years after a gastrectomy (77).

FUNCTIONAL DYSPEPSIA

There have been numerous studies evaluating the effectiveness of *H. pylori* eradication treatment in patients with functional dyspepsia who are *H. pylori*-positive, and the results have been conflicting. The most recent Cochrane review concluded that there is a small benefit in improving symptoms, with 14 patients needing to be treated to benefit 1 patient (78). Eradication rates for *H. pylori* infection in patients with functional dyspepsia are lower than that in patients with duodenal ulcer disease (79). Also, most patients will still have symptoms after completing the eradication treatment (78). For patients with functional dyspepsia who continue to have symptoms after their *H. pylori* infection is eradicated, it is reasonable to offer them a short trial of a PPI (1).

For patients with functional dyspepsia who are *H. pylori* negative, antisecretory therapy with a PPI or H_2RA is more effective than placebo (NNT for PPIs = 10.0 to 14.6) (80,81). PPIs were slightly more effective than H_2RAs, but the effect was not significant (80). A recent randomized controlled study demonstrated the effectiveness of itopride, a dopamine D2 antagonist with anti-acetylcholinesterase effects, but this medication is not currently available in the United States (82).

For patients with functional dyspepsia who do not respond to *H. pylori* eradication or a PPI, if symptoms are suggestive consider other conditions such as biliary or pancreatic disease, celiac disease, or gastroparesis (1). Psychological approaches and psychiatric medication have also been investigated in patients with functional dyspepsia. There is insufficient evidence to determine if psychological approaches such as psychotherapy, relaxation techniques, or hypnotherapy are useful (83). Reviews suggest that antianxiety or antidepressive medication (primarily tricyclic antidepressants) may be useful in patients with functional dyspepsia, but more study is needed (84,85). A more recent randomized controlled trial showed no benefit of using venlafaxine (a selective serotonin and norepinephrine uptake inhibitor) in patients with functional dyspepsia compared with placebo (86).

KEY POINTS

- Perform a history and physical examination to evaluate the patient's dyspepsia and to rule out other causes of abdominal pain.
- Patients with alarm symptoms or with symptoms starting after 55 years of age should receive an endoscopy as the initial diagnostic test. Unstable patients should be admitted to the hospital for stabilization and further evaluation.
- Patients without alarm symptoms who present with heartburn or other GERD symptoms may be offered a PPI as the initial therapy.
- Patients without alarm symptoms may be offered a test and treat strategy, with testing for an *H. pylori* infection as the first step and eradication offered to those with an infection. A PPI may be offered if there is no *H. pylori* infection.
- For patients in communities with a low prevalence of *H. pylori* infection, a PPI may be given empirically as the initial therapy.
- Most patients with dyspepsia have functional dyspepsia. These patients may be offered *H. pylori* eradication therapy if indicated or a PPI. Some patients with functional dyspepsia will be difficult to treat.

CHAPTER

22

Lower Intestinal Symptoms

Charles M. Kodner

Lower abdominal symptoms are caused by a wide range of conditions, from innocent to life-threatening, many of which may initially present with subtle symptoms. Diagnosis involves judicious selection of imaging studies to complement the history and physical examination, balancing the need to avoid overtesting this large population of patients against the need to accurately diagnose specific conditions. Although specific management is available for many conditions, empiric or symptomatic care for functional intestinal symptoms is often appropriate. The aim of this chapter is to discuss efficient diagnostic and management strategies for some of the most common lower abdominal complaints: lower gastrointestinal (LGI) bleeding, acute and chronic diarrhea, and constipation.

LOWER INTESTINAL BLEEDING

CLINICAL OBJECTIVES

1. List common causes of lower intestinal bleeding in adults.
2. Describe an initial diagnostic evaluation strategy for patients who have evidence of lower intestinal bleeding.
3. Describe a diagnostic approach for adult patients with lower intestinal bleeding and no evident source on initial endoscopic evaluation.

Acute LGI bleeding is one of the most common reasons for hospital admission, estimated at 20 to 30 per 100,000 population, with increasing rates in older age (1). LGI bleeding may present in different ways, depending on the underlying pathology and on the rate of intestinal blood loss. With slow, chronic bleeding, patients may be asymptomatic and are often identified through an incidentally abnormal Hemoccult test, hemoglobin, or hematocrit. Upper gastrointestinal (UGI) blood loss, with slower transit through the colon, classically presents with dark or tarry stools (melena), although more rapid transit or brisk UGI bleeding may present as red blood per rectum. Initial or recurrent episodes of bright red blood per rectum (hematochezia) may indicate lower intestinal pathology, and patients may present with complaints of varying amounts of blood loss, from droplets on toilet tissue to more brisk bleeding. Finally, patients may present with acute, massive rectal bleeding requiring urgent intervention, including transfusion.

After LGI bleeding has been identified, colonoscopy is typically the initial step to identify a LGI bleeding source. Exceptions include patients in whom an upper GI source is clinically suspected, who should undergo esophagogastroduodenoscopy first, and young patients with an apparent perianal source such as a hemorrhoid for whom anoscopy with close clinical follow-up may be sufficient. Improvements in endoscopic techniques have prompted a shift in terminology for GI bleeding; rather than classify bleeding as upper or lower (proximal or distal to the ligament of Treitz), some experts recommend classifying bleeding as upper (above the ampulla of Vater), mid (small intestinal, from the ampulla of Vater to the terminal ileum), or lower (colonic) GI bleeding (2).

DIFFERENTIAL DIAGNOSIS

Among adult patients undergoing diagnostic evaluation, the most common causes of LGI bleeding are diverticular disease, ischemic colitis, angiodysplasia, neoplasm, and benign anorectal bleeding (1) (Table 22.1). The causes of LGI bleeding in children are different, and include disorders such as juvenile polyposis (including hereditary polyposis syndromes), inflammatory bowel disease, Meckel diverticulum, Henoch-Schönlein purpura, and intussusception. The remainder of this discussion will focus on bleeding in adults.

CLINICAL EVALUATION

History and Physical Examination

The history should identify previous episodes of GI bleeding and any associated workup; attempt to quantify the amount of blood lost and the frequency of bleeding; and identify patient symptoms such as abdominal pain, diarrhea, passage of mucus, perianal discomfort, fever, or other complaints that will help to localize the source of bleeding. Patients should also be asked specifically about contributory medical conditions, including: peptic ulcer disease; liver disease or alcohol use; bleeding disorders or bruising; and use of any medications such as nonsteroidal anti-inflammatory drugs, warfarin, aspirin, clopidogrel, or other antiplatelet agents.

The role of the physical examination is primarily to assess the degree of hemodynamic compromise (blood pressure, orthostatic vital signs, overall clinical appearance, signs of anemia, or volume loss), although some clinical conditions causing LGI bleeding also have physical exam findings. Examples include stigmata of cirrhosis (spider angiomas, hepatomegaly, jaundice), bruising, and malnutrition from colorectal cancer. Perianal examination should be performed to evaluate for fissures, hemorrhoids, or fistulae. The role of Hemoccult testing in patients who already complain of rectal bleeding is unclear, and a negative Hemoccult test should not impede further investigation of a reliable history of rectal bleeding.

TABLE 22.1 Common Causes of Lower Intestinal Bleeding in Hospitalized Patients

Diagnosis	Typical Presentation	Frequency (%)*
Diverticulosis	Painless bleeding, possibly constipation	24
Other colitis (infectious, antibiotic-associated)	Bloody diarrhea, abdominal pain, fever	14
Ischemic colitis	Maroon-colored stools, abdominal pain, other vascular disease	12
Benign anorectal disease (hemorrhoids, anal fissure, fistula)	Fissures: perianal itching or tearing Internal hemorrhoids: painless bleeding, possibly external hemorrhoids or perianal itching or burning Fistula: history of inflammatory bowel disease, perianal discharge, visible fistula opening	12
Colorectal cancer	Microscopic blood (positive Hemoccult), microcytic anemia, weight loss, altered bowel habits	7
Postpolypectomy	Bleeding following procedure	5
Inflammatory bowel disease	Diarrhea with bleeding, abdominal pain, weight loss	3
Arteriovenous malformation (angiodysplasia)	Painless bleeding, may be recurrent without previously identified cause	2
Any small bowel or upper gastrointestinal cause	Chronic gastritis: alcohol use, nonsteroidal anti-inflammatory drug (NSAID) use Variceal bleeding: chronic liver disease Peptic ulcer: gnawing abdominal pain, NSAID use Small bowel disorders: angiodysplasia, vascular disease, small bowel tumors, Meckel's diverticulum	7
Unknown		12

*This is a nonweighted average frequency from studies in Reference 1, consisting primarily of patients hospitalized for lower gastrointestinal bleeding.

Diagnostic Testing

Patients with LGI bleeding should have a complete blood count performed to evaluate for anemia or thrombocytopenia. Serum ferritin, reticulocyte count testing, and other studies as indicated should be ordered if the cause of anemia remains unclear. Routine chemistry testing (including serum albumin if poor nutritional status is suspected) and coagulation studies may provide diagnostic clues in some patients. Many imaging and functional tests are available to assess for LGI bleeding; the indications and use of these tests is summarized here and in Table 22.2.

Recommended Diagnostic Strategy

The first diagnostic step should be to attempt to exclude UGI bleeding. Approximately 2% to 15% of patients presenting with LGI bleeding will have an UGI source (1). Nasogastric lavage containing gross blood, 25% blood-tinged fluid, or strongly Hemoccult positive dark fluid is highly specific for an UGI source of bleeding, but is not very sensitive (approximately 40%); this test is no longer commonly performed because of limited diagnostic impact, and is best reserved for patients with brisk bleeding in whom esophagogastroduodenoscopy (EGD) is not already planned (1,5). The blood urea nitrogen-to-creatinine ratio is not sufficiently accurate to guide clinical decision making. Although highly specific if >36, it is insensitive at that level (approximately 10%) (6). Diagnostic approaches for different patient presentations are outlined below.

OBSCURE BLEEDING

Obscure GI bleeding, or bleeding from the GI tract that persists or recurs without an obvious cause after diagnostic evaluation, is categorized as obscure-overt bleeding (if bleeding is clinically evident) or occult bleeding (if it is not). Approximately half of occult bleeding cases remain undiagnosed; depending on age, colon cancer is identified in 2% to 17% of patients (2). Patients with occult GI blood loss and no anemia should have colonoscopy performed, as well as upper endoscopy if upper GI tract symptoms are present (2). No additional testing is recommended in most patients if these investigations are negative.

Previous guidelines for patients with persistent bleeding and initially negative upper and lower endoscopy recommended stepwise testing with red blood cell scans, angiography, enteroclysis, small bowel series, or other tests. However, in light of current technologic advances and the low diagnostic yield of these tests, wireless capsule endoscopy should be considered the "third test" in many patients if bleeding recurs. Overall, lesions in the small intestine account for roughly 5% of causes of obscure LGI bleeding (2).

In those with occult GI blood loss, iron deficiency anemia, and negative EGD and colonoscopy, small intestinal bleeding from angiodysplasia or small bowel tumors is a common diagnosis and capsule endoscopy is indicated (2). In patients with obscure GI bleeding, anemia, and overt melena or maroon blood per rectum, repeat endoscopy may be revealing, particularly if cap-fitted or side-viewing endoscopic methods are used.

TABLE 22.2 Diagnostic Studies for Lower Intestinal Bleeding*

Test	Description	Clinical Diagnostic Role
EGD	Direct visualization of the upper GI tract	Often an initial test for LGI bleeding where an upper source is suspected; may be repeated in cases of obscure LGI bleeding particularly in patients with hematemesis or NSAID use
Colonoscopy	Direct visualization of entire colon	Preferred test for initial and recurrent bleeding, allows biopsy and local treatment as well as diagnosis; may be repeated in cases of obscure LGI bleeding, especially in elderly patients
Capsule endoscopy	Swallowed radiotelemetry capsule allows visualization of entire small intestine	Preferred test for obscure LGI bleeding with negative EGD and colonoscopy; more sensitive than push enteroscopy
Anoscopy	Direct visualization of distal rectum and anus	Evaluate for internal hemorrhoids especially if history of constipation or external hemorrhoids on examination
Double-contrast barium enema	Air injected into bowel to contrast with residual barium to visualize bowel mucosa	Option if colonoscopy cannot be performed
Small bowel "push" enteroscopy	Extension of upper endoscopy to visualize 15–160 cm of small bowel distal to Treitz ligament	Potentially long procedure times and patient discomfort but higher diagnostic yield than small bowel radiography
SBFT	Timed radiographic imaging following ingestion of contrast dye	May identify signs of colitis or structural lesion causing small bowel bleeding
Enteroclysis	Barium delivered via tube directly to small intestine with radiographic imaging	More uncomfortable but higher diagnostic yield and sensitivity than SBFT
Technetium-99m-tagged red blood cell scan	Nuclear medicine imaging 12–24 hours after injection of labeled RBCs, no bowel preparation required	May be helpful to localize site of bleeding exceeding 0.1–0.4 mL/min
Meckel scan	Nuclear medicine imaging of abdomen following intravenous radioactive isotope	Helpful to identify small bowel bleeding only if positive; does not rule out small bowel bleed if negative*
Arteriography	Intravenous contrast agent with subsequent imaging of vascular supply, no bowel preparation required	Identifies bleeding into gut lumen if rate >0.5 mL/min; may identify typical vascular patterns in non-actively bleeding angiodysplasia or neoplasia Allows therapeutic interventions but some risk for complications
Abdominal computed tomography scan	Contrast two-dimensional imaging of abdomen	May identify larger neoplasms or nonspecific inflammatory changes, but cannot identify source of bleeding

EGD = esophagogastroduodenoscopy; GI = gastrointestinal; LGI = lower GI; NSAID = nonsteroidal anti-inflammatory drug; SBFT = small-bowel follow-through; UGI = upper GI.
*Information drawn from References 1 through 4.

The rebleeding rate for angiodysplasia lesions is not known, but approximately half may not rebleed (2); thus, patients without a diagnosis after initial upper, mid and lower endoscopy may be followed conservatively, with monitoring for worsening anemia or grossly evident bleeding. Such patients might be cautiously reassured that no small or large intestinal cancer was identified on initial testing and further testing can be avoided, though regular colonoscopic surveillance may be indicated. Fortunately, <1% of patients younger than age 40 with nonacute rectal bleeding have cancer (7).

NONMASSIVE GROSS BLEEDING (HEMATOCHEZIA)

The evaluation of patients with grossly evident rectal bleeding should begin with an assessment of vitals and fluid status, physical examination for benign anorectal disease, abdominal examination, and complete blood count. A nontender abdominal examination actually increases the risk of severe bleeding because vascular and diverticular bleeding are typically more severe but are nonpainful and nontender to examination. Patients should undergo EGD for suspected UGI bleeding and colonoscopy if the diagnosis remains unclear, or if LGI bleeding seems most likely. Patients who are younger than age 40 have a very low incidence of colorectal cancer (8), but evaluation of the entire colon may still be necessary for cases of undiagnosed, severe, or recurrent LGI bleeding.

The timing of a colonoscopy can be determined by stratifying patients into high- or low-risk groups for severe bleeding after initial presentation. A validated clinical decision rule has identified key risk factors for "severe bleeding," defined as continued bleeding within 24 hours of hospital admission and/or recurrent bleeding after 24 hours of stability (Table 22.3). Patients with three or more of these risk factors have a high (approximately 80%) risk of severe bleeding, and patients with no risk factors have a much lower risk (approximately 10%) (9). Whereas patients at high risk for severe bleeding have improved outcomes with urgent colonoscopy (within 12 hours of admission), patients at low risk might safely be referred for less urgent evaluation.

In cases of continued active bleeding, American Gastroenterological Association (AGA) guidelines recommend (2) small bowel visualization via capsule endoscopy or enteroscopy (4), which may confirm the small bowel as the site of bleeding. Other tests, including nuclear red blood cell scan, angiography, enteroscopy, enteroclysis, or small bowel series have declined in use in recent years, though may be indicated in specific circumstances. For example, patients with LGI bleeding, other vascular disease, and strong suspicion for ischemic colitis might require only noninvasive vascular imaging to confirm the diagnosis with conservative management of the GI bleeding.

If bleeding persists after this degree of evaluation, physicians should discuss with patients in detail the risks versus benefits of continued diagnostic evaluation. It may be appropriate in such patients to observe, transfuse, or treat empirically with iron supplementation, with relative confidence that worrisome causes of bleeding have been ruled out.

TABLE 22.3 Clinical Risk Factors for Severe Acute Lower Gastrointestinal Bleeding*

Heart rate ≥100 beats/minute
Systolic blood pressure ≤115
Syncope
Nontender abdominal examination
Bleeding per rectum during first 4 hours of evaluation
Aspirin use
More than two active comorbid conditions (heart failure, ischemic heart disease, renal failure, liver failure, cancer, etc.)
Interpretation: • ≥3 risk factors: high (approximately 80%) risk of severe bleeding • 1–3 risk factors: moderate (approximately 45%) risk of severe bleeding • 0 risk factors: low (approximately <10%) risk of severe bleeding

*Data are from Reference 9.

MASSIVE LOWER INTESTINAL BLEEDING

Angiodysplasia and diverticular disease are the most common causes of acute, massive LGI bleeding. Colonoscopy remains the diagnostic study of choice in these cases, with its high diagnostic yield limited only by poor visualization in cases of active, profuse bleeding. In patients who are hemodynamically stable, colonoscopy may be performed urgently (within 12 hours of admission) to identify the source of bleeding. Colonic preparation, ideally with colonoscopy within 1 hour of the colon prep, improves visualization. Earlier colonoscopy has been associated with a shorter hospital length of stay, due primarily to diagnostic yield rather than treatment interventions (10). Second-line investigations of massive bleeding include capsule endoscopy, arteriography, tagged red blood cell scan, and helical computed tomography scan. Emergent exploratory laparotomy (with or without intraoperative endoscopy) may be indicated in patients with continued bleeding, hemodynamic compromise, and no identified source with the above tests.

Management

Many cases of LGI bleeding resolve spontaneously with supportive care (11). Diverticular bleeding may be controlled endoscopically (2,12) with epinephrine injection, bipolar probe coagulation, or metallic clips; medical therapy includes stool softeners and other measures to control constipation, and if possible avoidance of aspirin or other antithrombotic or anticoagulant medications. Although avoidance of small, hard seeds or nuts has traditionally been recommended for patients with diverticular disease to prevent rebleeding, evidence for this recommendation is limited and a recent large cohort study (13) showed no association between nut, corn, or popcorn consumption and incidence of diverticular disease. Surgical resection of bowel prone to profuse bleeding may be required in patients with recurrent or massive hemorrhage.

Colonic angiodysplasia may be managed endoscopically by epinephrine injection or bipolar laser coagulation. Transcatheter embolization or vasopressin infusion may also be helpful. Medical therapy is indicated for patients with diffuse vascular lesions, lesions inaccessible to endoscopic therapy, recurrent bleeding despite local therapy or surgical resection, or an unknown diagnosis, with vascular bleeding suspected (2). Options include hormonal therapy, vasopressin, octreotide, and others. Octreotide has been shown effective for variceal bleeding, and has been reported to be effective in obscure lower intestinal bleeding (14,15), but has not been evaluated in randomized trials for this purpose. Various superselective embolization treatment options are evolving (2).

The option of blind surgical resection for obscure bleeding in patients with recurrent bleeding and continued requirements for transfusion is a complex decision. Every effort should be made to identify the source of bleeding, and the likelihood of rebleeding following resection, from multifocal mucosal angiodysplasia or other lesions, should be considered (2). Wireless capsule endoscopy and double-balloon enteroscopy have markedly improved the ability to identify specific bleeding

TABLE 22.4 Key Recommendations for Practice

Recommendation	Strength of Recommendation
LGI	
Urgent colonoscopy should be the initial diagnostic step for massive LGI bleeding (2,9).	B
Colonoscopy is the initial diagnostic test for occult LGI bleeding (1,2).	A
Repeating upper and lower endoscopy may be preferred before other diagnostic tests for colonic or small bowel bleeding (2,9).	C
Classify LGI bleeding as upper, mid, or lower GI tract.	C
Capsule endoscopy is the preferred test for obscure LGI bleeding with negative EGD and colonoscopy (2).	C
Clinical criteria can accurately identify patients at lower and higher risk for severe LGI bleeding (9).	C
Acute and Chronic Diarrhea	
Manage acute infectious diarrhea primarily by initiating rehydration, using the oral route when possible (16).	A
Classify chronic diarrhea as inflammatory, watery, or fatty to guide further diagnostic studies (26).	C
Diagnose irritable bowel syndrome based on clinical criteria, reserving testing for patients with "alarm symptoms" (30).	B
Constipation	
Routine laboratory testing and plain abdominal radiographs have limited evidence to support or reject their use, but may be useful to exclude secondary causes in selected patients (41).	C
Patients with rectal bleeding, iron deficiency, weight loss, or other concerning symptoms should have colonoscopy (42).	B
Constipated patients without "alarm" symptoms or signs suggesting neoplasm do not routinely need colonoscopy or other imaging studies unless indicated for routine screening purposes because of age (42).	B
Treatment of idiopathic normal-transit constipation should begin with fiber or other bulk-forming agents and inexpensive saline laxatives (41).	B

A = consistent, good-quality patient-oriented evidence; B = inconsistent or limited-quality patient-oriented evidence; C = consensus, disease-oriented evidence, usual practice, expert opinion, or case series; EGD = esophagogastroduodenoscopy; GI = gastrointestinal; LGI = lower GI.
For information about the SORT evidence rating system, see *http://www.aafp.org/afpsort.xml*.

sites in the small bowel, and blind resection should be reserved for a very small subset of patients. Table 22.4 summarizes key recommendations regarding LGI bleeding.

ACUTE DIARRHEA

CLINICAL OBJECTIVES

1. Describe key clinical features of common infectious and noninfectious causes of acute diarrhea, primarily in adults.
2. Describe a clinically useful role for stool cultures and other diagnostic testing in patients with acute diarrhea.
3. Describe appropriate treatment options for adult patients with "traveler's diarrhea."

Diarrhea is an alteration in normal bowel movements characterized by an increase in frequency, water content, or volume of stools. Evidence-based guidelines from the Infectious Disease Society of America (IDSA) (16) cite infectious diarrheal diseases as the second leading cause of morbidity and mortality worldwide, and the cause of 1.8 million hospitalizations and 3,100 deaths in the United States annually. Some causes of infectious diarrhea may result in long-term complications such as hemolytic-uremic syndrome or renal failure (Shiga toxin-producing *Escherichia coli*), Guillain-Barré syndrome (*Campylobacter jejuni* infection), or malnutrition with a variety of enteric infections. In the United States, an estimated $23 billion is spent annually on diarrhea, including $6 billion on foodborne illnesses, which account for 250,000 patients requiring hospitalization and 80% of cases of bacterial diarrhea (17).

The first step in evaluating patients with diarrhea is to establish the severity of the symptoms and to classify the presentation as acute (presumably infectious) diarrhea lasting <14 days, or chronic intermittent diarrhea (discussed in the next section of this chapter) (18). The differential diagnosis, evaluation, and management strategies are very different for these two scenarios.

Differential Diagnosis

The differential diagnosis for adults with acute diarrhea focuses primarily on infectious agents. The most common infectious disorders among adults in industrialized nations are listed in Table 22.5, along with their most common epidemiologic settings or modes of transmission. Particularly for persistent diarrhea (lasting longer than 2 weeks, but not chronic) there are a number of noninfectious causes that should also be considered. These include drug-induced diarrhea, particularly non-*Clostridium difficile* antibiotic-associated diarrhea; toxin-induced diarrhea; laxative abuse or factitious diarrhea; and postinfectious irritable bowel syndrome (19). These can usually be identified from the patient's history. Other noninfectious causes of persistent diarrhea include first presentations of causes of "chronic" diarrhea, including irritable bowel syndrome (IBS), inflammatory bowel disease, ischemic bowel disease (especially in older patients with vascular disease), malabsorption syndromes including gluten enteropathy (celiac sprue), or other causes.

Postinfectious irritable bowel syndrome (19) presents as typical diarrhea-predominant IBS, following an episode of acute infectious (usually bacterial) diarrhea with no residual evidence of active infection.

CLINICAL EVALUATION

Initial evaluation of the patient with acute diarrhea should include an assessment of the need for intravenous rehydration and the need for symptomatic treatment. Although detailed recommendations for oral versus intravenous rehydration are beyond the scope of this chapter, every attempt should be made to rehydrate the patient using oral rehydration solution. Symptomatic relief with bismuth subsalicylate or loperamide for noninflammatory diarrhea should be initiated as the diagnostic workup proceeds.

TABLE 22.5 Exposures and Symptoms Suggesting Specific Infectious Diarrheal Disorders*

Finding	Infectious Organism Suggested
Epidemiologic	
Consumption of undercooked poultry or employment in poultry industry	*Campylobacter*
Recent use of antibiotics	*C. difficile*
Community outbreak during winter in clusters or on cruise ships	Norovirus
Ingestion of untreated water by traveler or hiker	*Giardia, Cryptosporidium*
Travel to tropical or semitropical area	Enterotoxigenic *Escherichia coli,* enteroaggregative *E. coli, Shigella, Salmonella, Campylobacter*
Travel to a developing area	*Cyclospora, Cryptosporidium, Entamoeba histolytica*
Daycare center attendance or employment	*Shigella, Giardia, Cryptosporidium*
Swimming in or drinking untreated fresh surface water from a lake or stream	*Giardia, Cryptosporidium*
Seafood	*Vibrio*
Visiting a farm or petting zoo, having contact with animals with diarrhea	*E. coli*
Community acquired, food borne transmission	*Salmonella, Yersinia, Campylobacter, E. coli* (including O157-H7), *C. perfringens, S. Aureus, B. cereus*
Community acquired, person-to-person transmission	*Shigella,* Norwalk, rotavirus, other enteric viruses
Receptive anal intercourse or oral-anal sexual contact	*Giardia, Clostridium histolyticum*
Clinical	
Incubation period <6 hours	*Staphylococcus aureus* or *Bacillus cereus* toxin-induced
Incubation period 6–24 hours	*Clostridium perfringens* or *B. cereus* more likely
Fever, abdominal pain, bloody stools	*Salmonella, Campylobacter, Shigella*
Afebrile, abdominal pain, bloody stools	Shiga toxin-producing *E. coli*

*Data are from References 16, 17, and 18.

History and Physical Examination

Most cases of acute infectious diarrhea are caused by self-limited viral gastroenteritis; the acute onset of vomiting, watery diarrhea, and mild abdominal pain in a healthy patient with no unusual exposures and no worrisome symptoms suggests such a routine viral infection. The patient history should focus on identifying features that (a) indicate a specific organism or other concerning cause of the diarrhea or (b) warrant further diagnostic evaluation. Public health measures may be required if a reportable infection is identified, and the history should include questions about possible disease outbreaks. A number of symptoms or other historical features can help to suggest specific causes of diarrhea (Table 22.5).

Fever, severe abdominal pain, bloody bowel movements, and vomiting are more likely to occur with infectious (especially bacterial) enteritis, but the predictive value of any single finding is low (16). Shigellosis, salmonellosis, and campylobacteriosis are "inflammatory diarrheas" typically characterized by fever, abdominal pain, bloody stools, fecal leukocytes, or occult blood. The physical examination, while useful and fairly reproducible in children, is not as helpful in adults. It is generally sufficient to think in terms of no, some, or severe dehydration rather than trying to assign a percentage dehydration in adults (McGee S, JAMA 1999).

Diagnostic Testing

Although many patients with acute diarrhea are asked to provide stool samples for culture, fecal leukocytes, and examination for ova and parasites in the stool, such testing may be overused. Most cases of acute infectious diarrhea are self-limited, and stool testing results are available only after the patient's illness has resolved (16). One study of stool samples tested by labs in the FoodNet foodborne diseases surveillance network (16) found only a 1% to 2% positive yield of stool studies for salmonella, shigella, campylobacter, and *E. coli* O157:H7, at a cost of more than $1,000 per positive result. In particular, the yield of diagnostic testing for routine stool cultures and ova or parasite examination is very low for patients hospitalized >3 days (many of whom have *Clostridium difficile* colitis). Diagnostic testing should be limited to patients with a higher likelihood of a specific organism (e.g., older than age 65, neutropenic, HIV positive), and where such testing will aid either treatment decisions or public health investigation (20).

Recommended Diagnostic Strategy

Diagnostic testing is not generally indicated for suspected viral, self-limited gastroenteritis, nor should broad stool testing be pursued without consideration for the specific organisms involved. IDSA guidelines (16) recommend the strategy outlined in Table 22.6. This strategy includes classifying the episode of diarrhea as community-acquired, acquired during travel, hospital-acquired, or persistent (21). Stool cultures are indicated for severe diarrhea (more than five stools per day), diarrhea lasting longer than 1 week, fever or dysentery, or when multiple cases are identified in a community (17).

One important challenge is distinguishing *C. difficile* colitis from other causes of antibiotic-associated diarrhea. *C. difficile* infection causes a toxin-mediated enteritis, and is most commonly associated with use of clindamycin, cephalosporins, and penicillins. However, other mechanisms and other antibiotics can cause diarrhea, and only 10% to 20% of stool specimens tested for *C. difficile* toxin are positive (22). The primary mechanisms for other antibiotic-associated, non-*C. difficile* diarrhea primarily include direct effects of antibiotics on the intestinal mucosa and the metabolic consequences of reductions in intestinal flora. Patients with antibiotic-associated, non-*C. difficile* diarrhea usually have a previous history of similar responses to antibiotics; typically have more moderate diarrhea without fever, cramps, fecal leukocytes, or rectal bleeding; and typically are not markedly ill, though they may be mildly dehydrated. Non-*C. difficile*-associated diarrhea usually readily resolves on withdrawal of the implicated antibiotic, whereas *C. difficile* colitis does not.

TABLE 22.6 Guidelines for Diagnostic Testing in Selected Patients with Acute Diarrhea

Clinical Situation	Tests
Suspected viral gastroenteritis	None
Community-acquired or traveler's diarrhea associated with significant fever or blood in stool	Culture for *Salmonella, Shigella, Campylobacter, E. coli* O157:H7
Diarrhea is bloody, associated with tenesmus, or part of a nosocomial outbreak	Perform stool culture and test for shiga toxin
Antibiotic use or chemotherapy in recent weeks	Test for *Clostridium difficile* toxins A and B
Nosocomial diarrhea, onset after 3 days in the hospital	Test for *C. difficile* toxins A and B
Persistent diarrhea >7 days (especially if immunocompromised)	Test for ova and parasites (*Giardia, Cryptosporidium, Cyclospora, Isospora belli*)
Patient is HIV positive	Test for *Microsporidia* and *M. avium* complex in addition to stool culture as above

*Data are from Reference 16 and 17.

MANAGEMENT

Oral rehydration and general supportive care remain the most important factors in patient management. Primary care physicians who suspect a disease outbreak should contact local public health authorities. Outbreaks might be suspected on the basis of diarrheal illness in a daycare attendee or employee, or a resident of an institutional facility (nursing home, hospital, military facility, prison), or similar presentations or diagnoses among a defined group of individuals.

The management of the full spectrum of infectious diarrheal illnesses is complex; the patient's immune status, age, duration of illness, and general medical conditions are all important factors in determining the need and duration of specific treatment. In general, antibiotics do not improve outcomes for acute diarrheal illnesses that are typically self-limited, but antibiotic therapy is important in cases of more severe diarrhea or dysentery. The antibiotic recommendations in Table 22.7 apply to immunocompetent adults; IDSA guidelines (16) or other resources (17) should be consulted before prescribing specific treatment. One important exception to antimicrobial treatment is dysentery caused by Shiga toxin-producing *E. coli*, which includes O157:H7 strains but is distinct from enteropathogenic, enterotoxigenic, and enteroinvasive *E. coli*. Shiga toxin-producing *E. coli*, which is identifiable on culture in cases of more severe diarrhea, can cause hemolytic uremic syndrome, and the risk of this may be increased with antibiotic therapy, though this increased risk is not fully proven. Treatment in such cases is primarily supportive (17).

Traveler's diarrhea is a specific case of acute diarrheal symptoms occurring in people who have crossed an international boundary; most cases are self-limited and resolve within 5 days. However, approximately 10% of patients (depending on destination) will develop more severe symptoms such as bloody diarrhea, which may be because of enterotoxigenic *E. coli* or other organisms. Fluid and electrolyte replacement remains the focus of treatment in patients who are dehydrated; early treatment with antibiotics has been proposed to limit the development of more severe illness, or to shorten the duration of symptoms. A Cochrane review (23) found that antibiotics for traveler's diarrhea shorten the duration and severity of symptoms, though with an increased risk of minor side effects. Another review found that probiotics are a useful adjunct to rehydration therapy in treating acute infectious diarrhea, though there is insufficient evidence to indicate which particular regimen might be most effect (24). Ciprofloxacin or other fluoroquinolones are often used for empiric treatment; concurrent use of loperamide with antibiotic treatment is considered safe and effective in reducing

TABLE 22.7 Selected Antibiotic Therapy for Specific Infectious Diarrheal Conditions*

Target Disorder	Intervention
Shigellosis or enteroinvasive *E. coli* infection	Levofloxacin 500 mg once daily for 3 days, or ciprofloxacin 750 mg once a day for 3 days, or azithromycin 500 mg once a day for 3 days, or trimethoprim/sulfamethoxazole 160/800 mg twice daily for 3 days if susceptible
Non-*typhi* salmonellosis	Treatment not routinely recommended† or levofloxacin 500 mg once a day for 7–10 days for severe cases
Campylobacteriosis	Erythromycin 500 mg twice daily for 5 days, or azithromycin 500 mg once a day for 3 days
Enterotoxigenic *E. coli* diarrhea, enteroaggregative *E. coli* diarrhea, or traveler's diarrhea	Ciprofloxacin 750 mg once a day for 1–3 days, or azithromycin 1,000 mg as a single dose, or rifaximin 200 mg 3 times a day for 3 days
Shiga toxin-producing *E. coli*	No antibiotic therapy recommended
Yersinia species	Treatment not routinely recommended
Vibrio cholerae	Doxycycline 300 mg single dose, or tetracycline 500 mg 4 times a day for 3 days (other regimens may also be effective, see detailed guidelines)
C. difficile colitis	Metronidazole 500 mg three times daily for 10 days, or vancomycin 125 mg four times a day for 2 weeks for more severe cases
Giardiasis	Metronidazole 250–750 mg three times daily for 7–10 days, or tinidazole 50 mg/kg body weight up to 2 g

*Data are from Reference 15 and 17.
†Patients <6 months old, >50 years old, or with valvular heart disease or other conditions may require specific treatment.

the duration of symptoms. Prophylactic treatment with antibiotics is not recommended, but bismuth subsalicylate may be a good prophylactic option in patients who are not taking aspirin or other salicylates.

CHRONIC DIARRHEA

CLINICAL OBJECTIVES

1. Describe key clinical features of common conditions causing chronic diarrhea symptoms in adults.
2. Describe an appropriate role for stool studies and other diagnostic testing to evaluate patients with chronic diarrhea.
3. Describe key diagnostic features in the patient history that suggest IBS, and recommend treatment options for most patients with IBS.

The point prevalence of chronic diarrhea in the United States, defined as increased stool frequency, is approximately 5% (25,26). For many patients, it is the liquidity or consistency of the stools that becomes abnormal and is described as diarrhea, rather than the quantity of stool (26). The impact on patients' quality of life, in terms of the effect of symptoms, lost time from work, and the need for treatment, can be considerable. Evaluation is driven primarily by a careful history to search for clues to the underlying diagnosis, with directed testing for specific disorders or to categorize the type of diarrhea. Most of the recommendations for evaluating and managing chronic diarrhea are based on expert opinion, rather than properly designed epidemiologic studies or controlled trials (26,27).

Differential Diagnosis

AGA guidelines (25,26) classify chronic diarrhea into four categories (Table 22.8). Secretory diarrhea is the most common type according to two case series from a tertiary referral center (27).

CLINICAL EVALUATION

History and Physical Examination

Physicians should elicit the onset, timing, pattern, and duration of symptoms, as well as any history of weight loss, travel or exposure to potentially contaminated food or water, abdominal pain, fecal incontinence, or recent medication use. Importantly, the history should clarify the quality of the stools, including whether stools are watery, bloody, or fatty.

The history alone can strongly suggest the diagnosis in patients with chronic diarrhea. Pain, weight loss, and bloody diarrhea suggest inflammatory bowel disease. Weight loss and fatty diarrhea suggest malabsorption. Celiac disease (celiac sprue) is a fairly common cause of chronic diarrhea; associated abdominal pain, a characteristic rash (dermatitis herpetiformis), or associated anemia or osteoporosis increase the likelihood of celiac disease (28). Travel or exposure to untreated water raises the possibility of chronic infectious colitis, such as that caused by *Giardia lamblia*. Medications, radiation, and cholecystectomy or colectomy can all lead to chronic diarrhea. Rarely, patients will also overuse laxatives, leading to a factitious diarrhea. The effect of stress or diet on symptoms should also be elicited. Microscopic colitis is increasingly recognized as a common cause of chronic diarrhea; a typical presentation is recurrent, episodic bouts of watery diarrhea several times a day without blood or mucus, with definitive diagnosis by biopsy if necessary (29). Finally, the history should include a review of systems to address symptoms of systemic illnesses,

TABLE 22.8 Causes of Chronic Diarrhea*

Mechanism	Disorder
Secretory diarrhea	Disordered motility (postvagotomy, hyperthyroidism, autonomic neuropathy, irritable bowel syndrome)
	Inflammatory bowel disease
	Nonosmotic laxative abuse
	Ileal bile acid malabsorption
	Neuroendocrine tumors (carcinoid syndrome, VIPoma, gastrinoma)
Osmotic diarrhea	Magnesium, phosphate, sulfate ingestion
	Carbohydrate malabsorption (lactose intolerance)
Fatty diarrhea	Malabsorption syndromes (short-bowel syndrome, postresection diarrhea, celiac and other mucosal disease, mesenteric ischemia)
	Maldigestion (pancreatic insufficiency, bile acid deficiency)
Inflammatory diarrhea	Inflammatory bowel disease
	Infectious disease (cytomegalovirus)
	Radiation colitis
	Neoplasia (colon cancer, lymphoma)

*Data are from References 25 and 26.

TABLE 22.9 Rome II Criteria for Irritable Bowel Syndrome*

At least 12 weeks (which need not be consecutive) in the preceding 12 months, of abdominal discomfort or pain that has two out of three of these features: • relieved with defecation; and/or • onset associated with a change in frequency of stool; and/or • onset associated with a change in form (appearance) of stool
Symptoms that cumulatively support the diagnosis of irritable bowel syndrome • abnormal stool frequency (for research purposes abnormal may be defined as greater than three bowel movements per day and less than three bowel movements per week) • abnormal stool form (lumpy/hard or loose/watery stool) • abnormal stool passage (straining, urgency, or feeling of incomplete evacuation) • passage of mucus • bloating or feeling of abdominal distension

*Data are from References 29 and 30.

such as hyperthyroidism, diabetes, acquired immunodeficiency syndrome, or collagen vascular diseases.

The diagnosis of IBS can be made on clinical grounds—the Rome II criteria (Table 22.9) have a high positive predictive value. Patients who meet these criteria and do not have "alarm symptoms" (e.g., bleeding, fever, family history of colorectal cancer, chronic severe diarrhea, weight loss, malnutrition) can be treated for IBS without further testing (29) and typical diarrhea-predominant IBS should not be considered a "diagnosis of exclusion."

The physical examination may occasionally offer clues to the diagnosis for a patient's diarrhea (e.g., thyromegaly suggesting hyperthyroidism, rash suggesting celiac sprue, perianal fistula suggesting Crohn disease), but typically the most important finding from the physical examination is an assessment of the extent of dehydration or nutrient deficiency.

Diagnostic Testing

Routine laboratory testing may provide additional clues to the underlying diagnosis and can help establish the severity of dehydration or nutrient-related anemia or electrolyte disorders. Complete blood counts may identify leukocytosis consistent with an infection, and eosinophilia may suggest neoplasm, allergy, parasitic infection, or other causes. An elevated sedimentation rate suggests inflammatory bowel disease (IBD) but is highly nonspecific. If celiac disease is suspected, serologic testing for antiendomysial antibodies and anti-tissue transglutaminase antibodies should be obtained (28); the older antigliadin antibodies are no longer considered sensitive or specific enough to diagnose celiac disease.

Colonoscopy is recommended when IBD or malignancy is suspected because of the presence of bleeding, other "red flags," patient age, or when persistent or worsening symptoms prompt suspicion for microscopic colitis. Anti-*Saccharomyces cerevisiae* antibodies and antineutrophil cytoplasmic antibodies are specific but nonsensitive tests for IBD, which are helpful when positive to rule in disease. Negative tests do not rule out IBD (31).

Recommended Diagnostic Strategy

AGA guidelines (25,26) recommend that chronic diarrhea be categorized as *watery* (either osmotic or secretory), *fatty*, or *inflammatory* to guide further evaluation and treatment. Gross inspection of the stool by physician or patient is often sufficient to establish this categorization (25), although a simple stool analysis provides more definitive information. Further stool evaluation should be guided by the physician's overall impression of the patient's most likely diagnosis and the need for further testing. Table 22.10 describes some available stool sample tests and their possible diagnostic impact. AGA guidelines (26) suggest that stool cultures be performed in many patients with chronic diarrhea, although they often provide little useful information. Chronic diarrhea because of infectious agents is rare in immunocompetent patients in the US (27), and microscopic examination for ova and parasites should be reserved for patients where such illness is clinically suspected.

MANAGEMENT

Management of chronic diarrhea primarily involves treating or correcting the underlying cause, such as IBS, IBD, or malabsorption syndrome. Empiric therapy is indicated for symptomatic relief pending additional testing, when testing has failed to reveal a diagnosis, or when no specific therapy is available (26). Opioids remain the most effective empiric medical therapy for diarrhea; loperamide or diphenoxylate are used for more mild cases of chronic diarrhea, although morphine is occasionally effective for severe, intractable cases. Cholestyramine, bismuth, or dietary fiber is also useful empiric treatments in some patients. None of these agents have been studied in randomized trials for this purpose, though extensive experience supports their benefit (26).

IBS is a common cause of chronic diarrhea; the management of this disorder requires a combination of patient education, dietary adjustments, and individualized pharmacologic treatment. Useful medications for diarrhea associated with IBS include (29,32):

- loperamide (Imodium), often prescribed regularly as 2 mg once or twice daily
- diphenoxylate and atropine (Lomotil), though patients may develop tolerance over time
- alosetron (Lotronex), a 5-HT3 antagonist, 1 mg twice daily improves symptoms and quality-of-life scores, but use should be limited to women with severe diarrhea-predominant IBS symptoms because of concerns about side effects
- medications for abdominal pain, such as antispasmodics (hyoscyamine or mebeverine) or tricyclic antidepressants, though evidence for efficacy is limited

Microscopic colitis should be treated with oral budesonide, which has the greatest proven efficacy; oral prednisolone, methotrexate, mesalamine, and other agents have not proven effective in smaller studies (33).

A detailed discussion of treatment of IBD is beyond the scope of this chapter. In general, Crohn disease and ulcerative

TABLE 22.10 Stool Specimen Testing and Suggested Diarrhea Category*

Stool Analysis	Disorder or Diarrhea Category Suggested	Clinical or Diagnostic Role
Occult blood	Celiac sprue, inflammatory diarrhea, neoplasm	50–70% of patients with celiac sprue are Hemoccult positive, unclear role for other conditions
Wright stain or microscopy for white blood cells	Infectious or inflammatory cause of diarrhea	Reported "few WBC" may be false positive
Latex agglutination test for neutrophil product lactoferrin	Acute infectious diarrhea including *Clostridium difficile* colitis	Unclear role in chronic diarrhea
Sudan staining for stool fat	Malabsorption syndrome	Semiquantitative measure for stool fat content provides similar information
Fecal culture	Bacterial colitis	Identify rare bacterial causes of chronic diarrhea, especially for *Aeromonas* or *Pseudomonas* species in patients exposed to untreated well water
Microscopic evaluation for ova and parasites	Protozoal or parasitic infection (e.g., giardiasis)	Multiple samples increases sensitivity; *Giardia*-specific stool antibody test or PCR are more sensitive and specific, but cost may be an issue
Stool pH and electrolytes	Osmotic or secretory diarrhea pH <5.3 suggests carbohydrate malabsorption	Osmotic gap elevated (>125 mOsm/kg) in pure osmotic diarrhea, and low (<50 mOsm/kg) in pure secretory diarrhea
Stool laxative testing	Factitious diarrhea, laxative abuse	Patient history and/or search of hospital room for laxatives may have higher sensitivity than stool testing

*Data are from Reference 26.

colitis should be considered in patients presenting with chronic diarrhea, especially if abdominal pain or rectal bleeding are present. These conditions can be effectively managed using a combination of oral and topical aminosalicylates, corticosteroids, antibiotics, and other agents. Recent evidence-based reviews provide additional details regarding the diagnosis and management of IBD (34,35). Table 22.4 lists key recommendations regarding acute and chronic diarrhea.

CONSTIPATION

CLINICAL OBJECTIVES

1. Describe common causes and contributing factors for chronic constipation.
2. Describe indications for colonoscopy or other diagnostic testing in adults with chronic constipation.
3. Describe management options for adults with chronic functional constipation.

There is no single definition of chronic constipation, although it is often defined in research studies (36) as the inability to evacuate stool completely and spontaneously three or more times per week. Patients may describe any of the following as constipation: small or hard stools, infrequent bowel movement (fewer than three per week), the need to strain to have a bowel movement, a sense of fullness or bloating, a sense of incomplete evacuation, or an inability to have a bowel movement without excessive straining or time on the toilet. Physicians and patients emphasize different symptoms in their definition of chronic constipation, and physicians should ask about this broader constellation of symptoms and not just stool frequency or consistency.

There are multiple physiologic steps required to achieve normal bowel movements. These include absorption of water; segmental bowel contractions that mix stool and move feces short distances; high-amplitude contractions that move fecal waste larger distances in the colon; unimpaired passage of stool through the colon and rectum; and synchronized voluntary striated muscle contraction and involuntary smooth muscle contraction for defecation.

Risk factors for chronic constipation in adults include female gender, non-white ethnicity, older age, physical inactivity, limited education, and depression. Constipation is also a frequently encountered symptom in palliative care settings, particularly when chronic opioid medications are used. Constipation in children has a different spectrum of disorders and may represent a neurologic disorder, a functional or emotional problem (particularly when associated with nocturnal enuresis), or a manifestation of sexual abuse. The diagnosis and management of

TABLE 22.11 Differential Diagnosis of the Patient with Chronic Constipation*

Diagnosis
Primary Constipation
Functional constipation†
• Idiopathic functional constipation†
• Irritable bowel syndrome†
• Pelvic floor dysfunction (anismus)
• Slow-transit constipation
Secondary Constipation
Medications*
• Iron supplements†
• Calcium channel blockers (verapamil)†
• Diuretics
• Opioids†
• Anticholinergics, antihistamines
• Anticonvulsants
• Antidepressants
• Antipsychotics
• Laxatives (chronic abuse)
• Nonsteroidal anti-inflammatories
• Calcium supplements
• Antacids
Metabolic/endocrine
• Hypothyroidism†
• Hypomagnesemia
• Hypercalcemia
• Hypokalemia
• Uremia
• Heavy metal poisoning
Mechanical obstruction
• Colon cancer†
• Compression by extracolonic tumor
• Stricture (diverticular, postischemic)
• Large rectocele
• Postsurgical changes
• Anal stenosis from anal fissure, etc.
• Crohn disease, megacolon
Neuropathies
• Spinal cord injury or tumor
• Parkinson disease
• Cerebrovascular disease
• Multiple sclerosis
• Hirschsprung disease
• Others (Chagas disease, congenital anal sphincter myopathy, hyperganglionosis)
Other conditions
• Depression
• Degenerative joint disease, immobility
• Autonomic neuropathy
• Cognitive impairment
• Cardiac disease

*Data are from References 29 and 30.
†Common causes.

chronic constipation in children at various ages is quite different from that in adults; this section will focus on adult patients.

Differential Diagnosis

Physiologically, constipation can be divided (36,37) into broad categories of normal-transit constipation (most common, affecting 59% of patients), defecatory disorders, or slow-transit constipation. However it is probably easiest for clinicians to classify causes of constipation by etiology, as shown in Table 22.11, rather than physiology. Among patients with severe, intractable constipation, the most common causes are IBS, pelvic floor dysfunction, isolated slow-transit constipation, or combinations of these (38). Factors such as inadequate fluid intake, decreased physical activity, and insufficient dietary fiber are important contributing factors to chronic constipation, but recent evidence (40) emphasizes that these should not be viewed as the sole cause of patients' constipation, which may be multifactorial.

Patients with normal-transit constipation ("functional" constipation) have a normal rate of stool passage through the colon and normal stool frequency, yet feel that they are constipated. The perception of constipation may be because of difficulty with evacuation, hard stools, abdominal pain or bloating, constipation, or other symptoms. Symptoms typically respond to treatment with dietary fiber, with or without an osmotic laxative.

Defecatory disorders may be caused by dysfunction of the pelvic floor or anal sphincter, structural abnormalities (e.g., rectal intussusception), or failure to effectively coordinate the muscular functions of defecation because of a variety of conditions.

Slow-transit constipation is a disorder occurring primarily in young women with chronic constipation beginning in adolescence. It is caused by abnormal function of myenteric plexus neurons. Symptoms of bloating and abdominal discomfort are the presenting symptoms rather than constipation.

CLINICAL EVALUATION

History and Physical Examination

Patients complaining of abdominal pain, back pain, rectal bleeding, nausea, early satiety, bloating, or other symptoms should be asked about constipation symptoms. If patients are directly asked, "Are you constipated?" the answer may vary depending on that patient's definition of this problem; likewise patients who complain of constipation may have many different symptoms and normal stool patterns. All patients complaining of constipation should be asked in detail about stool frequency, consistency, discomfort, straining, bleeding, and any need for medical or manual assistance to have an effective bowel movement.

TABLE 22.12 Red Flags for Patients with Chronic Constipation Indicating More Serious Disease

Red Flags	Suggested Cause
Progressive symptoms	Obstruction because of colon cancer or extracolonic mass
Lower intestinal bleeding	Colon cancer, Crohn's disease
Weight loss >10 lb	Colon cancer
Anemia	Colon cancer
Family history of colon cancer or inflammatory bowel disease	Colon cancer, inflammatory bowel disease
Rectal pain, urinary stress incontinence	Defecatory disorder
Need to manually remove stool, apply perineal pressure, or strain excessively to have a bowel movement	Pelvic floor dysfunction
Age >50 years	Colon cancer

Functional constipation, IBS, medications (especially opioids), neurologic or spinal cord injury, marked physical inactivity, and symptoms of thyroid disorders are readily identified in the patient history and may be sufficient to establish the diagnosis. Patients should be specifically asked about their use of over-the-counter laxatives, including which agents are used, how often, and for how long. A typical pattern of alternating diarrhea with constipation may suggest IBS (Table 22.9); recent changes in medication may suggest an adverse effect of medication. The history should also focus on specifically inquiring about "alarm" symptoms (Table 22.12) that may suggest specific secondary causes; these patients and any patient over age 50 years may require colonoscopy to rule out malignancy or other serious causes.

The physical examination does not usually provide additional information to confirm the diagnosis or the cause of chronic constipation. However, the exam may help to identify a few specific abnormalities, including: thyromegaly; marked abdominal distension suggesting obstruction; local perianal abnormalities such as hemorrhoids or fissure; altered rectal tone suggesting neurologic impairment; or obstructing masses such as tumors or rectocele.

Pelvic floor dysfunction is an important cause of chronic constipation, and it is helpful to identify this problem early because symptoms do not respond to, and may be worsened by, routine dietary changes, stool softeners, and laxatives. The primary defect is the inability to evacuate stool from the rectum because of inappropriate contraction or relaxation of the pelvic floor muscles and external anal sphincter. Symptoms may include prolonged or excessive straining before defecation, the need for perineal or vaginal pressure to allow bowel movement, difficulty passing even liquid stools or enema liquid, or the need for manual removal of stool by the patient. Suggestive findings on physical examination of the rectum may include abnormal descent of the anal verge or "ballooning" of the perineum while the patient bears down, or tenderness on palpation of the puborectalis muscle at the posterior rectal wall (37).

Diagnostic Testing

The role of diagnostic tests for chronic constipation in selected patients is summarized in Table 22.13. However, evidence-based guidelines do not recommend obtaining these tests routinely for all or even most patients. Plain abdominal radiographs may help identify large amounts of stool in the colon, confirming the presence of chronic constipation, and may show evidence of obstruction or ileus. Typically these films do not help identify the cause of constipation, however. No high-quality studies have evaluated the role of routine plain films in patients with chronic constipation (41). Although barium enema testing may provide additional anatomic information and has the potential to identify obstructing lesions or narrowed bowel segments, it adds little to information that can be obtained from plain radiographs. Compared with colonoscopy, barium enema testing may not be sufficiently accurate to exclude small polyps or other concerning lesions (41).

Recommended Diagnostic Strategy

Current guidelines (42) indicate that in the absence of alarm signs or symptoms (including age 50 years or older), there is no evidence to recommend the routine use of flexible sigmoidoscopy, colonoscopy, barium enema, thyroid function tests, serum calcium, or other diagnostic tests in patients presenting with constipation.

Adult patients older than 50 years of age with chronic constipation may need to be evaluated by colonoscopy to rule out colon cancer, IBD, or other obstructing lesions. Guidelines for using colonoscopy in patients with constipation (43) report that the yield of colonoscopy in identifying neoplasm in patients with chronic constipation but no concerning symptoms is comparable to that in asymptomatic patients. Therefore, colonoscopy may not be necessary in such patients, unless age or other factors indicate a need for such testing. A systematic review (41) of diagnostic modalities for chronic constipation identified a yield of 2.0% for colonoscopy in detecting colon cancer in a large retrospective

TABLE 22.13 Role of Diagnostic Tests for Selected Patients with Chronic Constipation

Test	Recommended Role
Routine blood counts, thyroid profile, and chemistry profile	To exclude metabolic or endocrine cause in patients with suggestive signs or symptoms
Plain abdominal x-ray	To confirm chronic constipation, but no role in determining diagnosis
Barium enema	To identify structural bowel lesions when colonoscopy cannot be performed
Colonoscopy	For patients who have "alarm" signs or symptoms, or who are older than 50 years of age
Colonic transit study*	For patients with symptoms suggesting slow-transit constipation
Anorectal manometry, balloon expulsion test, or defecography*	To identify pelvic floor dyssynergia or other defecatory disorder

*Used primarily in patients referred to tertiary care centers for severe chronic idiopathic constipation, unresponsive to other therapy (41).

study of patients with constipation and a yield of 1.0% for flexible sigmoidoscopy.

Guidelines from the American Society for Gastrointestinal Endoscopy (ASGE) (43) recommend that patients with constipation undergo colonoscopy if they have rectal bleeding, heme-positive stool, iron deficiency anemia, weight loss, obstructive symptoms (such as excessive straining), recent onset of constipation, rectal prolapse, or change in stool caliber. Patients older than age 50 with constipation who have not had colon cancer screening should have a colonoscopy; flexible sigmoidoscopy may be adequate in younger patients, although colonoscopy allows dilation of benign colonic strictures in some patients.

Chronic constipation has been investigated as a risk factor for colorectal cancer, and patients may express this as a concern about "toxic substances" building up in the colon because of constipation, and increasing the risk of cancer. Epidemiologic studies are older, limited, and conflicting; the most recent evidence suggests that there is no increased risk of cancer from chronic constipation (46). Additional testing for defecatory and pelvic floor dysfunction, or other testing suggested by suspected or likely diagnosis, are usually pursued in consultation with a gastroenterologist.

MANAGEMENT

Initial management of patients with chronic constipation should address resolving correctable factors, such as removing offending medications, treating metabolic or endocrine conditions, improving hydration, increasing physical activity or mobility, or surgically removing obstructing tumors, as much as possible.

Patients with symptoms suggesting pelvic floor dysfunction should be referred for appropriate diagnostic testing. Patients with this condition do not respond well to increasingly aggressive regimens of stool softeners and laxatives, and should be referred for intensive pelvic floor retraining or biofeedback programs.

In most patients with idiopathic, normal-transit constipation, management should begin with recommendations for dietary fiber and/or the routine use of stool softener agents (Table 22.14). The prescription for dietary fiber should be specific—the target dosage should be 20 to 25 g of dietary fiber daily beyond usual intake, and patients should be instructed to begin with a lower, twice-daily dose and slowly increase to the target dose over 2 to 4 weeks. Patients should be warned that fiber supplements increase gaseousness, but symptoms may improve over several days (39).

Obtaining sufficient dietary fiber through fruits and vegetables may be difficult (typically 1 g per serving or less), and dietary changes should emphasize bran cereals (4 to 10 g per serving), raspberries or blackberries (4 to 5 g per serving), bran muffins, or beans (2 to 3 g per serving). Other over-the-counter bulk-forming agents may be used according to patient preference; these should be taken with water, and patients should be advised of likely side effects. For all these agents, patients should be instructed that improvement may take some weeks. Fair evidence suggests that psyllium increases stool frequency in patients with chronic constipation, but there is insufficient evidence regarding the efficacy of other bulk-forming agents. Likewise there is insufficient evidence for the efficacy of stool softeners in patients with chronic constipation (42), although all of these agents may be effective in some patients.

Patients who do not respond to these measures should next try inexpensive saline laxative agents to achieve soft, but not liquid, stools. These agents promote osmotic retention of fluid in the intestinal lumen. Patients with persistent symptoms should be prescribed either more expensive hyperosmolar laxatives, or stimulant laxatives, such as those listed in Table 22.14. Polyethylene glycol (PEG) and lactulose have been shown to be effective at improving stool frequency and consistency in patients with chronic constipation (42); there is insufficient evidence for the efficacy of saline laxatives, although their low cost may make their use more acceptable to patients. Patients may need to try multiple agents to find the most effective regimen. Dietary changes and stool softener

TABLE 22.14 Treatment Options for Chronic Constipation*

Drug	Comments, Cautions, Adverse Effects	Dosage	Relative Cost*
Bulk-forming Agents			
Dietary fiber (bran, Benefiber)	Bloating, flatulence, diminished iron and calcium absorption	1 cup bran per day, 2 teaspoons Benefiber up to three times per day	$
Psyllium (e.g., Metamucil, Konsyl, Perdiem with fiber)	Bloating, flatulence	1 teaspoon up to three times a day with water	$
Methylcellulose (e.g., Citrucel)	Less bloating	1 teaspoon up to tid with water	$
Calcium polycarbophil (e.g., Fibercon)	Bloating, flatulence	2–4 tablets daily	$
Stool Softener			
Docusate sodium (e.g., Colace)		100 mg twice a day	$
Saline Laxatives			
Magnesium (e.g., Milk of Magnesia, Haley's MO)	Dehydration, abdominal cramps, magnesium toxicity	15–30 mL once or twice daily	$
Hyperosmolar Laxatives			
Lactulose (e.g., Chronulac)	Transient abdominal cramps, flatulence	15–30 mL once or twice daily	$$
Polyethylene glycol (e.g., GoLYTELY, Colyte, MiraLAX)	Stool incontinence because of potency	8–32 oz daily	$$
Stimulant Laxatives			
Bisacodyl (e.g., Dulcolax)	Incontinence, abdominal cramps, rectal burning with daily use	10 mg suppositories up to three times per week	$
Sennosides (senna) (e.g., Senokot)	Unproven degeneration of Meissner's and Auerbach's plexus, malabsorption	2 tablets daily up to 4 tablets twice a day	$
Newer Agents			
Lubiprostone (Amitiza)	Nausea, headaches, diarrhea; approved for chronic idiopathic constipation up to 12 weeks	24 mcg twice a day	
Methylnaltrexone (Relistor) (44)	Indicated for opioid-induced constipation in patients with advanced illness who are receiving palliative care	12 mg (for patients 62–114 kg; otherwise 0.15 mg/kg) given subcutaneously every other day	
Prucalopride (Resolor) (45)	nausea, headache	2 or 4 mg once daily	

Relative cost: $ = <$33.00; $$ = $34.00–$66.00; $$$ = >$67.00.
*Information from Reference 38 unless otherwise indicated.

treatment should be continued as laxatives are tried. Stimulant laxatives (including enemas or suppositories), such as those listed in Table 22.14, should be recommended only for intermittent, as-needed use of severe flare-ups of chronic constipation. There is insufficient evidence to make firm recommendations regarding their use in patients with chronic constipation, but for some patients these agents seem to be highly effective in alleviating constipation symptoms.

The safety of long-term laxative use, especially stimulant laxatives, has been questioned for many years, with concerns of possible damage to the colonic myenteric system, increased risk of cancer, and tolerance or even addiction to these laxatives. It is true that some patients with chronic constipation may depend on these agents over a long period for appropriate stool frequency, and some patients may abuse laxatives by using many times the recommended dose. However, available evidence suggests that there are no harmful effects on the colon and no significantly increased risk for addiction or colorectal cancer from using laxatives at recommended doses on a chronic basis to control symptoms (47).

A number of newer medications show promise in treating chronic constipation, but do not have an established place in routine treatment. Tegaserod, a 5-HT1 agonist previously used for constipation, was removed from the US market in 2007 because of possible increased risk of cardiovascular events. These agents should be considered when other treatments have been unsuccessful, and are listed in Table 22.14.

Patients with truly intractable constipation or slow-transit constipation ("colonic inertia") represent a complex management challenge—these may include patients with inoperable obstructing tumors, scleroderma, neurologic injury, amyloidosis, or other conditions. Aggressive use of laxatives (stimulant, saline, PEG solutions, lactulose) may be effective (38), or patients may be candidates for surgical intervention, such as total colectomy with ileorectal anastomosis, continent sigmoid colon conduit, or other procedures. Key recommendations for chronic constipation are listed in Table 22.4.

CHAPTER

23

Cognitive Impairment

Philip D. Sloane, Christine Khandelwal, and Daniel I. Kaufer

CLINICAL OBJECTIVES

1. List the signs, symptoms, and diagnostic approach to the following common cognitive disorders of older people: delirium, Alzheimer disease (AD), vascular dementia, frontotemporal dementia (FTD), Lewy body dementia (LBD), and Parkinson dementia.
2. Conduct and interpret a screening examination for cognitive impairment, using the Mini-Cog and the AD-8, on a patient.
3. Conduct and interpret a diagnostic evaluation of a patient with cognitive impairment using cognitive testing, laboratory studies, and brain imaging.
4. Implement basic principles of dementia management, including medication use, nonpharmacological management of behavioral symptoms, and working with community resources with a patient.

Complaints about cognitive problems, such as memory loss, slowed thinking, or reduced mental capacity, are commonly brought to physicians by older people or their family members. Some slowing in mental processing and function is normal as people age; however, the incidence of diseases causing progressive cognitive loss also increases with advancing age. Therefore, the family physician must be prepared to:

- efficiently screen patients to determine if cognitive impairment is present;
- efficiently and comprehensively diagnose patients with cognitive impairment; and
- effectively manage patients with dementia and other causes of cognitive impairment

Cognitive impairment results from altered brain function that affects one or more intellectual abilities. Currently, isolated short-term memory deficits that go beyond mild forgetfulness, but do not otherwise interfere with functional abilities are referred to as "mild cognitive impairment" (MCI). Dementia is defined as cognitive impairment that involves multiple domains and is associated with a decline in the ability to carry out everyday activities. The most common cause of dementia in the elderly is AD, and many affected individuals exhibit isolated memory problems before developing full-blown AD. Besides AD, which can also occur as a mixed dementia in conjunction with cerebrovascular disease, there are many other potential causes, ranging from reversible medication effects to rapidly progressive and fatal diseases.

Approximately three million people in the United States have dementia (1). Dementia increases dramatically with age, so that the frequency of dementia among people ages 65 to 70 is approximately 2%, whereas for people over 85 it is more than 30% (1). Not all cognitive complaints reflect dementia, however; in fact, nearly twice as many people with cognitive impairment have milder symptoms that do not meet criteria for dementia (2).

Normal aging is associated with an increase in reported memory problems (typically forgetting names) and small declines in memory test performance (3). Among older people with memory complaints, some may be overly concerned about minimal memory dysfunction, whereas people with more severe memory deficits seen in AD are often unaware of or tend to minimize their symptoms. Therefore, the family physician must systematically evaluate cognitive complaints.

As the US population grows older, assessing cognitive impairment and diagnosing and managing dementia will be an increasingly important component of primary care medicine. The family physician must be adept at assessing and monitoring patients who have mild cognitive symptoms, and identify those who develop a progressive dementia. Particularly challenging is the fact that the onset of dementia is insidious and the transition from normal age-related cognitive lapses to diagnosable dementia is gradual and, therefore, difficult to detect. Consequently, every family physician needs to develop a systematic approach to dementia screening and evaluating patients with cognitive impairment, and have a working knowledge of the common dementias.

DIFFERENTIAL DIAGNOSIS

The differential diagnosis of cognitive impairment includes normal aging changes, mild cognitive impairment, delirium, and a number of different dementia diagnoses. Table 23.1 summarizes these conditions.

AD

AD is the most common cause of cognitive impairment in the elderly. Its course tends to be insidious in onset, slowly progressive, and to eventually lead to impairment of even basic bodily functions, and finally—if no other illness intervenes—to death. Figure 23.1 provides a graphic timeline of the typical course of AD, along with some of the common symptoms, signs, and clinical markers of disease progression.

The earliest symptoms in AD are difficulty with higher cognitive functions such as memory, language, problem solving, and reasoning. Memory loss is usually prominent early in

TABLE 23.1 Common Diagnoses among Older Persons with Cognitive Complaints

Dementia Diagnosis	Primary Anatomic Location	Clinical Presentation		Key Laboratory and Radiological Findings	Prognosis
		Typical History	Typical Physical Examination Findings		
Normal aging changes	None	Occasionally forgetful of names	None	Mild generalized cortical atrophy, nonspecific white matter changes	Good
Mild cognitive impairment	Medial temporal	Impaired short-term memory for events	None	Variable medial temporal lobe atrophy	Increased risk of AD
Delirium	Cortical/subcortical	Often toxic/metabolic/infectious etiology	Impaired attention, may be fidgety and tremulous, or apathetic/obtunded	EEG slowing, evidence of drug or metabolic toxicity, signs of infection	Depends on etiology and severity
Alzheimer disease (AD)	Cortical (temporal and parietal)	Gradually progressive short-term memory and other cognitive deficits	Generally normal neurological examination (may be apraxic)	Medial temporal and parietal lobe atrophy	Course 4–20 years (average 8 years)
Vascular dementia	Cortical and/or subcortical	Often a history of multiple strokelike events and/or vascular risk factors	Variable, may see limb or face weakness, sensory loss, aphasia, visuospatial disturbance, incoordination	Evidence of significant cerebrovascular disease (infarcts, small vessel disease) on brain imaging	Course static or progressive (often coexists with AD)
Frontotemporal dementia	Cortical (frontal and temporal	Typically presents with change in behavior/personality (apathy, disinhibition) or language	Variable, may see limb apraxia, gait difficulties, frontal release signs	Brain imaging may show severe atrophy in frontal and/or temporal lobes	Variable, progressive, speech/swallowing difficulties
Lewy body dementia	Cortical and subcortical	Fluctuating attention, visual hallucinations, parkinsonian motor signs, sleep disturbance	Limb rigidity, bradykinesia, may see intention tremor and gait disturbance	No specific brain imaging features	Variable, may see more rapid functional decline compared to Alzheimer's
Parkinson dementia	Subcortical	Parkinson disease with later-onset cognitive dysfunction	Limb rigidity, bradykinesia, resting tremor, gait disturbance	No specific brain imaging features	Variable, may have severe motor disability when dementia occurs

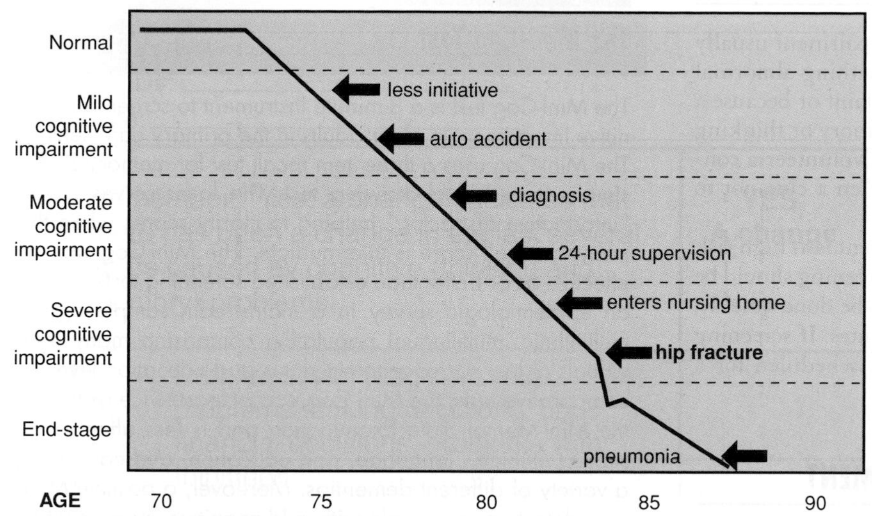

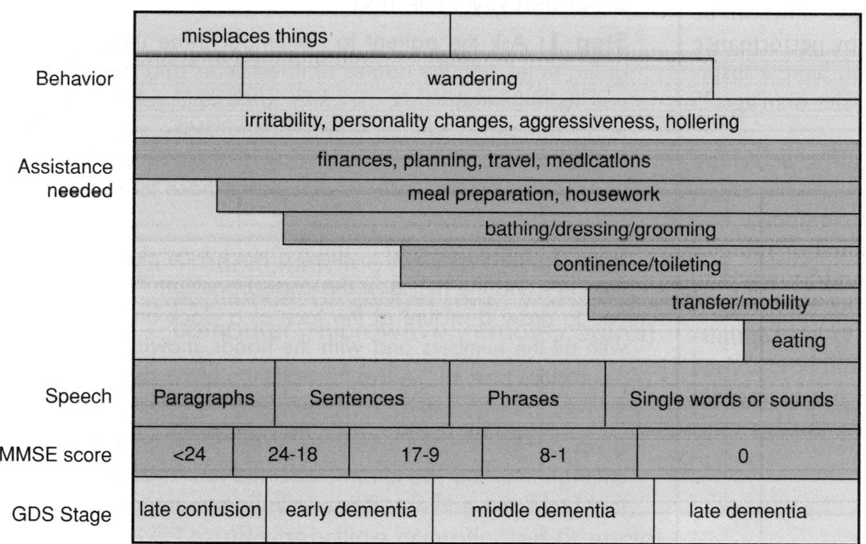

Figure 23.1 • Graphic timeline of a typical case of Alzheimer disease. **(A)** The slow progression of clinical features over more than a decade, beginning with less initiative noted by the family several years prior to diagnosis, progressing to need for 24-hour supervision, and ending with death from pneumonia after several years in a nursing home. **(B)** Correlates the common clinical measures of dementia (cognition, behavior, and stages of illness) with the course of the disease in the same patient.

the disease and typically progresses over time. Also, patients with early AD often are disproportionately impaired in category fluency (e.g., naming as many animals as they can in a minute) compared with letter fluency (e.g., naming words that begin with F) (4). Other findings seen with AD or other disorders with more focal cortical involvement from strokes or degeneration include: agnosia (inability to recognize and identify objects or people despite having knowledge of the characteristics of those objects or people), aphasia (either a partial or total loss of the ability to communicate verbally or using written words), and/or apraxia (total or partial loss of the ability to perform coordinated movements or manipulate objects in the absence of motor or sensory impairment) (4).

Other Common Dementias

Besides AD, the two most common dementias are vascular dementia and Lewy body dementia (including people with Parkinson disease and later-onset dementia). These "subcortical" dementias typically show less severe memory dysfunction, particularly early in the disease course, and tend to have greater deficits in attention, visuospatial skills, and executive function (initiation, planning, behavioral apathy) (4). Other dementias are profiled in Table 23.1.

Mild Cognitive Impairment

Mild cognitive impairment (MCI) is present when cognitive function is impaired more than one would expect based on the individual's age and education level, but is not severe enough to interfere with activities of daily living. MCI is classified into two subtypes: amnestic and nonamnestic. Amnestic MCI is present when the person has isolated memory loss; nonamnestic MCI involves impairment in other areas than memory (5). Amnestic MCI has a more ominous prognosis and is associated with a high risk of progression to AD (6). The annual rate of progression to dementia among healthy community-living adults age 55 and older is about 1% to 2% per year; in contrast, the annual conversion rate from MCI to dementia is 6% to 22% per year, with about 50% having dementia within 5 years (7,8).

negative predictive value >70%) in detecting early cognitive changes associated with many common dementing illness, including AD, vascular dementia, Lewy body dementia, and frontotemporal dementia (11,12). Scores in the impaired range (see the following section) indicate a need for further assessment. Scores in the "normal" range suggest that a dementing disorder is unlikely, but a very early disease process cannot be ruled out. More advanced assessment may be warranted in cases where other objective evidence of impairment exists.

The AD-8 is based on an informant ratings (present/absent) of changes from a previous level of functioning. The format of the AD-8 as a written questionnaire facilitates communicating sensitive information about the patient by the informant without the risk of overt embarrassment. A score of 2 or more positive items is a positive screen and indicates that a formal cognitive evaluation is needed.

Evaluation of Suspected Cognitive Impairment

The Diagnostic and Statistical Manual of Mental Disorders (DSM) IV identifies the following criteria for dementia: (i) memory impairment, (ii) aphasia and/or apraxia, agnosia or an impairment in executive function, and (iii) a significant reduction in social or occupational function from a previous level of performance, which is not explained by another psychiatric or neurological disorder (13). These criteria accurately identify AD on clinical grounds, whereas diagnostic criteria for other dementias (e.g., vascular dementia, Lewy body dementia, frontotemporal dementia) are not as robust (14). Compared with AD, other dementias tend to have more variable clinical presentations, which makes defining diagnostic criteria more difficult.

Dementia, as defined in DSM IV, stands in contrast with delirium, which is distinguished by a primary alteration in attention. Although dementia syndromes tend to be chronic, progressive, and irreversible, and delirium states tend to be acute or subacute, fluctuating, and reversible, though these distinctions are more relative than absolute. Toxic, metabolic, and infectious disturbances associated with delirium are more likely to be potentially reversible than degenerative disorders. Brain dysfunction associated with dementia may render the patient more vulnerable to delirium-producing factors, highlighting the clinical challenge posed by the combination of dementia and superimposed delirium. Careful evaluation of people referred for dementia can identify treatable or reversible disorders in up to 20% of cases (15).

Distinguishing cognitive impairment associated with an underlying brain disorder from potentially reversible cognitive symptoms (e.g., associated with depression) often demands ongoing evaluation, including appropriate diagnostic tests and perhaps therapeutic challenge with an antidepressant drug. Abrupt onset of thinking changes in temporal relation to a psychological stressor, poor effort on cognitive testing (particularly with demanding tasks), and prominent neurovegetative signs such as insomnia and anorexia are characteristic of depression-associated cognitive impairment. Drug-induced cognitive impairment occurring as a result of anticholinergic agents, sedative-hypnotic drugs (e.g., benzodiazepines), or opiate analgesics is common in the elderly and may variably cause or contribute to symptoms of dementia or MCI. A temporal association of cognitive symptom onset with the initiation or increase in dosing of such drugs should prompt withdrawal of any potentially offending agent. Accurately diagnosing dementia usually requires a systematic, longitudinal approach and, in many cases, targeted therapeutic additions or deletions. Multiple etiological factors are common, and the search for potentially reversible or modifiable conditions should be pursued vigorously.

Although poor spontaneous retrieval memory is common to both Alzheimer and other dementias, preserved recognition is characteristic of non-Alzheimer dementias (16), such that learning impairment can be partially corrected by providing more conspicuous cues to encourage learning and promote recognition (17). Selective deficits on verbal fluency testing may also help distinguish frontosubcortical disorders from AD, as the former tend to exhibit greater difficulty with phonemic (letter) fluency tasks, which is relatively preserved in AD (4).

Therefore, a general approach to dementia differential diagnosis can be outlined using short-term memory deficits (primary or secondary) and the presence of associated clinical or laboratory signs.

- AD is characterized by early, severe short-term memory difficulties that become worse over time. On testing, individuals with AD typically do poorly on memory recall tests, and are not usually helped when given recognition cues (e.g., "fruit" for apple).
- By contrast, individuals with vascular cognitive impairment/dementia, Lewy body dementia, or frontotemporal dementia tend to have less severe short-term memory deficits and often are aided by poor performance on category testing (e.g., naming as many animals as they can in one minute), category clues (e.g., giving the hint "fruit" when the answer is "apple") or multiple choice recognition (offering several choices, including the word to be recalled).

Other features that may help distinguish non-AD are the presence of focal neurological or motor signs, prominent psychiatric features, and a history of one or more strokes.

HISTORY AND PHYSICAL EXAMINATION

The clinical history of the person who screens positive for cognitive impairment should be taken systematically, evaluating function (and changes in function), looking for risk factors, evaluating the family history, identifying potential comorbid or complicating conditions, identifying behavioral manifestations, and taking a careful history of symptom onset and progression. Table 23.2 displays the elements to include in this history.

In taking a history, the clinician should be on the alert for symptoms and signs that suggest the presence of a rapidly progressive, treatable, or potentially reversible condition that would be important not to miss diagnostically. These conditions include delirium, depression, hypothyroidism, vitamin B12 deficiency, neurosyphilis, a brain tumor, normal pressure hydrocephalus, and a subdural hematoma. Key signs and symptoms and next diagnostic steps for these conditions are displayed in Table 23.3.

DIAGNOSTIC TESTING

A diagnostic evaluation for dementia should also include one or more formal diagnostic tools. These fall into two general categories: Tools to diagnose dementia, and tools to identify comorbid conditions or reversible factors that may mimic dementia or coexist with dementia.

Several formal tools to evaluate dementia are appropriate for primary care physicians. Primary care physicians should be familiar with one of these tools and have preprinted forms in

TABLE 23.2 Historical Features of a Dementia Evaluation

Core Feature
Change from a previous level of functioning
Individual Factors
Cultural background Educational level Social/occupational demands Life circumstances (social, financial, occupational, living arrangements) Premorbid personality characteristics
Hereditary Factors
Familial risk factors (stroke, hypertension, diabetes mellitus) Genetic: family history suggesting autosomal dominant inheritance or multiple cases in family
Associated Medical/Neurological Conditions
General medical conditions (hypothyroidism, hypertension, diabetes mellitus, heart disease) Neurological conditions (transient ischemic attacks, strokes, seizures, syncope, head trauma) Associated motor features (tremor, gait difficulties, speech/swallowing disturbance, ataxia) Sleep disturbances (sleep apnea, insomnia, sleep-associated movement disorder)
Initial Manifestations
Impaired recent memory (repeats self, forgets what was heard or read, misplaces things) Poor decision making, judgment, or problem solving; decreased organizational skills Difficulty learning new tasks or performing routine tasks Problems managing money (balancing checkbook, forgetting to pay bills) Difficulties expressing self (word finding) or participating in conversation Getting lost in familiar areas, forgetting known routes while driving Change in personality (apathetic, disinhibited), mood (sad, irritable), or behavior (odd or bizarre)
Behavioral Manifestations (specifically ask spouse of caregiver about these)
Sleep disturbance Suspiciousness, irritability or paranoia Repetitive behaviors (asking questions repeatedly, pacing, doing things repeatedly) Driving patterns and driving safety Delusions or hallucinations Agitated or aggressive behaviors toward caregiver or others Depression or anxiety Impulsive, disinhibited, or socially inappropriate behaviors Changes in appetite or eating pattern
Course
Static Progressive Fluctuating

the office or on a downloadable computer file for ready use when such an evaluation is needed. Dementia evaluation tools especially appropriate for primary care include the following:

- the Saint Louis University Mental Status Examination (SLUMS) (18);
- the Montreal Cognitive Assessment (MoCA) (19,20); and
- the Mini-Mental State Examination (21) or, to better detect early dementia and mild cognitive impairment, the expanded MMSE (22).

Clinicians should be aware that the MMSE is copywritten, whereas the SLUMS and the MoCA are in the public domain and can be used without a fee.

Several additional formal tools are useful for clinicians in evaluating patients for comorbid conditions that may complicate or mimic dementia. Among the more useful are:

- A depression screen, such as the Geriatric Depression Scale (23) or the PHQ-9 (24,25), both of which have been well validated in geriatric populations.
- A measure of the anticholinergic burden of the medications the patient is taking. Because AD involves a cholinergic deficit within the brain, cumulative anticholinergic effects from multiple medications can worsen cognitive impairment and interfere with the action of pharmaceutical agents such as donepezil. Several anticholinergic burden scales are available (26–28).

TABLE 23.3 Red flags Suggesting Potentially Treatable and/or Reversible Causes of Cognitive Impairment

Potential Cause	Key Characteristics	Diagnostic Method
Delirium	Acute change in mental status Fluctuating course Inattention Disorganized thinking or altered level of consciousness	History and physical Cognitive status examination Laboratory testing as appropriate (e.g., complete blood count, electrolytes, renal function)
Depression	Apathy Frustration or giving up during testing with cognitive assessment tools	Depression screening and diagnosis Response to treatment
Hypothyroidism	Fatigue, cold intolerance, constipation, weight gain, bradycardia, and non-pitting edema (myxedema) Classical signs often absent in elderly	History and physical Thyroid function tests
Vitamin B12 deficiency	Paresthesias Peripheral neuropathy (loss of vibratory and positions sense in lower extremities) Ataxia	Vitamin B12 level
Neurosyphilis	Delusions of grandeur Emotional lability Argyll Robertson pupils	Serum FTA Spinal fluid FTA
Brain tumor	Headache Seizures Nausea/vomiting Focal neurological signs	MRI or CT
Normal-pressure hydrocephalus	Triad of incontinence, wide-based gait, and dementia	MRI or CT Radioisotope flow studies of CSF Therapeutic lumbar puncture
Subdural hematoma	History of trauma (often minor) Fluctuating level of consciousness Headache Hemiparesis Focal neurologic signs	MRI or CT

CT = computed tomography; MRI = magnetic resonance imaging; FTA = fluorescent treponemal antibody test (screen for syphilis).
Adapted from Langois J, Boorson S: Cognitive Impairment. In: Sloane, PD, et al (eds): *Essentials of Family Medicine, 5th Edition*. Baltimore: Lippincott, Williams & Wilkins, 2007.

Numerous laboratory tests are recommended to rule out causes of delirium and of conditions that may mimic dementia. Generally considered routine tests include: a complete blood count, a thyroid stimulating hormone level, a vitamin B12 level, serum electrolytes, serum calcium, serum glucose or glycosylated hemoglobin, and a noncontrast computerized tomography scan or magnetic resonance imaging scan of the brain (29).

RECOMMENDED DIAGNOSTIC STRATEGY

Figure 23.3 outlines a general diagnostic strategy for addressing cognitive impairment in primary care. Suspicion is initially raised when the patient appears to not remember well or to be confused during a routine office visit, or when a family member mentions concerns about memory. At such times, one can often conduct a rapid screen such as the Mini-Cog and/or the AD-8 on the spot, and then set up a more detailed visit if the screen is positive. At other times, memory concerns will be the chief complaint, in which case, depending on the clinical situation, the physician may screen or directly enter into a more formal diagnostic evaluation.

The diagnostic process outlined above will often identify whether the patient's clinical picture fits a diagnosis of AD or of vascular dementia. If the diagnosis is not clear, if atypical signs and symptoms are present, or if a less common diagnosis (e.g., frontotemporal or Lewy body dementia) is suspected, then referral to a memory disorders clinic, a neurologist, or a geriatrician is recommended.

MANAGEMENT

Management of dementia and related cognitive disorders involves careful attention to cognitive status, general health, behavioral and family issues, and connection with community

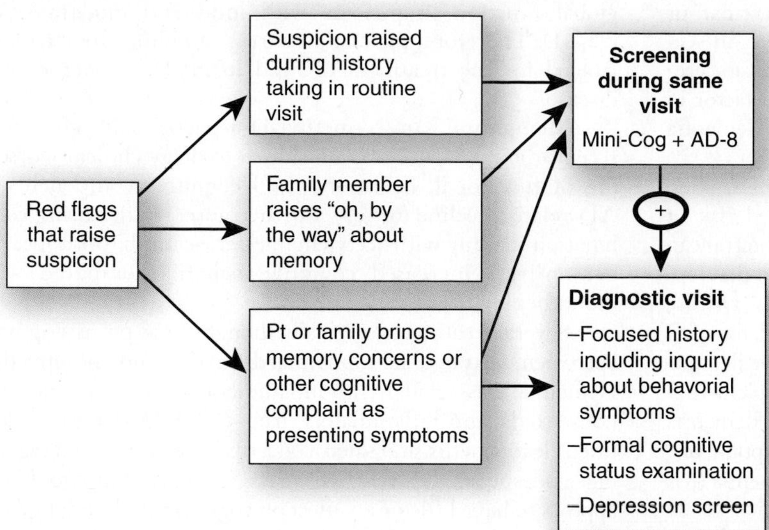

Figure 23.3 • Primary care approach to the detection and diagnosis of dementia.

resources. The approach must be individualized, because the needs and capabilities of the individual vary widely according to the stage of the disease (see Fig. 23.1) and the background, interests and living situation of the person with the disease and those who are providing care.

Prevention

People with a strong family history of dementia, including many family caregivers, are concerned about what they can do to prevent the disease. Most of the strategies that appear effective involve healthy lifestyle and prevention of cardiovascular disease (30). These strategies have been divided into three areas: treatment of vascular risk factors, diet and increasing neuronal reserves; they are summarized in Table 23.4.

High blood pressure in midlife is a risk factor for cognitive impairment and dementia/AD in late life, but results are inconsistent for the effects of late-life blood pressure (31). Several longitudinal observational studies showed significant reductions in the incidence of dementia in treated versus non-treated hypertensive patients (32,33); in addition, the double-blind, placebo-controlled Systolic Hypertension in Europe (Syst-Eur) trial concluded that long-term antihypertensive

TABLE 23.4 Strategies for Prevention of Dementia

General Strategy	Specific Actions and Goals	Strength of Recommendations
Treatment of vascular risk factors	• Treat hypertension to ≤140/90	A
	• Treat hypercholesterolemia to LDL ≤100	C
	• Treat diabetes to HbA1c ≤7	C
	• Prescribe aspirin in people with established cardiovascular disease	C
	• Manage heart failure optimally	C
	• Smoking cessation	C
Neuroprotection	• Folate and vitamin B12	C
	• Mediterranean Diet	B
	• Moderate alcohol consumption	B
Building up neuronal reserves	• Cognitive activity	B
	• Physical activity	B
	• Social and leisure activity	B

A = consistent, good-quality patient-oriented evidence; B = inconsistent or limited-quality patient-oriented evidence; C = consensus, disease-oriented evidence, usual practice, expert opinion.
For information about the SORT evidence rating system, see *http://www.aafp.org/afpsort.xml.*
Adapted with modifications from Purandare N, Ballard C, Burns A. Preventing dementia. *Advances in Psychiatric Treatment.* 2005;11:176–183.

treatment decreased the incidence of AD and vascular or mixed dementia by 55% (34,35). Similarly, primary and secondary prevention of stroke reduces dementia related to cerebrovascular disease either directly or as a comorbid factor in AD (36). The relationship between cholesterol and dementia risk is less clear, as study results have been inconsistent (37).

Diet appears to have a role in prevention. Fish consumption is related to lower cognitive decline and a decreased risk of dementia (38–45). Studies also suggest that the Mediterranean Diet is associated with a trend for reduced risk of both developing MCI and of MCI conversion to Alzheimer's Disease (40–43,45). Nutritional supplements such as vitamin E, omega 3 fatty acids, and other antioxidant nutrients do not have demonstrable benefits; however, vitamin B12 and folate supplementation in mid-late life may have a beneficial effect on dementia incidence or decline (31). In regard to alcohol consumption, one to three drinks daily appears to lower the risk for dementia (RR 0.58), largely by reducing vascular dementia (46,47).

Social, cognitive, and physical activities are linked in longitudinal studies with reduced risk of cognitive decline and dementia (48). Whether these represent cause-and-effect or an association with other factors (e.g., socioeconomic status or education) is unclear. However, though the evidence is modest, a mentally, physically, and socially active lifestyle is recommended in late life, because even if the cognitive benefits are not yet entirely clear, this lifestyle should bring about improved quality of life and overall health (31).

Management of MCI

Current recommendations for management of MCI are similar to those presented above for prevention: healthy lifestyle and vascular risk factor reduction. In addition, careful medication review to minimize or eliminate drugs with sedative and anticholinergic properties is indicated.

However, once a patient has been diagnosed with MCI, the patient and their family often ask if any treatment can be provided to prevent the further progression of MCI to dementia. Unfortunately, numerous clinical studies testing the acetylcholinesterase inhibitors have been undertaken and none has been demonstrated to prevent progression from MCI to AD (49–51). Consequently, no drug treatments are approved for MCI.

Management of Dementia

The primary management strategy for dementia is to preserve function and independence, minimize risk factors, and to help maintain quality of life for as long as possible. Pharmacologic interventions may be effective for improving cognitive function for certain dementias and useful in treating depression. Nonpharmacologic interventions, including measures to manage behavioral symptoms and ensure safety at home, are critically important, as is family support. Attention to long-term decisions regarding finances, nursing home placement, and caregiver stress are also important in the management of dementia. Table 23.5 summarizes the available evidence on key treatment strategies for dementia.

MEDICATION FOR COGNITIVE SYMPTOMS

Based on several randomized controlled trials and recent Cochrane reviews, cholinesterase inhibitors (donepezil, rivastigmine, galantamine), modestly improve cognition and global function in patients with mild and moderate AD (52–61). Therefore, the cholinesterase inhibitors are currently labeled for the treatment of mild to moderate Alzheimer's disease.

Memantine, an N-methyl-D-aspartic acid glutamate receptor antagonist, has been shown to delay clinical worsening of functional, behavioral, and cognitive components of AD-related decline (62–65). Furthermore, studies using combination therapy with acetylcholinesterase inhibitors appear to demonstrate increased cognitive benefits compared with monotherapy (64,66).

Several treatments originally thought to be promising have been demonstrated in randomized trials to not be effective. Dementia is associated with inflammation; however, studies of nonsteroidal anti-inflammatory drugs (NSAIDs) have not identified clear benefits, and safety concerns have been raised regarding widespread NSAID use (31). Similarly, Ginkgo biloba appears to have little or no effect on cognitive decline (31,67).

BEHAVIOR (NONPHARMACOLOGICAL) TREATMENT OF SYMPTOMS IN DEMENTIA

AD and the related dementias are primarily behavioral disorders. It is the behavioral symptoms that cause the most challenges for families and professional caregivers, and whose management is the key to effectively maintaining someone with dementia living in the community. Unfortunately, although there are numerous medications available to treat behavioral symptoms (see the next section), none is very effective, and all have significant toxicity. Therefore, nonpharmacological approaches are the mainstay of management and can often make a huge difference in terms of quality of life for people with dementia and those who surround them.

People with dementia will often express themselves using agitation, aggression, or resistance to care. These behaviors should be understood as primarily a form of communication, as they tend to result from a mismatch between environmental demands and the individual's ability to understand or cope with what is happening. Therefore, the first step in approaching these symptoms is to look for provoking factors, such as pain, infection, anxiety, or caregiver behaviors that are perceived as threatening. A good strategy to approach such problems is to evaluate what happened before the behavior, and how care providers reacted to the behavior, since it is much easier to change how caregivers (and the environment) change than to change the people with dementia.

Behavioral interventions for dementia can be placed in several categories (68). In each category the interventions must be chosen to match the stage of dementia.

- Creating a facilitative physical environment. Here the goal is to structure the environment so the person with dementia is safe, has easily interpretable cues to know where he or she is, can make correct choices, and is not bombarded with unpleasant stimuli. Interventions in this category include such things as eliminating hazards, making the toilet visible from the bed, having lighting that reduces glare, and eliminating confusing noises.
- Stimulating cognitive function without overchallenging the individual. Cognition-focused interventions, such as cognitive stimulation (engagement in a range of group activities and discussions aimed at general enhancement of cognitive

TABLE 23.5 Key Treatment Approaches for Common Symptoms in Patients with Dementia and Related Disorders

Target Conditions and/or Symptoms	Intervention	Efficacy	Strength of Recommendation (References)*
Mild cognitive impairment	Cognitive enhancers (e.g., donepezil, memantine)	No consistent evidence of effect; most studies fail to show benefit	B (49–51,55,57)
Dementia: Cognitive symptoms	Cholinesterase inhibitors (donepezil, rivastigmine, galantamine, memantine)	Effective for mild, moderate, and severe dementia. Effect size equivalent to slowing cognitive decline by 6 months	A (50,52,55–65, 94–96)
	Cognitive training	Improved ability specific to the abilities trained	B (75,97)
	Physical activity	Improved physical health and reduced depression	B (87,98)
Caregiver stress, burden, and depression	Caregiver support group programs and educational programs; use of respite services	Caregiver support groups and counseling can reduce psychological morbidity and delay nursing home placement. More intense and longer programs have greater effect	A (87,90,91,99,100)
Depression in people with dementia	Selective serotonin reuptake inhibitors (SSRIs) (sertraline, citalopram)	Mild to moderate effects in reducing depressed mood; no effect on neuropsychiatric symptoms	A (76,77,82,83)
	Physical activity/exercise	A combination of exercise and caregiver education improved depression	B (87)
Agitation, aggression, and delusions in people with dementia	Caregiver training in dementia management skills	Customized programs for caregivers focusing on non-pharmacologic interventions decrease agitation	A (69,85,86,101)
	Antipsychotic drugs	Statistically significant effects in a minority of recipients, but unclear if benefits outweigh adverse effects	A (76,80,102)
	Benzodiazepine medications	Little evidence to support use in light of risk of worsening memory loss, confusion and falls	C (103,104)
	Anticonvulsants	Carbamazepine has been found to reduce agitation, anxiety, and restlessness but the efficacy in the long-term use is unknown; ataxia and hematologic toxicity occur. Valproic acid does not appear to be effective for neuropsychiatric symptoms	B (76,77,105)
	Cognitive enhancers (e.g., donepezil, memantine)	Donepezil and galantamine have been demonstrated to significantly improve agitation; effects are modest	A (61,72,73)
	Environmental modification	Music reduces agitation, aggression, and mood disturbance during eating and bathing	B (71,106–108)
	Physical activity	Physical activity and exercise programs significantly reduce agitation and aggressive events	A (87,88)

A = consistent, good-quality patient-oriented evidence; B = inconsistent or limited-quality patient-oriented evidence; C = consensus, disease-oriented evidence, usual practice, expert opinion.
For information about the SORT evidence rating system, see *http://www.aafp.org/afpsort.xml*.

and social functioning), cognitive training, and cognitive rehabilitation, are of great interest to people with early stage disease and can improve quality of life.

- Facilitating success in performing everyday activities. Depending on the stage of the disease, a variety of strategies can be helpful in facilitating success. Examples include laying clothes out in the order they need to be put on, providing written reminders (for those who can read), and providing finger foods (for people with significant apraxia but who want to feed themselves).
- Providing activities that allow the individual to experience pleasure and success. Examples of such interventions include having pleasant, stimulating surroundings such as gardens, bird feeders, picture albums, and familiar books; having structured activities that are suited to the cognitive level of the individual; and providing a mix of activities that provide for overall physical and cognitive health (e.g., dancing, going for a walk outside, preparing and eating a snack, reminiscence).
- Providing care in a manner that is quiet, gentle, nonforceful, and respectful. Care provision is a skill that requires both sensitivity to the individual and a toolkit of strategies to help avoid or abort agitated behaviors and resistance to care.

The implementation of an individualized, nonpharmacological intervention for residents appears to decrease agitation (69). Small studies have shown that music seemed to reduce agitation, aggression, and mood disturbance during eating and bathing (70,71).

PHARMACOLOGICAL TREATMENT OF BEHAVIORAL SYMPTOMS

When nonpharmacological methods are insufficient, physicians are often asked to provide a prescription to aid in management of behavioral symptoms. No drug is effective in even as many as 50% of cases; however, the following agents have some evidence supporting their use in selected cases:

- Cholinesterase inhibitors appear to provide some improvement in behavior, especially in confusion-related symptoms, and these effects may persist even into advanced AD (61,72–75).
- Selective serotonin reuptake inhibitors as a class have shown efficacy in the treatment of depression but not in the treatment of behavioral symptoms (76,77). However, citalopram has demonstrated efficacy in treating behavioral symptoms (78,79).
- Antipsychotic medications have clear sedating properties, but their effectiveness in treating behavioral symptoms in dementia is modest at best. The atypical antipsychotics (clozapine, olanzapine, risperidone, quetiapine, ziprasidone, aripiprazole) have shown statistical significance with probable clinical significance, but there is concern for adverse events such as strokes (76,80), because this class of drugs is associated with a threefold increase in the risk of CV adverse events compared to placebo. Typical antipsychotics (haloperidol, chlorpromazine, thioridazine, thiothixene, trifluoperazine, acetophenazine), on the other hand, have no clear evidence of benefit in treating neuropsychiatric symptoms, except for haloperidol, which may improve aggression, but it is unclear if this benefit outweighs adverse effects such as sedation and extrapyramidal symptoms (76,77,81).
- So-called mood stabilizers such as carbamazepine and valproic acid, which are generally used to treat seizures, have been associated with modest reductions in agitation, anxiety, and restlessness, but the efficacy in the long-term use is unknown and the risk of ataxia and hematologic toxicity in the elderly is a concern (76,77).
- There is little evidence to support the use of benzodiazepines for behavior management, especially since they have been lined to worsening memory loss, confusion, and falls.

MANAGEMENT OF DEPRESSION IN DEMENTIA

Overall, selective serotonin reuptake inhibitors appear to be effective for the treatment of depression in dementia patients. In particular, sertraline and citalopram appear to have the most favorable effectiveness-to-toxicity profiles and suggest it improved emotional bluntness, confusion, irritability, confusion, anxiety, fear, restlessness, and depressed mood (76,77,82). There is little evidence for trazodone to be effective in depression in dementia, though it may be used for sleep disturbances (83). Agents with substantial anticholinergic effects, such as amitriptyline and imipramine, should be avoided because of the adverse cognitive effects (84).

In terms of nonpharmacological therapy for patients with dementia and depression, there have been several small studies looking at exercise, education, and light therapy. An important aspect in dementia care is also providing caregivers with the skills and information to manage dementia symptoms, including helping their loved one with depression.

WORKING WITH FAMILIES AND COMMUNITY RESOURCES

Families, not institutions, provide the majority of care to people with AD and related dementias (*http://www.caregiver.org*). Care provided by family and friends often makes the difference between remaining at home and being placed in a long-term care facility.

Providing support for the caregivers is an important aspect of the care for patients with dementia. The TAP program (Tailored Activity Program), a customized program tailored for patients and their families to reduce behavioral symptoms was effective for families to learn how to react to behavioral symptoms (85). In another study, community consultants implemented a behavioral intervention with family caregivers, resulting in improvements in depression, burden, and reactivity to behavioral problems, and a reduction in the frequency and severity of care recipient behavior problems (86).

Exercise training combined with teaching caregivers behavioral management techniques appeared to improve physical health and depression in patients with AD (87). A walking program demonstrated an average reduction of aggressive events by 30% in dementia residents who participated (88).

Community support services play a critical role in the lives of many caregivers. Research has shown, for example, that counseling and support groups, in combination with respite and other services, can assist caregivers in remaining in their caregiving role longer, with less stress and greater satisfaction (89). Extended involvement in counseling and support for caregivers of people with mild to moderate dementia can improve caregiver mood and coping skills and may delay nursing home (NH) placement by as much as 12 to 24 months (87,90).

TABLE 23.6 How Physicians Can Partner with Community Resources to Address Common Management Problems in People with Dementia

Management Problem	What the Physician Can Do	Resources for More Information
Caregiver support	Refer to community caregiver support groups; refer to local county Department on Aging or Alzheimer's Association for education and support groups. For families who can afford to pay for services, especially if they live some distance away from the person with dementia, an option is to hire a geriatric care manager.	Eldercare Locator, a public service of the U.S. Administration on Aging. The Eldercare Locator call 800-677-1116, website: *www.eldercare.gov.* Alzheimer's Association call 800-272-3900, website: *http://www.alz.org.* National Center on Caregiving call 800-445-8106, e-mail: info@caregiver.org. National Association of Professional Geriatric Care Managers. Website: *http://www.caremanager.org/*).
Driving concerns	Write a prescription for a driving evaluation. Write a letter to local to state department of motor vehicles expressing driving concerns and recommending an evaluation.	The Hartford (2000). At the Crossroads: A Guide to Alzheimer's Disease, Dementia, and Driving. *www.thehartford.com/alzheimers.* The Mayo Foundation for Medical Education and Research (2001). Dementia: Should Your Patient be Driving? *www.mayo.edu/geriatrics-rst/driving.html.*
Need for in-home help	Refer to physical therapy/occupational therapy for an in-home safety evaluation. Refer to a family caregiver specialist, local social service agency, or geriatric care manager.	Eldercare Locator, a public service of the US Administration on Aging. The Eldercare Locator call 800-677-1116, website: *www.eldercare.gov.*
Competency and legal issues	Encourage assignment of health care and financial power of attorney early in the disease (before diagnosis is ideal). Locate an elder attorney for documentation for advance directives, conservatorship issues/guardianship, financial and health power of attorney.	*The Conservatorship Book*, Lisa Goldoftas and Elizabeth A. Hendrickson, fifth edition, 2002, Nolo Press, 950 Parker St., Berkeley, CA 94710, (510) 549-1976.
Concern about safety at home	Make a home visit. Refer to an occupational therapist for an in-home safety evaluation.	Centers for Disease Control and Prevention National Center for Injury Prevention and Control (NCIPC) call 800-232-4636, e-mail: cdcinfo@cdc.gov.
Need for palliative, end-of-life care	Plan ahead and document discussions about end of life wishes. Know criteria for hospice referral of people with dementia.	Center to Improve Care of the Dying *www.medicaring.org.* Palliative Excellence in Alzheimer's Care Efforts (PEACE) (773) 702-0102. National Hospice Foundation (800) 338-8619 *www.hospiceinfo.org.*

Short-term programs have little to no effect on patient outcomes; however, they improve caregiver knowledge and coping ability (91).

For the primary care physician, an important element of dementia care is helping family caregivers gain access to home and community-based services such as counseling, support groups, transportation, meals, home care, and caregiver support services. Family caregivers can ask the physician about a wide variety of concerns that can often be addressed by community resources, so the family physician should be able to direct caregivers to the appropriate assistance. Table 23.6 provides guidelines and suggestions.

TAILORING TREATMENT TO THE TYPE OF DEMENTIA

Therapeutic approaches to AD and other dementias have to date been only modestly successful. Currently approved pharmacologic agents enhance neurotransmission, enhancing acetylcholine function. This has been proven to provide modest benefit in AD and more recently, in Parkinson disease with dementia, where cholinergic dysfunction is prominent (92). Several studies of cholinesterase-inhibitor agents in vascular dementia suggest potential symptomatic benefit, although these findings are likely confounded by the frequent coexistence of Alzheimer and vascular dementia.

By contrast, cholinergic deficits are not present in frontotemporal dementia, and common experience suggests that cholinesterase-inhibitor agents generally are not beneficial and may exacerbate behavioral disturbances in this disease. Memantine (Namenda), a partial antagonist of the n-methyl-d-aspartate glutamate receptor, initially developed for Parkinson disease in Europe, was later demonstrated to be effective in moderate to severe AD, and is now being tested as a potential therapeutic agent for frontotemporal dementia. Combination therapy with a cholinesterase-inhibitor combined with memantine has been shown to provide more benefit than monotherapy in a longitudinal clinical cohort of Alzheimer patients (93). Selective-serotonin reuptake inhibitors are also commonly used to treat behavioral disinhibition and obsessive-compulsive ritualistic behaviors in frontotemporal dementia, although data supporting their use from rigorous placebo-controlled trials is lacking.

Quetiapine (Seroquel) is widely regarded as a treatment of choice for addressing severe visual hallucinations and delusions that are common in Lewy body dementias, if measures such as eliminating anticholinergic drugs or antiparkinsonian dopaminergic agents are not successful. As with the treatment of any behavioral disturbance in the setting of dementia, there are currently no Food and Drug Administration–approved indications.

Eventually, the prevailing approach of treating common symptoms across different diseases will gradually give way to therapeutic agents that target specific disease-specific mechanisms.

LONG-TERM MONITORING AND FAMILY SUPPORT

AD and other degenerative dementias pose unique challenges from the standpoint of therapeutic monitoring. Although the AD course typically spans 8 to 10 years, therapeutic trials that establish the safety and efficacy of proven agents are typically conducted over a 6 to 12 month period. Moreover, the main effect of current therapies for AD is to slow progression over time, which becomes increasingly difficult to evaluate after 6 to 12 months of treatment. As symptomatic treatments, cholinesterase-inhibitors and memantine do not have any cumulative benefit beyond ongoing exposure. For example, after 5 years of treatment and discontinuation, an individual patients' residual functional status would settle out to be where they would otherwise have been if never exposed to treatment.

One of the most vexing challenges to clinical therapeutic monitoring of dementia is the absence of convenient metrics. Whereas clinical trials for antidementia agents typically employ a comprehensive test battery, such extensive assessment protocols are impractical in general care settings. However, clinical response can be partially measured by performing brief cognitive assessments and directed interviews regarding problematic behaviors on a regular basis.

An essential role of the clinician in providing long-term dementia care is to shape appropriate expectations. This includes educating patients and families about disease manifestations and course, while emphasizing the existence of individual variability. Although some patients may transiently improve with cholinesterase inhibitor or memantine therapy, the primary effect, based on placebo-controlled clinical trials, is to slow the progression of disease *symptoms*. To educate patients and families that therapeutic benefit may be associated with clinical decline, albeit at a slower rate, is a critically important cornerstone of current dementia care. Similarly, it is also helpful to keep the focus on the individual person as a whole, and to make explicit comments about retained abilities, particularly those that help maintain social roles. Also, it is helpful to emphasize that the person with dementia can have many pleasant experiences in spite of severe cognitive impairment.

Important issues to address over the disease course often include vocational activities, driving competency, financial capacity, the need for supervision, and, ultimately, provision for increasing care needs in a residential care facility. For children caregivers, gauging their own risk for developing a particular dementia affecting a parent or sibling may be important, as are ways to potentially lower their risk. Over the long term, making decisions about whether to stop taking one or more antidementia agents is couched in uncertainty about current benefit that may be addressed by a gradual therapeutic withdrawal and rechallenge, if clinically indicated, based on perceived impact on quality of life. In many cases, the primary focus of care gradually shifts away from the patient to the caregiver over time, as caregiver burden increases to a point where it may adversely affect their own health. At such times, balancing the growing dependency needs of the patient with the increasing strain imposed on the care provider can help guide difficult decisions regarding placement.

KEY POINTS

- Evaluation of people with concerns about cognitive function must include a rapid screening method such as the Mini-Cog and AD-8, followed by a more in depth evaluation of people who screen positive.
- An in-depth evaluation of someone with suspected cognitive impairment must determine whether mild cognitive impairment or dementia is present and rule out or identify the existence of treatable conditions such as delirium and depression.
- The common dementias include AD, vascular dementia, frontotemporal dementia, Lewy body dementia, and Parkinson dementia. Each has its own distinct presentation, clinical course, and treatment approach, though general therapeutic principles of dementia apply to all of these diagnoses.
- Family education and support over time is a critical element of dementia care, and should be done in partnership with available community resources.
- Medications currently play a relatively minor role in dementia care, in comparison to behavioral management techniques and family support; however, the primary care physician should be familiar with the available agents to treat cognitive and behavioral symptoms and prepare to prescribe and monitor them when appropriate.

CHAPTER

24

Palliative and End-of-Life Care

Gregg K. VandeKieft

CLINICAL OBJECTIVES

1. Define palliative care and describe the relationship between palliative care and curative care along the continuum of advanced illness.
2. Describe the Medicare hospice benefit, including appropriate timing and clinical criteria for referral.
3. List common symptoms in dying patients and effective treatment options for each.
4. Describe key psychosocial considerations in establishing patient-centered care plans.

Modern palliative care promotes aggressive symptom management at all stages of treatment for a serious illness, from early disease treatment through end-of-life care. According to the American Academy of Hospice and Palliative Medicine, "The goal of palliative care is to achieve the best possible quality of life through relief of suffering, control of symptoms, and restoration of functional capacity while remaining sensitive to personal, cultural, and religious values, beliefs, and practices" (1). This concept has been echoed by the Institute of Medicine, which also notes that "Palliative care in this broad sense is not restricted to those who are dying. . . . It attends closely to the emotional, spiritual, and practical needs and goals of patients and those close to them" (2).

Viewed from this context, it is clear that palliative care is a cornerstone not just of end-of-life care but also of chronic disease management. After all, diseases such as congestive heart failure (CHF), chronic obstructive pulmonary disease (COPD), arthritis, and Alzheimer disease are largely incurable, but much can be done to help the patient, and the goal of treatment is not only to extend life (a curative care principle) but also to maximize comfort, function, and quality of life. The difference at the end of life (i.e., in very advanced, terminal disease states) is that palliative care principles become paramount, and prolongation of length of life becomes much less important than quality of life.

Ideally, the transition from a curative care mentality to a palliative one should be gradual, with care of serious chronic illness being a blend of both approaches. For instance, American College of Chest Physicians clinical practice guidelines for the palliative care of lung cancer list 35 specific clinical interventions supported by Grade 1A to 1C evidence, all of which can be appropriately implemented when the goal is curative treatment, not just when the goal is comfort care (3).

A false dichotomy exists in the current US health care system between "curative care" and "comfort care." This attitude misses the more holistic approach of palliation throughout the course of care, leads to undertreatment of symptoms and ultimately results in late referrals to palliative care services such as hospice. A growing body of evidence demonstrates that patient satisfaction is improved, symptoms are better controlled, treatment choices are better aligned with patients' goals of care, and overall medical expenditures are decreased when palliative care is engaged early in the course of treatment and/or offered as a home-based alternative to patients who are either not yet eligible or psychologically ready to enroll in hospice care (4–7).

The National Consensus Project, a multidisciplinary coalition of professional organizations dedicated to hospice and palliative care, established a comprehensive overview of the conceptual foundations of palliative care, as well as a set of clinical practice guidelines, which are available for download at *http://www.nationalconsensusproject.org/Guidelines_Download.asp* (8). This chapter will focus on how to work within today's complex health care delivery environment to most effectively implement those guidelines, thereby delivering patient-centered, comprehensive palliative and end-of-life care.

PATHOPHYSIOLOGY OF SERIOUS ILLNESS AND THE DYING PROCESS

The dying process is accompanied by numerous common symptoms that must be managed well to provide the patient with maximal quality of life before they die. The most prominent symptoms include:

- **Pain.** Patients can experience both acute and chronic pain at the end of life. Pain may be *nociceptive*, which presumes normally functioning pain receptors and nerves, or *neuropathic*, which presumes abnormal function of either the peripheral or central nervous system (CNS). Nociceptive pain generally responds well to opioid analgesics; neuropathic pain often requires adjuvant analgesics in addition to opioids. (See Chapter 41 for further discussion of the physiology of pain.)
- **Dyspnea.** Dyspnea is the subjective sensation of breathlessness or difficulty in breathing. For dying patients and their families, dyspnea can be one of the most frightening and anxiety-provoking symptoms. If a treatable cause for dyspnea can be identified, the first step is to optimize treatment for that condition. Potentially treatable causes of dyspnea

include anxiety, airway obstruction, thick airway secretions, hypoxemia, pleural effusion, pneumonia, pulmonary edema, pulmonary embolism, anemia, or metabolic causes.

- **Nausea and Vomiting.** These symptoms may result from the patient's underlying medical condition or from medical therapy (e.g., chemotherapy). Four different neurotransmitters mediate stimulation of the vomiting center in the medulla: serotonin, dopamine, histamine, and acetylcholine.
- **Fatigue.** Tiredness is one of the most distressing symptoms associated with end-of-life care (9). Treatable causes such as anemia and medication adverse effects should be sought and corrected.
- **Constipation.** Differential diagnosis for constipation includes: medication effect, decreased gastrointestinal motility, ileus, mechanical obstruction, metabolic abnormalities, spinal cord compression, dehydration, autonomic dysfunction, and malignancy. Constipation is a frequent adverse effect of opioid analgesics, calcium channel blockers, and anticholinergic medications.
- **Anxiety.** Anxiety is a common response to the uncertainty associated with confronting one's impending death. However, anxiety also may reflect inadequate control of pain or dyspnea, a more longstanding psychiatric condition, or a medication adverse effect.
- **Depression.** The notion that terminally ill patients are inherently depressed or desire a prompt death is a misconception (10). Most patients with a terminal diagnosis will experience feelings of sadness, anger, and helplessness that are either temporary or moderate and intermittent. However, clinical depression may indeed be associated with terminal illness. In patients with depression, early diagnosis and intervention improves the likelihood that treatment will be helpful. Risk factors for depression include refractory pain, comorbid conditions, significant physical limitations, medication adverse effects (e.g., corticosteroids, benzodiazepines), family dysfunction, substance abuse, and a previous history of depression.
- **Delirium.** Delirium may develop rapidly, and is characterized by disorientation, cognitive impairment, and/or fluctuating levels of consciousness. Causes may include infection, medication adverse effects or withdrawal, and metabolic or hypoxic encephalopathy.

DIAGNOSIS AND ASSESSMENT

Serious illness requires an ongoing assessment of the appropriate balance between treatments that are palliative (i.e., whose goal is to minimize symptom burden and maximize quality of life), and those whose goal is to cure or prolong life. Negotiating these competing yet complementary treatment goals can be a significant challenge for clinicians, yet providing the best mix of treatments over time allows patients and families the greatest opportunity to pursue reasonable opportunities for cure or prolongation of life while minimizing iatrogenic suffering.

Clinical Assessment to Determine the Need for Palliative Care

Curative and palliative efforts ideally go hand in hand at each stage of the patient's treatment, with curative care predominating early in the illness and palliative care predominating near the end (Fig. 24.1).

THE HOSPICE BENEFIT

Medicare, most Medicaid programs, and most private insurers provide a hospice benefit. Patients receiving the Medicare hospice benefit sign a statement choosing the Medicare hospice benefit in place of standard Medicare-covered benefits for their illness, and enroll in a Medicare-certified hospice program. Hospice programs use an interdisciplinary team, including nurses, social workers, home health aides, pastoral care, and volunteers to assist the family and provide respite

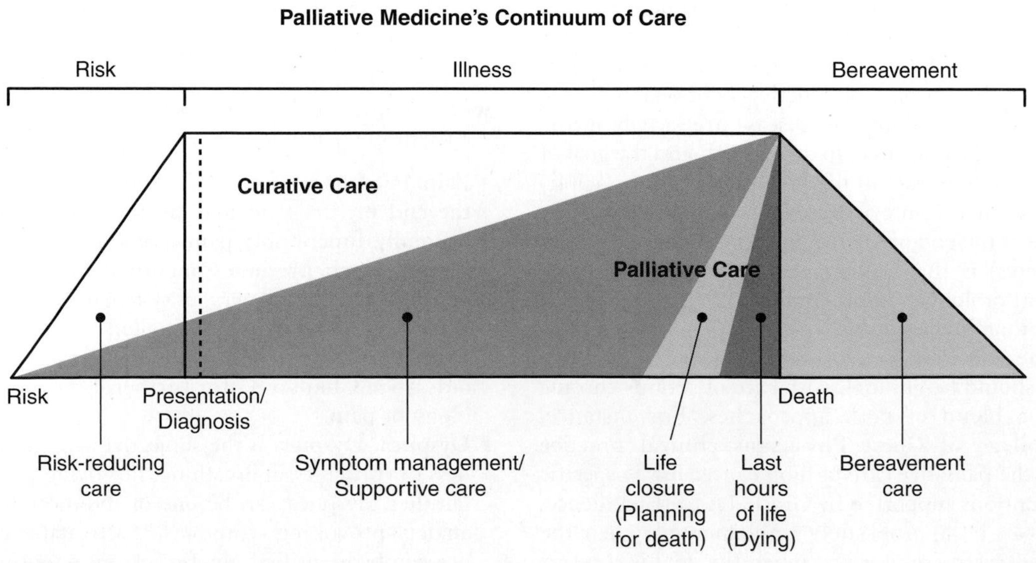

Figure 24.1 • Continuum of curative to palliative care.

care, and bereavement programs for the family after the patient's death. Ideally, most end-of-life care is carried out in the patient's home setting (which may be a nursing home or assisted-living facility). In addition, many hospices offer a residential facility for patients unable to remain at home. Hospitalization is occasionally indicated to manage symptoms that are too complex to manage at home or in a lower acuity facility, and Medicare offers a General Inpatient benefit to cover these services as a part of the patient's hospice care plan. Regardless of location, the basic principles of end-of-life care can be carried out provided adequate support and services are available.

As an example: Mary P is a 65-year-old woman with end-stage COPD who has been hospitalized five times in the past 2 years, including intubation and mechanical ventilation during two admissions. She is readmitted with a COPD exacerbation, managed overnight in the critical care unit with noninvasive positive pressure ventilation, stabilizes, and is transferred to a general medical floor. The following day, she tells her family physician, "I am so tired of this. I really don't want to come back to the hospital again, and I *never* want to be on a ventilator again." Her doctor speaks at length with Mary and her husband. After inquiring about their hopes for her future given the limits of her illness, and clarifying her specific treatment goals, they all agree that a home-based comfort-focused plan of care is most appropriate. A hospice referral is arranged. The hospice team spends extensive time with Mary and her family reviewing the high likelihood of recurrent COPD exacerbations, including possible acute bronchitis or pneumonia, and devises "sick day" plans to address symptoms during times of urgent need. Over the ensuing 5 months, Mary has three acute episodes that trigger urgent calls to her hospice nurse. On two occasions, Mary's family is able to manage her symptoms with telephone support from the hospice nurse, who obtains medical orders from Mary's family physician. On the third occasion, an on-call hospice nurse goes out to Mary's home and with support from Mary's physician is again able to adequately treat her symptoms. As time progresses, Mary becomes increasingly somnolent, eventually remaining obtunded independent of sedating medications. After 3 days of progressive respiratory decline, including Cheyne-Stokes respirations (which the hospice team had advised Mary's family to anticipate during the active dying process), Mary dies peacefully at home with her family at her bedside. Although her family finds it difficult to lose her, with hospice support her symptoms remain adequately treated and they are pleased that she is able to live out her final months on her own terms. After Mary's death, the hospice's bereavement coordinator makes a follow-up phone call to her family and tells them how to enroll in the hospice's bereavement support group if they are interested.

DETERMINING WHEN A PATIENT QUALIFIES FOR HOSPICE

Hospice eligibility criteria require the attending physician to certify that the patient's life expectancy is 6 months or less, if the disease follows its anticipated course. However, hospice patients may remain on service beyond the 6-month life expectancy provided there is adequate documentation that they met hospice eligibility criteria upon initiation of hospice services, and their condition remains hospice appropriate at the time of recertification.

Unfortunately, many patients miss out on hospice care or are referred very late in the course of a terminal illness because physicians feel uncomfortable predicting a life expectancy of <6 months. Scientific evidence lends support to this concern, because prognosis is an inexact science and the rate of error is high (11–13). One approach that can be helpful is to ask the question differently. Rather than asking if a patient will die in 6 months or less, a more appropriate question might be: "Would you be surprised if this patient died in the next 6 months?" This approach has been demonstrated to more effectively engage hospice benefits earlier in a patient's decline (14). Also, Medicare has approved a preelection benefit, which provides a nominal professional fee for a hospice medical director to consult with the primary physician about a patient regarding their eligibility for hospice care and their treatment alternatives. Palliative care consultations also provide this function.

DETERMINING HOSPICE ELIGIBILITY FOR COMMON ILLNESSES

To meet Medicare hospice eligibility, the attending physician must attest that: (i) the patient's condition is life-limiting and the patient and/or family have been informed of this determination; (ii) the patient and/or family have elected treatment goals directed toward relief of symptoms rather than cure of the underlying disease; and (iii) the patient has either documented disease progression or documented recent impaired nutritional status related to the terminal process. The National Hospice and Palliative Care Organization has published guidelines for determining prognosis for a variety of noncancer diagnoses, including heart disease, pulmonary disease, liver disease, kidney disease, dementia, stroke, and HIV/AIDS (15). Guidelines for conditions commonly managed on hospice by family physicians are outlined in Table 24.1.

Assessment of Common Symptoms during Palliative and End-of-Life Care

An important part of the palliative care physician's role is active patient assessment to identify whether the patient is experiencing symptoms, and, if so, the severity of those symptoms. These include pain, dyspnea, nausea and vomiting, fatigue, constipation, anxiety, depression, and delirium. Each of these symptoms should be formally looked for at each patient visit. Below are tips on how to evaluate each:

- **Pain.** Patients need to be *asked* about pain. It should not be assumed that patients will spontaneously report pain. A simple approach to pain assessment is listed in Table 24.2. Clarifying the underlying cause of pain (e.g., tumor, bony metastasis, neuropathic pain) will help plan optimal treatment. Patients with advanced dementia, who cannot verbally report their pain, require clinical observation. A 10-point scale, scoring five observable indicators (breathing, vocalization, facial expression, body language, and consolability) from 0 to 2, can assist in pain assessment for patients with dementia (16). Further details about assessment of pain are provided in Chapter 41.
- **Dyspnea.** Few symptoms are more distressing than uncontrolled breathlessness. Identifying the underlying cause of dyspnea is critical for treatment planning; common etiologies include cardiac or pulmonary disease (e.g., COPD, CHF), pleural effusions, ascites, anemia, and superior vena

TABLE 24.1 National Hospice and Palliative Care Organization Medical Guidelines for Hospice Eligibility in Selected Non-cancer Diagnoses*

Heart Disease
Symptoms at rest (New York Heart Association Class IV)
Optimal diuretic and vasodilator treatment
Ejection Fraction of ≤20% (helpful, but not required)
Not a revascularization or transplant candidate
Additional predictors of increased mortality risk: refractory angina, symptomatic ventricular or supraventricular dysrhythmias, unexplained syncope, prior cardiac arrest, cardiogenic stroke, HIV
Pulmonary Disease
Dyspnea at rest, unresponsive to treatment
Hypoxemia at rest while on supplemental oxygen (pO_2 ≤55, O_2 sat ≤88%)
Hypercapnia (pCO_2 ≥50)
Cor pulmonale or right heart failure (not due to valve disease or left heart failure)
Progressive decline in FEV1 (>40 mL per year)
Frequent hospitalizations or emergency room visits (no specific number, but an overall trend)
Not a lung transplant candidate
Liver Disease
Impaired synthetic function: e.g., PT >5 seconds over control, INR >1.5, serum albumin <2.5 mg/dL
Ascites despite maximal diuretic therapy
Bacterial peritonitis
Hepatic encephalopathy
Hepatorenal syndrome
Recurrent variceal bleeding
Kidney Disease
Creatinine clearance <10 mL/min (<15 mL/min with diabetes or CHF; ≤20 with diabetes *and* CHF)
Serum Cr >8 (>6 for diabetics)
Signs or symptoms of uremia
No longer on dialysis
Not a kidney transplant candidate
Dementia
Unable to walk, dress, or bathe without assistance
Urinary and fecal incontinence
No meaningful verbal communication (≤6-word sentence)
Co-morbid medical conditions that indicate increased mortality risk: severe dysphagia, aspiration pneumonia, pyelonephritis, septicemia, stage 3–4 decubitus ulcers, recurrent fever despite antibiotics
With feeding tube: documented signs of nutritional impairment (e.g., serum albumin ≤2.5 mg/dL, weight loss ≥10% over 6 months)
Without feeding tube: inability or refusal to maintain adequate oral intake

Source: Stewart et al. (15).
*These are not Medicare guidelines, but provide guidelines for general prognosis. This table does not represent the NHPCO guidelines in their entirety—the original guidelines should be consulted for clinical application.

cava syndrome. If the patient has adequate potential to benefit from interventions, a basic work-up for these causes is warranted. However, in actively dying patients the burden of evaluation may outweigh possible benefits, and a definitive cause cannot be identified for approximately a quarter of dyspneic patients at the end of life (17).

- **Nausea and Vomiting.** When nausea and vomiting occur, diagnostic evaluation should consider gastrointestinal, CNS, pharmacologic, metabolic, and psychological causes, as well as medication adverse effects. Different antiemetics work via different physiologic pathways, so clarifying the underlying cause of nausea is critical to choosing an agent or nonpharmacologic modality that addresses the underlying cause of the nausea (18).
- **Fatigue.** Decreased energy levels are ubiquitous in terminal illness. In cardiac or pulmonary disease, palliative treatments differ little from disease-specific interventions. Cancer cachexia or asthenia, however, is unique in that disease-specific treatments often worsen functional status, and symptoms progress regardless of caloric intake. Functional assessments such as the Palliative Performance Scale provide a general overview of a patient's clinical status and can also provide valuable information regarding hospice eligibility and overall prognosis (19,20).

TABLE 24.2 Pain Assessment

Quality of pain: What does the pain feel like? What words would you use to describe it?
Severity: How bad is the pain? At its worst? At its best? Use rating scales (e.g., numerical scale from 1–10, or a scale that depicts facial expressions)
Temporal course: When did the pain start? How often does it hurt? Has it gotten better? Worse? Is it worse at certain times of the day?
Radiation: Where is the pain? Does the pain go anywhere else? Does it spread? Can you put one finger in the center of the pain?
Provocative factors: What makes the pain worse? What brings it on? What aggravates it?
Palliating factors: What makes the pain better? What do you do to get relief? What helps you?
Treatment: What have you tried to relieve the pain? How effective was it? Why did you stop it?

- **Constipation.** Constipation remains one of the most common distressing symptoms for patients receiving palliative or end-of-life care. Contributing factors include metabolic derangements from the underlying illness itself, immobility and decreased fluid intake associated with declining functional status, and medical treatments (especially opioid analgesics). When patients are treated with chronic opioids, standard practice is to initiate regular administration of a stimulant laxative.
- **Anxiety.** When anxiety arises, it is important to try to distinguish whether it is a primary psychological disorder (including distress resulting from familial or spiritual factors), a symptom of the underlying illness (such as anxiety from pain), or a medication adverse effect. Anxiety and dyspnea have the potential to create a "vicious cycle" where increased dyspnea exacerbates anxiety, which in turns further exacerbates the dyspnea. Further details about assessment of anxiety are provided in Chapter 48.
- **Depression.** Diagnosis of depression in end-of-life care is made more difficult by the fact that many somatic symptoms of depression in physically healthy adults, such as sleep disturbance, loss of appetite, and fatigue, can be caused by the underlying disease rather than by depression. Therefore, psychological criteria for depression (i.e., dysphoria, anhedonia, and feelings of worthlessness or guilt) become more important in end-of-life care. Further details about assessment of depression are provided in Chapter 50.
- **Delirium**. Delirium or agitation should not be confused with anxiety or dementia. Delirium is characterized by an acute, fluctuating, change in cognition not attributable to dementia, with diminished ability to focus or maintain attention. Precipitating factors include metabolic derangements, infection, CNS lesions, and medication adverse effects. Treatable causes should be sought out and addressed. Tools such as the Memorial Delirium Assessment Scale can aid in evaluation (21). Clinicians should also be aware that many terminally ill patients experience hypoactive delirium rather than the more characteristic agitated delirium (22).

MANAGEMENT

Family physicians who have longstanding relationships with patients and their families are ideally positioned to provide end-of-life services as the culmination of "cradle-to-grave" care. At times, however, patients are referred to subspecialists to manage serious illness, and the patient and family develop sufficient relationships with the subspecialist that their needs may be most appropriately met by having that physician continue as their attending physician during end-of-life care. At other times, they may prefer to have their long-standing primary care physician resume their care when palliative care is the goal. Substantial variation takes place among individual physicians, geographical regions, and local community practices, in terms of who provides end-of-life care.

When a patient enters hospice, there is an increasing trend for the hospice medical director to become the attending physician. Ideally, however, the hospice medical director serves in a consulting capacity, providing oversight of the hospice interdisciplinary team and, when warranted, providing specialized medical consultations and/or direct management in support of the patients attending physician.

Communication Issues

Patients and physicians often find it difficult to discuss death as a possible outcome of a serious illness, even when death is inevitable. This creates a major barrier to establishing patient-centered, goal-directed care plans. In one survey of physicians caring for cancer patients, less than half would discuss code status with an asymptomatic terminally ill patient with a prognosis of 4 to 6 months, and less than one quarter of respondents would discuss hospice or the patient's preferred site of death. Most physicians indicated that they would wait to discuss these matters until the patient was overtly symptomatic from the illness or there were no additional treatments to offer (23). This is unfortunate, however, because families who have lost loved ones report a significant reduction of stress when a proactive communication strategy is used (24).

Patients' needs range from basic information about their prognosis and what symptoms to expect to help with complex issues such as unresolved family conflicts or making final arrangements. These conversations are critical to helping patients make treatment choices about how they want to live their lives. Patients express a strong preference for clear discussions of prognosis and treatment options, especially when the time remaining becomes limited (25). Appropriate consultation and collaboration with social workers, counselors, or chaplains are often the most effective means of addressing more complex needs.

Even something as simple as the name of the program providing the service can become a barrier to accessing a service in a timely manner. In one comprehensive cancer center, clinicians were unlikely to consider their patients eligible for palliative care services, but they felt the exact same services would be very helpful for their patients when the program was introduced as "supportive care" rather than palliative care (26).

TABLE 24.4 Key Therapies for Symptom Relief in Palliative Care

Symptom	Intervention	Strength of Recommendation*	Comments and Cautions
Pain	Physical and psychosocial interventions	B	Numerous modalities available as components of multimodal therapy. Caution: Exclusive reliance on complementary or alternative therapies may lead patients to forego curative or life-prolonging conventional treatments; a collaborative approach is advised.
	Acetaminophen and nonsteroidal anti-inflammatory drugs (NSAIDs)	A	For mild pain, or as co-analgesic with opioid analgesics. Caution: Chronic or terminal illness may increase risk for acetaminophen induced hepatotoxicity or NSAID induced gastropathy and renal toxicity.
	Opioid analgesics	A	For moderate to severe pain. Multiple routes of delivery. Caution: Monitor for adverse effects, especially in opioid-naïve patients; treat preventively for constipation. Although risk of addiction is low in terminal illness, monitor for potential abuse or diversion.
	Tricyclic antidepressants	A	Effective for neuropathic pain. Caution: amitriptyline has high risk of anticholinergic adverse effects; nortriptyline is equally efficacious but better tolerated.
	Anticonvulsants	A	Effective for neuropathic pain; gabapentin best-studied. Caution: Risk of adverse effects greater in elderly or debilitated patients; start at low dose and titrate to effective dose. Reduce dosage if renal impairment.
	Corticosteroids	C	Effective for bony metastases or tumor mass effect. Caution: Adverse effects with prolonged use; most advantageous with limited life expectancy or for short duration of therapy.
	Radiation therapy	A	Effective for bony metastases or direct compression/obstruction from tumor mass. Caution: Substantial potential adverse effects; carefully consider benefits/burdens. Prognosis must be of sufficient duration to allow time to benefit from treatment.
Dyspnea	Physical and psycho-social interventions	B	Relaxation therapies and simple measures such as an oscillating fan may reduce medication usage.
	Oxygen	B	Effective for symptomatic hypoxemia. Caution: Can be drying to nasal mucosa, and nasal prongs or face mask can be uncomfortable; titrate to comfort during active dying phase. Over-reliance on oximetry rather than direct observation of patient's comfort level increases likelihood oxygen will be used even when there is no palliative benefit.
	Opioids	A	Morphine is gold standard for dyspnea relief. Short-acting agents confer greater symptom relief than long-acting agents. Caution: Balance dyspnea relief with acceptable level of sedation. If sedated, monitor closely for respiratory depression.
	Diuretics	A	For relief of pulmonary congestion or to reduce ascites. Caution: Electrolyte derangements a possible adverse effect.
Nausea and Vomiting	Metoclopramide	B	Has both promotility effect on GI tract and antidopaminergic effect in chemoreceptor trigger zone (CTZ). Caution: may cause extrapyramidal adverse effect.
	Phenothiazines	B	Caution: Higher adverse effect rate than metoclopramide.
	5-HT3 Receptor Antagonists (e.g., ondansetron)	B	Highly effective for chemotherapy or radiation therapy induced nausea. Caution: Very costly.

TABLE 24.4 *(Continued)*

Symptom	Intervention	Strength of Recommendation*	Comments and Cautions
Fatigue	Cause-specific treatment	B	Treat electrolyte derangements, anemia, anorexia, etc. Diagnostic evaluation and treatments should be considered within context of prognosis, functional status, and goals of care.
	Corticosteroids	A	Dexamethasone, methylprednisolone. Caution: Weigh short-term therapeutic benefits against risk of adverse effects with prolonged use.
	Psychostimulants	C	Caffeine, methylphenidate, modafinil, dextroamphetamine. Start at low dose and titrate upward as needed. Typically given in morning and mid-day. Caution: monitor for adverse effects of appetite suppression, insomnia, agitation.
Constipation	Dietary interventions	B	Increased dietary fiber and adequate hydration can improve laxation.
	Stool softeners	C	Should not be used as sole agent; use in conjunction with laxative.
	Laxatives	A	Initiate early in course of long-term opioids.
	Methylnaltrexone	B	Reverses opioid effects on gut without reversing analgesic effect. Caution: do not use in bowel obstruction.
Anxiety	Psychosocial interventions	A	Multiple anticipatory and responsive modalities; individualize to identifiable sources of anxiety.
	Benzodiazepines	A	Most effective when used with psychosocial interventions. Short-acting agents best for acute anxiety. Caution: habituation and tolerance are concerns; for long-term use, consider antidepressant as primary agent.
	Buspirone	B	Less habituating than benzodiazepines, fewer adverse effects in elderly. Caution: Less effective in patients with prior benzodiazepine treatment.
	SSRI antidepressants	A	Effective for long-term treatment.
Depression	Psychosocial interventions	B	Multiple modalities available; less evidence of effectiveness in end-of-life care.
	SSRI antidepressants	A	Effective, safe. Caution: May take weeks to achieve therapeutic effect; prognosis must be of sufficient duration to allow effect.
	Tricyclic antidepressants	A	Equally effect as SSRIs, less costly. Caution: Higher adverse effect rate. Greater risk if suicide attempted.
	SNRI antidepressants	B	Effective for depression, may also be effective for neuropathic pain.
	Other antidepressants	C	Mirtazapine effective for sleep disorder, comorbid anxiety, and as an appetite stimulant.
Delirium	Psychosocial interventions	C	Environmental changes to minimize disorientation key.
	Phenothiazines	A	Haloperidol gold standard, efficacy well documented. Caution: Regulatory limitations to use in long-term care setting.
	Atypical antipsychotics	B	Mixed evidence, but often helpful for patients needing a longer-acting agent. Caution: "Black Box" warnings about cardiac risks; for patients at the end-of-life, weigh risks and benefits.

*A = consistent, good-quality patient-oriented evidence; B = inconsistent or limited-quality patient-oriented evidence; C = consensus, disease-oriented evidence, usual practice, expert opinion.
For information about the SORT evidence rating system, see *http://www.aafp.org/afpsort.xml.*

TABLE 24.5 Equianalgesic Doses of Opiate Analgesics*

Opiate Agonist	Oral	Parenteral	Dosing Interval
Morphine	30 mg	10 mg	q3–4h
Hydromorphone	7.5 mg	1.5 mg	q3–4h
Meperidine†	300 mg	75 mg	q2–3h
Methadone	10 mg	5 mg	q6–8h
Fentanyl	Variable‡	—	Patches, every 3 day§
Oxycodone	15 mg	N/A#	q3–4h
Codeine	120 mg	N/A	q3–4h
Hydrocodone	30 mg	N/A	q3–4h

*Equianalgesic dosages are approximations only; more precise dosage corrections will be required based on the patient's clinical response.
†Meperidine is not recommended for chronic use because of seizure risk from normeperidine metabolite.
‡Fentanyl should not be used in an opiate naïve patient. Equivalent ranges have been developed for morphine, but many physicians feel that they do not accurately reflect actual experience with the medication. Careful clinical observation is needed to establish the correct equianalgesic doses when changing to or from fentanyl patches.
§Also available as a lozenge and parenterally with dosing intervals specific to the products.
#Not available.

changes in humidity or temperature of the ambient air, or relaxation techniques. Supplemental oxygen is effective for some patients. However, the majority of terminally ill patients experiencing dyspnea are not hypoxemic, and there is no evidence that they benefit symptomatically from the use of oxygen. Nebulized saline for thick secretions, or nebulized opioids for certain conditions or dyspnea refractory to standard treatments, are reported as effective alternatives, although well-controlled trials demonstrating their efficacy are lacking (36).

For conditions where severe dyspnea can be anticipated, such as end-stage COPD or CHF, patients and families need to educated regarding its probable occurrence and given treatment plans. Otherwise, they are at high risk for calling 911 and potentially ending up intubated and/or admitted to critical care, even if they have expressed a strong desire to avoid such a scenario.

NAUSEA AND VOMITING

If an underlying medical cause can be identified, appropriate treatments should be initiated. Palliative measures to alleviate nausea and vomiting include both nonpharmacologic and pharmacologic therapies. Prokinetic agents such as metoclopramide are especially useful and warrant being considered as first line therapy. Pharmacologic therapies are listed in Table 24.6.

TABLE 24.6 Pharmacologic Management of Nausea

Cause	Drug Class	Recommended Agents and Dosage
Movement-related nausea	Antihistamine	Meclizine 25–50 mg orally every 6 hours Hydroxyzine 25–50 mg orally every 6 hours
Tumor-related elevated intracranial pressure	Glucocorticoids	Dexamethasone 6–20 mg orally once daily
Gastric stasis	Prokinetic agent	Metoclopramide 10–15 mg orally every 6 hours, 30 minutes before meals/food and at bedtime
Stimulation of chemoreceptor trigger zone (drugs, uremia)	Dopamine	Prochlorperazine 5–20 mg orally every 6 hours, or 25 mg rectally every 12 hours, or 5–10 mg intravenously every 4 hours (maximum IV dose 40 mg/day) Promethazine 25 mg orally or rectally, or 12.5–25 mg intravenously, every 4–6 hours Haloperidol 0.5–2 mg orally, intravenously, or subcutaneously every 6 hours, then titrate
	Serotonin antagonist	Ondansetron 4–8 mg orally three times per day
Constipation	Laxative	See Table 24.7

FATIGUE

Fatigue at the end of life warrants a different approach than during recovery from acute illness. Specific recommendations should focus on energy conservation and optimizing fluid and nutritional status, concordant with the patient's stage of illness and goals for therapy. Patients wishing to maintain maximal functional status for as long as possible should remain physically active, and treatable causes such as anemia should be corrected. Medical interventions are of limited effectiveness, but some patients benefit from low-dose glucocorticoids (e.g., dexamethasone 2 to 8 mg by mouth daily) or psychostimulants (e.g., methylphenidate 2.5 to 5 mg each morning and noon initially, titrated to effect).

Eventually many diseases progress such that patients cannot do much more than remain at bed rest. In such situations, physicians can help by validating the patient's fatigue to family members, who may see the symptom as simply "mind over matter." Supportive care at this stage should focus on maximal quality of life within the context of their progressing debility.

CONSTIPATION

A common problem when treating constipation is the failure to titrate to an effective dose of a given agent, leading to the sense that "nothing works." Fecal impaction should also be ruled out if constipation does not respond to standard treatments. Treatment alternatives are listed in Table 24.7.

ANXIETY

Nonpharmacologic therapy includes counseling (both psychological and spiritual), social services consultation, and family support. With chronic use, short-acting agents (e.g., alprazolam), may not provide smooth symptom relief and may also induce withdrawal symptoms if a dose is missed. For acute anxiety, short or intermediate acting benzodiazepines (e.g., lorazepam) are the drug of choice. Chronic anxiety often responds well to selective serotonin reuptake inhibitors (SSRIs) or tricyclic antidepressants. Anxiolytics should be started at low doses and titrated to effect. Remain vigilant for adverse effects of sedation, confusion, or memory disturbance.

TABLE 24.7 Constipation Management

Treatment	Recommended Agent and Dosage	Comments
Stimulant laxatives	Prune juice 120–240 mL orally once or twice daily Senna 2 tablets or 5–10 mL of syrup orally at bedtime, titrate to effect Docusate 2 tablets orally at bedtime, titrate to effect Bisacodyl 5–15 mg orally or 10 mg suppository rectally at bedtime, titrate to effect	Irritates the bowel and stimulates peristalsis. Prolonged use can lead to laxative dependency and loss of normal bowel function.
Osmotic laxatives	Milk of magnesia 5–15 mL orally 1–3 times per day Lactulose 15–30 mL orally up to every 4–6 hours, then titrate to effect Magnesium citrate 1 (240 mL) orally as needed	Attracts water into the intestinal lumen, maintaining or increasing the moisture content and volume of the stool, distending the bowel, and inducing peristalsis. Use caution with magnesium containing products in patients with renal insufficiency.
Detergent laxatives (stool softeners)	Docusate sodium 100 mg capsule orally daily, titrate to effect Docusate calcium 1–4 orally once daily, titrate to effect	Promotes water retention in stool. Most effective for hard stools. Onset of effect can take 3 days. For opiate-related constipation that does not respond to the above, use in combination with a stimulant laxative.
Prokinetic agents	Metoclopramide 10–20 mg orally every 6 hours	Stimulates the bowel's myenteric plexus, increasing peristalsis.
Lubricant laxatives	Mineral oil 5–30 mL at bedtime Glycerin suppositories	Lubricates intestinal mucosa and softens stool.
Large-volume enemas	Tap water enemas Soap suds enemas	Softens the stool and distend the bowel, inducing peristalsis. Soap suds function like a stimulant laxative.
Opioid receptor antagonist	Methylnaltrexone 8–12 mg subcutaneously every other day	Blocks opioid effect on *mu* receptors, but only minimally crosses blood–brain barrier so reverses constipating side effect without adversely affecting analgesia.

Benzodiazepines can also trigger paradoxical agitation, particularly in the frail elderly, and also frequently worsen delirium.

DEPRESSION

Treatment alternatives for depression include counseling, spiritual support, and medication. Medical management may include SSRI or tricyclic antidepressants. In general, start with low dosages and titrate upward to effect. Psychostimulants are a useful adjunctive treatment for patients with severe depression or those very close to death, where the time needed to reach antidepressant effect is an issue.

DELIRIUM

If a reversible cause of delirium is identified (e.g., hypoxemia or opioid toxicity), it should be addressed specifically. If medical treatment is needed to relieve agitation, haloperidol remains the mainstay for treatment of acute delirium, with the atypical antipsychotics playing a key role as longer-acting agents. Anxiolytics can exacerbate delirium or agitation, particularly in the frail elderly. In long-term care settings, regulations regarding the use of antipsychotics as "chemical restraints" need to be taken into account, working collaboratively with the facility's director of nursing regarding the unique issues in end-of-life care can allow for optimal management of patients who are dying while respecting the regulatory limitations.

Patients nearing death may experience terminal delirium, which includes day/night reversals, agitation, restlessness, and moaning/groaning. At this time, the goal of management is to relieve distress for both patient and family, and longer acting, more sedating agents may be used.

Psychosocial Issues

Impending death presents patients and physicians with challenges in multiple domains. Patients confront their mortality, the process of dying, and their sense of the transcendent within a context of psychosocial, cultural, and spiritual factors that are both deeply personal and shared within families and communities. Although few physicians can have expertise in all psychosocial dimensions of end-of-life care, each should cultivate a basic awareness of and sensitivity to the unique psychosocial needs of patients for whom death is imminent. Making timely referrals to community resources that support patients' and families' spiritual and psychosocial needs will foster optimal end-of-life care across all domains.

SPIRITUAL ISSUES

When aware that the end of life is approaching, most patients develop a heightened sense of the transcendent. Spiritual concerns are most commonly addressed via religious traditions, but many patients address spiritual concerns independent of organized or formal religion. The extent to which individual physicians wish to engage spiritual issues will depend on the comfort with which they can communicate with the patient on this topic. This can range from simple inquiries into the patient's spiritual needs and support system to actually praying with and for patients.

Patients generally want their physicians to address spiritual issues during serious illness (37), but this does not mean that physicians should go beyond their own comfort or expertise, nor is it a license to evangelize or proselytize. Often, consultation with a spiritual or pastoral care advisor will be helpful. Hospitals and hospice programs have trained chaplains who are generally quite skilled at working with patients from diverse spiritual backgrounds on the patient's terms.

FAMILY ISSUES

Caring for a loved one during his or her final days can present a substantial burden for families but can also be very rewarding. Family responsibilities can range from coordinating chores to bathing a dying parent or navigating the emotional minefield of adult children who had been physically or sexually abused by the dying parent. Families often need outside help, including respite care (often provided under the Medicare hospice benefit), financial support, spiritual and psychological counseling, and arrangements for disposition of the body after death. Caregiving includes a substantial physical component to fulfill activities of daily living (e.g., mobility, bathing, toileting, dressing). Caregiving intensity tends to increase in the last 3 months of life and for many families exceeds 1 year (38). Because caregiving responsibilities are most often provided by women in our society, these issues also raise significant gender equity concerns, including impact on employment and fair distribution of work in the domestic setting.

Grief and Bereavement

Supportive preparation before the death will ease the family's burden and facilitate grieving. However, even with excellent preparation, a prolonged death can be physically and emotionally draining for the family and caregivers. "Tasks" of grieving include accepting the loss, experiencing the pain of the loss, adjusting to one's environment after the loss, and building a new life.

Normal grief does not require medical intervention. When agitated grieving impairs basic functions of daily living (e.g., unremitting crying, not eating or sleeping), a brief and carefully monitored course of benzodiazepines may be helpful. Later on, the judicious use of antidepressants is indicated if grief is accompanied by prolonged or incapacitating depression. It bears repeating that pharmacologic management is *not* indicated for "normal" grieving, but should be reserved for situations when basic functions of daily living are impaired, or protracted grieving appears to have evolved into a clinical depression.

The extent of a physician's involvement with the family will vary based on the prior relationship with the family. Personal expressions of condolence range from a phone call or card, to visiting the family at their home, to attending the formal visitation or funeral. Primary care physicians often care for other family members and should offer professional follow up to assess grief and personal issues after the death of their loved one. Additional resources may be available through the interdisciplinary hospice team.

CONCLUSION

The amazing technological progress of modern medicine comes with an unfortunate drawback: the desire to cure disease often overshadows the obligation to care for the patient.

Eric Cassell observed, "The relief of suffering and the cure of disease must be seen as twin obligations of a medical profession that is truly dedicated to the care of the sick. Physicians' failure to understand the nature of suffering can result in medical intervention that (though technically adequate) not only fails to relieve suffering but becomes a source of suffering itself" (39).

Physicians active in hospice and palliative care are often asked if their work is depressing. Most respond that the opposite is true: the work itself is very gratifying, because the prospect of patients not receiving the best available care at their time of greatest need is far more depressing. Caring for patients and families through the entire spectrum of the natural life cycle, including the time of bereavement following the death of a loved one, is an integral role for the family physician. Hospice and palliative care are not the last resort when medicine fails, but the completion of whole person care.

KEY POINTS

- Palliative care should not be limited to end-of-life care, but is ideally incorporated throughout curative and life-prolonging treatments.
- Rather than delaying hospice referrals until one is certain that a patient is in their 6 months of life, hospice referral may be appropriate once one can legitimately answer that they would not be surprised if the patient dies within the next 6 months if their illness follows its anticipated course.
- Ask patients what they understand their current situation to be, to facilitate the provision of appropriate information sharing. Then ask what they are hoping for, based on their current clinical status. Clarification of these questions is crucial to matching available treatment options to the patients' hopes and goals, and provide the foundation for patient-centered care planning.

CHAPTER 25

Breast Problems

Kendra L. Schwartz

CLINICAL OBJECTIVES

1. Describe the most important aspects of history and physical exam for diagnosing and managing breast pain.
2. Summarize what you should tell a patient about the possible causes of her nipple discharge.
3. Assess the amount of workup that should be completed in the office for nipple discharge and what testing should be referred to a consultant.
4. Cite what you should tell a patient with a breast mass regarding the possibility of cancer.
5. Describe which tests you should order for a breast mass that does not disappear with aspiration.

The three most common presenting problems related to the female breast are breast pain, nipple discharge, and a palpable mass (1). A woman with one or more of these problems is often concerned whether it represents a malignancy. This concern may be openly stated, but is often left unspoken, and an important part of the management involves acknowledging and appropriately addressing her fear.

BREAST PAIN

Mastalgia is a symptom complex of breast pain and tenderness, with or without nodularity. Among presenting breast complaints in primary care, mastalgia is at least as common, if not more common, than finding a lump (1–3). Most women are concerned about cancer. However, in a study of 987 women whose only complaint was breast pain, <1% had a malignancy on mammogram (4). Mastalgia is either cyclic or noncyclic, and the management depends on this categorization. Reassurance, after appropriate evaluation, that the pain is not due to cancer will be sufficient for most women; roughly 15% will require additional treatment (5).

Pathophysiology and Differential Diagnosis

Approximately two-thirds of women presenting with breast pain have cyclic mastalgia, which is bilateral pain varying in intensity throughout the menstrual cycle with the premenstrual time often the most painful. It is thought to be hormonally mediated although studies of circulating levels of progesterone, estrogen, prolactin, or quantity of hormone receptors have yielded conflicting results (6,7); however, altered hormone receptor sensitivity remains a possibility. The usual age at presentation is 33 to 35 years; the condition also has been reported by postmenopausal women on hormone therapy.

Noncyclic mastalgia is usually unilateral, typically occurs in women over the age of 40 years, and is not temporally related to the menstrual cycle. The differential diagnosis and relative frequency of causes of mastalgia are summarized in Table 25.1.

Postsurgical breast pain may occur at the site of an incision, particularly if the lines of Langer have been crossed. Mondor's disease (phlebitis of the thoracoepigastric vein) may be related to a history of breast surgery, trauma, or radiation (8). Costochondritis (Tietze syndrome) reportedly accounts for approximately 7% of noncyclic mastalgia (9). Ruptured breast implants may also be a cause of localized breast pain. Although subclinical operable breast cancer may present with noncyclic breast pain of recent onset, it is rare that pain is the only presenting symptom in malignancy (4).

Clinical Evaluation

A thorough history will help classify the mastalgia as cyclic or noncyclic. The physical examination is also important in determining the appropriate management strategy. A finding of recent onset of unilateral noncyclic pain in a postmenopausal woman should raise concern of malignancy. If a dominant mass or unilateral nipple discharge accompanies the mastalgia, cancer must be strongly considered.

HISTORY

Cyclic mastalgia is typically most severe premenstrually and subsides during the menses. It is usually bilateral, in the upper outer breast quadrants, and associated with nodularity. Women often characterize the pain as dull, aching, or heavy. The range of severity can be from mild to severe enough to limit clothing selections, sleep positions, or hugging. Patients should, therefore, be questioned regarding the effect on their lives. Obtain a history of current hormone therapy or oral contraceptive therapy, and previous history of breast problems or surgery. You should also ask about a family history of breast problems, including cancer.

Women with noncyclic mastalgia are more likely to describe their pain as unilateral, with no temporal relationship to their menstrual cycle. It may be constant or remitting, but the periods without pain are not related to the menses. The pain is often described as sharp, burning, or drawing and is more commonly located in the subareolar or medial portion of the breast. Non-breast causes may result in symptoms such as radiation to the arm or axilla, or pain with deep inspiration. As

TABLE 25.1 Differential Diagnoses in Patients with Mastalgia

Diagnosis	Frequency	History and/or Physical Examination Features
Cyclic	Common (67%)	Age <40 years, bilateral, pain related to menstrual cycle
Noncyclic	Somewhat common (33%)	Age >40 years, unilateral, pain unrelated to menstrual cycle
Musculoskeletal other than costochondritis	Uncommon	Reproduction of pain with palpation
Cancer	Rare	Persistent pain in same location Palpable mass on examination
Cervical radiculopathy	Rare	Arm and neck pain present
Costochondritis	Rare	Costochondral junction tenderness
Duct ectasia	Rare	Subareolar pain; discharge may be present
Trauma	Rare	History of trauma or previous surgery

with cyclic mastalgia, ask patients about previous breast problems or surgery and any family history of breast problems or cancer. If a nipple discharge is present, it should be evaluated as described in the next section of this chapter.

PHYSICAL EXAMINATION

The clinical breast examination (CBE) includes both inspection and palpation. Further information on clinical breast exam can be found on the American Cancer Society Website (*http://caonline.amcancersoc.org/cgi/content/full/54/6/327*). Inspection of the breasts focuses on evidence of trauma or old surgical scars; both are related to noncyclic mastalgia. Whether the history is consistent with cyclic or noncyclic mastalgia, you should thoroughly palpate the breasts. Nodularity is common with both complaints, but if a dominant mass is found, the appropriate management protocol should be followed to rule out malignancy.

Pain reproduced by palpation of the costochondral junction or the lateral chest wall suggests a musculoskeletal etiology such as costochondritis. Pain exacerbated by specific neck movements suggests cervical radiculopathy. If pain accompanies nipple discharge or a palpable mass, management should follow the guidelines outlined in those sections of this chapter.

LABORATORY TESTS

Diagnostic tests are not necessary unless a dominant mass is found. Only 4 of 987 women with mastalgia and no other symptoms or signs were found to have breast cancer in one study, a number similar to that in asymptomatic women (4).

Management

For 85% of women with breast pain, whether cyclic or noncyclic, reassurance from the physician after evaluation that the pain is not from cancer is sufficient treatment (5). For the remaining women, additional treatment will be needed. Management depends on whether the pain is cyclic or noncyclic.

CYCLIC PAIN

Behavioral Approaches

Objective evidence is lacking regarding the efficacy of most therapies for cyclic mastalgia. Before starting pharmacologic therapy, the physician should consider recommending a patient pain diary (including severity scale), a well-fitted brassiere (10), and diet modification.

- Keeping a daily record of the amount of pain for a minimum of 2 months helps to determine whether the pain is cyclic and its severity.
- In a small study of patients with breast pain, 75 women found relief after being professionally fitted with a brassiere.
- Although not of proven benefit by randomized trials, removing dietary methylxanthines (caffeine has been studied the most) and adopting a very low-fat diet may be helpful. There is no evidence of effectiveness of vitamin B or E, and high doses of these vitamins may increase mortality (11).

Pharmacotherapy

One herbal supplement and five medications (Table 25.2) have shown benefit in controlled studies. Three of the medications: bromocriptine, tamoxifen, and goserelin—a luteinizing hormone-releasing hormone analogue, are not generally recommended because of their adverse effects. Some studies have noted a significant placebo effect, with 20% or more women on placebo reporting improved symptoms (12,13). There is no evidence to support the use of thyroid hormones, progesterone, diuretics, or oral analgesics in the treatment of cyclic mastalgia.

Evening primrose oil, which is rich in gamma-linolenic acid, is thought to exert its effect by normalizing blood levels of essential fatty acids. In several trials, it was found to be effective (7,14); yet a recent placebo controlled trial showed no improvement in pain (13). It is well tolerated, has few adverse effects (nausea and bloating being the most common) (14), and is available over the counter.

The topical nonsteroidal gel, diclofenac, demonstrated significant pain reduction compared with placebo when used on the breast skin every 8 hours for 6 months (15). A smaller uncontrolled study, using diclofenac or piroxicam gel, also demonstrated improvement in pain symptoms after 2 months' use (16). There were no side effects reported in either study.

Danazol, a synthetic androgen, is the only drug approved by the US Food and Drug Administration for mastalgia. It is thought to act by inhibiting the midcycle luteinizing hormone

TABLE 25.2 Management of Mastalgia

Treatment	Common Dose	Possible Adverse Effects	Relative Cost	SORT Rating
Cyclic Mastalgia				
Proper-fitting brassiere	N/A	No adverse effects	$	B
Evening primrose oil	1 gram every 8 hours	None	$	B
Topical nonsteroidal anti-inflammatory	50 mg diclofenac gel every 8 hours	None	$	A
Danazol	50–100 mg every 12 hours	Weight gain, menstrual irregularity	$$	A
Bromocriptine	1.25–2.5 mg orally at bedtime	Nausea, vomiting, headache, postural hypotension	$$	B
Tamoxifen (short-term use only)	10 mg orally per day	Long-term use associated with endometrial cancer and osteoporosis	$$$	A
Goserelin	3.6 mg subcutaneous per month	Depression, vaginal dryness, hot flushes, oily hair/skin	$$$	B
Noncyclic Mastalgia				
Topical non-steroidal anti-inflammatory	50 mg diclofenac gel every 8 hours	None	$	A
Evening primrose oil	1 g every 8 hours	None	$	B

A = consistent, good-quality patient-oriented evidence; B = inconsistent or limited-quality patient-oriented evidence; C = consensus, disease-oriented evidence, usual practice, expert opinion, or case series.
For information about the SORT evidence rating system, see *http://www.aafp.org/afpsort.xml.*

surge and by competitively binding estrogen and progesterone receptors in the breast. Its overall improvement rate is estimated at 70% (7). The starting dosage is 50 mg twice a day, with titration upward as needed and tolerated (Table 25.2). Prescribing danazol only during the luteal phase has been studied in a randomized trial of 100 women, and was found to be effective. It may be associated with fewer adverse effects than continuous dosing (17). Risks include thrombotic or thrombophlebitic events as well as peliosis hepatitis and pseudotumor cerebri with long-term use.

Bromocriptine, the prolactin inhibitor, has been successfully used in treating cyclic breast pain (18). The relatively high incidence of adverse effects (20% to 33%) has limited its use (Table 25.2).

Tamoxifen also is effective for cyclic mastalgia (19,20). However, because of concerns regarding its effect on bone density and possible association with endometrial cancer, it is only recommended for short-term use in the treatment of severe mastalgia, and then only if all other therapies have failed.

In a randomized trial, goserelin, a luteinizing hormone-releasing hormone analogue, improved breast pain during treatment (21). Sixty-seven percent of women receiving a monthly goserelin depot injection compared with 35% of women receiving a sham injection reported an improvement in their pain during the treatment period. However, at 6 months posttreatment, the two groups had similar pain scores. There are numerous adverse effects associated with goserelin injection (Table 25.2).

NONCYCLIC BREAST PAIN

Noncyclic breast pain is managed by treating the underlying cause. If the pain is localized to the breast tissue, topical nonsteroidal drugs or evening primrose oil can be tried (6). If the pain is found to be musculoskeletal (as many as 90% of unilateral noncyclic cases), analgesics and/or anti-inflammatory drugs are recommended. Local injections of combined steroids and anesthetics have proven beneficial in prospective studies (22). Figure 25.1 is an algorithm for the diagnosis and treatment of mastalgia.

In general, surgical intervention is not recommended for treatment of mastalgia, except in the case of a dominant mass or mammary duct ectasia (both are addressed later in this chapter). In the past, procedures such as a subcutaneous mastectomy were used to treat pain, often resulting in a painful scar.

NIPPLE DISCHARGE

Nipple discharges, secretions from the breast(s) of a woman who is not lactating, are often categorized as either physiologic or pathologic (nonphysiologic). Physiologic discharges are described as nonspontaneous, bilateral, and arising from multiple ducts, whereas pathologic nipple discharges are typically spontaneous, unilateral, and arise from a single duct.

Most nipple discharge is caused by benign conditions (Table 25.3), but it is understandably a cause of concern. Once a discharge is discovered, the anxious patient may manipulate

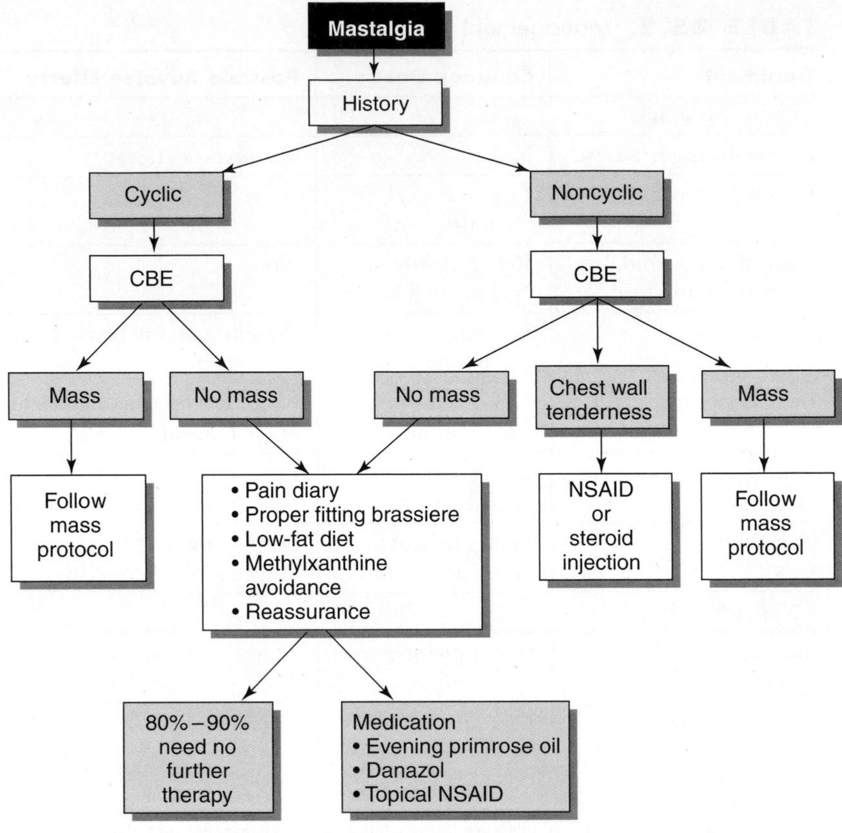

Figure 25.1 • Algorithm for mastalgia. CBE = clinical breast examination; NSAID = nonsteroidal anti-inflammatory drug. [permission needed]

TABLE 25.3 Differential Diagnosis of Nipple Discharge

Diagnosis	Frequency in Office Primary Care (% Within Physiologic or Pathologic Category)	Typical Presentation
Physiologic		
Idiopathic	Common (40%–45%)	Bilateral, milky or watery
Galactorrhea	Somewhat common (25%–30%)	Bilateral, milky (prolonged lactation)
Medication	Uncommon (10%–15%)	Bilateral, milky or watery
Anovulatory syndromes	Rare (1%–2%)	Bilateral, milky or watery, irregular menses
Sella turcica lesions	Rare (1%–2%)	Bilateral, milky or watery, irregular menses
Pathologic		
Duct papilloma	Common (40%–45%)	Unilateral, serous or bloody
Fibrocyst	Uncommon (15%–25%)	Usually unilateral, greenish or serous
Duct ectasia	Uncommon (15%–20%)	Usually bilateral, multicolored, sticky
Eczema	Rare	Usually unilateral, bloody, crusting
Paget disease	Rare	Usually unilateral, bloody, crusting
Early ductal carcinoma	Rare (5%–10%)	Unilateral, serous or bloody
Infection/inflammation	Rare (5%–10%)	Usually unilateral, purulent

Adapted from: Newman HF, Klein M, Northrup JD, et al. Nipple discharge: frequency and pathogenesis in an ambulatory population. *NY State J Med*. 1983;83:928–933; Seltzer MH, Perloff LJ, Kelley RI, et al. The significance of age in patients with nipple discharge. *Surg Gynecol Obstet*. 1970;131:519–522; Fung A, Rayter Z, Fisher C, et al. Preoperative cytology and mammography in patients with single-duct nipple discharge treated by surgery. *Br J Surg*. 1990;77:1211–1212.

the breast and nipple frequently to see if the discharge is still present, which may provoke more discharge. The prevalence of nipple discharge is about 10% based on a study of 2,685 women undergoing a routine health examination that included breast compression toward the nipple (23). The significance of the finding of nipple discharge depends on the age, gravidity, parity, and menopausal status of the woman, as well as the characteristics of the discharge itself.

Pathophysiology and Differential Diagnosis

Physiologic breast secretions are related to hormonal influences (i.e., prolactin) on breast tissue and are typically bilateral, involve multiple ducts, and require some form of manipulation to be expressed. Galactorrhea, a milky discharge, is the most common physiologic discharge and requires investigation for an endocrine abnormality or a pharmacologic cause if the woman is not pregnant or lactating. Precipitators may include nipple stimulation, sexual orgasm, sleep, exercise, and food ingestion. Galactorrhea may occur for 1 to 2 years or longer after childbirth and the discharge may be unilateral.

Pathologic reasons for increases in prolactin include hypothalamic lesions, pituitary tumors, chest wall trauma, hypothyroidism, renal failure (decreased prolactin clearance), and anovulatory syndromes, such as polycystic ovaries. Medications that may cause hyperprolactinemia or increase prolactin secretion are listed in Table 25.4. Other physiologic peptides that have prolactin-releasing activity include thyroid releasing hormone, serotonin, vasoactive intestinal peptide, and vasopressin.

Pathologic discharges can originate either from the nipple and areola region or from a breast duct. Eczema, nipple adenoma, and Paget disease can cause erythema and ulceration of the nipple skin, with an associated bloody discharge (Table 25.3). Ductal diseases associated with nipple discharge are duct ectasia (periductal mastitis), duct papilloma, and early ductal carcinoma. Duct papilloma is a benign condition of epithelial hyperplasia within the ducts. Papillomas that occur more peripherally are usually multifocal and have an increased risk for breast cancer.

Infection and abscess can lead to a purulent discharge (Table 25.3). Mastitis is more common in the puerperium, but can occur after weaning.

Clinical Evaluation

HISTORY

As Table 25.4 illustrates, important points to cover in the history of a woman presenting with nipple discharge include whether the discharge is bilateral, the characteristics of the secretion, recent pregnancy, current medications, menstrual cycle, menopausal status, exercise and sleep habits, sexual activity, and recent surgery or trauma.

A serous, watery, bloody, or serosanguineous discharge from one breast, especially in a postmenopausal woman, is the most concerning presenting complaint for cancer.

PHYSICAL EXAMINATION

A CBE should be completed including inspection of the skin and four quadrant palpation for masses to see if the discharge appears to be confined to a single duct (as in ductal papilloma or carcinoma). You should pay special attention to the subareolar region to identify the area at which pressure produces the discharge, and palpate for masses. A careful breast examination takes at least 5 minutes.

LABORATORY TESTS

If the history and physical examination are consistent with galactorrhea, and all physiologic and pharmacologic causes have been excluded, use a prolactin level to rule out hyperprolactinemia (Fig. 25.2). For women who are experiencing

TABLE 25.4 Key Elements of the History and Physical Examination for Nipple Discharge

Question/Maneuver	Purpose
Spontaneous or expressed discharge	Spontaneous is more indicative of cancer
Bilateral or unilateral discharge	Unilateral is more indicative of cancer
Characteristics of discharge	Milky suggests galactorrhea Serous, bloody, watery increases suspicion for cancer Multicolored suggests duct ectasia
Irregular menses in premenopausal woman	Suggests hyperprolactinemia
Headaches, amenorrhea, visual disturbances	Increase suspicion for pituitary or hypothalamic problem
Medications*	May be the cause of discharge
Palpable mass	Increases suspicion for cancer
Recent pregnancy or weaning	Suggests galactorrhea or mastitis
Sexual, exercise, and sleep patterns	Nipple stimulation, sexual orgasms, increased exercise and sleep may cause discharge
Skin changes	May suggest adenoma, eczema, Paget disease

*Medications associated with increased prolactin levels include amphetamines, cocaine, H2-receptor antagonists, hallucinogens, haloperidol, methyldopa, metoclopramide, opiates, oral contraceptives, phenothiazines, reserpine, tricyclic antidepressants, and verapamil.

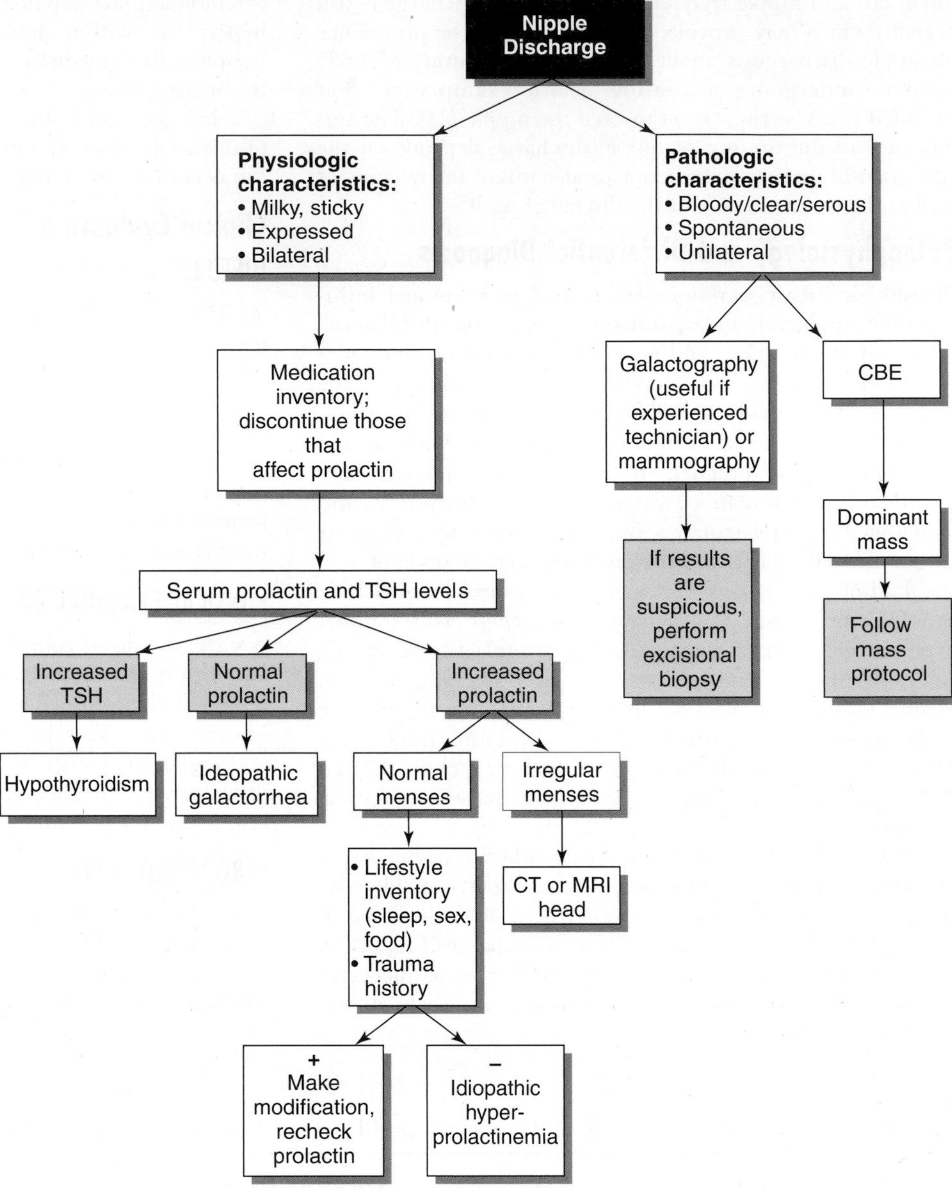

Figure 25.2 • Algorithm for nipple discharge. CBE = clinical breast examination; TSH = thyroid-stimulating hormone; CT = computed tomography; MRI = magnetic resonance imaging. [permission needed]

amenorrhea or other symptoms indicating pituitary or hypothalamic dysfunction, the prolactin and thyroid-stimulating hormone levels should be checked to rule out hyperprolactinemia and hypothyroidism, respectively. A β-human chorionic gonadotropin test for pregnancy should also be considered.

If both the prolactin and thyroid-stimulating hormone are normal and the patient is having regular cycles, a diagnosis of idiopathic galactorrhea can be made, and no further testing is indicated. If the patient has irregular menses or an elevated prolactin level, magnetic resonance imaging (MRI) of the posterior fossa of the brain is warranted to look for pituitary tumor. The higher the prolactin level, the greater the chance of pituitary adenoma; levels over 150 ng/mL are rare for causes other than prolactinoma (24).

Discharges that are more suspicious for cancer (i.e., unilateral, spontaneous, occurring in an older woman, bloody, serosanguineous, or watery) can first be tested with a guaiac card for the presence of blood, although reports are inconsistent regarding the predictive value of this test. The percentage of cancers whose discharges tested positive for hemoglobin ranges from 53% to 100% (25–27). Fluid cytology can also be obtained, although its clinical utility is debatable. The sensitivity of cytology is low (up to 45% in patients with carcinoma have normal cytology) and the specificity is high (96% to 97%) (27–29). Thus, it is useful when positive but does not rule out malignancy when negative. If cytology is negative and a bloody nipple discharge persists, an excisional biopsy should be performed. Cytology cannot differentiate between in situ and invasive cancer.

IMAGING

Surgical duct excision, which is the most specific diagnostic test, has traditionally been the method of choice for evaluating pathologic discharges. Galactography (or ductography), a radiographic procedure that involves injecting a radiopaque dye into a suspicious duct, may be helpful in differentiating between a benign and malignant neoplasm. An advantage of galactography is better localization of the lesion, which allows a more conservative surgical excision; however, the procedure is not always available. Mammary endoscopy (ductoscopy), also not consistently available, is an option to directly observe intraductal pathology, obtain biopsy samples, lavage fluid, and ductoscopically guided duct excision (30).

Mammography should be ordered in women whose history and CBE raise suspicion of cancer. Although the sensitivity of mammography for detecting cancer in patients with a nipple discharge varies considerably, from 13% (25) to 90% (31), the specificity is higher than 95%. Given the potentially high false-negative rate, the best use of mammography may be to determine if other nonpalpable abnormalities are present, which would increase the suspicion for cancer. Ultrasound may be more appropriate for younger women (younger than age 35 years) because of their dense breasts.

Management

If the history, CBE, and discharge indicate galactorrhea, a cause for hyperprolactinemia should be sought; if found, begin remedies such as a change of medication or lifestyle or evaluation for pituitary tumor. If the only abnormal result is an elevated prolactin level in a normally menstruating woman, a diagnosis of idiopathic hyperprolactinemia can be made. However, the patient should be followed closely for further increases in the prolactin level and signs or symptoms of pituitary tumor.

If the galactorrhea is bothersome or the hyperprolactinemia is associated with diminished libido, amenorrhea, and infertility, a dopamine agonist can be used for treatment (24). Bromocriptine and cabergoline are approved by the US Food and Drug Administration for this purpose.

In the case of clear or blood-related (serous, serosanguineous, or sanguinous) spontaneous discharges, especially if unilateral, a mammogram and/or galactogram or ductoscopy (if available) should be ordered. If the result is suspicious or discharge persists, surgical excision of the abnormal area is necessary for definitive diagnosis. If a mass is palpable in a woman with a pathologic discharge, she should be treated as described in the following section.

PALPABLE BREAST MASS

Breast cancer is the most common malignancy in women and the second leading cause of cancer death. The majority of cases present as a palpable mass, usually found by the patient. For this reason, most women are understandably frightened on discovering a breast mass. Among the common presenting breast complaints, breast mass ranks second to breast pain (1). A complaint of finding a breast mass must always be taken seriously.

TABLE 25.5 Differential Diagnosis of Breast Mass

Diagnosis	Age Group (y)	Diagnosis (%)	Usual Characteristics of the Mass
Breast cancer	25–40	<10	Unilateral, hard, and immobile
	41–50	10–20	
	51–70	50–80	
	>70	>80	
Breast cyst	25–40	<5	Unilateral, soft, and well-defined
	41–50	10–20	
	51–70	7–12	
	>70	<10	
Fibroadenoma	<25	50–75	Unilateral, smooth, and mobile
	26–50	10–30	
	51–70	<5	
	>70	<1	
Fibrocystic changes	<25	10–25	Bilateral, soft, and irregular; change with cycle
	26–40	30–40	
	41–70	Uncommon*	
	>70	Rare	
Duct papilloma	Uncommon for all ages, but most frequent at ages 30–50		Unilateral subareolar mass with discharge

Adapted from: Byrne C. Breast. In: Harras A, Edwards BK, Blot WJ, et al., eds. *Cancer Rates and Risk*. Washington, DC: National Cancer Institute. NIH publication no. 96–691. 1996:120–126; Devitt JE. Benign breast disease in the postmenopausal woman. *World J Surg.* 1989;13:731–735; Hindle WH. Other benign breast problems. *Clin Obstet Gynecol.* 1994;37:916–924; Ligon RE, Stevenson DR, Diner W, et al. Breast masses in young women. *Am J Surg.* 1980;140:779–782; Ferguson CM, Powell RW. Breast masses in young women. *Arch Surg.* 1989;124:1338–1341.

*More frequent in women on hormone therapy.

TABLE 25.6 Red Flags Suggestive of Breast Cancer

Symptom	Characteristics
Pain	Unilateral, noncyclic
Nipple discharge	Unilateral Watery, serous, serosanguineous, bloody Single duct
Breast mass	Unilateral Hard, immobile Noncystic Skin retraction, dimpling, or edema (peau d'orange)
History	Postmenopausal Previous patient history of breast cancer Family history of breast cancer

Pathophysiology and Differential Diagnosis

The risk of breast cancer increases with age, and postmenopausal women presenting with a mass are much more likely to have cancer than premenopausal women. Other causes of a breast mass are shown in Table 25.5. Fibroadenoma and fibrocystic masses are the most common causes of a breast mass in women younger than age 25 years (32), whereas duct papillomas typically occur in the late menstrual years.

Clinical Evaluation

HISTORY

The provider should assess breast cancer risk factors in every woman with a breast mass. Family history of breast cancer in a first-degree relative increases the risk two times; if three first-degree relatives have been affected, the risk increases up to fourfold (33). A personal or family history of breast or ovarian cancer diagnosed before age 40 years increases the risk of breast cancer and should raise suspicion of a hereditary cancer syndrome (34). A previous diagnosis of atypical hyperplasia on breast biopsy is a risk factor (35). History of pregnancy before age 30 years is protective, as is a fewer number of years menstruating (35).

In addition, the patient should be questioned regarding nipple discharge and pain in the affected breast. Nipple discharge may accompany duct papilloma or cancer. If pain is present, the patient should be asked if it coincides with her menstrual cycle, because masses associated with fibrocystic changes are often painful in the premenstrual period.

PHYSICAL EXAMINATION

The clinical breast examination should include inspection and palpation of both breasts as well as palpation of the axillary and supraclavicular lymph node regions (*http://caonline.amcancersoc.org/cgi/content/full/54/6/327*). Table 25.6 outlines red flags suggestive of breast cancer. Skin retraction, dimpling, edema (peau d'orange), and bloody nipple discharge should raise suspicion for malignancy. If a mass is found, carefully palpate the opposite breast to determine if a symmetric mass is present. If a mirror-image mass or thickening is found, the risk of cancer is very low.

The typical malignant mass is immobile and rock hard with irregular borders. With this finding on CBE, especially in the presence of enlarged axillary nodes, an immediate referral to a surgeon for biopsy should be made. Table 25.7 lists key elements of the history and physical examination for palpable mass and suggested diagnosis. However, physical characteristics of a breast mass alone should not dictate the workup. The test characteristics of clinical breast exam are shown in Table 25.8; physical examination is accurate ([true positive + true negative]/total patients) in only 60% to 80% of cases (36,37) Malignant masses can resemble all other types of breast masses and reexamination of any breast mass is recommended within the next month, during the time of least hormonal influence (3 to 10 days after the onset of menses) (32). An effective office tracking system is necessary to ensure that these patients are not lost to follow-up; if that possibility exists, the woman should be referred to a surgeon rather than told to return for reexamination.

LABORATORY TESTS

The first step in evaluating a breast mass, especially in a perimenopausal or older woman, is to determine whether the mass is cystic or solid (Fig. 25.3). Breast cyst aspiration can be performed in the office using a 22-gauge needle and syringe. The location of the mass should be carefully documented in case of a bloody aspirate. To rule out the rare intracystic carcinoma, you should send all bloody aspirates and any aspirate obtained from a postmenopausal woman not on hormone therapy for cytology.

Alternatively, an ultrasound can be obtained to determine if the mass is cystic. Aspiration has the advantage of therapeutically draining the cyst and providing a more expedient diagnosis. If the ultrasound shows a cyst, the cyst should still be

TABLE 25.7 Key Elements of the History and Physical Examination for Palpable Mass

Question/Maneuver	Purpose
Age; previous or family history of breast, endometrial, or ovarian cancer; menstrual history	Determine whether there is an increased risk of breast cancer
Pain or tenderness	Suggests fibrocystic mass or fibroadenoma
Nipple discharge	Suggests duct papilloma or carcinoma
Mirror image mass in opposite breast	Suggests fibrocystic changes

TABLE 25.8 Characteristics of Diagnostic Tests Used to Identify Malignancy in a Woman with a Breast Mass

Test	Sensitivity	Specificity	LR+	LR−
Clinical breast examination	0.92	0.65	2.6	0.1
Mammography	0.89	0.65*	2.5	0.2
Fine-needle aspiration	0.83[†]	0.90[‡]	27	0.2
Ultrasound	0.78	0.89	7.1	0.3
Clinical breast examination + fine-needle aspiration + mammography (positive result on one or individual tests is a positive triple test result; all test results negative is a negative triple test result)	0.99	0.98	50	0.02

Adapted from: van Dam PA, Van Goethem MLA, Kersschot E, et al. Palpable solid breast masses: retrospective single- and multimodality evaluation of 201 lesions. *Radiology*. 1988;166:435–439; Wolberg WH, Tanner MA, Loh WY. Fine-needle aspiration for breast mass diagnosis. *Arch Surg*. 1989;124: 814–818; Kaufman Z, Shpitz B, Shapiro M, et al. Triple approach in the diagnosis of dominant breast masses: combined physical examination, mammography, and fine-needle aspiration. *J Surg Oncol*. 1994;56(4):254–257; Hammond S, Keyhani-Rofagha S, O'Toole RV. Statistical analysis of fine-needle aspiration cytology of the breast. A review of 678 cases plus 4,265 cases from the literature. *Acta Cytol*. 1987;31:276–280; Butler JA, Vargas HI, Worthen N, et al. Accuracy of combined clinical-mammographic-cytologic diagnosis of dominant breast masses. *Arch Surg*. 1990;125:893–895.
Abbreviation: LR, likelihood ratio.
*Range, 0.55–0.74.
†Range, 0.65–0.99.
‡Range, 0.55–0.97, but more recent work suggests a higher specificity.

aspirated and cytology performed as indicated previously. In a study of 174 patients with palpable cystic masses, characteristics detected on ultrasound that were significantly correlated with malignancy included thick wall, mural tumor, internal septae, and size >3 cm (38).

IMAGING

Mammography is obtained to evaluate for clinically occult malignancies, not to characterize the mass. It is not recommended in women younger than 25 to 30 years of age or in pregnant women because the increased density of the breast tissue in these women renders the mammogram difficult to interpret. In addition, the breast is more radiosensitive in younger women, theoretically increasing risk of cancer from mammograms. An interval of 2 weeks between a mammogram and cyst aspiration is recommended because aspiration can sometimes result in hematoma formation, which could confuse mammographic interpretation.

A negative mammogram should not be interpreted as reassuring in the presence of a breast mass. The test characteristics for mammography in women with a palpable mass are shown in Table 25.8. Particularly in premenopausal women, mammography is more likely to yield a false-positive result (a cancer scare) rather than a true positive (cancer) or a false negative (missed cancer).

DIAGNOSTIC PROCEDURES

Fine-needle aspiration (FNA) is recommended as the third component of the triple approach (along with CBE and mammography) in a breast mass workup. FNA should be performed by a clinician comfortable with and experienced in the procedure, usually a surgeon. One review (39) found that the sensitivity and specificity of FNA ranged from 77% to 99% and from 55% to 99%, respectively, although recent publications show improved specificity (see Table 25.8).

Common reasons for a false-negative reading are an inadequate sample and a well-differentiated tumor. In such cases, the procedure must be repeated, or an open biopsy must be performed. If there is any question of atypia, an excisional biopsy should be done. If the results of the FNA show malignancy, you should discuss treatment options with the patient and plan definitive surgery.

Excisional biopsy is the gold standard for diagnosis of a breast mass. However, it has been estimated that if all "lumps" were biopsied, only 20% to 25% would be malignant (40). Consequently, the triple approach to a breast mass (as outlined in the following section) has gained popularity in recent years.

Management

The management recommendations for the evaluation of a breast mass are consistent. A triple approach (CBE, mammography, and FNA) is recommended to minimize both the number of excisional biopsies done for benign disease, and the number of missed cancers. In a series of 234 patients who underwent an excisional biopsy in addition to this triple approach, all patients who had breast cancer had at least one positive test result (41). Although the specificity for the triad of tests was only 57%, the negative predictive value was 100%—all patients who had negative findings for malignancy in the three tests had benign lesions on excisional biopsy. Another study of 259 women with palpable breast masses confirmed these findings (42). Dynamic MRI is a procedure that may have accuracy similar to that of the triple test (43); however, the triple test remains the gold standard. Figure 25.3 is an algorithm for the management of a palpable breast mass.

If a cystic mass recurs after aspiration, mammography and excisional biopsy should be recommended. Intracystic or partially cystic cancers should be suspected if the aspirate is bloody, or if a residual mass persists directly after aspiration. In those cases, you should recommend mammography and excisional biopsy. All patients should be rechecked in 4 to 6 weeks after the initial aspiration.

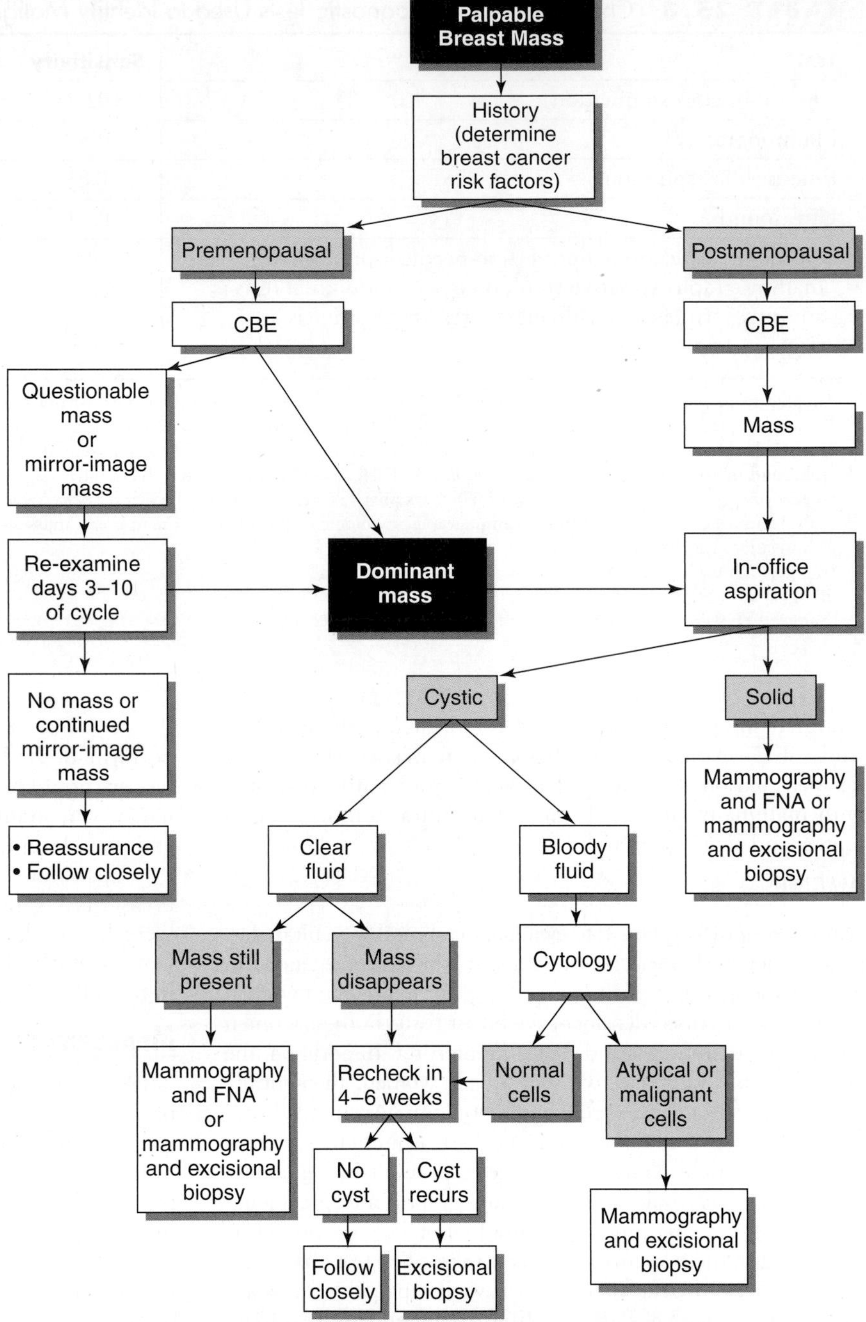

Figure 25.3 • Algorithm for palpable breast mass. CBE = clinical breast examination; FNA = fine-needle aspiration.

If any of the components of the triple approach are suspicious or consistent with malignancy, the mass should be biopsied. If all three results are negative, the mass can be closely followed with CBE by the same examiner every 3 months for two visits, then again in 6 months to determine if it is stable. Benign breast masses may spontaneously resolve over time.

SPECIAL CONSIDERATIONS

The Lactating Breast

Mastitis is a cellulitis of the interlobular connective tissue within the mammary gland. The clinical spectrum can range from focal inflammation to systemic flulike symptoms of fever, chills, and muscle aches. The affected breast will usually exhibit a tender, erythematous, wedge-shaped swelling. Estimates of the incidence of mastitis range from 2.5% to 33% of breastfeeding women; the actual value is probably closer to 10% (44,45). Most cases occur within the first 2 months postpartum. The infection is bacterial, usually staphylococci; the breast skin and the infant's mouth have been proposed as the source.

The key to the management of mastitis is complete emptying of the breast, warm compresses, early antibiotics, and bed rest. The patient should be advised to continue breastfeeding (46,47); stopping breastfeeding would put her at increased risk of abscess formation. In fact, some experts recommend increased feedings on the affected side to minimize stasis. Others recommend starting feedings with the unaffected breast to allow the affected breast to "let down," thereby diminishing any pain accompanying feeding. Antibiotic coverage of gram-positive organisms with an agent such as dicloxacillin or erythromycin for at least 10 days will usually control the infection and is safe for the infant.

The Abnormal Screening Mammogram

The management of nonpalpable mammographic abnormalities is a common concern of family physicians. The American College of Radiology has published recommendations to facilitate decision making when a screening mammographic abnormality is detected (48). The American College of Radiology's Breast Imaging Reporting and Data System classifies lesions into five categories: benign, likely benign, intermediate, likely malignant, and malignant. Additional imaging studies, such as spot compression or ultrasound, may be recommended to characterize the abnormality on the screening mammogram. If the results of the screening mammogram or the additional studies are benign or likely benign, a final recommendation is made of: normal screening interval, shorter follow-up interval, or biopsy (options for which include fine-needle, core, and excisional).

An abnormal mammogram report should prompt you to perform a history and CBE, if it has not already been done. If an abnormal physical finding (e.g., dominant mass) is present, that algorithm should be followed. A previous mammogram for comparison is very helpful. Lesions classified as probably benign have a low risk (<2%) of cancer and can be followed with mammographic surveillance. Reports of intermediate, suspicious, or malignant lesions should be aggressively managed to obtain a final diagnosis. If a report provides ambiguous recommendations, it is advisable to consult a surgeon.

KEY POINTS

- Breast pain can be classified as cyclic (bilateral pain, most severe premenstrually and subsiding during menses) or noncyclic (often unilateral, sharp, burning, or drawing); the former is managed using a well-fitted brassiere, a trial of diet modification and medications including evening primrose oil, topical nonsteroidal gel, and hormonal therapy (e.g., danazol) and the latter by addressing the underlying cause (e.g., musculoskeletal, tender mass).
- A focused examination for a breast complaint includes a clinical breast examination (inspection, palpation) and chest wall examination. Additional testing is needed for identification of a dominant mass or nipple discharge.
- Women with a physiologic nipple discharge (nonspontaneous, bilateral, milky, arising from multiple ducts) should undergo a medication review and get a prolactin level to rule out hyperprolactinemia; if elevated, an MRI of the posterior fossa of the brain is obtained to look for a pituitary tumor. If serum prolactin is not elevated (or following negative imaging), women can be offered a dopamine agonist (e.g., bromocriptine, cabergoline) if the galactorrhea is bothersome or associated with diminished libido, amenorrhea, and infertility.
- Women with a pathologic discharge (spontaneous, unilateral and arising from a single duct) should have the discharge tested for blood and possibly for malignant cells (cytology). Surgical duct excision is the most specific diagnostic test, but galactography (or ductography) may be helpful. Most are due to benign conditions; cancer is identified in 5% to 10% of cases.
- For women with a breast mass, clinicians should perform a risk assessment for cancer, a clinical breast exam with breast cyst aspiration if the mass is cystic, mammography or ultrasound (the latter used for women younger than age 30 years or to assist with identifying a cyst), and an FNA.
- Red flags suggestive of breast cancer include a mass that is unilateral, hard, immobile, with skin retraction, dimpling, edema (peau d'orange), and bloody nipple discharge; especially in a postmenopausal woman.

CHAPTER

26

Pregnancy Prevention, Contraception, and Medical Abortion

Leslie A. Shimp and Mindy A. Smith

CLINICAL OBJECTIVES

1. Describe an appropriate evaluation for a woman before prescribing a contraceptive method.
2. Summarize an approach to discussing contraceptive options based on patient's age and smoking status.
3. Identify key points for patient education that will promote optimal use of contraception.
4. Describe the role of emergency contraception for patients seeking contraception.
5. Cite the benefits (contraceptive and noncontraceptive) and risks of commonly used contraceptives.

It is estimated that 95% of sexually active women use contraception at some time during their life and that each woman uses up to three different methods. The typical US woman wants only two children and to achieve this goal she and her partner must use a contraceptive method for about 30 years (1). Although most contraceptive methods have side effects and potential adverse effects, the morbidity and mortality associated with pregnancy and childbirth are higher than for any single contraceptive method (2).

About 7% of all office visits by women of reproductive age are for contraception (3). Despite the variety of contraceptive methods available, about 50% of all pregnancies in the United States are unintended, regardless of a woman's age (4). Teenagers are a high-risk group for unintended pregnancy; 25% of women and 18% of men use no method of contraception at first intercourse (5). Use of contraceptives dramatically reduces the likelihood of pregnancy (Table 26.1).

Of sexually active women not using a contraceptive method, approximately 85% will become pregnant over 1 year. The probability of conception is 15% to 33% per cycle depending on the frequency of sexual intercourse (3). The ovum is able to be fertilized for only 12 to 24 hours after ovulation (6). Sperm usually remain viable for 3 days after intercourse. The most fertile period for women is the several days before ovulation and ends 24 hours after ovulation (6). After the egg is fertilized, it is transported to the uterine cavity in about 2 to 3 days. Implantation occurs approximately 6 to 7 days after fertilization following cell division that forms a blastocyst (6). Pregnancy, as defined by the National Institutes of Health, the American College of Obstetricians and Gynecologists, and the Food and Drug Administration (FDA) is implantation of the blastocyst in the endometrium (2).

BARRIERS TO USE OF CONTRACEPTIVES

Many factors are involved in the high rate of unintended pregnancy in the United States. In addition to lack of knowledge about contraceptives (and reproductive health in general) and financial barriers, it is critical to address attitudes, motivation, and feelings of individuals and couples that influence the successful use of contraceptives (7). For example, common reasons women report discontinuing a contraceptive include side effects (expected and unexpected), difficulty with use, and safety concerns (3). Misinformation about the risks and benefits of contraceptives is common.

Many pregnancies occur when a woman discontinues a contraceptive method and does not begin use of another method before intercourse (8). For example, within 6 months of being prescribed an oral contraceptive (OC), 28% of women have discontinued its use; almost half without consulting a health care provider (8). Women should therefore know about a second method they can use if the chosen method proves unsatisfactory and about the availability of the emergency contraceptive (EC).

CONTRACEPTIVE METHODS

Both reversible and permanent forms of contraception are popular in the United States. Methods used by women practicing contraception in 2002 were: OC 30.6% (used by 11.6 million women 15 to 44 years of age), female sterilization 27% (10.3 million women), male condom 18% (6.8 million women), and male sterilization (vasectomy) 9.2% (3.5 million) (9). The OC and female sterilization have been the two leading methods in the United States since 1982. During their lifetimes, 82% of women who have ever had intercourse have used the OC and 90% have used a male condom (9).

Hormonal Contraceptives

There are two types of hormonal contraceptives used by women: combined contraceptives and progestin-only contraceptives. The methods of delivery include oral, intramuscular/subcutaneous injection, subdermal implant, vaginal, and transdermal routes.

TABLE 26.1 Contraceptive Methods

Method	Effectiveness (% Unintended Pregnancy/Year)	Noncontraceptive Benefits	Common Side Effects/Complications
Oral contraceptive	8	Protection against ovarian, endometrial and colorectal cancer, benign breast tumors, ovarian cysts, dysmenorrhea and blood loss Reduces acne Suppresses endometriosis Treats hot flashes	Amenorrhea, spotting and BTB, nausea, acne, breast pain/tenderness, increased vaginal discharge, melasma, decreased libido VTE, risk of MI or stroke (<2 events /100,000 women years) Hyperkalemia (Yasmin) Benign hepatic tumor
Patch (Ortho Evra)	8	Similar to OC	Similar to OC; possible increased risk of VTE Local skin irritation
Vaginal ring (NuvaRing)	8	Similar to OC except less spotting and BTB	Similar to OC except vaginal discomfort (2%–3%) and discharge (5%)
Progestin-only oral contraceptive	8	Protection against ovarian and endometrial cancer and PID Compatible with breastfeeding; Reduced risk of PID and VTE vs. estrogen containing OC	Menstrual changes (unpredictable, frequent or prolonged bleeding) and amenorrhea Narrow margin of error for contraceptive efficacy (late or missed pills)
Injectable medroxyprogesterone acetate (Depo-Provera and Depo-subQ Provera 104)	3	Protection against uterine cancer Compatible with breastfeeding Reduced risk of PID and VTE vs. estrogen containing OC	Menstrual changes and amenorrhea Weight gain (15 lb over 4 years), headaches Transient decrease in bone density Adverse effect on lipids Slow return of fertility (average 10 months)
Implanon	0.38	Compatible with breastfeeding	Menstrual changes (unpredictable, frequent or prolonged bleeding) and amenorrhea Minor surgery needed for implantation and removal
IUD Tcu380A (ParaGard) LNG-IUS (Mirena®)	 0.8 0.1	Protection against endometrial cancer Decreased menstrual blood loss and pain	Menstrual cramping and increased or irregular bleeding* Rarely PID Occasional oily skin with LNG-IUS
Diaphragm with spermicide	16	Possible protection against some STIs Reduced cervical cancer risk Reversible and inexpensive	Vaginal and UTI risk TSS risk Latex allergy Cervical irritation
Today Sponge Nulliparous Parous woman	 16 32	Possible protection against some STI (GC, chlamydia, trichomonas)	Difficulty with removal Increased vaginal infection and UTI and TSS risk
Condom Male Female	 15 21	Protection against STIs, Nonprescription, low cost	Regular use with spermicide may cause skin irritation or tiny abrasions (increases risk for STI) Latex allergy or contact dermatitis
Spermicide	29	Ease of use, nonprescription, low cost Lubrication	Skin, vaginal or penile allergy or sensitivity Messy May cause skin irritation or tiny abrasions (increases risk for STI)

TABLE 26.1 *(Continued)*

Method	Effectiveness (% Unintended Pregnancy/Year)	Noncontraceptive Benefits	Common Side Effects/Complications
Natural family planning	13%–20%	Low cost (unless barrier method used during fertile days)	No protection against STIs
Sterilization Female Male	 0.5 0.15	Female: reduced risk of ovarian cancer and PID	Short-term post-surgical pain and infection risk (both)

BTB = breakthrough bleeding; GC = gonococcus; LNG = levonorgestrel; LNG-IUS = levonorgestrel intrauterine system; MI = myocardial infarction; OC = oral contraceptive; PID = pelvic inflammatory disease; STI = sexually transmitted infections; TSS = toxic shock syndrome; UTI = urinary tract infection; VTE = venous thromboembolism.

*Users of the Tcu390A typically have heavier menses, and irregular bleeding is common in the initial months of use. Women using the LNG-IUS typically have irregular, light bleeding or spotting during the initial months of use. After several months, about 20% of women using the LNG-IUS experience amenorrhea.

COMBINED OC

Description

The "pill" contains two hormones: an estrogen and a progestin. In most OCs, the estrogen is ethinyl estradiol (EE) 20 to 35 mcg. There are nine progestins contained in OCs marketed in the United States. Progestins vary by selectivity (preferential binding to the progesterone receptor rather than the androgen receptor). Third-generation progestins (norgestimate and desogestrel) are more selective and thus have fewer androgenic side effects such as acne and adverse lipid effects. OCs with second-generation (levonorgestrel, norgestrel) and third-generation progestins are more acceptable to users than OC containing first-generation progestins (e.g., norethindrone) (10).

Drospirenone, a spironolactone analogue, is a unique progestin that has antiandrogenic and antimineralocorticoid effects. These actions can improve acne and seborrhea and counteract fluid retention caused by estrogen; however, drospirenone may increase potassium levels. Although this is unlikely (11), the manufacturer recommends caution if women are taking other medications that increase serum potassium and to obtain a potassium level during the first month of use.

OCs are also described as monophasic (same dose of estrogen and progestin in each pill) or multiphasic (amounts of hormones in tablets can vary across the cycle/month). There is no convincing evidence that multiphasic OCs offer any advantages compared to monophasic OCs (12). Most OC products contain 21 active tablets and a total of 21 or 28 tablets. Extended cycle products (Seasonale, Seasonique) provide 84 active tablets and continuous use Lybrel is used daily without interruption.

Mechanism of Action

The primary contraceptive action of the OC is suppression of ovulation. Additional contraceptive actions are primarily the result of progestins and include creation of thickened cervical mucus that blocks sperm from the uterus, inhibition of capacitation (ability of sperm to fertilize an egg), interference with transport of the egg and sperm, and endometrial changes that interfere with implantation. Most of these actions precede fertilization; all precede implantation. The OC does not disrupt an established pregnancy or harm a developing fetus.

Efficacy

In general, all OCs are equally effective (Table 26.1). Use of the lowest dose of estrogen is recommended to reduce adverse effects. Users of OCs containing 20 mcg may experience breakthrough ovulation (8). One study found that heavier women (>70 kg or 154 lb) may have higher failure rates when using OCs containing <35 mcg of EE (13).

Benefits

In addition to high efficacy, OCs are reversible, safe, and an option throughout all reproductive years. OC use may decrease a woman's risk for certain cancers (Table 26.1) (14, 15); however, long duration of use (>8 years) may increase overall cancer risk (15).

Side Effects

The OC also has some disadvantages and risks (Table 26.1). It must be taken daily and does not protect against sexually transmitted infections (STI).

Among OC users, both smoking and hypertension increase the risk for some cardiovascular diseases (myocardial infarction, stroke, and venous thromboembolism [VTE]) by as much as ninefold (8,16). Among women who smoke, the mortality attributable to OC use is approximately 1 per 10,000 for women >35 years, but only 1 per 100,000 for women <35 years of age (17). Among higher risk women, progestin-only contraceptives or OCs containing third-generation progestins may be safer options.

There is an increased risk for stroke for women with migraine headaches who experience auras and OCs are contraindicated in these women; also, any woman >35 years with migraines should not use OCs (18,19).

VTE is the most common cardiovascular risk associated with OCs. For users of low-dose OCs, the rate is increased three- to sixfold (baseline 3 to 6 per 100,000 reproductive-age women). Risk for VTE is highest during the first year of OC use (8,17).

The relationship between breast cancer and OC use is unclear. A well-designed case-control study found no

TABLE 26.2 Contraindications to Use of Contraceptives

Contraindication	Potential Risk
Combined (Estrogen-Progestin) Hormonal Contraceptives (Tablets, Patch, Ring)	
Breastfeeding <6 weeks postpartum	Infant exposure to contraceptive steroids
Breastfeeding >6 weeks to <6 months postpartum*	Decreased quantity of breast milk and shortened duration of lactation
Immediately postpartum (<21 days)*	Thrombosis
Smoking plus age >35 years*	CVD, especially MI
CVD (HTN[†], CHD, stroke,) or high risk for CVD[‡]	CVD events MI, stroke
Presence of DVT/PE or history of DVT/PE	Thrombosis
Major surgery with prolonged immobilization	Thrombosis
Thrombogenic mutations (e.g., Factor V Leiden)	Thrombosis
Migraine headache (with aura or age >35 years)	Ischemic stroke
Breast cancer or history of breast cancer	May worsen prognosis
DM with end-stage organ involvement[§], or with other vascular disease, or if >20 years' duration	CVD and thrombosis
Gall bladder disease; past OC-related cholestasis	Worsening gall bladder disease
Liver disease (viral hepatitis, cirrhosis, tumor)	Increasing tumor growth
Medications that affect liver enzymes[‖]	Increase or decrease hormone bioavailability Decreased effectiveness of OCs
Progestin-only Contraceptives (POP, DMPA, Implant)	
Breastfeeding <6 weeks postpartum	Infant exposure to contraceptive steroids
CVD (HTN[†]) or high risk for CVD[‡], (DMPA) CHD, stroke (all)	CVD, MI, stroke, decreased HDL Possible increase in thrombosis (less than OCs)
Acute DVT/PE	Thrombosis
Migraine headache (with aura)—all	Headaches may worsen and persist after discontinuation of contraceptive
Unexplained vaginal bleeding (DMPA, implant)	Irregular bleeding of contraceptive may mask underlying pathological condition
Breast cancer or history of breast cancer	May worsen prognosis
Liver disease (severe cirrhosis, tumor)	Increasing tumor growth
Anticonvulsants[‖] (POPs, possibly implant) (DMPA – no drug interactions)	Decreased effectiveness of contraceptive*
Allergy to implant components (Implanon)	Allergic reaction
Intrauterine Device	
Breastfeeding (LNG-IUS only)	Infant exposure to contraceptive steroids
Insertion >48 hours, <4 weeks postpartum	Higher expulsion rates
Acute DVT/PE (LNG-IUS only)	Thrombosis
CHD–current, history of CHD (LNG-IUS only)	Adverse effect on lipids (potential)
Migraine headache (with aura) (LNG-IUS only)	Headaches may worsen and persist after discontinuation of contraceptive
Unexplained vaginal bleeding	Need to evaluate for pregnancy, irregular bleeding of contraceptive may mask underlying pathological condition (prior to insertion); if IUD in place no need to remove to evaluate
Current cervical, endometrial, or ovarian cancer	Postpone insertion; if IUD in place no need to remove

TABLE 26.2 *(Continued)*

Contraindication	Potential Risk
Breast cancer/history of breast cancer (LNG-IUS)	May worsen prognosis
Current PID	Postpone insertion; if IUD in place no need to remove – treat with appropriate antibiotics
Anatomical abnormalities (e.g., distorting fibroids)	Inability to safely insert or retain
STI current or increased risk of STI, AIDS[#]	Increased risk of IUD complications/infection; with AIDS monitor closely for pelvic infection
Serious liver disease (LNG-IUS only)	Increasing tumor growth
Diaphragm	
Allergy to latex or spermicides (either partner)	Allergic reaction
History of TSS	Recurrence
Physical anatomic obstructions to placement	Inability to insert or retain
At risk for or HIV infected, AIDS	Repeated use of the spermicide nonoxynol-9 increases the risk of acquiring HIV infection
Spermicide	
At risk for or HIV infected, AIDS	Repeated use of the spermicide nonoxynol-9 increases the risk of acquiring HIV infection
Latex Male Condoms	
Allergy to latex	Allergic reaction

CHD = coronary heart disease; CVD = cardiovascular disease; DM = diabetes mellitus; DVT = deep venous thrombosis; HTN = hypertension; MI = myocardial infarction; PE = pulmonary embolism; PID = pelvic inflammatory disease; STI = sexually transmitted infection; TSS = toxic shock syndrome.
*Combined OC effect only.
†Women with controlled HTN are at less risk for CVD events than women with untreated HTN.
‡Multiple risk factors such as age, smoking, DM, HTN.
§Nephropathy, neuropathy, retinopathy.
||Medications include antiretroviral therapy (ritonavir-boosted protease inhibitors) and anticonvulsants (phenytoin, barbiturates, carbamazepine, primidone, topiramate, oxcarbazepine, lamotrigine, Rifampicin, rifabutin).
#WHO does not classify HIV-infected or at risk as a contraindication to use.
Information from: World Health Organization. Medical Eligibility Criteria for Contraceptive Use, 2009. Available at *http://www.who.int/reproductivehealth/publications/family_planning*. Accessed February 23, 2010.

increased risk of breast cancer for current or former OC users (20). Women with first-degree relatives with breast cancer do not need to avoid OCs (21). Among women at high risk for breast cancer because of BRCA1 genetic mutation, use of the OC for longer than 5 years, and use before age 30 years, increased the risk of breast cancer (OR 1.33, 95% CI 1.11–1.6 and OR 1.29, 95% CI 1.09–1.52, respectively). Nonetheless, use of OCs to prevent ovarian cancer, especially after age 30 years, is supported (22).

Contraindications

Contraindications to OC use are shown in Table 26.2. Because thrombotic complications are the most common serious side effects, providers should refrain from providing OCs to women with current or past deep vein thromboses (DVT) or pulmonary emboli (PE), major surgery with immobilization, structural heart disease, diabetes mellitus long-standing (>20 years) or with complications (presence of nephropathy, neuropathy, retinopathy), hypertension, or for women who are older than 35 years and heavy smokers.

Drug Interactions

Drug interactions are common with OCs (Table 26.3). Most interactions interfere with contraceptive efficacy and are contraindications to use of the OC. Health providers should carefully consider potential drug interactions and recommend use of a backup method if there is concern about reduced efficacy during short-term use of the drugs listed in the table.

Key Points for Patient Education

- Women should be counseled about symptoms that may indicate serious health problems potentially associated with OCs. These can be remembered by the mnemonic ACHES: Abdominal pain (gallbladder or liver disease, blood clot), Chest pain (myocardial infarction, PE), Headaches (stroke, hypertension, migraine), Eye problems (migraine, stroke, or TIA, blood clot in the eye), and Severe leg pain (DVT).
- Cessation of tobacco smoking should be strongly encouraged and may preclude use of the OC for women >35 years (see Chapter 47). The World Health Organization suggests that for women >35 years who are light smokers, OCs

TABLE 26.3 Selected Clinically Significant Interactions with Oral OCs*

These Drugs May Reduce the Efficacy of OCs	
Antibiotics (e.g., penicillins, tetracyclines)	Reduced efficacy unlikely but failure possible For women taking a 20–35 mcg OC, use BUM during antibiotic therapy or for 14 days (whichever is shorter) PLUS 7 days
Aprepitant, barbiturates, bosentan, carbamazepine, felbamate, griseofulvin, modafinil, nevirapine, oxcarbazepine, phenytoin, primidone, protease inhibitors (nelfinavir, ritonavir, lopinavir, tipranavir), rifampin, topiramate	Use an alternative contraceptive or an additional nonhormonal BUM during concurrent therapy
OC May Increase The Adverse Effects or Toxicity of These Drugs	
Cyclosporine, troleandomycin	Avoid concurrent use
Alprazolam (and perhaps other benzodiazepines), prednisone (corticosteroids), selegiline, theophylline, tizanidine	Monitor for adverse effects and reduce the dose as needed
Decreased Effect of Non-OC Medication	
Lamotrigine	Potential for elevated blood pressure and fluid retention; monitor and stop licorice use if blood pressure increases
Herbal and Nutrition Interactions with the OCs	
St. John's wort (*Hypericum perforatum*) Chasteberry (*Vitex agnus*) Red clover (*Trifolium pratense*) Licorice (*Glycyrrhiza glabra*)	Possible loss of contraceptive efficacy or increased estrogen toxicity Avoid concurrent use
Licorice (herbal) *Glycyrrhizae glabra* Caffeine	Increase in adverse effect Monitor blood pressure May result in increased central nervous system stimulation; decrease caffeine intake if this occurs

BUM = back-up method; OC = oral contraceptive.
*Also presumed to occur with the progestin-only pill, contraceptive patch and vaginal ring.

should be used cautiously but are not contraindicated. For women >40 years, any tobacco use is a contraindication to OC use (8).

- Timing of start for OCs (e.g., immediate, first Sunday of the month) makes little difference in outcome. For example, in one study, immediate start was associated with better initiation but not continuation of OC, and had no influence on pregnancy rate (23). A backup method of contraception should be used for 7 days after beginning OCs for best pregnancy prevention.
- Missed pills are a common use error. Management depends on when in the cycle the pill is missed and how many tablets are missed. Refer to manufacturer prescribing information for management of missed pills.

Nonoral Combined Hormone Contraceptives

Although the OC is very effective, it requires daily ingestion of the tablet and 47% of users miss one or more pills per month (2). Two newer hormonal contraceptive products, Ortho Evra patch and NuvaRing, were designed to avoid the need for daily patient action while providing a contraceptive efficacy similar to that of the OC.

TRANSDERMAL PATCH (ORTHO EVRA)

Ortho Evra is a thin transdermal patch that contains EE (20 mcg is released every 24 hours) and norelgestromin. As with the OC, inhibition of ovulation is the primary mechanism of action.

The patch is believed to have similar efficacy, health benefits, health risks, and drug interactions as the OC, although patches may be less effective for women who weigh more than 198 lb (Table 26.1) (24). However, a recent comparison of the patch and OCs found similar efficacy but more side effects with the patch (25). Women OC users who switched to a patch in one randomized controlled trial (RCT) had a low (27%) continuation rate likely because of side effects including longer periods (38%) and mastalgia (25%) (26). The FDA has required the addition of a warning to the labeling for the contraceptive patch because of the possibility of a higher incidence of venous thromboembolic events (VTE) compared with other estrogen-progestin contraceptives (24).

Key Points for Patient Education with Use of the Contraceptive Patch

- The patch should be applied once a week for 3 weeks; then there is a patch-free week. There is enough medication in

TABLE 26.4 Comparison of the Three Formulations of Progestin-only Contraceptives

Progestin-only Contraceptive (Progestin)	Mechanism of Action	Long-term Effectiveness	Drug Interactions	Return to Fertility After Discontinued	Weight Gain
Progestin-only pill (POP); Minipill (Norethindrone)	Thickening of cervical mucus Endometrial changes	No	Yes	Immediate	Minor
Long-acting Injection Depo Provera (IM) and Depo-SQ-Provera 104 (medroxyprogesterone acetate)	Prevention of ovulation (primary action)	Yes 3 months per injection	No	Delayed, on average, 10 months after last injection	Significant (5– 15 lb); not all users gain weight
Subdermal Implant Implanon (Etonogestrel, an active metabolite of desogestrel)	Prevention of ovulation (primary); thickening of cervical mucus; endometrial changes	Yes 3 years per implant	Yes	Immediate	Minor

the patch for 2 additional days so if the patch is changed late within this timeframe no backup contraceptive is needed.

- The patch should be applied to clean dry skin of the upper outer arms, abdomen, buttocks, or the torso (except for breasts) and changed on the same day each week.
- When a patch is removed the next patch should be applied to a different area of the body.
- If a patch becomes detached (1% to 3% of users), it can be firmly pressed back on. If the patch will not stick, it should be removed and another patch should be applied immediately.

VAGINAL RING (NUVARING)

NuvaRing is a soft, flexible and transparent ring that releases EE (15 mcg/day) and etonogestrel (active metabolite of desogestrel; 120 mcg/day). The efficacy, drug interactions, side effects, and risks/benefits of this device are thought to be similar to the OC (27). Contraceptive action begins the first day of use. The acceptance rate was high in one RCT where 71% of previous OC users chose to continue using the ring rather than return to OC use (26).

Key Points for Patient Education with Use of the Vaginal Contraceptive Ring

- The vaginal ring should be kept refrigerated until use.
- The vaginal contraceptive ring should be compressed and inserted high into the vagina (exact placement not necessary).
- One ring is left in the vagina for 3 weeks. It is *not* removed for sexual intercourse. At the end of 3 weeks, the vaginal ring is removed and there is a ring-free week. Menses will occur during this week.
- Use of a backup method of contraception is necessary for the first 7 days the ring is inserted unless a woman has switched from another hormonal method of contraception (see prescribing information for the ring to determine when the ring should be inserted).
- The vaginal ring should be discarded in the trash (not flushed).
- The next vaginal ring should be inserted on the same day of the week as the previous ring was inserted even if menses are continuing.
- If expulsion of the vaginal ring occurs, the device should be rinsed in cool or warm water and re-inserted as soon as possible but within 3 hours. Use of a backup method of contraception will be necessary for 7 days if the ring is out of the vagina for >3 hours.
- Tampons, vaginal antifungals, and vaginal spermicides can all be used when the vaginal ring is in the vagina.

Progestin-only Contraceptives

DESCRIPTION

There are three progestin-only contraceptives: the progestin-only pill (POP), also known as the minipill, DMPA (intramuscular medroxyprogesterone acetate; Depo-Provera and DMPA-SC 104, subcutaneous medroxyprogesterone acetate; Depo-subQ Provera 104) and a subdermal implant, Implanon (28).

The progestin-only contraceptives have the advantage of eliminating exposure to estrogen making these contraceptive methods particularly useful for women who have contraindications to use of estrogen. They are also more suitable for women who want to breastfeed as they do not impair lactation. Efficacy of these contraceptives is shown in Table 26.1. Table 26.4 shows a comparison of the three formulations.

PROGESTIN-ONLY PILL

The POP is a tablet that is taken daily with no interruptions. Because the thickened cervical mucus is critical to its efficacy, the POP must be taken the same time every day as this effect is lost if the pill is taken "late" (3 or more hours later than its usual administration time).

Although it is common for women taking the POP to experience menstrual irregularity including absence of menses (amenorrhea), a woman should be instructed to see her physician if she experiences severe lower abdominal pain while taking the POP; this may be caused by an ectopic pregnancy or an ovarian cyst.

MEDROXYPROGESTERONE INJECTIONS

DMPA is a long-acting contraceptive administered via intramuscular or subcutaneous injection every 3 months. DMPA-SC 104 is a low-dose formulation of DMPA that is similar in onset of action, efficacy, and safety to DMPA-IM (29). The slower rate of absorption of the subcutaneous formulation allows for the lower dose of DMPA (29).

DMPA-IM is injected into the deltoid or gluteus muscles every 11 to 13 weeks. DMPA-SC 104 is injected into subcutaneous fat in the upper thigh or abdomen over the same interval. DMPA-SC 104 can be self-administered by women, decreasing the need for quarterly clinic visits. A back-up method of contraception needs to be used for 1 week after the first injection of DMPA-IM. No backup method is required for DMPA-SC 104 if the initial injection occurs within the first 5 days of menses (29). If a woman is late for her DMPA injection, she should begin use of a backup method of contraception immediately. If she had unprotected sexual intercourse and has not had an injection within the past 13 weeks, she should consider use of the emergency contraceptive.

Both formulations of DMPA are very effective contraceptives and efficacy of DMPA-SC 104 is not reduced among women with higher body mass index (29) (Table 26.1). DMPA is a useful contraceptive for women taking Accutane and other potentially teratogenic drugs.

Side effects and potential complications are listed in Table 26.1. It is common for women using DMPA to experience menstrual irregularity and about half will experience amenorrhea after one year of use; eventually almost all users stop bleeding. This is not harmful. Although there is a slow return to fertility upon discontinuing DMPA, by 12 months after the last injection of both formulations of DMPA about 95% users have resumption of ovulation.

SUBDERMAL IMPLANT

Implanon is a single contraceptive rod (4 cm long, 2 mm in diameter) that is inserted subdermally in the groove between the biceps and triceps muscles in the upper nondominant arm. It provides very effective continuous contraception for three years but is rapidly reversible; within 3 months of removal the majority of users have resumed ovulation (30) (Table 26.1). Implanon may be less effective in heavier women (>130% of ideal body weight). Chronic use of medications that induce liver enzymes (e.g., carbamazepine, HIV [antiretroviral] medications) are contraindications to the use of Implanon (30).

SIDE EFFECTS AND CONTRAINDICATIONS

All progestin-only contraceptives are associated with irregular bleeding, spotting, and amenorrhea especially compared with the combined OC (Table 26.1) (28). DMPA has two side effects that can decrease patient satisfaction: menstrual disturbances and weight gain (Table 26.1); bleeding disturbances (as above) are also the most common reason for discontinuation of the implant (30). Treatment of prolonged and/or frequent bleeding may be accomplished with use of low-dose estrogen, doxycycline, or NSAIDs (30).

Because of the potential for bone loss with DMPA, ACOG recommends counseling DMPA users about the possible adverse effects on bone and use of calcium and vitamin D supplements to offset any negative bone effects. Although alternative contraceptives without these potential effects on BMD (e.g., implants, IUDs) may be considered as preferred agents for adolescents, ACOG supports the continued use of DMPA, even for adolescents (31). Evidence suggests partial or full recovery of bone occurs after discontinuation of DMPA; further, bone loss slows with continued use. Limiting use to two years is not recommended, nor is monitoring of BMD (31). Contraindications for the progestin-only contraceptives are shown in Table 26.2.

DRUG INTERACTIONS

Some medications interact with the POP and Implanon. Medications known to interact with the POP are shown in Table 26.2. In addition, it would be prudent to consider the potential drug interactions listed in Table 26.3 as possible interactions for the POP and Implanon because progestins provide the major contraceptive action for the OCs.

KEY POINTS FOR PATIENT EDUCATION

- Progestin-only contraceptive methods are compatible with breastfeeding. These contraceptives do not decrease milk volume nor do they have adverse effects on child growth or development when started after 6 weeks postpartum (32).
- Women should not begin their use sooner than 6 weeks postpartum to avoid early exposure of the infant to hormones. Neonates possess a limited ability to metabolize and excrete drugs and there is the potential for adverse effects on developing organs (33).
- A backup method of contraception is generally recommended for the first 7 to 28 days of use of the POP; if the POP is taken 3 or more hours late, use of a backup method is advised for 48 hours to reestablish thickened cervical mucus.
- Women using DMPA should be encouraged to consume a healthy diet with adequate calcium (usually 1,000 mg a day through diet or supplements) and vitamin D and engage in weight-bearing exercise to help maintain a healthy weight and bone density.
- A woman should see her physician if she experiences severe lower abdominal pain while using DMPA. This may be caused by an ectopic pregnancy. She should also contact her physician if she experiences severe headaches, depression, heavy bleeding or signs of infection (e.g., pus) at the injection site.
- A woman using Implanon should be able to feel the device after insertion; if she cannot the device may not have been inserted correctly and it may not provide a contraceptive effect.

Hormonal Emergency Contraceptives

Although informing patients about the availability of EC and/or offering a prescription is suggested as part of contraceptive care/counseling by the AAP and ACOG (34,35), few clinicians include this information or a prescription when providing (regular) contraceptives, as they should. Ready access to this agent would increase the number of women using it. Plan B is now available as a nonprescription product for women 17 years of age and older; for women 16 years of age and younger it is only available as a prescription medication. A consumer purchasing the nonprescription EC must obtain it from a pharmacist and show personal identification with proof of age (of the purchaser). In addition, pharmacists can provide the EC without a prescription, via protocol or collaborative practice agreement, in 9 states (36).

DESCRIPTION

EC are used after intercourse to prevent pregnancy. The risk for an unintended pregnancy is often apparent (contraceptives are forgotten or fail, unprotected sexual intercourse occurs). In these cases, use of EC offers the opportunity to avoid unintended pregnancy.

There are two commonly used types of oral EC: levonorgestrel and OCs containing EE plus either levonorgestrel or norgestrel known as the Yuzpe regimen (6). Two regimens are available for the levonorgestrel EC: two 750-mcg (0.75 mg) doses of levonorgestrel or a single 1.5-mg dose. For the two dose regimen, one tablet is taken as soon as possible and the second is taken 12 hours later. Since 2009, a single tablet version (Plan B One-Step) and a generic version (Next Choice) of the levonorgestrel EC have been available. The two regimens have the same efficacy and similar side effects (37).

The Yuzpe regimen uses two doses of OC pills taken 12 hours apart over 1 day of treatment. Each dose contains ≥100 mcg of EE and either ≥1 mg of norgestrel or ≥0.5 mg of levonorgestrel. Total hormone doses are 200 mcg of EE and either 2 mg of norgestrel or 1 mg of levonorgestrel. For example, if using Alesse (20 mcg EE plus 0.1 mg levonorgestrel), a prescriber would instruct a woman to take five tablets for each of two doses. Using Lo-Ovral, a norgestrel product (30 mcg EE plus 0.3 mg norgestrel), a woman would be instructed to take four tablets for each of the two doses.

MECHANISM OF ACTION

The primary contraceptive action of the EC is to inhibit the mid-cycle LH surge and thus ovulation. If given at least 2 days prior to ovulation, prevention or delay of ovulation occurs. If ovulation occurs, the contraceptive action is prevention of fertilization; no data show that the EC prevents implantation (38). The EC does not impair the development of an embryo or disrupt an already established pregnancy. Furthermore, there are no known adverse effects to the fetus from inadvertent exposure to EC and a recent trial found no association between use of the levonorgestrel EC and risk of major congenital malformations, pregnancy complications, or other adverse pregnancy outcomes (39). The EC is also regarded as safe for use in breastfeeding woman after 6 weeks postpartum (37).

EFFICACY

The effectiveness EC is highly dependent on timing. The pregnancy rate is only 0.5% if taken within 12 hours but 4.1% if taken 61 to 72 hours after unprotected intercourse. Use of the levonorgestrel EC within 72 hours of unprotected intercourse can reduce the likelihood of pregnancy by 89%. The use of OCs in the Yuzpe regimen has been shown to decrease the likelihood of pregnancy by 75%.

SIDE EFFECTS AND CONTRAINDICATIONS

It is common for users of EC to experience nausea and vomiting. About 50% of users of the Yuzpe regimen experience nausea and 20% experience vomiting. Users of the levonorgestrel EC experience only half as much nausea and vomiting. Use of an antiemetic before taking the EC can reduce the associated nausea and vomiting. There are no evidence-based medical contraindications to use of the EC.

DRUG INTERACTIONS

Information about drug interactions with the EC is very limited. Broad-spectrum antibiotics do not interact with the levonorgestrel EC but theoretically drugs that induce hepatic enzymes may decrease the effectiveness of the EC (40).

KEY POINTS FOR PATIENT EDUCATION

- Take the first (or only) EC tablet (or tablets for the Yuzpe regimen) as soon as possible after unprotected sexual intercourse; for the two-dose regimen take the second tablet(s) 12 hours later.
- Use of the EC can delay ovulation; therefore, the risk of pregnancy may be greater than usual just after use of EC. It is important that a regular method of contraception be started immediately; they are more effective than EC at preventing pregnancy.
- Vomiting is a common side effect of EC. If vomiting occurs within 1 to 2 hours of the dose, repeat the dose as soon as possible. Use of an antinausea medication 1 hour before the EC (e.g., dimenhydrinate [Dramamine], meclizine hydrochloride [Bonine]) should be considered, especially if taking an oral contraceptive as an EC.
- Use of an EC may cause a delay in the time of menses, usually 1 week or less. If menses are delayed over 1 week past the usual time or do not occur within 3 weeks after use of the EC, a pregnancy test is advisable.

Intrauterine Device (IUD)

DESCRIPTION

There are two types of IUDs available in the United States: the Copper T-380A (TCu380A; ParaGard) and the levonorgestrel intrauterine system (LNG-IUS [Mirena]) (41). Both of these IUDs provide very effective and long acting but reversible contraceptive action (Table 26.1); the TCU-380A has a 10-year duration of use while the LNG-IUS provides 5 years of use.

MECHANISM OF ACTION

The IUDs contraceptive action is to prevent fertilization of the egg. The TCu380A alters tubal and uterine fluids thus impairing sperm function and preventing fertilization. The LNG-IUS has several contraceptive actions including thickening of cervical mucus, inhibiting sperm capacitation and survival, and suppression of the endometrium; in some women it also inhibits ovulation. Importantly, in contrast to common erroneous (consumer) information, IUDs are not abortifacients. In fact, studies have found no fertilized eggs in women using the IUD (41).

EFFICACY

Both IUDs are highly effective with similar, very low failure rates (Table 26.1).

INSERTION

Detailed instructions on placing an IUD can be found in *Contraceptive Technology* (41) or the manufacturer's prescribing information. Providers are encouraged to read and follow the manufacturer's instructions on insertion. Before insertion and after a discussion of safety and efficacy, explain the insertion procedure to the patient. Consider administration of an oral analgesic agent at least 30 to 60 minutes before the procedure to minimize pain. The IUD should be inserted slowly and gently.

IUDs may be placed at any time during the menstrual cycle, provided the woman is reasonably certain she is not pregnant, as well as immediately following childbirth (within 10 minutes of expulsion of the placenta), 4 to 6 weeks postpartum in a woman who is breastfeeding and has had no menses, and immediately after or up to 3 weeks after a first trimester abortion. Nulliparity, severe dysmenorrhea, heavy menstrual flow, and insertion 1 to 2 days after childbirth or after a second-trimester abortion are associated with higher expulsion rates (41). The copper IUD may also be used as an EC within 7 days of unprotected intercourse.

There is little risk of infection following correct insertion of an IUD in an otherwise healthy woman and prophylactic antibiotics are generally not needed; ACOG notes that in women who test negative for gonorrhea and chlamydia, prophylactic antibiotics appear to provide no benefit (Strength of Recommendation, SOR=A) (42).

Following the procedure, the woman should be given the IUD user identification card (provided in the IUD packet) including the name of the IUD, date of insertion (completed by the provider), and date of recommended removal. The woman should also be instructed to check for the IUD string to verify retention.

BENEFITS

Benefits of the IUD are displayed in Table 26.1. IUDs are an especially good choice for women who cannot use OCs for medical reasons and for women who want long-term contraception but are not candidates for sterilization.

SIDE EFFECTS AND CONTRAINDICATIONS

Both IUDs may cause changes in uterine bleeding, although they differ with regard to their effect. A common adverse effect of the TCu380A is heavy menses and irregular bleeding during the initial 3 to 6 months of use (12). In contrast, the LNG-IUS tends to cause irregular light bleeding which stops after several months due to suppression of the endometrium. About 20% of LNG-IUS users develop amenorrhea after a year of use.

Contraindications for both IUDs are listed in Table 26.2. New data have shown that two conditions previously linked to IUD use, PID and tubal infertility, are not increased by IUD use but rather by the insertion process. One study found that salpingitis occurred in only about 1 in 1,000 women who had an IUD inserted (41). In addition, the IUD is not contraindicated for women with heart valve abnormalities because IUD insertion is not associated with bacteremia.

KEY POINTS FOR PATIENT EDUCATION

- IUDs are a long-acting, highly effective, and cost-effective method of contraception.
- Menstrual bleeding patterns are likely to change with IUD use. Users of the Copper T 380A will likely experience an increase in menstrual blood loss while users of the LNG-IUS have a significant decrease in menstrual bleeding and about 20% experience amenorrhea (41).
- Cramping and discomfort are common for about 15 minutes after IUD insertion. If cramping continues or is severe, uterine perforation should be considered.
- Expulsion of the IUD occurs in a small number of women (2% to 10%). A woman should be told to contact her prescriber if she cannot feel the strings of the IUD, the strings feel long or if she can feel the IUD near the cervix. She should check for the strings periodically for the first few months.
- Cramping, pelvic pain, purulent discharge, and/or fever occurring within the first 3 weeks after insertion may indicate uterine infection. The IUD will need to be removed and antibiotics prescribed.
- A follow-up visit should be planned at about 3 to 6 weeks after insertion to verify that the IUD is still in place, no infection has occurred, and to address any questions or concerns.

Barrier Methods

Barrier methods include the diaphragm, contraceptive sponge, and condoms (male and female). The contraceptive action of these methods is achieved by physical and/or chemical (spermicide) barriers to passage of sperm into the uterus and upper reproductive tract. Barrier methods have a higher failure rate than hormonal contraceptives or IUDs; correct usage is critical to their effectiveness.

DIAPHRAGM

Description

The diaphragm is a dome-shaped (rim) reusable barrier contraceptive made of latex.

Mechanism of Action

The diaphragm acts as a physical barrier, covering the cervix, and the spermicide provides a chemical barrier.

Efficacy

The most important factor in effectiveness is correct and consistent use. Pregnancy rates are similar for parous and nulliparous women who use the diaphragm (Table 26.1).

Fitting and Insertion

There are three basic types of diaphragms: arcing, coil, and flat spring. Most providers use the arcing rim style in sizes 60 to 80 mm. An estimate of the correct size is obtained by measuring the distance along the examiner's index finger from the posterior vaginal wall to about 1 cm before the inside of the pubic arch. This distance should correspond to the diameter of the device.

Spermicide is applied to the diaphragm so that the cup holding the spermicide faces the cervix. One to three teaspoonfuls of spermicide is spread throughout the cup and some additional spermicide is spread around the rim. Jelly/gel spermicides are preferred as they adhere best to the diaphragm and are not as easily diluted by cervical secretions.

The diaphragm is inserted by pinching the sides together and gently inserting it into the vagina with a small amount of lubricant on the leading edge. Once inserted, it should cover the cervix and fit snugly but comfortably in place with the rim in contact with the posterior and lateral vaginal walls and the anterior edge about one fingerbreadth before the public arch. It should be easily removable. The woman (or her partner) should be encouraged to practice insertion and removal in the office, after the fitting, until comfortable with the procedure.

Benefits

Possible benefits are listed in Table 26.1. There are no data from trials supporting a decrease in STIs; however, several studies have found a decreased risk for cervical dysplasia and cancer among women using the diaphragm which was postulated to be due to cervical protection from HPV (43).

Side Effects and Contraindications

Colonization of the vagina with *Escherichia coli* occurs in women using the diaphragm which likely increases the risk of bacterial vaginosis and urinary tract infections (UTIs) (43). Women who experience frequent UTIs should urinate before inserting the diaphragm and after intercourse. It may also be appropriate to have the fit of the diaphragm checked. Contraindications to use of the diaphragm are shown in Table 26.2.

Key Points for Patient Education

- Women or their partners can insert the diaphragm while standing, squatting, or lying down. Women usually find it easiest to insert the diaphragm by pinching it together with the thumb and third finger of their dominant hand, introducing the device into the introitus, and using the first finger (or opposite hand) to push the back edge inside the vagina. The device should slide easily into place but it may spring out of a woman's hand on initial attempts; she should be warned that this may happen and to not be discouraged.
- The diaphragm is removed by inserting the first finger under the rim and pushing forward or by rotating the wrist (so that the knuckles of the hand are visible) allowing the device to be hooked by the index finger and pulled out of the vagina.
- A diaphragm can be inserted up to 6 hours before intercourse and must remain in position for at least 6 hours after intercourse; it should not remain in the vagina for >24 hours.
- If intercourse occurs more than once during the 6 hours, the diaphragm should be left in place but additional spermicide should be inserted vaginally.
- The diaphragm should not be used until at least 3 days after use of a vaginal antifungal; oil-based lubricants such as massage oil, hand lotion or Vaseline should not be used with the diaphragm.

Contraceptive Sponge (Today Sponge)

DESCRIPTION

The contraceptive sponge is a soft, one-size polyurethane foam device containing the spermicide nonoxynol-9. It is a single-use device.

MECHANISM OF ACTION

There are three actions that provide a contraceptive benefit: spermicide, sponge absorption of sperm, and physical blocking of sperm (holds spermicide against cervix and blocks cervical os).

EFFICACY

The sponge is more effective for women who have never had a child. The failure rate for nulliparous women (16%) is half that for parous women (32%) (Table 26.1).

BENEFITS

The sponge is a relatively low-cost nonprescription device providing 24-hour protection.

SIDE EFFECTS AND CONTRAINDICATIONS

The sponge should not be used while menstruating as this increases the risk of toxic shock syndrome (TSS) (Table 26.1).

KEY POINTS FOR PATIENT EDUCATION

- To use the sponge, moisten with 2 tablespoons of water, squeeze once, and then insert so that dimple is pressed over the cervix; the loop should be away from the cervix.
- The sponge provides a contraceptive action for 24 hours, including multiple acts of intercourse, and can be inserted well before intercourse.
- The sponge should remain in place for at least 6 hours after last act of intercourse but should be removed within 24 hours. Extending the time can result in a bad odor and a risk of TSS.
- The sponge is removed by pulling on the loop. When the sponge is removed it should be checked to be sure it is intact; all pieces should be removed from the vagina.
- The sponge should be discarded into the trash.
- The sponge should not be used concurrently with a vaginal antifungal; this may result in dilution of the spermicide and decrease contraceptive effectiveness.
- The sponge should not be used during menstruation.

Male and Female Condoms

DESCRIPTION AND MECHANISM OF ACTION

The male condom is a sheath that covers the penis and acts as a physical barrier contraceptive. Male condoms are made of three different materials: latex, polyurethane, and lamb caecum (natural skin). Useful characteristics of condoms are lubrication (reduces tearing) and a receptacle end to hold the semen. There is no contraceptive advantage to the use of condoms lubricated with spermicide and they are higher in cost, have a shorter shelf life, and have been associated with higher risk of UTI among female partners (44).

The female condom is a device that is comprised of a polyurethane sheath spanning two rings—one inserted vaginally and the other lying outside the vagina partially covering the labia—that provides a physical barrier. The device is coated on the inside with a lubricant. The female condom is more expensive than the male condom with a typical cost of $3.

EFFICACY

The male condom is more effective than the female condom, although effectiveness of the condom is highly dependent upon correct use (Table 26.1).

BENEFITS

Latex condoms are superior to polyurethane and natural skin condoms for protection against STIs either transmitted by infected secretions or by contact with infected skin. Natural skin condoms have small pores through which viruses and bacteria can pass; polyurethane condoms are more prone to slippage than the latex condoms.

SIDE EFFECTS AND CONTRAINDICATIONS

Side effects are listed in Table 26.1.

KEY POINTS FOR PATIENT EDUCATION

- The male condom is applied over the erect penis. It should be unrolled a short distance over a finger to be certain that it is unrolling properly. If the condom does not have a receptacle/reservoir end, users should pinch the tip of the condom to leave about one-half inch of space at the end when putting the condom on the penis to hold the semen.
- The penis should be withdrawn soon after ejaculation, while still erect, holding the rim of the condom against the base of the penis to prevent slippage. Remove the condom away from the partner's genitals without spilling the semen, check for visible damage, and discard.
- The female condom is inserted into the vagina by pinching together the smaller ring, introducing the device into the vagina. This end of the condom is not anchored. The large ring should be placed over the vaginal opening to protect the genitalia from infection. It can be inserted up to 8 hours before intercourse. It should not be used in combination with a male condom as the friction between the two condoms may displace one or both.
- Only water-based lubricant products (e.g., K-Y jelly, Astroglide, Replens) should be used along with latex male condoms. Oil based lubricants (e.g., baby oil, hand lotion, Vaseline) and vaginal antifungals can damage latex condoms. Latex condom use should be avoided until at least 3 days after use of a vaginal antifungal.
- Polyurethane female and male condoms are not adversely affected by oil-based lubricants or vaginal antifungal preparations.
- If an allergic or other skin reaction occurs, switching to another type of condom may eliminate the problem.
- Condoms should be used before their expiration date and should be stored in a cool dry location to avoid deterioration caused by heat, light, and air.

Spermicide

DESCRIPTION AND MECHANISM OF ACTION

Spermicides, which contain the agent nonoxynol-9, come in a variety of forms (cream, gel, foam, film, suppository/insert) and can be used alone or in combination with other contraceptives such as diaphragms and condoms. Nonoxynol-9 is a surfactant that destroys the sperm cell membrane.

EFFICACY

Although not highly effective (Table 26.1), efficacy is dependent on use of an adequate amount of spermicide. In addition, a spermicide product with at least 100 mg of nonoxynol-9 per dose should be used as lower doses may provide less contraceptive efficacy (45). Spermicides should be inserted close to the time of intercourse to avoid dilution. Only some (foam or gels) offer immediate protection; suppositories and film must be inserted at least 15 minutes before intercourse. When used alone or with a condom, a foam product is preferred as foams spread more completely and also offer the benefit of bubbles as a physical barrier. Viscous gels can also provide a physical barrier.

BENEFITS

The benefits are listed in Table 26.1. These products can also be used in conjunction with condoms to increase contraceptive effectiveness and can be used as a backup method by women using another contraceptive such as the OC.

SIDE EFFECTS AND CONTRAINDICATIONS

Common side effects are displayed in Table 26.1. The spermicide nonoxynol-9 does not protect against STIs and may facilitate transmission of HIV via irritation of vaginal mucosa (46, 47). According to the WHO, spermicide use is contraindicated for women at high risk of HIV, with HIV infection, or who have AIDS (48).

DRUG INTERACTIONS

Concurrent use with vaginal lubricants and vaginal antifungal products may dilute the spermicide and decrease effectiveness.

KEY POINTS FOR PATIENT EDUCATION

- Follow the directions on the package labeling.
- Use of an adequate amount of spermicide is important for contraceptive effectiveness.
- If shaking of a foam product is required, be sure to shake for the suggested time. Shaking creates bubbles that assist in the contraceptive action.
- Allow the time for certain spermicides (15 minutes for suppository or film) to dissolve or melt before intercourse; all are effective when inserted <1 hour before intercourse.
- Insert the spermicide high into the vagina, near the cervix.
- If more than 1 hour has elapsed since insertion of spermicide before intercourse, more spermicide should be inserted vaginally. Additional spermicide should be inserted before each act of intercourse.
- The spermicide must remain in the vagina for at least 6 hours after intercourse.
- If your product has a plastic reusable applicator, wash the applicator with soap and water after each use.
- Be sure to have an extra container of spermicide on hand. It is hard to determine when a container is almost empty.

Natural Family Planning/Fertility Awareness Methods

DESCRIPTION

There are several methods of natural family planning (NFP). These methods depend on identifying days during each menstrual cycle when intercourse is most likely to result in pregnancy. In the calendar method, a woman determines her period of fertility based on previous menstrual cycles over 1 year. Fertile days are calculated by subtracting 18 days from the length of the shortest cycle (first fertile day) and 11 days from the longest cycle (last fertile day). Intercourse is avoided

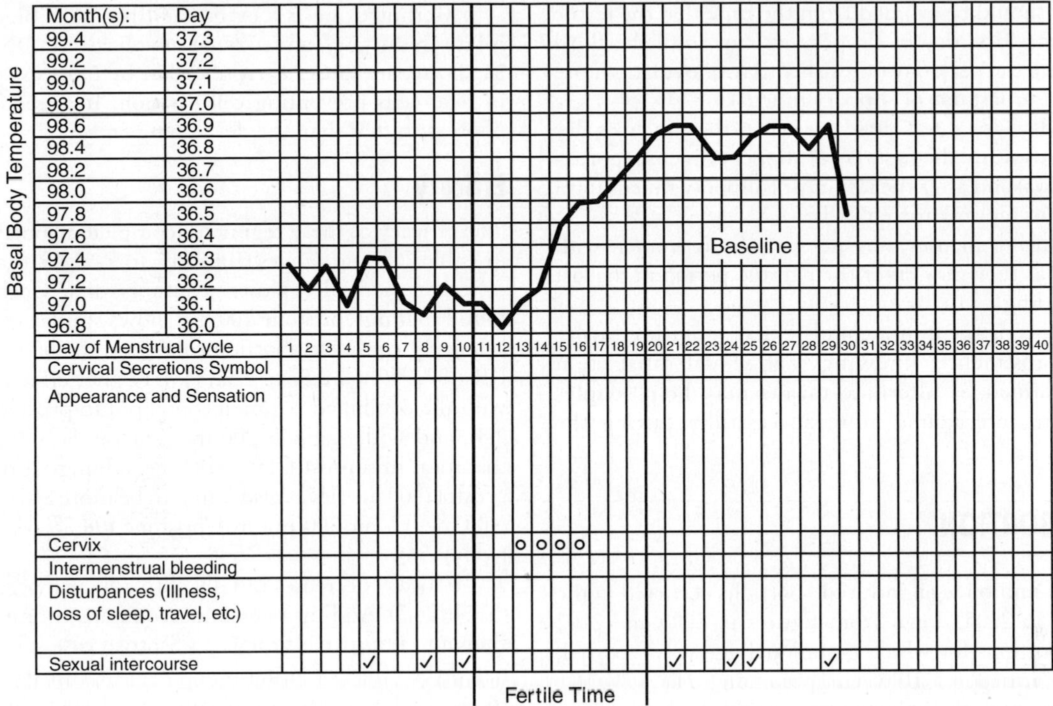

Figure 26.1 • Symptothermal variations during a model menstrual cycle. From Figure 16-4 in Jennings VH, Arevalo M. Fertility Awareness-Based Methods, in: Hatcher RA, Trussell J, Nelson AL, et al., eds. Contraceptive Technology, 19th ed. New York: Ardent Media, Inc., 2008:343–360. Used with permission.

or a barrier method is used during these days. High cycle variability makes this method less effective.

The temperature method is based on the rise in basal body temperature (BBT) that occurs just after ovulation (0.4°F to 1.0°F). The mucus method is based on the change in consistency of cervical mucus from thick and dry to clear, thin, and sticky at ovulation. Both are used to predict the time of ovulation; intercourse is avoided or a barrier method is used for several days before and after presumed ovulation.

In the symptothermal method, couples use a combination of two or more fertility indicators. An example of a chart used to document the rise in BBT, cervical mucus changes, and other symptoms that may assist women in determining fertile days is shown in Figure 26.1.

MECHANISM OF ACTION

Based on knowledge of female reproductive physiology—that a woman's egg survives <1 day and sperm survive up to 5 days inside the female genital tract—the actual fertile period lasts for about 6 days each cycle (6). By avoiding intercourse for a number of days before and after the time that an individual women is likely to ovulate each month, the couple can avoid pregnancy.

EFFICACY

Typical use efficacy rates vary from 13% to 20% (Table 26.1); authors of a Cochrane review were unable to determine the comparative effectiveness of fertility-awareness–based methods because of poor quality of studies and limited continuation rates by subjects (49).

BENEFITS

In addition to benefits listed in Table 26.1, NFP can be used to conceive and to detect impaired fertility.

SIDE EFFECTS AND CONTRAINDICATIONS

In addition to lack of STI protection, a woman must have fairly regular ovulatory cycles to use this method. Certain conditions may make it difficult to use this method including recent menarche or childbirth, breastfeeding, perimenopause, persistent genital tract infections, or recent discontinuation of a hormonal contraceptive.

KEY POINTS FOR PATIENT EDUCATION

Couples need careful instruction, often over several sessions with a trained instructor, to use this method effectively.

- A woman should record her basal temperature before rising each morning from bed. A special BBT thermometer can assist in documenting the small rise that follows ovulation.
- The cervical mucus should be checked following menses. When the mucus becomes slippery (resembling raw egg white), a woman is entering her most fertile days that continue until 3 days after the last day that the slippery mucus appears. Women may notice other symptoms of ovulation such as adnexal pain (mittelschmerz) or low backache, abdominal bloating, vulvar swelling, spotting, or a widening of the cervical os.
- Test kits to detect the LH surge that triggers ovulation are available, but expensive.

- Intercourse should be avoided from the time that the fertile period begins (first day of slippery mucus) until the third day following the peak day of fertility (day of ovulation, rise in BBT, and/or last day of slippery mucus).
- The safest days for intercourse are when the mucus is dry between menses and the first day of slippery mucus (approximately 4 days) and after the last day of slippery mucus until menses begins (approximately 8 days).
- The days during menses may not be safe in women with short cycles as they may enter their fertile period in the last days of bleeding.
- Couples may engage in noncoital sexual activities during periods of abstinence; knowing that sexual satisfaction may be obtained by alternate means may help couples abstain from intercourse more successfully during the fertile time.

MEDICAL ABORTION

A total of 1.21 million legal induced abortions occurred in the United States in 2005, down from figures in 2000 and 2002 (50). Of all abortions for which gestational age was reported, 79% were performed at ≤10 weeks' gestation (51).

For many years, the only option available was aspiration abortion (commonly called surgical abortion). However, aspiration abortion is not available to many women in part because the number of abortion providers continues to decline, leaving 87% of all US counties without an abortion provider (51). Integration of abortion care into the primary care setting allows for improved access, greater privacy, and improved continuity of care for women and families facing this health crisis (52).

Medical abortion refers to the use of medications to induce an abortion. Medical abortions accounted for 13% of all abortions in the United States in 2005 and 22% of abortions before 9 weeks' gestation (51). Medical abortion is an option for women who wish to terminate a pregnancy up to 63 days' gestation (calculated from the first day of the last menstrual period).

Description

Medications and the regimens currently used in medical abortion are shown in Table 26.5. Administration of oral mifepristone followed by a vaginal prostaglandin analogue (usually misoprostol) is the most commonly used medical abortion regimen.

Mechanism of Action

Mifepristone (RU-486) is a derivative of norethindrone that has a high affinity for progesterone receptors, binding to them and preventing activation (acts as a progesterone antagonist). It also stimulates prostaglandin synthesis by cells of the early decidua. It causes decidual necrosis, cervical softening, increased contractility (24 to 36 hours after its administration), and increased sensitivity to prostaglandins.

Misoprostol is a prostaglandin analogue that causes uterine contractions. It may be given orally or vaginally, the later route of administration causing greater uterine contractility.

Methotrexate is a cytotoxic drug that blocks dihydrofolate reductase, an enzyme involved in DNA synthesis. Methotrexate causes early abortion by blocking the folic acid in fetal cells preventing cell division. It acts on the cytotrophoblast rather than the developing embryo.

Efficacy

The efficacy of these regimens (completed abortion) is shown in Table 26.5 and ranges from 88% to 99%. With respect to the different medical regimens, authors of a Cochrane review found that mifepristone 200 mg shows similar effectiveness in achieving complete abortion compared to 600 mg (four trials, RR 1.07, 95% CI 0.87 to 1.32) (53). Higher effectiveness is seen with the combined regimen compared to prostaglandin alone (53), and with vaginal (800 mcg) or buccal (800 mcg) rather than oral misoprostol (53–55). The sublingual route of misoprostol (400 mcg) was also found to be more effective than oral (400 mcg) after 200 mg mifepristone (98.7% vs. 94%, respectively) (56).

Efficacy decreases rapidly with advancing gestational age (Table 26.5). Adding a possible second dose of misoprostol was shown to improve efficacy in a Scottish case series, and eliminated the effect of gestation on overall efficacy (57). A RCT (n = 2,181 women) comparing the efficacy of 100 mg and 200 mg doses of mifepristone and 24- and 48-hour intervals to administration of 800 mcg vaginal misoprostol for termination of early pregnancy found similar efficacy rates for all regimens (range 91.7% to 93.5%) (58).

Procedure

Recommended laboratory tests prior to medical abortion are hemoglobin or hematocrit and blood typing (54). Anti-D immune globulin should be administered if indicated. Confirmation of pregnancy by ultrasound or pregnancy testing is necessary (SOR=B). Ultrasound confirmation and dating is recommended as all the US trials have used ultrasound; however, results from French trials suggest that selective use of ultrasound is sufficient when patients are managed by highly experienced clinicians (54).

Administration of a regimen from Table 26.5 should proceed based on gestational age, efficacy, and physician experience. Pain can be reduced by administration of oral acetaminophen, acetaminophen with codeine, or an NSAID. Although NSAIDs reduce the synthesis of endogenous prostaglandins, they do not interfere with the action of preformed prostaglandins; in one study, ibuprofen (600 mg as needed) was more effective than acetaminophen and did not appear to reduce the efficacy of misoprostol (59).

Follow-up in 1 to 2 weeks is recommended, but there is no consensus on whether an office visit is necessary. Methods to verify abortion include ultrasound, a history of bleeding with uterine involution on physical examination, and human chorionic gonadotropin testing (54). β-hCG should decrease by 50% within 1 week for regimens including mifepristone or methotrexate and misoprostol administered between 2 and 5 days afterward (54). However, a 75% decrease in hCG is needed to assure completed abortion; total disappearance of hCG may take as long as 90 days after the procedure. If hCG remains elevated, consider ectopic pregnancy.

TABLE 26.5 Comparison of Medical Abortion Regimens

Regimens	Success Rates (%)	Advantages	Disadvantages	Gestational Age
*Mifepristone, 600 mg orally + misoprostol, 400 μg orally (48 hours later)	92	FDA-approved regimen	Must remain in office or clinic 4 hours after administration	Up to 49 days
*Mifepristone, 200 mg orally + misoprostol, 800 μg vaginally (up to 72 hours later)	95–99	More effective[†] Less time to expulsion Fewer side effects Improved complete abortion rates	Requires vaginal medication administration	Up to 63 days
Mifepristone, 100 *or* 200 mg orally + misoprostol, 800 μg vaginally (24 *or* 48 hours later)	91.7–93.5	No differences by dose or timing	No differences in adverse effects	Up to 63 days
Mifepristone, 200 mg orally + misoprostol, 800 μg buccal (24–36 hours later)	96.2	More effective than oral misoprostol	Fever and chills 10% more often with buccal administration	Up to 63 days
Mifepristone, 200 mg orally + misoprostol, 400 μg sublingual (24 hours later)	98.7	More effective than oral misoprostol	Fever and chills more often with sublingual	Up to 63 days
*Methotrexate, 50 mg/m^2 IM or 50 mg vaginally, + misoprostol, 800 μg vaginally 3–7 days later	92–96	Readily available medications[‡] Low drug cost	Takes longer for expulsion	Up to 49 days
*Misoprostol only, 800 μg vaginally repeated for up to three doses	88	Low drug cost	Requires complicated dosing regimen Higher incidence of side effects than other regimens More painful than surgical abortion	Up to 56 days

FDA = US Food and Drug Administration; IM, intramuscularly.
*ACOG bulletin (see below).
[†]Compared with first listed regimen.
[‡]Compared to mifepristone and misoprostol.
Information from: *ACOG practice bulletin. Clinical management guidelines of obstetrician-gynecologists. Number 67, October 2005. Medical management of abortion. *Obstet Gynecol*. 2005;106(4):873; Winikoff B, Dzuba IG, Creinin MD, et al. Two distinct oral routes of misoprostol in mifepristone medical abortion: a randomized controlled trial. *Obstet Gynecol*. 2008;112(6):1303–1310; Raghavan S, Comendant R, Digol I, et al. Two-pill regimens of misoprostol after mifepristone medical abortion through 63 days' gestational age: a randomized controlled trial of sublingual and oral misoprostol. *Contraception*. 2009;79(2):84–90; von Hertzen H, Piaggio G, Wojdyla D, et al. Two mifepristone doses and two intervals of misoprostol administration for termination of early pregnancy: a randomised factorial controlled equivalence trial. *BJOG*. 2009;116(3):381–389; Say L, Kulier R, Gülmezoglu M, et al. Medical versus surgical methods for first trimester termination of pregnancy. *Cochrane Database Syst Rev*. 2005;(1):CD003037.

Benefits

Medical abortion affords a woman both privacy and autonomy. Most women will be able to avoid surgical intervention with its small risk of uterine or cervical injury, infection, and the risk of anesthesia. Medical abortions are less painful and may be emotionally easier. In addition, in a systematic review of seven cohort studies, the incidence of miscarriage and postpartum hemorrhage was significantly lower in the pregnancy following a medical versus surgical abortion (60). A Cochrane review, however, found insufficient evidence to comment on the acceptability and side effects of medical versus surgical first-trimester abortion (61). Finally, both aspiration and medical abortion in the first trimester are safer than carrying a pregnancy to term.

Side Effects and Contraindications

Medical abortion causes more bleeding than surgical abortion although the amount is rarely clinically significant. Less than 1% of women require emergent curettage because of excessive bleeding (54). Cramping may be severe. With all medical regimens, there is some degree of waiting and uncertainty (expulsion may take days to weeks) and an extra clinic visit required.

Infection has also been reported after medical abortion including four deaths from endometritis and TSS associated with *Clostridium sordellii* that occurred within 1 week after medically induced abortions (62); this infection has also been reported in cases of death after childbirth and miscarriage. A review of the literature shows that the overall rate of infection following medical abortion is very low (0.92%, n = 46,421) (63).

Side effects of medical abortion using mifepristone and misoprostol include nausea (20% to 52%), thermoregulatory dysfunction (i.e., warmth, fever, chills, hot flash; 9% to 56%), dizziness (12% to 37%), headache (10% to 37%), vomiting (5% to 30%), and diarrhea (1% to 27%) (54). Use of vaginal misoprostol decreases the time to expulsion and limits gastrointestinal side effects. Methotrexate may rarely cause oral ulcers (<1%).

Medical abortion is contraindicated in women whose pregnancies are more advanced than 63 days. Medical abortion is also contraindicated in women with ectopic pregnancy, IUD in place, severe anemia, or known coagulopathy, long-term steroid use or allergy to abortion medications (54). Women with uncontrolled seizure disorder should not receive misoprostol. Women with cardiovascular disease, uncontrolled hypertension, or chronic liver, renal, or respiratory disease have been excluded from clinical trials so less is known about the safety of medical abortion for these women. Medical abortion should not be attempted where there is not immediate access to surgical abortion. Other considerations include a woman's interest in participation in her care, keeping follow-up appointments, and her ability to understand the instructions because of limited cognition or a language barrier.

Patient Education

All abortion care counseling should include a discussion of whether the woman is certain about her decision to terminate the pregnancy. Once she has made the decision, the method to be used may be selected. Counseling should include benefits and risks of both medical and aspiration procedures and the woman should be questioned about potential contraindications. If there are no medical or other contraindications (above) and her pregnancy is 63 days' or less gestation, she is a candidate for medical abortion. Contraception should be discussed following an abortion.

Women with continuing pregnancies following medical abortion should have their abortion completed by aspiration. Opinions vary with respect to management of persistent gestational sac without cardiac activity in which expectant management or the use of repeated doses of misoprostol is likely to be effective. Other reasons for a subsequent aspiration procedure include heavy bleeding (patients monitor for excessive bleeding and should be evaluated if they experience two soaked maxipads per hour for 2 or more hours in a row) and patient intolerance of the procedure.

There do not seem to be long-term psychological ill affects attributable to abortion. However, Bradshaw and Slade found 10% to 20% of women experienced sexual problems in the first weeks and months after an abortion, with 5% to 20% reporting sexual difficulties a year later (64).

CHOOSING A METHOD: ASSISTING PATIENTS WITH OPTIMAL DECISION MAKING

The health care provider has an important role in screening for health conditions that may influence the choice of a birth control method or require treatment before initiating contraception. The first visit for this purpose also presents an opportunity to offer periodic health screening services if not already obtained (see Chapter 6). During this visit, the following aspects of the history and physical examination will provide useful risk information for patients to consider in choosing an initial birth control method.

Key History and Physical Exam

- A medical history should be obtained focusing on current and past illnesses that constitute cautions or contraindications to the use of a particular method (Table 26.2).
- Because hormonal methods may alter menstrual patterns, a review of a woman's current menstrual pattern is helpful.
- Consider the patients need for protection against STIs and for high method effectiveness.
- Prior success with a method, frequency of intercourse, and motivation to use a method at the time of intercourse will also help direct choice.
- A blood pressure measurement demonstrating uncontrolled hypertension (see Chapter 11) is a relative contraindication for combined OCs.
- A clinical breast examination may be useful in identifying breast cancer (see Chapter 25), a finding which precludes use of hormonal contraceptives.
- A pelvic examination demonstrating evidence of STI on the skin, vulva, and cervix (see Chapter 32) is a contraindication for an IUD and structural abnormalities of the vagina may preclude use of a diaphragm.

For female adolescents, it may be more important to provide a method of contraception and defer the pelvic examination if the examination itself poses a barrier to initiating contraception. The examination may be performed at a follow-up visit once trust has been established (65). Figure 26.2 incorporates many of these considerations in an algorithm to guide selection of a method.

Ancillary Tests

A Pap smear should be obtained if the woman is sexually active and has never had one or has not had one in the past 3 years (see Chapter 6). Cultures for gonorrhea and *Chlamydia* should be performed, following informed consent, in women <25 years of age (SOR=A) and culture or serum for VDRL or HIV encouraged in others, based on history and examination findings (see Chapter 32). Additional laboratory investigations including liver function, lipid profile, or coagulation profile may be reserved for patients with risk factors.

Putting it All Together

Selecting a contraceptive method that the patient is willing to use consistently and correctly and one that is medically appropriate is essential. Remember that no one method of contraception is suitable for each person or couple and various contraceptive methods may be appropriate over a lifetime.

The algorithm shown in Figure 26.2 can be useful in assisting couples or individuals in selecting a method. Condoms should be encouraged for new partnerships, teenage partners, patients at high risk of STIs, and for couples where one partner has a viral STI and the other partner is not infected. For those requiring maximal protection, methods

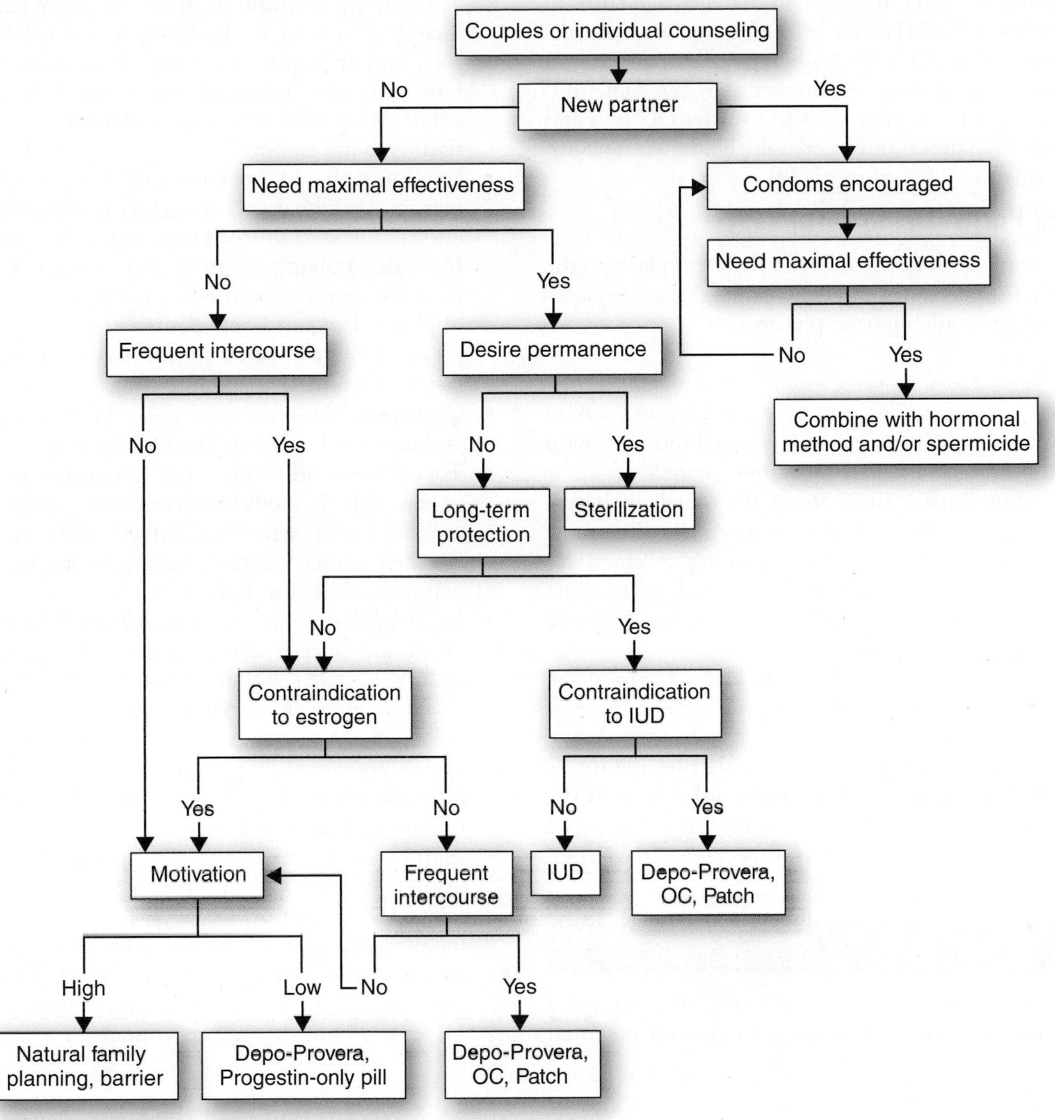

Figure 26.2 • Algorithm to guide in the selection of a contraceptive method. (Adapted from Smith MA, Shimp. Family planning. In Smith MA, Shimp LA, eds. Common Problems in Women's Health Care. New York: McGraw-Hill Companies, 2000. Used with permission.)

with the least opportunity for user error should be employed (e.g., IUD, DMPA, implant). Women engaging in frequent intercourse should consider OCs or DMPA; those who have less frequent intercourse or a contraindication to estrogen use might consider vaginal barrier methods or NFP. Finally, the progestin-only contraceptives are an option for older women with contraindications to estrogen and for lactating women. Patients should be encouraged to consider or choose a second method of contraception in case the chosen method proves unacceptable.

FOLLOW-UP AND MANAGING CONTRACEPTIVE SIDE EFFECTS

Many women experience side effects that require intervention. The following is a list of options for patients who wish to continue use of a chosen method.

ORAL CONTRACEPTIVES (OC)

Of women choosing an OC, approximately 25% experience minor side effects during the first 3 months after initiation (19).

- Nausea—likely to resolve within the first 3 months of use; take the OC with food and/or at bedtime. Alternatively, use a pill with lower or no estrogen.
- Breast tenderness—use a proper fitting bra or a pill lower in estrogen and/or progestin.
- Menstrual changes, typically a decrease in menses or amenorrhea—reassure or change to an OC with increased estrogen activity, a third-generation progestin pill, or a pill with higher progestin potency.
- Spotting and bleeding—likely to resolve within the first 3 months of use; assess for missed pills, erratic timing of

administration, or drug interactions. If heavy menstrual bleeding occurs, a NSAID may be used to reduce bleeding. Alternatively, try a pill with higher progestin potency, a third-generation progestin, or increased estrogen content.
- Weight gain is not common with use of the OC (66) and negative mood changes and decreased libido are uncommon, occurring in <20% of users (19).

Transdermal Patch (Ortho Evra)

- Irritation—apply each new patch to a different place on the skin than that used for the previous patch. Single replacement patches are available from pharmacies.

IUD

- Heavy periods—usually decrease over time; try an NSAID during the first few days of menses. Vaginal bleeding with pain should prompt evaluation for ectopic pregnancy.
- Expulsion—symptoms include unusual vaginal discharge, cramping or pain, spotting, dyspareunia or male discomfort during intercourse, absence or lengthening of the IUD string, and presence of the IUD in the cervical os or vagina (41). If the IUD is partially expelled, remove the IUD and consider insertion of a new IUD.
- IUD strings may be missing, too short, or too long—if the string is missing and the woman is unaware of expulsion of the IUD, an ultrasound or x-ray may be obtained. If the string is within the canal, it may be brought through the os with a cotton swab or endometrial biopsy instrument. If the IUD is in place, nothing more needs to be done. If the male partner complains of penile discomfort because of the string, strings may be cut shorter.

KEY POINTS

- Before prescribing a contraceptive method, clinicians should complete a medical history (focused on potential cautions or contraindications to a particular method), including current medications, menstrual and sexual history, history of prior method use (problems or successes), blood pressure measurement, clinical breast exam, and pelvic exam; the latter may be deferred if a barrier to initiating contraception.
- Condoms should be encouraged for new partnerships, teenagers, and patients at high risk of STIs with consideration of OCs or DMPA if engaging in frequent intercourse. If maximal pregnancy protection is needed, methods with least user error should be considered (e.g., IUD, DMPA, implant). Progestin-only contraceptives are a good option for older women with contraindications to estrogen and for lactating women.
- Cessation of tobacco smoking should be strongly encouraged and may preclude use of the OC for women >35 years.
- To optimize adherence and minimize accidental pregnancy, patients should receive contraception education, be familiar with potential side effects (and their management) for their chosen method, have a second (backup) method planned, and know about EC.
- EC, available nonprescription as Plan B for women 17 years of age and older, is safe and highly effective (pregnancy rate of 0.5% if taken within 12 hours and 4.1% if taken 61 to 72 hours after unprotected intercourse). There is likely an increased risk of conception immediately following EC use; use/resumption of a regular contraception method is critical after use of the EC. EC may cause a delay of menses onset, usually by 1 week or less.
- Major contraindications for specific methods include immediate post-partum (hormonal methods including LNG-IUS), cardiovascular disease (hormonal methods including LNG-IUS), breast cancer and liver disease (hormonal methods including LNG-IUS), STI or PID (IUD), latex allergy (latex condom, diaphragm), at risk for or HIV/AIDS (diaphragm, spermicide).

CHAPTER 27

Dysuria

George R. Bergus

CLINICAL OBJECTIVES

1. Describe an approach to the evaluation of dysuria in women, men, and children.
2. If dysuria is from a urinary tract infection (UTI), summarize how to determine whether the infection involves the upper or lower urinary tract.
3. Cite the treatment options for upper and lower UTIs.

Dysuria is pain or discomfort associated with urination that is localized to the bladder or urethra. This is a common chief complaint in the primary care office setting (1). Approximately 3% of all office visits are in response to this symptom (2,3). Most patients with dysuria are otherwise healthy women who have an uncomplicated urinary tract infection (UTI) requiring only minimal evaluation and a short course of antibiotics. However, physicians need to approach the complaint of dysuria with care so that the appropriate workup and treatment can be selected based on location of infection, age and gender of the patient, the patient's underlying health, and any factors signaling a more complicated infection.

This chapter focuses on UTIs. These infections can be divided into four very broad categories: (i) acute uncomplicated lower tract infection in women, (ii) recurrent uncomplicated lower tract infection in women, (iii) acute upper tract infection (pyelonephritis) in women, and (iv) UTIs in children, men, and geriatric patients. Each of these categories should be further divided into simple and complex infections, as there are important differences in their evaluation and treatment.

PATHOPHYSIOLOGY AND DIFFERENTIAL DIAGNOSIS

Pathophysiology

Most UTIs are caused by bacteria that normally inhabit the colon; 80% to 90% of community-acquired UTIs in adults and children are from *Escherichia coli* (4,5). The predominance of a single species of bacterium is important because it allows empiric therapy to have a high probability of success. Other gram-negative organisms (*Proteus* species, *Klebsiella pneumoniae,* and *Pseudomonas aeruginosa*) cause infections but are much less common except among people who are hospitalized, live in long-term care facilities, are immune compromised, or have undergone recent genitourinary catheterization or instrumentation. Gram-positive organisms (*Staphylococcus saprophyticus, Staphylococcus aureus*, group B *streptococcus*, and *Enterococcus faecium*) are also uropathogens, but are much less common causes of UTI. Anaerobic bacteria predominate in the gut but almost never cause UTI.

The usual route of infection involves bacteria invading the bladder by ascending from the perineum and passing through the urethra. Only a small number of *E. coli* strains in the colon are involved in these infections. These strains have a variety of virulence factors, including adhesive fimbriae, which allow these bacteria to adhere to the uroepithelium and resist the flushing action of urine flow. Infections usually remain within the bladder but bacteria sometimes ascend through the ureters to invade the upper urinary tract. When the renal parenchyma becomes infected, the infection is called pyelonephritis. Infections within the urinary tract are only rarely caused by a bloodborne source.

Differential Diagnosis

Although UTI is the most common cause of dysuria, this symptom can be from noninfectious causes or from infections outside of the urinary tract. For example, among menopausal women dysuria can be from vaginal atrophy from the loss of estrogen stimulation of vaginal mucosa. Other causes of dysuria are listed in Table 27.1 along with distinguishing symptoms and signs. Additional information can also be found in the chapters on vaginitis (Chapter 33), menopause (Chapter 29), prostate infection (Chapter 30), and sexually transmitted infections (STIs) (Chapter 32).

Dysuria is sometimes attributed to the poorly understood "urethral syndrome." This syndrome of pain on urination without a clearly identifiable cause has been ascribed to trauma, chemical irritation, low levels of urinary pathogens, or infection of periurethral tissue by unknown microorganisms (6). The diagnosis of urethral syndrome is made only after the symptomatic patient has had normal findings on physical examination, and normal urinalysis and culture.

Risk Factors and Clinical Epidemiology

With the exception of the neonatal period, women have a higher risk for UTI than men. During the third and fourth decades, this gender difference is at its maximum, with women at 40 to 50 times greater risk of UTI. Young adult women have the highest incidence of UTI of any group, and average one infection every other year (7). Elderly men develop UTI at a rate approaching that observed in elderly women, particularly when they are living in long-term care facilities.

TABLE 27.1 Differential Diagnosis of Dysuria in Otherwise Healthy Women and Men

Diagnosis	Frequency	Distinguishing Symptoms and Signs
Women of Reproductive Age		
Lower tract UTI	Very common	Nocturia, cloudy or malodorous urine
Vaginitis	Common	Vaginal discharge, perineal pruritus
Upper tract UTI	Uncommon	Fever, flank pain, CVA tenderness
Urethritis	Uncommon*	
Perineal trauma	Uncommon	Evidence of trauma and tenderness on exam
Interstitial cystitis	Uncommon	Frequency and urgency for 6 months with negative workup
Older Women		
Vaginal atrophy	Common	Vaginal mucosal atrophy on examination
Men		
Prostatitis	Common	Hesitancy, urgency with decreased urine flow, tender prostate
Urethritis	Uncommon	Urethral discharge, dysuria localize to penis

CVA = Costovertebral angle; UTI = urinary tract infection.
*May be more common in college health centers and reproductive health clinics.

Not all women are prone to UTI; only 50% to 60% report ever having an infection. Individuals with certain genetic, physiologic, or behavioral risk factors are more prone to develop UTI. For example, 10% to 20% of women have an epithelium to which uropathogenic *E. coli* adhere more easily. A history of at least two previous UTIs is a marker for this type of epithelium and is a strong predictor of subsequent infections. Another high-risk group is women with colonization of the vagina by uropathogens. The use of a contraceptive cream or jelly with nonoxynol-9 is associated with this colonization and subsequent UTI. Some barrier contraceptives (i.e., diaphragm, sponge) also increase the risk of UTI (see Chapter 26).

Other risk factors for women include sexual intercourse and a shorter distance from urethra to anus (8). Fecal incontinence and stasis of urine in the bladder are risk factors in both men and women. Incomplete or infrequent bladder emptying are common causes of stasis.

Risk factors for pyelonephritis in healthy women are very similar to those reported for lower tract infection and are listed in Table 27.2 (9).

TABLE 27.2 Risk Factors for Acute Pyelonephritis in Healthy Women (9)

- Recent urinary tract infection
- Diabetes mellitus
- Recent incontinence
- New sexual partners
- Use of spermicide
- Mother with history of urinary tract infection

CLINICAL EVALUATION

The extent of clinical evaluation of urinary symptoms varies and depends largely on the clinical setting. In some cases, management by telephone may be appropriate, whereas in others, a detailed physical examination supplemented by laboratory investigation is required.

History

UTIs in healthy adults are typically accompanied by urinary frequency, nocturia, pain on urination, and suprapubic discomfort. The clinician can use the history to determine the probability of UTI, and to exclude other causes for symptoms. When a healthy adult woman complains of moderately severe dysuria and nocturia, there is about a 65% probability that UTI is the cause (10). If the same woman also reports cloudy or malodorous urine and nocturia or urgency or recurrence of symptoms following a diagnosis of UTI, the probability of UTI increases to around 90% (10). In this setting, little further clinical evaluation is needed if there are no risk factors for a complicated infection (11). If vaginal complaints are also present or the dysuria is described as external, a more thorough evaluation is needed to exclude STIs and vaginitis. It is important to remember the complaint of dysuria is not as diagnostic of UTI in children, men, or elderly women.

The key elements of the history and physical examination of the patient with dysuria, including test characteristics when known, are listed in Table 27.3. Note that no single element of the history and physical exam is very accurate. Elements of the history that suggest infection of the upper urinary tract (pyelonephritis) include fever, chills, abdominal pain, flank pain, and vomiting. Pyelonephritis can be further divided into

TABLE 27.3 Key Elements of the History and Physical Examination for Dysuria

Diagnosis	Question or Maneuver	Sensitivity	Specificity	LR+	LR−
UTI					
	Moderate severe nocturia	0.54	0.64	1.8	0.53
	Moderate severe dysuria	0.80	0.57	1.6	0.40
	Moderate severe urgency	0.24	0.90	1.3	0.86
	Frequency	0.87	0.32	1.3	0.41
	Malodorous urine	0.24	0.90	1.3	0.94
	Cloudy urine	0.46	0.79	2.3	0.68
Pyelonephritis					
	Chills and rigors	0.32	0.87	2.5	0.78
	Fever	0.44	0.80	2.2	0.70
	Nausea and vomiting	0.24	0.84	1.5	0.90
	Flank pain	0.48	0.67	1.5	0.78

Information from: Dobbs FF, Fleming DM. A simple scoring system for evaluating symptoms, history and urine dipstick testing in the diagnosis of urinary tract infection. *J R Coll Gen Pract*. 1987;37:100–104; Österberg E, Aspevall O, Grillner L, et al. Young women with symptoms of urinary infection. Prevalence and diagnosis of chlamydial infection and evaluation of rapid screening of bacteriuria. *Scand J Prim Health Care*. 1996;14:43–49; Little P, Turner S, Rumsby K, et al. Developing clinical rules to predict urinary tract infection in primary care settings: sensitivity and specificity of near patient tests (dipsticks) and clinical scores. *Br J Gen Pract*. 2006;56(529):606–612.

simple and complex episodes. "Red flags" for these more serious infections are summarized in Table 27.4.

Fever and dysuria can be from conditions other than pyelonephritis. For example acute prostatitis or genital herpes can also cause dysuria and fever. Similarly, the lack of upper tract symptoms such as fever and flank pain does not eliminate the possibility of infection of the upper urinary tract. Such an infection is termed "occult pyelonephritis" Risk factors for these infections include dysuria for more than 7 days, an immunosuppressing condition, prior episode of acute pyelonephritis within the past year, known anatomic abnormality, a history of recurrent infections, and diabetes mellitus (3).

Physical Examination

The physical examination in adults with dysuria should be focused, whereas in children it should be more comprehensive. You will need to obtain the patient's vital signs, palpate the mid and lower abdomen, and percuss the flanks of the patient. Tenderness over a flank or in the midabdomen suggests upper tract disease; however, suprapubic tenderness with an uncomplicated lower tract infection is common. In men, the penis should be gently milked to elicit a urethral discharge, and a rectal exam performed to feel for a tender or boggy prostate; these findings suggest urethritis and prostatitis, respectively (see Chapter 30). You should perform a vaginal examination on women who report vaginal discharge or irritation (see Chapter 33).

TABLE 27.4 "Red Flags" for a Complicated Infection (3)

- Male gender
- Infant or geriatric age
- Symptoms for more than 7 days
- Immunosuppressing condition
- Episode of acute pyelonephritis within the past year
- Known anatomic abnormality
- Diabetes mellitus
- Fever
- Flank pain or tenderness

Laboratory Tests

COLLECTING A SPECIMEN

Most adults and toilet-trained children can provide non-contaminated specimens by catching a midstream specimen of urine in a sterile container (the first few seconds of urine is not collected, as it can contain bacteria from the distal urethra). Giving the patient thorough instructions about cleansing the urethra and genitalia has been stressed, but controlled studies have not demonstrated any advantage to this practice (12).

Catheterization is the most frequently used method for obtaining urine specimens from infants and young children. This method has a high success rate of obtaining a noncontaminated specimen and is safe (13). Suprapubic aspiration of the bladder can also be used, but is more invasive, requires more physician time, and is no more successful. A urine sample obtained by placing a plastic collection bag over a child's genitalia often provides confusing data, because this technique results in many false-positive cultures. Contamination of the collected urine with bacteria from the skin is common. Collection of urine using diapers or absorbent pads has promise but has not been adequately studied (14).

TABLE 27.5 Characteristics of Urine Tests for Primary Care Patients with Dysuria (16,48,56)

Test	Sensitivity	Specificity	LR+	LR−
Dipstick				
LE	0.87	0.36	1.4	0.36
Nitrite	0.53	0.88	4.4	0.53
Either LE or nitrite	0.90	0.65	2.6	0.15
Sediment Microscopy				
1 bacterium/HPF	0.95	0.85	6.3	0.06
10 bacteria/HPF	0.85	0.99	85	0.15
5 WBC/HPF	0.91	0.48	1.7	0.19
10 WBC/HPF	0.82	0.65	2.3	0.28
5 RBC/HPF	0.44	0.88	3.7	0.60

HPF = high-power field; LE = leukocyte esterase; RBC = red blood count; WBC = white blood count.

URINALYSIS

The urinalysis includes a dry reagent test strip (the dipstick) and microscopy of a centrifuged urine sample. The dipstick, which detects blood, nitrite, and leukocyte esterase in the urine, is simple to perform and takes <5 minutes from sample collection to test result. The sensitivity, specificity, and likelihood ratios for these tests are summarized in Table 27.5.

The leukocyte esterase (LE) test detects the presence of an esterase from white blood cells and is positive in about three-quarters of all UTIs. False-positive results are not uncommon because of contamination by vaginal leukocytes or leukocytes from chlamydial urethritis, high urine pH, high levels of urine glucose, and certain drugs in the urine including tetracycline, cephalexin, gentamicin, imipenem, or clavulanic acid (15).

Nitrite is found in the urine when dietary nitrates are excreted into the urine and converted to nitrite by bacteria. In a primary care setting only about 50% of patients with UTI will have a positive nitrite test (16). There are three reasons why the sensitivity of this test for UTI is not very high. Gram-positive and *Pseudomonas* species will not be detected with this test because these bacteria do not convert urinary nitrates to nitrites. Those gram-negative bacteria, including *E. coli*, that convert nitrates to nitrites need several hours of contact with the urine to complete the conversion. Last, patients who excrete few nitrates into their urine, such as vegetarians, are especially likely to have a false negative result. Although a negative nitrite test is not very helpful at ruling out UTI (LR− 0.53), a positive nitrite test in a person with dysuria is fairly suggestive of UTI (LR+ 4.4) (16). Using the leukocyte esterase and nitrate in combination (the dipstick is considered positive if either test is positive and negative only if both tests are negative) is a better predictor of UTI than either test individually. When both are positive, UTI is likely in either adults or children.

Blood is detected by a dipstick using the peroxidase-like activity of hemoglobin in the urine. False-positive reactions can occur from the peroxidase-like activity of myoglobin or the presence of bacteria that produce peroxidase. Many patients with UTI do not have blood in the urine, but when present is useful for ruling in the diagnosis.

Direct microscopy of the urinary sediment is used to look for white cells (pyuria), red cells (hematuria), bacteria (bacteriuria), and white cell casts. The sediment is prepared by centrifuging a 10-mL tube of freshly voided urine, decanting the urine, and then resuspending the sediment with the residual urine adhering to the inside of the tube. The microscopy results are influenced by how long the urine is allowed to sit after collection, the duration and speed of centrifugation, the technique used to decant the urine and resuspend the sediment, and the technique of the individual performing the microscopy.

Although the number of leukocytes per high-power field (400× magnification) in the resuspended urine sediment is commonly used to diagnose UTI, there is disagreement about how many leukocytes identify the presence of infection. It is most appropriate to use the number of WBC/HPF in combination with the patient's probability of UTI before testing (17). For example, in a woman with typical symptoms of UTI and a high probability of UTI, 2 WBC/HPF can be considered positive. In men with dysuria, who have a lower risk of UTI, a more stringent cutpoint of 5 WBC/HPF is appropriate to define a positive test. This Bayesian approach will reduce the number of incorrect diagnoses. With children, because symptoms are less predictive of UTI, a cutoff of 10 WBC/HPF has been suggested (18).

The presence of bacteria at high power (400×) is also suggestive of UTI. If no bacteria are found in the sediment, a UTI is ruled out (LR− 0.06), and if 10 or more bacteria are seen per high-power field, the infection is ruled in (LR + 85). Intermediate bacterial counts are less helpful diagnostically. White cell casts can also be found in the urine sediment and are identified by their tubelike granular appearance. Their presence suggests inflammation within the kidney, with white blood cells collecting within the renal tubules. Infection is the primary cause of these casts, although interstitial nephritis can also produce them.

URINE CULTURE

The reference standard for the diagnosis of UTI is a "positive" urine culture meaning that a urine culture grows at least 100

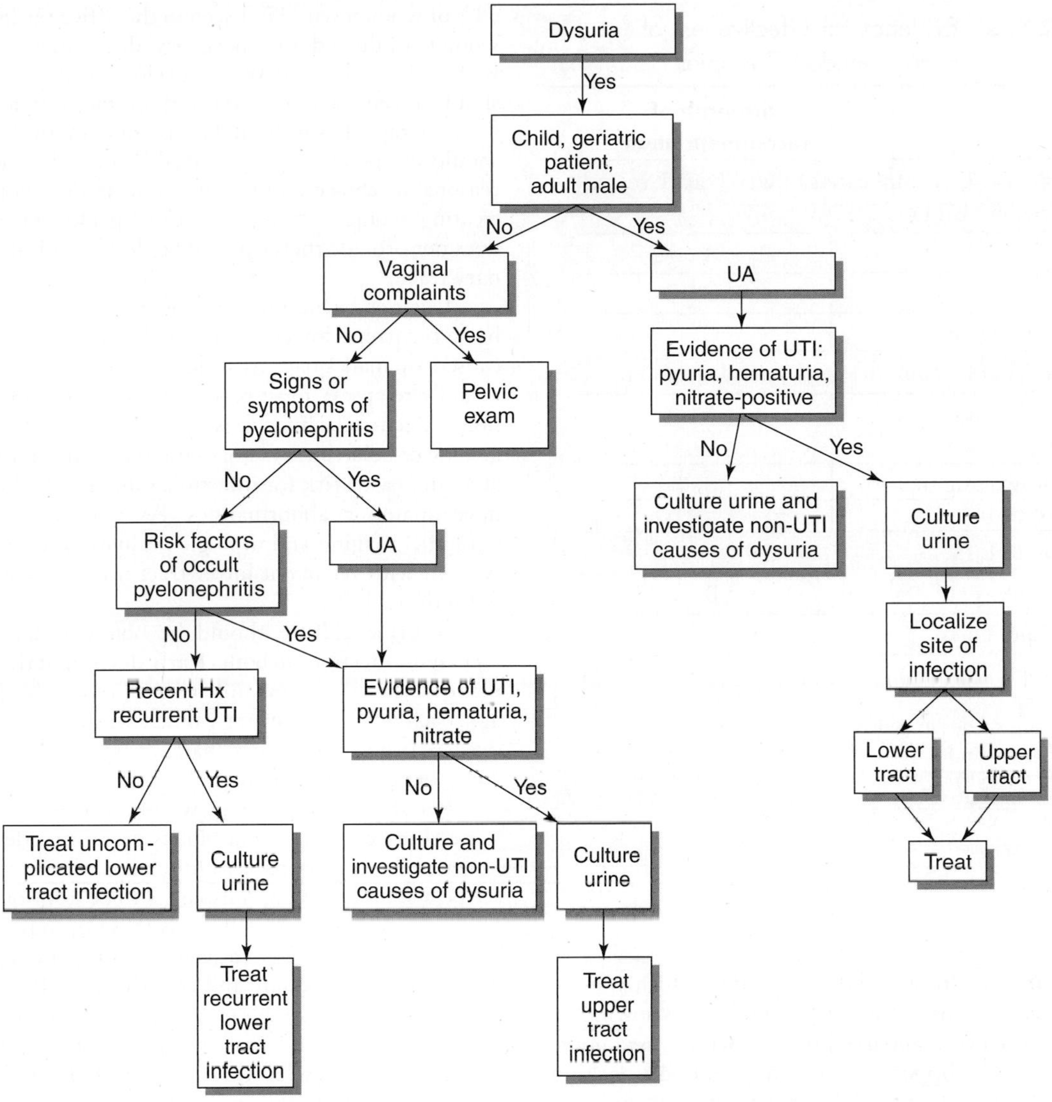

Figure 27.1 • Algorithm for the management of dysuria.

colony-forming units (cfu) of pathogenic bacteria per milliliter of urine (19,20). Urine cultures are not cost-effective in the routine care of UTI in healthy women because of time delay for results and lack of prediction of the clinical response to antibiotic treatment in this group of patients (21). Urine cultures are useful to confirm the infection and identify the organism and its antibiotic susceptibilities when evaluating dysuria in children, men, and older women, and in younger women who have either a significant probability of an upper tract infection or infection with bacteria not likely to respond to first-line antibiotics.

MANAGEMENT

In managing a patient with UTI, you should tailor the treatment plan to the characteristics of your patient and his or her infection. An algorithm for management appears in Figure 27.1.

Because UTI is very common in young, healthy women with dysuria, and because much of the required clinical data about women with dysuria can be collected over the telephone, some health providers and health care organizations manage suspected UTI in selected women without an office visit. This approach is supported by research (22) and by a retrospective study of more than 4,000 women managed through telephone contact, in which only 0.5% was subsequently diagnosed with an upper tract infection (23). A concern about telephone-based treatment of dysuria is that this results in needless use of antibiotics by 25% of women who receive symptom-directed treatment (24).

Acute Uncomplicated Lower Tract Infection in Otherwise Healthy Younger Women

Many uncomplicated lower tract UTIs in women are self-limited or respond to home remedies. Table 27.6 lists the strength of recommendations for different therapies. More than 40% of lower tract infections will clear within a week without

TABLE 27.6 Evidence for Effectiveness of Recommended Therapies

Intervention	Strength of Recommendation*
Management of Uncomplicated Lower Tract Urinary Tract Infection (UTI)	
Oral antibiotics	A
Cranberry juice	C
Increased fluid intake	C
Management of Uncomplicated Upper Tract UTI	
Oral antibiotics (in healthy women)	A
No need for imaging (in healthy women)	B
Prevention of UTI	
Cranberry juice	B
Increased fluid intake	C
Behavioral interventions	C

*A = consistent, good-quality patient-oriented evidence; B = inconsistent or limited-quality patient-oriented evidence; C = consensus, disease-oriented evidence, usual practice, expert opinion, or case series; UTI = urinary tract infection.
For information about the SORT evidence rating system, see *http://www.aafp.org/afpsort.xml.*

antibiotic treatment, although how to predict which women will clear their infections without treatment is unknown (25). Drinking unsweetened cranberry juice is a widely used home remedy but research support for this intervention is lacking (26). Because of these uncertainties, a short course of antibiotic therapy for UTI is the standard of care and is supported by the best evidence.

The antibiotic should be selected after considering the antibacterial spectrum, safety, and cost. Trimethoprim/sulfamethoxazole (TMP/SMX), TMX alone, nitrofurantoin, or a fluoroquinolone, such as ciprofloxacin, are frequently used for initial treatment of a lower tract UTI. Amoxicillin is not a good choice, since as many as 20% to 30% of the gram-negative organisms that cause UTI are resistant. Antibiotics for UTIs are summarized in Table 27.7. A urinary analgesic, phenazopyridine, is useful for patients with significant dysuria to quickly provide symptomatic relief.

Three days of antibiotic treatment is optimal for most acute uncomplicated cases of UTI. Three-day therapy results in a cure rate similar to that achieved with 7 to 10 days of treatment but with fewer antibiotic complications (27). An exception is that 7 days of treatment are needed when nitrofurantoin is used. Single-dose therapy has a lower cure rate and a higher recurrence rate. Generally, a follow-up visit is not required if the urinary symptoms resolve.

Women with occult pyelonephritis form an important subgroup of women with symptoms typical of uncomplicated lower tract infections. Occult pyelonephritis is present in up to 30% of women with UTI seen in the office setting, and 50% of women evaluated in emergency departments (28). Women with risk factors for occult pyelonephritis (see Table 27.2) should receive at least 7 days of antibiotic treatment. Single-dose therapy has a high failure rate in these patients and should not be used (29). TMP/SMX or a fluoroquinolone are reasonable choices. Nitrofurantoin should not be used for treating women at risk for occult pyelonephritis because it does not provide therapeutic drug levels within the upper urinary tract.

It is not uncommon for some young, healthy women to have recurrent lower UTIs. Although recurrences may be caused by inadequate treatment of a UTI (and are therefore actually relapses), most repeat infections represent new infections. Recurrent infections typically occur in women with genetic or behavioral factors, discussed earlier, that place them at an increased risk for infection. Only rarely do these women have anatomic abnormalities. As a result, extensive radiographic imaging and urologic evaluation have a low yield in women with recurrent lower tract infections and are usually not indicated.

A urine culture should be obtained for women with recurrent infections to both clearly document the infection and identify the organism and its antibiotic susceptibility. This approach will also prevent women with recurrent episodes of dysuria from causes other than UTIs from being inappropriately treated with antibiotics.

Recurrent infections in women can be treated with the same short courses of antibiotics recommended for isolated lower tract infections. Additionally, physicians often prescribe a short course of antibiotics to be kept on hand for use when a woman develops her typical symptoms. This "patient initiated treatment" is convenient for patients, and studies have shown it to be safe and effective (30). Prevention can be attempted by advising daily consumption of unsweetened cranberry juice and increasing fluid intake (see Table 27.6) (31,32). If a woman has three or more UTIs in a year that are related to sexual intercourse, she can be prescribed a single dose of antibiotics to be used routinely after intercourse. Commonly advised behavioral interventions (e.g., wiping front to back, not using pantyhose, postcoital voiding) have not been shown to prevent UTI.

Acute Pyelonephritis in Younger Women

Acute pyelonephritis is a systemic disease and requires different management than used for a lower tract infection. Women with pyelonephritis should be placed into one of three groups:

1. Women who are medically stable and maintaining hydration with oral intake.
2. Women who, because of severity of infection or underlying disability, are not medically stable or are unable to take oral fluids or medications.
3. Women who have infection complicated by abscess or obstruction, regardless of ability to take fluids by mouth.

Medically stable women who maintain hydration on oral fluids can be treated as outpatients; these women do as well as if they are treated with parenteral antibiotics (33,34). More than 90% of healthy women who develop pyelonephritis fall into this group. The choice of antibiotic, the duration of

TABLE 27.7 Initial Drug Therapy for Urinary Tract Infection

Drug	Dosage	Comments
Lower Tract Infections		
Amoxicillin/clavulanate (Augmentin)	Adult: 875 mg twice daily Child: 45 mg of amoxicillin component divided twice daily	Only if gram-positive organism suspected[1]
Cefixime (Suprax)	Adult: 400 mg daily Child: 8 mg/kg/d divided twice daily	
Cefpodoxime (Vantin)	Adult: 100 mg twice daily Child: 10 mg/kg/d divided twice daily	
Ciprofloxacin (Cipro)	Adult: 250 mg twice daily	Similarly priced as TMP/SMX
Nitrofurantoin (Macrodantin,	Adult: macrocrystals 50 or 100 mg	
Macrobid, Furadantin)	4 times daily, macrocrystals 100 mg twice daily Child: macrocrystals 5–7 mg/kg/day; divided 4 times daily	
Trimethoprim (Trimpex, Proloprim, others)	Adult: 300 mg daily	
Trimethoprim/sulfa-methoxazole (TMP/SMX) (Septra, Bactrim, others)	Adult: DS (160/800 mg) twice daily Child: 8 mg TMP/40 mg SMX/kg/day; divided twice daily	Not used if <2 months of age
Upper Tract Infections		
Amoxicillin/clavulanate (Augmentin)	Adult: 875 mg twice daily Child: 45 mg of amoxicillin component divided twice daily	Only if gram-positive organism suspected)*
Cefotaxime	Adult: 1–2 g IV every 8 hours until afebrile then oral cephalosporin Child: 100–200 mg/kg/day IV given 2 or 3 times daily until afebrile then oral cephalosporin	
Ceftriaxone	Adult: 1–2 g IV/day Child: 50–75 mg/kg/day, maximum of 2 g IV until afebrile then oral cephalosporin	
Cefixime (Suprax)	Adult: 400 mg daily Child: 8 mg/kg/d divided twice daily	
Cefpodoxime (Vantin)	Adult: 100 mg twice daily Child: 10 mg/kg/day divided twice daily	
Ciprofloxacin (Cipro)	Adult: 500 mg twice daily or 400 mg IV twice daily Child: 20–40 mg/kg/day to max of 1500 mg divided twice daily or 18–30 mg/kg/ day to maximum of 800 mg IV divided twice daily	Not first line and used only for resistant gram-negative infections
Levofloxacin (Levaquin)	Adult: 500 mg oral or IV daily	
Piperacillin/tazobactam	Adult: 3.375–4.5 g IV every 6 hours	
Trimethoprim/sulfa-methoxazole (TMP/SMX) (Septra, Bactrim, others)	Adult: DS (160/800 mg) twice daily Child: 8 mg TMP/40 mg SMX/kg/day divided twice daily	Not used if <2 months of age

[1]Hooton TM, Scholes D, Gupta K, et al. Amoxicillin-clavulanate vs ciprofloxacin for the treatment of uncomplicated cystitis in women: a randomized trial. *JAMA*. 2005;293(8):949–955.

Note: Length of treatment of outpatient:

Lower tract infection (oral antibiotics): female adult 3 days; male adult 7–10 days; healthy geriatric female 3 days; all other geriatric patients 7–14, child older than 2 months 7–14 days.

Upper tract infection outpatient (oral antibiotics): female adult 14 days, male adult 14 days; geriatric patient 14 days or child 14 days.

Upper tract infection hospitalized with initial IV antibiotics (switch to oral antibiotics when stable): female adult 14 days; male adult, geriatric patient, 21 days or child 7–14 days.

treatment, and the patient's ability to return for frequent follow-up are all important for successful outpatient management of pyelonephritis. Fourteen days of antibiotics are generally effective for outpatient treatment of otherwise healthy women with pyelonephritis (Table 27.7) (35). Parenteral ceftriaxone is widely used as a "loading" dose followed by oral antibiotics, but it has not been shown to offer an advantage over oral therapy alone. Regardless of the initial antibiotic selection, because pyelonephritis is a tissue infection, it is crucial to adjust antibiotic coverage with the aid of the urine culture and antibiotic sensitivity report.

Women with pyelonephritis need hospitalization if they have evidence of severe sepsis, are unable to take oral medication, or have an infection complicated by obstruction or renal abscess. For women with severe illness or urosepsis, the initial choice of parenteral antibiotic should be a fluoroquinolone, piperacillin/tazobactam, or a third-generation cephalosporin. Fifteen percent of these patients will have bacteremia, so blood cultures should be obtained prior to starting parenteral antibiotics (36). Intravenous antibiotics should be continued until the patient has been afebrile for 24 hours; the patient can then be switched to an oral agent to complete the 14 days of therapy. It is not necessary to observe patients as inpatients for 24 hours after switching to oral antibiotics (37).

When patients do not improve after 72 hours of parenteral therapy, imaging is indicated to identify a perinephric or intrarenal abscess, an unrecognized anatomic abnormality, or ureteral obstruction; either sonography or computed tomography can be used to identify these complications. Abscess or obstruction is an indication for urologic consultation. Complicated infections should be treated for at least 21 days.

To confirm cure after clinical resolution of pyelonephritis, a follow-up culture should be obtained 2 to 4 weeks after the end of antibiotic treatment. Imaging of the urinary tract after successful treatment is not recommended except in women with more than one episode of pyelonephritis, a slow response to parenteral antibiotics, abnormalities on their follow-up urinalysis, or a history of childhood UTI without previous imaging.

SPECIAL CONSIDERATIONS

Adult Men with UTIs

A more extensive evaluation is warranted in men with dysuria because they are more likely to have a complicated infection. As with women, men should be identified as having either an upper tract or a lower tract infection. Other causes of dysuria, including prostatitis (Chapter 30) and urethritis, need to be excluded as causes of urinary symptoms.

The initial choice of antibiotic for men with a suspected lower tract infection is typically a fluoroquinolone. Pretreatment culture is recommended, and antibiotic treatment should be continued for 7 to 10 days. Shorter duration treatment is not well studied in men. Men with pyelonephritis can be treated as outpatients with a fluoroquinolone or in hospital with parenteral antibiotics if their symptoms are severe. Those managed as outpatients should be treated for 14 days, whereas hospitalized patients should receive a total of 14 to 21 days of antibiotic therapy. After a second lower tract infection or a single episode of pyelonephritis, the adult male patient should undergo imaging to identify an anatomic abnormality or nephrolithiasis. Ultrasonography and plain abdominal radiograph appear to be comparable to intravenous pyelogram as the initial imaging study (38).

UTIs in Older Adults

In older patients, UTI can present without urinary symptoms but with mental status changes, tachypnea, tachycardia, fever, gait instability, or falls. These symptoms are not specific and can be caused by many other conditions, including other infections, hypoxia, an adverse reaction to medications, or metabolic abnormalities. Diagnosis of UTI in this age group is challenging because the symptoms are nonspecific and asymptomatic bacteriuria is common, affecting 10% of elderly men and 20% of elderly women (39).

Lower tract UTI in nonfrail elderly women should be treated for 3 days, although duration of 7 to 14 days has been traditionally recommended for older women (40). Urine culture should be obtained before treatment because the organism or its antibiotic sensitivity is not as predictable as in younger women. Pending culture results, these patients can be started on a fluoroquinolone or TMP/SMX. Older patients with upper tract infections should be treated using the same guidelines given for men in the preceding section.

Some elderly women get repeated UTIs. If these are from documented relapses occurring after short course therapy, subsequent infections should be treated for 14 days with an oral antibiotic, which is selected based on the culture and susceptibility testing. After frequent relapses, the patient should be evaluated for undiagnosed nephrolithiasis and for an abnormally large residual volume after voiding. If one of these predisposing problems is not found, a trial of topical estrogens can be tried to reduce UTI frequency. A nightly application of estrogen cream to the vaginal area for 2 weeks followed by biweekly application diminishes vaginal colonization by gram-negative uropathogens and typically reduces episodes of symptomatic UTI (41).

UTIs in Children

Approximately 5% to 8% of girls and 1% to 2% of boys have at least one symptomatic UTI during childhood (42). As with adults, children can be at increased risk for UTI because of perineal colonization by uropathogens or urine stasis in the bladder. Young children are prone to perineal colonization because of fecal incontinence. Several studies have also shown that non-circumcised male infants are at a higher risk for UTIs compared with their circumcised peers, perhaps because they are more likely to harbor *E. coli* on their genitalia (43). Older children can be prone to urine stasis because of infrequent voiding. Between 30% and 50% of young children with UTI will have vesicoureteral reflux, which places young children at high risk for recurrent upper tract infections and progressive renal scarring from lower tract infection (44).

CLINICAL EVALUATION

You should always elicit a thorough history and perform a physical examination in a child with suspected UTI to exclude other causes of the symptoms. In addition, children can have UTI without the dysuria or other urinary symptoms typically seen in adults. The presence of a UTI should always be considered in infants and young children in the first year of life with unexplained fever (45). Neonates with UTI might present only with late-onset jaundice, poor weight gain, irritability, or hypothermia. In infants, diarrhea, vomiting, or failure to thrive might be the only presenting complaint. In infants with fever, history of a previous UTI, temperature higher than 40°C and suprapubic tenderness are the findings most useful for identifying those with a UTI (46). In girls younger than age 2 years presenting to the emergency department with fever, approximately 5% will have a culture positive UTI as the cause (47).

As discussed earlier, classic urinary symptoms that typify UTI in adults are relatively uncommon in preschool children, with only 10% of UTIs generating these complaints. In school-age children, UTI can present with back pain, abdominal pain, or urinary incontinence instead of dysuria (46). Urethral irritation from bubble bath soap, vaginitis, pinworms, and trauma resulting from masturbation or sexual abuse are more common causes of dysuria in children than is UTI.

LABORATORY TESTS

No rapid test can detect UTI in all infants and young children. The dipstick and microscopic urinalysis has limited sensitivity. Nor are these tests specific for UTI because young children can develop pyuria after viral immunization or with non-urinary foci of infection. Therefore, urine culture is a routine part of the evaluation of these patients, regardless of the result of the urinalysis. In older children, the dipstick and microscopic urinalyses are more useful tests for assessing infection and have similar sensitivity and specificity to those reported in adults (48) (see Table 27.5).

MANAGEMENT

After 3 months of age, children with lower tract UTI are treated along the same general guidelines as UTIs in women. When symptoms are mild and the urinalysis suggests an infection, 3 days of oral antibiotics should be prescribed after a urine sample is obtained for culture (49). TMP/SMX, amoxicillin/clavulanate, nitrofurantoin, or third-generation cephalosporins are reasonable first choices for treating these infections. Fluoroquinolones are not routinely used in children because of concern of toxicity to growing cartilage. Although large studies have not confirmed this toxicity, fluoroquinolones are usually reserved for UTIs in children when the first-line antibiotics are not effective (50) (see Table 27.7). Acute pyelonephritis in this age group is routinely treated with parental antibiotics although there is growing evidence that oral antibiotics can be as effective (51).

All children younger than 3 months of age with UTI need hospitalization and parenteral antibiotics. For these children, parenteral ampicillin and gentamicin or a third-generation cephalosporin should be used as initial coverage, with therapy later adjusted based on the urine culture and sensitivity results. Single daily dosing of gentamicin is safe and effective.

A urine culture should be obtained after completion of therapy in children to confirm successful treatment. Renal function should also be evaluated by measuring the serum creatinine. Imaging studies to detect anatomic or functional abnormalities, such as vesicoureteral reflux, are indicated for children with UTI with any of the following: any UTI in a child <2 years of age, recurrent lower tract infections in children >2 years of age, or a single episode of pyelonephritis in children >2 years of age (44).

Catheter-associated UTI

Catheter-associated UTI is a common source of iatrogenic gram-negative bacteremia because catheters are frequently used in patients with diminished resistance to infection and provide an easy portal of entry for bacteria. Catheter-related infections can be prevented by removing the urinary catheter as soon as possible, or by not inserting one in the first place. The infection rate for people with urinary catheters is about 5% per day regardless of whether the catheter is used short-term or long-term. Prophylactic antibiotics may reduce the risk of catheter-related infections in patients who have only a short-term need for a catheter, such as postoperative patients (52,53), but prophylaxis is not routinely used because when infections do occur they involve resistant organisms (54).

Prophylaxis does not work with long-term catheter placement; almost all catheterized patients will develop bacteriuria within 30 days. Maintaining a closed drainage system and adhering to appropriate catheter care techniques will limit infection and complications in the short run. But as duration of catheterization is the principal determinant of infection with long-term indwelling catheters, it is not clear that any interventions can decrease the prevalence of bacteriuria in this setting. Intermittent catheterization will markedly reduce the risk of UTI and is preferable to a chronic, indwelling catheter. However, many people using intermittent catheterization will develop UTI, and most will develop asymptomatic bacteriuria (55).

Many catheter-associated infections occur in long-term care facilities because 5% to 10% of residents in these institutions have long-term indwelling catheters. Nearly all of these patients are bacteriuric and will have colonization with multiple organisms. Catheter flushing or daily perineal care does not prevent infection. Patient's urine should be cultured and they should be treated only if symptoms develop. Antibiotic therapy of culture positive but otherwise asymptomatic patients will only enhance the emergence of resistant pathogens that cause urinary infections. Evaluation is a challenge because symptoms may only consist of low-grade fever, decreased appetite, weight loss, increased confusion, or problems with falling.

When the infection is mild, treatment with an oral fluoroquinolone is usually successful and hospitalization is not necessary. The catheter should be replaced if it has been in place for more than 2 weeks. Bacteria adhere to the surface of the urinary catheters and create a biofilm, which prevents antibiotics from reaching the embedded bacteria. Although there are no studies that define the optimal duration of therapy, 7 days of therapy are often used with patients who clinically respond within 72 hours to treatment. Parenteral antibiotics are indicated for moderately severe infections. In all cases of catheter-associated UTI, it is important to remember that most patients with catheters are elderly or medically compromised, and are usually less able to tolerate an infection than young adults.

KEY POINTS

- The extent of clinical evaluation of dysuria depends largely on the clinical setting; symptoms in an otherwise healthy adult woman without vaginal complaints are likely from a UTI requiring minimal workup, whereas vaginal atrophy should be considered in older women and prostatitis in men.
- A urine culture should be obtained when infection of the upper urinary tract (pyelonephritis) is suspected because of the presence of fever, chills, abdominal pain, flank pain, vomiting, and a urine sample suggestive of infection.
- A short course of antibiotic therapy for UTI is the standard of care and is supported by the best evidence; trimethoprim/sulfamethoxazole trimethoprim alone, nitrofurantoin, or a fluoroquinolone are commonly used. A urinary analgesic is useful for patients with significant dysuria to quickly provide symptomatic relief.
- Medically stable women with pyelonephritis who maintain hydration on oral fluids can be treated as outpatients with oral antibiotics (adjusted based on culture results) for 14 days; women requiring hospitalization are usually treated with parenteral antibiotics (fluoroquinolone, piperacillin/tazobactam, or a third-generation cephalosporin) until afebrile for 24 hours then be switched to an oral agent to complete the 14 days of therapy.
- After a second lower tract infection or a single episode of pyelonephritis, the adult male patient should undergo imaging to identify an anatomic abnormality or nephrolithiasis usually with ultrasonography and plain abdominal radiograph.
- Imaging studies to detect anatomic or functional abnormalities, such as vesicoureteral reflux, are indicated for children with UTI with any of the following: any UTI in a child <2 years of age, recurrent lower tract infections in children >2 years of age, or a single episode of pyelonephritis in children >2 years of age.

CHAPTER

28

Menstrual Syndromes

Elizabeth A. Burns, Louise Parent-Stevens and
4th Edition Author: Barbara Supanich, RSM, MD

CLINICAL OBJECTIVES

1. Describe an appropriate clinical, laboratory, and radiologic evaluation for a woman with dysmenorrhea.
2. Cite the best course of treatment for a woman with dysmenorrhea.
3. Summarize the steps in evaluation (clinical, laboratory or radiologic) of a woman with premenstrual syndrome.
4. Discuss the therapeutic options for a patient with premenstrual syndrome.
5. Describe the appropriate evaluation for a perimenopausal woman with menstrual irregularity.
6. Summarize an approach to management of a patient with menorrhagia.

Menstrual complaints are common and concerning to women. In a study of women referred to hospital-based gynecology clinics for menstrual issues, the top three complaints were pain with menstruation (33%), perimenstrual mood changes (32.8%), and increasing menstrual flow (29.1%) (1); other concerns included prolonged menstruation (25.3%) and experiencing premenstrual pain (17.5%).

Menstrual problems present throughout the reproductive years and should be evaluated with care keeping in mind that women, especially adolescents, may present with this concern when other issues (e.g., undesired pregnancy, sexually transmitted infection [STI], or sexual assault) are the real reason for the visit (2). A careful history, respecting the privacy of the patient and addressing issues of confidentiality, will enable a patient to provide accurate answers and voice her concerns fully.

Three of the most common problems related to menstruation will be covered in this chapter. Dysmenorrhea affects up to 60% of menstruating women and can be mild or extremely debilitating (3). While premenstrual symptoms affect most women, premenstrual syndrome (PMS) is diagnosed in approximately 30% of women; premenstrual dysphoric disorder (PMDD) is the most severe form and uncommon (4). Abnormal uterine bleeding is a presenting complaint in 20% of primary care gynecology visits and accounts for approximately 25% of gynecologic procedures (5).

DYSMENORRHEA

Dysmenorrhea, defined as painful menstrual periods, can be classified into primary or secondary. Primary dysmenorrhea, the more common presentation, is menstrual pain in a patient with normal pelvic anatomy and no underlying pathology. It has a usual onset between menarche and 20 years of age. Pain typically begins 24 to 36 hours before the onset of menses and can continue for the first 3 days of menstruation. The pain is cyclical and often described as crampy. Associated symptoms may include headache, nausea, inner thigh pain, and lower back pain. Secondary dysmenorrhea is associated with underlying pelvic pathology and often has its onset after age 20 years. The pain of secondary dysmenorrhea is usually progressive with age and not always synchronous with menses.

Pathophysiology

The pathophysiology of primary dysmenorrhea is linked to increased prostaglandin (PG) activity in the uterus, which causes uterine contractions and ischemia (6). The prostaglandin, PGF2α, is produced by the endometrium during ovulatory cycles and mediates pain sensations and stimulates smooth muscle contractions. Studies have also shown that women with primary dysmenorrhea secrete an increased amount of vasopressin and leukotrienes, which may potentiate uterine contractions and pain (6,7).

The pathophysiology of secondary dysmenorrhea varies with the underlying cause. The differential diagnosis for secondary dysmenorrhea is shown in Table 28.1. The most likely etiology in an individual patient depends on her age, history, and physical examination findings.

Clinical Evaluation

The evaluation of a woman with dysmenorrhea should focus on her age, sexual history, clinical presentation, and physical examination. Some patients, especially adolescents, may be reluctant to discuss their sexuality with a health care provider. It is important that all patients be questioned in a comfortable and private setting. If legally and ethically possible (e.g., patient is not engaging in dangerous or life-threatening behavior), patient confidentiality should be maintained.

HISTORY

The initial evaluation of dysmenorrhea should include a complete menstrual history from menarche, including the type of

TABLE 28.1 Differential Diagnosis of Menstrual Problems

Category	Diagnosis	Frequency in Primary Care
Primary Dysmenorrhea		Very common
Secondary Dysmenorrhea	Cervical stenosis, cervical polyps, ovarian cysts, pelvic inflammatory disease, endometriosis, leiomyomas/fibroids	Common
	Intrauterine device complications, endometrial cancer	Uncommon
	Imperforate hymen, uterine synechiae, Tubo-ovarian abscess	Rare
Premenstrual syndrome		Common
	Major depressive and anxiety disorders, chronic medical conditions (e.g., diabetes, thyroid disease, autoimmune disorders), oral contraceptive use	Common
	Substance abuse, eating disorders	Uncommon
	Personality disorders	Rare
Abnormal uterine bleeding		Common
	Anovulatory bleeding, hormonal medication use, intrauterine pregnancy, spontaneous abortion	Common
	Thyroid disease	Fairly common
	Ectopic pregnancy, infections, coagulopathies, blood dyscrasias, medication (nonhormonal) use, cervical, uterine cancer	Uncommon
	Molar pregnancy, trauma, foreign body, systemic disease (adrenal, hepatic, renal), vaginal or vulvar cancer	Rare

symptoms experienced, the age of onset, the timing of symptoms in relationship to her menstrual cycle, and the severity and duration of symptoms. A sexual history should be obtained from all women. In a woman with mild to moderate cramps that began before age 20 years, which occur up to 48 hours before the onset of menses in the presence of a normal pelvic and abdominal exam, the most likely diagnosis is primary dysmenorrhea. New onset of pain after age 20 years or pelvic pain at times other than the menstrual cycle requires further evaluation for a secondary cause of dysmenorrhea. Key elements in the history for causes of dysmenorrhea are shown in Table 28.2.

Endometriosis, a common cause of secondary dysmenorrhea, should be considered if the patient has pain at the time of ovulation or risk factors for endometriosis, including early menarche, heavy menses, nulliparity or a family history of endometriosis (8). The presence of back pain and diarrhea is suggestive of endometrial implants on the bowel.

Any sexually active woman who presents with pelvic pain, with or without vaginal discharge, should be evaluated for pelvic inflammatory disease (PID). Pelvic pain accompanied by fever, chills or symptoms of systemic illness may be indicative of PID or tubo-ovarian abscess.

Cervical stenosis, leiomyomas, and endometrial cancer should be considered in women who are perimenopausal, menopausal or postmenopausal. In a postmenopausal woman with vaginal bleeding, with or without accompanying pain, endometrial cancer must be ruled out (Tables 28.2 and 28.3).

PHYSICAL EXAMINATION

The physical examination for the assessment of dysmenorrhea generally includes an abdominal and pelvic exam. However, in a young woman who has never been sexually active, the pelvic exam can be omitted if her presentation is consistent with a diagnosis of primary dysmenorrhea (7). You should perform an abdominal examination to evaluate the uterus and ovaries for enlargement or masses. The pelvic examination is also used to evaluate the uterus and adnexal areas for masses or areas of tenderness. Findings of pelvic tenderness, cervical motion tenderness, uterosacral nodularity, enlarged ovaries, or a fixed uterus are suggestive of endometriosis (9). Exquisite pain on palpation of the adnexal area or an area of adnexal fullness is consistent with tubo-ovarian abscess, especially if accompanied by fever. Unfortunately, physical examination is neither specific nor sensitive for diagnosing endometriosis.

DIAGNOSTIC TESTING

As the diagnosis of primary dysmenorrhea is based chiefly on history and presentation, confirmatory tests are not necessary. In the evaluation of secondary dysmenorrhea, tests should be guided by the clinical evaluation. Cultures for sexually transmitted infections (STIs), including gonorrhea and chlamydia, should be obtained in women with a history of vaginal or cervical discharge, multiple sex partners, unprotected intercourse, or recent onset of symptoms (<14 days).

TABLE 28.2 Key Elements in the History and Physical Examination for Dysmenorrhea and Abnormal Uterine Bleeding

Question/Maneuver	Diagnosis
Dysmenorrhea	
Information about age, duration and description of symptoms, prior history of dysmenorrhea, prior treatments and response to treatments, previous prescribed and OTC medications for dysmenorrhea, other key medical conditions, general health	Assist in creating and narrowing the differential diagnosis
Look for red flags (see Table 28.3)	Screen for PID, endometrial cancer, ectopic pregnancy, and tubo-ovarian abscess
Dysmenorrhea that is more intense at the time of ovulation or persists as menstrual flow diminishes	Endometriosis
History of multiple colposcopies and surgical (including cryosurgical) treatments of the cervix	Evaluate for cervical stenosis
No history of menses in presence of severe pelvic pain	Evaluate for imperforate hymen
Obtain sexual history, history of STIs	PID, dyspareunia
History of gynecologic surgery	Pelvic adhesions, cervical stenosis
Psychosocial history	Assist in understanding the patient's perception(s) of pain, coping skills, and formulation of a treatment plan
Temperature	Infectious causes
Focused abdominal and pelvic examinations:	
Palpable/enlarged uterus	Leiomyomas, pregnancy, malignancy
Cervical stenosis on speculum examination	Cervical stenosis
Thick purulent cervical discharge	Cervicitis, PID
Tender and enlarged adnexal area	PID
Bleeding from cervical os in postmenopausal woman	Malignancy
Abnormal Uterine Bleeding	
Determine if woman is ovulatory	Determines which diagnostic pathway to follow (Fig. 28.2)
Information about age, ob/gyn history, menstrual history, description of symptoms, rating of pain, response to prior treatments, and general health	Assist in creating and narrowing the differential diagnosis
Look for red flags (see Table 28.3)	Screen for uterine cancer, ectopic pregnancy, threatened or missed abortion
Medications	Warfarin sodium or aspirin
Focused abdominal and pelvic examination: speculum and bimanual examination, observe for petechiae, palpate thyroid	If abnormalities are elicited, focuses examiner on particular differential diagnosis

ob/gyn = obstetric and/or gynecologic; OTC = over the counter; PID = pelvic inflammatory disease; STIs = sexually transmitted infections.

If warranted, HIV testing should also be offered to the patient (see Chapter 32).

Patients with pain at time of ovulation should have a transvaginal ultrasound (TVU) which is useful in diagnosing as well as excluding ovarian cysts or tubo-ovarian abscess (10). Magnetic resonance imaging (MRI) has a low sensitivity (69%) and specificity (75%) for the diagnosis of endometriosis, best diagnosed by history, ultrasound (endometriomas) and laparoscopy (11).

RECOMMENDED DIAGNOSTIC STRATEGY

A general approach to the patient with menstrual-related pain is outlined in Figure 28.1. The initial goal is to distinguish between primary and secondary dysmenorrhea, as this will guide the management strategy in an individual patient.

Management

When treating a patient with dysmenorrhea, it is important to remember that the perception and experience of pain is highly individual and may not correlate with clinical findings. The goals of dysmenorrhea management are to identify the cause of the patient's pain, relieve her symptoms, and restore functioning to the greatest extent possible. The strength of recommendation (SOR) rating for different management strategies is listed in Table 28.4.

(text continues on page 342)

TABLE 28.3 Red Flags Suggesting Progressive or Life-threatening Disease in Patients with Pelvic Pain or Abnormal Uterine Bleeding

Diagnosis	Red Flags Suggestive of the Disease
Uterine cancer	Any vaginal bleeding in a postmenopausal woman or intermenstrual bleeding in a perimenopausal woman, >5 mm of thickness of endometrium on transvaginal ultrasound, palpable pelvic mass, or endometrial cells on Pap smear
Ectopic pregnancy	Missed period, or abnormal previous period, with unilateral pelvic pain; may have vaginal bleeding; may have adnexal fullness palpated on pelvic examination
Missed or threatened abortion	Missed or abnormal previous period, with severe pelvic cramping/pain and vaginal bleeding
Pelvic inflammatory disease	Fever, purulent vaginal discharge, abdominal or pelvic pain, exquisitely tender on palpation of pelvic organs, malaise, septic appearance
Tubo-ovarian abscess	Fever, malaise, septic appearance, palpable fullness in the adnexa, or exquisite tenderness on pelvic examination

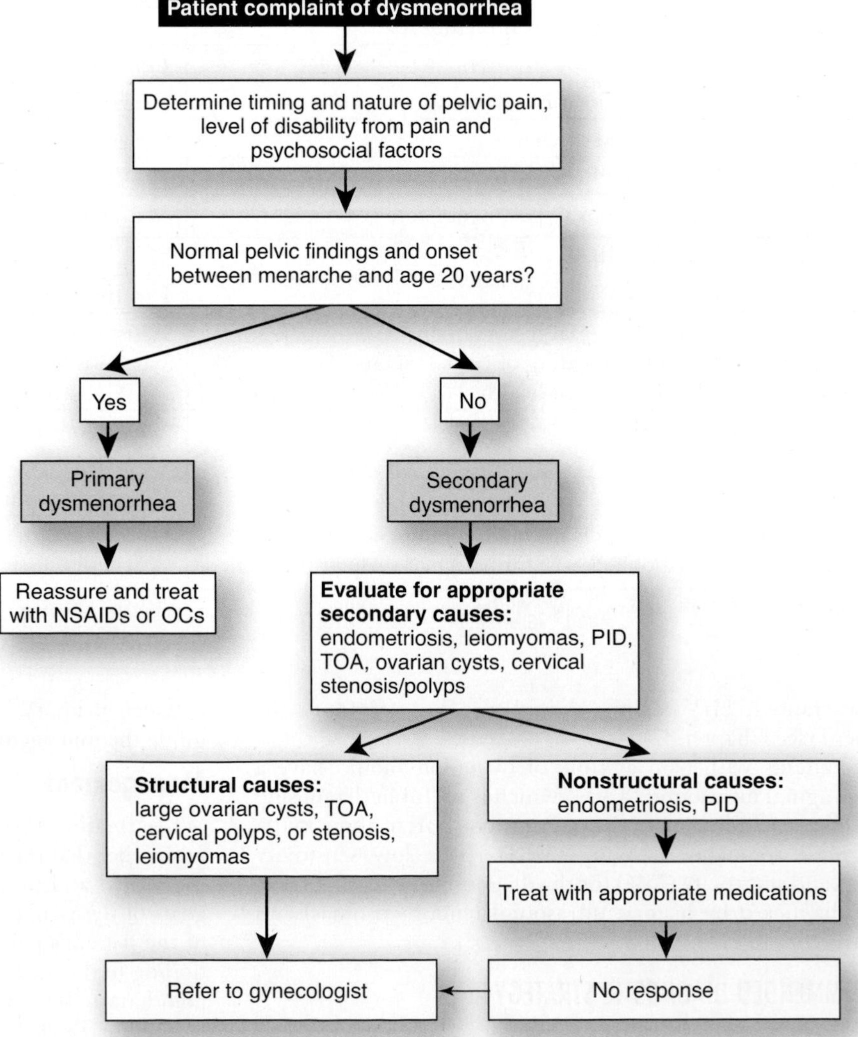

Figure 28.1 • General approach to the patient with dysmenorrhea. NSAIDs = nonsteroidal anti-inflammatory drugs; OCs = oral contraceptives; PID = pelvic inflammatory disease; TOA = tubo-ovarian abscess.

TABLE 28.4 Management of Dysmenorrhea, Premenstrual Syndrome, and Abnormal Uterine Bleeding

Target Disorder	Intervention	Strength of Recommendation*	Comments
Dysmenorrhea	NSAIDs	A	See Table 28.5 for specific agents and dosing
	OCs	A	
	Medroxyprogesterone acetate	B	
	Levonorgestrel-releasing IUD	B	
Endometriosis	NSAIDs	B	First line for mild-moderate disease
	OCs	A	Continuous (noncyclic) use may be beneficial
	Medroxyprogesterone acetate	A	
	Danazol	A	Antiestrogenic/androgenic effects
	GnRH agonists	A	Antiestrogenic effects area concern—combination with low-dose estrogen/progestin may limit side effects
	Levonorgestrel-releasing IUD	B	May limit recurrence of symptoms after surgery
PMS	SSRIs	A	See Table 28.6 for specific agents and dosing
	Calcium supplementation	A	1,200 mg/day of elemental calcium
	Drospirenone-containing OC	A	
	Other serotonergic antidepressants	B	Not as well studied as SSRIs. See Table 28.6 for specific agents and dosing
	Buspirone	B	Primary effect is to reduce anxiety. See Table 28.6 for dosing
	Alprazolam	B	Primary effect is to reduce anxiety. See Table 28.6 for dosing
	Spironolactone (26)	B	Intermittent dosing during luteal phase. Primary effect is to limit bloating and fluid retention
	Pyridoxine (vitamin B6) (28)	B	Usually 50 mg daily. Primary effect is on depression and generalized symptoms
	Magnesium (29)	B	Generally felt to be safe in the absence of renal or cardiovascular disease
	NSAIDs	B	Mefenamic acid and naproxen best studied. Primary effect is for relief of pain and headache
	Chasteberry (*Vitex agnus castus*) (36–38)	B	Herbal remedy
	Vitamin E	C	Generally felt to be nontoxic
	Lifestyle modifications	C	Low risks and non-PMS benefits

(*continued*)

TABLE 28.4 (*Continued*)

Target Disorder	Intervention	Strength of Recommendation*	Comments
Abnormal uterine bleeding	NSAIDs	B	As effective as other alternatives; taken during menstrual flow
	OCs, cyclic progesterone, HT (56)	B	Effective for AUB; need to caution about side effects and proper administration; may take several cycles to be effective
	Levonorgestrel intrauterine device (57)	A	Effective in decreasing AUB
	Endometrial ablation (58)	A	Effective in decreasing AUB; not for women who wish to maintain fertility; many methods now available, but no evidence to recommend one over another

AUB = abnormal uterine bleeding; GnRH = gonadotropin releasing hormone; HT = hormone therapy; NSAIDs = nonsteroidal anti-inflammatory drugs; OCs = oral contraceptive pills; PMS = premenstrual syndrome; SSRIs = selective serotonin reuptake inhibitors.
*A = consistent, good-quality patient-oriented evidence; B = inconsistent or limited-quality patient-oriented evidence; C = consensus, disease-oriented evidence, usual practice, expert opinion, or case series.
For information about the SORT evidence rating system, see *http://www.aafp.org/afpsort.xml.*

PRIMARY DYSMENORRHEA

Nonsteroidal anti-inflammatory drugs (NSAIDs), the most common initial treatment for primary dysmenorrhea, are effective in 80% to 85% of cases (6,12) (see Table 28.5 for a listing of agents commonly used). The NSAID should be initiated with the onset of pain or menses and continued on a scheduled regimen for the first 2 to 3 days of menstrual flow. Because there is similar efficacy but wide patient variability in response and side effects between NSAIDs (12), if one NSAID is ineffective at adequate doses, the patient can try an NSAID from a different class.

Oral contraceptives (OC); which are effective in 50% to 80% of cases, are an alternate therapy for patients who also need contraception. There is inadequate evidence to recommend one OC over another for treating dysmenorrhea (13,14). Use of an NSAID with an OC provides additional pain relief (15). The levonorgestrel-IUD and depot medroxyprogesterone have also been shown to reduce symptoms of dysmenorrhea (6,16) (see Chapter 26). For women who prefer nonpharmacologic management, use of a low-level heat patch is helpful (17,18).

After treatment of primary dysmenorrhea has been initiated, its efficacy should be assessed after several months and annually. After successful treatment has been achieved, the patient should be reevaluated if her symptoms recur.

SECONDARY DYSMENORRHEA

The choice of treatment for secondary dysmenorrhea will be dictated by the underlying etiology. Management approaches for several causes are outlined below.

Endometriosis

The management of endometriosis is dependent on the treatment goals. For control of pain, the patient can be treated with OCs and NSAIDs. OC cycles, given consecutively without a placebo week, can be tried if standard dosing of OCs provides inadequate relief (19). Alternative treatments include LNG-IUD and depot medroxyprogesterone (8). If these interventions are unsuccessful, the patient should be referred to a gynecologist for possible surgical ablation or treatment with other forms of medical management, such as danazol, and GnRH agonists. If restoration of fertility is the desired outcome, the patient should be referred to a gynecologist as surgical interventions may produce better outcomes (20).

Pelvic Inflammatory Disease

Most patients with PID can be treated as outpatients (see Chapter 32). If the patient appears septic, is pregnant, is unlikely to follow-up appropriately, or has failed to respond to appropriate oral antibiotics, she should be admitted for intravenous antibiotic treatment.

Ovarian Cysts and Cervical Polyps

If ovarian cysts are unilocular, <6 cm in diameter on ultrasound, and the CA-125 level is normal, the patient can be managed expectantly or NSAIDs can be initiated. Although OCs have commonly been used for the management of ovarian cysts, evidence does not support this approach (21). If the cysts are ≥6 cm, multilocular, bilateral, solid, or mixed cystic/solid or if the CA-125 is elevated, you should refer the patient to a gynecologist for further evaluation (10).

If cervical polyps are the cause of pelvic pain, referral to a gynecologist should be provided if the family physician is not trained in cervical curettage or hysteroscopy.

Tuboovarian Abscess

Tuboovarian abscess is a medical emergency and the patient should immediately be stabilized and referred to a gynecologist.

TABLE 28.5 NSAIDs for the Treatment of Dysmenorrhea

Drug	Contraindications (CI)/ Cautions/Adverse Effects (AE)	Dosage	Relative Cost†
Dysmenorrhea			
Traditional NSAIDs	CI: Aspirin-induced bronchospasm AE: dizziness, drowsiness, headache, gastric irritation/ ulceration, exacerbation of HTN, renal disease		
Diclofenac		50 mg 3 times/day or 100 mg stat then 50 mg 3 times/day, max 150 mg/day	$
Ibuprofen*		200–800 mg every 4–6h, max 3,200 mg/day	$
Ketoprofen		12.5–50 mg every 6–8h, max 300 mg/day	$
Meclofenamate		100 mg 3 times daily (not to exceed 6 days), max 400 mg/day	$
Mefenamic acid		500 mg stat, then 250 mg every 4h (not to exceed 1 week)	$$$$
Naproxen		500 mg stat, then 250 mg every 6–8h, max 1,250 mg/day	$
Naproxen sodium‡		440–550 mg stat, then 220–275 mg every 6–12h	$
COX-2 selective NSAIDs	CI: sulfa allergy AE: May increase risk of CVD in persons with or at risk for CVD		
Celecoxib¶		400 mg stat, then 200 mg 2 times/day	$$$$
Mild-Moderate Pain§			
Etodolac	Same as for traditional NSAIDs	200–400 mg every 6–8h, max 1,000 mg/day 64 (180)	$
Fenoprofen		200 mg every 6–8h, max 3,200 mg/day	$$

COX = cyclooxygenase; d = daily; NSAIDs = nonsteroidal anti-inflammatory drugs.
*Available in OTC strength.
†Relative cost for 5-day course: $, <$10; $$, $10–$20, $$$: $20–$30; $$$$, >$40.
¶Do not use as first-line treatment—may be used as alternates if first-line NSAIDs are ineffective or not tolerated.

PREMENSTRUAL SYNDROME

PMS is the term for a constellation of physical, emotional, and behavioral symptoms that occur during the luteal phase of the menstrual cycle. PMDD, defined as a severe form of PMS, significantly affects a patient's ability to function. (For the purposes of this chapter, the term PMS will be inclusive of both PMS and PMDD unless otherwise specified.)

The presentation of PMS varies significantly between women and can also vary from cycle to cycle in an individual woman. The most common and distressing symptoms are emotional lability, anger, irritability, anxiety, depression and "feeling out of control." Other common symptoms include fluid retention, edema, breast tenderness, headaches, and dietary cravings (22). By definition, symptoms begin during the luteal phase and must abate with the onset of menses. The patient must be symptom free during the follicular phase and the symptoms cannot be attributable to other physical or psychological causes.

The etiology of PMS is unclear and numerous theories have been postulated and then discarded. Currently, research suggests that in susceptible women, the normal hormonal fluctuations of the menstrual cycle trigger an altered sensitivity to serotonin and possibly other neurotransmitters, including γ-amino butyric acid and allopregnanolone (22,23).

Surveys show that approximately 85% of menstruating women experience at least one symptom associated with PMS, whereas PMDD is reported to occur in 5% to 20% of menstruating women (4,22).

Differential Diagnosis

Many medical and psychiatric conditions may be exacerbated by the hormonal fluctuations of the menstrual cycle, causing symptoms that mimic PMS. Table 28.1 lists some of these conditions.

Clinical Evaluation

PMS is a diagnosis of exclusion; therefore a thorough history and focused physical examination are vital to making an appropriate diagnosis.

HISTORY

Initially, the interview should focus on the patient's symptoms, including age at onset, onset and severity in relation to her menstrual cycle, and when, if ever, the symptoms abate. The patient should be asked to what degree her symptoms cause distress or impair her functioning. If the patient does not experience a symptom-free interval during the follicular phase, menstrual exacerbation of a chronic condition should be considered rather than a diagnosis of PMS.

A thorough medical history should be taken to look for medical conditions that may mimic PMS symptoms. A patient with rheumatoid arthritis who reports increased fatigue and joint pains during the luteal phase is experiencing an exacerbation of her underlying disease rather than true PMS. Patients should be questioned about any personal or family history of depressive/anxiety disorders as these may predispose to PMS. However, mood disorders may be aggravated premenstrually so a clear history of absence of symptoms during the follicular phase should be elicited before making a diagnosis of PMS. A history of similar symptoms during pregnancy, the postpartum period, or while on hormonal contraception is suggestive of PMS (4).

PHYSICAL EXAMINATION

In an otherwise healthy woman, there are no physical abnormalities associated with PMS. If a patient has no specific physical complaints related to her symptoms, the physical exam may be brief; however, the patient should be up to date on her gynecologic exam. Presence of symptoms that may indicate a medical condition, such as joint pains, should be assessed.

DIAGNOSTIC TESTING

There are no laboratory tests or imaging studies that confirm the diagnosis of PMS. If the patient has symptoms of or risk for a medical condition, such as thyroid disease or an autoimmune disease, that may be exacerbated premenstrually, appropriate diagnostic testing should be done prior to a diagnosis of PMS. In women over age 40 years, a follicle-stimulating hormone (FSH) level should be measured to assess if perimenopause is a factor in the patient's symptoms (4).

RECOMMENDED DIAGNOSTIC STRATEGY

Several organizations, including the American Congress of Obstetricians (ACOG) and the American Psychiatric Association (APA) have published diagnostic criteria for PMS and PMDD, however, there is no consensus on this issue (4). Both sets of criteria require that symptoms occur during the luteal phase, remit during the follicular phase, and cause some degree of dysfunction. The ACOG criteria for PMS are broad, requiring a sole symptom, whereas the APA's criteria for PMDD, published in the DSM-IV and commonly utilized for research purposes, are more strict, requiring a minimum of five symptoms, one of which must be dysphoric in nature (4,24) (see *http://www.medscape.com/viewarticle/551199_2* for the AGOG criteria and *http://www.web4health.info/en/answers/bipolar-depr-pmdd-cri.htm* for the APA criteria).

For an accurate diagnosis of PMS, the patient should ideally log her daily symptoms for a minimum of two menstrual cycles. Although the patient can record her symptoms on a calendar or in a notebook, use of a standardized daily symptoms calendar can facilitate the process. Examples of such tools include as the Daily Symptom Report, the Daily Record of Severity of Problems, the Calendar of Premenstrual Experience, or the Prospective Record of the Impact and Severity of Menstruation (25). (See *http://women.webmd.com/pms/premenstrual-syndrome-pms-home-treatment* for an example of a menstrual diary.) A record that shows a pattern of moderate to severe symptoms during the luteal phase that are absent or significantly minimized during the follicular phase is consistent with a diagnosis of PMS. In reality, it may be difficult for patients to provide such a log. Less cumbersome diagnostic strategies may include use of abbreviated monitoring forms or having the patient schedule an evaluation during the late luteal phase at which time she is most likely to be experiencing her symptoms (4).

Given the lack of diagnostic agreement and the difficulty in obtaining good prospective data, failure of an individual to meet the strict criteria for PMDD, as outlined in DSM-IV, should not preclude a clinical diagnosis of PMDD and initiation of appropriate therapy.

Management

Women who seek medical attention because their premenstrual symptoms interfere with normal work, personal activities, or relationships should be offered therapeutic intervention. The focus of therapy should be guided by the patient's specific symptoms, with emphasis on the symptom(s) that cause the patient the most distress. The patient should understand that no single therapy is effective for all symptoms and that identifying the best treatment may require the trial of several agents for several months each. Many treatment modalities have been suggested for PMS; however, there are few well-controlled clinical trials. The treatment recommendations for PMS and the strength of recommendation supporting their use are listed in Table 28.4.

NONPHARMACOLOGIC MANAGEMENT

Education and supportive measures are important in the management of PMS and have been reported to improve symptoms and a patient's sense of control. Lifestyle modifications, including relaxation techniques, regular aerobic exercise, sodium and caffeine restriction and increased intake of complex carbohydrates, are widely recommended although lacking in supportive evidence; the limited risks and other benefits of these interventions warrant their use (26). In patients with mild symptoms, a 2-month trial of lifestyle modification is reasonable. For women with moderate to severe symptoms, addition of a pharmacologic agent to lifestyle modification is appropriate.

PHARMACOLOGIC THERAPY

Dietary Supplements

Calcium supplementation (1 to 1.2 g/day) has been shown in several studies to improve the physical and mood symptoms of PMS (26,27) (SOR=A). Pyridoxine (vitamin B6) has been widely studied in PMS. A systematic review of these studies suggests that pyridoxine may provide some benefit for irritability, breast tenderness, fatigue and bloating (28) (SOR=B). Because of the risk of neurotoxicity with chronic use of higher doses, pyridoxine dose should be limited to 50 mg/day. Magnesium, 200 to 360 mg/day may provide improvement in symptoms (SOR=B) but there are inadequate data to support a recommendation for the use of vitamin E (29,30) (SOR=C).

Psychotherapeutic Agents

There is good clinical evidence that selective serotonin reuptake inhibitors (SSRIs) are effective for improving mood symptoms related to PMS (SOR=A). Fluoxetine, sertraline, and

TABLE 28.6 Psychotropic Drugs for the Management of PMS

Drug	Contraindications (CI)/ Cautions (C)/Adverse Effects (AE)	Dosage*	Relative Cost†
SSRIs	CI: MAOI use AE: anxiety, insomnia, decreased libido		
Citalopram (Celexa)		20 mg daily or 10–30 mg intermittently	$$
Fluoxetine (Prozac, Sarafem)		20 mg daily or 20 mg intermittently	$
Fluvoxamine (Luvox)		100 mg daily	$$
Paroxetine (Paxil, Paxil CR)		5–30 mg daily 12.5–25 mg daily (CR) or 12.5–25 mg CR intermittently	$ $$ (CR)
Sertraline (Zoloft)		50–150 mg daily or 100 mg intermittently	$
Other serotonergic antidepressants			
Nefazodone	CI: MAOI use CI: multiple drug interactions AE: Hepatoxicity, constipation, hypotension	200–600 mg daily	$–$$
Venlafaxine (Effexor)	CI: MAOI use AE: HTN	50 mg daily	$$
Duloxetine (Cymbalta)	CI: MAOI use C: narrow angle glaucoma AE: CNS, GI	60 mg daily	$$$$ (brand only)
Tricyclic antidepressants	CI: MAOI use C: H/O seizures, narrow angle glaucoma, CV disease AE: Sedation, urinary retention		
Clomipramine		25–75 mg daily or 25–75 mg intermittently	$
Nortriptyline		50–125 mg daily	$
Anxiolytic			
Alprazolam	C: Drug interactions; taper the dose over 2 days after the onset of menses AE: Drowsiness, dependence	1–2 mg intermittently	$
Buspirone	CI: MAOI use AE: Drowsiness, dizziness	25–60 mg intermittently	$

MAOI = monoamine oxidase inhibitor; SSRI = selective serotonin reuptake inhibitor; HTN = hypertension; CNS = central nervous system; GI = gastrointestinal; H/O = history of; CV = cardiovascular.
*Intermittent dosing begins on day 14 of cycle and continues until onset of menses.
†Relative cost for month supply: $, <$30; $$, $30-$60, $$$: $60-$90; $$$$, >$90.

paroxetine carry a Food and Drug Administration–approved indication for treatment of PMS. Limited clinical trial data support a similar effect with other SSRIs and non-SSRI serotonergic antidepressants (see Table 28.4). Because data support their efficacy, these agents are considered first-line therapy in patients with significant psychological PMS symptoms (31,32). Intermittent treatment (dosing during the luteal phase only) with SSRIs has been shown to be effective, although less so than continuous daily dosing (33). Because of fewer side effects and lower cost, however, an intermittent regimen is a good choice for patients with moderate symptoms.

If anxiety is the primary complaint and the patient has not responded to an appropriate trial of an SSRI, an anxiolytic can be tried. Luteal phase dosing of either buspirone or alprazolam has been shown in small trials to be effective in managing anxiety related to PMS (SOR=B). Because of concerns regarding the addictive potential of alprazolam and the relative lack of data on use of these agents in PMS, they are considered second-line therapy (28) (Table 28.6).

Diuretics and Nonsteroidal Antiinflammatory Drugs

Some women experience marked fluid retention and bloating during the premenstrual period. Spironolactone, a mild diuretic with antiandrogenic properties, has been shown in clinical trials to improve the subjective symptom of bloating (26) (SOR=B). It is dosed at 100 mg daily during the luteal phase. Other diuretics have not been well studied in the management of PMS. NSAIDs are useful for menstrual headaches and the joint and muscle aches that can occur with PMS.

Hormonal Therapy and Menstrual Cycle Modulation

There are very limited data on the efficacy of OCs for PMS. Anecdotally, some women report improvement in PMS symptoms on OCs; however, OCs may cause PMS-like adverse effects, including fluid retention and mood changes. An OC containing drospirenone, a progestin with spironolactone-like effects, is Food and Drug Administration–approved for the treatment of PMDD. It is not clear if this agent is effective for less severe PMS symptoms or if it is more effective than other OCs (34). If a woman with PMS desires OCs for contraception, she can be given a drospirenone-containing OC. She should monitor her symptoms closely and consider switching to alternate contraception if an exacerbation is noted. Despite a theory that PMS is caused by progesterone deficiency, studies do not support a benefit of progesterone therapy (35).

Elimination of the hormonal fluctuations of the menstrual cycle has been shown to improve PMS and the condition generally abates once menopause occurs. Bilateral oophorectomy and drugs that eliminate menstrual cyclicity, such as danazol and the GnRH agonists, have been shown to effectively treat PMS but are associated with significant risks (22,26). Patients with severe PMS who have failed other therapies should be referred to a gynecologist.

Herbal Medicine

In several small trials, chasteberry (*Vitex agnus castus*), has been shown to reduce both physical and psychological symptoms of PMS (36–38) (SOR=B). Evening primrose oil has not been shown to be of benefit (30,39). There are limited data supporting use of other herbal agents for PMS.

ABNORMAL UTERINE BLEEDING

Definitions

It is important to understand the range of normal when it comes to a woman's menstrual cycle. Variability in the menstrual cycle has been noted at the beginning and end of a woman's reproductive life. An analysis of menstrual records from more than 1,000 women reveals that most women set their own menstrual interval by age 19 years and that the length and variability change imperceptibly between ages 19 and 49 years (40). Between the 5th and 95th percentiles, the menstrual cycle ranges from 24 to 42 days. The majority of women will have cycles between 21 and 35 days, but only about 15% have an actual cycle length of 28 days (41). Bleeding days range from 4 to 8 days. Between ages 15 and 43 years, most women will have no more than a 3-day variation in cycle length. Variability increases to 4 to 5 days after age 44 years for the majority of menstruating women (40).

The traditional definitions of abnormal menstrual patterns are as follows (40,41):

- Oligomenorrhea—intervals >35 days; <2 bleeding episodes in a 90-day period
- Polymenorrhea—intervals <24 days; >4 bleeding episodes in a 90-day period
- Menorrhagia—regular normal intervals with excessive flow or duration of >10 days
- Metrorrhagia—irregular intervals

Menorrhagia has been difficult to determine quantitatively in the clinical setting. Traditionally defined as blood loss of ≥80 mL per bleeding episode, methods to measure or approximate this degree of blood loss have been cumbersome and impractical. A recent study reported a model for determining menorrhagia based on clot size (>1.1 inch in diameter), low ferritin level, and rate of change of sanitary protection (every 1 to 2 hours or more frequently). This model correctly identified 76% of women with measured menstrual blood flow of ≥80 mL and supports the idea that the subjective judgment of the patient, long thought to be unreliable, should be used in the assessment of heavy menstrual bleeding (42) (SOR=A). Menorrhagia occurring in the absence of structural uterine disease is referred to as dysfunctional uterine bleeding (DUB).

Pathophysiology

Normal uterine bleeding is the result of cyclic, sequential stimulation of the endometrium by estrogen and progesterone, and occurs after withdrawal of the hormonal effect. This pattern is mimicked pharmacologically by OCs and some HT (hormone therapy) regimens. Abnormal uterine bleeding (AUB) can result from hormonal disturbances such as estrogen withdrawal (estrogen only HT, missed pill) or unopposed estrogen with breakthrough bleeding (anovulatory cycles). Women on progesterone only medications (contraceptive pill, implant, and injections) can have abnormal bleeding patterns due to progesterone withdrawal or breakthrough bleeding (41).

Anovulatory cycles can be due to many etiologies including PCOS (polycystic ovary syndrome), eating disorders, endocrinopathies (i.e., thyroid disease or prolactinoma), obesity, or the suppression of ovulation from weight loss or excessive exercise. Menstrual abnormalities in women with thyroid disease occur in just under 25% of women with either hyper- or hypothyroidism; the most common complaint in both groups is oligomenorrhea (43). Anovulation is also seen at the extremes of a woman's reproductive life. In reproductive age women, anovulatory bleeding and hormonal medication use are the most common causes of noncyclic bleeding (5,41).

Other possible causes of AUB are listed in Table 28.1. Risk factors for endometrial cancer include age (>40 years), anovulatory cycles, obesity, nulliparity, diabetes, and tamoxifen therapy. Endometrial cancer has been reported in women younger than age 40 years; women with chronic anovulation and obesity who present with AUB should be considered at risk (44).

Medications such as antipsychotics, anticoagulants, SSRIs, corticosteroids, and tamoxifen have been known to cause AUB, as have certain herbal supplements (e.g., ginseng, ginkgo, soy). Renal, hepatic, adrenal, and thyroid disease and blood dyscrasias may cause AUB. Other causes for AUB include foreign objects, including IUDs, trauma, and congenital (Müllerian) structural abnormalities (5,45). Coagulopathies, once thought to be a rare cause of abnormal bleeding, have been shown to be present in 13% of women with heavy uterine bleeding (46).

Some causes of AUB vary with age. The incidence of structural lesions and endometrial cancer increases with age. Pregnancy-related causes occur during the reproductive years. Anovulation can occur throughout the reproductive years.

Clinical Evaluation

Although many women presenting for an evaluation of a menstrual problem will give a straightforward history, clinicians should remember that for some, such a complaint may be an acceptable way to obtain a medical evaluation. The pelvic exam can be very traumatic to adolescent patients coming for a first evaluation or for women who have a history of sexual assault. The patient's cultural background or personal comfort level may also result in a limited (abdominal only) exam. In these cases, the history and further laboratory and pelvic ultrasound investigations can assist in identifying the most likely diagnosis.

HISTORY

The initial evaluation of AUB should include a complete menstrual history from menarche in order to understand if this is a chronic or newly acquired bleeding pattern. The bleeding episodes should be quantified and characterized. A history of clots >1.1 inch and a report of changing sanitary pads or tampons every 1 to 2 hours or more frequently supports a diagnosis of menorrhagia (42). Cyclical periods associated with premenstrual symptoms suggestive of a progesterone effect (breast tenderness, dysmenorrhea) provide more than a 95% probability that the woman is ovulating (5). Timing of the bleeding episodes (postcoital, intermenstrual, mid-cycle) should be noted. A history of pregnancy symptoms and/or abdominal pain, even in the presence of reported previous period-like bleeding, should raise suspicion that the patient is having a complication of pregnancy. Inquiring about associated symptoms and complaints, such as dyspareunia, galactorrhea, and hirsutism will help complete the patient's history and direct further workup.

A sexual history; reproductive history; and medication review, including nonprescription supplements and herbals, are also essential to making a diagnosis. A review of systems should help evaluate for systemic diseases (adrenal, renal, hepatic, and thyroid) or coagulopathies.

A screening test developed to detect underlying coagulation disorders includes the following: a history of excessive menstrual bleeding since menarche; or history of one of the following—postpartum hemorrhage, surgery related bleeding, or bleeding associated with dental work; or a history of two or more of the following—bruising >5 cm once or twice a month, epistaxis once or twice a month, frequent gum bleeding, family history of bleeding symptoms (SOR=B). These symptoms occur statistically more often in women with von Willebrand disease and a positive screen will help determine further workup (47).

In addition, the woman's medical and surgical history and previous exam findings and evaluations may help in establishing the etiology of AUB.

PHYSICAL EXAMINATION

To evaluate the severity of bleeding, patients should be screened for orthostatic hypotension and an elevated pulse rate. Other vital signs of importance are pain, weight, and body mass index. The patient should be observed for signs of systemic disease (bruising, petechiae, and jaundice). The physical exam, based on the history, should be performed. The thyroid gland should be examined. Careful attention should be given to the abdominal and pelvic exam, to evaluate for hepatosplenomegaly and uterine enlargement due to fibroids or pregnancy.

On pelvic exam, evidence of infection, trauma, foreign body, IUD string, cervical polyps or neoplasia may help identify the source of the bleeding. Trauma or foreign bodies may indicate sexual assault or self-mutilation. Cervical cultures, a pap smear and a biopsy of any visible lesion should be done at the time of the initial exam if possible. Uterine size, shape, and consistency should be assessed. Adenomyosis is strongly suspected in a uterus that is enlarged, diffusely tender, and soft to boggy to palpation. Irregular contours are more likely with fibroids. The adnexal exam can help identify any masses or localized pain suggestive of an ectopic pregnancy or abscess. A recto-vaginal exam may be helpful in assessing structural abnormalities (5).

LABORATORY TESTING

Laboratory testing should be systematic and based on the information from the history and the physical exam. Initial testing should be directed at eliminating life-threatening or serious conditions, such as pregnancy (serum hCG) or severe anemia (hemoglobin or hematocrit). Thyroid-stimulating hormone and prolactin levels should be obtained if history (oligomenorrhea, galactorrhea) or physical exam (enlarged thyroid, galactorrhea) is suggestive. Women with known or suspected systemic illness should have appropriate laboratory evaluation (5,45). If a coagulopathy is suspected, hemostasis testing should be done in consultation with a hematologist, as the accurate diagnosis of von Willebrand disease is dependent on appropriate testing conditions. Tests, beyond the initial hemoglobin and platelet count, include a prothrombin time, partial thromboplastin time, Von Willebrand factor antigen, ristocetin cofactor, Factor VIII, ABO type, Ivy bleeding time, and/or platelet function analyzer-100 closure time. Iron studies should be obtained for the anemic patient (47).

PCOS (the most common cause of oligomenorrhea in adolescents) should be suspected if there is a history of irregular menses 2 years after menarche, clinical hyperandrogenism, or biologic hyperandrogenism (elevated plasma testosterone, LH/FSH ratio >2), evidence of insulin resistance, and polycystic ovaries. Serum testosterone, DHEA-S, and 17-α hydroxyprogesterone should be obtained in patients with hirsutism and hyperandrogenism (2,48).

The next step in the evaluation of AUB is to determine the need for further investigation, such as an endometrial biopsy, transvaginal ultrasound (TVU), or hysteroscopy to evaluate for endometrial cancer and structural abnormalities. Which investigation to begin with may be a matter of what is available and acceptable to the patient. A meta-analysis of studies to assess the accuracy of endometrial sampling devices showed that the Pipelle had the best detection rate for endometrial cancer in both pre- (91%) and post- (99.6%) menopausal women (Table 28.7). The detection rate for atypical hyperplasia is also high (49) (SOR=A). A meta-analysis of TVU studies showed that an endometrial thickness ≥5 mm is a useful test for endometrial disease; use of HT, however, lowers specificity (50) (SOR=A) (Table 28.7).

For the evaluation of postmenopausal bleeding, TVU is considered the first step, if available. Endometrial sampling will alter TVU findings and should be deferred until after the TVU, as the study results may render it unnecessary. It should be noted that some investigators use 4 mm rather than 5 mm

TABLE 28.7 Characteristics of Diagnostic Tests Useful in Patients with Abnormal Uterine Bleeding

Diagnosis	Test	Sensitivity	Specificity	LR+	LR−
Menorrhagia	Low ferritin, clots over 1.1 inch, changing pad every 1–2 hours (40)	60	86	4.28	0.46
Atypical hyperplasia	Endometrial biopsy	81	98	40.2	0.19
Uterine cancer	Endometrial biopsy—premenopausal women (47)	91	98	45.5	0.09
	Endometrial biopsy—postmenopausal women (47)	99.6	98	49.8	0.004
	TVU endometrial thickness ≥5 mm (no HT) (48)	96	92	12	0.04
	TVU endometrial thickness ≥5 mm (on HT) (48)	96	77	4.17	0.05

HT = Hormone Therapy; LR = likelihood ratio; TVU = Transvaginal ultrasound.

for the cutoff for further evaluation (51). A small study (144 premenopausal women) used 8 mm endometrial thickness as a cut off with a sensitivity of 83.6%, specificity of 56.4% and negative predictive value of 95.6% for detection of abnormal endometrium (52).

Ultrasound is more likely to identify structural abnormalities that would be missed with the biopsy alone or hysteroscopy approach and is more acceptable to patients. In a recent cost analysis, initial TVU was most cost effective in pre- and perimenopausal women where the prevalence rate of benign disease is high. However, 5% to 10% of the time, the endometrium cannot be visualized. This would necessitate follow-up with biopsy and/or hysteroscopy or saline infusion sonography (SIS) (53–55). MRI and saline infusion sonography can be used to further evaluate patients for leiomyomata and adenomyosis (5). Hysteroscopy should be used to assess focal structural lesions and as a next step when SIS is not definitive (51).

Management

Once life-threatening complications have been ruled out, management can proceed according to the cause of the bleeding. Women who are older than age 35 years, at increased risk for endometrial cancer, or who have abnormal findings on exam require further testing. A suggested systematic workup for AUB is shown in Figure 28.2. Detection of structural abnormalities, such as an endometrial thickness >5 mm, endometrial atypia or adenocarcinoma will usually result in a referral to a gynecologist for further evaluation. The clinician's challenge, after the initial diagnosis is made, is to effectively bring the bleeding under control with a minimum of side effects. This can be done using medication, a levonorgestrel-releasing IUD (LNG IUD), or surgical interventions.

MEDICATIONS AND THE IUD

Medications have been shown to effectively control AUB, both by regulating the menstrual cycle (i.e., OCs, cyclical progesterone) and decreasing the amount of blood flow (i.e., NSAIDs, oral luteal progesterone, OCs, Danazol, tranexamic acid, ethamsylate, LNG IUD) (see Table 28.4). NSAIDs have been shown to be less effective than tranexamic acid or Danazol, but the latter medications are less frequently used due to risks, side effects, and cost. There were no statistical differences in effectiveness between naproxen and mefenamic acid, or between NSAIDs and oral luteal progestogens, LNG IUS, ethamsylate, and OCs (56) (SOR=B).

In a study of LNG IUD compared with cyclical 21-day oral progesterone therapy for menorrhagia, the LNG IUD was more effective, had greater patient satisfaction, and its use led to a higher proportion of women who deferred surgery when compared with oral medication use (57) (SOR=A). In a study comparing medical and surgical therapy, surgery reduced menstrual bleeding more than medical treatments, but the LNG IUD appeared equally effective in improving quality of life (SOR=A). Long-term oral medication was useful for a minority of women (58).

OVULATORY AUB

As shown in Figure 28.2, consideration should be given to an evaluation for coagulopathy. If no abnormalities are detected, a trial of hormonal therapy (OC, cyclic progesterone, HT, LNG IUD) can be initiated. Therapy should be directed toward control of bleeding. If there is no or minimal response in 3 months, reevaluation (with additional studies such as hysteroscopy, saline infusion sonography) should take place.

ANOVULATORY AUB

Anovulatory bleeding is common in adolescents and often reassurance and education is all that is needed. In adolescents with anovulatory menorrhagia (i.e., DUB), OCs, if not contraindicated, will effectively control the bleeding and have the added advantage of establishing a predictable bleeding pattern and providing contraception. For those adolescents unable to tolerate or unwilling to take cyclical hormonal (estrogen/progesterone or progestin only) therapy, NSAIDs at the time of menses will decrease the bleeding and may be an acceptable alternative (see Table 28.4). Women with anovulatory bleeding who are <35 years old without risk factors for endometrial cancer can be treated using a similar approach. Women >35 years or those with risk factors for endometrial cancer should have an endometrial biopsy or TVU as part of the initial workup. Management of the underlying cause of anovulatory cycles should be considered. Adolescents with PCOS will

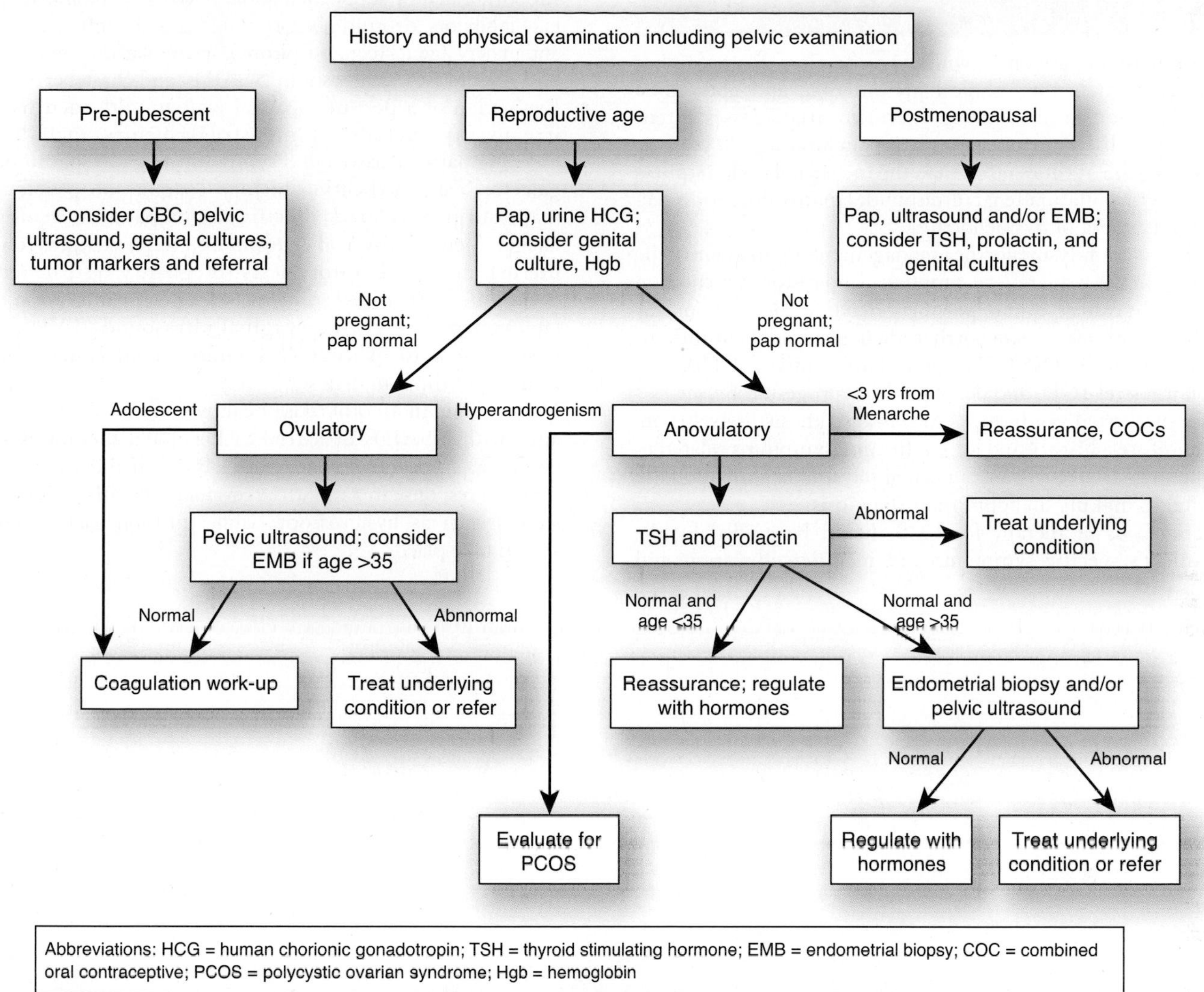

Figure 28.2 • General approach to the patient with abnormal uterine bleeding. From: Keehbauch J, Hill A, Burns EA, et al. Abnormal Uterine Bleeding, FP Essentials™, Edition No. 353, AAFP Home Study. Leawood, Dan: American Academy of Family Physicians, October 2008.

have their menorrhagia controlled by OCs, but issues of obesity and insulin resistance must also be addressed (2,48).

If there is no response to the treatment for menorrhagia after 3 months, further evaluation should be undertaken, either at the primary care office or through gynecological referral. Irregular bleeding/spotting may occur in the first 3 months of OC use, especially with progestin-only pills, so care should be taken to provide counseling on how to take the medication (same time every day). Intermenstrual spotting in women using OCs can be treated with NSAIDs, supplemental estrogen, or a change in the pill formulation. However, if the bleeding continues, the woman should be evaluated for structural abnormalities and other causes of bleeding (59).

The same stepwise approach can be taken for women in the reproductive age range after appropriate evaluation. Use of the LNG IUD, which can be placed for 5 years, is cost-effective and may be more acceptable for women in this age group. It preserves fertility, unlike the surgical approaches, and insertion can be done in a primary care office. Progestogen side effects do occur, which may lead to early discontinuation. When compared with endometrial resection, a 3-year study showed that both treatments reduced menstrual bleeding (60) (SOR=A).

SURGICAL OPTIONS

Surgical endometrial destruction techniques have been developed as alternatives to hysterectomy. Newer techniques (balloon ablation, bipolar radiofrequency ablation) do not require use of hysteroscopy and outcomes compare favorably with transcervical resection of the endometrium (61) (SOR=A). Hysterectomy, however, continues to have the advantage in cessation of AUB and high satisfaction rates when compared to endometrial ablation (SOR=A). The quality of life scales for both are similar; there was some evidence of greater improvement in health measures (energy, pain, overall health) for women who underwent hysterectomy. With the retreatment that is often necessary after endometrial ablation, the cost differential narrows over time (62).

KEY POINTS

- Evaluation of a woman with dysmenorrhea focuses on her age, sexual history, clinical presentation, and abdominal and pelvic examination (e.g., uterine/ovarian masses or tenderness, discharge); new onset of pain after age 20 years or pelvic pain at times other than the menstrual cycle requires further evaluation (e.g., ultrasound, laparoscopy) for a secondary cause of dysmenorrhea.
- The goals of dysmenorrhea management are to identify the cause of the pain, relieve symptoms, and restore functioning to the greatest extent possible; effective medications for pain in primary dysmenorrhea are nonsteroidal antiinflammatory drugs (NSAIDs), oral contraceptives (OCs), levonorgestrel-IUD, and depot medroxyprogesterone.
- Premenstrual syndrome (PMS) is a diagnosis of exclusion; therefore a history and log confirming symptoms related to the menstrual cycle and a normal physical examination are vital to making an appropriate diagnosis.
- The focus of therapy for PMS should be guided by the patient's specific symptoms and includes education and support, calcium supplementation, selective serotonin reuptake inhibitors, drospirenone-containing oral contraceptives, antianxiety agents (e.g., buspirone), spironolactone, pyridoxine (vitamin B6), magnesium, NSAIDs, and chasteberry.
- Evaluation of a perimenopausal woman with menstrual irregularity includes a menstrual history including bleeding pattern, associated symptoms (e.g., dyspareunia, galactorrhea), medication history, coagulation problems (e.g., surgery-related bleeding, postpartum hemorrhage), focused physical examination (e.g., skin, thyroid, uterus), initial laboratory tests (pregnancy test, hematocrit, other tests directed by exam), and consideration of endometrial biopsy, transvaginal ultrasound (TVU), or hysteroscopy to evaluate for endometrial cancer and structural abnormalities.
- Menorrhagia in an otherwise healthy woman can be managed with NSAIDs or a trial of hormonal therapy (OC, cyclic progesterone, levonorgestrel IUD); if there is no or minimal response in 3 months, reevaluation (with additional studies such as hysteroscopy, saline infusion sonography) should take place.

CHAPTER

29

Promoting Health for Women at Menopause

Linda French

CLINICAL OBJECTIVES

1. Summarize the additional history that would you obtain from a perimenopausal woman experiencing bothersome hot flashes.
2. Describe the treatment options for menopausal symptoms.
3. Discuss preventive services should you offer a woman following menopause.

Menopause is defined as permanent amenorrhea in a previously cycling woman. Natural menopause is the permanent cessation of menstrual cycles caused by the exhaustion of the ovaries. Medical intervention that removes or terminates ovarian function also leads to menopause. If a premenopausal woman has a hysterectomy without oophorectomy, her ovaries may still produce hormonal cycles and she is considered premenopausal until ovarian cycles stop.

Perimenopause or climacteric, the period around menopause, begins with the onset of symptoms attributed to the menopausal transition. Common climacteric symptoms, in order of frequency, are: vasomotor symptoms (hot flashes), mood disturbances, sleep disturbances, decreased libido, and vaginal dryness.

In addition to menopause, there are other changes that affect women in the middle years. These include personal issues of sexuality and aging, the "empty nest" response generated by children becoming fledgling adults, aging parents who may be ill or disabled, and health problems of friends and spouses. These developmental life changes can provoke symptoms similar to those of menopause or aggravate ones that already exist. On the other hand, there are many women who find "menopausal zest." Their children are out of the home, financial security may be reached, and there no longer is a fear of pregnancy.

NATURAL HISTORY

A woman's hormonal rhythm changes gradually beginning typically in her early to middle 40s. As ovarian mass decreases so does production of ovarian hormones, including inhibin. Reduced levels of inhibin, even without a corresponding reduction in estrogen level, may cause the follicle-stimulating hormone (FSH) level to rise. Ovarian production of progesterone diminishes as the corpus luteum, formed after ovulation, decreases in size. Menstrual cycles become somewhat shorter, and estrogen changes are more variable. Estrogen levels can be higher than in former years because of recruitment of more ovarian follicles by higher FSH levels. Estrogen tends to predominate over progesterone, promoting fibroid changes in the uterus and breasts.

Before menopause, the ovary produces most of the body's circulating estrogen, which consists of three types: estriol (E3), estradiol (E2), and estrone (E1). Total estrogen decreases by about 60% after menopause, and the major reduction is in E2. Obese women have higher postmenopausal estrogen based on E1 production by the adipose cells. This may contribute to the increased risk for endometrial and ovarian cancers among obese women.

The mean age at menopause in the United States is 51 years (1). Smokers experience menopause about 2 years earlier than nonsmokers. Perimenopausal menstrual irregularity begins typically 4 years before menopause (range 1 to 7 years). For 10% of women, menses simply cease without previous menstrual irregularity. Premature menopause is defined as cessation of menstrual periods before 40 years of age. About 10% of women are menopausal by age 46, 30% to 35% by age 50, and 90% by age 56. There is a familial tendency toward similarity in age at menopause.

History and Physical Exam

The patient-centered medical history can be divided into three areas: menstrual, urogenital, and climacteric symptoms and relevant additional history (Table 29.1). The physical examination focuses on evaluation of general appearance, and breast and pelvic examinations (Table 29.1).

DIAGNOSIS OF MENOPAUSE

Menopause is traditionally diagnosed retrospectively—1 year after the LMP. An FSH level >40 mIU/mL is also often used to diagnose menopause if testing is indicated. However, a high FSH may not be reliable to diagnose menopause because the level can drop again, accompanied by further ovulatory cycles. Further ovulatory cycles are not expected if FSH is >60 mIU/mL (2). In women receiving estrogens, either as oral contraceptives or for treatment of perimenopausal symptoms, FSH levels should be measured 7 to 10 days after stopping estrogens.

TABLE 29.1 Key Elements in the History and Physical Examination of the Perimenopausal Woman

Area of Concern	Questions	Purpose
Key History		
Menstrual history	Last menstrual period Cycle length Regularity Amount of bleeding Associated symptoms	Monitor change through menopause, assess risk for anemia
Contraception	Need for and type(s) used	Prevent pregnancy
Urogenital symptoms	Change in sexual activity/libido Dyspareunia Urinary frequency or incontinence Symptoms of cystitis and vaginitis	Assess need for further diagnosis and treatment
Climacteric symptoms	Hot flashes (frequency, timing, triggering stimuli, successful relief measures) Mood Sleep patterns Skin and hair texture	Explore treatment options Assess for mood or sleep disorder
Health Maintenance (See Well Adult Care, Chapter 6)	Health habits Diet and vitamin supplements Pap smear and mammogram	Opportunity for improvement Sufficient calcium/vitamin D Up to date
Relevant past medical history	Osteoporosis Heart disease Cancer (e.g., breast, genital)	Need for therapy Added risk for hormone therapy
Focused Physical Examination		
General appearance	Evidence of dry skin or fatigue condition of hair Affect Weight and distribution of fat Height and spine (change in height, kyphosis, or cervical hump)	Assess need for further diagnosis and treatment (e.g., depression, hypothyroidism, osteoporosis)
Neck	Thyroid	Detect goiter
Breast	Texture Masses Tenderness Nipple discharge Axillary lymph nodes	Detect breast cancer or need for additional testing
Pelvic examination	External genitalia, urethra, vagina Cervix Uterus/ovaries	Assess for urogenital atrophy Detect cancer Assess size, abnormalities (ovaries should not be palpable by menopause)

Climacteric Symptoms

VASOMOTOR SYMPTOMS

Vasomotor symptoms or hot flashes are the most common symptom associated with the menopause transition. Hot flashes are sensations of warmth, frequently accompanied by skin flushing and perspiration. A chill may follow. This is the consequence of a sudden change in the hypothalamic control of temperature regulation, although the precise triggers have not been elucidated. Between 50% and 80% of women in Western countries experience these symptoms beginning several years before menopause. The prevalence of hot flashes peaks in the year that menses cease and most often decrease gradually after that (1). By 4 years after the

TABLE 29.2 Nonestrogen Treatments for Vasomotor Symptoms

Generic (Trade)	Side Effects with More Than 10% Incidence	Usual Dose	Relative Cost per Month*
Gabapentin (Neurontin, generic)	Somnolence Dizziness Fatigue	300 mg three times daily	$$
Paroxetine (Paxil, generic)	Insomnia Somnolence Dizziness Tremor	20 mg daily	$$
Venlafaxine (Effexor)	Nausea Headache Somnolence Dry mouth Dizziness Insomnia	75 mg daily or 37.5 mg twice daily	$$$
Clonidine (Catapres, generic)	Dry mouth Somnolence Dizziness Constipation	0.1 mg twice daily	$
Megestrol (Megace, generic)	Weight gain Caution: small risk of thromboembolism	20 mg twice daily	$
Black cohosh (Remifemin, generic)	Not documented	40 mg twice daily	$

*Relative cost: $ = <$25.00; $$ = $26.00–$66.00; $$$ = >$67.00.

final menstrual period, about 20% of women still have hot flashes and they can be lifelong.

Numerous well-controlled studies have shown the effectiveness of oral or transdermal estrogen-containing therapy for hot flashes, with 70% to 90% of women experiencing good relief (3,4). The weight of evidence regarding phytoestrogens is that they are not effective therapy (5,6). Alternatives to estrogen for treatment of hot flashes include gabapentin, venlafaxine, paroxetine, clonidine, and megestrol acetate (Table 29.2). However, doses of gabapentin <300 mg 3 times are no different than placebo (7). Transdermal progesterone cream, available over the counter as a health supplement, may improve vasomotor symptoms. Megestrol appears to be nearly as effective as estrogen with a 70% reduction in symptoms (8). Although long-term use of megestrol acetate by cancer survivors for the treatment of hot flashes has been shown to be effective and well tolerated (9), it is not customary to use it for other women at menopause. Small studies of relaxation techniques have also shown symptom reduction (10).

MOOD DISTURBANCES

Irritability and mood swings are common climacteric complaints. Women often compare them with what they experienced previously as premenstrual symptoms. However, studies of depressive symptoms in menopausal women indicate that menopause is not associated with increased rates of major depression. Women with a previous history of postpartum depression may be at increased risk for recurrence of depression in perimenopause. Stressful life context and poor health status appear to be more important risk factors for depression than symptoms of menopause in climacteric women.

Women with mild psychological and predominantly vasomotor symptoms may benefit from a trial of hormone therapy (HT) before using psychotropic medication (11). For important dysphoric symptoms, antidepressants are indicated (See Depression, Chapter 50). Androgens have a positive effect on mood, but safety with long-term use has not been established.

SLEEP DISTURBANCE

Many perimenopausal women complain of poor sleep, often attributed to nocturnal hot flashes. High body mass index and increased age are associated with polysomnographic abnormalities, not hot flashes (12). Treatment, as described previously for vasomotor symptoms, may improve poor sleep due to night sweats. Other approaches to insomnia, such as sleep hygiene measures and progressive relaxation techniques, also can be used. If sleep apnea is suspected, a sleep study may be indicated.

UROGENITAL SYMPTOMS

Urogenital symptoms are reported by up to 40% of postmenopausal women. Premenopausal vaginal tissues are normally elastic and rugated with a high glycogen content, which helps maintain the bacterial flora dominated by *lactobacilli* and a vaginal pH between 3.5 and 4.5. After the decline in estrogen postmenopausally, the mucosa thins with loss of collagen support and fibrous transformation of the elastic fibers, the *lactobacilli* become less prominent, and vaginal pH increases to 5.5 to 6.8. The genital tract atrophies gradually. The labia shrink, the mucosa loses its rugae and becomes smooth and pale, and the introitus and vagina may contract.

Atrophic vaginitis refers to associated symptoms of vaginal discomfort, including dryness, burning, and itching. Urinary symptoms may coincide, such as frequency, urgency, dysuria, and stress incontinence. Some women develop recurrent urinary tract infection (UTI) or symptomatic bacterial vaginosis (see Vaginitis, Chapter 33).

Low-dose topical estrogen is effective treatment for atrophic vaginitis (Table 29.3). In a Cochrane review of treatments for vaginal atrophy, creams, pessaries, estradiol vaginal ring and tablets were all effective but women appeared to favor the ring (13). Ultra-low-dose therapy is also effective for many women (14). Different preparations appear to be equally effective. Serum estrogen levels with topical therapy are approximately one tenth that of systemic therapy. For women who develop recurrent UTI, topical estrogen is likely to reduce recurrences (15).

Another class of treatment shown to be effective is vaginal lubricants including liquid and gel products to coat and moisturize the vaginal epithelium. There is some evidence that the gel product (Replens) used three times weekly may be as effective as a topical estrogen. Vitamins D and E have also been studied and may be helpful (16).

Continuing sexual activity is associated with maintaining elasticity and lubrication. A causal relationship is difficult to determine because better elasticity may allow some women to continue intercourse. On the other hand, semen may help maintain lower pH.

SEXUAL FUNCTION

Dyspareunia is a frequent complaint related to genital dryness and involution. For sexual dysfunction caused by urogenital atrophy, a low dose of intravaginal estrogen generally provides good symptom relief within 6 months without altering the endometrium.

Women's sexual interest usually declines gradually during the late reproductive years with an additional drop at the time of menopause (17). Testosterone and dehydroepiandrosterone (DHEA) seem to increase sexual interest when added to estrogen therapy. In a study of sildenafil (Viagra), there was no benefit to middle-age women with sexual arousal difficulties (18).

OSTEOPOROSIS PREVENTION AND TREATMENT

Maximum bone density is attained in young adulthood. Women then typically lose 50% of cancellous and 30% of trabecular bone mass over their remaining lifetime. (Men lose 30% and 20%, respectively.) Cancellous bone is concentrated in the spine and ends of long bones. Bone loss begins in the premenopausal years and accelerates in the early postmenopausal years. Lack of estrogen causes a release of osteoclastic inhibition. Increased osteoclastic activity in the immediate postmenopausal period leads to an imbalance between bone resorption and formation. This is more damaging than that caused by decreased osteoblastic activity. The net result is that bone turnover increases, with more resorption than formation of bone.

Poor intake of calcium and vitamin D, sedentary lifestyle, low body fat, and Caucasian race (especially Northern European ancestry) increase the risk of osteoporosis (Table 29.4). Smoking is a significant risk for osteoporotic hip fractures (19% of current smokers vs. 12% of those who have never smoked, with a dose-response gradient) (19). Certain medical conditions and medications also cause bone loss (Table 29.4). Recent studies have demonstrated an increased risk of osteoporotic fractures among older women who take proton-pump inhibitors or selective serotonin reuptake inhibitors SSRIs (20,21). Prolonged functional amenorrhea, brought on by competitive athletic training or excessive weight loss, and other ovulatory disturbances can also contribute to bone loss in younger women.

Prevention is the least costly approach to osteoporosis and should begin in youth (see Table 29.5). Primary prevention should include smoking cessation, weight-bearing exercise, and sufficient intake of calcium and vitamin D. Screening for osteoporosis is recommended routinely at age 65 years by the US Preventive Services Task Force and at ages 60 to 64 years with risk factors (Table 29.4).

The most appropriate way to diagnose osteoporosis is by dual-energy x-ray absorptiometry of both spine and femur. If bone density is less than 2.5 standard deviations (SD) below the mean for young women (T-score), a diagnosis of osteoporosis is confirmed. If bone mineral density (BMD) is less than 1 SD but not less than 2.5 SD below the mean for young women, a diagnosis of osteopenia is made and measures for prevention of further bone loss should be instituted. Evidence to support the value of retesting is lacking and testing intervals less than 2 years not recommended because they are too short to assess interval change.

Pharmacologic Treatments

Estrogen produces a dose-response gradient for bone maintenance in postmenopausal women (see Table 29.3). HT decreases fractures while treatment continues. Discontinuation leads to a phase of accelerated bone loss like that following natural menopause (22). Protection against fractures is lost within 5 years after cessation of HT (23,24). Concerns about cardiovascular and breast cancer risks of combined estrogen-progestogen HT have led to a decrease in use of HT for prevention and treatment of osteoporosis. ET has been shown to decrease risk of osteoporosis, but progesterone alone is not an effective therapy. Ultra-low-dose estrogen-only therapy has been found to improve bone density without endometrial stimulation (25,26). Androgens also have a positive effect on bone mass.

Other pharmacologic treatments available for treatment of osteoporosis are presented in Table 29.6. They include bisphosphonates, salmon calcitonin, and human parathyroid hormone analog; all treatments are relatively expensive. Sufficient intake of calcium (1,000 to 1,500 mg calcium carbonate or 400 mg daily calcium citrate) and vitamin D (800 IU daily or 50,000 IU every 2 months) should be concurrent with the administration of any of these drugs. However, excessive calcium supplementation increases risk for cardiovascular events in older women (27).

Bisphosphonates are the most commonly used therapies for osteoporosis. They are potent inhibitors of bone resorption. The long-term effects of inhibiting bone resorption with

TABLE 29.3 Hormone Preparations for Perimenopausal Women (Estrogens)

Generic (Trade)	Form	Doses Available	Usual Dose	Relative Cost*
Estrones				
Conjugated estrogen (Premarin, generic)	Oral	0.3, 0.45, 0.625, 0.9, 1.25	One tablet daily, lower doses most commonly used	$$
	Vaginal cream	0.625 mg/g	1/2–1 applicator	$$$
Esterified estrogens (Menest)	Oral	0.3, 0.625, 1.25, 2.5 mg	0.3–1.25 mg	$
Estropipate (Ogen, Ortho-Est, generic)	Oral	0.625, 1.25, 2.5, 5 mg	0.625–1.25 mg	$
Ogen vaginal	Vaginal	1.5 mg/g	1/2–1 applicator	$
Estradiols				
Micronized estradiol (Estrace, generic)	Oral	0.5, 1, 2 mg	0.5–1 mg	$$
	Vaginal cream	0.1 mg/g	1/2–1 applicator	$$$
Estradiol	Oral	0.45, 0.5, 0.9, 1, 1.5, 1.8, 2 mg	One tablet daily	$
Conjugated B estrogen (Enjuvia)	Oral	0.625, 1.25 mg	One tablet daily	$$$
17β-estradiol	Transdermal	0.025, 0.05, 0.075, 0.1 mg/ 24-hour patches		$
Climara	Transdermal	0.025, 0.0375, 0.05, 0.06, 0.075, 0.1 mg/day	Once weekly	$$
Alora	Transdermal	0.025, 0.05, 0.075, 0.1 mg/day	Twice weekly	$$
Vivelle/Vivelle Dot	Transdermal	0.025, 0.0375, 0.05, 0.075, 0.1 mg/24 hours	Twice weekly	$$
Menostar	Transdermal	0.014 mg/24 hours	Once weekly	$$
Estradiol Topical Emulsion (Estrasorb)	Transdermal	1.74 g package with 2.5 mg estradiol hemihydrate/g	One package to each leg daily	$$
Gel 0.06% (EstroGel)	Transdermal	1.25 g per pump with 0.75 mg estradiol	One pump once or twice daily	$$
Estradiol ring (Estring) (Femring)	Vaginal ring	7.5 mcg/24 hours for 90 days 50 or 100 mcg/ 24 hours for 90 days	One ring every 90 days	$$$ $$$
Estradiol vaginal tablet (Vagifem)	Vaginal tablet	0.025 mg	1 tablet twice weekly	$$$
Progestins				
Micronized progesterone (Prometrium)	Oral	100 mg, 200 mg	200 mg/day	$$
Medroxyprogesterone acetate (Provera, generic)	Oral	2.5, 5, 10 mg	2.5 mg daily, or cyclic use of higher doses	$
Combined Estrogen and Progestin				
Conjugated estrogens plus medroxyprogesterone acetate (Prempro Premphase)	Oral	0.625/5 mg, 0.45/1.5 mg, 0.3/1.5 mg	Once daily	$$
	Oral	0.625 mg 0.625/5 mg	Day 1–14 Day 15–28	$$
17β-Estradiol plus norethindrone acetate (CombiPatch)	Transdermal	0.05 mg estradiol plus 0.14 or 0.25 mg norethindrone acetate	Twice weekly	$$

(*continued*)

TABLE 29.3 *(Continued)*

Generic (Trade)	Form	Doses Available	Usual Dose	Relative Cost*
Ethinyl estradiol/ norethindrone acetate (Femhrt)	Oral	2.5 mcg ethinyl estradiol/ 0.5 mg norethindrone acetate or 5 mcg ethinyl estradiol/ 1 mg norethindrone acetate	Once daily	$$
Estradiol plus Norgestimate (Prefest)	Oral	1 mg estradiol in all tablets plus norgestimate 0.09 mcg pulsed (3 tablets with, then 3 tablets without)	Once daily	$$
Androgens				
Testosterone	Transdermal			
1% gel (AndroGel, Testim)	Transdermal	2.5, 5 g tube, or packet	0.5 g daily (5 mg)	$$$
Combination Estrogen and Androgen				
Esterified estrogens and methyltestosterone (Estratest, or Estratest HS)	Tablet	1.25 mg E/2.5 mg M	1 per day	$$
	Tablet	0.625 mg E/1.25 mg M	1 per day	$$

*Relative cost: $ = <$33.00; $$ = $34.00–$70.00; $$$ = >$71.00.

bisphosphonates are uncertain, however, making it advisable to avoid routine screening and treatment of women <60 years old.

Alendronate (generic, Fosamax) was the first bisphosphonates approved by the US Food and Drug Administration (FDA) for the treatment of postmenopausal osteoporosis. It is taken orally on an empty stomach (with clear fluids while standing or sitting), 5 mg daily or 35 mg weekly for prevention, 10 mg daily or 70 mg weekly for treatment. It reduces the incidence of vertebral and non-vertebral fractures by about half. Gastroesophageal reflux is common and esophageal ulcer, myalgia, and arthralgia are also possible adverse drug events. Jaw bone necrosis is a rare, but serious, adverse effect. Risk is also increased for atrial fibrillation with number-needed-to-harm of 100 (28). Both of these are likely class effects of the bisphosphonates and are more likely when used at higher than usual doses. Treatment lasting at least 5 years is recommended for osteoporosis, but the optimal duration of treatment has not been established. Alendronate can also be used on a quarter-year cycle, 14 days on and 76 off, as preventive treatment for high-risk or osteopenic women.

Risedronate (Actonel) reduces vertebral and nonvertebral fractures over a 3-year period in women with osteoporosis (29). Adverse effects are similar to those of alendronate, but may be milder. BMD improves from baseline less than with alendronate, but a difference in incidence of fracture between the two has not been demonstrated (30).

Ibandronate (Boniva) is also effective and can be given once monthly (150 mg) or as a daily dose of 2.5 mg. One study suggested that the once monthly regimen of this drug was preferred by 75% of the women compared with alendronate weekly dosing, based on convenience and less frequent side effects (31). Pamidronate (Aredia) 30 to 60 mg intravenously every 6 months and zoledronic acid (Zometa) are other FDA-approved choices for treatment of osteoporosis after fractures.

Three other classes of medications may be used to treat osteoporosis. Raloxifene, a selective estrogen receptor modulator (SERM), has been shown in short-term studies to prevent

TABLE 29.4 Risk Factors for Osteoporosis

Risk Factors
Genetic predisposition Caucasian, especially Northern European
Lifestyle factors Smoking Sedentary Poor calcium intake Poor vitamin D intake
Reproductive history Early premenopausal vasomotor symptoms History of functional amenorrhea Ovulatory disturbances (oligomenorrhea) Premature ovarian failure Premenopausal hysterectomy Premenopausal oophorectomy
Medications Glucocorticoids (e.g., prednisone) Excess thyroid hormone Depo-medroxyprogesterone acetate Chemotherapeutic agents Proton pump inhibitors Selective serotonin reuptake inhibitors

TABLE 29.5 Preventing Osteoporosis

Intervention	Strength of Recommendation*	Comments
Smoking cessation	A	
Weight-bearing exercise	A	
Calcium	A	1,000 mg or more daily
Vitamin D	A	400 IU for all women, 800 IU for elderly
Estrogen or bisphosphonate therapy	B	Especially in high-risk women
Testosterone	C	Evidence of long-term safety is lacking
Dehydroepiandrosterone	C	Evidence of efficacy is lacking

*A = consistent, good-quality patient-oriented evidence; B = inconsistent or limited-quality patient-oriented evidence; C = consensus, disease-oriented evidence, usual practice, expert opinion, or case series.
For information about the SORT evidence rating system, see *http://www.aafp.org/afpsort.xml.*

vertebral fractures. Intranasal calcitonin (Miacalcin) may also be used. Data on fracture incidence with this treatment are not available. Human parathyroid hormone, teriparatide (Forteo), is the first approved drug for osteoporosis treatment that acts by stimulating osteoblastic activity. It can be used to treat severe osteoporosis, but is quite expensive. It is generally given in a daily dosage of 20 mcg subcutaneously for up to 2 years. It increases bone density and decreases back pain associated with recurrent vertebral fractures. Interestingly, the combination of teriparatide with alendronate does not increase bone density more than either one alone, although their mechanisms of action differ (32).

MENOPAUSAL HORMONE THERAPIES

The once popular term "hormone replacement therapy" has been largely dropped in the medical literature following release of results from the Women's Health Initiative study (WHI) in 2002 (33), when it was realized that it is not acceptable practice to routinely treat menopause as a hormone deficient state. The favored terms are hormone therapy (HT), which may be divided into estrogen-only therapy (ET) or combined estrogen-progestogen hormone therapy (CHT).

TABLE 29.6 Pharmacological Therapies for Osteoporosis

Generic (Trade)	Formulations	Usual Dosing
Alendronate + cholecalciferol (Fosamax Plus D)	70 mg + 2,800 IU	70/2,800 once weekly
Ibandronate (Boniva)	2.5 mg, 150 mg	2.5 mg daily or 150 mg once monthly, treatment or prevention
Risedronate (Actonel)	5 mg, 30 mg, 35 mg	Prevention and treatment 5 mg daily or 35 mg weekly (30-mg dosage recommended for treatment of Paget)
Risedronate and calcium (Actonel with calcium)	35 mg + 1250 mg calcium carbonate	Once weekly
Others		
Salmon calcitonin (Miacalcin)	2 mL bottles of 15 activations, 200 IU per activation for intranasal use	One activation daily in alternating nostrils for treatment but not prevention, also effective for pain management of osteoporotic fracture
Raloxifene (Evista)	60 mg tablet	One daily for prevention or treatment
Human parathyroid hormone (Forteo)	750 mcg/3 mL pen injector device	20 mcg subcutaneously daily

TABLE 29.7 Risks and Benefits of Combined Hormone Therapy in the Women's Health Initiative Study

Outcome	NNH* for 1 Year	NNH for 5 Years
Myocardial infarction	1,429	286
Stroke	1,250	250
Venous thromboembolism	555	111
Deep venous thrombosis	1,000	200
Pulmonary embolism	1,250	250
Breast cancer	1,250	250
Balance of risks versus benefits	500	100
Outcome	**NNT† for 1 Year**	**NNT for 5 Years**
Hip fracture	2,000	400
Vertebral fracture	2,000	400
Colon or rectal cancer	1,667	333

*NNH means "number needed to harm." It stands for the number people getting treatment when one person gets the harmful effect.
†NNT means "number needed to treat." It stands for the number of people getting treatment when one person gets the beneficial effect.

HT continues to be prescribed frequently for symptomatic relief as described above.

A woman without a uterus can take ET continuously. To reduce the risk of endometrial cancer, a woman with a uterus should receive CHT, with progestin to protect against the endometrial cancer risk with unopposed estrogen. CHT may be taken either continuously or cyclically as described in the following section; the latter allowing for withdrawal bleeding. To avoid unpredictable uterine bleeding, a woman should generally be at least 3 years postmenopause to use a continuous regimen. Lower dose continuous formulations have better rates of amenorrhea (34). Table 29.3 lists options for hormone preparations.

There are several ways of prescribing CHT. Increasingly transdermal formulations are used to limit the risk of venous thromboembolism, the most common adverse effect (35). A common oral combination is estrogen with medroxyprogesterone (Provera), which can be taken cyclically or continuously. Oral micronized progesterone (Prometrium) derived from yams is FDA approved for cyclic administration with a usual dose of 200 mg daily for 14 days in each cycle, given at bedtime because it may cause drowsiness. If used continuously the usual dose is 100 mg daily. For women who complain of symptoms on the days off of estrogen with cyclic treatment, estrogen can be given continuously, adding a progestogen for 10 to 14 days each month. Continuous estrogen, with use of progestogen for 14 days each quarter, (i.e., every 3 months) has also been shown to provide adequate endometrial protection (36).

Some vendors promote "bioequivalent" HT giving the impression that it is safer. Usually women provide saliva samples for customization of dosing. However, saliva samples are a poor method of determining systemic levels. There is no evidence other than lower breast cancer risk with yam-derived progesterone compared with synthetic progestogens to suggest that this approach is safer.

Cardiovascular Effects

The WHI was conducted with a principle objective to answer the question of whether HT was cardioprotective as suggested by observational data. To the contrary, there were small increases in the CHT group of myocardial infarctions, strokes, and venous thromboembolism, with a mean of 5.2 years follow-up (see Table 29.7). Among women beginning CHT who were <10 years' postmenopause there was no increase in coronary events (37). The ET portion of the study reported in 2004 had almost 2 years longer follow-up. It showed no increase in myocardial infarctions and similar increases in stroke and venous thromboembolism. Transdermal estrogen for secondary prevention of coronary events is not of benefit (38).

Risk of Breast Cancer

The WHI study of CHT was stopped when the increase in risk of breast cancer with active treatment became statistically significant, with a mean duration of treatment of about 5 years. Previous studies of CHT showed similar increases. There is still some uncertainty about whether ET increases breast cancer risk. If so, it is of much smaller magnitude than with CHT. The WHI showed a nonsignificant decrease in breast cancer with almost 7 years ET use (39). A meta-analysis of large observational studies suggests an increase in breast cancer risk of smaller magnitude than with CHT (40). A large French cohort study showed no increase in breast cancer risk among women taking estrogen plus progesterone, but increased breast cancer risk with synthetic progestogens (41).

Memory

Although observational studies suggested benefit of HT for cognitive function, the WHI showed a slight increase in risk of the diagnosis of Alzheimer disease as well as a more important risk of at least a 2-point decline in Mini-Mental Status Exam score (42,43). Another clinical trial showed no benefit from adjunctive treatment with estrogen in women with Alzheimer disease (44). ET did not slow Alzheimer disease progression or improve global cognitive or functional outcomes for women with mild to moderate disease.

Other Effects

There is an increase in risk of gall bladder surgery of about 1% among women who use HT for 5 years (45). In addition, about one in eight women has worsening of urinary incontinence with use of HT (46). Ethanol causes a delay in the initial degradation of sex hormones. Appropriate dosing for women with regular alcohol consumption may be less than that for nondrinkers (47). Grapefruit juice also delays the degradation of estrogen (48). Several studies have documented that there is not an increase in weight or body fat with use of HT in perimenopausal women.

Androgens

Endogenous production of testosterone decreases gradually during a woman's reproductive years. Exogenous testosterone has a beneficial effect on bone density and libido in perimenopausal women (49). However, long-term safety data are lacking and caution with use is warranted. Testosterone is available either alone or in combination with conjugated estrogen (Estratest and Estratest HS) (Table 29.3). It is also available in a topical gel formulation intended for men (AndroGel). A topical formulation intended for women was not given FDA approval because of safety concerns. Testosterone can be compounded in a cream and used topically on the skin or vulva.

The adrenal glands are the main source of endogenous androgens in postmenopausal women. The principal hormones are DHEA and dehydroepiandrosterone sulfate. Higher dose oral estrogen treatment significantly reduces the bioavailability of endogenous androgens by increasing sex hormone-binding globulin, thereby creating a hypoandrogenic state. A review of 11 studies (50) suggests that 50 mg per day of DHEA may be helpful treatment for sexual dysfunction; risks should be assessed for individual patients. DHEA is available as a dietary supplement.

SERMs

SERMs act differently at estrogen receptors in various organs. On some receptors, they may have an estrogen-like effect, and on others an antiestrogen effect. There are three products available in the United States: tamoxifen, raloxifene, and toremifene. The last is only approved for treatment of metastatic breast cancer and will not be reviewed here. Approval for tibolone, available in many other countries, was expected about the time WHI results were published, but has been delayed.

Tamoxifen is FDA approved for the prevention of breast cancer in high-risk women. The National Cancer Institute Trial showed a 45% decrease in relative risk of breast cancer in the tamoxifen-treated group (51). Two smaller European studies showed no protective effect. Concerns about increased risk of endometrial cancer have largely limited its use. Treatment risks also include deep vein thrombosis (about three times normal) and stroke, which are similar to risk with ET. Hot flashes and depressive symptoms are common.

Raloxifene has been approved for treating osteoporosis, although it is less effective than estrogen or alendronate (52). To date, raloxifene has been proven helpful in preventing vertebral fractures but not fractures of the hip, ankle, or wrist. The Study of Tamoxifen and Raloxifene (STAR) showed that raloxifene is as effective as tamoxifen for breast cancer risk with fewer adverse events (53). It is FDA approved for this purpose.

Other SERMs are in development. The hope is to find drugs that are tailored to produce a better balance of estrogenic and antiestrogenic effects, thus providing the benefits of estrogen while reducing its risk to the breast and uterus, and minimizing side effects. The publication of results from the WHI has led to greater caution in the introduction of such drugs.

Phytoestrogens

There are several classes of plant substances that are functionally similar to E2, including isoflavones (legumes), lignins (linseed), coumestans, and resorcylic acid lactones. Known as phytoestrogens, they include at least 20 compounds from 300 plants. They are weaker than natural estrogens, and are not stored in tissues. Common phytoestrogen-containing foods are parsley, garlic, soybeans, wheat, rice, dates, pomegranates, cherries, and coffee. Soy is the legume highest in isoflavones. Some phytoestrogens have been isolated and are sold over the counter.

Women report fewer menopausal symptoms in parts of the world where the staple diet includes foods high in phytoestrogens. The incidence of breast and other cancers, as well as coronary artery disease, is lower for Japanese women, who excrete far more isoflavonoids in their urine than do European or American women. Phytoestrogens may be among the dietary factors affording protection against cancer and heart disease in vegetarians in general. There is some evidence that isoflavones do not increase endometrial thickness. However, the effect of pharmacological doses of isolated isoflavones on breast and endometrial cancer risks are uncertain, and caution is warranted.

Most trials of phytoestrogens have failed to find a significant effect of soy or isoflavones on vasomotor symptoms versus placebo (5,6). No differences have been found compared with placebo for cognitive function, bone mineral density, or plasma lipids (54).

Black cohosh is an herbal preparation often used for treating menopausal symptoms. In Germany, a standardized preparation is approved for short-term (6 months) use. A well-designed RCT found no difference in hot flashes with black cohosh compared with placebo (55). A systematic review (56) of herbal preparations for treating menopausal symptoms found that the available studies were too few and too weak to provide clear evidence of benefit.

EDUCATIONAL INTERVENTIONS

Patient education has been shown to improve women's knowledge and beliefs about menopause (57). Written information is nearly as effective as a lecture-discussion format (58). There are many books available for the lay public about menopause. The quality of information about pharmacotherapy and nonpharmacotherapy options is variable. Many publications promote herbal products that are not effective or for which evidence of

TABLE 29.8 Resources for Patient Education Regarding Menopause

Organization	Contact Information	Description
North American Menopause Society	*www.menopause.org*	Menopause guidebook *Menopause: A New Beginning* (5th grade reading level) Web site also has list of frequently asked questions and answers, and suggested reading list
American Academy of Family Physicians	1-800-944-0000	*Menopause: What to Expect When Your Body is Changing* *Osteoporosis: Keeping Your Bones Healthy and Strong*
American Congress of Obstetricians and Gynecologists	1-800-410-ACOG	Brochures *Midlife Transitions: A Guide to Approaching Menopause* *The Menopause Years* *Preventing Osteoporosis*
Office on Women's Health, US Department of Health and Human Services	*www.4woman.gov/owh/pub/menoguide.htm*	Resource guide including agencies, institutions, reports, and books

benefit is lacking. Two books with objective information are: *A Woman's Guide to Menopause and Perimenopause* by Minkin and Wright, and *The Greatest Experiment Ever Performed on Women* by Seaman. The latter traces the history of menopausal hormone use through the results of the WHI. Other resources are listed in Table 29.8.

KEY POINTS

- Additional history useful for tailoring management in a woman experiencing bothersome hot flashes includes last menstrual period and bleeding pattern; need for contraception; frequency, timing, triggering stimuli, successful relief measures for the hot flashes; and other symptoms (mood, sleep, urogenital, skin and hair texture); physical examination focuses on evaluation of general appearance, and breast and pelvic examinations.
- Options for treating hot flashes include oral or transdermal estrogen-containing therapy, transdermal progesterone cream, gabapentin, venlafaxine, paroxetine, clonidine, relaxation therapy, and possibly megestrol acetate; data are conflicting on phytoestrogens but they do not seem to be effective.
- Atrophic vaginitis (symptoms of vaginal discomfort, dryness, burning, and itching) can be managed with low-dose topical estrogen, estradiol vaginal ring, and oral estrogen (ultra-low-dose therapy is effective for many women); vaginal lubricants are also helpful as is continuing sexual activity which helps maintains vaginal elasticity and lubrication.
- Risk factors for osteoporosis include poor intake of calcium and vitamin D, sedentary lifestyle, low body fat, and Caucasian race whereas smoking, proton-pump inhibitors, and selective serotonin reuptake inhibitors increases fracture risk; screening is recommended routinely at age 65 years and at ages 60 to 64 years with risk factors.
- Diagnose osteoporosis by dual-energy x-ray absorptiometry of both spine and femur and consider treatment with estrogen, bisphosphonates, salmon calcitonin, or human parathyroid hormone analog; the latter three treatments are relatively expensive; sufficient intake of calcium and vitamin D should be concurrent with the administration of any of these drugs.
- Preventive services to offer women following menopause are a review and counseling for health habits (e.g., diet, exercise, smoking), adequate intake of calcium and vitamin D, and a discussion of needs for Pap smears and mammography interval.

CHAPTER

30

Men's Health Concerns

Larissa S. Buccolo and Anthony J. Viera

BENIGN PROSTATIC HYPERPLASIA

CLINICAL OBJECTIVES

1. Discuss how to make the diagnosis of benign prostatic hyperplasia (BPH).
2. Describe factors that should be considered when managing BPH.
3. List reasons for referring a man with BPH to a urologist.

Benign prostatic hyperplasia (BPH) refers to neoplastic, nonmalignant proliferation of the prostatic tissue surrounding the urethra. BPH is a condition that occurs in aging men as the prostate gland undergoes exposure to androgenic and estrogenic stimulation over time (1). While a genetic component to development of BPH exists, only increasing age and androgenic stimulation are well-established etiologic factors.

The prevalence of BPH is estimated to be 8% in men in their 30s, 50% in men in their 50s, and 80% in men older than 80 years (2). These estimates correlate with histologically defined BPH discovered at autopsy (3). BPH is clinically important when it leads to lower urinary tract symptoms (LUTS) or bladder outlet obstruction (Table 30.1). Potential complications of bladder outlet obstruction include renal failure, urinary retention (acute and chronic), recurrent urinary tract infections (UTIs), bladder calculi, and bladder dysfunction.

Per year, acute urinary retention (AUR) develops in 1% to 2% of men with symptoms of BPH (4). However, the symptoms of BPH do not necessarily progress in every man who initially presents with LUTS or AUR. In one study of 212 men who presented with either LUTS or AUR and were followed for 4 to 7 years, 48% of those not undergoing surgery no longer had symptoms of BPH (5). In another study, 52% of men who did not have surgery had no change in their BPH symptoms over 5 years, 32% had improvement, and only 15% developed worsening symptoms (5). In addition to increasing age, three risk factors predict progressive BPH: change in size and force of urinary stream, sensation of incomplete emptying, and enlarged prostate on digital rectal examination (3).

Symptoms

The symptoms of BPH result from a combination of factors. The increased tone of the richly innervated prostatic smooth muscle fibers creates a dynamic (reversible) obstruction. As the prostate itself enlarges, it creates a mechanical (fixed) obstruction as it encroaches on and impinges the urethra (central hypertrophy). The bladder, in response to the increased outlet resistance, begins to increase the force of its contractions. Eventually, the detrusor muscle develops hypertrophy and fibrosis. Collagen deposition in the bladder wall leads to loss of bladder elasticity and compliance. Loss of normal control over the reflex detrusor response can ensue, and if left untreated, can progress to severe bladder dysfunction.

Symptoms that may develop throughout this process are shown in Table 30.1. Importantly, these symptoms are not specific for BPH, and not all patients with BPH develop them. Patients with symptoms attributable to BPH usually have some combination of irritative and obstructive symptoms. Other disorders that can cause similar symptoms are also shown in Table 30.1.

Initial Evaluation

The goals of the history are to clarify symptoms consistent with BPH and exclude conditions that mimic BPH. Ask the patient if he has a history of prostate problems or other urologic disease. Note any recent or remote urethral or bladder trauma (including instrumentation). Ask about the symptoms described in Table 30.1, but also ask questions to help exclude other conditions that might cause LUTS. Inquire about sexually transmitted infections (STIs). A history of erectile dysfunction (ED) is also important to consider for both diagnostic as well as therapeutic reasons. Pelvic pain, back pain, or weight loss are not due to BPH.

The examination for suspected BPH focuses on the abdomen, genital area, and rectum. Bladder distension can sometimes be detected by palpating and percussing the suprapubic region. Digital rectal examination (DRE) is performed to assess the size, consistency, and shape of the prostate. Ability to estimate prostate size might be improved by training using a three-dimensional prostate model (6). The size of the prostate does not correlate with BPH symptoms and the degree of central hypertrophy cannot be assessed with the DRE. Table 30.1 shows DRE findings that can help determine the cause of LUTS.

Diagnostic Testing

The only laboratory test needed in the initial evaluation of men suspected of having BPH is a urinalysis. The presence of hematuria should prompt consideration for referral for cystoscopy. The presence of white blood cells might signify infection (cystitis or prostatitis). A serum creatinine is no longer recommended in the initial evaluation of BPH because there are no data demonstrating a relationship between severity of

TABLE 30.1 Differential Diagnosis for Lower Urinary Tract Symptoms in Men

	BPH	Prostate Cancer	Prostatitis	Bladder Tumor or Stone	Neurogenic Bladder	Urethritis	Urethral Stricture
Common Symptoms	Irritative: Urinary frequency, urgency, nocturia, urge incontinence	Often asymptomatic	Infectious: Fever, chills	Gross hematuria	Incontinence, dribbling, loss of sensation of full bladder, frequency/urgency, small volume voiding	Irritative: Dysuria, frequency, urgency	History of urethral trauma or instrumentation, frequent urethritis
	Obstructive: Reduced stream, hesitancy, straining to void, interruption of stream, terminal dribbling, prolonged urination, incomplete emptying	Obstructive: Difficulty urinating Other: Erectile dysfunction (new), back or hip pain	Other: Dysuria, pelvic or perineal pain	Irritative: Frequency, urgency, dysuria (tumor, or with concomitant UTI in case of stone) Other: Flank pain (stone)	Other: Neurologic symptoms: paresthesias, numbness, weakness	Other: Penile drainage, history of unprotected intercourse	Obstructive: Weak stream, straining to void Irritative: Frequency, urgency, dysuria, incontinence
	May have history of UTI (from retained urine)	Induration, nodularity, or asymmetry of prostate	History of UTI	History of UTI	Decreased sphincter tone	Leukocytosis on urinalysis	Stricture seen on imaging studies
	Microscopic hematuria	Elevated PSA	Tender, boggy prostate	Gross or microscopic hematuria	Gait abnormalities	Positive gonorrhea or chlamydia cultures	Blood in urine or semen
	Prostate enlarged, rubbery		Leukocytosis on urinalysis	Abnormal urine cytology (bladder cancer)	Lower extremity neuromuscular abnormalities		Large PVR
	Large PVR			Stone present on imaging			

UTI = urinary tract infection; PSA = prostate-specific antigen; PVR = postvoid residual; UTI = urinary tract infection.

TABLE 30.2 American Urological Association BPH Symptom Score*

CIRCLE THE ONE BEST ANSWER TO EACH QUESTION

Questions	Never	<1 Time in 5	<Half the Time	About Half the Time	>Half the Time	Almost Always
Over the past month, how often have you had the feeling that you did not empty your bladder completely after you finished urinating?	0	1	2	3	4	5
Over the past month, how often have you had to urinate again <2 hours after you finished urinating?	0	1	2	3	4	5
Over the past month, how often have you found that you stopped and started again several times when you urinated?	0	1	2	3	4	5
Over the past month, how often have you found it difficult to postpone urination?	0	1	2	3	4	5
Over the past month, how often have you had a weak urinary stream?	0	1	2	3	4	5
Over the past month, how often have you had trouble getting your urine stream started?	0	1	2	3	4	5
Over the past month, how many times have you averaged getting up to urinate from the time you went to bed at night until the time you got up in the morning?	None	One time	Two times	Three times	Four times	Five times

Total score: ____________ (sum of circled numbers)

Key: 0–7, absent/mild symptoms; 8–19, moderate symptoms; 20+, severe symptoms.
*Modified from Barry MJ, Fowler FJ, O'Leary MP, et al: The American Urological Association Symptom Index for benign prostatic hyperplasia. *J Urol* 1992;148:1549–1557.

symptoms and impaired renal function. Additionally, baseline renal insufficiency is no more common in men with BPH than similarly aged men in the general population (7,8).

Optional tests in the evaluation of BPH include urine cytology, postvoid residual (PVR) volume, and a maximal urinary flow rate. Urine cytology may be useful in men with predominantly irritative voiding symptoms who have a history of smoking or other risk factors for bladder cancer. A large PVR volume (>350 mL) may be associated with bladder dysfunction and predict a less favorable response to treatment. While a PVR volume can be determined in the family physician's office by simple in-out catheterization or a bladder scanner, maximal urinary flow rate and tests such as uroflowmetry (uroflow) are generally performed in a specialist's office. A uroflow test is used to estimate the volume urinated as well as duration and velocity of urination. Such tests are probably most useful in men contemplating invasive treatment options, as patients with lower baseline flow rates typically have better postsurgical outcomes.

Management

AMERICAN UROLOGIC ASSOCIATION SYMPTOM SCORE

The American Urologic Association (AUA) Symptom Score is a valid and reliable tool to evaluate the severity of BPH (Table 30.2). It consists of seven items and can be self-administered or interviewer-administered. In addition to documenting initial severity of BPH, it can be used to guide treatment decisions, monitor treatment effectiveness, and track progression.

TREATMENT DECISIONS

The rates of transurethral surgery for BPH declined significantly from the mid-1980s to the mid-1990s (9). This decline was partly due to increasing availability of effective medical therapies. As a result, family physicians and other primary care providers have an important role in helping men make informed decisions regarding treatment.

The management of BPH is guided by symptoms. Men without bothersome symptoms are best managed by a strategy

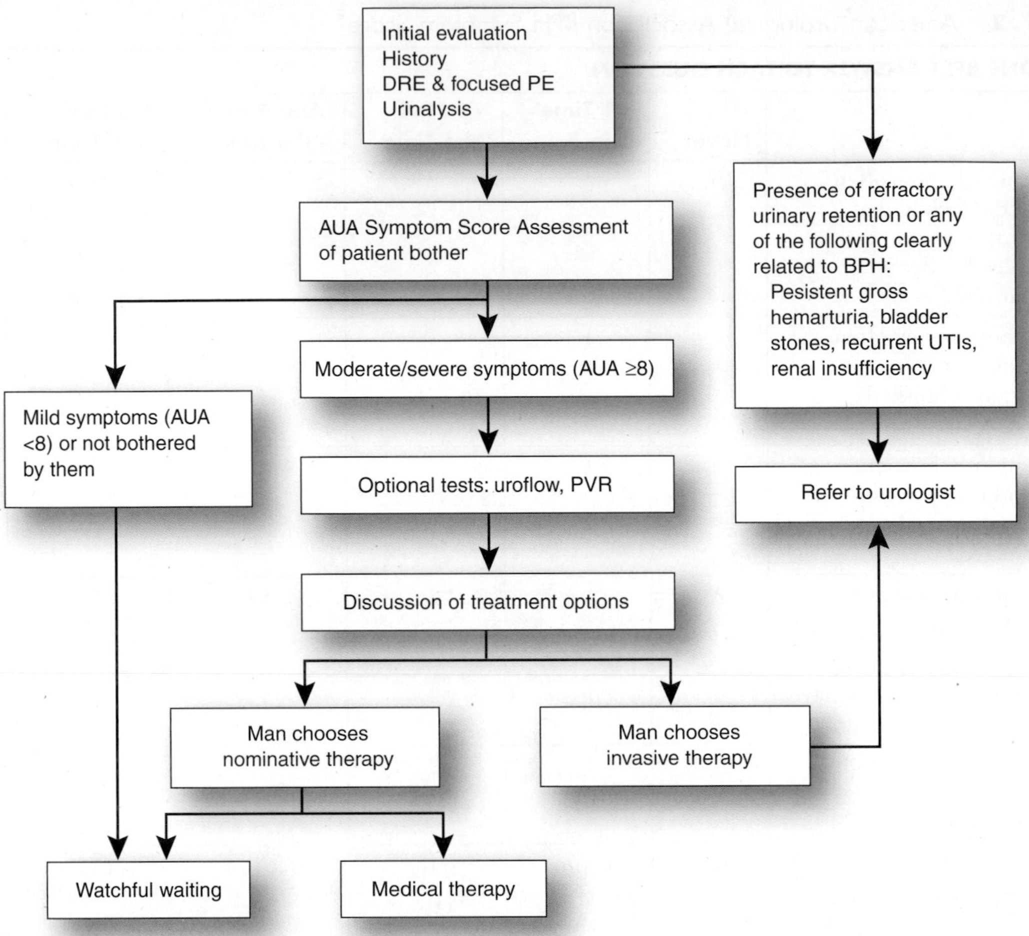

Abbreviations: DRE, digital rectal examination; PE, physical examination; AUA, American Urologic Association; PVR, post-void residual

Figure 30.1 • Benign Prostatic Hyperplasia (BPH) Diagnosis and Treatment. Adapted from: Management of BPH. *American Urological Association.* Available at: *http://www.auanet.org/content/guidelines-and-quality-care/clinical-guidelines/main-reports/bph-management/chapt_1_appendix.pdf.* Accessed November 20, 2009.

of watchful waiting (no active treatment). Men bothered by moderate to severe symptoms (AUA Symptom Score ≥8) could opt for watchful waiting, medical treatment, minimally invasive therapy, or surgery (Figure 30.1).

If the patient is to be managed expectantly (watchful waiting), additional general measures that might be helpful include avoiding caffeinated and alcohol-containing beverages (SOR B) and eliminating medications that can exacerbate urinary symptoms (e.g., diuretics, anticholinergics, tricyclic antidepressants). These men should be reevaluated yearly.

PHARMACOTHERAPY

α-Blockers

α-adrenergic blockers have been well studied and are generally the first-line medications used for BPH (Table 30.3). They reduce symptoms by relieving the dynamic component of bladder outlet obstruction. The currently used α-blockers are similarly effective and produce on average a 4- to 6-point improvement in the AUA Symptom Score (8).

5-α-Reductase Inhibitors

The 5-α-reductase inhibitors suppress the conversion of testosterone to dihydrotestosterone, which plays an important role in prostate growth. These medications reduce symptoms by relieving the fixed component of bladder outlet obstruction and are an option for men with BPH who have demonstrable prostatic enlargement. They are not effective—and thus not appropriate—for men who do not have enlarged prostates. They also must be taken for 3 to 6 months before a benefit is observed.

Combination Therapy

The combination of an α-blocker with a 5-α reductase inhibitor is slightly more effective than either agent alone in delaying the progression of symptomatic BPH in men who have enlarged prostates. The most well-studied combination is doxazosin with finasteride. Of 100 men with an average AUA Symptom Score of 17 treated for 1 year, monotherapy will help one to two men avoid clinical progression and combination therapy will help 3 men avoid clinical progression (10). Added cost and potentially more adverse effects are issues with combined therapy.

TABLE 30.3 Medications for BPH

α-blockers*
- Alfuzosin (Uroxatral)
  - Dose: 10 mg daily; take with food
  - Common adverse effects: orthostatic hypotension, dizziness, headache, weakness, rhinitis
  - Comments: May have less cardiovascular effects than doxazosin and terazosin
- Doxazosin (Cardura)
  - Dose: Start 1 mg at bedtime; titrate to 8 mg
  - Common adverse effects: orthostatic hypotension, dizziness, headache, weakness, rhinitis
  - Comments: May be useful in men with concomitant hypertension
- Tamsulosin (Flomax)
  - Dose: Start 0.4 mg daily; titrate to 0.8 mg
  - Common adverse effects: orthostatic hypotension, dizziness, headache, weakness, rhinitis
  - Comments: May have less cardiovascular effects than doxazosin and terazosin
- Terazosin (Hytrin)
  - Dose: Start 1 mg at bedtime; titrate to 10 mg
  - Common adverse effects: orthostatic hypotension, dizziness, headache, weakness, rhinitis
  - Comments: May be useful in men with concomitant hypertension

*The effects of doxazosin, tamsulosin, and terazosin are dose-dependent, and doses should be titrated gradually as side effects (e.g., orthostatic hypotension, dizziness) are also dose-dependent. Alfuzosin does not require titration. Because of increased incidence of side effects, neither the short-acting α-blocker prazosin (Minipress) nor the nonselective α-blocker phenoxybenzamine is recommended.

5α-Reductase Inhibitors
- Dutasteride (Avodart)
  - Dose: 0.5 mg daily
  - Common adverse effects: erectile dysfunction, decreased libido, decreased ejaculate volume
  - Comments: Consider checking PSA after 3 to 6 months for new baseline
- Finasteride (Proscar)
  - Dose: 5 mg daily
  - Common adverse effects: erectile dysfunction, decreased libido, decreased ejaculate volume, gynecomastia, orthostatic hypotension
  - Comments: Consider checking PSA after 3 to 6 months for new baseline; may increase risk of high-grade prostate cancer although lowers overall risk*

*Thompson IM, Goodman PJ, Tangen CM, et al. The influence of finasteride on the development of prostate cancer. *N Engl J Med.* 2003;349(3):215–224.

Plant Extracts

A Cochrane review concluded that saw palmetto (*Serenoa repens*) preparations are no more effective than placebo for treatment of BPH symptoms (11). Other plant extracts that have been studied include *Pygeum africanum* and B-sitosterol (12,13). The lack of standardization of herbal products must be considered when discussing them with patients. Dosages vary and adverse effects are generally mild. The current AUA Guideline does not recommend plant extracts for treatment of BPH.

INDICATIONS FOR UROLOGIC REFERRAL

Men with bothersome symptoms who are considering invasive therapy, either as an initial therapeutic option or because of symptoms refractory to medical management, should be referred to a urologist. Men who develop acute urinary retention should be referred for consideration of definitive therapy. Additional indications for referral are shown in Table 30.4. The evidence supporting pharmacologic and surgical treatments is summarized in Table 30.5.

TABLE 30.4 Indications for Referral for Men with Benign Prostatic Hyperplasia

- Acute urinary retention (especially if failed attempt at catheter removal)
- Bladder stones (although rarely from benign prostatic hyperplasia)
- Diagnosis is uncertain
- Man requests referral
- Recurrent gross hematuria
- Recurrent urinary tract infections
- Renal insufficiency (especially if responds to period of bladder catheterization)
- Symptoms refractory to medical management (most common reason)

TABLE 30.5 Evidence for Pharmacologic and Surgical Treatments

Intervention	Efficacy	SORT Rating*	Comment
TURP	10-point reduction in AUA Symptom Score	A	Surgical risks
α-blocker	4–6 point reduction in AUA Symptom Score	A	First-line medication
5α-reductase inhibitor	Combined with α-blocker, 6-point reduction in AUA Symptom score	A	Only in men with enlarged prostates

TURP = transurethral resection of prostate; AUA = American Urological Association.
*A = consistent, good-quality patient-oriented evidence; B = inconsistent or limited-quality patient-oriented evidence; C = consensus, disease-oriented evidence, usual practice, expert opinion, or case series.
For information about the SORT evidence rating system, see *http://www.aafp.org/afpsort.xml*.

SURGERY

Transurethral resection of the prostate (TURP) is considered the gold-standard surgical treatment for BPH. Symptom reduction is generally quite substantial. A large Veterans Administration study comparing TURP with watchful waiting showed a nearly 10-point reduction in symptom score in the TURP group compared to a 5.5-point reduction in the watchful waiting group. There was also a significant increase in urinary flow rate in men undergoing TURP (14).

Other surgical or invasive options include transurethral incision of the prostate (TUIP), transurethral needle ablation (TUNA), electrovaporization, and several techniques of laser prostatectomy. TUIP is an outpatient procedure generally limited to prostates of smaller size. TUNA is minimally invasive and performed under local anesthesia but is less effective than TURP. Both TUIP and TUNA are associated with high rates of secondary procedures. Prostatic stents might be used in certain high-risk patients with urinary retention but are associated with significant complications. Open prostatectomy is rarely performed for BPH in the United States and would generally be reserved for men with excessively large prostates.

PROSTATITIS

CLINICAL OBJECTIVES

1. Describe the differences between various prostatitis syndromes.
2. Discuss the management of the prostatitis syndromes.

Prostatitis is a common problem that tends to affect young and middle-aged men. Acute prostatitis is generally caused by ascending infection of the urinary tract and is the most easily recognized but least common of the prostatitis syndromes (Table 30.6). Approximately 7% of men with prostatitis have chronic bacterial prostatitis. It may occur as a complication of acute prostatitis or may manifest as recurrent UTIs. Chronic prostatitis/chronic pelvic pain syndrome (CP/CPPS) may present with similar symptoms, but no demonstrable bacterial source. It is the most common of the prostatitis syndromes.

Acute and Chronic Bacterial Prostatitis

The man with acute prostatitis will usually complain of urinary symptoms (irritative and obstructive), perineal or pelvic pain, and fever. Acute cystitis rarely occurs in men who have normal urinary tract anatomy and function. Thus, a lower UTI in a man should suggest prostatitis as the diagnosis. A DRE usually reveals a tender, boggy prostate. Prostatic massage for purposes of obtaining expressed prostatic secretions is not indicated (15). Urinalysis reveals leukocytes. A urine culture should also be ordered.

Acute prostatitis is treated with antimicrobials active against common infecting organisms, typically gram-negative rods (e.g., *Escherichia coli*, Proteus spp.), but also gram-positive cocci (e.g., enterococcus). Broad-spectrum antibiotics are begun while the urine culture is pending. Antibiotics can be tailored based on culture results and are continued for 4 to 6 weeks. Nonsteroidal anti-inflammatory drugs (NSAIDs), if not contraindicated, may be useful for pain relief.

Infection of the prostate gland, particularly if early treatment is not initiated, can be a source of severe systemic infection, or sepsis, which would necessitate hospitalization. A man who cannot tolerate oral antimicrobials also requires hospitalization.

A man who has recurrent UTIs not attributable to bladder catheterization or another urinary tract abnormality may have underlying chronic bacterial prostatitis. Such a patient may have had preceding acute bacterial prostatitis or may present de novo with urinary symptoms (e.g., dysuria, frequency) or low back, perineal, or groin discomfort. However, there is no evidence of acute prostatitis (e.g., no fever and normal DRE). Antibiotics are prescribed for a minimum of 6 weeks (Table 30.6).

Chronic Prostatitis/Chronic Pelvic Pain Syndrome (CP/CPPS)

CP/CPPS encompasses both the disorders previously referred to as nonbacterial (or abacterial) prostatitis and prostatodynia. The etiology is unknown, and studies do not support causative roles of infectious agents. Furthermore, it is not clear that the prostate is involved in all cases of CP/CPPS.

Symptoms are similar to those of chronic bacterial prostatitis (Table 30.6), but there is no identifiable source of infection. The "four-glass test," which includes postprostatic massage analysis of expressed prostatic secretions and urine, has been described for use in diagnosing CP/CPPS. However, its clinical usefulness is minimal (15). Treatment is with α-blockers and NSAIDs.

TABLE 30.6 Prostatitis Syndromes

Diagnosis	Symptoms	Physical Exam and Labs	Management
Acute prostatitis	Acute onset fever, chills, dysuria, pelvic or perineal pain	Tender, boggy, warm prostate Urinalysis reveals pyuria, bacteriuria, occasionally hematuria	Avoid prostatic massage and urethral catheters. Order urine culture and blood cultures, consider gonorrhea/chlamydia testing. Hospitalize if systemically ill and begin IV antibiotic (e.g., ampicillin/sulbactam or ampicillin plus aminoglycoside, fluoroquinolone). Oral antibiotic options: TMP/SMX DS or fluoroquinolone for 4–6 weeks. NSAIDs may help relieve pain and inflammation.
Chronic bacterial prostatitis	Gradual onset mild to moderate urinary symptoms; pain in low back, perineum, lower abdomen, genitals; painful ejaculation or hematospermia	Minimally tender or normal prostate exam Urinalysis consistent with UTI	Order urine culture. Consider gonorrhea/chlamydia testing. TMP/SMX DS or fluoroquinolone for 6 to 12 weeks. If recurrent, second course of antibiotics (for longer duration if the first course was 6 weeks).
Chronic prostatitis/chronic pelvic pain syndrome (CPPS)	Similar to symptoms of chronic bacterial prostatitis.	Prostate normal or minimally tender Urinalysis not consistent with UTI	Urine culture (should be negative). Consider gonorrhea/chlamydia testing. α-blockers (e.g., terazosin) for minimum of 6 months. NSAIDs and/or sitz baths may help pain.

IV = intravenous; TMP/SMX DS = trimethoprim/sulfamethoxazole double-strength; UTI = urinary tract infection; NSAIDs = nonsteroidal anti-inflammatory drugs.

PROSTATE CANCER

CLINICAL OBJECTIVES

1. Discuss prostate cancer screening and its effect on morbidity and mortality.
2. Cite problems with using PSA as a prostate cancer screening test.
3. Describe important elements of discussion with a patient who asks about prostate cancer screening.

Excluding nonmelanoma skin cancer, prostate cancer continues to be the most common cancer in American men and is second only to lung cancer as the leading cause of cancer death in men (16). The cause of prostate cancer is unknown. Of the most important known risk factors (Table 30.7), only diet is mutable.

Prostate cancer is generally slow growing, which contributes to the complexity of prostate cancer screening and the adage, "Many more men die *with* prostate cancer than *from* prostate cancer." Autopsy series have shown that among men who die from causes other than prostate cancer, up to one-fourth of those 50 to 59 years old have prostate cancer and two-thirds of men more than 80 years old have prostate cancer (17). Although an American man's lifetime risk of developing prostate cancer is 16%, his risk of dying from prostate cancer is 1% (16).

Occasionally, prostate cancer is diagnosed as a result of evaluation for symptoms such as difficulty urinating, new onset erectile dysfunction, or back or hip pain (advanced prostate cancer can metastasize to bone). Patients diagnosed in this manner are more likely to have advanced disease. Most prostate cancer, however, is diagnosed as a result of measuring blood levels of prostate-specific antigen (PSA) in asymptomatic men.

TABLE 30.7 Risk Factors for Prostate Cancer

Age
- Rare before age 45 years; risk increases with age

Race/ethnicity
- More common in black men than whites or Hispanics

Genetic Factors
- Men with a first-degree relative with prostate cancer have a twofold increased risk
- BRCA mutations may increase risk

Diet
- High in animal fat or low in vegetables increases risk

TABLE 30.10 Relative Risk of Lifestyle Variables and Co-morbid Conditions Associated with Sexual Dysfunction

Variable	Relative Risk	95% Confidence Interval
Physical activity*	0.7	0.6–0.7
Obesity†	1.3	1.2–1.4
Smoking	1.3	1.1–1.4
Television viewing time‡	1.2	1.1–1.3
Diabetes	1.5	1.2–1.9
Nonprostate cancer	1.4	1.1–1.6
Stroke	1.4	1.0–1.9
Antidepressant use	1.7	1.2–2.2
B-blocker use	1.2	1.1–1.5
Thiazide diuretic use	0.9	0.7–1.2
Finasteride use	1.2	0.7–2.3

*≥32.6 metabolic equivalent hours (METs) per week (equivalent of running 3 hours per week).
†Body mass index >28.7 kg/m^2.
‡>20 hours per week.
Data from: Bacon CG, Mittleman MA, Kawachi I, et al. Sexual function in men older than 50 years of age: results from the health professionals follow-up study. *Ann Intern Med.* 2003;139:161–168.

with a follow-up phase in 1995 through 1997 (39). Of men in their 40s, 40% admitted to some degree of sexual dysfunction, and this increased approximately 10% with each decade advance in age. Overall, 35% of men had moderate to complete ED (40). The follow-up study confirmed these age-associated declines and showed that these changes were nonlinear. In other words, the magnitude of change was larger with increasing age in all areas of sexual functioning (39). These changes included frequency of intercourse, erectile function, sexual desire, satisfaction with sex, and frequency of orgasm; notably, not all these variables are physically demanding, so there is no simple explanation for this decline (39).

This age-associated decline in sexual dysfunction was further confirmed in a prospective study in 31,742 men ages 53 to 90 years, 33% of whom (after men with prostate cancer were excluded) admitted to ED in the preceding 3 months. Other aspects of sexual functioning such as sexual desire and ability to achieve orgasm were again shown to sharply decline each decade after age 50 years (41).

Risk Factors

Several modifiable health factors have been linked with ED. Smoking, inactivity, and obesity are all associated with an increased risk of sexual dysfunction (Table 30.10) (41). Interestingly, alcohol intake did not appear to be a negative risk factor, and moderate intake appeared to be beneficial (relative risk 0.9) (41). Common comorbidities (e.g., diabetes) and medications including antidepressants, α-blockers, and β-blockers also have a negative effect on sexual functioning (41).

Problems with sexual functioning are not confined to the older population. In a 1992 study of adults aged 18 to 59 years, 31% of men had sexual dysfunction. Risk factors for this group were history of a STI, stress, recent decrease in household income, nonmarital status, history of same-sex activity, and history of adult–child sexual contact (42).

Normal Physiology

Normal penile erection is a vascular event that is triggered by neurologic stimuli in the presence of appropriate hormonal and psychologic influences. An erection begins with neural stimulation, which includes tactile and psychologic stimuli. Neural impulses enter the spinal cord and proceed via the parasympathetic pathway to the pelvic vascular bed, allowing for increased blood flow into the corpus cavernosa of the penis. A sacral reflex arc is activated by tactile stimulation, which also allows for redirection of blood flow into the penis.

With the proper stimuli, acetylcholine and nitric oxide (NO) are released by the nerves innervating the smooth muscle of the corpus cavernosum. NO enters the smooth muscle cells and, through a pathway involving cyclic guanosine monophosphate (cGMP), causes relaxation of the smooth muscle of the corpus cavernosum. The smooth muscle of the penile arteries also relaxes, allowing for increased arterial blood flow from the hypogastric artery into the penis. As the lacunar spaces within the corpus cavernosum fill with blood, they expand and pressure within the penis builds inhibiting venous outflow and producing an erection. Detumescence is mediated by sympathetic pathways and occurs when NO levels decrease, and the enzyme phosphodiesterase type 5 (PDE5) metabolizes cGMP (43,44).

Testosterone is not only an important factor in sexual desire, but is also thought to have a local effect on the penis. Testosterone receptors are present on the smooth muscle of the corpus cavernosum and appear to aid in maintaining NO levels in the penis. Thus, an adequate androgen supply is also necessary for an erection to occur (44).

Causes of Erectile Dysfunction

The cause of ED is usually multifactorial and can involve disruption anywhere in the spectrum of the vascular, neurologic, hormonal, and psychologic mediators of normal erectile physiology. It is important to remember that ED is not the sole manifestation of sexual dysfunction. Frequency of intercourse, sexual desire, ability to achieve orgasm, and overall satisfaction with sex are all important for the quality of an individual's sexual functioning.

An estimated 70% of cases of ED are vascular in origin (43). Normal arterial blood flow is an absolute requirement to sustain an erection. Failure to store blood in the venous system can also cause vasculogenic impotence. Many of the risk factors and comorbidities associated with ED are factors associated with poor circulation (Table 30.11).

NO activity and adrenergic stimulation are two factors involved in smooth muscle relaxation of the corpus. Thus, smokers, diabetics, and patients with testosterone deficiency are at additional risk due to lower levels of NO synthetase in their corpus cavernosum (38).

Depression was discovered by the MMAS to be the second most common risk factor for ED (40). Other psychogenic factors such as interpersonal conflict, stress, and anxiety, also play a role. Performance anxiety is common after a man experiences even one episode of ED; sex becomes an anxiety provoking experience and much of the man's focus becomes whether or not he will be able to perform. Adrenergic release due to stress during intercourse further perpetuates the problem by its effect on smooth muscle in the penis.

A complicating issue is that many of the medicines used to treat the risk factors for ED can themselves cause ED. Antidepressants, particularly selective serotonin reuptake inhibitors, can cause problems with libido and ejaculatory function as well as ED (43). Antihypertensives are probably the next most common class of drugs causing ED.

Initial Evaluation

A careful history and physical exam has a 95% sensitivity and a 50% specificity for diagnosing organic ED (45). Discussion of sexual function often needs to be initiated by the physician. In one survey, 71% of patients thought their doctor would dismiss their sexual concerns if brought up, and 68% thought that discussing the problem with their doctor would embarrass the physician (46).

TABLE 30.11 Risk Factors for Erectile Dysfunction

Age	Hyperthyroidism
Androgen deficiency	Hypothyroidism
Anxiety	Ischemic heart disease
Chronic renal failure	Medication use*
Cycling (prolonged pressure on pudendal and cavernosal nerves)	Metabolic syndrome Multiple sclerosis Obesity
Depression	Peripheral vascular disease
Diabetes mellitus	Prostate surgery
Dyslipidemia	Sedentary lifestyle
Genitourinary trauma	Substance abuse
Herniated discs	Tobacco use
Hyperprolactinemia	Unresolved patient/
Hypertension	partner conflict

*Common medications include α-blockers, antidepressants, β-blockers, cimetidine, clonidine, finasteride, ketoconazole, methadone, methyldopa, nicotine, spironolactone, thiazide diuretics.

Screening questionnaires such as the Sexual Health Inventory for Men (47) given at well-male visits can be useful tools to identify men who are having sexual issues; they can also provide the physician with a way of broaching the subject. Important questions in the history include the timing of the problem (rapid versus gradual), ability to achieve an erection and orgasm during masturbation, the presence of morning erections, and whether or not there are any marital problems. Sudden loss of erectile function with every attempt is almost always psychogenic in origin. The presence of nocturnal and morning erections means that neurologic reflexes and penile blood flow are intact; presence of these usually points to a psychogenic cause. The physician should assess for the presence of risk factors for ED.

A physical examination should include assessment of secondary sexual characteristics, a testicular exam (noting size and any masses or other abnormalities), assessment for normal penile anatomy, and a prostate exam to evaluate for evidence of prostatitis or malignancy. The physician should also be sure to note any evidence of poor circulation elsewhere in the body, the presence of gynecomastia, and any neurologic signs that could point to a pituitary tumor or spinal cord lesion.

The results of the history and physical examination should be used to guide the remainder of the evaluation. Laboratory studies may be done to assess for risk factors such as diabetes, hypercholesterolemia, hypogonadism, and endocrine abnormalities. One study of 1455 men with ED found abnormalities on laboratory testing in 28% of the patients (48). Low plasma testosterone was found in 6.9% of subjects, hyperprolactinemia in 1.2%, elevated random glucose in 9.3%, elevated ferritin in 1.6%, and hypercholesterolemia in 15%. Although glucose and lipid testing had the highest yield in this study, therapy was more effective for the conditions identified by the lower yield tests (testosterone and prolactin). Diabetes has been correlated with low testosterone levels, so elevated glucose levels should prompt further evaluation of androgen levels (49).

If history, physical exam, and laboratory testing fail to reveal an etiology, further testing is available but will usually require referral to a urologist. Nocturnal penile tumescence testing can be useful, particularly if the patient or his partner is unable to give a good history of nocturnal and morning erections. Portable devices such as the Rigi-Scan can be used to quantify the number and rigidity of nighttime erectile episodes. Rigi-Scan is up to 93% accurate for classifying ED as organic verus psychogenic, although there is a 12% false negative rate (45). Other special tests such as duplex ultrasound, angiography, and penile plethysmography are obtained less often, and should be left to the discretion of the consulting urologist. Typically these tests are reserved for patients who fail conservative management and are considering an invasive procedure.

Hypogonadism

Declining testosterone level is common as men age and is associated with both decreased libido and ED. Studies have shown a prevalence of 38.7% in men age 45 (50), and up to 50% of men in their 80s (51). In addition to sexual dysfunction, hypogonadism is associated with decline in cognitive functioning

TABLE 30.12 Contraindications to Androgen Replacement

Breast or prostate cancer
Abnormal prostate exam or elevated PSA without urologic evaluation
Hematocrit >50%
History of hyperviscosity syndrome
Severe LUTS
Class III or IV heart failure
Untreated obstructive sleep apnea

Seftel AD, Miner MM, Kloner RA, Althof SE. Office evaluation of male sexual dysfunction. *Urol Clin North Am.* 2007;34(4):463–482.
PSA = prostate-specific antigen: LUTS = lower urinary tract symptoms.

and general well-being, mood and sleep disturbances, and has been linked with metabolic syndrome (52).

Difficulties with the diagnosis and treatment of hypogonadism include lack of consensus on normal testosterone levels and the optimal method of measurement (total versus free testosterone). The US Food and Drug Administration cites 300 ng/dL as the lower limit of normal for total testosterone, although this arbitrary level has been challenged (52). There is a large overlap in testosterone levels in men with normal and abnormal libido (49). Consensus statements suggest that a total testosterone level <231 ng/dL or free testosterone <52 pg/mL requires treatment, while total testosterone >346 ng/dL or free testosterone >250 pmol/L should be considered normal (52).

Testosterone replacement in men with hypogonadism improves sexual function (49). Symptoms of hypogonadism should be present before supplementation is considered, regardless of testosterone level. Other causes of ED should be explored, as discussed previously. In the case of decreased libido, men should be screened for depression, a common finding in men presenting with sexual dysfunction.

Approved forms of testosterone supplementation to treat androgen deficiency, include intramuscular, oral, transdermal, and buccal preparations. Treatment goals should generally include a testosterone level in the mid-normal range and improvement in symptoms. Contraindications to starting or continuing treatment are listed in Table 30.12 (52).

Management

Of the 30 million American men currently estimated to suffer from ED, only 3 million are being treated (44). Treatment of any man with ED should follow a stepwise approach, beginning with the least-invasive therapies and continuing until an effective treatment is found (Figure 30.2). Lifestyle modifications such as weight loss, smoking cessation, and personal or marital counseling when indicated, should be considered first-line therapy. In one study, increased physical activity and reduction in BMI independently improved ED in obese men ages 35 to 55 years (53). Among men in the intervention group, 31% had regained sexual function after 3 years of lifestyle changes.

Modification of drug therapy when an offending agent is present is also an initial step. Treatment for comorbid conditions and androgen replacement should also be performed when indicated. If these changes are either ineffective or not feasible, the next line of treatment is usually oral medications. Figure 30.2 shows an algorithm that can guide evaluation and management.

PHARMACOTHERAPY

Oral Medications

The PDE5 inhibitors, sildenafil (Viagra), tadalafil (Cialis), and vardenafil (Levitra) are successful for the treatment of ED in 85% of cases, although they are less effective in men with diabetes (Table 30.13) (43,54). PDE5 inhibitors selectively inhibit the catabolism of cGMP, allowing the erectile response to occur in the presence of appropriate stimulation (54). It is important to emphasize to patients that PDE5 inhibitors work to enhance an erection rather than cause one. In other words, sexual stimulation is required in order to cause the NO release in the corpus cavernosum, which then works through cGMP to cause smooth muscle relaxation.

All of the PDE5 inhibitors are contraindicated in patients taking nitrates. Nitrates act as a donor of NO, which increases cGMP. Because PDE5 inhibitors prevent the breakdown of cGMP, the combination can cause an overload of cGMP and subsequently significant vasodilation and hypotension (55). A washout period for sildenafil and vardenafil of 24 hours (48 hours for tadalafil) is recommended before nitrate administration (55).

Table 30.13 compares the currently available PDE5 inhibitors with respect to dose, onset of action, and duration. Effectiveness is similar for these drugs; however, one study demonstrated that vardenafil was effective in 60% of men who

TABLE 30.13 Comparison of the PDE-5 Inhibitors

	Sildenafil	Tadalafil	Vardenafil
Doses (mg)	25, 50, 100	5, 10, 20	2.5, 5, 10, 20
Onset (min)	14–30	16–45	20–30
Duration (hours)	4	36	4
Active metabolite	Yes	No	Yes
Half-life (hours)	3–4	17.5	4–5
Side effects	Flushing, dyspepsia, headache, rhinitis, transient blue vision, hypotension		

Adapted from Carson CC. Erectile dysfunction: evaluation and new treatment options. Psychosomatic Medicine. 2004;66:664–671.

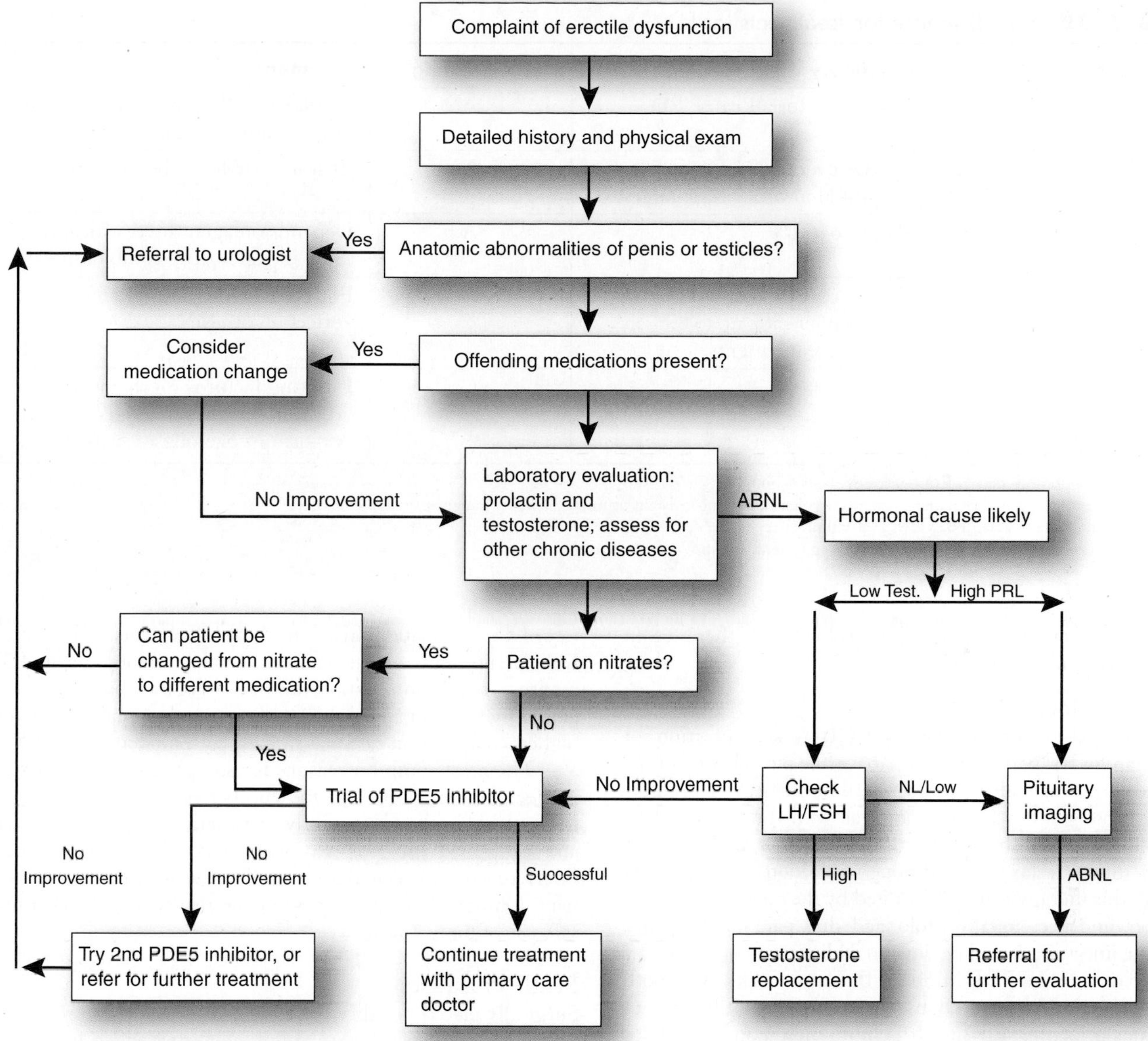

Abbreviations: ABNL, abnormal; NL, normal; PRL, prolactin; LH, luteinizing hormone; FSH, follicle stimulating hormones; PDE5, phosphodieterase-5

Figure 30.2 • Algorithm for management and treatment of erectile dysfunction.

did not respond to sildenafil (56). Thus, if a patient fails one PDE5 inhibitor, he may respond to another. Men should allow 6 to 8 trials to assess adequacy of PDE5 inhibitor treatment. Most PDE5 inhibitor's absorption may be affected by high-fat meals.

α-antagonists such as yohimbine are still prescribed by some physicians for the treatment of ED. Although some benefit has been reported in meta-analyses, controlled trials have shown lack of benefit (43).

Transurethral Drugs

After a patient has undergone an adequate trial of the PDE5 inhibitors, second-line therapy is usually either transurethral drugs or penile injections. Intraurethral alprostadil (MUSE) is prostaglandin E1 in pellet form that is inserted with an applicator about 3 cm into the urethral meatus. It is placed 5 to 10 minutes before intercourse and effects last about 1 hour. A randomized controlled trial of 1,511 men with various organic causes of ED showed successful intercourse in 43% versus 12% of the placebo group. Of the responders, 7 of 10 applications resulted in successful intercourse. Eighty-eight percent of men did not think that application of the pellet was uncomfortable. Side effects, the most common of which was penile pain, were mild and rarely resulted in discontinuation (57).

Unlike the oral agents, alprostadil will cause an erection even without sexual stimuli. Prostaglandin E1 works by stimulating intracellular production of cAMP. The combination of alprostadil plus sildenafil may be effective in patients not responding to monotherapy, but this should only be done

TABLE 30.14 Evidence for Treatments for ED

Intervention	Efficacy	SORT Rating*	Comment
PDE5 inhibitor	60–95% for all-cause ED	A	Similar for all agents; less effective for certain etiologies
Intraurethral alprostadil	43% overall; 67% among initial in-office responders	A	Efficacy rate for at home coitus
Intracorporeal injection therapy	Up to 97.6%	A	Depends on agent used; efficacy rate includes drug combinations
Vacuum-assist device	35% overall; includes high dropout rate; up to 89% in adherent patients	B	For rigidity only; no evidence for effect on orgasm
Penile prosthetic surgery	64%–93%	C	Limiting factor is mechanical dysfunction; for erection only, not orgasm or overall satisfaction

PDE5 = phosphodiesterase-5; ED = erectile dysfunction.
*A = consistent, good-quality patient-oriented evidence; B = inconsistent or limited-quality patient-oriented evidence;
C = consensus, disease-oriented evidence, usual practice, expert opinion, or case series.
For information about the SORT evidence rating system, see *http://www.aafp.org/afpsort.xml*.

under the recommendation of a urologist, as there is an increased risk of priapism (58).

Penile Injections

Intracorporeal injection therapy (ICI) is self-injection of prostaglandin E1, papaverine, or papaverine plus phentolamine into the corporeal body of the penis 10 minutes prior to intercourse. Prostaglandin E1 injections, as with the transurethral suppositories, work by direct stimulation of cAMP, causing smooth muscle relaxation. Although injections are generally painless, this therapy is usually limited by the man's fear of self-injection, and occasionally prolonged dull pain in the penis. Only one injection should be done in 24 hours.

Papaverine is a PDE inhibitor that also works by smooth muscle relaxation. It is rarely used as a single agent because of high rates of penile scarring. It is more often combined with phentolamine, which is a direct α-1-antagonist (43).

One study comparing 22 men on ICI and 31 men on sildenafil showed equal patient satisfaction with both treatments (59). Another study showed a 97.6% positive response rate with one of four ICI protocols, including combinations of drugs (60). Some men have even had a return of spontaneous erections after long-term treatment with ICI, particularly alprostadil. In one study, 85% of men were having spontaneous erections after 12 months of treatment compared with 37% at baseline (61). The most feared side effect of ICI is priapism, occurring in about 11% with papaverine and about 1% with alprostadil (62,63). For this reason, before issuing a prescription, urologists often administer the first dose of ICI in the office to monitor the patient for a prolonged erection.

OTHER TREATMENTS

Vacuum Assist Devices

Vacuum assisted erection devices are often the last step before invasive therapy. Several of these devices exist, which are engineered to increase arterial flow by vacuum pressure and use a tourniquet device to prevent venous outflow. The problems with these devices are a low patient satisfaction rate and high rate of discontinuation. In one study of 129 patients with organic ED given training on the device and followed for a mean of 37 months, the discontinuation rate was 65%, including all of the patients with mild ED and 70% of men with complete ED; the highest continuation rate was in men with moderate ED (64).

The most common reasons for stopping were that it was ineffective, too painful, or too cumbersome. Overall, 35% of the patients in the above study were satisfied with the device and continued use (64). Problems with the device include interference with ejaculation due to the tourniquet component, a hinge effect at the base of the penis, and a maximum safe use of up to 1 hour.

Penile Prostheses

Surgically placed prosthetic devices include malleable rods and inflatable prosthetics. These are usually reserved for last resort treatments. After a patient has failed oral agents, referral to a urologist is appropriate to determine further therapy. The evidence for these treatments of ED is summarized in Table 30.14.

KEY POINTS

- Benign prostatic hypertrophy is extremely common among aging men. When symptoms interfere with a man's quality of life, treatment options include medications or surgery.
- A urinary tract infection in a man is a clue to possible prostatitis. Treatment usually consists of several weeks of antibiotics. However, some types of prostatitis are not due to bacterial infection.
- It is unclear whether prostate cancer screening reduces mortality from prostate cancer. Before a man undergoes prostate cancer screening, clinicians should discuss the potential but uncertain benefits, possible harms, and gaps in the evidence.
- Most erectile dysfunction is vascular in origin. The first line pharmacologic treatment for erectile dysfunction in men not on nitrates who have no contraindication for sex is an oral phosphodiesterase-5 inhibitor.

CHAPTER

31

Relationship Issues

Sandra C. Clark and Timothy P. Daaleman

One of the joys of family medicine is the privilege of working with families. To follow a couple through pregnancy and delivery, and then to care for their growing family—helping them to manage acute and chronic illnesses, celebrating their successes, and guiding them through the various psychosocial stresses that inevitably arise during their individual and family life cycles—is satisfying and beneficial for both family and care provider. As a consequence of continuity of care, the bonds of mutual trust and affection increase exponentially. Many experienced primary care providers will agree that the most comprehensive and effective way to treat illness and stress in an individual is to understand the dynamic it has created within the patient's family.

In the past, the term "family" was restricted to married couples and their children; now we apply the term to those individuals who serve as someone's primary interpersonal network. The American Academy of Family Physicians defines family as a group of individuals with a continuing legal, genetic, and/or emotional relationship. This definition recognizes the fact that families now come in all shapes and sizes. The most recent census bureau report (2008) shows that 70% of children live with both parents (not necessarily biologic parents); 26% of children live with a single unmarried parent, usually a single mother; and 5% of children live with neither parent; the majority of these children are being raised by grandparents (1).

Increasing trends toward domestic and international adoption and same sex couples who raise children also affect the composition of today's family. It should also be noted that the percentage of women ages 40 to 44 years who are childless increased from 10% in 1976 to 20% in 2006, a consequence of higher infertility rates in women who defer childbearing for career, more couples deciding to forgo children, and more women remaining single and childless in life (2). It is a necessary challenge for the primary care provider to keep up with the evolving family as it grows, branches, and divides. Devoting a section of the medical chart or the electronic medical record to a family description or genogram can be extremely helpful.

The intent of this chapter is to explore issues relevant to primary care providers as they follow families coming together, expanding, breaking apart, and regenerating. The number and variety of relationship issues that present in the family care provider's office is vast; thus, in this chapter we will discuss some common problems with further information available in the recommended readings.

SEXUALITY AND SEXUAL IDENTITY

CLINICAL OBJECTIVES

1. Summarize how you might counsel a patient who is homosexual.
2. Analyze whether a person with a non-heterosexual sexual orientation should tell their family.

Sexual exploration and the struggle for sexual identity are important steps towards establishing a stable relationship. Results from the 2002 National Survey of Family Growth of 12,571 men and women aged 15 to 44 years provide normative data about sexual behavior:

- Multiple partners over the life span are common. Men ages 30 to 44 years reported a median of six to eight female sexual partners in their lifetimes; the median for women was about four.
- Oral sex without vaginal intercourse is common among heterosexual teenagers (13% of young men and 11% of young women at ages 15 to 17 years).
- Same sex activity is not uncommon. 6% of men reported having had anal or oral sex with another man (2.9% in the preceding 12 months); for women, 11% reported having a sexual experience with another woman (4.4% in the preceding 12 months). The proportion who considers themselves homosexual and bisexual is lower than the proportions who report ever having same-sex experiences. Among adults aged 18 to 44 years, 2.3% of men consider themselves homosexual, and 1.8% bisexual; for women, the corresponding proportions are 1.3% and 2.8%, respectively (3).

These data reflect both a certain amount of confusion and openness to experimentation on the part of teens and young adults regarding sexuality. When a young adult presents to a primary care practice, sexuality needs to be explored in a sensitive, nonjudgmental manner, with an emphasis on confidentiality. Also keep in mind that many teens and young adults do not include touching and fellatio in the category of "sex." The primary care provider should be comfortable discussing the possibility of sexual experimentation and the risks that experimentation might carry in terms of sexually transmitted infections and anxiety. Birth control and emergency contraception need to be a part of any discussion about sexuality. Patients may also need support and guidance if they plan to discuss their homosexuality or bisexuality with family and friends.

It is important to ask about a history of rape or childhood sexual abuse as part of a discussion on sexuality. A survey in 2001 showed a prevalence rate of 13.5% for women and 2.5% for men for sexual abuse, either by rape or molestation (4); other studies have put the rate of sexual abuse as high as 25% for women and 17% for men (5). Rape and childhood sexual abuse are strong predictors of depression, anxiety, substance abuse, and posttraumatic stress disorder (4). In addition, a history of rape or molestation, especially when penetration is involved, is a strong predictor of sexual dysfunction, including conditions such as anorgasmia, pelvic pain, or hypoactive sexual desire. These patients may benefit from psychotherapy (6).

For a homosexual teen or young adult, coming out to friends and family is probably one of the most stressful events of his or her life. This may be particularly difficult for children of immigrant families if there is a strong cultural bias against homosexuality and extramarital sexual intercourse. Family reactions vary widely, from acceptance to banishment from the family. Studies have shown that some parents go through a grief process when they discover that their child is homosexual which parallels the grief process for death—shock, denial, sadness, anger, and eventual acceptance. Some parents will attempt to bargain with their child, withholding love or financial resources until he or she "changes back" to a heterosexual orientation.

Nevertheless, most experts agree that coming out is a way to maintain honesty and intimacy within a family, and that admitting to a homosexual orientation ultimately benefits all involved. For patients who anticipate coming out to their family, primary care providers should caution patience and restraint in the face of their parents' or others' initial reaction. For example, if a parent's initial response is anger and rejection, he or she should avoid responding with more anger. Calmly reaffirming his position, or giving his parents more time to reconsider their position, is a far better response. In cases where parents react in an extreme manner, the provider should work to get the patient and his or her family into therapy (7).

THE INFERTILE COUPLE

CLINICAL OBJECTIVES

1. Describe how you manage a couple presenting with infertility at the first office visit.
2. Cite which aspects of an infertility evaluation can be performed by the family care provider.
3. Summarize when referral to a specialist is warranted and the type of specialist.

For couples wanting children, infertility can be a devastating blow to their view of who they are and what they want to achieve in life. Studies show that infertile women are significantly more depressed than their fertile counterparts, with depression and anxiety levels equivalent to those of women with heart disease, cancer, or HIV-positive status. In one study, 11% of infertile women studied met the criteria for major depressive episode.

Infertility is defined as 12 months of appropriately timed intercourse that does not result in conception. Only 20% of couples actively trying to conceive will be successful in a given month, but 85% will become pregnant within a year. Thus, by definition, the infertility rate for couples is about 15%. The likelihood of infertility increases as a woman ages. By the time a woman is 35 years old, the live birth rate is half that of the younger population (8).

The family care provider can play a very active role in the workup of infertility, especially in the early stages. Some problems, such as metabolic syndrome, can be entirely managed by the primary care provider. For persistent fertility problems, however, the primary care provider and the patient need to negotiate the point at which specialty care is needed. After referral, the primary care provider continues to offer psychosocial support to the family, and can help them with decision making.

Clinical Evaluation

When one considers all of the factors that must be in place and functioning to achieve conception, it is a wonder that the infertility rate is so low. A man needs an adequate quantity of high-quality sperm, which demands a functioning pituitary-gonadal axis and normal male anatomy. A woman needs functioning ovaries, high-quality ova, patent fallopian tubes, a receptive uterus, and a functioning pituitary-gonadal axis. In infertile couples, up to 40% involve a male factor, 30% to 40% are caused by female pelvic conditions (endometriosis, tubal disease, pelvic adhesions) and an additional 10% to 15% are attributed to ovulatory dysfunction and cervical factors. Roughly 10% of infertility cases remain unexplained after a thorough workup (8).

HISTORY AND PHYSICAL EXAMINATION

An infertility workup initially consists of a careful history and examination of both partners. Table 31.1 provides an overview of infertility history (9). Although women frequently present to the office alone to discuss infertility, having both partners present will provide more useful information for the provider, including direct observation of how the couple is interacting.

The physical examination and laboratory evaluation of men and women presenting with infertility are displayed in Table 31.2. Examination of men for varicoceles is best done with the patient standing and performing the Valsalva maneuver. Genetic testing should be considered if a disorder is suspected. For example, Klinefelter syndrome (XXY karyotype) is found in approximately 1 in 700 to 1,000 men and causes small, firm testes, low serum testosterone levels, and azoospermia (10).

Management

AMENORRHEA AND ANOVULATION

A woman older than age 16 years who has never had a menstrual cycle carries the diagnosis of primary amenorrhea and should be referred to an endocrinologist or gynecologist. Obtain lab tests for women with secondary amenorrhea or irregular menses (Table 31.2). To assess for hypogonadism, a

TABLE 31.1 Highlights of History-Taking for an Infertile Couple

Family history	Is there a family history of genetic disorders?
	Is there a family history of diabetes?
Sexual history	What is the timing of intercourse with the fertility period?
	Does the patient know the time of her fertility period during the cycle?
	Is there a history of erectile dysfunction or ejaculatory dysfunction?
	Is intercourse painful?
	Is there a history of sexually transmitted diseases?
Menstrual history	Are the patient's menstrual periods regular?
	Are her menses heavy or painful?
Toxin exposure	Has the patient been exposed to radiation?
	Does the patient use marijuana or alcohol? How much?
	Does the patient smoke?
Social history	How important is conception to both partners?
	How strong is the relationship at this point?
	How has the inability to conceive so far affected your relationship?
	What diagnostic testing or assisted reproductive technologies would you be willing to try?

Source: Trantham P. The infertile couple. *Am Fam Physician.* 1996;54(3):1001–1010.

progesterone challenge can be done with 10 mg of medroxyprogesterone acetate daily for 13 days. If there is menstrual bleeding after the progesterone challenge, estrogen production is adequate. A negative result (i.e., no withdrawal bleeding) suggests premature ovarian failure; a follicle stimulating hormone and estrogen level would confirm this diagnosis (10).

A common cause of anovulation is polycystic ovary syndrome (PCOS) (see Chapter 28), defined as the presence of oligo or anovulation in combination with hyperandrogenism. It has been estimated that 5% to 7% of women of reproductive age suffer from this disease. Endovaginal ultrasound can be helpful, especially if the patient has pelvic pain or a palpable ovary on exam, but it is not necessary to make the diagnosis of PCOS. Ultrasound will typically show ovaries with multiple small cysts.

Clomiphene and metformin are the most common treatments used by family care providers to treat ovulatory dysfunction. They can be used alone or in combination. Clomiphene is usually started at 50 mg per day for five days on days 3 to 7 of the menstrual cycle; the cycle either coming on its own, or induced using progesterone withdraw as described previously. Clomiphene induces ovulation in 8% to 30% of cases. A home ovulation kit can help guide the timing of intercourse. Metformin (at doses as high as 2,000 mg per day) is another option, especially when PCOS is suspected. A 2007 study showed a live birth rate of 22.5% in clomiphene users, 7.2% in metformin users, and 26.8% in the combination therapy group, demonstrating the superiority of clomiphene (11).

NORMAL MENSES

Women with a history of normal menses can be assumed to ovulate. Their workup should be directed toward anatomic problems, such as tubal patency, endometrial receptivity, the presence of scar tissue or endometriosis involving the pelvic organs, or inhospitable cervical mucus. This workup is usually done by a gynecologist. Performing a hysterosalpingogram involves injecting dye through the cervix and into the endometrial cavity, which then passes into the fallopian tubes. The hysterosalpingogram gives useful information regarding the shape and lining of the uterus, and the patency of the fallopian tubes. Hysteroscopy is used to directly view the endometrial lining to look for irregularities, such as scar tissue or polyps. Laparoscopy is used to visualize the pelvic organs.

GENERAL APPROACH

For most young couples with normal histories and exams, it is reasonable to get a semen analysis, document ovulation with a home kit, and wait up to 2 years before beginning more extensive testing. Couples with unexplained infertility have a pregnancy rate of 60% to 70% within 3 years. Because of their declining fertility rate, women who present at age 35 years for infertility require immediate evaluation and management. Women who are taking clomiphene, metformin, or both should be given a 3- to 6-month trial before referral to an infertility specialist for more aggressive therapies. Intrauterine insemination generally has a success rate of 17% per cycle, and in vitro insemination has a success rate of 44% per cycle (12).

Throughout the infertility workup the primary care provider needs to follow the mental health of the couple. How are they managing as a couple and individually? Is there a perception of blame by one partner towards the other? How is their sex life? Are they both in agreement with the workup and the increasingly expensive options for conception? Would they consider adoption and at what point? There are no easy answers for these questions, but the primary care provider can serve as an

TABLE 31.2 Physical Examination and Laboratory Evaluation for Infertility

Examination of Men Presenting with Infertility
Maneuver
Estimate volume of testes (normal >10 mL)
Check for varicoceles
Screen for sexually transmitted infection, if appropriate
Laboratory Tests
Semen analysis
Chromosomal testing if disorder suspected
Examination of Women Presenting with Infertility
Maneuver
Pelvic examination for anatomic abnormalities, evidence of infection, and adnexal tenderness
Thyroid exam (goiter)
Breast exam (galactorrhea)
Skin and hair (excess androgen)
Laboratory Tests
Secondary amenorrhea: thyroid stimulating hormone, prolactin, progestational challenge
If hirsutism, acne, and clitoromegaly: dehydroepiandrosterone sulfate level (DHEA-S) (congenital adrenal hyperplasia)
If hirsutism, obesity, male pattern baldness, or acanthosis nigrans: serum testosterone, fasting insulin, glucose, DHEAS, 17a hydroxyprogesterone (PCOS)

important facilitator for these discussions. The presence of marital stress and depression needs to be assessed and managed in the office, or by referral to a mental health specialist.

THE CHILD WITH SPECIAL CARE NEEDS

CLINICAL OBJECTIVE

1. Beyond listening and expressing empathy, describe what you can do to help parents with a child who has special needs.

Children with special health care needs (CSHCN) are defined as having medical, behavioral, or other health care needs for more than 1 year. According to the 2002 National Survey of CSHCN, almost 13% of US children meet this definition, including 4% who have chronic emotional, behavioral, or developmental problems (13).

In working with CSHCN, the concept of the "medical home" is critical. A medical home is an office or clinic where a patient can receive routine sick and well care, can identify a personal doctor or nurse as his or her own, has no difficulty in obtaining needed medical referrals, can get needed care coordination, and can have family-centered care. According to the National Survey, only half of CSHCN receive care that meets all five of the components established for medical home, and access to a medical home is significantly affected by race and ethnicity, and poverty (14).

The family care provider is ideally suited to provide the medical home for CSHCN. Because family care providers and their office staff can provide ongoing relationships with an entire family, the family medicine office is in an excellent position to help parents adjust to the grief and the altered circumstances that having a CSHCN can bring, and to make medical care a supportive part of their parenting of the child. Family-oriented health care providers can help coordinate and explain the results of the specialty care that is necessary. This is particularly true of families with cultural and language barriers.

Clinical Evaluation and Management of CSHCN

Caring for CSHCN requires that the primary care provider be well trained in detecting developmental and emotional problems at an early stage. Age-appropriate pediatric exam sheets or templates, which list developmental milestones for particular ages, should be available at the time of exam. Pediatric screening tools, such as the Child Development Inventory, the Pediatric Symptom Checklist for mental health problems, the Checklist for Autism in Toddlers, the Vanderbilt for attention deficit disorder are increasingly being used to detect problems early. Also, the primary care provider should be knowledgeable about the resources available in his or her area, and how to access these resources.

Practices that care for a large number of children may want to consider onsite psychological services or having a social worker on call to assist them with coordinating the care for CSHCN. For children with complicated mental and/or physical handicaps, a typical team might include a social worker who would work with the family to find resources in the community to assist the patient and family, a therapist for counseling, physical therapists, speech therapists, and occupational therapists. School aged children get many of these services through the school system.

INTIMATE PARTNER VIOLENCE

CLINICAL OBJECTIVES

1. Cite when you should consider a diagnosis of intimate partner violence.
2. Describe an appropriate evaluation for a victim of intimate partner violence.

Intimate partner violence (IPV) is defined as actual or threatened physical or sexual violence or emotional or psychological abuse by a current or former spouse or dating partner (15). It is the most extreme manifestation of relationship dysfunction, and is one of the more frustrating problems facing the primary care provider. Screening for and managing IPV is time consuming, requires frequent follow up, and often has an unsatisfactory outcome. But one has only to get past the front-page headlines of the local newspaper to see the consequences of IPV. Each year it is estimated that 1,200 women die as a consequence of IPV (16). This figure does not include the far greater number of victims who live in constant fear.

The victims of IPV are overwhelmingly female, women being abused 4.3 times more often than men (15,17). One in four women in the United States has reported being physically and/or sexually abused by a current or former partner, and 1.5% report being abused within the last year (18). A recent study of four community-based primary care internal medicine clinics confirms these figures, and stresses the need for screening. In that study, 21.4% of women who completed the self-administered survey in the clinic reported having experienced domestic violence sometime in their adult lives, and 5.5% had experienced domestic violence in the year before presentation (19). The study administered several psychological tests to women who had recently been abused, and to women who had not been abused. In comparison with women not recently abused, women suffering abuse within the last year were more likely to be younger than 35 years; single or separated; had more physical symptoms (e.g., headache, back pain); had higher scores on measures of depression, anxiety, and somatization; were more likely to be abusing drugs and alcohol; and were more likely to have attempted suicide (19).

Pregnancy is a particularly susceptible time for women to be abused, with estimates as high as 17% of women being physically or sexually abused at this time (20).

Clinicians must be familiar with the typical cycle of abuse. The cycle begins with a gradual increase in tension between the victim and the abuser. This can take the form of name calling, increasing jealousy, suspicion of infidelity, and/or controlling behavior. The tension mounts until the victim is physically or sexually assaulted. A period of remorse on the part of the abuser then follows during which time he or she will ask forgiveness and promise change; the victim will frequently forgive and take back the abuser. A variable period of relative stability will ensue, followed by increasing tension as before. Not all IPV follows this cycle, however, because some abuse will end after the first cycle; for others the violence is either unpredictable or not mitigated by periods of tranquility.

Clinical Evaluation

All women should be screened for IPV. It is reasonable to screen during annual exams and during urgent visits that involve injuries consistent with IPV, multiple somatic complaints, or depression. However, it is dangerous for a victim of IPV to be asked about domestic violence when the abusing partner (or someone who might report to the abusing partner) is present. Therefore, all screenings, whether written or oral, must be done with only the patient present. Getting the patient alone should, however, be approached with caution, creativity, and diplomacy, because a controlling partner will often not let the patient out of sight in a clinic, for fear that they will admit to abuse.

There are several screening tools available to detect IPV in a primary care setting:

- The Conflict Tactics Scale (CTS) and the Index of Spouse Abuse (ISA) are the gold standards of detection, but are time consuming and impractical in an office setting; the ISA consisting of 30 items on a scale of 1 to 5, and the CTS consisting of 19 items on a 7-point ordinal.
- The Partner Violence Screen (PVS) consists of the following four questions: (i) Have you been hit, kicked, punched, or otherwise hurt by someone within the past year?; (ii) If so, by whom?; (iii) Do you feel safe in your current relationship?; and (iv) Is there a partner from a previous relationship who is making you feel unsafe now? The PVS shows sensitivity of 71.4% and specificity of 84.4 (21).
- The Abuse Assessment Screen, is designed to assess IPV in pregnancy and consists of the following three questions: (i) Within the last year have you been hit, slapped, kicked, or otherwise physically hurt by someone?; (ii) Since you've been pregnant have you been hit, slapped, kicked, or otherwise physically hurt by someone?; and (iii) Within the past year, has anyone forced you to have sexual activities? This questionnaire also has a body map for marking injuries (20).
- The Hurt, Insulted, Threatened, and Screamed (HITS) scale is a paper and pencil instrument that comprising the following four items that are scored on a 5-point scale: How often does your partner physically hurt you, insult you or talk down to you, threaten you with harm, and scream and curse at you? One study has shown a sensitivity of 96% and a specificity of 91%, using a cutoff of greater than 10.5 as indicative of abuse (22).

After the primary care provider determines that a patient is the victim of IPV, the next step is to assess the acuity of the situation. Is it safe for the patient to go home? Should the police be called?

Two states require reporting domestic violence: Kentucky and California, whereas eight states require the reporting of nonaccidental or intentional injuries: Alaska, California, Colorado, Florida, Georgia, Michigan, Ohio, and Pennsylvania. Reporting is controversial. Some opponents state that it discourages some women from seeking treatment for IPV, and that it increases the risk of retribution by the abusing partner. Proponents feel that it takes the burden of the decision from an often conflicted victim, and that it leads to more arrests and treatment of abusing partners (23).

If a patient is thought to be in imminent danger of further abuse, whether or not the police are involved, the provider and patient should negotiate a safety plan by placing her in a shelter for battered women, a hotel, or with a trusted relative or friend. If the patient decides to return home, prompt follow up by office visit or phone call should be completed.

HISTORY AND PHYSICAL EXAMINATION

After the acuity of the situation is resolved, the provider needs to perform a thorough history, and a focused exam. The history should include:

- **Time frame:** When did the abuse start?
- **Manner:** How is the partner being abused?
- **Frequency:** How often is the patient being abused?
- **Past Plan:** What are the actions and resources that the victim has used in the past to **deal** with the abuse?
- **Future Plan:** Does the patient have a **plan** for dealing with future abuse?
- **Safety:** Are there others in the home, particularly children, who are at risk for abuse?

If the patient presents with physical evidence of abuse, the mechanism of injury must be fully detailed. A body map or photograph demonstrating the location and severity of the injuries is a very useful supplement to written notes.

Management

One of the most important roles that a primary care provider can play when dealing with a victim of IPV is to listen. Admitting to abuse is often painful and embarrassing. Many victims blame themselves for the abuse. It is important to dispel this myth. Simply stating "nobody ever deserves to be abused by their partner" can be very powerful and affirming for the patient. The primary care provider needs to have a good understanding of community resources to discuss options, such as alternative living situations or local shelters. Handouts with important numbers, including crisis hotlines, legal resources, and emergency shelters, should be given. Close follow-up is important.

In addition to dealing with IPV issues, comorbidities should be addressed. Alcohol, drug addiction, and depression are frequently present in abused women. Both conditions impair the victim's ability to make decisions and plan for the future, and treatment can make a tremendous difference in their ability to cope (19).

Finally, primary care providers need to consider the management of IPV as an ongoing process. Many women will repeatedly return to an abusive situation, often for years, before leaving their partners; some women never leave; and sometimes the abuse stops with or without intervention. The provider needs to constantly reassess the situation and guide the patient toward a safe and positive outcome. It is also critical to realize that women are particularly susceptible to abuse when they leave a relationship. In fact, many women will refuse to leave an abusive partner for fear of retaliation. In a 2003 study of women who survived a homicide attempt by an intimate partner, two-thirds of the attempts happened around the time of a relationship change, and half of the women did not realize that their lives were in danger. Thus primary care providers need to make sure patients have a safety plan when they intend to leave their abusive partner (24).

INFIDELITY

CLINICAL OBJECTIVES

1. Demonstrate how you would discuss the results of a newly positive test for sexually transmitted infection with a patient who is unaware of possible infidelity.
2. Summarize how you might counsel such a patient.

Infidelity is a common challenge faced by couples, which has lasting effects on a relationship because once discovered, it causes mistrust and a reevaluation of the core values shared by the couple. It is estimated that between 20% to 25% of Americans will have sex with someone other than their spouse while they are married. In the past, the male partner was more likely to engage in extramarital sex (EMS), but as women have entered the workforce the difference between the sexes has narrowed. Studies have shown that, compared to faithful partners, perpetrators of EMS are less satisfied with their marriage, have a higher level of education and socioeconomic status, and were married at a younger age. Infidelity occurs most often when one partner works, and the other is unemployed (25).

EMS most often presents in primary care in the context of a sexually transmitted infection (STI). Whether or not the infection is suspected, discussing the implications of an STI is akin to walking through a mine field—one never knows when or if an explosion will occur. Therefore, first and foremost, do not discuss the implications of an STI with a patient until you have the results in hand. Many relationships have been ruined based on the suspicion of an STI, which later turned out to be a nonsexually transmitted infection. Discussing a positive test for an STI should preferably be done face-to-face with the infected patient—alone. The implication of infidelity should be frankly but tactfully discussed. If the patient is the perpetrator, discussions need to center around informing all partners involved, so that they will also seek treatment. If the patient is the "victim" of EMS, guiding the patient through the basics of how to confront his or her partner can be very helpful. The safety of both the accusing party and the accused needs to be assessed.

Primary care providers should routinely ask about infidelity during physical exams. "How strong is your relationship with your current partner?" will occasionally elicit a discussion on actual or suspected EMS. A more telling question is "Would you like to be tested for sexually transmitted infections as part of the exam?" A positive answer should be followed up and discussed.

Not surprisingly, infidelity frequently leads to long-term problems within a relationship. In one sampling of psychotherapists, 34% of couples seeking treatment where EMS was involved ended up divorcing, and only about 15% of relationships remained intact and were characterized by improvement and growth (26). Couples therapy or individual therapy should be encouraged to guide patients through decisions about recommitting to versus ending their relationship.

MARITAL SEPARATION AND DIVORCE

CLINICAL OBJECTIVES

1. Describe how you would counsel a married patient in an increasingly distant and unsatisfactory relationship.
2. Summarize how the primary care provider can anticipate and guide young couples early in a relationship.
3. Cite how divorce impacts families.

Throughout the family cycle, the primary care provider needs to be aware of the usual stresses that marriages go through and provide anticipatory guidance. For example, the years after the first child's birth are both some of the best years of a couple's life and the most stressful for the parents, placing a strain on the marriage. A newborn brings many sleepless nights, adjustments of work schedules and careers, constant negotiation and relegation of parental duties, and less intimacy. Mothers and fathers who decide to quit their jobs to stay at home with the baby may feel underappreciated and socially isolated. During this critical time, the provider might initiate

TABLE 31.3 Tips on Working with Individuals and Couples

Schedule or choose a time to talk when there will be little distraction.
Keep your discussions private; avoid having them in front of family or friends.
Start with a positive statement. For example: "I love you and I see that you have been working very hard to help me, but I am feeling . . . "
Use "I" statements instead of "YOU" statements. For example: "I" get upset when I'm not consulted on how we should handle our finances" instead of "You never include me in big financial decisions."
Do not walk out in the middle of a conversation, unless you feel that you are on the verge of doing or saying something you will regret. If you do leave a discussion, try to continue it as soon as possible.
It is okay to initiate a difficult or complicated conversation with a letter, but the letter must be followed with face-to-face conversation.
Discussions are not "won" or "lost." Both parties should feel they have gained something.
Try to understand and accept a patient or couples belief system and values; don't impose yours on them. Many couples and families may function quite harmoniously with a very different concept from yours of how a family should work. Focus on the problem that they specifically bring to you.
Try to give patients an easy, concrete task to complete before the next visit. For example, if the couple was arguing about how to divide up child care responsibilities, for the next visit have them separately draw up a list of things they would be willing to do.

Source (first 7): Starling BP, Martin A. Improving marital relationships: strategies for the family physician. *J Am Board Fam Pract.* 1992;5(5): 511–516.

a conversation by asking how the couple is dealing with the demands of having a baby, and then, depending on the response, the provider could discuss proper communication techniques, the need for a part-time baby sitter on a regular basis, or local resources for stay-at-home parents. Other examples of stresses that may occur within a family include job changes, illness, or financial issues. Table 31.3 provides a number of tips for physicians working with individuals and couples, including counseling couples who are having difficulty (27).

The scope of divorce in the United States is far reaching. Consider these statistics from 2001:

- Approximately 45% of marriages end in divorce.
- Only 50% of single parent households headed by the mother have child support agreements from the father, and of those, only 50% receive the full amounts due.
- An employed mother in a two-parent home is in contact with the children 25 hours a week. After the divorce, this number decreases to 5.5 hours a week. A housewife spends 45 hours a week with her children; after divorce she spends 11 hours a week with them.
- The employed father pre-divorce spends an average of 20 hours a week with his children, but only 2 hours a week after the divorce.
- Five years after a divorce, one of three children found themselves still embroiled in the ongoing bitterness of their two battling parents. At 10 years, half of the women and a third of the men studied were still intensely angry at their former spouses (28).

These are grim statistics; divorce takes a toll on both parents and children. Divorce usually involves the betrayal of an ideal for marriage followed by a breakdown in effective communication. What once was a relationship built on trust and shared goals becomes a dysfunctional and angry set of individuals (29).

Children can suffer before, during, and after divorce. Parents in a high conflict relationship often have no emotions or time left over for their children, and they frequently project their anger and frustration toward their partner onto their children. Children are often witnesses to verbal and at times physical abuse. They will often be drawn into alliances with one parent against the other and begin distancing themselves from one parent. As a result, studies have shown that children of divorce have more behavioral, academic, and conduct problems than children with intact families. In fact, approximately half of these problems are detectable as early as 4 years before parents actually separate. In these families, divorce might actually be better for the children, rather than staying in a high conflict situation (30).

Several recent studies support the trend towards joint custody (31). Children spend more time with both parents in this situation. When both parents continue in the parenting role—helping with homework and setting limits for example, instead of using their time for special trips and entertainment—children appear to adjust better. Children whose parents decide on mediation instead of a prolonged and occasionally ugly legal battle tend to do better as well.

Half of divorced people remarry within 5 years (28). If one or both of the parents bring children into the new relationship, a "blended" family begins. Living in a blended family requires flexibility and many adjustments by everyone in the family. Depending on custody arrangements, children may or may not be in the home at any given time. New alliances have to be established, and the prickly issues of respect and authority have to be negotiated.

Primary care providers are ideally positioned to help a struggling family. As discussed earlier, interventions early in the conflict, done in the office or by a family therapist, should be aimed at reestablishing effective communication. The "Ten Commandments of Divorce" (Table 31.4) is a helpful tool that can be provided as part of primary care-based counseling (28).

Throughout a separation or divorce, comorbidities such as depression and insomnia need to be addressed, and the family, separately or together, should be followed closely for problems related to the conflict. It is crucial for the family care provider to recognize that the parents' psychological health and the strength of the parent-child bond are important factors for a family in this transition.

TABLE 31.4 The Ten Commandments for Divorcing Parents

1. Inform the children of the divorce and explain the reason for the divorce in terms that are appropriate for the ages of the children, and are neutral. Both parents should be present and all children should be told at the same time, unless it is impossible. 2. Reassure the children (especially the younger children) that the divorce is not their fault. Repeat this explanation over and over and over. 3. Except for cases of abusive relationships or concerns of immediate safety, inform the children well in advance of anyone moving out of the house. 4. Clearly inform the children of the expected family structure after the divorce, and who will live where. Discuss visitation clearly. 5. Do not make children be adults. 6. Do not discuss money. Children do not comprehend money or the true costs of maintaining a household. If they ask, do not lie, but be aware that $200 seems like a small fortune to a school-aged child.	7. Children need rules. Be consistent in this area, even if it is the only area in your entire life that is consistent. 8. Children must never be forced into taking sides. Both parents love them, and they can love both parents. 9. Belittling your ex-spouse should be avoided within earshot of the children. They believe everything you say, even when it is out of anger or frustration. But do not lie to cover up irresponsible behavior by the other parent. Children will see through it quickly and your credibility will suffer in other areas. 10. Never, ever put your children in the middle between you and your spouse. They are not buffers or pawns or messengers or prizes to divide like property. They are your children. They are the most precious things in the world to any parent. They are the one best things that came out of the marriage.

Source: Bryner CL. Children of divorce. *J Am Board Fam Pract*. 2001;14:201–210.

THE IMPACT OF DISABLING CHRONIC ILLNESS ON FAMILY RELATIONSHIPS

CLINICAL OBJECTIVES

1. Describe your clinical roles and responsibilities to both the patient with dementia and his or her caregiver(s).
2. Summarize your screening approach for family stress or emotional distress in patients or other family caregivers as chronic illnesses progress.
3. Cite some clinical interventions and approaches to caring for a patient's illness that are inclusive of family caregivers.

Chronic diseases, such as heart disease, stroke, cancer, and dementia are among the most prevalent and serious health conditions today, accounting for 70% of all deaths in the United States (32). These diseases disproportionately affect older adults; approximately 80% of elders have at least one chronic condition resulting in pain, loss of function, or limited activity (33).

The scope of care delivered to these patients by family members is staggering: an estimated 27.6 million family caregivers provide care to patients, and the economic value of their care is estimated to be $196 billion (34). There is wide variation in the amount of care needed depending on the disease. For example, annual care costs for patients with Alzheimer disease are estimated at $65 billion; for depression, however, these costs total only $9 billion (35,36). Patients with Alzheimer disease are dependent on caregivers for long periods, greatly impacting family caregivers' time and taxing their financial resources (37,38).

Caregiving generally connotes informal and unpaid care, which is usually provided by family members, and goes beyond the support provided in social relationships (39). The primary family caregiver is most often the spouse (70%), followed by an adult child (20%), and friends or distant relatives (10%); 70% of caregivers are women (40,41).

Clinical Evaluation

Caregiving exerts a substantial strain, so primary care providers should be attentive to stressors that impact the emotional and physical health of family caregivers. The patient-provider continuity in a longstanding provider-family relationship offers the provider familiarity with the patient's social and cultural context, which impacts the illness trajectory (42). With this understanding as a foundation, clinicians can gauge the impact of illness on family caregiving by monitoring stressors and resources (34). Stressors include caregiving tasks and conflicts (e.g., family conflict, employment strains, financial burden) that occur as a result of caregiving (37).

Providers should be attentive to physical complaints that may indicate caregiver burden or burnout. Poor sleep, increased irritability, and depressed mood or affect can be indicators of worsening emotional strain (37). Community-based resources, such as area agencies on aging and faith communities, can provide respite and other supportive services to help reduce the physical and emotional burden of caregiving.

Management of Family Relationships in the Context of Chronic Illness

A family-focused approach to chronic illness emphasizes several areas: (i) defining and assessing the relational context in which care takes place; (ii) including the caregiver, other family members, and friends as potential targets for interventions; (iii) addressing the relational, personal, and educational needs of the patient and family members; (iv) viewing disease as an ongoing process that requires continuity of care between the health care team and the family; and (v) including the patient, caregiver, and other family members in outcomes assessment (42).

Interventions to help manage family relationships and reduce potential negative outcomes for the family system include support groups, addressing family relationships, and psychotherapy (42). Support groups target coping, decision making, and problem solving among family members. Family relationship interventions use a variety of behavioral and educational techniques to foster emotional expression and collaboration among family members. Psychotherapy is usually reserved for families with severe dysfunctional relationships caused by the disease burden or preexisting family dynamics (42).

It is inevitable that as patients get sicker, primary care providers will increase their interaction with caregivers. Providers can help caregivers:

- Obtain health care power of attorney. This is especially important if the caregiver is not the patient's spouse. When many decisions need to be made quickly, a family needs one voice, and legally that voice is the person with the health care power of attorney.
- Know the patient's end-of-life wishes and help caregivers feel comfortable carrying out those wishes.
- Know about existing community resources to help care for the patient at home.
- Consider in advance, at what point, if any, the caregiver would wish to have the patient placed in an alternative living situation.
- Determine how the caregiver is faring with the stress.

Another tool the primary care provider can use to help a family understand and better care for an ill family member is the family meeting. When done properly, the family meeting serves to update the family on the patient's condition, discuss the course of the patient's disease, and answer questions about past and future testing and therapies. It is also a great opportunity to observe how the family interacts, to mediate differences in opinion, and to negotiate a path that hopefully is agreeable to all. Ultimately, the family meeting is most helpful to the primary caregiver who will feel more supported and less overwhelmed with the patient's ongoing care. The primary care provider can encourage this process by asking each family member or friend how they can help the caregiver and patient.

Death, Dying, and Bereavement

Chronic illness often leads to a transition from active care to palliative care. Primary care providers need to keep in mind four major areas in providing palliative care: effective communication and establishment of care goals; coordination of care; pain and symptom care; and social, spiritual, and bereavement support (43).

TABLE 31.5 Summary of Key Evidence-based Recommendations Regarding Management of Relationship Issues

Recommendation	Strength of Recommendation*
Sexuality	
Screening annually for chlamydia in adolescents	A
Screening for HIV, RPR, GC annually in adolescents	B
Counseling adolescents on birth control	C
Counseling homosexuals on coming out	C
Infertility	
Metformin for the use of polycystic ovary disease	B
Clomiphene for the use of ovulatory dysfunction	B
Assisted technologies for couples with infertility	C
Intimate Partner Violence	
Screening women for domestic violence	C
Divorce	
Counseling on effective communication between couples	C
Self-Management of Chronic Illness	
Effectiveness of using self-management in chronic illness	B

*A = consistent, good-quality patient-oriented evidence; B = inconsistent or limited-quality patient-oriented evidence; C = consensus, disease-oriented evidence, usual practice, expert opinion, or case series HIV = human immunodeficiency virus; RPR = rapid plasma reagin; GC = gonococcus.
For information about the SORT evidence rating system, see *http://www.aafp.org/afpsort.xml*.

2008. This increase is likely due to increased screening, more sensitive screening tests, and increased emphasis on reporting.

Overall, chlamydia infection is seen more often in minority populations and in women, especially young women. Women aged 24 years or younger are 5 times more likely to be infected than those older than 30 years. The greater risk among young women is probably from behavioral characteristics, as well as physiological factors such as increased exposure of cervical columnar epithelium. Other risk factors for infection include: (i) sexually active adolescents (5% to 10% prevalence), (ii) multiple sex partners, (iii) a partner with other partners during last three months, (iv) a recent new partner, (v) inconsistent use of barrier contraception, (vi) unmarried status, (vii) trading sex for drugs or money, (viii) history of prior STIs, (ix) living in urban areas and lower socioeconomic status, (x) education not beyond high school, (xi) patients attending sexually transmitted disease (STD) clinics, (xii) those with mucopurulent discharge form cervix or urethra, and (xiii) incarceration.

Pregnant women are at increased risk of acquiring chlamydia because of physiological immunosuppression and/or cervical ectopy. When left untreated, this infection during pregnancy increases the risk of miscarriage, premature rupture of membrane, prematurity, intrauterine growth retardation, and postpartum endomyometritis.

Clinical Evaluation

C. trachomatis and *Neisseria gonorrhea* cause similar clinical syndromes, but the former tends to cause fewer acute manifestations and more significant long-term complications. Chlamydia is transmitted through infected secretions and mucous membranes of urethra, cervix, rectum, conjunctiva, and throat. In addition, an infected mother can infect her baby during vaginal delivery (vertical transmission). The incubation period ranges from 1 to 2 weeks. Asymptomatic infection occurs in approximately 70% of women and 50% of men; however, in women it can produce insidious pathological damage of the upper genital tract without providing protective immunity (2).

Presenting symptoms vary depending on gender, age, and site of infection. Lower genital tract infection (endocervix) is the most common in women; they can present with a mucoid vaginal discharge without odor, abnormal menstrual bleeding, and lower abdominal pain.

Physical findings include cervicitis (inflammation of the cervix) with a yellow or cloudy mucoid discharge from the cervical os. Chlamydia infections in the lower genital tract do not cause vaginitis so if vaginal discharge is present without cervical discharge, look for a different diagnosis or co-infection (see Chapter 33). The infected cervix is often friable (tends to bleed easily) when touched with a swab or spatula. One can also see ectocervical erythema, ulceration, or both. Cervicitis, however, is due to documented gonorrhea or chlamydia infection in only 25% of women so signs and symptoms alone cannot be used to predict chlamydia infection.

Urethritis is the most common manifestation of chlamydia infection in heterosexual men. Approximately 30% to 40% of urethritis in men is secondary to *C. trachomatis;* the prevalence decreases as men age (3,4). Dysuria or perimeatal tingling are the most common symptoms. A mild to moderate, clear to white urethral discharge may be present, best observed in the morning before voiding. In order to observe the discharge, the penis may need to be milked.

Diagnostic Testing

Wet mount and the amine test (significant odor release with addition of potassium hydroxide to vaginal secretions) on vaginal discharge helps differentiate chlamydia infection from other infections such as urinary tract infection, bacterial vaginosis, and trichomoniasis. In the wet mount, the presence of >10 white blood cells per high-power field is a predictor of endocervical infection.

The diagnosis of nongonococcal urethritis can be confirmed by the presence of >5 white blood cells per high power field in a Gram stain of penile discharge in the absence of intracellular gram-negative diplococci. Other tests that support the diagnosis of urethritis are a positive leukocyte esterase test or presence of >10 white blood cells per high-power field in a first void urine specimen.

C. trachomatis infections can be detected using culture of epithelial cells (it is an obligatory intracellular organism) and nonculture techniques. Culture is considered the gold standard (near 100% specificity). Because viable infectious chlamydia elementary bodies are detected only by culture, this is the method of choice for medicolegal cases and for conducting antibiotic susceptibility testing with persistent infection following treatment. Otherwise, the highly sensitive and specific nonculture techniques—nucleic acid amplification tests (NAAT)—have replaced the chlamydia culture (3,4).

The Centers for Disease Control and Prevention (CDC) recommends using one of the several available NAAT assays when screening for chlamydia infection in both men and women. Their advantages include: (i) high performance (sensitivity >90% and specificity >99%), (ii) ability to detect *N. gonorrhoea* from the same specimen, and (iii) ability to produce reliable results with noninvasive (self-collected) specimens such as urine, vulvovaginal swabs, and tampons, making them acceptable to most patients. They do, however, cost more than culture methods and can remain positive for up to 3 weeks after the pathogen's death because of its ability to amplify the genetic material of the nonviable organism. Thus, early retesting within 3 weeks should not be performed.

Although NAAT testing is now recommended, same-day results are not available. Chlamydia rapid testing (immunoassay) provides a result within 30 minutes (5). This test is also inexpensive and easy to interpret with similar test characteristics compared with NAAT (6).

The source of the swab testing depends on the site of infection; in patients with suspected cervicitis and urethritis it is collected from cervix and urethra, respectively, and in people who engage in receptive anal intercourse a rectal swab specimen is obtained. Because of the significant number of co-infections, any patient receiving testing for chlamydia should be tested for gonorrhea.

Treatment of Chlamydia

The treatment for *C. trachomatis* infections depends on several factors including site of infection, age of the patient, and whether the infection is complicated or uncomplicated. The primary goals of treatment are eradication of pathogens, resolution of symptoms, and prevention of complications.

Advise the patient that all sexual partners should be evaluated, tested, and treated if they had sexual contact during the 60 days preceding the patient's onset of symptoms or diagnosis.

TABLE 32.1 Treatment Regimens for Uncomplicated Urogenital Chlamydia Infection

Recommended Regimens	Alternative Regimens
Men and Nonpregnant Women	
• Azithromycin 1 g orally single dose • Doxycycline 100 mg orally 2 times/day for 7 days	• Erythromycin base 500 mg orally 4 times/day for 7 days • EES 800 mg orally 4 times/day for 7 days • Ofloxacin 300 mg orally 2 times/day for 7 days • Levofloxacin 500 mg orally once/day for 7 days
Pregnant Women*	
• Azithromycin 1 g orally single dose	• Amoxicillin 500 mg 3 times/day for 7 days • Erythromycin base 500 mg 4 times/day for 7 days or 250 mg 4 times/day for 14 days • EES 800 mg 4 times/day for 7 days or 400 mg 4 times/day for 14 days

EES = erythromycin ethylsuccinate.
*Doxycycline, ofloxacin, erythromycin estolate, or levofloxacin are contraindicated during pregnancy.
Information from: Workowski KA, Berman SM. Sexually transmitted diseases treatment guidelines, 2006. *MMWR Recomm Rep.* 2006; 55(RR-11):1–94.

The most recent sex partner should be evaluated and treated even if the time of the last sexual contact was >60 days before symptoms onset or diagnosis (4). If sexual partners are not likely to seek evaluation and treatment, then delivery of antibiotic therapy by the patient to their partners is an option. Patient delivered therapy is not routinely recommended for men having sex with men because of a high risk for coexisting infections, especially undiagnosed HIV infection, in their partners.

Evidence-based guidelines from the CDC for the treatment of uncomplicated genital chlamydia infections are shown in Table 32.1 (4). Either azithromycin or doxycycline is acceptable for men and non-pregnant women and pregnant women are usually treated with azithromycin (4). In patients who are allergic or intolerant to the first-line drugs, an alternative regimen recommended by CDC should be used (Table 32.1). When possible, medications should be given on site with the first dose directly observed. To minimize transmission, instruct patients treated for chlamydia to abstain from sexual intercourse for 7 days after single dose therapy or until completion of a 7-day regimen and to abstain from sexual intercourse until all of their sex partners are treated.

Empiric treatment is recommended when follow up cannot be assured and there are no available results from STI testing. It is also considered for patients with gonococcal infection with no definite exclusion of chlamydia infection, men with nongonococcal urethritis, and men younger than 35 years with epididymitis. One should target both gonorrhea and chlamydia in prescribing empiric treatment. Like other STIs, a number of adjunctive measures are crucial in the management of patients with chlamydia including evaluation for other STIs, HIV counseling and testing, safer sex counseling and condom provision, and contraception provision and referral.

Follow-up

The CDC does not recommend test of cure for chlamydia after completion of a recommended antibiotic regimen as cure rates are high (4); the exceptions include: (i) those with persistent or recurring symptoms, (ii) nonadherent patients, (iii) patients treated with an alternative regiment, and (iv) pregnant women. When repeat testing is indicated, culture to verify susceptibility is preferred, and retreatment directed accordingly. Three weeks after completion of treatment, a test of cure is needed for pregnant women with repeat screening for high-risk women during third trimester (4).

The majority of posttreatment infections result from reinfection because the patient's sex partners were not treated or the patient resumed sex with a new infected partner. Because reinfection is common and repeat infections confer an elevated risk for PID, CDC recommends that patients with chlamydia infections should be rescreened (technically, not a test of cure) 3 to 4 months after antibiotic completion (4). Patients who present within 12 months of their initial infection and have not been screened should be reassessed for infection. Limited evidence is available on retesting infected men; however some specialists suggest retesting approximately 3 months after treatment.

Screening and Prevention

Primary prevention starts with education, and is the same as for all STIs. The CDC has stressed behavioral changes (e.g., delaying the age of first intercourse, reducing the number of sexual partners, using barrier contraception) and annual screening of sexually active women age 25 years or younger and sexually active older women with risk factors. The United States Preventive Services Task Force (USPTF) has a similar recommendation for these patients; however it did not explicitly recommend annual screening (7).

Both the CDC and USPTF recommendation screening all pregnant women at increased risk of infection (including women age 25 years or younger) at the first prenatal visit (see Chapter 4). In addition, CDC recommends repeat testing in the third trimester for those at increased risk. This helps reduce maternal postnatal complications and chlamydial infection in the newborn.

While there is insufficient evidence to recommend routine screening of sexually active men, routine screening of men is appropriate in settings of high prevalence such as correctional facilities and STD clinics. In men having sex with men, one should routinely screen for STIs (at least yearly) and offer patient-centered prevention counseling.

Chlamydia Infections in Children

Chlamydia should be considered for all infants ages younger than 30 days of age with conjunctivitis (ophthalmia neonatorum), especially if the mother has a history of untreated chlamydia infection; nearly 20% to 50% of newborns of infected mothers developing conjunctivitis (8). These infants present within 5 to 12 days of birth with swelling and mucopurulent drainage of one or both eyes.

Commonly used prophylaxis with silver nitrate or antimicrobial ointment at birth reduces the risk of gonococcal eye infections but not chlamydia conjunctival infections. Ophthalmia neonatorum is treated with erythromycin base or ethylsuccinate 50 mg/kg/day orally, divided into 4 doses per day, for 14 days. Topical treatment alone or with systemic treatment is not effective.

Chlamydia pneumonia develops in 10% to 20% of infants' ages 1 to 3 months who are exposed to *C. trachomatis* during delivery. The characteristics include a protracted onset of symptoms, a staccato cough usually with no wheezing, and no temperature elevation. Peripheral eosinophilia occurs frequently. Initial treatment and diagnostic tests should include *C. trachomatis* for all infants aged 1 to 3 months with possible pneumonia. For these infants, a nasopharyngeal swab is sent for chlamydia testing and they are treated with erythromycin base or ethylsuccinate 50 mg/kg/day orally divided into 4 doses per day for 14 days.

The mothers of infants who have chlamydia infection and their sex partners should be evaluated and treated for chlamydia and other STIs. When this infection is acquired after the neonatal period, sexual abuse must be considered; however, perinatally transmitted infection of the nasopharynx, urogenital tract, and rectum can persist for more than 1 year.

Complications

PID occurs in 20% to 40% of untreated women with chlamydia; in men untreated chlamydia infections occasionally result in epididymo-orchitis. Other complications include chronic prostatitis (see Chapter 30) and Reiter syndrome. Persistence of pain, discomfort, and irritative voiding symptoms beyond 3 months from the onset should alert the clinician to the possibility of chronic prostatitis and chronic pelvic pain syndrome in men.

Reiter syndrome is the constellation of reactive arthritis, urethritis, and conjunctivitis. The reactive arthritis occurs in approximately 1% of men with chlamydia infection, and even fewer in women, with a male to female ratio of 5:1. It is seen 1 to 3 weeks from the infection onset. Besides this triad of symptoms, patients with Reiter's syndrome may have painless papulosquamous mucocutaneous lesions that tend to occur on the palms and soles. The initial episode usually lasts 3 to 4 months but in rare cases the synovitis lasts up to one year.

GONORRHEA

Gonorrhea is the second most common reportable bacterial STI in the United States and remains a significant cause of preventable and treatable morbidity in both men and women. *Neisseria gonorrhea* is a gram negative, intracellular diplococcus. Its incubation period is 2 to 6 days. Urethritis and cervicitis are the most common presentations in men and women, respectively.

Epidemiology

In the United States, more than 300,000 cases of gonorrhea are reported annually (1). Unfortunately, an equal number of cases go unreported. Overall rates have declined since the mid-1970s with 111.6 cases per 100,000 reported in 2008 (1). The distribution among women and men is similar. The highest reported rates are seen among adolescents and young adults (women aged 15 to 19 years and men aged 20 to 24 years), minorities (20 times greater frequency in blacks than whites), men having sex with men, and people living in southeastern United States.

Risk factors are similar to those for chlamydia. Gonorrhea is acquired by both sexual and vertical transmission. The attack rate is 50% to 73% after one documented exposure to an infected male sexual partner and increases to 93% after repeated exposure (9).

Clinical Symptoms

Like chlamydia, gonorrhea infection in women is often asymptomatic. The cervix is the most common site of mucosal infection. Symptomatic infection typically manifests as vaginal pruritus, postcoital bleeding, deep dyspareunia, and/or odorless mucopurulent discharge.

On examination, the cervix may appear friable with mucopurulent drainage from the cervical os. *N. gonorrhea* does not affect vaginal epithelium so a second infection should be sought if vaginitis is present (see Chapter 33). Besides cervicitis, the other common infections from *N. gonorrhea* include infection of Bartholin's and Skene's glands. Urethritis with dysuria and yellowish penile discharge is the most common presentation of symptomatic gonorrhea in men. On examination, the penis may be erythematous with a purulent discharge at the meatus. When absent, the discharge may be expressed by milking the penis.

Gonorrhea infections can be present in the rectal area in men and women. In women it can occur because of perianal contamination from a cervical infection or from direct infection from anal intercourse. In men this infection occurs because of direct exposure through anal intercourse. Most individuals with rectal gonococcal infections have few if any symptoms; although anal pruritus, mucopurulent anal discharge, anal fullness, painful defecation, and rectal bleeding can occur. In severe cases, it is difficult to differentiate from inflammatory bowel disease.

Pharyngeal infections caused by *N. gonorrhoeae* usually occur after orogenital exposure to an infected individual. Pharyngeal erythema with or without exudates and anterior cervical lymphadenopathy may be present. Most cases will spontaneously resolve without treatment and do not usually result in adverse sequelae but treatment reduces the transmission risk.

Diagnostic Testing

Both culture and nonculture methods for detecting *N. gonorrhoeae* are available. As for chlamydia, NAAT testing has replaced culture (4). The Food and Drug Administration (FDA) has approved these tests for specimen types including male urine, male urethral swabs, vaginal swabs, and endocervical swabs. In contrast to male urine specimens, female urine has a high level of inhibitory substances that can impair test performance and NAAT is not approved for the detection of

N. gonorrhoeae in female urine specimens. Overall these tests have better sensitivity (92% to 96% vs. 65% to 85% for culture) and similar specificity (98% to 100% vs. 100% for culture) to culture and the results are obtained faster.

Because of high specificity (>99%), a gram stain of a male urethral specimen that demonstrates polymorphonuclear leukocytes with intracellular gram negative diplococci can be considered diagnostic for infection with *N. gonorrhoeae* in symptomatic men. However, as it has lower sensitivity (95%), a negative gram stain is not sufficient for ruling out infection in asymptomatic men. For the same reason, gram stain of endocervical, pharyngeal, and rectal specimens also are not sufficient to detect gonococcal infection and are not recommended.

In general, culture is the most widely available option for the diagnosis of gonorrhea infection in nongenital sites such as rectum and pharynx. NAATs are not FDA approved for these sites. Culture is preferred in patients with persistent infection to provide antimicrobial susceptibility results. Finally, one should not forget to screen for other major STIs in patients with gonorrhea.

Treatment

Due to increasing resistance to antimicrobials for uncomplicated gonorrhea (10), CDC no longer recommends fluoroquinolones for treating this infection. Currently, cephalosporins (single dose ceftriaxone 125 mg IM or single dose cefixime 400 mg orally) are the only class of drugs still recommended for treatment of gonorrhea (4) including pregnant women.

In the case of type 1 hypersensitivity to β-lactam antibiotics, the best option is cephalosporin treatment after desensitization. Otherwise, use of culture with susceptibility testing to fluoroquinolones can be employed to direct therapy (except pregnancy). High-dose azithromycin (2 g) also may have a role for these unusual but important cases. Patients should refrain from sexual contact until both they and their sexual partners have been treated, and all symptoms have resolved.

Because dual infection with chlamydia is common (10–30%), concurrent empiric treatment for both organisms is recommended, especially if chlamydia infection has not been ruled out by NAAT. Azithromycin or doxycycline is used to treat chlamydia (Table 32.1). Increasing the dose of azithromycin to 2 g potentially cures gonorrhea but is not recommended by the CDC because of cost, increased side effects and rising mean inhibitory concentration (MIC) documented over the last 10 years. All sexual partners who had contact with the infected patient within the past 60 days should be evaluated and treated. If contact occurred beyond 60 days, the most recent sexual partner should be evaluated and treated.

Follow-up

Patients treated with a recommended regimen for uncomplicated gonococcal infection do not need a test of cure given the high clinical efficacy (97%). However, if symptoms persist or recur shortly after treatment, a test of cure is indicated by culture to verify susceptibility, and direct retreatment. A test of cure is advised in 3 weeks following treatment for pregnant women.

Rescreening should be performed within 3 months of treatment of all patients with gonorrhea irrespective of treatment failure given the high rates of reinfection. If patients do not seek medical care for retesting in 3 months, providers are encouraged to test these patients whenever they next seek medical care within 12 months, regardless of treatment of sexual partners.

Screening

Routine annual screening for gonorrhea is recommended by CDC for all sexually active women 25 years of age or younger and for older women at increased risk for infection. The CDC and USPSTF do not recommend screening for low-risk men as men are usually symptomatic when infected.

All pregnant women should be routinely screened for gonorrhea at their first prenatal visit. In presence of risk factors, rescreening is advised in the third trimester. Screening is important during pregnancy as many women with gonorrhea are asymptomatic and, left untreated, at risk of pre-term rupture of membranes, preterm labor, chorioamnionitis, and postpartum endomyometritis.

Gonorrhea in Children

Gonococcal infection among infants usually results within 3 to 5 days of delivery from exposure to infected cervical exudates at birth. After age 1 year, almost all gonococcal infections are due to child abuse. The most severe manifestations in the newborn are ophthalmia neonatorum and sepsis. The later may include arthritis and meningitis. Less severe manifestations are rhinitis, vaginitis, urethritis, and infection at the site of fetal monitoring.

Gonococcal ophthalmia neonatorum is rare in the United States, but early diagnosis and treatment is important to reduce globe perforation and blindness. Common findings include inflammation of the conjunctiva and mucopurulent eye discharge. Gram stain and culture of the exudates help establish the diagnosis. To prevent this eye infection, routine prophylaxis is recommended at birth; options include single application of 0.5% erythromycin or 1% tetracycline ophthalmic ointment into the eyes. Topical antibiotics do not work for established infection. In this case, parenteral administration of a single dose of ceftriaxone is recommended.

Complications

Gonorrhea results in PID in approximately 10% to 40% of cases if left untreated. Rarely *N. gonorrhea* left untreated in men results in epididymitis or prostatitis (see Chapter 30).

Disseminated gonococcal infection is a rare complication of *N. gonorrhoeae* infection and occurs in 1% to 3% of adults who do not receive treatment. In disseminated disease, the organism spreads by septic emboli causing polyarticular tenosynovitis and dermatitis. Symptoms may be mild (slight joint pain, few skin lesions, no fever) to severe with overt polyarthritis and high fever. These patients have no urogenital signs and symptoms. It is extremely rare to see severe adverse effects of disseminated gonorrhea such as endocarditis, meningitis, and myocarditis due to use of antibiotics.

PELVIC INFLAMMATORY DISEASE

PID is an acute infection in a woman of any or all of her upper genital tract structures (i.e., uterus, fallopian tubes, and ovaries). It may manifest as endometritis, salpingitis, oophoritis, peritonitis, perihepatitis, and/or tubo-ovarian abscess. PID is a polymicrobial infection typically initiated by the ascent of a sexually transmitted agent, most commonly *N. gonorrhoeae* or *C. trachomatis,* from the endocervix to the upper genital structures. However, up to 70% of cases are nongonococcal and non-chlamydial (11,12). Other micro-organisms isolated from the fallopian tubes in acute PID include: *Mycoplasma hominis, Streptococcus* sp., *Staphylococcus* sp., *Haemophilus* sp., *Escherichia coli, Bacteroides* sp., *Peptostreptococcus* sp., *Peptococcus* sp., *Clostridium* sp., and *Actinomyces* sp. (13).

It is estimated that more than 1 million women experience an episode of acute PID annually in the United States, and more than 100,000 become infertile as a result (14). In 2008, there were an estimated 168,837 women ages 15 to 44 diagnosed with PID in emergency departments. Visits to physician's offices for PID have declined from 254,000 in 2000 to 104,000 in 2008 (13). This decline in numbers is primarily from aggressive chlamydia screening and treatment.

Clinical Evaluation

PID diagnosis can be elusive; no set of signs or symptoms is pathognomonic (15). Recent onset of lower abdominal pain that worsens during coitus or with jarring movement may be the only presenting symptom. Other symptoms include fever, malaise, vaginal discharge, irregular bleeding, nausea, and vomiting. The symptoms usually develop during menses or in the first 2 weeks of the menstrual cycle (4). PID is less likely if symptoms referable to the bowel or urinary tract predominate. It is rare to have PID during pregnancy as following the first trimester of pregnancy the mucus plug and decidua seal off the uterus from ascending bacteria.

Women who develop PID have a 20% chance of becoming infertile, 18% chance of developing pelvic pain, and 9% lifetime chance of a tubal pregnancy (16). Because untreated mild or subclinical PID is often responsible, one should have a low threshold for making the diagnosis. The CDC recommends empiric PID treatment in sexually active women at risk for STIs who complain of acute (30 days or less) lower abdominal or pelvic pain and uterine, adnexal, or cervical motion tenderness, for whom no other cause can be identified (14).

Diagnostic Testing

PID is a clinical diagnosis. Most laboratory tests are nonspecific. In a symptomatic, at-risk patient, the sensitivity of signs or symptom for diagnosis of PID versus laparoscopy ranges from 10% to 74% except for tenderness of pelvic organs on bimanual exam (sensitivity of 99%) (15).

Begin evaluation for women suspected of PID with a pregnancy test to rule out ectopic pregnancy or intrauterine pregnancy complications. Other recommended tests include: gonorrhea and chlamydia, microscopic exam of vaginal discharge, complete blood counts (fewer than one-half of patients with exhibit leucocytosis), urinalysis, and ESR or CRP.

Diagnostic imaging with transvaginal ultrasound, computed tomography, or magnetic resonance imaging is used to evaluate PID in women who have an adnexal mass on palpation, if the diagnosis is uncertain, or if inpatient treatment is necessary because of infection severity (16).

Endometrial biopsy and laparoscopic examination of the pelvis should be considered for patients with PID who are not responding to therapy or are severely ill; with a specificity approaching 100%, laparoscopy has substantial value in confirming the diagnosis of PID (17). Laparoscopy, however, is not sensitive (50%) enough to be considered a diagnostic gold standard (17). Patients with acute PID should also be tested for other major STIs (4).

TABLE 32.2 Criteria for Hospitalization Patients with Pelvic Inflammatory Disease

- Patient does not respond clinically to oral antimicrobial therapy
- Patient is pregnant
- Severe illness such as nausea and vomiting or high fever
- Surgical emergencies (e.g., appendicitis) cannot be excluded
- Tubo-ovarian abscess present
- Unable to follow or tolerate outpatient oral regimen

Adapted from Workowski KA, Berman SM. Sexually transmitted diseases treatment guidelines, 2006. *MMWR Recomm Rep* 2006; 55(RR-11):1.

Treatment

The differential diagnosis for PID is extensive. However, a trial of antibiotics should not be withheld when clinical suspicion of PID is high. Outpatient treatment is as effective as inpatient treatment in clinical trials (17). The CDC has published guidelines for when inpatient therapy is most appropriate (Table 32.2) (4).

The options for outpatient treatment include two equally effective regimens (Table 32.3). If patients with PID meet hospitalization criteria and parenteral antibiotic therapy is indicated, the preferred regimen is cefotetan or cefoxitin plus doxycycline; the latter given orally whenever possible because it causes venous sclerosis. Fluoroquinolones are no longer recommended if *N. gonorrhoeae* is a proven or suspected pathogen (10).

One should counsel patients with PID on safe sex practices, the need for partner treatment, and the need to screen for other STIs. To decrease the risk of reinfection, male sex partners should be examined and treated if they had sexual contact with the patient during the previous 60 days before the patient's onset of symptoms. Women at risk of an STI should be educated about PID symptoms and to seek immediate treatment.

HUMAN PAPILLOMAVIRUS

Human papillomavirus (HPV) is the most common viral STI in the United States (18). It causes anogenital warts and cervical cancer, as well as a portion of other anogenital and head and neck cancers. There are more than 100 HPV subtypes, differentiated primarily by the genetic sequence of the outer capsid protein L1. Types 6 and 11 ("low-risk" types of HPV) cause common venereal warts and recurrent respiratory papillomatosis. Low- and high-grade cervical dysplasias and anogenital cancers are associated with types 16, 18, 31, 33, and 35 ("high-grade" or "oncogenic" types of HPV) (19). HPV types 16 and 18 account for about 70% of cervical cancers worldwide (20).

TABLE 32.3 CDC Recommended Pelvic Inflammatory Disease Treatment Regimens

Outpatient Regimens (all oral regimens for 14 days' duration)	**Inpatient Regimens***
• Ceftriaxone 250 mg IM single dose PLUS • Doxycycline 100 mg orally twice a day WITH OR WITHOUT • Metronidazole 500 mg orally twice a day	• Cefotetan 2 g IV every 12 hours OR • Cefoxitin 2 g IV every 6 hours PLUS • Doxycycline 100 mg orally or IV every 12 hours
• Cefoxitin 2 g IM PLUS • Probenecid 1 g orally single dose PLUS • Doxycycline 100 mg orally twice a day WITH OR WITHOUT • Metronidazole 500 mg orally twice a day	• Clindamycin 900 mg IV every 8 hours PLUS • Gentamicin loading dose IV or IM (2 mg/kg of body weight), followed by a maintenance dose (1.5 mg/kg) every 8 hours. Single daily dosing may be used.
• Other parenteral third-generation cephalosporin (e.g., ceftizoxime) PLUS • Doxycycline 100 mg orally twice a day WITH OR WITHOUT • Metronidazole 500 mg orally twice a day	• Ampicillin/sulbactam 3 g IV every 6 hours PLUS • Doxycycline 100 mg orally or IV every 12 hours

*Parenteral and oral therapy have similar clinical efficacy when treating women with pelvic inflammatory disease of mild or moderate severity. Inpatient regimens may be discontinued 24 hours after the patient shows clinical improvement with continuation of an oral regimen for at least 14 days.
Adapted from Update to CDC's sexually transmitted diseases treatment guidelines, 2006: fluoroquinolones no longer recommended for treatment of gonococcal infections. *MMWR Morb Mortal Wkly Rep* 2007;56:332.

About 29% of the general population is infected with high-risk viral types, with the highest prevalence in 14 to 19 year olds (14). Risk factors for HPV are primarily related to sexual behavior (number of partners, new partners, lifetime partners, and partner's sexual history) (20).

Clinical Evaluation

The majority of HPV infections are asymptomatic, unrecognized, or subclinical. The most common clinical manifestation of genital HPV infection is genital warts (condylomata acuminate). Genital warts may appear as single or multiple papules on the vulva, cervix, vagina, perineum, penis, scrotum, or perianal region. External HPV lesions are frequently associated with cervical lesions. HPV infection may also manifest as recurrent respiratory papillomatosis and cancers (anal, vulvar, vaginal, cervical, penile, and a subset of head and neck cancers) (20,21). As many as 15% of HPV cervical infections will progress to cervical intraepithelial neoplasia or carcinoma within 2 to 3 years if left untreated (22).

HPV can be transmitted easily by contact between infected individuals and their partners. Condoms reduce the risk of transmission but because the HPV virus can be present at multiple sites, condoms do not provide 100% protection. The infection tends to be transient with a significant number of individuals having spontaneous resolution of the virus without treatment; 70% of cases resolve spontaneously within 1 year and 91% within 2 years (23,24).

Diagnostic Testing

A definitive diagnosis is based on detection of viral nucleic acid (i.e., DNA or RNA) or capsid protein. Anogenital HPV infection is usually a clinical diagnosis based on appearance of lesions and their locations. If a lesion is present and the diagnosis uncertain, a biopsy of the site can confirm HPV. It is otherwise unnecessary to biopsy an obvious genital lesion.

Cervical HPV can be diagnosed by Pap smear, which correlates well with the presence of HPV DNA by polymerase chain reaction (PCR). Viral typing, using a DNA probe, to look for high-risk HPV types is used in the triage of women with atypical squamous cells of undetermined significance and in screening women age >30 years in conjunction with the Pap test (4). The presence of genital warts does not necessitate HPV testing, a change in the frequency of Pap tests, or colposcopy.

Treatment

Treatment is not recommended for subclinical genital HPV infection as there is no cure. Treatment options are shown in Table 32.4. Success of treatment does not depend on the regimen used but on the number and size of warts (4). Because of uncertainty regarding treatment effect on transmission and the high rate of spontaneous resolution, some patients may choose to forego treatment (4). Women should be counseled to undergo regular Pap screening (4).

The management of individuals with HPV does not necessarily include examination of sexual partners because treating partners' HPV does not reduce transmission or play a role in recurrences (4). However, sexual partners may benefit from an evaluation for other STIs and counseling concerning implications of their partner's HPV.

HPV Screening and Vaccination

Most HPV infections are asymptomatic and clear spontaneously. As a result, HPV DNA testing is not recommended except in specific settings related to cervical cancer screening and management (as discussed previously). There is no indication for HPV testing among men as identifying infection does not prevent HPV-associated diseases no therapy eradicates infection.

HPV vaccines may have a significant impact on the prevalence and incidence of HPV infection and its sequelae. Two HPV vaccines are currently in use: the Merck quadrivalent

TABLE 32.4 Treatment for External Genitalia Human Papillomavirus (HPV)

Medication/Modality	Instructions	Comments
Patient Applied		
Podofilox 0.5% solution or gel	Patient applies to warts twice daily for 3 days followed by 4 days of no therapy. May repeat for up to 4 cycles.	• Total area treated should not exceed 10 cm^2 or total volume used per day not >0.5 mL. • Safety not proven during pregnancy
Imiquimod 5% cream	Patient applies to warts once daily at bedtime, 3 times per week for up to 16 weeks	• Treatment area should be washed with soap 6–10 hours after application • Safety not proven during pregnancy
Provider Administered		
Cryotherapy with liquid nitrogen or cryoprobe	Follow appropriate directions based on system used	• Repeat application usually needed every 1–2 weeks • Must be trained in technique because over or undertreatment can reduce the efficacy or increase complication rates
Podophyllin resin 10%–25% in a compound tincture of benzoin	Small amount applied to each wart and allowed to air dry	• Weekly treatments until resolution • Total area treated should not exceed 10 cm^2 or total volume used per day not >0.5 ml • Safety not proven during pregnancy
Trichloroacetic acid (TCA) or bichloracetic acid (BCA) 80%–90%	Apply small amount only to warts and allow to dry	• Treatment may be repeated weekly until resolved • Easy to apply excessive amounts and cause skin irritation
Surgical removal	Tangential scissor or shave excision, curettage, or electrosurgery	• Advantage of warts being eliminated in one treatment • Disadvantage is the potential complication from surgery
Intralesional interferon	Interferon injected directly into warts	• Repeat treatment usually necessary • Causes significant systemic adverse effects so not recommended for routine treatment
Laser surgery	Based on equipment	• Usually only requires one treatment • Reserved for more extensive lesions because of potential complications

Adapted from Centers for Disease Control and Prevention. Sexually transmitted diseases treatment guidelines, 2006. *MMWR Recomm Rep* 2006; 55(RR-11):1.

vaccine (HPV-6, -11, -16, and -18) and GlaxoSmithKline bivalent vaccine (HPV-16 and -18). Both vaccines have high efficacy among girls and women not previously exposed to the HPV vaccine types. They are recommended for girls and women ages 9 to 26 years.

GENITAL HERPES

Genital herpes is caused by herpes simplex virus (HSV). This virus has two serotypes (HSV-1 and HSV-2). About 50 million people in the United States are presumed to have the genital HSV infection (14). The infection is usually transmitted by people unaware that they have herpes or who are asymptomatic when transmission occurs. In the United States, only 20% of those patients who present to physicians with genital symptoms receive a correct diagnosis of genital herpes (25).

Clinical Evaluation

Genital herpes has three clinical presentations: (i) first-episode primary infection (new infection), (ii) first-episode nonprimary infection (unrecognized HSV), and (iii) recurrent episodes. First-episode primary infection usually causes significant symptoms including a prodrome of fever, malaise, headache, myalgia, and genital paresthesias before the breakout of cutaneous lesions. Multiple, painful vesicles develop 1 to 3 days after the prodrome in the genital or perianal area which later ulcerate. Often there is associated painful inguinal lymphadenopathy. Patients are most infectious during this early phase of prodromal symptoms or open ulcers.

The first-episode nonprimary genital HSV infection tends to be less severe with fewer lesions, faster healing, and a shorter period of viral shedding. In patients with recurrent HSV infection (any episode of HSV infection in patients with prior diagnosis of genital herpes) there is usually a prodrome of tingling, pruritus, or dysesthesias before the outbreak of genital lesions. The lesions normally erupt in the same site as the primary episode and crust over in 4 to 5 days. Viral shedding can occur at anytime during this process.

Up to 50% of patients with first-episode genital herpes have HSV-1 as the cause (26). The majority of recurrences and subclinical shedding are caused by genital HSV-2 infection (27,28). This has important prognostic implications because patients with HSV-1 genital infections are less likely to have recurrent episodes than those with HSV-2. According to the CDC (4), type-specific HSV serologic assays might be useful in the following scenarios: (i) recurrent genital symptoms or atypical symptoms with negative HSV cultures; (ii) a clinical diagnosis of genital herpes without laboratory confirmation; and (iii) a partner with genital herpes.

Diagnostic Testing

The clinical diagnosis of genital herpes is insensitive and nonspecific. The classical painful, multiple, vesicular or ulcerative lesions are absent in many infected people (4). According to the CDC, isolation of HSV in cell culture is the preferred virologic test for patients who seek medical treatment for genital ulcers or other mucocutaneous lesions (4). The sensitivity of culture is low, especially for recurrent lesions and declines rapidly as the lesions heal. Therefore, the culture needs to be performed in the first few days of a breakout. Both viral culture from the lesions and the type specific antibodies help distinguish between subtypes.

The presence of serum antibodies to HSV-2 is usually indicative of genital herpes whereas HSV-1 antibodies do not differentiate between genital and oropharyngeal infection. HSV DNA detection by PCR increases HSV detection rates by 11% to 71% compared with viral culture (25). PCR tests, however, are not FDA approved for testing genital specimens and routine screening for HSV-1 or HSV-2 in the general population is not recommended (4).

Treatment

The treatment regimen depends on the type of infection. Antiviral drugs offer clinical benefits to the majority of symptomatic patients with genital infections. However, these drugs neither eradicate latent virus nor affect the frequency or severity of recurrences after treatment (4).

Three antiviral medications provide clinical benefit for genital herpes: acyclovir, valacyclovir, and famciclovir (29–31). Most patients also need analgesics for pain control. One should be careful using topical anesthetic agents such as 5% lidocaine ointment, because of the potential for sensitization (25).

First-episode genital HSV should be treated within five days of onset while new lesions are still forming (25) (Table 32.5). There is no evidence of benefit from courses longer than five days (25). Topical antiviral agents are of no benefit, alone or in combination with orals (25).

Frequent recurrences of genital herpes are common but tend to diminish over time. These episodes are self-limiting and generally cause minor symptoms (25). Recurrences could be treated with episodic or suppressive therapy; decisions are made in partnership with the patient. Patients should understand that intermittent asymptomatic shedding of virus occurs.

TABLE 32.5 Treatment for Genital Herpes

First Clinical Episode of Genital Herpes*
• Acyclovir 400 mg orally three times a day for 7–10 days OR
• Acyclovir 200 mg orally five times a day for 7–10 days OR
• Famciclovir 250 mg orally three times a day for 7–10 days OR
• Valacyclovir 1 g orally twice a day for 7–10 days
Suppressive Therapy for Recurrent Genital Herpes
• Acyclovir 400 mg orally twice a day OR
• Famciclovir 250 mg orally twice a day OR
• Valacyclovir 500 mg orally once a day OR
• Valacyclovir 1.0 g orally once a day
Episodic Therapy for Recurrent Genital Herpes
• Acyclovir 400 mg orally three times a day for 5 days OR
• Acyclovir 800 mg orally twice a day for 5 days OR
• Acyclovir 800 mg orally three times a day for 2 days OR
• Famciclovir 125 mg orally twice daily for 5 days OR
• Famciclovir 1000 mg orally twice daily for 1 day OR
• Valacyclovir 500 mg orally twice a day for 3 days OR
• Valacyclovir 1.0 g orally once a day for 5 days

*Treatment might be extended if healing is incomplete after 10 days of therapy.
Adapted from Workowski KA, Berman SM. Sexually transmitted diseases treatment guidelines, 2006. *MMWR Recomm Rep* 2006; 55(RR-11):1.

Effective episodic treatment of recurrent herpes requires initiation of therapy within 1 day of lesion onset or during the prodrome. This therapy should be patient initiated (Table 32.5) and a prescription for an antiviral medication with instructions should be provided. All drugs are equally efficacious and selection is based on ease of administration and cost (4).

Suppressive therapy reduces the frequency of genital herpes recurrences by 70% to 80% in patients with frequent recurrences (>6 per year), and is also effective in those with fewer recurrences (4) (Table 32.5). Safety and efficacy have been documented for daily acyclovir for as long as 6 years and with valacyclovir or famciclovir for 1 year (4). Patients with >10 recurrences per year may not respond as well to 500 mg of valacyclovir so other regimens should be used.

There are no vaccines currently approved for prevention of genital herpes (25). The HSV-2 glycoprotein-D adjuvant vaccine has shown limited efficacy in preventing clinical disease and only in women who were seronegative for both HSV-1 and HSV-2 at baseline.

SYPHILIS

Syphilis is a chronic systemic STI caused by the spirochete *Treponema pallidum*. It initiates infection by accessing subcutaneous tissues via microscopic abrasion during sexual intercourse. Virtually all new syphilis infections are sexually acquired.

Less common modes of transmission include nonsexual personal contact, infection in utero, blood transfusion, and organ transplantation. The disease is most infectious during its early stages (primary and secondary syphilis) with a transmission rate of approximately 30%. When it manifests clinically, the presenting features vary depending on the infection stage (primary, secondary, tertiary, and latent) (Table 32.6).

Although the rate of primary and secondary syphilis in United States declined 90% between 1990 and 2000, the annual rate has been on the rise since 2001. This increase was mainly attributed to men having sex with men accounting for 63% of reported primary and secondary syphilis cases. The incidence of early syphilis in 2008 was 7.6 cases per 100,000 population in men and 1.5 cases per 100,000 population in women (4). In 2007, 11,181 new cases of early syphilis were reported (4).

Syphilis remains an important problem in the south and in urban areas of other parts of the United States. It affects mostly young adults (20 to 30 years of age) who are black or Asian/Pacific Islanders. Syphilis is also associated with an increased risk of HIV acquisition and transmission.

Clinical Evaluation

Following acquisition of *T. pallidum,* the initial clinical manifestations are termed primary syphilis. A 3-week (range 10 to 90 days) incubation period usually occurs between the inoculation of *T. pallidum* and development of a primary lesion called a chancre (Table 32.6). Because of its location, primary syphilis often goes unrecognized in women and homosexual men. If left untreated, the lesion heals spontaneously in 3 to 6 weeks.

Four to eight weeks later, approximately 25% of patients with untreated primary syphilis develop a systemic illness called secondary syphilis (32) (Table 32.6). Patients with secondary syphilis may not have a history of preceding chancre. Most lesions of secondary syphilis resolve spontaneously in 3 to 6 weeks without treatment; about 25% relapse within the first year.

Latent syphilis is a period where patients have no signs or symptoms of syphilis except abnormal serology but are at risk of spontaneous mucocutaneous relapse; this period has classically been divided into early and late latent syphilis (Table 32.6). Left untreated, one third of patients with secondary syphilis will develop late complications of syphilis, a diverse group of manifestations termed tertiary syphilis. Tertiary syphilis along with late latent syphilis constitutes late syphilis. It is not necessary for individuals to experience primary or secondary syphilis prior to developing tertiary syphilis. Complications of tertiary syphilis are rare outside of resource poor countries.

Diagnostic Testing

T. pallidum cannot be detected by culture. Serological tests are used initially to make a presumptive diagnosis of syphilis. Common indications for testing include routine screening in pregnancy, patients with suspected disease, and screening high-risk patient populations.

Serological tests are nontreponemal (Venereal Disease Research Laboratory test (VDRL) and Rapid Plasma Reagin (RPR) tests) or more specific, treponemal. Both types of tests are reactive in people with any treponemal infection, including yaws, pinta, and endemic syphilis. Nontreponemal tests are limited by decreased sensitivity in both early primary and late syphilis, where up to one third of untreated patients may be nonreactive. In addition, false positive tests can occur in patients with autoimmune conditions, vaccination, chronic liver disease, endocarditis, HIV, tuberculosis, other infections, pregnancy, increasing age (about 10% among those age >70 years), and injection drug use. Nontreponemal tests usually become nonreactive after treatment although low titers of antibodies can persist for long periods.

In the presence of a positive nontreponemal test, the treponemal tests (e.g., fluorescent treponemal antibody absorb [FTA-ABS]) are used to confirm the diagnosis. They are more difficult and expensive to perform, which limits their usefulness as screening tests. Treponemal tests remain positive forever regardless of disease activity or treatment. Treponemal antibody titers do not correlate with disease activity and should not be used to assess treatment response.

A spinal tap for cerebrospinal fluid (CSF) analysis to rule out neurosyphilis is recommended for all children (>1 month of age) with syphilis, patients with treatment failure, patients with nervous system or eye involvement, those with evidence of tertiary syphilis, and those infected with both HIV and late latent syphilis/syphilis of unknown duration. Similarly all patients with syphilis should be screened for other major STIs including HIV. Involvement of central nervous system is detected by examination of CSF for pleocytosis (>5 white blood cells/mm^3), increased protein concentration (>45 mg/dL), or VDRL reactivity. The CSF VDRL test is highly specific (rules in disease) but is insensitive. In contrast, a reactive FTA-ABS test reflects passive transfer of serum antibody into CSF and has low positive predictive value. A nonreactive FTA-ABS test, however, may be used to rule out neurosyphilis (high negative predictive value).

Treatment

Penicillin G, administered parenterally, is the preferred drug for treatment of all patients, including pregnant women, in all stages of syphilis (4) (Table 32.6). Adequate treatment of a pregnant woman before 16 weeks' gestation should prevent fetal damage, and treatment before the third trimester should adequately treat the infected fetus. No proven penicillin alternatives are available for treating neurosyphilis, congenital syphilis, or syphilis in pregnant women (4). When alternatives are unavailable, penicillin is prescribed following desensitization in the presence of penicillin allergy.

After treatment, clinical and serological follow-up with a quantitative nontreponemal serological test is recommended at 6 and 12 months for early syphilis, at 6, 12, and 24 months for late syphilis, and at 1, 3, 6, 12, and 24 months for pregnant women (4). A fourfold decrease in titer by 6 months after therapy is considered an adequate response to treatment.

Patients with persistent or recurrent signs and symptoms of syphilis, a sustained fourfold increase in nontreponemal titer, or failure of initial high (>1:32) nontreponemal titers to decline fourfold within 6 months after therapy for early syphilis, are considered treatment failures. For retreatment, most prescribe weekly injections of benzathine penicillin G 2.4 million units IM for 3 weeks if the CSF result is normal (4).

A Jarisch-Herxheimer reaction is an acute febrile reaction frequently accompanied by headache, fever, and myalgia that can occur within the first 24 hours after therapy for early syphilis. Patients should be informed about this possible reaction. Antipyretics are used but do not prevent the reaction.

TABLE 32.6 Stages and Treatment Regimens for Syphilis

Early Stage	Characteristics	Treatment
Primary syphilis	• Single, painless macule at inoculation site becoming a papule that ulcerates • Lesion usually on the penis (heterosexual men); anal canal, rectum, mouth or penis (homosexual men); cervix or labia (women) • Nontender inguinal lymphadenopathy	• First line: Penicillin G benzathine 2.4 million units IM once • Second line: Doxycycline 100 mg orally every 12 hours for 14 d OR tetracycline 500 mg orally every 6 hours for 14 days
Secondary syphilis	• Preceding constitutional symptoms (e.g., fever, anorexia, headache, meningismus) • Widespread, nonpruritic, scaly and usually symmetrical maculopapular rash that may be pustular, annular or follicular • Rash may involve the palms and soles • Nontender lymphadenopathy, especially epitrochlear nodes • Intertriginous papules can enlarge into broad, moist, pink or gray-white, highly infectious lesions called condyloma lata • Rarely vasculitis with hepatitis, iritis, uveitis, arthritis, nephritis, and neurological involvement (e.g., cranial nerve palsy or auditory nerve)	• As above
Early latent	• No signs or symptoms, abnormal serology • Infection duration less than one year • Risk of mucocutaneous relapse • Potentially infectious	• As above
Late Stage	**Characteristics**	**Treatment**
Late latent	• No signs or symptoms • Abnormal serology • Infection duration one year or more • Risk of mucocutaneous relapse	• First line: Penicillin G benzathine 2.4 million units IM weekly × 3 doses • Second line: Doxycycline 100 mg every 12 hours for 28 days OR tetracycline 500 mg every 6 hours for 28 days

Tertiary syphilis	• Onset 1–30 years after primary infection
	• Manifestations include:
	  • CNS involvement (neurosyphilis, general paresis, tabes dorsalis)
	  • Cardiovascular syphilis (saccular aneurysm of ascending aorta, aortic incompetence, stenosis of coronary ostia)
	  • Gummas involving skin and bone
		• As above
		• Neurosyphilis
		  • Penicillin G 3-4 million units IV every 4 hours OR 18–24 million units IV continuous infusion over 24 hours for 10–14 days OR penicillin G procaine 2.4 million units IM daily PLUS probenecid 500 mg every 6 hours orally for 10–14 days

Congenital syphilis	• Early: rhinitis or snuffles, mucocutaneous lesions, bones changes (e.g., osteitis), hepatosplenomegaly, lymphadenopathy, anemia, jaundice, and thrombocytopenia • Late: subclinical or interstitial keratitis, eighth nerve deafness, arthropathy, neurosyphilis, and gummatous periostitis • Stigmata: Hutchinson teeth, mulberry molars, saddle nose, and saber shins	• Penicillin G 50,000 units/kg every 12 hours for first 7 days of life, and every 8 hours thereafter for a total of 10 d OR penicillin G procaine 50,000 units/kg IM daily for 10 days

CNS = central nervous system.
Adapted from: Centers for Disease Control and Prevention. Sexually transmitted diseases treatment guidelines, 2006. *MMWR Recomm Rep* 2006;55(RR-11): 1–94.

Among pregnant women, it may induce early labor or cause fetal distress.

In addition to treating people with the disease, it is also important to treat the exposed partners. Sexual transmission of *T. pallidum* usually occurs from contact with mucocutaneous syphilitic lesions, uncommon after the first year of infection. However, people exposed sexually to a patient with syphilis irrespective of its stage, should be evaluated and treated as follows (4):

- People who were exposed within 90 days preceding the diagnosis of early syphilis in a sex partner should be treated presumptively, even if seronegative.
- People who were exposed >90 days before the diagnosis of early syphilis in a sex partner should be treated presumptively if serological test results are not available immediately and the opportunity for follow-up is uncertain.
- Long-term sex partners of patients who have late syphilis should be evaluated clinically and serologically for syphilis and treated on the basis of evaluation findings.

Screening

CDC and USPSTF recommend syphilis screening at the first prenatal visit. In the absence of therapy, fetal infection acquired early in pregnancy could result in miscarriage, stillbirth, growth restriction, hydrops fetalis, premature delivery, congenital syphilis, and neonatal death. In addition, pregnant women who remain at increased risk for syphilis or where the prevalence of syphilis is high should have repeated testing for syphilis in the third trimester and at delivery. Seropositive pregnant women are considered infected unless an adequate treatment history is documented and sequential antibody titers have declined.

CDC recommends routine screening for populations at increased risk of infection including: men who have sex with men, commercial sex workers, people who exchange sex for drugs, those in correctional facilities, and STD clinic patients (see *www.cdc.gov* for a complete list) (33).

Congenital Syphilis

Nearly four of every five pregnancies complicated by syphilis, especially early syphilis, are at increased risk for adverse outcomes. Damage to the fetus depends on the developmental stage at the time of infection and the infection duration but generally does not occur until after the fourth month. Congenital syphilis can be divided into three types: (i) early (within the first 2 years of life), (ii) late (after 2 years of age), and (iii) residual stigmata (see Table 32.6).

Newborns of mothers with a reactive serological test may have reactive tests because of transplacental transfer of maternal IgG antibodies. Therefore, asymptomatic infants born to adequately treated pregnant women get monthly quantitative nontreponemal serology to monitor for appropriate reduction of antibody titers. Rising or persistent titers indicate congenital infection and these infants should receive treatment. Other indications for treatment, particularly at birth, include: (i) unknown treatment status of a seropositive mother, (ii) mother has received inadequate or nonpenicillin therapy, (iii) treatment given to the mother in the third trimester, and (iv) the infant is difficult to follow. Penicillin is the only recommended drug (Table 32.6).

HUMAN IMMUNODEFICIENCY VIRUS (HIV)

HIV is a retrovirus that produces a broad spectrum of disease from asymptomatic to acquired immunodeficiency syndrome (AIDS). After infection, the virus enters, replicates, and then destroys the CD4 lymph immune cells (also called T-helper cells); after disabling the body's immune system, a wide range of illnesses can result. The transition from initial HIV infection to AIDS takes a median of 10 years. During this time, viral replication occurs and accelerates as the immune system deteriorates. Transmission can be sexual, vertical, through the use of shared/contaminated needles, through exposure to contaminated blood, and via breast milk.

Up to 45 million people are infected worldwide, most in sub-Saharan Africa. In 2006, it was estimated that over 1 million people in the United States had HIV infection, with 21% undiagnosed. HIV screening is aimed at finding those unaware of their infection and initiating treatment to preserve their immune systems, avoid opportunistic and immunodeficiency illness, and reduce transmission.

Clinical Evaluation

Most individuals with HIV infection are asymptomatic; a portion of newly infected individuals will develop an acute retroviral syndrome with fever, pharyngitis, weight loss, adenopathy, and nausea/vomiting. HIV testing during this acute illness can be misleading as it takes from 3 weeks to 6 months for individuals to develop detectable HIV antibodies. If clinical suspicion is high, an ultrasensitive HIV viral load test can be used to diagnose HIV infection before antibodies develop.

AIDS is defined as a positive HIV blood test with either a major opportunistic condition or a CD4 count of less than 200/mm^3 (4). The opportunistic conditions could include certain infections, cancers, or syndromes that are often linked to AIDS (Table 32.7).

TABLE 32.7 Cancers, Opportunistic Infections, and Syndromes Associated with HIV

Cancers
- Invasive cervical cancer, Kaposi sarcoma, Burkitt lymphoma, immunoblastic lymphoma, and brain lymphoma

Infections
- Coccidioidomycosis, cryptococcosis, cryptosporidiosis, cytomegalovirus disease, herpes simplex, histoplasmosis, isosporiasis, *Mycobacterium avium* complex or *M. kansasii, M. tuberculosis, Pneumocystis pneumonia,* recurrent pneumonia, recurrent salmonella septicemia, toxoplasmosis of brain, or candidiasis of bronchi, trachea, lungs or esophagus

Syndromes
- Encephalopathy (HIV-related or AIDS dementia), progressive multifocal leukoencephalopathy, and HIV wasting syndrome

Diagnostic Testing

Initial testing for HIV is performed using an enzyme immunoassay for antibodies to HIV (4). If the initial test is positive, confirmatory testing using the Western blot assay is performed. If the confirmatory test is positive, the patient is diagnosed with HIV and considered infectious.

Rapid office testing using a drop of blood or a buccal swab is available. Turnaround time is less than an hour so almost all patients tested leave the office with the result. This relatively inexpensive test plays an important role in areas with high HIV prevalence, in patients at high risk, and in pregnant women with unknown HIV status in labor. Although when positive, these patients need a confirmatory Western Blot test, rapid tests have sensitivity and specificity close to 100%.

The current guidelines for initial laboratory evaluation of patients with newly diagnosed HIV disease include CD4 cell count, plasma HIV RNA (viral load), complete blood count, liver and renal functions, and urinalysis. The following tests should be performed to identify opportunistic infections: (i) RPR or VDRL for syphilis; (ii) tuberculin skin test unless a history of previous tuberculosis or positive skin test; (iii) *Toxoplasma gondii* immunoglobulin G; (iv) hepatitis A, B, and C serology; and (v) cervical Pap testing. Some authorities also advise rectal Pap screening, because of a higher incidence of HPV and higher rates of anal cancers (34).

Treatment

The current recommendation is to begin antiretroviral therapy in all patients with a history of an AIDS-defining illness or severe HIV infection regardless of the CD4 count, and in those whose CD4 counts are <200 cells/mm^3 (34). Patients should be offered antiretroviral therapy if they are asymptomatic and have CD4 counts of 201 to 350 cells/mm^3. If patients with HIV have a CD4 count of >350 cells/mm^3, treatment is more individualized, though some authorities now recommend treatment for any patient whose CD4 drops below 500 cells/mm^3. Additionally, prophylaxis for opportunistic infections must be advised for patients whose CD4 is <200 cells/mm^3. These drugs can be safely discontinued after the CD4 cell counts have increased above the thresholds for initiating prophylaxis.

Because treatment of HIV and AIDS has changed dramatically over the last few years, current treatment recommendations by the National Institute of Health (NIH) are kept at its website (*http://AIDSinfo.nih.gov*) and not in a printed document (34). Treatment recommendations are also available at the NIH website: *http://aidsinfo.nih.gov/Guidelines/Default.aspx*

Screening

Because individuals with HIV can be asymptomatic, the CDC recommends: (i) HIV screening for patients in all health care settings after the patient is notified that testing will be performed unless the patient declines (opt-out screening), (ii) people at high risk (multiple partners, men who have sex with men, needle use, sex workers, and others) should be screened for HIV at least annually, (iii) separate written consent for HIV testing should no longer be required, and (iv) prevention counseling should no longer be required. Even though the CDC published revised guidelines recommending that all individuals between 13 and 64 years of age be screened for HIV regardless of recognized risk factors, the USPSTF maintains that there are inadequate data to support screening all adolescent and adults for HIV (35). For pregnant women, HIV screening should be included in the routine panel of prenatal screening tests for all pregnant women.

KEY POINTS

- A focused history for a woman with a suspected STI includes inquiring about vaginal discharge, vaginal bleeding particularly after intercourse, pelvic or abdominal pain, menstrual cycles, any possibility of pregnancy, and the presence of any painful or painless genital lesions. PID is suspected in women with recent onset of lower abdominal pain that worsens during coitus or with jarring movement with or without associated constitutional symptoms such as fever and malaise. In men, the history should include presence and character of any penile discharge, dysuria, scrotal or testicular pain, and the presence of any painful or painless genital lesions.
- A pelvic examination should be performed on a woman who may have an STI. At the time of this exam one should observe the external genitalia, perirectal area, inner aspects of thighs and suprapubic areas for lesions and/or visible discharge. The appearance of the cervix and any discharge present should be documented. Usually a swab is taken from the cervix to test for chlamydia and gonorrhea. A bimanual exam is very important to document cervical motion tenderness and to feel for any adnexal enlargement or mass.
- The genital examination in men includes observation of the penis (including the glans), scrotum, perirectal, inner thigh, and suprapubic areas for any lesions or discharge. If there is penile discharge present or the patient has had a recent STI exposure, screen for both chlamydia and gonorrhea; the penis can be milked if discharge is not apparent.
- Though not commonly used, culture is the gold standard. It still plays a role in medicolegal cases and in patients with persistent infection following treatment. Otherwise, NAAT has replaced culture for diagnosing chlamydia and gonorrhea. Specimen types for this test include male urine, male urethral swabs, vaginal swabs, and endocervical swabs. Unlike male urine, female urine has a high level of inhibitory substances that can impair test performance. For that reason, NAAT is not approved for the detection of *N. gonorrhoeae* in women by checking their urine specimens.
- Azithromycin or doxycycline is used for treating uncomplicated chlamydia infection in men and non-pregnant women; of these two drugs, doxycycline is contraindicated during pregnancy. Single-dose cephalosporins are the recommended treatment for gonorrhea irrespective of pregnancy status.
- One should counsel patients with chlamydia, gonorrhea, or PID on safe sex practices, the need for partner treatment, and the need to screen for other STIs. To decrease the risk of reinfection, sex partners should be examined and treated if they had sexual contact with the patient during the 60 days before the patient's onset of symptoms.

CHAPTER

33

Vaginitis

Vani Selvan and Timothy J. Benton

CLINICAL OBJECTIVES

1. Cite the most common causes of infectious vaginitis.
2. Summarize the key parts of the history and physical examination that differentiate between the three most common causes of vaginitis.
3. Describe the bacterial, chemical, and cellular makeup of the normal vaginal contents.
4. Identify the diagnostic tests and office microscopy useful in elucidating the cause of vaginitis.
5. Describe treatment options for acute and recurrent cases of the common causes of vaginitis.
6. Outline the evidence-based preventive strategies for vaginitis.

Vaginitis is an inflammatory response of the vaginal mucosa most often caused by a fungal, bacterial, or parasitic infection and resulting in discharge, itching, and/or vulvovaginal discomfort. Primary care providers frequently encounter adolescent and adult women with these complaints making vaginitis one of the most commonly seen conditions, approximating 10 million office visits annually (1,2). Costs associated with treatment and missed work are about $1.8 billion annually for *Candida* vulvovaginitis (CVV) alone (3). Unfortunately, the symptoms related to vaginitis are similar despite differing etiologies, making diagnosis challenging.

The simple macroscopic anatomy of the vagina belies a complex microscopic and chemical environment that serves as a defense mechanism. Alterations of the normal vaginal flora and the existing acidic chemical milieu are the precursors to vaginitis. The clear physiologic vaginal discharge contains three general categories to consider as the foundation for the diagnostic algorithm presented below: bacterial, chemical, and cellular.

- The bacterial flora consists predominantly of Lactobacillus acidophilus, facultative long rod diphtheroids, Staphylococcus epidermidis, beta hemolytic streptococci, and coliforms (4). Vaginitis can result from introduction of organisms (e.g., *Gardnerella, Mobiluncus anaerobes, Trichomonas*) (5) not typically predominant in the vagina or from an overgrowth of organisms otherwise found in an asymptomatic state (e.g., *Candida* and lactobacilli).
- Commensal microorganisms maintain the chemical makeup of the vagina at a desired pH <4.5. Changes in the normal bacterial content (e.g., antibiotic use, douching, introduction of pathogenic organisms via sexual intercourse, or hormonal changes of pregnancy or menopause) may change the pH balance leading to vaginitis.
- The cellular component of the vagina consists only of desquamated vaginal epithelial cells. The presence of other cells, such as white blood cells indicative of an inflammatory process or stippled-appearing epithelial cells (clue cells, Fig. 33.1) confirming bacterial vaginosis (BV), assists in diagnosis.

DIAGNOSIS

Not only are there three categories to consider in the diagnostic approach to patients with vaginal symptoms but also three most common etiologies that account for two-thirds of cases: BV, CVV, and *Trichomonas* vaginitis (TV) (Table 33.1) (2,5).

Differential Diagnosis

BV occurs most frequently among women of childbearing age. Estimates of prevalence differ among populations studied and range from 4% to 10% in student health clinics, 17% to 19% in family planning clinics, and up to 24% to 40% in sexually transmitted infection (STI) clinics (6). Additionally, as many as 30% of pregnant women and women attending infertility clinics harbor BV (6). BV has an ethnic distribution in descending order of frequency: African American, Hispanic, Caucasian, and Asian women (6).

Second in frequency is fungal infection; in one study, 6.5% of telephone survey respondents reported having CVV within the previous 2 months (3). One in 10 of these women will go on to develop recurrent infection (3).

TV occurs least frequently with an estimated prevalence of 3% among 14- to 49-year-old women. TV has the same ethnic distribution as BV (7). Unlike BV, which can occur in the absence of sexual intercourse, TV is an STI with a prevalence of 5% in family planning clinics and 75% among prostitutes (1,8).

The remaining one third of diagnosed cases include atrophic vaginitis in postmenopausal women; dermatologic conditions such as lichen sclerosus or lichen planus, vulvodynia, lactobacillosis, and allergic vaginitis (5,9).

Despite a standard evaluation, up to 30% of women with vaginal complaints remain undiagnosed. Some of these women may have chronic vaginitis, typically not caused by an infection; others fail conventional therapy despite a clear diagnosis.

History and Physical Examination

The initial history and physical exam will help direct further testing of the bacterial, chemical, or cellular vaginal contents. Each of the three common causes of vaginitis has unique

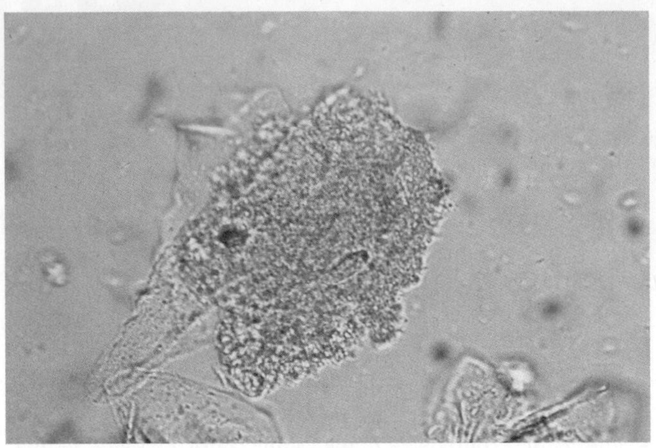

Figure 33.1 • Clue cell: from left to right: normal epithelial cell; clue cell low power field; clue cell high power field.

findings useful in directing confirmatory laboratory or in-office testing.

The history begins with open-ended questions followed by more specific inquiry into the description of symptoms such as burning, swelling or cracking of the skin; external dysuria; itching; odor; the presence and character of discharge (type, duration and timing); a risk factor analysis including sexual history; recent and current medications; and medical history. A summary of the likelihood of the disease being present based on specific symptoms and examination findings are shown in Table 33.2.

Localizing whether or not the symptoms involve the external (vulva) or internal (vagina) genitalia also helps to distinguish the causes of vaginitis. Vulvar symptoms (itching or burning) may suggest either TV or CVV, but vulvar pruritus, swelling, pain, and external dysuria have high specificity for CVV (10). In severe cases, prominent pain may exist externally because of fissuring; this does not occur in TV or BV. In contrast, itching and burning without the other skin changes suggests TV. Patients with BV rarely have symptoms related to the vulva; in fact, BV is completely asymptomatic in 50% of women (2,5).

If the primary complaint centers on vaginal odor the woman probably has BV. The characteristic "high cheese" or "fishy" odor is one of the diagnostic criteria for BV noted by Amsel (Tables 33.2 and 33.3) (11). Women may complain that they notice the smell after intercourse, as semen often accentuates the odor. Absence of a fishy odor increases the likelihood of CVV (2). TV can produce a non-fishy smell and is further distinguished from BV by external itching and burning, although to a lesser extent than CVV.

TABLE 33.1 Differential Diagnosis of Vaginitis

Very common	Bacterial vaginosis
	Candida vulvovaginitis
Common	Trichomonas vaginitis
	Cervicitis
	Vulvodynia
Uncommon	Allergic vaginosis
	Atrophic vaginitis
	Lichen sclerosus
	Lichen planus
	Lactobacillosis

All three of the major causes of vaginitis are associated with vaginal discharge but there are specific features that can guide the health care provider (Table 33.2). The presence of a thick "curdy" discharge strongly suggests CVV (10). Similarities exist between TV and BV discharge in amount and general character; however, a grayish white color (Amsel Criteria, Tables 33.2 and 33.3) is more typical of BV while yellow or green and "frothy" signals TV (11). Another distinguishing feature is that a complaint of discharge itself, excluding those with the characteristic CVV discharge, will more specifically signal BV since TV is less in amount and usually just introital (12).

Beyond identifying the specific symptoms and character of the discharge, eliciting risk factors including sexual history, recent and current medications, and medical history help to identify the cause. Sexual transmission of BV remains controversial and research is hampered by the lack of a clinical correlate in the male; however, evidence suggests increased incidence among partners with BV and multiple sexual partners. There is also an association of BV with STIs, including *Chlamydia trachomatis, Neisseria gonorrhoeae*, herpes, and syphilis (2,13,14). Risks for BV also include smoking and douching. TV is an STI, preventable using male or female latex condoms, making a detailed history of the patient's sexual practices relevant (15,16). Approximately 30% or more of women with TV have other STIs and this co-infection may increase the risk of urinary tract infection, upper genital tract disease, and Bartholin gland infection (17,18). Thus, women with TV should be routinely tested for other STIs.

For women with suspected CVV, a previous history of CVV, diabetes, oral contraceptives, intrauterine devices, steroid use, and antibiotic therapy predispose women to infection. Despite isolation of *Candida* from the penis, semen, rectum, and oral cavity of sexual partners, a clear pattern of transmission does not exist, but risk is increased with cunnilingus (5,19). However, neither eradication of these sources, stopping oral sex, nor treatment of the partner decreases recurrence of symptomatic CVV (19,20). This is also true for the approximately 50% of women who are asymptomatic vaginal carriers of *Candida*; therefore, screening is not recommended (5).

The first step of the physical exam includes an inspection of the external genitalia for mucosal breakdown, swelling, or erythema, as well as evidence of scratching with pruritus. Throughout the examination, pay particular attention to odor as this too is partly diagnostic. The traditional next step is to use a speculum to inspect the vaginal walls and the cervix. Although a speculum exam allows for visualization of the vagina and cervix, it may not be necessary in all cases because a specimen can be obtained from the vagina using just a cotton swab either by patient or by the provider during the exam (21). If the cervix is visualized, punctate hemorrhages with vesicles or papules on the surface, a so-called "strawberry cervix" (colpitis macularis), confirms TV (22) (Table 33.2). Appropriate cultures for STI tests may also be indicated, but the primary basis for diagnosis is in analysis of a sample from the pooled vaginal contents acquired using a cotton swab.

TABLE 33.2 Likelihood of Disease Based on Signs, Symptoms and Diagnostic Tests

Strength of Recommendation (SOR) History & Physical (H&P) or Diagnostic Test (Dx)	Probability of Vaginitis When Finding is	
Bacterial Vaginosis (BV)		
Helpful for ruling in BV when present	Present (%)	Absent (%)
SOR* B; H&P → Increased vaginal discharge (LR+ 1.8)[2]	43.5	20.7
SOR A; Dx− → Vaginal pH >4.5 (LR+ 3.4)[2]	69.4	9.1
SOR A; Dx− → Wet mount Clue cells (LR+ 30)[19]	81.8	5.7
SOR A; Dx− → Wet mount Clue cells >20% (LR+ 5.3)[2]	77.9	16.7
SOR A; Dx− → Positive Whiff test (LR+ 9.6)[2]	86.5	18.9
SOR A; Dx− → Amsel criteria (3/4 or more) (LR+ 9.9)[2]	86.8	18
Helpful for ruling out BV when absent		
SOR B; H&P → Fishy odor (LR− 0.3)[2]	57.8	11.4
SOR A; Dx− → Gram stain (LR− 3.1)[2]	75.6	9.1
SOR A; Dx− → Fem Card pH or amine+ (LR− 0.2)[2]	60.5	10.7
For Recurrence		
Affirm VPIII Microbial Identification Test (LR+ 190)[35]	99.2	3.2
Candida Vulvovaginitis (VVC)		
Helpful for ruling in CVV when present		
SOR B; H&P → Chief complaint of pruritus/burning (LR+ 3.4)[10]	45.9	16.5
SOR B; H&P → Thick Curdy vaginal discharge (LR+ 18)[10]	81.8	17.2
SOR B; H&P → Vulvar edema (LR+ 2.4)[10]	37.5	17.4
SOR B; Dx− → Yeast forms on a KOH preparation (LR+ 2.7)[2]	72.6	33.6
SOR B; Dx− → Yeast rapid antigen tests (LR+ 4.56)[2]	75.3	17.6
Helpful for ruling out CVV when absent		
SOR B; H&P → Vulvar pain/burning (LR− 0.91)[10]	29.8	18.5
SOR B; H&P → Vulvar erythema (LR− 0.84)[10]	33.3	17.4
SOR B; H&P → Vulvar pruritus (LR− 0.78)[10]	25.9	16.3
SOR B; Dx → Vaginal pH <4.9 (LR− 0.32)[2]	75.3	12.1
For Recurrence		
Affirm VPIII Microbial Identification Test (LR+ 41)[35]	95.8	9.4
PCR – Genzyme (LR+ 48.5)[34]	97	2
Trichomonas Vaginitis (TV)		
Helpful for ruling in TV when present		
SOR C; H&P → Pruritus (LR+ 3.8)[12]	62	23.1
SOR C; H&P → Burning (LR+ 12)[12]	83.7	25.5
SOR C; H&P → Vulvar edema (LR+ 2.4)[12]	37.5	17.4
SOR A; Dx− → Frothy discharge (LR+ 2.9)[12]	55.4	11.4
SOR A; Dx− → Trichomonads in wet prep (LR+ 58)[12]	96.1	14.6
SOR A; Dx− → pH >4.5 (LR+ 2.5)[12]	51.7	8.7
SOR A; Dx− → Trichomonads in Pap smear (LR+ 19)[12]	37	1.2

(*continued*)

TABLE 33.2 *(Continued)*

Strength of Recommendation (SOR) History & Physical (H&P) or Diagnostic Test (Dx)	Probability of Vaginitis When Finding is	
For Recurrence		
Affirm VPIII Microbial Identification Test (LR+ 92)[35]	98.4	5.1
Helpful for ruling out TV when absent		
SOR C; H&P → Introital discharge (LR− 0.3)[12]	55.4	11.4
SOR C; H&P → Odor (LR− 0.4)[12]	51.7	14.6
SOR A; Dx− → Inflamed cervix (strawberry cervix) (LR− 0.4)[12]	47.4	14.6

LR+ = positive likelihood ratio; tests with higher values, especially >5, are good at ruling in disease.
LR− = negative likelihood ratio; tests with lower values, especially <0.2, are good at ruling out disease.
*A = consistent, good-quality patient-oriented evidence; B = inconsistent or limited-quality patient-oriented evidence; C = consensus, disease-oriented evidence, usual practice, expert opinion, or case series.
For information about the Strength of Recommendation Taxonomy evidence rating system, see *http://www.aafp.org/afpsort.xml*.
Adapted from Anderson, MR, Klink, K, Cohrssen, A. Evaluation of vaginal complaints. *JAMA* 2004;291:1368–1379.

Diagnostic Testing

After a complete history and physical the health care provider will likely have a good idea of the cause of vaginitis as detailed in the algorithm presented in Figure 33.2; however, confirmation occurs by pH testing, in-office microscopy of a wet mount slide, and a 10% potassium hydroxide (KOH)-prepared slide of the vaginal discharge.

The pH is normal with CVV and elevated (5 to 7) in TV and BV. This simple test of applying the vaginal discharge to litmus paper directly from the swab specimen (or during the speculum exam place the litmus paper against the lateral vaginal wall) requires some care in performing as blood and cervical mucus can cause inaccuracy due to their alkalinity (23).

TABLE 33.3 Amsel and Nugent's Criteria for Bacterial Vaginosis

Amsel Criteria*	Nugent's Criteria (Gram Stain)*
Positive result is presence of at least three criteria	Positive test is total score of seven or higher
1. Adherent grayish-white discharge	1. Presence of lactobacillus (many = zero and none = four)
2. Positive whiff test	2. Gardnerella and Bacteroides (none = zero and many = four)
3. Vaginal pH greater than 4.5	3. Curved gram-variable rods (none = zero and many = two)
4. Presence of clue cells	

*Amsel criteria have 70% sensitivity and 94 % specificity (49). Nugent's criteria are 89%–100% sensitive and 83%–97% specific with a score of seven or more (37).

After completing pH testing, place the swab in a saline solution for further analysis by microscopy (Table 33.2).

With just two slides prepared for examination under the microscope, wet mount and KOH in-office testing will identify most cases of vaginitis (2). A Gram stain has usefulness in diagnosing BV (Table 33.2) in the laboratory using Nugent's criteria (Table 33.3), but it is rarely performed in the office (17,24). If necessary, the wet mount slide can be sent for Gram stain.

Preparation of a wet mount includes adding saline to the vaginal discharge on a slide or placing the swab in a 2-mL test tube of saline solution then applying a drop to a microscope slide with a cover slip. If the slide contains clue cells (Fig. 33.1), the single most reliable predictor, the patient has BV (Table 33.2) (5,25). The presence of an "abnormal background flora" described as either a lack of long-rod predominance and/or the presence of a large proportion of short rods, cocci, or curved rods, also suggests BV. Moving organisms under low or high power likely represent motile trichomonads (Fig. 33.3) confirming TV (Table 33.2) (5,26). Finally, noting white blood cells (WBCs) may help only to confirm a suspicion of TV, CVV, or STI.

The second slide (KOH) provides a basis for the diagnosis of CVV but when preparing the slide it may indicate BV. After placing some of the discharge on a microscope slide, application of one or two drops of 10% KOH will release aromatic amines resulting in the characteristic "fishy odor" characteristic if BV is present, the whiff test (Amsel Criteria, Table 33.3). Following 10 minutes of air-drying, the staining will show hyphae or budding yeast of *Candida* (22). Identifying single yeast forms is less accurate than budding yeast; otherwise, a KOH test is positive in 50% to 70% of women with CVV due to *C. albicans*, but in only 7% to 16% of women with Torulopsis glabrata—a non–hyphae-forming fungus (27,28). If available, a rapid antigen test can be used, but cannot be relied on if negative (Table 33.2) (29).

If difficulty arises in performing these tests, the US Food and Drug Administration has approved the FemExam pH and Amine Test Card for testing vaginal discharge. It has a high level of accuracy and reproducibility (Table 33.2) (30).

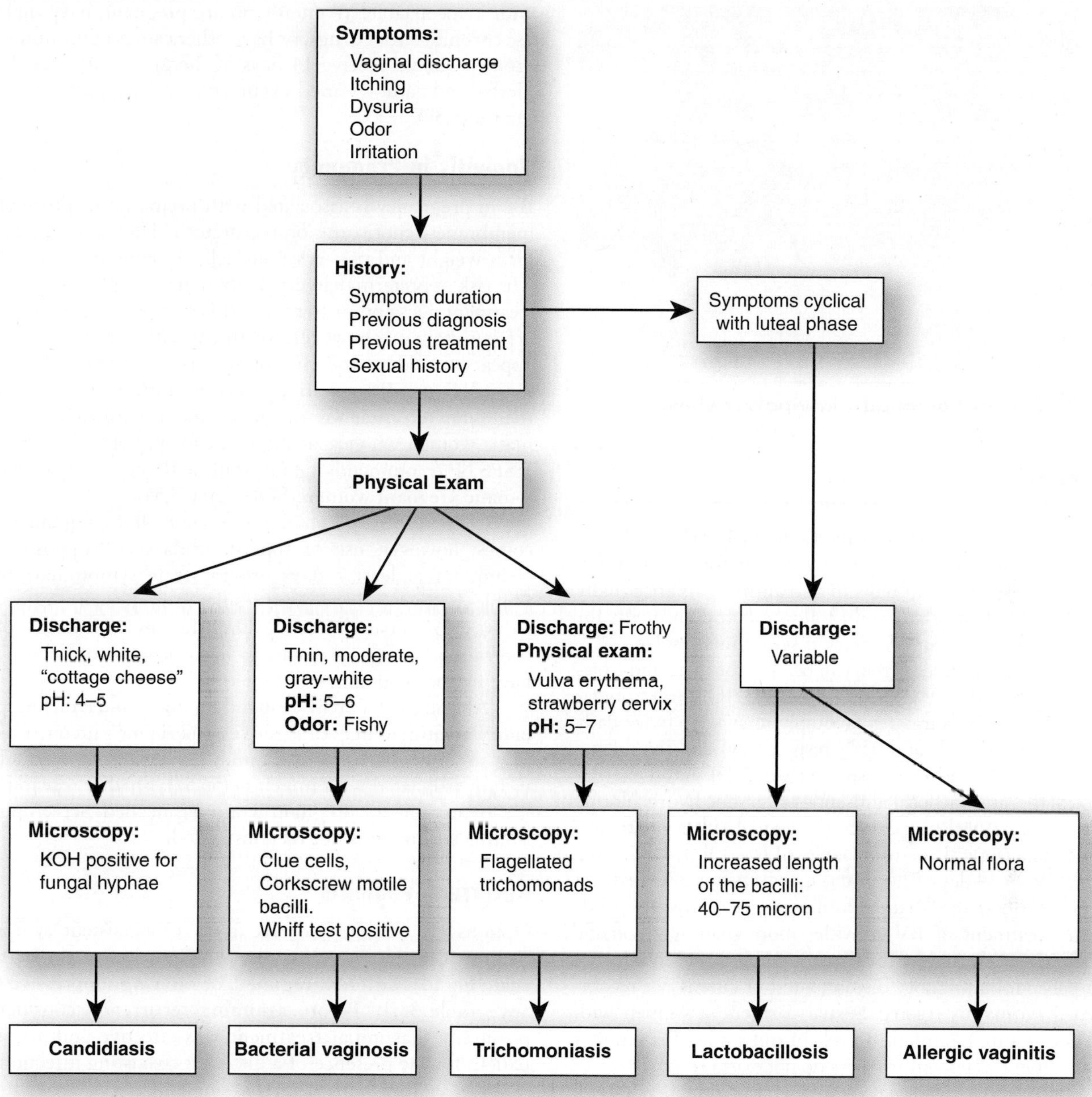

Figure 33.2 • Diagnostic algorithm (5).

In summary, the use of the history and physical exam along with simple in office tests outlined in the algorithm (Fig. 33.2) will identify the cause of vaginitis in the majority of cases. Additional testing as described below may occasionally be necessary.

Additional Testing

Additional testing options include culture of the vaginal discharge; enzyme-linked immunosorbent assay, polymerase chain reaction, and DNA probe each with specific indications. Culture will identify any of the common three causes of vaginitis and is indicated for women with treatment failures or a high index of clinical suspicion with inconclusive initial tests and/or treatment failure. For example, in a patient with persistent TV symptoms, a high pH, and leukocytes without trichomonads on wet mount, culture can be used as the "gold standard" to identify TV (SORT B) (20). Culture can also confirm CVV for the 50% of women with CVV who have negative microscopy (31,32).

Gene-based or enzyme assays are useful secondary tests for practitioners unable to perform microscopy (33). A DNA probe (Affirm VPIII Microbial Identification Test) has a high sensitivity (90% to 100%) for *Trichomonas*, *Gardnerella*, and *Candida* but is expensive (34). Another widely available and accurate option is a rapid (10 minute) polymerase chain reaction–based trichomonas detection called Genzyme (33,35). Last, *Gardnerella* species produce the cytotoxin vaginolysin identifiable by an enzyme-linked immunosorbent assay antibody-based technique with reasonable accuracy; however, further trials are needed to identify proper use in the clinical setting (35).

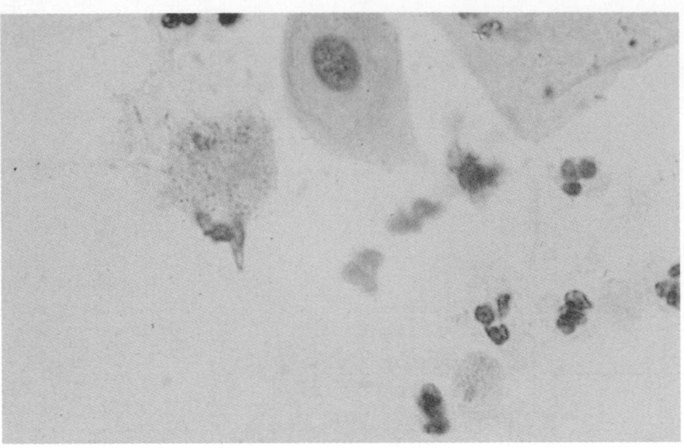

Figure 33.3 • Trichomonads: low-power view.

TREATMENT

Treatment options are shown in Table 33.4. Metronidazole (oral or intravaginal) is first-line treatment for BV and TV (36,37). For CVV, intravaginal and oral antifungals are equally efficacious (38). Test of cure and follow-up appointments for BV, CVV, and TV are unnecessary if symptoms resolve.

For BV, topical clindamycin can be used for metronidazole-allergic patients; efficacy exceeds 80% (36,38). Oral metronidazole as a single dose compares favorably to a 7-day twice daily regimen (cure rate 87% and 92%, respectively) and the relapse rate is similar (53% and 44%, respectively) (37,39). As an alternative topical therapy, the local antiseptic octenidine hydrochloride phenoxyethanol (OHP) appears to have equal efficacy to topical metronidazole (topical metronidazole: 61.0%, OHP for 7 days: 57.6%, OHP for 14 days: 71.0%) and may be better tolerated and easier to use; Food and Drug Administration approval is pending (40). Treatment of BV provides more than symptomatic relief because it reduces the incidence of subsequent endometritis and pelvic inflammatory disease; a test of cure is not recommended if symptoms resolve. Sexual partners of women with BV do not require treatment (Level Ib) and studies for simultaneous treatment of lesbian partners do not exist (41,42).

TV is treated using oral metronidazole as either a one-time dose or as a 7-day course with an expected cure rate of 90% (43). In contrast to the other two primary causes of vaginitis, all sexual partners of women with TV require treatment and a test of cure is recommended if symptoms recur or do not resolve (SOR=C) (43). Although a single oral dose of tinidazole (2 g) has equal efficacy, expense limits its use. Allergy to metronidazole poses a significant problem, as potential cross-reactivity to tinidazole exists; therefore, in-hospital desensitization with either an oral or intravenous protocol is recommended for symptomatic and pregnant women with hypersensitivity to metronidazole (44,45). If desensitization is impossible, 6.25% paromomycin cream (250 mg of paromomycin per 4-g applicator intravaginal daily for 2 to 3 weeks) provides an effective option. Paromomycin can cause severe vaginal ulceration that appears to be self-limiting and resolves with discontinuation of therapy (46).

CVV treatment options have a greater than 80% cure rate in uncomplicated cases, so cost, convenience, and patient preference should guide the choice. Oral medication while offering convenience has potential for systemic side effects, particularly with ketoconazole. Women who are pregnant, have diabetes, use chronic steroid drugs, or have other causes of immunocompromise should receive 14 days of therapy (SOR=A) (38,47). Herbal and natural remedies currently lack supporting data for their use (39).

Vaginitis in Pregnancy

BV in pregnancy is associated with premature rupture of the membranes, chorioamnionitis, preterm labor and birth, low birth weight and post-cesarean delivery endometritis (47–50). The risk of preterm delivery doubles in asymptomatic cases but treatment does appear to reduce this risk. Among women who are symptomatic, however, treatment with oral metronidazole appears to reduce the risk of preterm delivery (51,52). The United States Preventative Services Task Force (USPSTF) therefore, recommends diagnosis and treatment of symptomatic women who are at high risk for preterm delivery. The USPSTF recommends against routine BV screening of asymptomatic pregnant women (SOR=B) (53,54).

CVV during pregnancy does not alter pregnancy outcomes; however, use of topical imidazoles (suppository or cream) for at least 7 days provides safe symptomatic relief (Table 33.4). A 7-day course results in higher cure rates than 4 days (90% versus 50%) (55). Oral therapy with imidazoles is contraindicated in pregnancy; butoconazole or terconazole have not been adequately studied.

Although TV will respond to metronidazole in pregnancy, treatment may cause adverse perinatal outcomes offsetting the potential risks of premature delivery and low birth weight associated with infection (56,57). Further research into TV treatments for pregnant women is needed. Screening and routine treatment is not recommended.

Recurrent Vaginitis

Options for treatment of recurrent or persistent symptoms include using the same medication for a longer time period, changing to a different regimen, or offering suppressive therapy (Table 33.4). Before assuming recurrence, consider the possibility that initial treatment was effective and assess the patient for the presence of a different coexisting infection.

For women with BV, recurrences occur in about 10% of women within 3 months; the presence of a different infecting organism such as Mobiluncus (curved rods on wet mount) is sometimes found (58,59). Alternative treatment for recurrent BV includes a different medication (clindamycin, amoxicillin/clavulanate, tinidazole) or 14 days of metronidazole (60,61). Suppressive therapy with twice weekly intravaginal metronidazole for 28 weeks after initial daily treatment for 10 days has shown success (number needed to treat = 6) but may cause pain or candidiasis (number needed to harm = 5) (62).

Management of recurrent TV involves metronidazole with higher dosing or as combination therapy of topical and oral (63). A second course of 500 mg twice daily for 7 days may be tried but a third recurrence warrants increased dosing to 2 g daily for 5 to 7 days (47). Culture and sensitivity can be useful in guiding therapy.

Recurrent CVV, defined as four episodes in 1 year with partial resolution between each, occurs in about one quarter of patients and is confirmed by at least two occasions having

TABLE 33.4 Treatment of Vaginitis*

Intervention	Efficacy	Strength of Recommendation†	Comments and Cautions
Bacterial vaginosis (BV)		A	Treatment is indicated for symptomatic women and asymptomatic women undergoing invasive gynecological procedures
Metronidazole 500 mg oral twice daily for 7 days	84%–97%	A	• Metronidazole is first line for non-pregnant women; intravaginal equals oral treatment • Avoid alcohol with metronidazole until 24 hours after use (72 hours for tinidazole) due to disulfiram-like effect • Clindamycin is regarded safe during pregnancy
Clindamycin 2% cream 1 applicator at bedtime for 7 days	72%–94%	A	
Metronidazole 500 mg—4 orally one time	87%–94%	A	
Metronidazole 0.75% cream 1 applicator twice daily for 5 days	75%–79%	A	
Clindamycin 300 mg oral twice daily, 7–14 days	79%	A	
Clindamycin ovules 300 mg intravaginal at bedtime for 3 days	54%	A	
Avoid douching, use of shower gel, antiseptic agents, or bath shampoo		C	
Trichomonas vaginitis (TV)		A	TV is sexually transmitted and women and their sexual partners should be treated even if asymptomatic; treatment during pregnancy may cause adverse perinatal outcomes offsetting potential benefit
Metronidazole 500 mg—4 orally one time	90%–95%	B	• Avoid alcohol with metronidazole until 24 hours after use (72 hours for tinidazole) due to disulfiram-like effect • Metronidazole as a single oral dose of 2 g is effective in pregnancy, but the effect on pregnancy outcome is uncertain • For recurrent infection increase duration of therapy to 14–21 days or add intravaginal gel as adjunct to oral therapy • Desensitization required if metronidazole allergic; if not possible, use paromomycin
Metronidazole 500 mg oral twice daily for 7 days	90%	B	
Tinidazole 500 mg—4 orally one time	86%–100%	B	
Paromomycin 6.25% 4 g intravaginal daily for 2–3 weeks	No data	C	
Candida vulvovaginitis (VVC)		A	Symptomatic women should be treated; intravaginal and oral antifungals are equally effective but potential systemic side effects and drug interactions may occur with oral medication

(*continued*)

TABLE 33.4 *(Continued)*

Intervention	Efficacy	Strength of Recommendation[†]	Comments and Cautions
Betaconazole 2% cream 1 applicator at bedtime for 7 days	81%–92%	A	• Intravaginal preparations of butoconazole, clotrimazole, miconazole, and tioconazole are available OTC; no agent is superior • For recurring VVC, use 10–14 days of induction therapy with a topical or oral azole, followed by fluconazole at a dosage of 150 mg once per week for 6 months [SORT A] • Creams and suppositories can weaken latex condoms and diaphragms, caution is advised • Treatment of sex partners is not recommended except with recurrence • Topical azoles, applied for 7–14 days, are recommended for pregnant women. [SORT A] • Avoid oral antifungals in pregnancy and breastfeeding [SORT A]
Clotrimazole 1% cream 1 applicator at bedtime for 7 days	72%–77%	A	
Clotrimazole vaginal suppository 100 mg at bedtime for 7 days	52%–72%	A	
Miconazole 2% cream 1 applicator for 7 days	No data	C	
Miconazole vaginal suppository 100 mg at bedtime for 7 days	No data	C	
Terconazole 0.8% cream 1 applicator at bedtime for 3 days	No data	C	
Nystatin 100,000 units at bedtime for 14 days	70%–90%	B	
Fluconazole 150 mg oral one time, may be repeated in 72 hours if still symptomatic	80%–95%	A	
Boric acid vaginal suppository 600 mg twice daily for 14 days	77%–81%	C	
Yogurt douching once daily for 3 days	55%	C	

d = days; PTB = preterm birth; SORT = strength of recommendation taxonomy; OTC = over-the-counter.
*Interventions in each section are listed by best to worst efficacy, if known, with SORT, comments and cautions.
†A = consistent, good-quality patient-oriented evidence; B = inconsistent or limited-quality patient-oriented evidence; C = consensus, disease-oriented evidence, usual practice, expert opinion, or case series.
For information about the Strength of Recommendation Taxonomy evidence rating system, see *http://www.aafp.org/afpsort.xml.*
Information from: Clinical Effectiveness Group, British Association for Sexual Health and HIV (BASHH). National guideline for the management of bacterial vaginosis. London (UK): British Association for Sexual Health and HIV (BASHH); 2006. 14 p; Clinical Effectiveness Group, British Association for Sexual Health and HIV (BASHH). United Kingdom national guideline on the management of trichomonas vaginalis. London (UK): British Association for Sexual Health and HIV (BASHH); 2007. 8 p; Clinical practice guidelines for the management of candidiasis: 2009 update by the Infectious Diseases Society of America. *Clin Infect Dis.* 2009;48(5):503–505; Workowski KA, Berman SM. Diseases characterized by vaginal discharge. Sexually transmitted diseases guidelines, MMWR 2006/vol 55/No.RR-11; Sobel JD, Nyirjesy P, Brown W. Tinidazole therapy for metronidazole resistant vaginal trichomoniasis. *Clin Infect Dis.* 2001;33:1341–1346; Marrazzo J. Vulvovaginal candidiasis. *BMJ* 2002;325:586.

heavy growth of *C. albicans* on microscopy (SOR=C) (64). These patients may respond to maintenance therapy for 2 to 4 months given as either pulses corresponding to the menstrual cycle or continuously as described in Table 33.4. Additional options for managing patients with recurrent CVV, which may result from unusual causes such as *Torulopsis glabrata* and *Candida tropicalis*, are to continue maintenance therapy for a longer period or try one of the following: boric acid suppositories, oral itraconazole or flucytosine given orally or topically (64–67). Suppressive therapy with once-weekly oral fluconazole will reduce recurrences but is expensive (64,68). Unfortunately, attempts to restore the protective bacterial flora by eating yogurt containing live cultures of Lactobacillus acidophilus or use of intravaginal preparations have limited success in preventing recurrences or post-antibiotic CVV (69,70). Patients can also try risk factor modification of dietary changes (increasing intake of dairy products), oral contraceptive discontinuation, or periodic intravaginal or oral culture-positive yogurt use (SOR=C) (70). These associations do not necessarily imply causation of CVV, and a change in risk factors or behavior may not prevent further infections.

Other Causes of Vaginitis

Vaginal symptoms may also due to non-infectious causes. Allergic vaginitis from chemical irritants like spermicides, douches, detergents, fabric softeners, soaps, bath oils, salts, sanitary napkins, and latex condoms results in mild to severe itching and/or burning of the vulva without discharge (71). Severe reactions may cause labial swelling and erythema resembling CVV. After ruling out infection as discussed previously, treatment consists of steroid ointment and avoidance.

Atrophic vaginitis may be found in menopausal women. These women typically have itching and discharge with nonspecific findings on wet mount such as WBCs and parabasal cells. This condition responds to estrogen replacement either topically or orally (see Chapter 29).

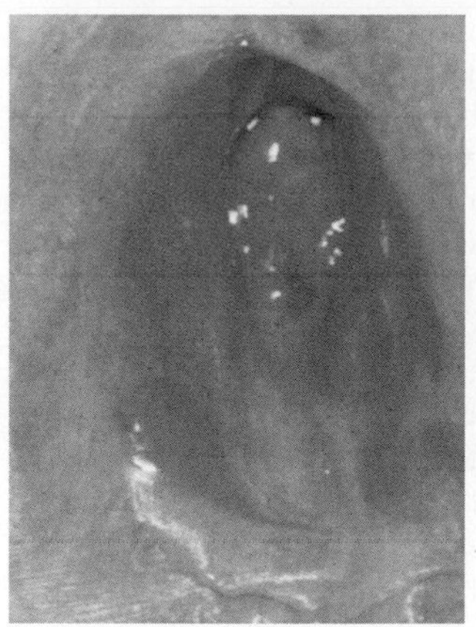

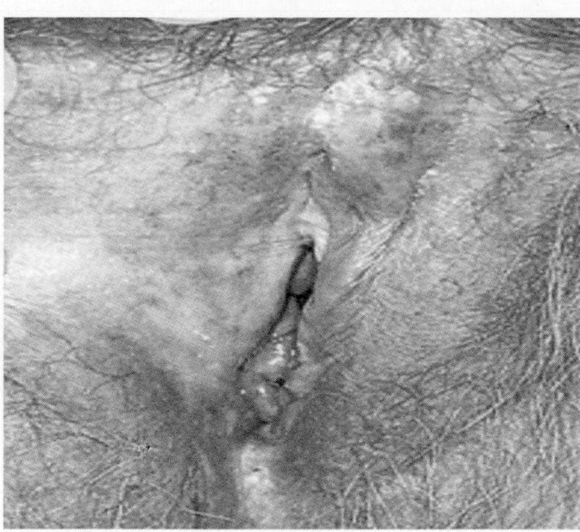

Figure 33.4 • Lichen planus (A) and lichen sclerosus (B).

Another noninfectious cause associated with WBC's and parabasal cells on wet mount is desquamative inflammatory vaginitis. This condition is further characterized by a purulent vaginal discharge demonstrating a lack of lactobacilli, high pH, and numerous epithelial cells. Women report vulvar irritation or itching and the treatment consists of intravaginal steroids and/or clindamycin (intravaginal or oral) (71).

Dermatologic conditions such as lichen planus and lichen sclerosus may cause vaginal symptoms but these problems are evident on physical exam (Fig. 33.4). Biopsy may be required for diagnosis. Lichen planus is usually self-limiting and lichen sclerosis responds to topical steroids. The etiology of these conditions is unknown.

Vulvodynia is a condition causing vulvar burning, stinging and soreness to touch, intercourse, tampon insertion, etc. that may be confused with vaginitis. The physical exam is normal other than tenderness to palpation. Vulvodynia is often mistaken for CVV and treated as such, but reconsidered after lack of treatment response.

Lactobacillosis is an overgrowth of lactobacilli resulting in cyclical discharge and discomfort, especially before menses. It is diagnosed by wet mount showing long filaments or lactobacilli organized into chains (Fig. 33.5). Treatment consists of amoxicillin/clavulanate 500 mg three times a day for 7 days, doxycycline 100 mg orally twice a day for 10 days, or azithromycin (72).

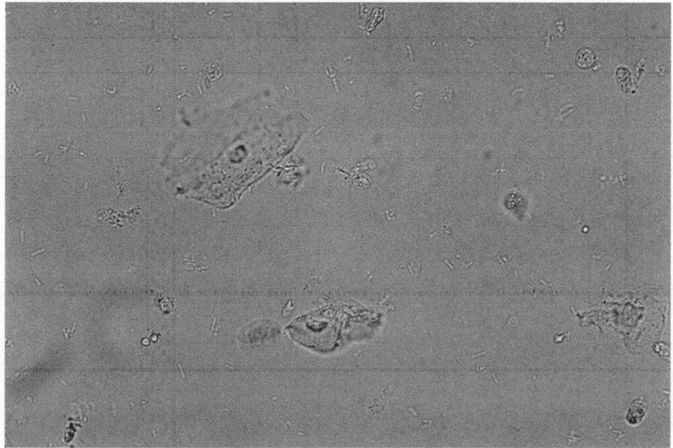

Figure 33.5 • Lactobacillosis. Lactobacilli in long filament chains.

EDUCATION AND PREVENTION

Abnormal vaginal discharge may develop in women who practice various routine hygiene habits, such as douching, daily use of panty liners, "feminine hygiene" sprays, powders, or rinses, bubble baths or other scented bath products, and tight or restrictive synthetic clothing (73–75). Avoiding these may lower risk of vaginitis. Douching is not recommended for the prevention or treatment of vaginitis (SOR=B).

With nonprescription treatment readily available, many women will self-diagnose often assuming they have CVV. Incorrect self-diagnosis leads to delay in diagnosis, unnecessary expenses, or worsening symptoms (76). Women with or without a history of CVV misdiagnose themselves 66% and 89% of the time, respectively; this is similar to a physician's inability to make the correct diagnosis by history alone (77,78). Patients need to be educated regarding inaccuracy of self-testing and diagnosis or telephone diagnosis. A clinical evaluation of women with vaginal symptoms is recommended, particularly for women who fail to respond to self-treatment with a nonprescription antifungal (SOR=C) (47).

KEY POINTS

- Vaginitis is an inflammatory response of the vaginal mucosa from either non-infectious or infectious causes. The most common causes of infectious vaginitis are bacterial vaginosis (BV), candida vulvovaginitis (CVV), and Trichomonas vaginitis (TV).
- The vaginal bacterial flora consists predominantly of Lactobacillus acidophilus, facultative long rod diphtheroids, Staphylococcus epidermidis, beta hemolytic streptococci, and coliforms; these microorganisms maintain the chemical makeup of the vagina at a desired pH less than 4.5. The cellular component of the vagina consists only of desquamated vaginal epithelial cells.

- Vulvar symptoms (itching or burning) suggest either TV or CVV while vulvar pruritus, swelling, pain, external dysuria, and the presence of a thick "curdy" discharge have high specificity for CVV. Patients with BV rarely have symptoms related to the vulva. "Fishy" odor is consistent with BV.
- Confirmation of vaginitis occurs by pH testing, in-office microscopy of a wet mount slide, and a 10% potassium hydroxide (KOH)-prepared slide of the physician or patient-collected vaginal discharge. The pH is normal with CVV and elevated (>4.5) in TV and BV. The presence of clue cells and abnormal background flora suggest BV. Under low or high power microscopy, motile trichomonads confirm TV. Addition of 10% KOH to the wet mount will release aromatic amines resulting in the characteristic "fishy odor" of BV (whiff test) and hyphae or budding yeast under microscopy are indicators of CVV. Microscopy of the vaginal discharge is the best test for determining an etiology for vaginitis due to CVV, BV, or TV.
- Metronidazole (oral or intravaginal) is first-line treatment for BV and TV. Intravaginal and oral antifungals are equally efficacious treatments for CVV. Follow-up is not needed if symptoms resolve. No test of cure is required for BV, CVV or TV.
- Abnormal vaginal discharge may develop in women who practice various routine hygiene habits, such as douching, daily use of panty liners, "feminine hygiene" sprays, powders, or rinses, bubble baths or other scented bath products, and tight or restrictive synthetic clothing; avoiding these may lower risk of vaginitis.

CHAPTER

34

Ankle and Knee Pain

Cathy Abbott and Henry C. Barry

ANKLE PAIN

CLINICAL OBJECTIVES

1. Describe the functional anatomy of the ankle
2. Provide a differential diagnosis for and know the common causes of lateral, medial, posterior, and anterior ankle pain
3. Describe the expected outcomes of the common treatments for ankle pain

Ankle pain is among the most common and important musculoskeletal complaints seen by primary care physicians, accounting for more than 750,000 outpatient visits each year (1). Additionally, ankle injuries are the most common injuries in sports, with about 5% of high school and college athletes spraining their ankle each year (2).

Ankle pain may be traumatic or nontraumatic. The painful ankle may be acute, chronic, an acute exacerbation of a chronic condition or a recurrent acute presentation. Traumatic disorders include sprains, strains, dislocations, fractures, and overuse syndromes, such as tendinitis and stress fractures. The terms "sprain" and "strain" are often used interchangeably; however, they are technically different. Sprains are injuries in which a ligament is stretched or torn, whereas strains are injuries that involve stretching or tearing of tendons or muscles. Nontraumatic disorders include degenerative joint disease (DJD), rheumatologic disorders, osteomyelitis, and neoplasms.

FUNCTIONAL ANATOMY

A solid knowledge of the functional anatomy of the ankle is imperative to understanding the nature of underlying problems and in facilitating rehabilitation. The ankle joint, depicted in Figure 34.1, is a hinge joint, which can also invert and evert in response to walking on irregular surfaces. It includes the distal fibula, talus, and distal tibia. The ankle mortise (combined joint structure) which is formed from these bones is stabilized on the lateral side by—from anterior to posterior—the anterior talofibular ligament, the calcaneal fibular ligament, the posterior talofibular ligament, and the peroneus longus and brevis tendons. The anterior talofibular ligament is part of the lateral joint capsule, running from the anterior distal fibula to the neck of the talus and is the most susceptible ligament to acute injury. In the frontal plane, the anterior tibiofibular ligament, posterior tibiofibular ligament and syndesmosis, a thickened sheet of interosseous membrane, stabilize the mortise and allow minimal motion between the distal tibia and fibula. Most importantly, they prevent separation of the tibia and fibula as the forces from the calcaneus and talus are transferred up the leg.

On the medial side, the deltoid ligament is composed of a superficial and deep layer. The thickness of this ligament medially along with the distant extension of the lateral malleolus providing boney stabilization makes the ankle quite resistant to eversion stress. The mortise of the ankle joint allows dorsiflexion, plantar flexion, and internal and external rotation. The subtalar joint formed by the talus and calcaneus allows true inversion, eversion, and internal and external rotation. The Achilles tendon attaches at the posterior portion of the calcaneus, and is the primary plantar flexor. The peroneus brevis and longus tendons are the primary everters of the ankle, and run posterior then inferior to the lateral malleolus. The peroneus brevis attaches to the distal fifth metatarsal, sometimes causing an avulsion fracture when it is strained. The posterior tibialis tendon runs posterior and inferior to the medial malleolus and attaches to the navicular, assisting in inversion and supporting the arch.

DIFFERENTIAL DIAGNOSIS

Acute injuries to the ankle can result in injuries to the lateral or medial ligaments or to the tibiofibular ligaments and syndesmosis (the "high ankle sprain"), tendinous injuries, or fractures of the ankle or midfoot. Ligamentous injuries to the ankle can be classified by grade according to the degree of instability and functional disability. This classification is important because it guides therapy. Grade I injuries have minimal swelling and partial ligament tearing, but no clinical instability. Grade II injuries usually result from a complete tear of the anterior talofibular ligament Grade III injuries result from complete ligamentous disruption of the anterior talofibular ligament and calcaneal fibular ligament.

Most ankle injuries result from forced inversion with the ankle in plantar flexion. The anterior talofibular ligament is the most commonly injured ligament. The anterior talofibular ligament is vulnerable during plantar flexion because it is aligned vertically (parallel to the fibula) and is under tension. This is commonly injured when a ball player lands on another's foot or when a person steps off a curb onto an uneven surface.

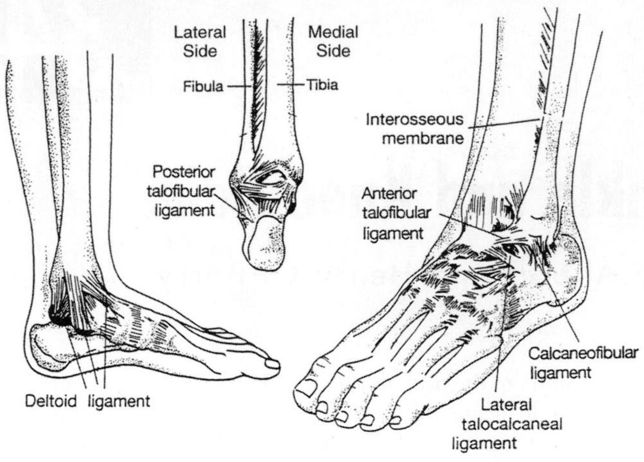

Figure 34.1 • Anatomy of the ankle joint. (Adapted from Leach RE. A nonsurgical approach to early mobility: acute ankle sprain, treat vigorously for best results. *J Musculoskel Med.* 1983;1[1]:69.)

Tendinosis involving the Achilles tendon, the peroneal tendons, or the posterior tibialis tendon is a common, often chronic condition, which can cause ankle pain. This previously was known as tendinitis however a more correct reflection of its chronic, overuse etiology has prompted it and other tendinopathies to be currently referred to as a tendinosis. The mechanism is repetitive microtrauma that stresses the peritendinous structures, resulting in inflammation and even partial tendon rupture. Training errors, running in improper shoes, running on hills, and running on uneven or hard surfaces are common causes of Achilles tendinosis (3). Achilles tendon rupture is a common hazard in jumping sports and can be a complication of steroid injections (4) or fluoroquinolone antibiotics (5). Table 34.1 summarizes the differential diagnosis of ankle pain.

CLINICAL EVALUATION

You should perform a careful history and physical examination in all patients with ankle pain. It is especially important to address potential red flags (see Table 34.2). These conditions are serious and require early referral. You should also ask all patients about their treatment and activity goals. For instance, an elderly patient with severe DJD may be satisfied to become independent in transferring out of bed and in getting to the bathroom. Others may desire to return to their previous performance level in full contact sports. Management should be individualized and congruent with the patient's goals.

History and Physical Examination

The history should address the location, duration, character, and intensity of pain. It should also include a description of the mechanism of the injury, ameliorating and exacerbating

TABLE 34.1 Differential Diagnosis of Ankle and Knee Pain

Diagnosis	Frequency in Primary Care	Frequency in Emergency Department
Ankle		
Inversion injury	Very common	Very common
Avulsion fracture	Common	Very common
Achilles tendonitis	Common	Common
Eversion injury	Uncommon	Uncommon
Fibular fracture	Uncommon	Common
Syndesmosis injury	Uncommon	Uncommon
Trimalleolar fracture	Rare	Rare
Knee		
Anterior knee pain*	Very common	Very common
Degenerative joint disease	Very common	Common
Patellar tendonitis	Common	Common
MCL/LCL strain or tear	Common	Common
Meniscal tear	Common	Common
ACL strain or tear	Common	Common
Patellar dislocation	Uncommon	Uncommon
Fracture	Uncommon	Common

*Also known as patellofemoral syndrome or chondromalacia patellae.

TABLE 34.2 Red Flags in Patients with Ankle or Knee Pain

Red Flag	Diagnosis Suspected
Hemarthrosis	Internal derangement, hemophilia
Knee pain and limp	Hip disorder (e.g. Legg-Perthes, in child with slipped capital femoral epiphysis, normal knee examination)
Poor response to treatment	Internal derangement, malignancy (rare)
Bony swelling	Tumor
Fever	Osteomyelitis, septic arthritis
Rash, joint swelling	Collagen vascular disorders, gonococcal arthritis

factors, previous injury, and current treatment. Further history should concentrate on whether a "snap" or "pop" was felt (suggesting ligament rupture), the time delay from injury to the onset of symptoms, and the initial treatment given. Symptoms such as an inability to bear weight immediately after the injury or a feeling that the ankle "gives way" are especially worrisome; the former is an important factor in distinguishing sprain from fracture (Fig. 34.2, Ottawa Ankle Rules [OAR]) (6). Inquiring about the chronicity of the symptoms and about changes in the level of activity, such as an increase in the number of miles run prior to symptoms or an increase in the intensity of workouts is also helpful particularly when the symptom is more chronic and insidious in onset.

The physical examination should include evaluation of gait, range of motion, strength testing, palpation, and finally, ought to include an assessment of stability (Fig. 34.3). To help distinguish an ankle sprain from a fracture, you should palpate the posterior edge and the tip of each malleolus and the base of the fifth metatarsal. You should also have the patient take four steps. This information is used in the OAR, and can be used to determine the need for radiography (see Fig. 34.2).

For lateral ankle pain, the *talar tilt test* evaluates the calcaneofibular ligament and is performed by stabilizing the distal lower leg in one hand while grasping each side of the foot at the talus and applying a varus stress (see Fig. 34.3). Asymmetric degrees of motion between the two ankles suggest instability although the specificity of this test is low. To perform the *anterior drawer test,* with the ankle slightly externally rotated and plantar flexed, grasp the calcaneus and try to slide the heel forward (see Fig. 34.3). A 3-mm difference between ankles suggests disruption of the anterior Talofibular ligament.

With anterior/lateral ankle pain, the *squeeze test* compresses the tibia and fibula together above the midpoint of the calf. Pain indicates a syndesmosis sprain, commonly called the "high ankle" sprain. The *Cotton test,* sometimes called a "rocker test," for syndesmosis sprains is performed like the talar tilt test, except mediolateral force is applied, and any degree of motion over 3 mm is considered abnormal. Side-to-side comparisons should be performed in both of these tests.

In medial ankle pain, injuries to the deltoid ligament result from dorsiflexion-eversion trauma, are relatively rare,

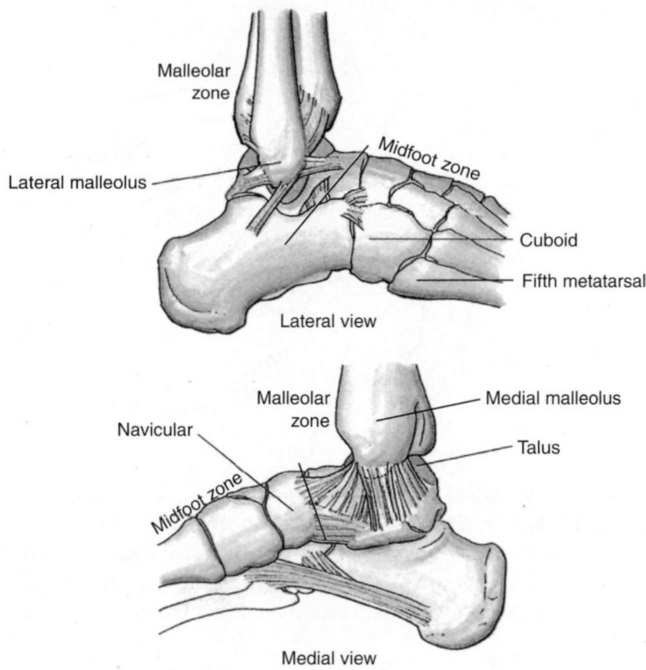

Figure 34.2 • Ottawa ankle rules for radiographic series in acute injuries. You should perform a radiograph if the patient has pain in the malleolar or midfoot zone and one of the following:

- Bony tenderness at posterior edge or tip of either malleoli
- Bony tenderness over the navicular
- Bony tenderness at the base of the fifth metatarsal
- Inability to bear weight both immediately and in the emergency department (four steps) (i.e., patient is unable to transfer weight twice onto each foot regardless of limping)

(Text adapted from Stiell IG, McKnight RD, Greenberg GH, et al. Implementation of the Ottawa ankle rules. *JAMA*. 1994;271. Illustration reprinted with permission from Moore KL, Agur AMR. *Essential Clinical Anatomy*. Baltimore, MD: Williams & Wilkins; 1995:276.)

and are often associated with fractures. Unlike each of the discrete lateral ankle ligaments, the deltoid ligament functions as a single unit and is *very* strong so, when it is injured, is therefore more frequently associated with fracture or posterior tibialis tendon injury.

Posterior ankle pain may be associated with the Achilles tendon. A visible defect in the Achilles tendon may occur in cases of complete or partial rupture. Palpation of the Achilles tendon may reveal crepitus, tenderness, swelling, or a gap. The *Thompson* (or midcalf compression) *test* assesses if the Achilles tendon is intact. With the patient lying prone on the exam table and the feet extended over the edge of the table, the gastrocnemius and the soleus are compressed by squeezing the calf. If the foot plantar flexes, the test is negative or normal. If the foot does not move, the test is positive, indicating complete or near complete rupture of the tendon.

Diagnostic Testing

Less than 10% of patients presenting with acute ankle injury in the family medicine setting have an ankle fracture. To

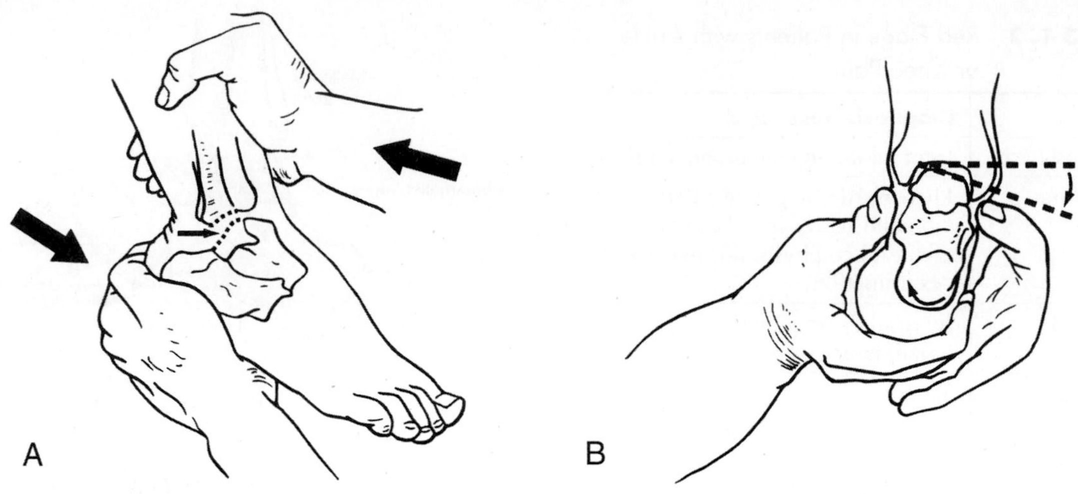

Figure 34.3 • Stress testing of the ankle. **(A)** Positive anterior drawer sign (small arrow). The anterior drawer sign test is used to evaluate the intactness of the anterior talofibular ligament. **(B)** Talar Tilt Test to evaluate the stability of the anterior talofibular and calcaneofibular ligaments. The ankle is unstable if the anterior talofibular and calcaneofibular ligaments are torn. (Reprinted with permission from American Osteopathic Association. Foundations for Osteopathic Medicine. Baltimore, MD: Williams & Wilkins; 1997:638.)

reduce unnecessary use of radiographs and make the treatment of ankle injuries more cost effective, the OAR (see Fig. 34.2) have been developed and prospectively evaluated. Prospective multicenter evaluation of the OAR has confirmed that it is highly sensitive compared with clinical examination alone of ankle and midfoot fractures, respectively (Table 34.3) (6,7). Thus, <1 in 300 family medicine patients with acute ankle injury and a negative evaluation using the OAR will have a fracture. The OAR are also valid in children older than 6 years of age with ankle injuries (8,9).

Keep in mind that the decision rule applies to an acutely injured ankle. You may wish to obtain radiographs when you find bone pain in the absence of injury or when the patient experiences night pain, or when symptoms do not fit conventional diagnoses or respond to treatment. These symptoms may indicate more serious conditions (see Table 34.2). Although radiographic stress testing, arthrography, and arthroscopy have been used in some centers to assess injury severity, the results of such testing rarely change the conservative treatment given, and they are not recommended.

Ultrasound (10–12) and magnetic resonance imaging (MRI) (11,13,14) have been used to evaluate suspected Achilles tendinosis or Achilles tendon rupture. Although ultrasound is reported to be fairly sensitive and specific, there is no accepted gold standard, and the published studies have included only patients with severe injuries. MRI has typically been studied in patients undergoing surgery. Most importantly, neither study is known to add significantly to the clinical examination. Nevertheless, the MRI, by demonstrating the extent of the defect, particularly for young athletes in high demand sports, can help with prognosis and the decision to allow the athlete to return to play.

TABLE 34.3 Key Elements of the History and Physical Examination in Patients with Ankle or Knee Pain

Ankle Pain					
Diagnosis	**Test**	**Sensitivity**	**Specificity**	**LR+**	**LR−**
Sprain versus fracture (6–9,60)	Ottawa ankle rule	0.93–1.00	0.39	1.5–1.7	0.01–0.05
Knee Pain					
Diagnosis	**Test**	**Sensitivity**	**Specificity**	**LR+**	**LR−**
Fracture (40,41)	Ottawa Knee Rule (see Table 34.7)	0.85–1.00	0.49–0.60	1.7–2.5	0.01–0.3
Anterior cruciate ligament tear (35)	Lachman test Composite examination	0.60–1.0 0.82	0.92 0.94	25.0 25	0.1 0.04
Meniscus injury (35)	Joint line tenderness McMurray test Composite examination	0.79 0.53 0.77	0.91 0.59 0.91	0.9 1.3 2.7	1.1 0.8 0.4

TABLE 34.4 Management of Ankle Sprain

Treatment	Efficacy	Strength of Recommendation*	Comment
Early mobilization (15,16)	Compared with those treated with bracing, patients treated with early mobilization are twice as likely to return to sport; return to activity 5 days sooner; 2.6 times less likely to experience instability; and 1.8 times more likely to be satisfied with their outcome.	A	Systematic review of clinical trials have found no studies showing harm, reduced function, or pain and most show improvement in patient-oriented outcomes with early mobilization.
Lace-up ankle brace (17)	Compared with semirigid braces, lace-up braces are 4 times less likely to cause disabling swelling	A	
Semirigid brace (17)	Compared with elastic bandage, patients return to activity 4 days sooner.	A	
Physical therapy (20)	Prevents subsequent sprains	B	

*A = consistent, good-quality patient-oriented evidence; B = inconsistent or limited-quality patient-oriented evidence; C = consensus, disease-oriented evidence, usual practice, expert opinion, or case series.
For information about the SORT evidence rating system, see *http://www.aafp.org/afpsort.xml*.

MANAGEMENT

As with many other conditions, management of ankle pain begins with an assessment of this individual patient's goals. You should then proceed to address symptom relief, as that is usually the reason the patient seeks care, and then restoration of function. Table 34.4 summarizes some treatment options and the level of evidence for each intervention, and Table 34.5 summarizes commonly used medications.

Ankle Sprains

INITIAL MANAGEMENT

The foundation for most injuries can be summarized with the mnemonic RICE: Rest, Ice, Compression, Elevation. Nonsteroidal anti-inflammatory drugs (NSAIDs) are commonly used in all sprains for analgesia and to reduce inflammation (see Table 34.5). Grades I and II lateral ankle sprains usually heal in approximately 8 to 15 days, respectively. Grade I sprains are treated symptomatically with ice, compression wraps, and elevation. Contrary to intuition, these sprains do not require immobilization. Early mobilization improves function, reduces pain and swelling, and speeds return to work and sports (15,16). Grade II sprains should be treated with ice, compression, and elevation for 48 to 72 hours, along with immobilization in a lace-up splint or an air-stirrup splint for 2 to 7 days (17). Crutches will help the patient avoid putting weight on the injured ankle.

The management of grade III lateral ankle sprains is similar to that of grade II sprains, although recovery is longer, and a small percentage of patients may require surgery. Most patients can be managed using an air-stirrup splint or a below-knee cast for up to 3 months followed by formal physical therapy. While one systematic review (18) suggests that patients with severe sprains do better with surgery, another more critical review suggests that the methodology supporting this conclusion was flawed and was unable to determine the relative effectiveness of surgical and conservative treatment for severe acute lateral ankle sprains (19). Therefore, current practice is to consider referring patients to a surgeon only if they have persistent functional impairment in spite of treatment and rehabilitation or if they have x-ray evidence of separation of the tibia and fibula.

The management of syndesmosis sprains is similar to that of third-degree sprains. In syndesmosis sprains, each time the patient steps, the body's weight is transferred upward, causing the syndesmosis to stretch, become more stressed and increase the pain and increase the instability. Healing time may be up to 6 to 8 weeks; often the patients need a longer period of immobilization. Removable splints (i.e., posterior splint, pneumatic splint, or a Bledsoe brace) or casting facilitates progressive weight-bearing. Progressive weight-bearing, as tolerated, should be allowed, and analgesics should be prescribed. Passive range-of-motion exercises (e.g., tracing the alphabet, drawing circles, etc. with the foot), especially dorsiflexion, should begin within a week of the injury.

LONG-TERM MANAGEMENT

Rehabilitation of the ankle joint is important in preventing future sprains, although the data are limited (16,20–22). Rehabilitation includes strengthening exercises, proprioception training, and functional exercises. The removable splints should be worn until the individual has been pain-free for at least 2 weeks. Patients with sprains treated with cast immobilization take longer to return to full activity and have worse outcomes unless patients receive intensive rehabilitation and are closely monitored. Recurrent ankle sprains and chronic pain after an ankle sprain are usually the result of inadequate

TABLE 34.5 Pharmacotherapy for Ankle or Knee Pain*

Drug	Dosage	Contraindications/Cautions/Adverse Effects	Relative Cost
Acetaminophen	325–650 mg q4–6h, up to maximum of 4000 mg daily	History of current ETOH abuse, liver dysfunction	$
Aspirin	Up to 4,000 mg/day (q4–6h)	NSAID allergy; third trimester of pregnancy; active ulcer; varicella or influenza infection in children and teenagers; caution in pregnancy, lactation, asthma, elderly, impaired renal or liver function, GI ulcers; adverse effects—prolonged bleeding time, life-threatening allergic reactions, salicylism	$
Ibuprofen	Up to 3,200 mg/day (TID–QID)	All NSAIDs have the same contraindications as aspirin.	$
Naproxen	250–550 mg BID–TID), maximum of 1,500 mg/day		$
Tolmetin	600–1,800 mg/day (TID), maximum 180 mg/day		$$$
Diclofenac	100–150 mg/day (BID–TID) maximum 200 mg/day BID		$
Indomethacin	25–150 mg BID–QID; maximum 200 mg/day	History of proctitis, rectal bleeding (suppository form); late pregnancy; adverse effects: frontal headache, fluid	$
Oxaprozin	1,200 mg once daily, maximum 1,800 mg/day	Avoid use in the elderly	$$$
Piroxicam	20 mg once daily	Depression; Parkinson disease; epilepsy; sepsis	$
Etodolac	600–1,200 mg/day (BID–QID), maximum 1,200 mg/day		$$
Nabumetone	1,000–2,000 mg/day (QD or BID)	Slow onset of action; most useful for chronic pain	$$
Celecoxib	100–200 mg QD–BID	Caution when used with patients with cardiovascular disease[†], reduced gastrointestinal bleeding (7%) in select populations, but it still can occur	$$$
Etodolac	600–1,200 mg/day (BID–QID), maximum 1,200 mg/day		$$
Nabumetone	1,000–2,000 mg/day (QD or BID)	Slow onset of action; most useful for chronic pain	$$
Celecoxib	100–200 mg QD–BID	Caution when used with patients with cardiovascular disease[†], reduced gastrointestinal bleeding (7%) in select populations, but it still can occur	$$$

BID = twice daily; ETOH = alcohol; GI = gastrointestinal; NSAID = nonsteroidal anti-inflammatory drugs; Q = every; TID = three times daily.
*$ = <$33, $$ = $34–$66, $$$ >$67.
*The degree of analgesic effect does not vary significantly among acetaminophen, nonsteroidal anti-inflammatory drugs, and COX-2 inhibitors.
[†]COX-2 inhibitors have been linked with increased risk of thrombotic events resulting in some having been withdrawn from the market.

rehabilitation. These individuals should receive more extensive supervised therapy. If pain persists after a ligamentous injury despite adequate rehabilitation, occult fracture should be suspected, especially talar dome fractures.

Ankle supports such as semirigid orthoses or Aircast braces have been shown to prevent ankle sprains during high-risk sporting activities in those with previous Grade II or III tears (e.g., soccer, basketball) (23).

Ankle Fractures

Many fractures can be managed in the office without referral. Avulsion or chip fractures are the most common and can occur at the distal fibula below the level of the mortise, the distal portion of the tibial plafond, and the anterior surface of the talus. Regardless of avulsion fracture size, these usually can be treated based upon the severity of the associated ankle sprain. For example, if the patient has an avulsion fracture but has a grade I sprain, treat the patient symptomatically with ice, compression wraps, and elevation. These do not require immobilization. If the fragments are displaced more than 2 mm, immobilize the patient in a cast or posterior splint and refer to an orthopedic surgeon. Avulsion fractures of the peroneus brevis insertion from the fifth metatarsal head will heal without treatment but should be immobilized until weight-bearing can be tolerated. Nondisplaced navicular and cuboid fractures should be casted. Fractures of the talus within the mortise, the fibula at or above the joint or mortise surface, the tibial plafond near the joint line, and bimalleolar, trimalleolar, and any displaced fractures should be immobilized and referred. You should refer patients with fractures of the base of the fifth metatarsal (Jones' fracture), the proximal second, third or fourth metatarsals (known as Lis Franc fractures) and of the growth plate (Salter-Harris fractures) to an orthopedic surgeon. Do not forget to provide analgesics for your patient (see Table 34.5).

Achilles Tendinosis

The evidence to support various management options for Achilles tendinosis is insufficient to suggest any one specific best approach (24). Conservative management until better data come along makes reasonable sense for most patients: relative rest, rehabilitation of the gastrocnemius and soleus muscles, ice, heel lifts, and analgesics. Rehabilitation of the calf muscles begins with progressive stretching and range-of-motion exercises followed by strength training. NSAIDs may be helpful in reducing pain and inflammation (see Table 34.5).

Steroid injection has been advocated by some into the Achilles tendon sheath, but its role is controversial (24) and it is considered a significant risk factor for subsequent rupture. Attempts should be made to correct foot biomechanical abnormalities. For example, patients whose feet pronate or supinate excessively should wear shoes matched to their gait. Patients with severe abnormalities should use orthotics. Surgery is recommended only for patients who fail conservative therapy and desire to continue activities that exacerbate tendinosis, and in those patients with Achilles tendon ruptures. The rate of re-rupture is about 13% in patients treated conservatively compared with about 4% in those treated surgically (number needed to treat to benefit one = 11; 95% confidence interval [CI], 7–29). However, complications such as adhesions, altered sensation, keloid scars, and wound infection occur in 10% to 16% in recent studies of patients treated surgically and in fewer than 3% of patients treated non-operatively (number needed to treat to harm one = 8–15) (25–27). These complications were less common when the repair was percutaneous rather than with open repair. Considering the potential risks and benefits, nonoperative treatment may be preferred in the sedentary patient, and surgery more reasonable in very active patients.

KEY POINTS

- The ankle joint is a hinge joint that is also capable of inversion and eversion to facilitate walking on irregular surfaces. It is this latter capability that also makes it vulnerable to injury.
- Ankle sprains, the most common sports injury, most often occur from forced inversion. Most can be treated conservatively with ice, compression, and elevation. Patients with more severe sprains should also use a lace-up splint or an air-stirrup splint.
- The Ottawa Ankle Rules help identify patients who will not need an x-ray.
- All patients with ankle injuries should undergo rehabilitation after the acute treatment to prevent future injuries and to avoid long-term impairment.

KNEE PAIN

CLINICAL OBJECTIVES

1. Describe the functional anatomy of the knee.
2. Provide a differential diagnosis for and describe common causes of chronic knee pain
3. Provide a differential diagnosis for and describe common causes of acute knee pain
4. Describe the expected outcomes of common treatments for knee pain

Although ankles are the most commonly injured joint in sports, patients see a physician twice as frequently for knee pain, accounting for nearly 2 million visits to family physicians annually (1). Unlike ankle pain however, knee pain is most commonly a chronic presentation caused by DJD. Acute injury and overuse, however, remain important causes of knee pain. Table 34.1 summarizes the differential diagnosis for knee pain.

The demands of everyday life, sports and recreation create stresses for knees: rotation, direct contact, and repetitive load. Although the history provides major clues to the diagnosis, knowledge of the anatomy and a careful examination of the knee are essential. Primary care physicians can manage most causes of knee pain. Some acute knee injuries and patients with severe DJD require surgery to restore function or to allow return to work or play. This underscores the importance of an accurate diagnosis.

In a population-based study of nearly 2,000 adults, about 30% reported knee pain in the previous month and 1 in 5 had degenerative changes on x-ray of the knee. Among the entire sample, including those without knee pain, one-third had evidence of meniscal damage (tear or destruction) on MRI (28). As with all other joints, the prevalence of DJD of the knee increases with age. Degenerative disease of the knee affects about 5% of adults younger than 45 years of age , 7% older than 45, and 12% of those older than 60 (29). Injuries to the knee ligaments and cartilage are common, although the exact frequency depends on the population and activity level. For example, downhill skiers, while having two to three knee injuries per 1,000 skier days, have approximately four anterior cruciate ligament (ACL) injuries per 100,000 skier days (30). Soccer players, on the other hand, have about 1 ACL injury per 10,000 player hours (31). Women are two to eight times as likely as men to sustain ACL injuries (32). Nordic skiers have a high rate of knee injury of any type (about two injuries per 1,000 skier days), even though many people consider this activity to be "easy on the knees." Most (58%) of these injuries, however, are to the medical collateral ligament (MCL) (33).

The knee joint (see Fig. 34.4) consists of the patella, tibia, and femur. The patella is a sesamoid bone with a keel-shaped undersurface that fits between the medial and lateral femoral condyles. The primary stabilizers of the knee are the ACL and posterior cruciate ligament (PCL), the MCL and lateral collateral ligament (LCL), the menisci, the joint capsule, and the medial and lateral retinacula that attach to the patella. Secondary stabilizers of the knee include the iliotibial band (also known as the tensor fascia lata) and the quadriceps, hamstrings, and popliteus muscles.

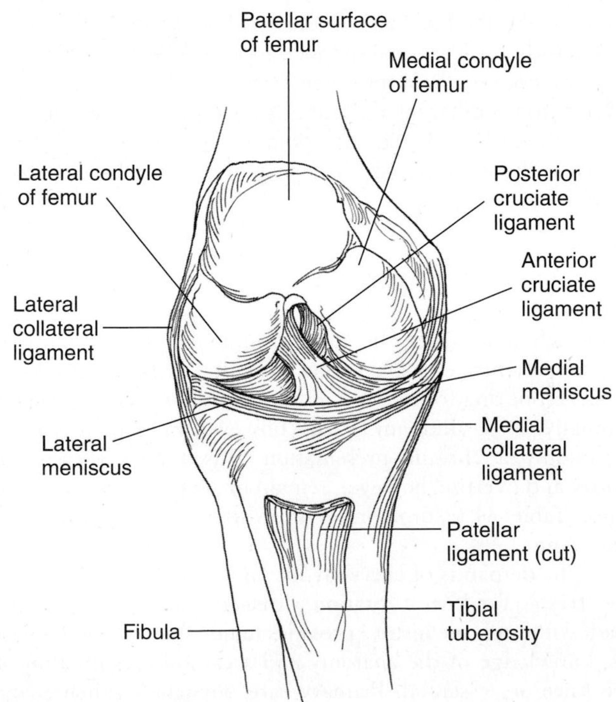

Figure 34.4 • Knee joint, anterior view. (Reprinted with permission from Rucker LM. *Essentials of Adult Ambulatory Care*. Baltimore, MD: Williams & Wilkins; 1997:556.)

The knee acts as a hinge joint that allows forward translation and internal rotation of the tibia during leg flexion and rearward translation and external rotation during extension. When the knee is flexed, the MCL and LCL provide stability to medially and laterally directed stress, respectively. The MCL and LCL also limit external and internal rotation during knee extension and flexion. The ACL is the only structure that prevents anterior movement of the tibia on the femur. It also helps the MCL stabilize the knee during lateral stress when the knee is flexed. The PCL resists posterior movement of the tibia on the femur. The crescent shaped medial and lateral menisci act primarily as shock absorbers but also stabilize the knee during movements such as pivoting. The popliteus muscle, also attached to the lateral meniscus, prevents the lateral meniscus from sliding forward and getting crushed between the tibia and femur during flexion. It also locks the knee in full extension, and unlocks the knee during the initiation of flexion.

Differential Diagnosis

The mechanism of injury is an important clue to the specific diagnosis in patients with acute knee pain. Collateral ligament injuries result from medially or laterally directed stress to a planted knee, such as in football or skiing. Posterior cruciate injuries are rare and usually occur in a motor vehicle accident when a flexed knee hits a dashboard. The ACL can be injured by many mechanisms such as: an external force applied to a planted knee (e.g., during a football tackle); hyperextension and internal rotation (e.g., a basketball or volleyball player landing on somebody's foot); sudden deceleration with a flexed knee that pivots or rotates (e.g., a skiing fall); landing and pivoting or cutting (e.g., in soccer); or falling backward with a ski boot, displacing the tibia anteriorly. These mechanisms are not specific for ACL injuries, as sudden twisting or pivoting can also injure the menisci or cause patellar dislocation.

Chronic knee pain may be a long-term sequela of previous injury, especially if it was incompletely rehabilitated. Chronic knee pain is often associated with weak quadriceps muscles from disuse, resulting in patellofemoral dysfunction (PFD) or anterior knee pain (AKP). AKP is a catch-all term that includes common conditions such as patellar tendonitis, PFD, and chondromalacia patellae. The causes of DJD are multiple. The primary problem may, in fact, be genetic, traumatic, or obesity rather than overactivity or exercise-related (34).

Clinical Evaluation

HISTORY

When evaluating a patient with knee pain, you should ask about the location, duration, character, and intensity of pain. You should also obtain a description of potential contributing factors. If there was an injury, you should ask about the mechanism, the position of the knee at the time of the injury, ameliorating or exacerbating factors, previous injury, and current treatment. Table 34.2 summarizes potential red flags, which are serious and may require early referral. Finally, you should determine the patient's treatment and activity goals, so management can be individualized.

The mechanism of injury and the presence of hemarthrosis are the two strongest indicators of internal derangement of the knee in the acutely injured knee. Patients with hemarthrosis are likely to complain of sudden swelling (<24 hours after the injury) and bruising. Hearing or feeling a "pop" suggests an ACL tear, whereas locking of the knee (where the knee gets "stuck" at some point in its range of motion) is typically associated with meniscus injuries or a loose joint body (usually cartilage). Inability to bear weight and persistent "giving way" of the knee indicate internal derangement but are not specific for any one injury. Patients with AKP often experience pain with specific actions such as climbing up or down stairs, squatting, or prolonged sitting with the knees flexed. They may also report snapping, popping, clicking, or catching sensations in the knee. Patients with degenerative joint disease (DJD) typically complain of stiffness with inactivity and pain with weight bearing activity. In contrast to the stiffness associated with rheumatoid arthritis, the stiffness of DJD often improves after a few minutes of activity. Swelling of the knee is not common in DJD except during an acute flare-up or in the presence of severe degeneration associated with bony changes.

PHYSICAL EXAMINATION

A thorough and complete knee examination for meniscus or ligamentous injury is better at diagnosis than any one specific maneuver (35). Table 34.3 summarizes the accuracy of various elements of the knee examination.

The *Lachman test* is very good at ruling in and ruling out anterior cruciate ligament tears in experienced hands (35). It is performed with the knee flexed to 20 to 30 degrees and with one top hand stabilizing the femur while the lower hand, with the thumb on top, wraps around the inside of the proximal tibia. Using the lower hand, smoothly and gently try to slide the tibia forward. When the leg is too large or the hands too small, place a knee or other firm support under the thigh and place both hands near the tibial plateau. A 3-mm side-to-side difference or the absence of a distinct stop (also called an "endpoint") indicates an ACL tear. Before the Lachman test is performed, flex the knee to 90 degrees and push the tibia in a posterior direction (*posterior drawer test*) to ensure PCL integrity. If the PCL is torn, the Lachman test is still accurate but must be done more carefully.

The presence of hemarthrosis suggests a significant knee injury that may require surgery. Patients with hemarthrosis usually have significant effusions and ecchymosis. Although it is difficult to distinguish between effusion and hemarthrosis without aspirating the joint, the presence of ecchymosis and the onset of swelling in <24 hours will favor hemarthrosis. Approximately 70% of knee injuries with hemarthrosis are ACL tears (36). Osteochondral fractures are seen in about 10% of knee injuries with hemarthrosis. Although many studies report the prevalence of derangement in a series of subjects with hemarthrosis, one cannot calculate diagnostic test characteristics (such as likelihood ratios, sensitivity, specificity) without knowing about the other injured patients who did not have hemarthrosis. This is a common problem in the orthopedic literature.

Joint line tenderness (JLT) is not very reliable for diagnosing meniscus tears (35). Posterolateral or posteromedial pain that occurs at the extremes of flexion or extension suggests meniscal injury. In a patient with anterior JLT, pain with squatting suggests chondromalacia rather than a meniscus tear. The *McMurray test* (see Fig. 34.5) is another physical examination maneuver used to detect meniscal damage. To perform this test,

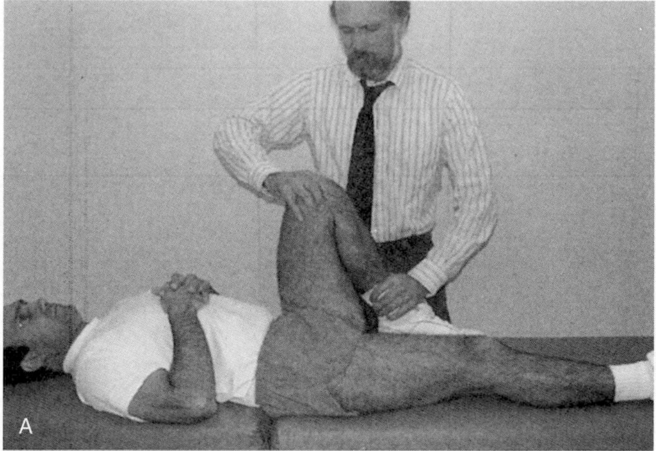

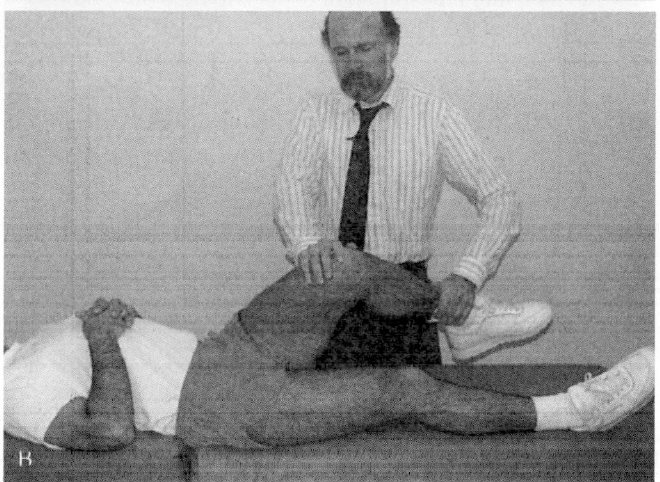

Figure 34.5 • McMurray test. **(A)** Starting position. **(B)** Extension of the leg with valgus and internal rotation evaluates the medial meniscus (shown in image), while extension of the leg with varus force and external rotation evaluates the lateral meniscus. (Reproduced with permission from Hyde TE, Gengenbach MS. *Conservative Management of Sports Injuries*. Baltimore, MD: Williams & Wilkins; 1997:392.)

place the knee in full flexion and place your fingers along the lateral joint line. Use your other hand to cup the heel. While applying a combination of external rotation and medially directed stress, bring the knee slowly into extension. A palpable click suggests a lateral meniscus tear. It is very likely that, in the presence of a tear, this will also cause an increase in pain. Now repeat the maneuvers with your fingers along the medial joint line and apply internal rotation and laterally-directed stress to the knee to detect medial meniscus tears. If the range of motion of the knee is restricted, a McMurray test cannot be performed accurately. By itself, the McMurray test is not very sensitive or specific (35).

When a patient's history suggests a collateral ligament injury, the severity is determined by the physical examination. Side-to-side comparisons are essential. Pathologic laxity is graded according to the amount of joint opening during valgus or varus stress, and is classified as grade I (<5 mm), grade II (5 to 8 mm), grade III (8 to 11 mm), and grade IV (more than 11 mm) (37). Grade I and grade II tears have definite end points, but grade III and IV tears have soft or mushy end points.

TABLE 34.6 Characteristics of Diagnostic Tests in Patients with Knee Pain

Diagnosis	Test	Sens (95% CI)	Spec (95% CI)	LR+ (95% CI)	LR− (95% CI)
Medial meniscus tear (42)	MRI	0.89 (0.83–0.95)	.80 (0.73–0.87)	4.5 (3.9–9.5)	0.14 (0.09–0.28)
Lateral meniscus tear (42)	MRI	0.79 (0.73–0.85)	0.91 (0.84–0.98)	8.7 (5.6–11.7)	0.23 (0.15–0.31)
Anterior cruciate ligament tear (42)	MRI	0.87 (0.83–0.91)	0.91 (0.88–0.94)	9.6 (4.5–14.6)	0.14 (0.09–0.19)
Posterior cruciate ligament tear (42)	MRI	0.75 (0.65–0.85)	0.93 (0.88–0.98)	11 (4.7–17.3)	0.27 (0.16–0.37)
Anterior knee pain (also called patella femoral dysfunction or chondromalacia patellae (49)	MRI MR arthrogram CT arthrogram	0.29 0.69 0.65	0.97 0.99 0.99	9.6 70 65	0.7 0.3 0.3

CT = computed tomography; MR = magnetic resonance; MRI = magnetic resonance imaging; Sens = sensitivity; Spec = specificity; LR+ = positive likelihood ratio; LR− = negative likelihood ratio; 95% CI = 95% confidence interval.

As summarized in Table 34.3, a combination of clinical exam maneuvers along with detailed history are better at diagnosing meniscal and ligamentous injuries of the knee rather than the use of specific individual physical exam tests separately, although for meniscal injuries, even the composite examination has only modest diagnostic accuracy (35).

If the diagnosis is uncertain (e.g., the patient is guarding too much or swelling prohibits adequate testing), application of ice, temporary immobilization, and the use of analgesics are common techniques for reducing the swelling and pain. The patient should return within a week for repeat evaluation.

Examination of the knee in patients with chronic AKP often reveals atrophy of the quadriceps and crepitus with manipulation of the patella. Several clinical tests for AKP have been reported although these are qualitative tests, and their accuracy has not been quantified. In the *patellar apprehension test,* the examiner applies inferiorly directed pressure at the superior portion of the patella. In the *patellar compression test,* the examiner firmly holds the patella in place while the patient contracts the quadriceps muscle. In either the patellar apprehension test or the patellar compression test, if the patient winces, grabs the knee, or otherwise voices displeasure, the test is considered positive. Patellar laxity is tested by manipulating the patella from side to side and determining the degree of movement in comparison with the opposite knee.

DIAGNOSTIC TESTING

Table 34.6 summarizes the accuracy of imaging studies for evaluating the injured knee. Stiell and colleagues developed and validated the Ottawa Knee Rules (Table 34.7) to assist in the evaluation of acute knee injuries, in patients 18 years of age and older (38,39). He found that the rule is nearly 100% sensitive for fracture, but other investigators have found somewhat lower sensitivity. The rule is easy to use, and clinicians correctly interpret it 96% of the time (40). If the rule is negative, there is <1% risk of fracture. The Pittsburgh knee rules, another clinical decision tool for acute knee injuries, is about 99% sensitive and 60% specific (41). The Pittsburgh knee rules recommend that you order an x-ray for patients with pain caused by a fall or blunt trauma, and who are younger than 12 years of age or older than age 50. For patients of other ages, x-rays are necessary only if patients are unable to walk four full weight-bearing steps.

In adolescents with open growth plates, take a more conservative approach because no validated clinical prediction rules exist for this population. Also, keep in mind that the decision rule applies only to an acutely injured knee. You may wish to obtain radiographs when you find bone pain in the absence of injury, when the patient experiences night pain, or when the patient's symptoms do not fit conventional diagnoses or respond to treatment. These symptoms may indicate the presence of more serious conditions (see Table 34.2).

In the absence of fracture, radiographs rarely alter the management of an acute knee injury. If you suspect internal derangement of the knee, the question whether to perform an MRI arises. Although MRI is sensitive and specific for ACL tears (42), several studies have found it to be less accurate than the clinical examination (41,43–45). The literature on diagnostic

TABLE 34.7 The Ottawa Knee Rules

Obtain a radiograph of the knee if the patient has any of the following characteristics:
- Age 55 years or older
- Tenderness at the head of the fibula
- Isolated patella tenderness
- Inability to flex to 90 degrees
- Inability to bear weight both immediately and in the emergency department (four weight transfers onto each leg, regardless of limping)

Adapted from Stiell IG, Greenberg GH, Wells GA, et al. Derivation of a decision rule for the use of radiography in acute knee injuries. *Ann Emerg Med.* 1995;26:405–413.

testing suffers from many flaws, including the lack of an accepted gold standard, the absence of a wide spectrum of injury severity, and failure to adequately account for the potential effect of examiner experience.

MRI should not be used to diagnose a suspected isolated ACL tear. If you are not certain that there is an ACL tear, referring the patient to a physician with greater experience is usually more cost effective than ordering an MRI (43). If meniscal damage is seen on the MRI along with the ACL tear, surgical repair should be strongly encouraged.

MRI can also detect meniscal lesions (see Table 34.6). An MRI can be helpful if a patient with a strongly suggestive history and persistent pain has a negative clinical examination and poor response to conservative therapy (several weeks of rest followed by physical therapy). However, up to 16% of asymptomatic patients may have meniscal abnormalities on MRI! (46,47) This emphasizes the importance of taking a good history and using clinical signs to determine a mechanism for injury and then using the MRI to *confirm* the clinical diagnosis, not using imaging to *make* the diagnosis. The data on ultrasound for confirming meniscal injuries is limited, having been studies in patients with symptoms and findings that led to arthroscopy (48).

Although AKP is best diagnosed clinically, several radiographic procedures, such as plain radiography, MRI, computed axial tomography (CT) scan, sonography, and scintigraphy, are also available. None are needed however in most patients with AKP. Imaging should be reserved for those who fail to respond to therapy or if the diagnosis is in doubt. The characteristics of these tests are summarized in Table 34.6. Although radiographs using Merchant's views have been a standard among some specialists for years, the findings rarely alter the initial conservative management. Merchant's views are performed with the knees flexed 45 degrees and the x-ray beam declined 30 degrees. More than 16 degrees of subluxation is considered abnormal.

Gagliardi (49) compared MRI, MR arthrography, and CT arthrography to surgical findings in patients with AKP ranging from mild to severe. Each procedure was very good at ruling in disease if positive but was less helpful when normal.

All of the following results may be found in radiographs of patients with DJD: normal findings; sclerotic joint margins; asymmetric joint space narrowing; subchondral cyst formation; osteophytes; and bone destruction. None of these findings are specific to degenerative joint management, and they may be found in many other arthritides.

MANAGEMENT

Begin by assessing the patient's goals and current level of function. Symptom relief should then be addressed, as that is usually the reason the patient seeks care, followed by helping the patient return to function. Table 34.8 summarizes the available treatment options and the level of evidence to support them; medications commonly used for management of knee pain are listed in Table 34.5.

The following are major reasons to refer a patient for additional evaluation or for surgery:

- hemarthrosis or rapid fluid accumulation;
- ACL or meniscus tears;
- third-degree collateral ligament injuries;
- severe functional impairment;
- uncertainty about the diagnosis (referral for second opinion);
- poor response to conservative treatment (referral for second opinion).

Appropriate surgical referral, therefore, depends on the ability of the primary care physician to perform an accurate and complete history and physical examination of the patient with knee pain.

TABLE 34.8 Management of the Most Common Causes of Knee Pain

Diagnosis	Treatment	Strength of Recommendation*	Comments
Knee pain (61)	Exercise: NNT = 13 to reduce pain by greater than 50%	B	2-year exercise program
Anterior cruciate ligament tear	Surgery: unclear benefit(51)	C	
Meniscus tear	Surgery	C	
Degenerative joint disease	Glucosamine (Rotta preparation), NNT = 5 to improve pain Intra-articular corticosteroid injection(57): NNT = 5 for improved pain at 6 months	A	
Severe degenerative joint disease	Arthroscopic debridement is no more effective than sham surgery	B	
Anterior knee pain	Patella taping (compared with sham taping, pain is reduced 1.9 points on 10 point scale) (53)	B	

NNT = number needed to treat.
*A = consistent, good-quality patient-oriented evidence; B = inconsistent or limited-quality patient-oriented evidence; C = consensus, disease-oriented evidence, usual practice, expert opinion, or case series.
For information about the SORT evidence rating system, see *http://www.aafp.org/afpsort.xml*.

Initial Management of Knee Injuries

The initial management of an acute knee injury depends on the type and severity of the injury. As with most other acute injuries, the foundation can be summarized with the mnemonic RICE: Rest, Ice, Compression, Elevation. Fractures should be immobilized in a long leg splint, patients referred immediately to an orthopedic surgeon, and appropriate analgesia given. Collateral ligament tears, whether grade I or grade II, should be treated with a knee immobilizer and crutches until the pain has subsided enough to permit weight-bearing. Ice, compression, and elevation also help reduce pain and swelling. When unable to adequately examine an acutely injured knee, you should begin symptomatic therapy and re-examine within a week. To prevent weakness of the quadriceps and secondary AKP, the patient should begin isometric and leg raise exercises (one leg at a time) while wearing the immobilizer. As the pain dissipates, range-of-motion exercises should be started, followed by a progression of stationary bicycle riding and resistance exercises before returning to sports specific training. Grade I sprains usually heal in a week or less, whereas grade II injuries may take 2 to 3 weeks to heal. You should refer patients with grade III injuries to an orthopedic surgeon. These injuries are usually treated with a brace that allows 30 degrees of flexion for 2 weeks; the brace is then unlocked to allow 30 to 90 degrees of flexion. Return to full activity may take up to 9 weeks.

The initial management of an acute ACL tear is immobilization and referral to an orthopedic surgeon. Factors associated with a greater likelihood of success with surgical reconstruction of the ACL include isolated injury (versus multiple derangements), younger patient age, and future activities that do not include jumping or cutting. Reduced likelihood of success may occur with greater degree of displacement of the tibia on the femur, physically demanding work activity or sports, and poor compliance with a rehabilitation program. Surgery is also indicated in an individual who initially elects not to have surgery but has repeated episodes of the knee "giving out" or is unable to perform daily activities.

The initial management of meniscus tears is controversial. In most cases, rest and protected weight-bearing combined with a short course of physical therapy comprise the initial treatment. If locking, pain, or inability to return to usual activities persists beyond 3 to 4 weeks, after imaging has confirmed the diagnosis, the patient should be referred.

Patellar dislocations are treated both surgically and conservatively, although the re-dislocation rate may be as high as 25% to 35% with conservative treatment. Children and adolescents, however, have similar rates of dislocation whether treated surgically or conservatively (50). There may be an associated tear of the medial retinaculum or of the insertion of the vastus medialis. Conservative therapy consists of a brief period of immobilization, ice, and compression, followed by bracing the patella with a lateral buttress knee sleeve and starting a functional rehabilitation program. Patients usually are able to return to full activity after recovery.

Long-term Management of Knee Disorders

For adult patients, it is unclear if the outcome of surgery for non-acutely diagnosed ACL tears is better than conservative treatment (51). Physical therapy is usually indicated for individuals undergoing casting or surgical procedures. Although physical therapy to strengthen the quadriceps and hamstrings in the ACL-deficient knee can allow the individual to return to sports or full activity, several prospective longitudinal studies have shown that the incidence of meniscal tears, DJD, pain, and disability are significantly greater in those who elect conservative treatment. This is particularly true for those who have meniscus tears associated with the initial ACL tear. Prophylactic bracing has not been shown to stabilize the anterior cruciate deficient knee, or prevent these unsuccessful outcomes (52).

AKP generally should be managed conservatively, with analgesics (see Table 34.5), quadriceps strengthening exercises, patellar taping (53), and ice. Particularly useful are eccentric exercises that strengthen the quadriceps near the patellar insertion (54). These are performed by having the patient stand on one leg and then squat partially. Ultrasound appears to be no more effective than sham ultrasound (55). Surgical intervention is usually not needed, and is reserved for patients who fail conservative therapy or have anatomic defects, such as patella alta or severe genu varum.

DJD is a chronic, degenerative condition. NSAIDs are commonly prescribed for it, but no studies have evaluated their impact on functional outcomes or disease progression. As DJD is not an inflammatory condition, NSAIDs may be no better than acetaminophen for long-term management of DJD. A short NSAID course (1 to 2 weeks) may be beneficial during an acute flare-up.

Glucosamine, a form of amino sugar that occurs naturally in the body, is used to treat DJD. It comes in two preparations, Rotta and non-Rotta. Only the Rotta preparation has shown any benefit for pain and function in patients with symptomatic DJD (56). Corticosteroid injections are rarely indicated. Although intra-articular steroids may provide pain relief (57), the effect is brief and does not alter the course of the disease, and recurrent steroid use can damage articular cartilage.

Physical therapy and flexibility and strength training may help to maintain function. Patients with refractory pain, impaired mobility, and severe DJD on radiograph should be referred to an orthopedic surgeon for possible joint replacement. To delay surgery, a course of intra-articular injections of viscous biosynthetic cartilage precursors (hyaluronic acid) is an option. However, arthroscopic debridement of the knee is no better than sham surgery or physical therapy plus medication in improving long-term pain and function (58,59). See Chapter 35 for further discussion of the management of DJD.

KEY POINTS

- The knee is a hinge joint with several structures that maintain alignment (MCL, LCL, ACL, PCL), cushion the joint during weight bearing (menisci) and protect the inner structures (patella)
- Key factors in determining the likely cause of knee pain include the location, duration, character, and intensity of symptoms and whether an acute injury occurred.
- In patients with acute knee injuries, the Ottawa Knee Rules or the Pittsburgh Knee Rules can identify which patients are unlikely to have a fracture and therefore not need x-rays.
- Most patients with an acute injury can be treated using rest, ice, compression wraps, and elevation.

CHAPTER

35

Arthritis and Rheumatic Diseases

John R. Gimpel

CLINICAL OBJECTIVES

1. Differentiate between the clinical presentation of patients with osteoarthritis and rheumatoid arthritis.
2. Evaluate a patient with joint pain and describe the diagnostic features of the common causes.
3. Educate patients with fibromyalgia syndrome.
4. Identify musculoskeletal "red flags" when encountering patients in clinical settings.
5. Discuss the management of patients with common forms of arthritis.

Rheumatic diseases are a variety of conditions and syndromes involving stiffness and pain in joints and/or muscles. Rheumatic diseases are the most prevalent chronic conditions in the United States, a leading cause of disability (1), and lead to costs that exceed 2.5% of the gross national product (2). Arthritis refers to rheumatic diseases involving pain and/or inflammation of one or more joints within the body. There are numerous types of arthritis, with differing causes and defined clinical features. One out of every five adults has a physician-diagnosed form of arthritis over their lifetime (3). In general, women suffer more frequently from rheumatic complaints than men, and the incidence of arthritic disorders increases rapidly over the age of 50 years. Most patients with rheumatic complaints are seen first by primary care physicians. With the advancing age of the United States and world populations, the prevalence of musculoskeletal conditions will continue to increase over time. The most common conditions are listed in Table 35. 1. Here the most common forms of arthritis and rheumatologic diseases that are managed by family physicians are reviewed.

DIFFERENTIAL DIAGNOSIS

It can be difficult to clearly distinguish several rheumatic presentations from each other and there may be overlap between differing conditions. Several patterns of presentation are well recognized and ultimately a diagnosis is often made based on that clinical pattern. An algorithm to assist in distinguishing different rheumatic and connective tissue disorders is shown in Figure 35.1. Table 35.2 shows common differences between osteoarthritis (OA) (*also known as* degenerative joint disease) and rheumatoid arthritis (RA). Table 35.3 lists Red Flags suggestive of systemic disease and nonarticular manifestations of common rheumatologic conditions.

A GENERAL APPROACH TO DIAGNOSIS AND MANAGEMENT

In rheumatic disorders, the history and clinical examination are the keys to effective diagnosis: laboratory tests and radiographs are used mainly to confirm an already strong suspicion of a specific diagnosis. Historical, clinical, and laboratory criteria have been developed by the American College of Rheumatology (ACR) for a wide range of joint and connective tissue disorders and these are applied here where available (4,5). These criteria are considerably more accurate than either laboratory testing or imaging alone in establishing a diagnosis in patients with musculoskeletal disorders. Many laboratory tests used in rheumatologic diagnosis perform adequately when the probability of disease is high, but are much less useful in the primary care office with patients where the prevalence of rheumatic diseases is much lower (5–7).

Two very commonly used laboratory tests are the erythrocyte sedimentation rate (ESR) and C-reactive protein (CRP). These are laboratory markers of inflammation, but their specificity is quite low. Up to the age of 50, the upper limit of normal for the ESR in most laboratories is 15 to 20 mm/hr in men and 25 to 30 mm/hr in women (8). However, ESR values generally increase by 5 mm/hr every decade in normal patients over the age of 40 so that for example, an ESR of 50 in a 60-year-old woman may not be abnormal. A very high ESR (>90 mm/hr), however, is typically associated with giant cell arteritis, advanced collagen vascular disease, and septic arthritis. The CRP level may be a more timely indicator of current disease activity than the ESR.

Immunologic tests should be ordered only if there already is a strong suspicion of the diagnosis and generally are more useful when performed serially than when obtained as a single battery of testing: for example, antibody to double-stranded DNA may be appropriate to order only in those patients who have a positive, clinically significant initial anti-nuclear antibody (ANA) result (6,7,9). The efficacy of lab tests for diagnosing patients with joint pain is shown in Table 35.4. A guide to interpreting synovial fluid analysis is presented in Table 35.5 and typical radiographic findings of common forms of arthritis are described in Table 35.6.

In taking care of patients with rheumatologic disease, the family physician should be able to:

- identify the major rheumatic disorders,
- arrange a program of pain relief (physical modalities, injections, and analgesics),
- advise on appropriate disease-specific therapy, and
- provide patient education and appropriate exercise programs as indicated.

TABLE 35.1 Prevalence of Rheumatic Disorders per 1,000 Population

Common Rheumatic Conditions	Prevalence per 1,000 Population
Non-articular	132
Bursitis, tendonitis, synovitis	11
Shoulder syndromes	7
Humeral (lateral or medial) epicondylitis	4
Fibromyalgia	30 women 5 men
Somatic dysfunction	200
Osteoarthritis (all ages)	
Any joints	250
Hip	13
Knee	15
Osteoarthritis (age >65 years)	
Any joints	750
Knee	95
Hip	55
Gout or pseudogout	3
All ages	3
Age >50 years	15
Inflammatory arthritis	
Rheumatoid arthritis	25
Systemic lupus erythematosus	0.04
Polymyalgia rheumatica (age >50 years)	0.2–0.7
Giant cell arteritis (age >50 years)	0.05–0.1

For many different forms of arthritis, there are similar broad goals of management that can be implemented by the family physician:

- Symptom relief—medication, rest, splinting, adjust footwear
- Restoration/maintenance of motion and function—physical therapy/occupational therapy/manipulative treatment, provide assistive devices
- Prevention/correction of deformities—physical therapy, surgery
- Suppression of symptoms—medication, complementary and alternative therapy
- Emotional health—patient education, weight loss if overweight, social work, physical conditioning, counseling on employment and sexuality.

Referral to a rheumatologist may be indicated when:

- the diagnosis remains unclear after initial workup,
- the disease is severe or progressive,
- the disease is potentially life-threatening and/or complex therapy is needed, or
- rarely performed or complicated diagnostic studies and procedures are required.

Referral to an orthopedic surgeon is indicated when the patient might benefit from joint replacement or reconstructive surgery. Involvement of other professionals (e.g., physical therapists, occupational therapists, podiatrists) may be an important adjunct to treatment for certain patients.

A GENERAL APPROACH TO THE USE OF ANTI-INFLAMMATORY MEDICATIONS

A similar approach to the use of medications can be followed in treating many forms of arthritis. Table 34.5 in Chapter 34: Ankle and Knee Pain summarizes the common anti-inflammatory medications currently used. Acetaminophen, up to 4,000 mg/day, is clearly superior to placebo, and has a similar safety profile, so it is generally considered first-line medical therapy in many forms of arthritis. At higher doses, acetaminophen can cause some gastrointestinal (GI) symptoms, and massive overdosages or when used with excessive alcohol (three drinks or more daily) has been associated with hepatotoxicity. Acetaminophen may not be as effective as nonsteroidal anti-inflammatory drugs (NSAIDs) for pain reduction in some

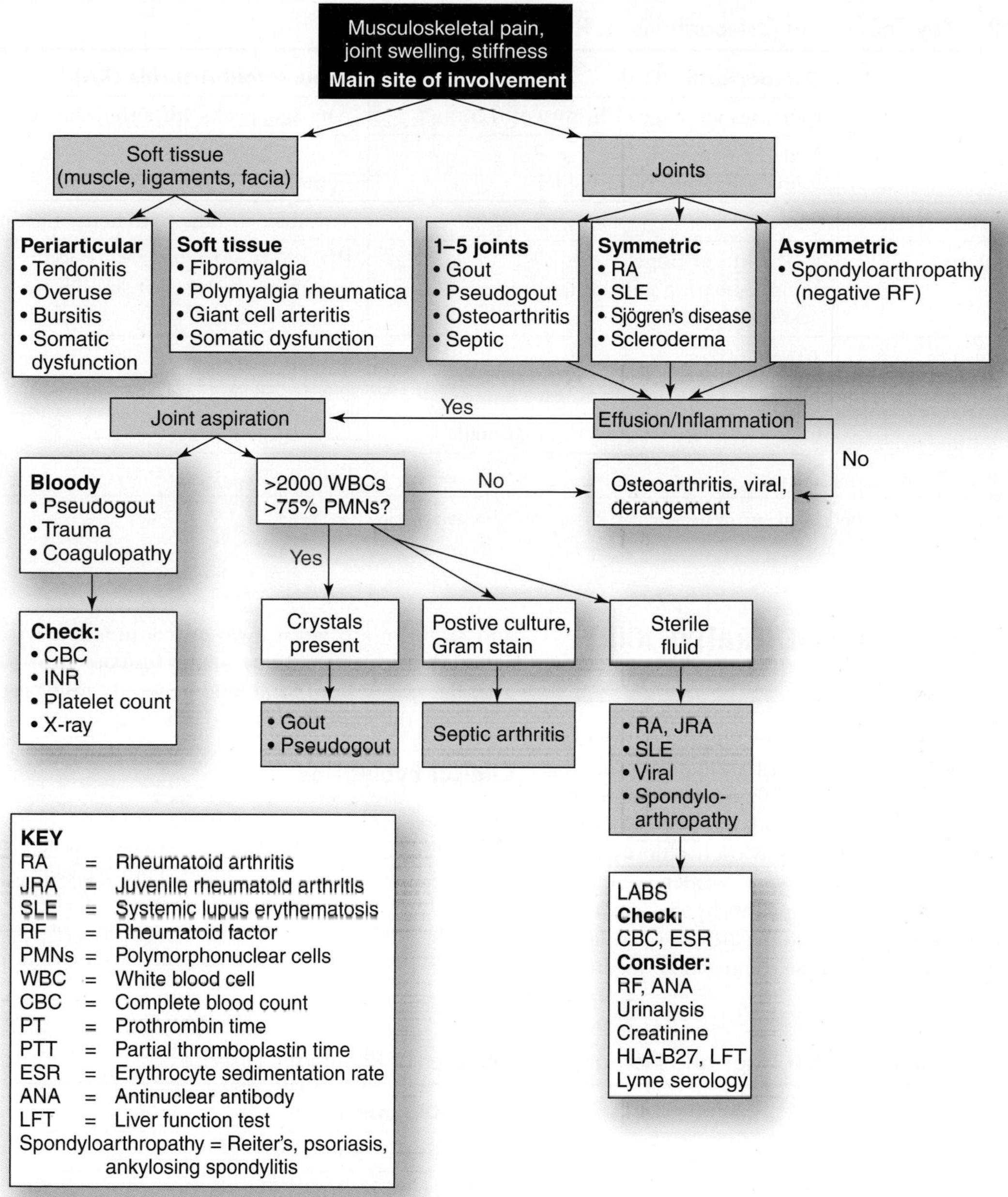

Figure 35.1 • Initial approach to joint problems. (Adapted and reprinted with permission from American College of Rheumatology, Ad Hoc Committee on Clinical Guidelines. Guidelines for the initial evaluation of the adult patient with acute musculoskeletal symptoms. *Arthritis Rheum*. 1996;39:1–8.)

patients (e.g., people with OA of the knee and hip), but may be equal in improving function (10). If there is an unacceptable response to acetaminophen, NSAIDs can be either added or substituted, basing the dose on the patient response (see Table 34.5). Consideration must be given to the risks of NSAID therapy, especially in the elderly or in those patients with a history of upper GI bleeding or renal dysfunction. Monitoring for potential adverse effects in patients on long-term NSAIDs may require baseline and annual monitoring of complete blood count, serum creatinine, and liver enzyme tests (9,11). NSAID-induced gastric ulcers can be prevented by prescribing misoprostol, an analogue of prostaglandin E, given 200 μg four times daily. Histamine-2 blockers and proton pump inhibitors are alternatives when misoprostol cannot be tolerated. Selective cyclooxygenase 2 (COX-2) inhibitors (e.g., celecoxib) are associated with fewer bleeding complications than other NSAIDs (0.5% versus 1.2% over 1 year of treatment); however, the cardiac safety of these agents remains controversial (12). In addition, COX-2 inhibitors are significantly more expensive than other NSAIDs (13). Tramadol, a nonopioid centrally acting analgesic, can be added to NSAID therapy for short-term use to help with severe pain (14).

TABLE 35.2 Key Features of Osteoarthritis vs. Rheumatoid Arthritis

	Osteoarthritis (OA)	Rheumatoid Arthritis (RA)
Age range	Increases with age or history of trauma	Any age; peaks 4th–6th decades
Gender	Male > Female before age 50 Female > Male 50 and older	Female ≫ Male
Clinical course	Chronic	Variable; chronic with acute flare-ups
Pattern of presentation	DIP joints of fingers; Weight-bearing joints (hips, knees especially)	PIP joints of fingers, MCP joints; Symmetric pattern of small joint involvement
Inflammatory features	Absent	Present
Early morning stiffness	Dissipates in 15–30 minutes	Dissipates in 45–60 minutes
Risk factors	Obesity, injury/trauma, occupational	Genetic, smoking
Systemic manifestations	No	Common

DIP = distal interphalangeal; PIP = proximal interphalangeal; MCP = metacarpophalangeal joints.

OSTEOARTHRITIS (OA) OR DEGENERATIVE JOINT DISEASE (DJD)

OA is the most common arthritic disorder, and is considered to be more of a degenerative than an inflammatory process. Risk factors include: age older than 50, injury to a joint, obesity, prolonged occupational or sports stress (especially competitive contact sports), and heredity. Most healthy asymptomatic people will have developed some evidence of this degenerative process in weight-bearing joints by the age of 55. Biomechanical and immune damage to the articular cartilage, bone, and synovium are thought to be the mechanism. Bone and cartilage are worn away in conjunction with increased synovial thickening. Bony spurs (osteophytes) form at the articular edges, with local (and generally mild) inflammation involving the joint capsule and adjacent ligaments.

Clinical Evaluation

Table 35.2 outlines the typical features of OA. It usually presents in middle-aged or older individuals as mild, dull, aching pain in one or a limited number of joints. Pain typically worsens with activity, improves with rest, and can be aggravated by damp, cold weather. There are no systemic symptoms or signs. Stiffness comes from inactivity but commonly improves after about 15

TABLE 35.3 Red Flags and Non-articular Features of Rheumatic Diseases

Feature	Possible Diagnosis
Fever, chills, monoarticular presentation	Septic arthritis
Weight loss	Malignancy with metastasis to bone; rheumatoid arthritis; systemic lupus erythematosus (SLE)
Headaches, loss of vision, scalp tenderness, jaw claudication	Giant cell arteritis
Skin and/or nail changes	Psoriasis, scleroderma, systemic lupus erythematosus, Reiter syndrome, Lyme disease (erythema migrans)
Constitutional symptoms along with multiorgan system signs and symptoms	SLE, collagen vascular disorder
Cutaneous/subcutaneous nodules	Gout, rheumatoid arthritis
Conjunctivitis/uveitis/dry eyes	Rheumatoid arthritis, Sjögren syndrome, Reiter syndrome
Chest pain, cough, dyspnea	Rheumatoid arthritis, SLE
Diarrhea/abdominal pain	Scleroderma, rheumatoid arthritis, reactive arthritis, arthritis of inflammatory bowel disease
Dysuria/urethral discharge	Reactive arthritis

TABLE 35.4 Diagnostic Tests for Different Rheumatic Disorders in Symptomatic Patients

Disease	Test	Sensitivity (%)	Specificity (%)	LR+	LR−
Reactive arthritis	HLA-B27	50–80			
Ankylosing spondylitis	HLA-B27 (white patients)	92	92	12	0.1
	HLA-B27 (black patients)	50	98	25	0.5
Rheumatoid arthritis	Rheumatoid factor	70–80			
Rheumatoid arthritis	ANA 1:40	49	68	1.5	0.8
	ANA 1:160	14	95	2.8	0.9
Systemic lupus erythematosus	ANA 1:40	97	68	3.0	0.0
	ANA 1:160	95	95	19	0.1
Sjögren's syndrome	ANA 1:40	84	68	2.6	0.2
	ANA 1:160	74	95	15	0.3
Scleroderma	ANA 1:40	100	68	3.1	0.0
	ANA 1:160	87	95	17	0.1

ANA = antinuclear antibody; LR = likelihood ratio.
Adapted and Reprinted with permission from Tan EM, Feltkamp TEW, Smolen JS, et al. Range of antinuclear antibodies in "healthy" individuals. *Arthritis Rheum*. 1997;40:1601–1611.

minutes of exercise. Morning stiffness typically lasts <30 minutes (14). Patients may have joint instability or buckling. The patient complains of pain and reduced function and, in the case of knee and hip disease, difficulty walking and climbing stairs. Usually the symptoms will wax and wane over time, with increasing involvement of more joints. However, the patterns and trajectory of the disease are highly variable and often cannot be predicted.

The distribution of joints affected in the hands and feet in OA is different from that in RA (see Fig. 35.2), and it is more likely than other arthritides to affect large joints such as the knee or hip, and often involves the hands and the spine as well. There are often boney enlargements and limitation of the range of motion of affected joints. Crepitus (cracking sounds heard or felt with movement of the joint) is a common and sensitive criterion for the disease. There may be effusions in large joints without associated marked inflammation (redness, warmth). OA of the wrists, ankles, and shoulders is often the result of trauma or other secondary causes. Specific clinical signs include:

TABLE 35.5 Findings in Synovial Fluid in Common forms of Arthritis

Diagnosis	White Cell Count	PMN (%)	Color/Clarity	Other
Normal	0–200	0–25	Clear/yellow	None
Trauma	5,000	50	Red/opaque	RBC ++
Osteoarthritis	500–2,000	<25	Clear to slightly cloudy/ yellow-white	Cartilage debris, Mucin clot firm
Acute rheumatic fever	2,000–15,000	50	Yellow-white	None
Gout	2,000–100,000	75	Yellow-white/translucent or opaque	Urate crystals
Pseudogout	2,000–100,000	75	Yellow-white/translucent or opaque	Pyrophosphate crystals
Septic arthritis	50,000–100,000, maybe >100,000	>95	Yellow-white/opaque	Positive culture in 80%, positive Gram stain in 70%, Mucin clot friable
Rheumatoid arthritis	2,000–100,000	>50	Yellow-white/translucent-opaque	Mucin clot, often xanthochromic

PMN = polymorphonuclear leukocytes; RBC ++ = red blood cell.

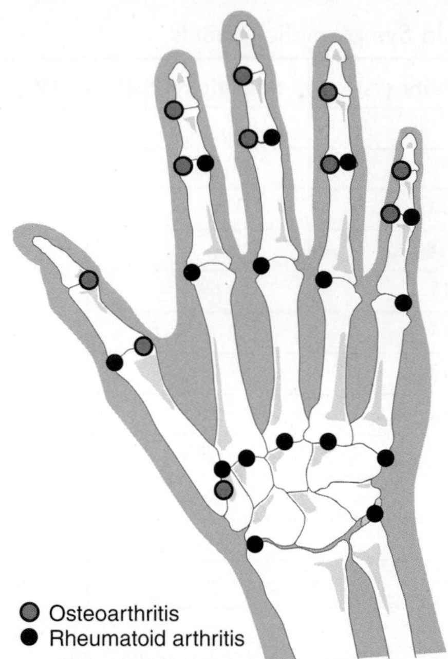

Figure 35.2 • Distribution of joint involvement in rheumatoid arthritis and osteoarthritis.

- hands—enlargement of the distal interphalangeal and/or proximal interphalangeal joints; carpometacarpal joint of the thumb often with some deviation of the phalanges; pain on motion (see Fig. 35.2)
- feet—swelling (possibly with bunion deformity-first metatarsal-phalangeal joint subluxation) of the big toe and distal interphalangeal joints
- knees and hips—pain and crepitus on passive motion; tenderness to palpation at the joint line; muscle atrophy. Hard swelling is caused by bone spurs, whereas soft swelling comes from effusions. There is significant limitation of range of motion on active and passive testing.
- spine—degenerative change is common, often with associated somatic dysfunction leading to limited motion and stiffness of the neck or lower back. Osteophytes (bony spurs) at the facet joints can produce local pain and compression of spinal nerve roots, causing neuropathy (weakness and sensory loss). When disc degeneration and osteophyte formation are severe, spinal canal stenosis can cause direct injury to the spinal cord in the neck or lumbar spine areas (see Chapters 36 and 37). Spinal stenosis can present with symptoms that mimic claudication.

Laboratory Tests and Imaging Studies

Synovial fluid analysis may be useful in ruling out possible inflammatory arthritis (see Table 35.5), but is often not necessary in patients with OA. The ESR is normal except in rare cases of erosive OA or primary generalized OA, which may have more of an inflammatory presentation similar to RA. Radiologic imaging is useful primarily when surgical intervention is considered and should not be used to make a diagnosis: radiographic changes of degeneration are routinely found in asymptomatic patients (see Table 35.6). Computed tomography and magnetic resonance imaging can be helpful in individual patients, such as to evaluate for possible cervical or lumbar spinal stenosis in patients with persistent symptoms that may need surgery.

Management

Twice-daily exercise programs and low-impact aerobic conditioning produce increased strength and pain reduction. Activity that causes pain lasting longer than 2 hours should be avoided. The use of braces, attention to supportive shoes, and other orthotics can relieve pain from asymmetric walking patterns. Exercise to the muscle group or groups that support particular affected joints (e.g., quadriceps for the knees) can be beneficial to reduce the wear and tear on the affected joints. Obese patients should lose weight, especially before orthopedic surgery for joint replacement; weight loss can improve long-term progression (Strength of Recommendation [SOR]=B) (14). Acupuncture can produce a measurable effect in some patients with OA of the knee (15). Other complementary or alternative therapies are widely used by patients with osteoarthritis with varying levels of supportive evidence (16). Findings supporting the efficacy of glucosamine sulfate, used alone or in combination with chondroitin sulfate, are highly variable but generally positive (17–20).

TABLE 35.6 Typical Radiographic Findings in Arthritic Conditions (71)

Disease	Finding
Rheumatoid arthritis	Osteopenia, joint surface erosions, subchondral bone cysts
Systemic lupus erythematosus	Minimal nonspecific changes
Gout	Bone cysts, punched out erosions on joint surfaces
Ankylosing spondylitis	Bilateral sacroiliitis, squaring of lumbar vertebrae, irregular bone erosion and sclerosis at the corners of the vertebrae, vertical syndesmophytes and loss of definition of apophyseal joints, juxta-articular osteoporosis, joint fusion
Osteoarthritis	Nonuniform joint space loss (may be minimal and reflect the only finding early in osteoarthritis), osteophyte formation, calcification of cartilage, cyst formation, and subchondral sclerosis

TABLE 35.7 Regimens for Corticosteroid Therapy*

Preparation	Schedule	Usual Dosage	Indication
Prednisone	Daily low dose oral	7.5 mg	Maintenance therapy
Prednisone	Short-term oral	20–30 mg/day (1–2 weeks) with taper over 7–14 days	Short flare
Prednisone	Maintenance oral	Alternating 5–10 mg 4 times daily	
Prednisone	High dose oral	60 mg daily	Severe, acute illness
Methylprednisolone sodium succinate[†] (Solu-Medrol)	Intravenous pulse	500–1,000 mg/day for 3 days	Severe flare
Triamcinolone	Intramuscular pulse	80 mg on alternate days 2 times	Severe flare
Methylprednisolone acetate[†]	Intra-articular		
	Interphalangeal	50–10 mg	25-gauge needle
	Wrist, ankle, Elbow	10–40 mg	20- to 22-gauge needle
	Knee, shoulder	40–80 mg	16- to 24-gauge needle

*Adverse effects: skin—thinning, striae, acne, hirsutism, bruising; cardiovascular—hypertension, edema; musculoskeletal—osteopenia, myopathy; personality—mood disorder, insomnia, euphoria; gastrointestinal—ulcer, bleeding; ophthalmic—glaucoma, cataract; endocrine—adrenal suppression, perforation, pancreatitis; metabolic—diabetes, obesity, menstrual disorders, hyperlipidemia.
[†]A variety of articular steroid preparations with different half-lives and costs are available.

Nonrandomized trials with the amino acid supplement S-adenosyl methionine (SAM-e) have shown some efficacy in OA, but the cost may be prohibitive for most patients (21). There is little evidence that the use of ginger is beneficial in OA; the same applies for the use of the antioxidant vitamins A, C, E, or selenium (22). The use of oral avocado and soybean unsaponifiables in 300 mg daily provided some symptom relief in patients with OA of the hip (21). Care should be exercised with herbal and dietary supplements, because there is increasing evidence that adverse effects and drug interactions can occur with oral supplements. Manipulative treatment and other manual modalities have been shown to be successful for select patients (23).

Medication can be given for pain relief in osteoarthritis as outlined in the general discussion previously (General Approach to Anti-inflammatory Medications). The use of topical capsaicin (0.025% cream applied four times daily for OA affecting the knee, ankle, finger, wrist, or shoulder) may be beneficial, with the minor side effect of a localized burning sensation (14). It is postulated to act as an irritant/counterirritant. In the same fashion, topical analgesic creams (salicylate cream) may be effective for focal joint pain, and can be applied four times daily (14). Intra-articular steroid injections can be used for joints with effusion and inflammation (Table 35.7).

Viscosupplementation is now widely used particularly for OA of the knees (24), with relatively low risks of adverse reactions: this is discussed further in Chapter 34. Patients with severe OA who are not responding to more conservative treatment and those with intractable pain or serious functional impairment should be referred to an orthopedic surgeon for osteotomy or arthroplasty. Arthroscopic surgery is no more effective for moderate to severe OA of the knee than optimal non-surgical approaches (25). Long-term outcomes for joint replacement/arthroplasty are good (26,27). Table 35.8 summarizes the level of evidence for the most effective therapies for OA.

PREVENTION

In both primary and secondary prevention of OA, the most important factor in protecting weight-bearing joints is maintaining an appropriate body weight (28). Exercise, especially of the supporting muscles (quadriceps for knees, abdominal muscles for lumbar spine), also has an important role.

RHEUMATOID ARTHRITIS (RA)

RA is a chronic inflammatory polyarthritis that primarily affects peripheral joints and related periarticular tissues. It usually starts as an insidious symmetric polyarthritis, often with nonspecific symptoms. Although RA is a systemic disease, it mostly affects the synovial membrane of joints. It is approximately three times more frequent in women than in men, and commonly (70% of cases) begins between 25 and 50 years of age. Its prevalence is 0.5% to 1.5% of the population in industrialized countries (29).

The exact cause of RA is unknown, but is likely multifactorial in people with a certain genetic susceptibility (HLA-DR shared epitope). Smoking is the major known environmental risk factor for RA, though little is known about the mechanisms involved. It is clear that persistent immune stimulation changes the synovial cell phenotype into one that invades articular cartilage and adjacent tissues. In the affected joint, the synovium forms a pannus of granulomatous tissue that erodes cartilage, ligaments, tendons, and eventually bone. These granulomas can also form subcutaneous nodules (rheumatoid nodules) and affect other organs such as lungs, heart, and bowel. Effusions may be present in joints, and surrounding muscles atrophy from disuse. Severe musculoskeletal deformities can eventually occur, ending in fibrous fusion (ankylosis) of joint surfaces. In the hands, these can be characterized by

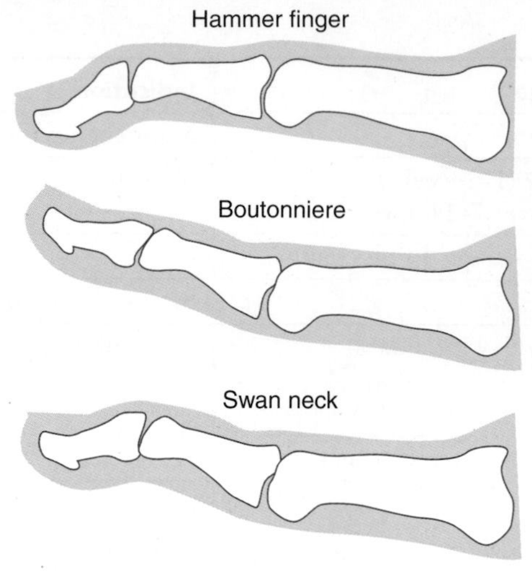

Figure 35.3 • Finger deformities in rheumatoid arthritis.

ulnar deviation, hammer fingers, boutonnière and swan-neck deformities of the fingers (Fig. 35.3), and sometimes tendon rupture in the extremities. The disease can cause flexion deformities of the toes, valgus deviation of the foot, and fixation of the ankle joint. Entrapment neuropathies in arms or legs are common (carpal, ulnar, and tarsal tunnel syndromes). Vasculitis and granulomas can lead to skin ulcers, scleritis in the eye, pleuritis, pulmonary nodules and fibrosis, pericarditis, osteoporosis, and splenomegaly. Sjögren syndrome (dry eyes and mouth) occurs in 20% of cases.

The differential diagnosis is extensive (see Fig. 35.1), and non-rheumatologic causes of the joint pain and swelling, myalgia, fatigue, fever, and weight loss must also be considered. The ACR has produced a set of criteria to promote diagnostic accuracy: criteria include arthritis lasting longer than 6 weeks (though evidence suggests that 12 weeks may be more specific), a positive rheumatoid factor (RF), and radiologic damage (9). Further criteria are presented in Table 35.9. When all are present, there is a sensitivity of 90% and specificity of 89% in making the diagnosis (likelihood ratio [LR]+ = 8.9; LR− = 0.11) (9,30).

TABLE 35.8 Level of Evidence for Different Therapies

Intervention	Strength of Recommendation*
Osteoarthritis	
Nonsteroidal anti-inflammatory drugs	A
Topical analgesics	A
Intra-articular hyaluronate	A
Manipulation and physical therapy	B
Acupuncture	B
Intra-articular steroids	B
Opioids	B
Aerobic exercise	B
Occupational interventions	B
Arthroplasty	B
Weight loss	B
Joint replacement	B
Rheumatoid arthritis	
Nonsteroidal anti-inflammatory drugs	A
Disease-modifying agents	A
Biologic agents	A
Self-help education, monthly telephone contact with counseling	A
3 months of physical therapy	A
Walking/conditioning program	A
Weight loss	C

*A = consistent, good-quality patient-oriented evidence; B = inconsistent or limited-quality patient-oriented evidence; C = consensus, disease-oriented evidence, usual practice, expert opinion, or case series.
For information about the SORT evidence rating system, see *http://www.aafp.org/afpsort.xml*.

TABLE 35.9 ACR Diagnostic Criteria for Gout and Rheumatoid Arthritis

Disease	Criteria	Interpretation
Rheumatoid arthritis	• Morning stiffness for at least 1 hour • At least three joints involved in soft tissue swelling or effusion (joints: PIP, MCP, wrist, elbow, knee, MTP) • At least one joint affected in wrist/MCP/PIP distribution • Symmetric involvement of the same joint, both sides of body • Nodules found subcutaneously or over bony points • Rheumatoid factor positive • Bone changes (erosions/decalcification) in hand/wrist radiographs	90% sensitive, 89% specific if all present. If pretest probability is 10%, patients meeting all of these criteria have 70% chance of RA.
Gout	In patients with more than one attack of acute arthritis and maximum inflammation within 24 hours • Monoarthritis • Redness over joints • First MTP joint involved • Unilateral first MTP joint attack • Unilateral tarsal joint attack • Tophus identified • Hyperuricemia • Asymmetric swelling in joint on radiograph • Subcortical cysts on radiograph • Urate crystals in joint fluid • Joint fluid culture negative	The presence of 6 of 11 of these criteria confirms gout (98% sensitive and 95% specific; LR+, 20; LR−, 0.02) (2).

LR = likelihood ratio; MCP = metacarpophalangeal; MTP = metatarsophalangeal; PIP = proximal interphalangeal; RA = rheumatoid arthritis.

Clinical Evaluation

Initially, there are aches and pains in the muscles and joints, sometimes accompanied by a low-grade fever, early morning stiffness, fatigue, and weight loss in 70% of patients. Although most rheumatic diseases involve morning stiffness, its' duration is a semiquantitative measure of degree of articular inflammation. Early-morning stiffness takes quite a bit longer to dissipate (45 to 60 minutes or more) in inflammatory arthritides such as RA, than in patients with OA (15 to 30 minutes). Other differences in presentation between OA and RA are summarized in Table 35.2. Subsequently, there is symmetric joint swelling, usually involving the proximal interphalangeal and metacarpophalangeal or metatarsophalangeal (MTP) joints of the hands or feet respectively (see Fig. 35.2). Wrists, knees, and ankles may also be affected. Rarely is only one joint involved. Activities of daily living are usually impaired. The patterns of progression and joint involvement are quite variable and include the following:

- Episodic—lasting a few months, then resolving only to return at shorter intervals
- One or two joints remain inflamed for several months before others are affected
- Morning stiffness and fatigue for many months, but with no pain
- Malaise, fever, weight loss for several months preceding joint involvement
- Progressive subtle swelling of the joints
- Severe onset, getting progressively worse without relief

Some patients suffer from RA for some years, and then the disease becomes inactive or "burned out." Patients may develop signs and symptoms of non-articular involvement that lead to pulmonary, cardiac, and bowel symptoms (see Table 35.3).

Physical examination findings can include weight loss, fever, joint swelling, tenderness to palpation, loss of range of motion, an enlarged spleen, muscle atrophy, inflammation of the tendons and tendon sheaths, and deformities in 20% of cases. Rheumatoid nodules can be found on the extensor aspects of the forearm in 25% of patients with RA. Vasculitis can cause peripheral neuropathy in the legs or arms. Similar neuropathy can occur from nerve entrapment by inflammatory tissue. Cardiac arrhythmias, pericarditis, and pleurisy are other results of vasculitis. Finally, a global assessment of function and emotional status should be undertaken (29).

Laboratory Tests and Imaging Studies

Rheumatoid factor (RF) test results only become positive some time (weeks to months) after the onset of RA. Up to 40% of patients with RA are seronegative early in the course of the disease, when they are also often likely to first present to their family physician. In fact, 25% of patients with RA will never have a positive RF test result: these patients are considered to have *seronegative RA*. A positive RF titer is generally considered significant at 1:160, and is more predictive of inflammatory disease at 1:320 (6). Non-rheumatic conditions that are also associated with a positive RF include bacterial endocarditis, tuberculosis, sarcoidosis, and malignancies. Elderly patients in the general population may have a positive RF 10% of the time, though usually at a very low titer—1:40 or less. In addition to RF, there may be variable results for antinuclear antibody, ESR, and CRP tests described earlier (and reviewed in Table 35.4). There is usually a hypochromic anemia with a normal white blood cell count, unless splenomegaly (which can cause leukopenia) is present. Joint fluid will show typical inflammatory changes (Table 35.5). Radiographic changes are specific but not sensitive (Table 35.6). More than half of patients have no detectable erosions on X-rays in the first 6 months, with the most rapid progression occurring over the first 2 years (31). Baseline studies include both hands and wrists on the same film, and both feet while standing. Early findings show peri-articular demineralization and swelling close to the joints. Joint spaces become narrowed, and erosions develop close to articular surfaces. Later changes show subluxation and deformities.

Management of RA

PHARMACOTHERAPY

The major treatment goals are to relieve symptoms (pain, swelling, fatigue), improve joint function, and reduce joint damage and disability. Because joint damage begins 6 months after the onset of RA, continued efforts to control the inflammatory process through disease modifying therapy has become the standard of care for patients with RA.

The first-line agents in acute disease are as outlined in the general approach to anti-inflammatory medications described earlier in this chapter. In RA, however, NSAIDs are initially preferred to acetaminophen because of their greater anti-inflammatory effects, despite higher risks of side effects (32). To reduce joint damage and disability, disease modifying antirheumatic drugs (DMARDs) however are generally also added early in the course of the disease, and usually no later than 6 months from onset of symptoms. Methotrexate, a dihydrofolate reductase inhibitor, is generally the first-line DMARD of choice for most patients with RA, because of its proven clinical benefits, well-understood long-term efficacy and toxicity profile, adaptability in that it can be combined effectively with most other DMARD agents, and cost (33). There is a high withdrawal rate with methotrexate, however, because of side effects, and it should not be prescribed to women who are pregnant or anticipate being pregnant (34).

Sulfasalazine or the antimalarial drug hydroxychloroquine are sometimes used first in patients with milder forms of RA. Tumor necrosis factor (TNF) receptor blockers (see the following section) are also now being widely used early in RA treatment but at significant cost. Other DMARDs include gold salts, D-penicillamine, and azathioprine and are reviewed in Table 35.10. Corticosteroid treatment options include low-dose, pulsed intravenous/intramuscular, or intermittent high-dose regimens and are reviewed in Table 35.7 (35). Auranofin (oral gold) has been shown to reduce disease activity, but not to significantly impact radiologic progression or long-term functional status, and therefore may be less effective than other DMARDs (36). Leflunomide, an inhibitor of pyrimidine synthesis, has a different mechanism of action than other DMARDS, and is a newer treatment option. Leflunomide has similar efficacy (SOR=A) and incidence of adverse effects as methotrexate, and it is more effective than, and as safe as, sulfasalazine, but its long-term safety profile is unclear (37). The costs of leflunomide treatment are also higher than treatment with methotrexate or sulfasalazine. Combination treatment with several DMARDs may enhance the efficacy over single-drug treatment, but balance of benefit and potential harm must be continually re-evaluated.

Uncertainty remains concerning therapeutic protocols for RA. There are three current approaches: the pyramid, the step-down bridge, and the sawtooth regimen (35). Initially, all patients are started on a program of patient education in a multi-faceted program that includes exercise, physical and occupational therapy, health care maintenance and psychological support.

PROTOCOL #1: PYRAMID MANAGEMENT

This is generally used for milder presentations and disease. If NSAIDs are not contraindicated, they are started primarily for symptom control. If the patient has not significantly improved in 2 to 3 weeks, treatment with a DMARD is initiated, usually methotrexate alone or in combination with sulfasalazine or hydroxychloroquine (38). Low-dose oral corticosteroids may be used to bridge the time period in which the peak response to DMARDs is developing (see Table 35.7). If DMARDs are ineffective, high-dose corticosteroids may be needed. TNF receptor blockers are now being used earlier in the course of RA.

PROTOCOL #2: STEP-DOWN BRIDGE MANAGEMENT

For very aggressive disease, treatment can be initiated with high-dose oral corticosteroids (60 mg prednisone daily), together with hydroxychloroquine, sulfasalazine, and methotrexate, along with folic acid. Medications are then withdrawn sequentially, and the corticosteroids tapered gradually, as control improves. TNF receptor blockers are typically also included here.

PROTOCOL #3: SAWTOOTH MANAGEMENT

In this regimen, single or combined DMARDs are given, usually including TNF receptor blockers, and agents are substituted if control deteriorates. Local joint flare-ups can be treated with intra-articular injections of corticosteroids.

SPECIFIC MEDICATIONS

Glucocorticoids

Corticosteroids are effective and widely used in rheumatic diseases, but 30% to 50% of patients on long-term steroids will develop osteoporosis (36). The most rapid bone mineral loss occurs in the first 6 to 12 months of therapy. When the long term oral dose is >30 mg/day, there is a 20% to 50% reduction in bone mineral density (39). When the dose is <10 mg/day, there is only a 10% reduction in bone mineral density.

To prevent bone loss, use the lowest dose of steroids for the shortest period of time, administer calcium (1,500 mg of elemental calcium/day) and vitamin D (800 IU/day), and consider adjuvant hormone replacement therapy for selected postmenopausal women. Bisphosphonates are effective in treating bone loss.

Biologic Response Modifiers (TNF Receptor Blockers)

Biologic response modifiers such as infliximab, etanercept, and adalimumab are injectable agents used for patients with moderate to severe RA that is refractory to NSAIDS, DMARDs, and low-dose corticosteroids. These agents block the action of TNF, which plays a major role in promoting joint inflammation. They produce substantial short-term improvement (30% to 50%) and slow RA progression; however, use is limited by side effects and risks (40,41).

TABLE 35.10 Treatment Regimens for Rheumatoid Arthritis

Drug	Peak Response	Maintenance Dose	Laboratory Checks
Antimalarials (hydroxychloroquine)	2–3 months	Hydroxychloroquine: start with 200 mg orally twice daily; after good response, long-term: decrease back to 200 mg orally daily	Ophthalmic check every 12 months, LFT, creatinine every 6 months
Sulfasalazine	4–5 months	500 mg/day with weekly increase to 2–3 g daily in two divided doses	LFT, CBC, creatinine every 3 months
Methotrexate	3–6 weeks	7.5 mg orally every week, increasing to 20 mg every week Daily folic acid to reduce oral and GI side effects	LFT, CBC, creatinine every 8–12 weeks
Gold salts (sodium thiomalate, aurothioglucose) Oral auranofin	5–8 months	IV/IM 50 mg/week, then monthly 6 mg daily, may increase after 4–6 months to 9 mg daily. If no response after 3 months at 9 mg, then discontinue	Urine, CBC, LFT every 4 months
Azathioprine	4–6 months	1 mg/kg/day; may increase by 0.5 mg/kg at 4-week intervals to a maximum of 2.5 mg/kg	CBC, differential every 2 months
Tumor necrosis factor receptor blockers			PPD screening before initiating treatment; periodic CBC monitor for CHF
Etanercept		25 mg injected subcutaneously twice weekly (72–96 hours apart)	
Infliximab		3 mg/kg infusion, repeated after 2 and 6 weeks, then every 8 weeks	
Adalimumab		40 mg injected subcutaneously weekly or every other week	
Leflunomide	3–6 weeks	100 mg/daily for 1–3 days, then 20 mg a day	LFT, CBC, creatinine every 8–12 weeks Monitor blood pressure

CBC = complete blood count; CHF = congestive heart failure; GI = gastrointestinal PPD = purified protein derivative; IM = intramuscularly; IV = intravenously; LFT = liver function test.

Tuberculosis, invasive fungal infections, and other opportunistic infections have been reported during therapy with these agents, so patients should be screened for tuberculosis prior to initiation of treatment, and the drugs should be discontinued at any sign of infection.

Table 35.8 summarizes the level of evidence for the most effective therapies for RA and Table 35.10 the doses and regimens of the most commonly used medications.

Complementary and Alternative Therapy

Alternative treatments similar to those employed for OA are commonly sought out by RA patients (16,42). Superficial moist heat and cryotherapy as palliative therapy as well as the use of paraffin wax baths, with or without therapeutic exercise, have shown short-term benefits, but there is inconsistency in the evidence. Likewise, balneotherapy and spa therapy, and bathing in warm water with or without minerals, have shown some positive results in patient symptoms in small studies, but the evidence is limited by the poor methodological quality of the studies.

Low-level laser therapy has been advocated as an alternative and non-invasive treatment for RA and has demonstrated short-term relief of pain and morning stiffness in small studies, with no side effects. The dosing, the length of treatment time, and the long-term effects are controversial (43). There is considerable variability in the evidence for the use of other alternative therapies for RA (44). Fish oil or other sources of omega-3 fatty acids may be a useful option in patients for pain from inflammation in RA (45).

Long-Term Care

For long-term RA care, every follow-up visit should include a patient-centered assessment of progress, a review of medications and adverse effects, consideration of general health promotion and disease prevention, and a review of functional abilities.

Possible surgical interventions include synovectomy to reduce further damage to the joint, resection arthroplasty, joint fusion, and joint replacement (46,47). Synovectomy is primarily palliative, with relief lasting only 1 to 3 years. Tenosynovectomy involves debriding tendon sheaths to improve motion. Resection arthroplasty removes the damaged part of a non-weightbearing joint, and arthrodesis relieves pain by fusing the joint. Joint replacement using silastic prostheses has been the major innovation in arthritis care in recent years, leading to significant pain relief and improved function; long-term outcomes are not known however.

Physical and occupational health specialists play an important role in helping patients with RA function maximally at home and at work. Dynamic exercise therapy at an appropriate intensity for approximately 3 months has been shown to improve aerobic capability, muscle strength, and joint mobility without increasing pain, joint damage, or disease activity (46). Manipulative treatment, especially for secondary areas of somatic dysfunction, may assist with symptoms and patient function (48). Supportive care includes splinting to preserve joint function (especially of the wrists), and to protect and rest inflamed joints. There is no evidence that this ultimately reduces deformities, however, and may in fact lead to permanent restriction of motion. Extra-depth shoes or insoles may be helpful, but there is some conflicting evidence supporting their use and their effect in the reduction in pain and deformity (49). Occupational therapy can assist patients by teaching them adaptive techniques for daily chores and assistive devices and modification of the home can help patients remain independent for a longer time (SOR=A).

Patients suffering from any form of chronic arthritis often have significant psychosocial problems involving body image, depression, social interactions, and sexuality. Individual and group therapy may be useful, and treatment for depression may be needed: the family physician is ideally suited to address these whole-person issues over time with patients and their families.

The course of RA is highly variable and unpredictable; generally it is associated with a shortened life expectancy (5). About 5% of patients will be in remission within 2 years of the first attack, 15% to 25% will have progressively deteriorating disease despite maximal therapy, and the remainder will follow a varying course of intermittent flare-ups and remissions. Almost 90% of the joints that will be affected over time in a patient are involved during the first year of the disease. In patients who do not undergo a spontaneous remission (usually within 1 to 2 years of onset), structural joint damage may occur, leading to articular deformities and functional impairment. The prognosis for these patients seems to depend on the severity of the synovial inflammation. About half will be unable to work in 10 years (5). A poor prognosis is also indicated by a high-titer RF result (a strongly positive RF result predicts 60% mortality at 8 years, compared with 18% mortality for patients with a negative RF result). Rheumatoid nodules, extra-articular involvement, persisting acute phase reactants, more than 20 joints involved, psychological helplessness, and significant functional disability within 1 year of onset are all poor prognostic indicators. If the ESR remains at approximately 30, the risk ratio for total joint replacement is 2.7, but this increases to 4.8 if the ESR remains above 60. Interestingly, RA commonly goes into remission during pregnancy for uncertain reasons.

SYSTEMIC LUPUS ERYTHEMATOSUS (SLE)

SLE is a rare multisystem disease with multiple auto-antibody formation, occurring mostly in women, especially of African American and Asian heritage. Arthritis occurs in 80% of cases, with a similar pattern to that outlined in RA. A variety of skin problems can occur, including the typical facial "butterfly" (malar) rash on cheeks and nose, discoid scaling lesions on the scalp and extremities, photosensitivity, alopecia, and oral ulcers. SLE most often manifests as a mixture of constitutional symptoms, with skin, musculoskeletal, and mild hematologic involvement (50,51). The patient may suffer from Raynaud phenomenon, nephritis, pleuro-pericarditis, GI involvement, and central nervous system damage. Less frequently, the patient may have predominantly hematologic, renal, or neuropsychiatric manifestations.

SLE is often difficult to diagnose. The antinuclear antibody (ANA) is positive in 90% of cases, but the specificity of this test is poor (i.e., there are often false positives), whereas the anti–double-stranded DNA and anti-Smith antibodies are positive in 50% and 30% of patients, respectively. The ACR recommends ANA testing only in patients with two or more unexplained signs or symptoms (SOR=C). Care should be exercised not to test patients with isolated myalgias or arthralgias because of the high degree of false positives and the potential emotional consequences of fear of this disease (51). ANA testing is positive in 5% of tested women and older patients but generally at a titer that is <1:320 (6,7). Four of the 11 diagnostic ACR criteria must be met for a diagnosis of SLE (5).

The ACR recommends referral to a rheumatologist for patients with characteristic signs and symptoms of SLE and a positive ANA, particularly in cases with more significant or unstable disease (SOR=C) (5). Treatment for SLE includes sunscreen (with UVB/UVA coverage) for skin problems, NSAIDs and a variety of medications similar to those used in RA: hydroxychloroquine, low- or high-dose steroids, methotrexate or azathioprine used as steroid-sparing drugs (50), and ultimately immunosuppressive agents (intravenous cyclosporine or cyclophosphamide). Identifying and treating cardiovascular risk factors is particularly important. Targeted biologic therapies are under development, which may alter treatment algorithms in the future.

Drug-related lupus refers to the development of a lupus-like syndrome after exposure to certain medications, and usually results in rapid resolution of the signs and symptoms on withdrawal from the drug. Autoantibodies may persist for 6 to 12 months. Although there are many drugs implicated in drug-related lupus, the two most probable drugs are procainamide and hydralazine (5).

GOUT

Gout is the most common form of inflammatory arthritis in men older than 40 years of age. It is more common in men and African Americans, has a genetic predisposition in 40% of patients and affects 5% of all men older than 65 years of age (1–3).

Symptoms are caused by the deposition of monosodium urate crystals in and around the tissues of joints, which induces local inflammation, necrosis, fibrosis, and subchondral bone destruction. The abnormal amounts of urates in the body results from defective metabolism of uric acid or can occur as a result of acquired causes of hyperuricemia, such as in cancers (multiple myeloma, polycythemia vera), chronic renal disease, psoriasis, alcoholism, and with certain medications (e.g., thiazide and loop diuretics, cyclosporine, niacin). The diagnostic criteria for gout are shown in Table 35.9.

Clinical Evaluation

Gout often starts as an acute attack developing over several hours. Sometimes there is a prodromal phase with arthralgias, fever, and chills. The attack will subside in a few days, often with desquamation of the skin overlying the affected joint. It usually affects one to three joints of the fingers and/or toes. Other joints in the feet, ankle, elbows, wrists, and, rarely, the sacroiliac joints, can be affected. The great toe is involved in 75% of cases and the knee and ankle in 50% of attacks. For many patients, the natural course of the disease is of increasingly frequent and severe episodes (60% recurrence in the first year, and 25% in the second year). For other patients, there may be no clear pattern. Patients who develop polyarticular gout usually have other complex medical problems such as hypertension, cardiac disease, obesity, and renal disease, which modify and complicate uric acid metabolism.

An affected joint typically is swollen, red, hot, and tender. The classic description depicts a patient who cannot even tolerate the weight of the bed sheets on the swollen tender big toe. Chronic gout may be associated with swollen, intermittently painful joints in the hands and feet as well as tophi (urate deposits in the soft and cartilaginous tissues of the metatarsophalangeal joint, elbow, tendons of the hands, and ears that cause local nodular swelling and may discharge white material).

Laboratory Tests

Although an elevated serum urate level is suggestive of gout, many patients with high serum urate levels are asymptomatic and will never develop gout. High levels are found in renal disease, blood disorders, lymphoma, diabetes, and hypertension in the absence of gout. Furthermore, the serum urate level will be normal in approximately 50% of gout patients during acute attacks, and may in fact lower with an acute attack (1,52). Serum urate levels are also notoriously variable from week to week in the same individual. However, measurement of serum urate levels 2 weeks or more after a suspicious episode of acute arthritis can be helpful in making the diagnosis: it likely will be elevated in patients with gout and low (<4 mg/dL) in patients without gout (SOR=B).

The definitive diagnosis of gout however is made by identifying the needle-like monosodium urate crystals from synovial fluid or a tophus that, on microscopy, are negatively birefringent in polarized light (yellow against red background); this finding is 85% sensitive (SOR=A). Imaging of joints early in the disease is often normal. Later, periarticular swelling is seen with punched-out areas on the surface of articular bone (most frequently on the first metatarsal).

Management

ACUTE GOUT

As with other forms of arthritis as outlined previously, acute gout is effectively treated with NSAIDs. Indomethacin 25 to 50 mg every 6 to 8 hours bas been traditionally preferred in gout because of its effectiveness, although it has a high side effect profile. A safer alternative is naproxen 500 mg two times daily) (SOR=A). A 10- to 14-day taper of oral prednisone (20 to 60 mg) can be substituted if the patient cannot tolerate NSAIDs (53). Corticosteroids can also be administered as an intra-articular injection (SOR=A). Oral colchicine, which has been used for centuries but was only approved by the US Food and Drug Administration in 2009 for the treatment of gout, has a narrow therapeutic window and cannot be used in patients with renal failure. Therefore, its use in acute gout is more limited. Opiates may be needed if the pain is excruciating. Allopurinol, febuxostat, and low-dose aspirin therapy are contraindicated in acute gout.

CHRONIC GOUT

Prevention is the cornerstone of treatment in chronic gout. Weight loss should be encouraged in overweight patients (54). Patients should avoid medications that may increase urate levels, such as diuretics and nicotinic acid. Recommend that the patient reduce purine-rich foods (e.g., red meat, seafood) even though these contribute only 1 mg/dL to urate level and the evidence is not completely clear that dietary modification will reduce gouty occurrences (54) (SOR=B). Likewise, increased consumption of low-fat dairy products may reduce their risk of gout flares, as may the addition of 250 to 500 mg daily of vitamin C (55). Patients should reduce their intake of sweetened soft drinks and fruit drinks, as well as alcohol in the form of beer and liquor but not wine; the former two contain purines and block renal excretion of urate. Instruct the patient to begin and then maintain a high clear fluid intake (56). This may be enough to control symptoms in patients who have only mildly elevated uric acid levels and have suffered only one or two attacks of gout. Many of these patients will not need prophylactic urate-lowering medication (5).

In patients with frequent acute episodes of gout who are willing to take a medication to prevent gout, the choice of drug used to lower the serum urate depends on the result of a 24-hour urinary uric acid study. Ideal candidates for urate-lowering treatment include urate *over* producers (24-hour urinary uric acid excretion >800 mg on a general diet, or >600 mg on a purine-restricted diet), those with 3 or more gout flares per year, those with recurring renal stones or tophi, and patients at risk for developing uric-acid nephropathy (e.g., those on treatment for myeloproliferative or lymphoproliferative disorders) (SOR=A). Xanthine oxidase inhibitors, allopurinol and, since 2009, febuxostat are appropriate for most of these patients, but should not be initiated during an acute gouty attack (SOR=A). During urate-lowering treatment, the target serum urate level is <6 mg per dL (SOR=B). For gout patients identified as urate *under* excretors (24-hour urinary uric acid excretion <800 mg on a general diet or <600 on a purine-free diet), the use of uricosuric drugs (e.g., probenecid, see below) would instead be first-line agents. These agents block tubular resorption of filtered urate in the kidney. However, these agents are contraindicated in patients with a history of nephrolithiasis and are ineffective in individuals with a GFR of <50 mL/minute.

Uricosuric drugs (probenecid, 250 mg twice daily, increasing to 2 or 3 g/day; or sulfinpyrazone, 50 to 100 mg twice daily, increasing to 200 to 400 mg twice daily) will also reduce the size of tophi. These drugs can also be used in combination with colchicine to reduce the frequency and severity of attacks. High clear fluid intake (2,000 mL/day) and oral potassium citrate (10–20 mEq three to four times daily) are also needed with these drugs to prevent crystal precipitation and calculus formation in the kidney. Adverse effects include rash (5%) and GI problems (10%).

SOFT-TISSUE SYNDROMES

This group of disorders consists of a collection of discernible patterns of local musculoskeletal pain, stiffness, and tenderness, which are often separate from joints. There may be an association with a systemic disease, rheumatic disorder, repetitive trauma, or stress, but usually the etiology is unclear. The tissues involved include fascia, muscle (typically with tender points, "trigger points" [areas of very localized muscle spasms, often involving only a few fibers], or myofascial points in the neck, shoulder, and low back region), ligaments, or tendons that become inflamed, and bursae that cause pain and swelling close to the joints (57).

Myofascial Trigger Points

The patient will describe pain and aching in muscles, sometimes after trauma, but most often arising spontaneously. The areas most affected are the neck and shoulder region, interscapular muscles, and the lower back and buttocks. Firm palpation of the muscle with the fingertips may reveal a trigger against the examining finger (57). Deep pressure on a trigger point will cause pain of reproducible distribution and quality. These problems may be secondary to poor posture and deconditioning and can be associated with underlying musculoskeletal or visceral pathology and can be associated with stress or psychosomatic disorders.

Trigger points will often respond to a graded exercise and conditioning program with local acupressure and deep massage. Acetaminophen or NSAIDs may give relief, although no strong evidence supports this approach. Muscle relaxants are not effective. Local injections of lidocaine, corticosteroids, or a combination of the two, or needle penetration of the trigger point without injection of any medication can produce immediate relief, but trigger points often recur. Spray and stretch techniques with ethyl chloride and manipulative treatment or massage may provide temporarily relief.

Somatic Dysfunction

Myofascial trigger points and similar impairments are described by osteopathic physicians as impairments of the somatic (body framework) system: somatic dysfunction. These areas can affect joints, skeletal and myofascial structures, and their related vascular, lymphatic, and neural elements. Somatic dysfunction is characterized by tissue texture abnormality, asymmetry, restriction of motion, and tenderness, one of which must be present for the diagnosis (58). Tissue texture abnormalities are palpable changes and include vasodilation, edema, hypertonicity, contracture, and ropiness that can be noted from the skin to periarticular structures. Somatic dysfunction is most commonly diagnosed in the spinal areas and trunk, but can also be found in the extremities or cranium. The physician uses one or more of a variety of manual techniques, depending on the patient and the problem, in an attempt to enhance movement and resolve the dysfunction. There have been many reports and small studies advocating for the efficacy of manipulative treatment to manage a host of diseases and disorders of structure and function; however, high-quality studies involving large numbers of human subjects are limited (23,59,60).

Fibromyalgia Syndrome

Fibromyalgia (FM), which occurs much more commonly in women, is characterized by widespread musculoskeletal pain and trigger points, often associated with extreme weakness or fatigue. FM is the most common cause of chronic widespread pain in the United States (5). There often is a history of anxiety, insomnia, depression, or previous physical abuse. It is not an inflammatory disorder, but may result from disordered brain processing, alterations in sleep patterns, and changes in neuroendocrine transmitters, such as serotonin, substance P, growth hormone, and cortisol (61). The patient may also complain of urethral syndrome (urinary frequency and painful urination). There is considerable overlap with chronic fatigue syndrome, adult attention deficit disorder, and possibly with food allergies (62). An associated non-restorative sleep disturbance with early morning waking often is present.

Evaluation of a patient with possible FM involves a detailed history and physical examination and testing to exclude other etiologies such as thyroid disease and anemia. Diagnostic criteria include a history of chronic widespread pain involving all four quadrants of the body and the axial skeleton, along with the presence of 11 of 18 tender points on physical examination (63,64).

Moderately effective treatments include patient education about the illness, exercise and supervised aerobic training, and correction of sleep disturbance using tricyclic antidepressants, other antidepressant medication, or cyclobenzaprine (65–67). Other approaches that have been successful in randomized trials include massage, manipulative treatment, heated pool/spa therapy, cognitive behavioral therapy, and acupuncture (64,65,68). Successful medications have been: pramipexole, pregabalin, tramadol, tropisetron. Partnering with the patient during regular follow-up and legitimizing their concerns is particularly important. Physicians can become frustrated with the patient's lack of response to treatment. Supportive counseling by the physician and the willingness to try novel strategies are exceedingly important.

Polymyalgia Rheumatica (PMR)

Polymyalgia rheumatica (PMR) affects older people, particularly women, and is characterized by pain and stiffness in the cervical spine and shoulder/hip girdles (5). Myalgias in these areas can be profound and are commonly accompanied by signs of systemic inflammation such as malaise, weight loss, sweats, and low-grade fever. Arthralgia can occur on occasion, and the presentation can be indistinguishable from that of acute, seronegative RA. The diagnosis is made on clinical grounds combined with an elevated sedimentation rate (often >60 mm/hour), anemia, and occasionally elevated liver function tests (particularly alkaline phosphatase). Treatment consists of low-dose steroids, starting with 10 to 15 mg and tapering to 5 to 7.5 mg daily for several weeks or months. The synovitis of PMR typically responds better to low doses of prednisone than does RA, which may help to differentiate the two.

Approximately 10% to 20% of patients may also have giant cell arteritis (temporal arteritis), an inflammatory swelling of the temporal arteries that can present with headaches, loss of vision, scalp tenderness, jaw claudication, and can lead to sudden blindness. The diagnosis is made on clinical grounds and confirmed by biopsy of the temporal artery. In a small percentage of patients with PMR and giant cell arteritis who have a normal ESR, positron emission tomography scanning may be helpful in diagnosis. Giant cell arteritis needs immediate therapy with high-dose steroids (69). Family physicians should remain alert for and play an active role in managing this medical emergency.

Infectious Disorders Affecting Joints

SEPTIC ARTHRITIS

The family physician must always consider septic arthritis in a joint that is acutely red and hot, especially in a patient who is febrile, unwell and has an extra-articular site of bacterial infection. Arthrocentesis is mandatory if a septic joint is suspected. If the patient has a diseased or prosthetic joint coupled with risk factors such as: older than 80 years of age, diabetes mellitus, hemodialysis, immunocompromised state, or intravenous drug abuse, the possibility of septic arthritis is even greater. Among non-gonococcal etiologies, *Staphylococcus aureus* and streptococci, including *Streptococcus pneumoniae*, are the most common organisms. *Staphylococcus epidermidis* infection is common in prosthetic joint infections, but rarely found in native joints. In young, otherwise healthy, sexually active adult populations, infection caused by *Neisseria gonorrhoeae* may be more common than non-gonococcal causes.

VIRAL INFECTIONS

Viral causes of polyarthritis are common. Infection with parvovirus B19, the cause of Fifth Disease (erythema infectiosum) in children, with characteristic "slapped cheeks," has been implicated in as many as 12% of adults presenting with polyarthritis or polyarthralgia, with or without the associated rash. The joint distribution is similar to that of RA, with prominent morning stiffness, and many patients with chronic symptoms may meet the diagnostic criteria for RA. Most patients, however, will have a negative or low-titer RF, and their symptoms will resolve spontaneously in 4 to 6 weeks.

LYME DISEASE

This is a chronic, inflammatory, multisystem disease caused by a tick-borne spirochete. Early in the disease, patients can experience arthralgias or a migratory polyarthritis. Late disease, occurring months to years after the tick bite, may include a chronic, monoarticular arthritis, typically affecting the knee. Diagnosis should be suspected in people with unexplained arthritis who live in areas where the disease is endemic, especially if the arthritis is preceded by the classic "bull's-eye" skin rash, termed erythema migrans, which occurs in 90% of patients infected and almost always within 1 month of the tick bite. Diagnosis can be confirmed by an enzyme-linked immuno-absorbent assay and false positives are reduced by secondary Western blot analysis; antibiotic treatment (doxycycline) in early disease prevents progression and is curative (70). There is no good evidence to support the benefit of long term antibiotics in patients with chronic symptoms who have been diagnosed with Lyme disease.

REACTIVE ARTHRITIS (REITER SYNDROME)

Reactive arthritis refers to a rheumatic presentation that follows shortly after certain infections of the GI tract (Shigella, salmonella, or campylobacter) or of the genitourinary tract (*Chlamydia trachomatis*). Most of the individuals affected are young men who are HLA B27-positive. There is also a higher prevalence in those with HIV infection. The classic clinical triad associated with reactive arthritis is: non-gonococcal urethritis, conjunctivitis, and arthritis, with the latter being an asymmetric, inflammatory, and oligo-articular arthritis usually of the knees, ankles, and small joints of the lower extremities. A papulosquamous skin rash (called keratoderma blennorrhagicum) that resembles mollusk shells or pustules on the soles or palms or other skin surfaces may be present; the rash can eventually coalesce to mimic the skin lesions of psoriasis. Synovial fluid analysis will show high inflammatory changes, but will not generally yield positive culture results because the joint inflammation is caused by immune complexes (see Table 35.5). Although the diagnosis is made on clinical grounds, urethral or cervical smears for *N. gonorrhoeae* and *C. trachomatis* should be performed; testing for HLA B27 shows a reasonable predictive value only if the clinical data support a strong likelihood of disease. The disease is self-limited in a majority of affected patients, but a few patients develop visual impairment from uveitis, or a chronic disabling foot arthritis or heel pain (enthesitis). Less likely complications from reactive arthritis include aortitis, cardiac conduction system abnormalities, amyloidosis, and neurologic conditions (5).

PATIENT EDUCATION

A great deal of information is available on self-care for patients with arthritis and rheumatologic conditions. The Arthritis Foundation publishes valuable educational materials as well as a regular newsletter. Physicians can also obtain useful information and catalogs of assistive devices for their patients (Arthritis Foundation, (800) 283-7800; *www.arthritis.org*). Other useful Web sites include the ACR (*www.rheumatology.org*), the American Academy of Family Physicians (*www.aafp.org*), Canadian guidelines (*www.arthritis.ca*), and the US Bone and Joint Decade 2002–2011 (*www.usbjd.org*).

KEY POINTS

- Arthritis and several rheumatologic diseases are common reasons for patients to see their family physician.
- Family physicians can manage many of the complaints of patients with arthritis and rheumatologic diseases.
- Most arthritis can be diagnosed clinically using history and physical exam and the role of laboratory testing is to confirm the clinical diagnosis.
- There are a number of different approaches to treating Rheumatoid Arthritis that physicians should be familiar with and a wide array of medications available.
- Temporal arteritis is a medical emergency that needs to be detected and treated promptly.
- It is important to have an interdisciplinary, team-based approach to managing many forms of arthritis, which lends itself to management within the patient-centered medical home.

CHAPTER

36

Low Back Pain

Scott Kinkade

CLINICAL OBJECTIVES

1. List the most common causes of back pain.
2. Apply the "red flag" screening questions to patients with back pain.
3. Perform a basic back exam.
4. Discuss appropriate treatments for common back problems.

Low back pain (LBP) is a self-reported symptom of pain that is experienced in the lower back region. It is important to recognize that LBP is a symptom and does not reflect any specific etiology or diagnosis and in fact there are multiple possible etiologies. It is typically considered to be acute or chronic (present >12 weeks) and both presentations usually have very different management plans.

The prevalence of LBP on any 1 day among adults in the United States is 5.6% (1), while 18% report having had back pain in the previous month (2). The lifetime prevalence of low back pain has been estimated to be at least 60% to 70% (3–5). The majority of patients with LBP self-treat their pain and only 25% to 30% seek medical care (6,7). However, back pain still ranks as one of the top reasons for visits to family physicians, and accounts for at least $26 billion in direct health care costs and 2.5% of total health care spending in the United States (8,9). Family physicians treat more patients with back pain than physicians from any other specialty and about as many patients with back pain as orthopedic surgeons and neurosurgeons combined (3). Back pain that becomes chronic is an economic burden in most industrialized countries. About half of the lost work days due to back pain are generated by the 15% of patients with chronic pain who require >1 month off work. The remaining other half of the lost work days are due to the 85% of patients who have self-limited back pain and are off work <7 work days (10).

A conservative approach to the diagnosis and management of LBP is warranted as most cases are self-limited and more serious cases can be detected by screening for the red flag conditions. The natural history of LBP overall is favorable with some studies showing that 60% of patients are better in 1 week, 90% are better in 6 weeks, and 95% are better in 12 weeks (11). A more conservative estimate is that one-third will be better in 1 week and two-thirds will be better in 6 to 7 weeks (12). However, relapses and recurrences are common in this condition, affecting about 25% to 40% of patients within 6 months (13,14).

DIFFERENTIAL DIAGNOSIS

The key elements of the spine are: the vertebral bodies that articulate with each other via posterior facet joints and the intervertebral disk; the spinal cord and nerves that exit via the neural foramina, and ligaments that stabilize the vertebral bodies and paraspinous muscles that stabilize the spine. Figure 36.1 reveals the most common ligaments of the lumbar spine. The intervertebral disk is composed of a thick outer annulus fibrosis and an inner gelatinous nucleus pulposus. Figure 36.2 shows a cross-section of a normal intervertebral disc unit with the associated spinal contents and nerve roots.

Most back pain does not have a clear etiology. Degenerative changes in any of the structures of the back can lead to pain. Strains of the muscles and ligaments can cause pain. The etiology of back pain can generally be divided into: mechanical conditions, non-mechanical causes, and non-spinal causes. Mechanical back pain implies an anatomic or functional abnormality that is exacerbated by movement. Patients with nonmechanical back pain typically have pain both at rest and with movement. Non-mechanical LBP is usually due to chemical irritation from causes of inflammation or infection. Table 36.1 summarizes the differential diagnosis for LBP.

Lumbar strain or sprain (reflecting soft tissue inflammation) is the most common cause of back pain and presents with pain in the lower back that can radiate into the buttocks or proximal lower extremities.

The syndrome of herniated disk or herniated nucleus pulposus with impingement of the nerve root (radiculopathy) is commonly known as sciatica. Figure 36.3 shows a diagram of a herniated disk impinging on a nerve root together with its associated magnetic resonance imaging (MRI) scan. This radicular pain typically radiates in a dermatomal pattern down the leg and below the knee. Whether or not symptoms radiate past the knee is a key distinguishing feature of sciatica since non-radicular causes of LBP typically do not radiate below the knee. The 30- to 55-year-old age group has the highest incidence of herniated disks (15). With increasing age, the disk becomes firmer (less gelatinous) and is less likely to herniate through the annulus fibrosis. The L4–L5 disk and L5–S1 disk account for 95% of herniations, the L3–L4 disk accounts for the remaining 5%. Herniation is very rare in disks above L3 (16).

Cauda equina syndrome is diagnosed when acute neurological impairment occurs in those structures supplied by the sacral nerve roots, notably causing bowel or bladder dysfunction or perineal ("saddle") anesthesia. This is a surgical emergency that requires urgent diagnosis and treatment. The most common causes are large paracentral disk herniations and

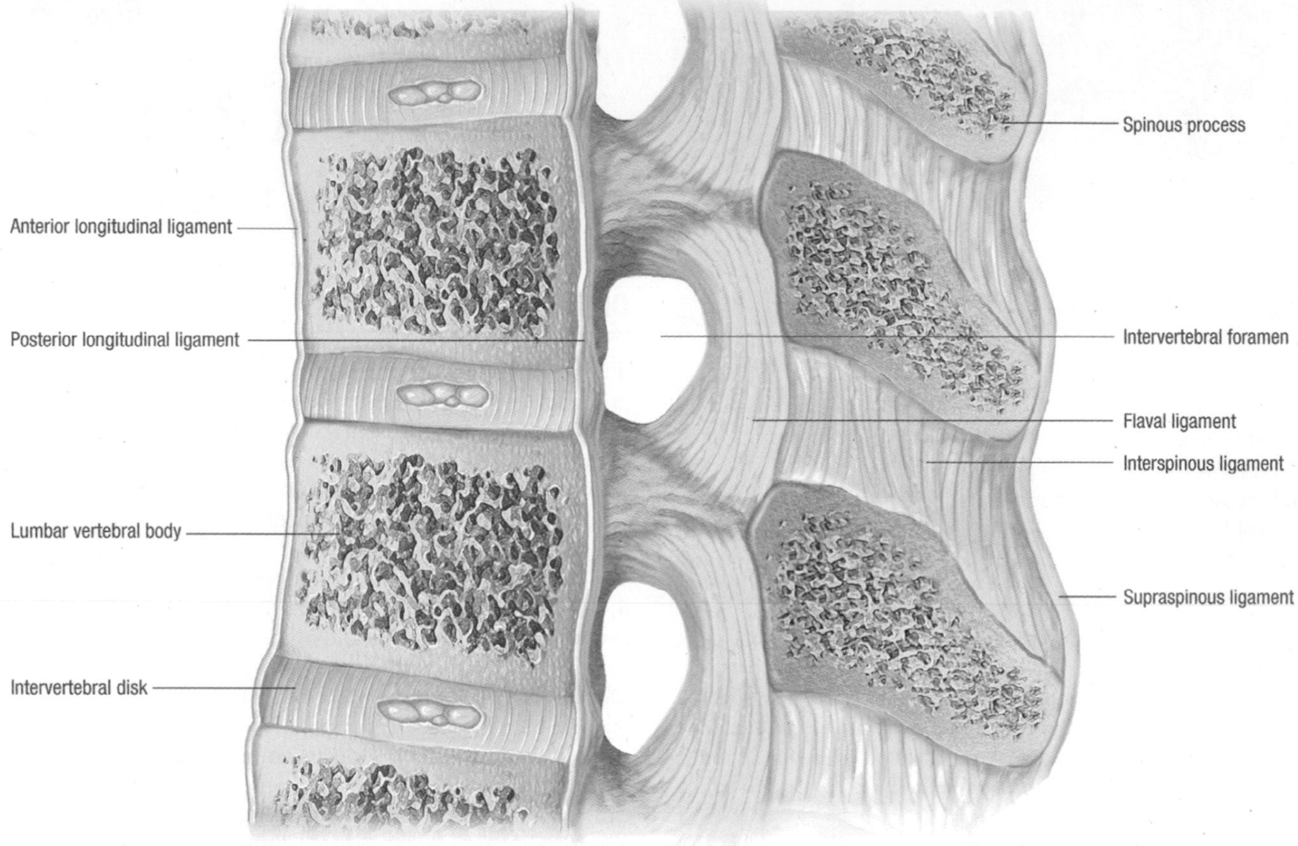

Figure 36.1 • Lateral view of ligaments of lumbar spine.

TABLE 36.1 Differential Diagnosis of the Patient with Low Back Pain*

I. Mechanical low back pain	97%
Lumbar strain or sprain/idiopathic low back pain	70%
Degenerative disk/facet process	10%
Herniated disk	4%
Spinal stenosis	3%
Osteoporotic compression fracture	4%
Spondylolisthesis	2%
II. Non-mechanical spinal conditions	~1%
Neoplasia	0.7%
Infection	0.01%
Inflammatory arthritis	0.3%
III. Non-spinal, visceral disease	2%
Pelvic organs (prostatitis, pelvic inflammatory disease, endometriosis)	
Renal (nephrolithiasis, pyelonephritis)	
Aortic aneurysm	
Gastrointestinal (pancreatitis, cholecystitis, peptic ulcer)	
Shingles *(Herpes zoster)*	

*Data from Deyo RA, Weinstein JN. Low back pain. *N Engl J Med*. 2001;344(5):363–370.

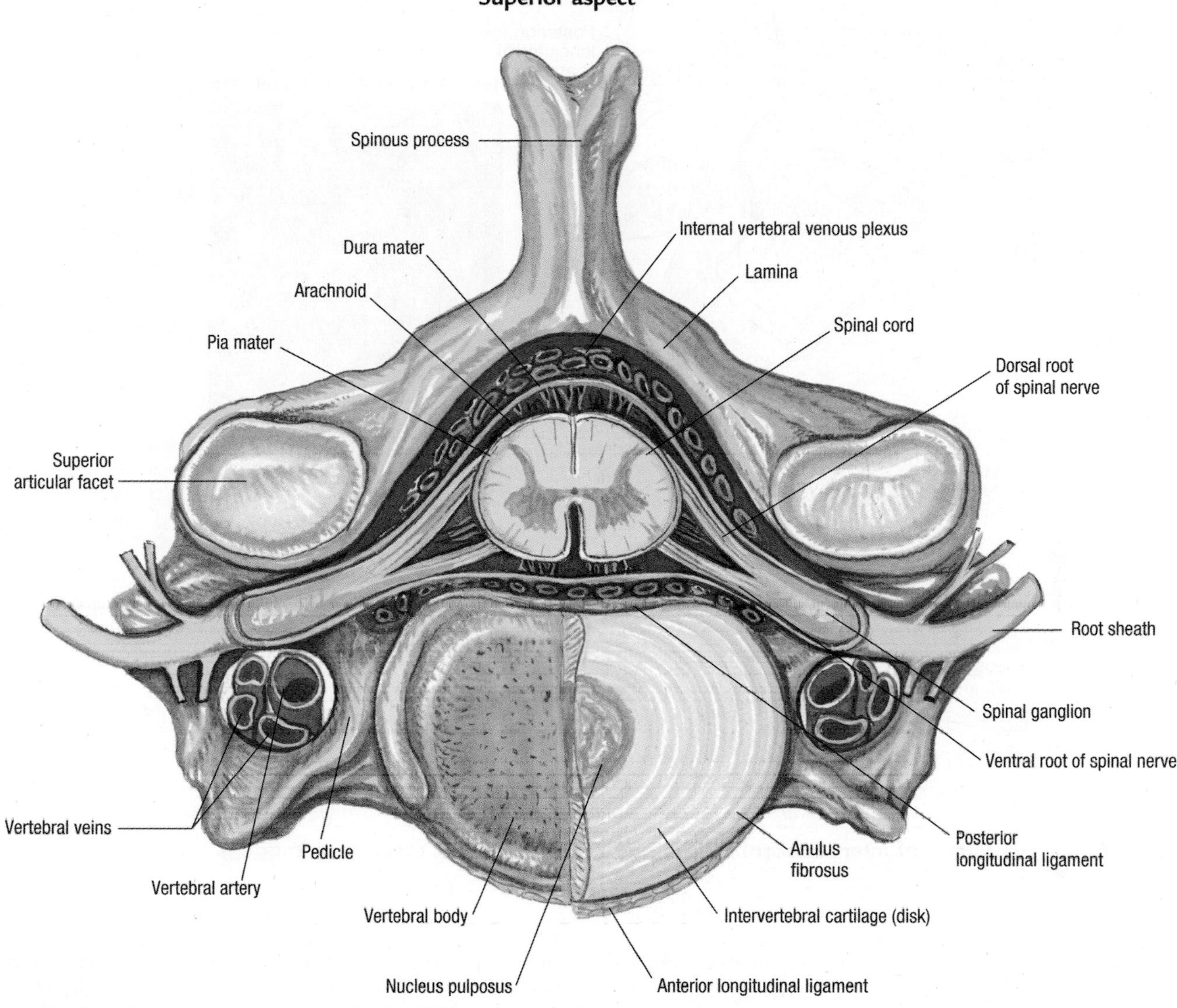

Figure 36.2 • Cross-section of lumbar inter-vertebral disk unit.

tumors. Even with prompt decompression, some patients do not recover completely.

Spinal stenosis occurs primarily in older individuals and is related to degenerative changes in the spine with resulting hypertrophy of the facet joints and ligamentum flavum. The diameter of the spinal canal or neural outlets is compromised, often at multiple levels.

Vertebral compression fractures typically occur in older individuals with osteoporosis. The traditional risk factors for osteoporosis are: female sex, early menopause, Northern European or Asian ethnicity, cigarette smoking, sedentary lifestyle, and chronic steroid use. An uncommon but often overlooked cause is neoplastic disease in the vertebra that leads to an insufficiency fracture.

CLINICAL EVALUATION

History

Use the same approach to taking a history that you would use with any patient with a chief complaint of "pain":

- Onset—Is the pain acute or chronic? Acute pain, especially after a precipitating event, suggests a disk problem or muscle strain. Can the patient recall the details of the onset? Pain that evolves slowly or insidiously is more likely with a degenerative process such as spinal stenosis or a rheumatologic process such as ankylosing spondylitis. Pain associated with trauma is worrisome for the possibility of a vertebral fracture.
- Character—Ask the patient to describe the pain. Is it sharp, dull, etc.? Chronic, constant dull pain may increase the probability of cancer. Burning, altered sensation or pain that is described as being like an "electric shock" is often typical of an irritated nerve or nerve root.
- Location and radiation—The typical pain of lumbar strain is usually in the paraspinous muscles, sometimes radiating into the buttock(s). Bone pain from metastatic disease or a compression fracture is often localized to the spine. Pain that radiates down below the knee suggests a herniated disk. As noted, cauda equine syndrome typically presents with "saddle" anesthesia and bilateral leg pains. Spinal stenosis also causes pain that radiates into the legs.

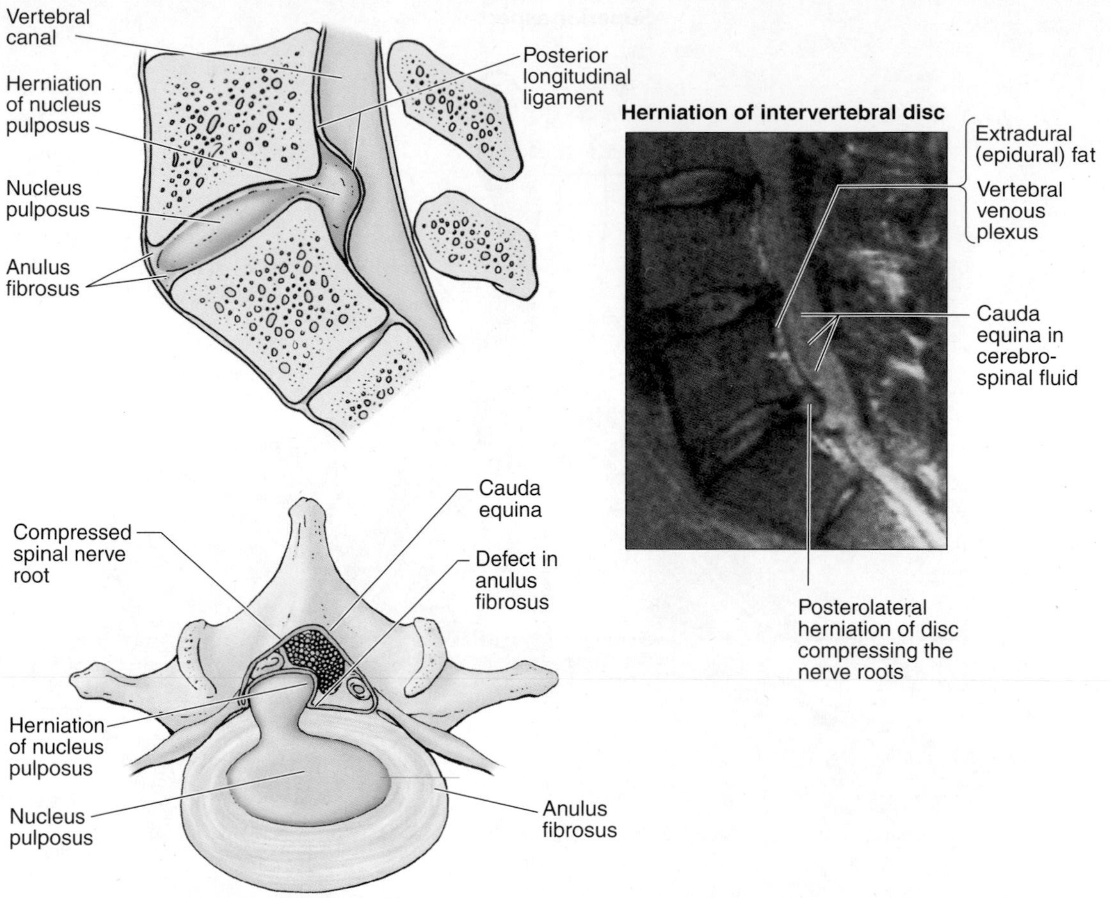

Figure 36.3 • Herniation of intervertebral disk, diagram and magnetic resonance imaging.

- Intensity—The intensity (or severity) of pain does not correlate well with the seriousness of the etiology. Individual patient reactions to pain are strongly influenced by psychosocial factors. However, it may be useful to gauge the patient's progress over time. The intensity of pain can be recorded on a visual analog scale (VAS). The VAS is usually a 10-cm line where zero represents no pain and 10 represents intense pain ("the worst ever experienced"). Using this or a similar tool at each visit can assist recognition of whether improvement is occurring. The severity of the pain can also be estimated from how it affects daily activities. For example, does the pain interfere with sleeping or with certain activities such as putting on shoes, driving, or walking?
- Duration—As noted, pain lasting longer than 12 weeks is usually classified as chronic. Pain lasting <12 weeks is acute, though some authors define 6 to 12 weeks of pain as subacute. Whether the pain is continuous or waxes and wanes with pain-free intervals can help determine the etiology. Rheumatic conditions tend to have initial stiffness and pain that decrease over a few hours. Diskogenic stiffness tends to decrease after 20 to 30 minutes. Pain from spinal stenosis tends to increase with increased activity.
- Associated symptoms—Particularly important associated findings are considered in the "red flag symptoms" section below. The presence of associated stiffness that takes time to resolve may indicate a systemic disorder such as ankylosing spondylitis. Coexisting urinary, gynecologic, or abdominal symptoms may help discern non–spine-related diagnoses.
- Aggravating factors—Pain from a herniated disk is usually worse with maneuvers that increase the intradiscal pressure such as valsalva, coughing, or bending forward. The leg pain from spinal stenosis is often called pseudoclaudication (or neurogenic claudication) because the symptoms tend to worsen with exercise. The lower leg pains in this case however are not due to ischemia as with typical vascular claudication, but rather to narrowing of the spinal canal causing radicular impingement. Because extension of the spine narrows the diameter of the canal and neural foramina, patients with spinal stenosis are more likely to have pain when walking downhill or down stairs. Figure 36.4 represents the posterior narrowing that occurs with extension of the lumbar spine. Patients with spinal stenosis typically feel better when they sit, crouch down, or if pushing a shopping cart, when leaning forward on the basket.
- Relieving factors—Has the patient tried prescription or over-the-counter medications or nonpharmacologic measures (massage, stretching, heat or ice, etc.) and found them helpful? Are there certain positions that relieve the pain? Remember to ask about the use of complementary and alternative therapies such

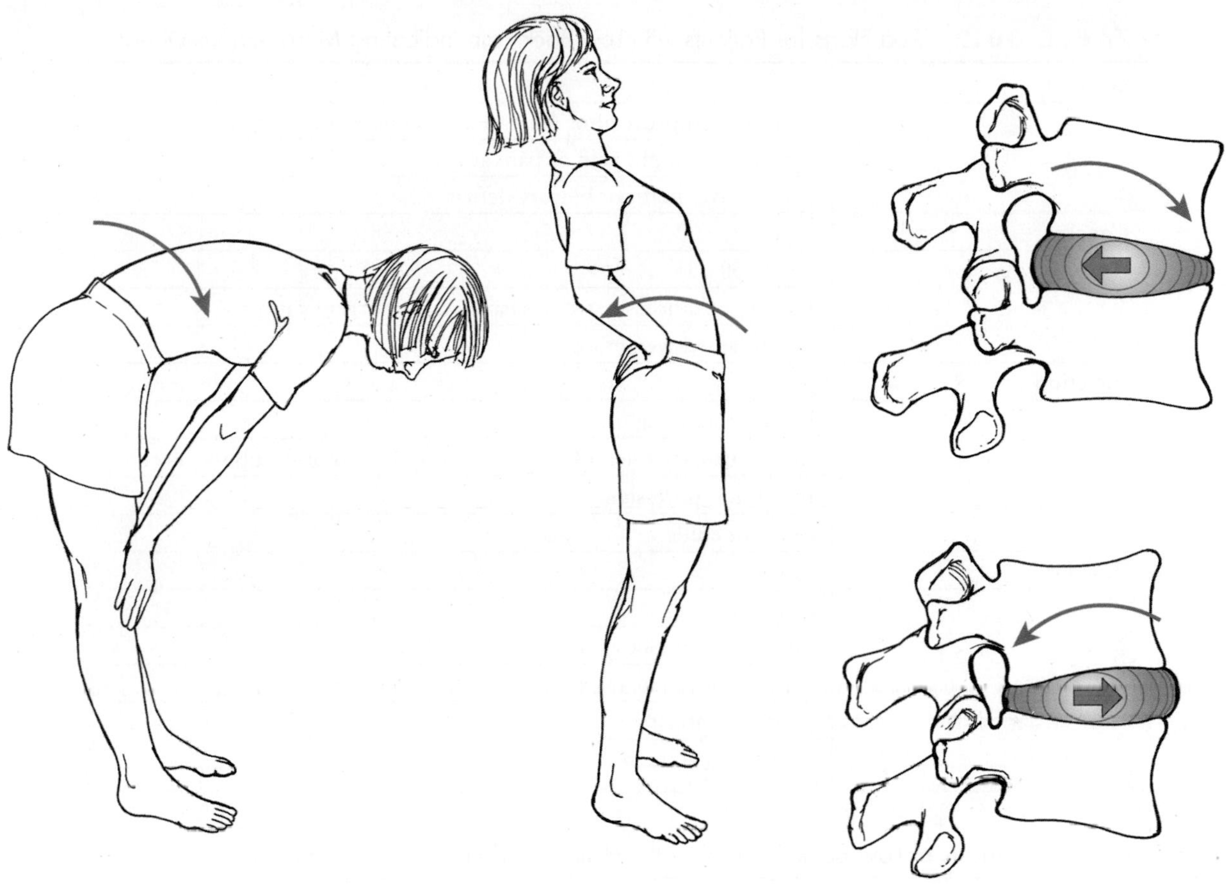

Figure 36.4 • Effects of flexion and extension on the intervertebral disk.

as chiropractic and acupuncture, as well as the use of dietary supplements.

- Psychosocial—It is critical to ascertain contextual details of how the pain is affecting the patient's lifestyle and other psychosocial factors, including beliefs about the pain and prognosis, coping strategies, and pending litigation or disability evaluation.
- "Red flag" symptoms:
  A focused assessment should be made to exclude serious underlying disease. Table 36.2 outlines several red flag symptoms for back pain that may indicate more serious disease. Negative answers to all four of these questions: (i) age >50, (ii) personal history of cancer, (iii) unexplained weight loss, and (iv) failed conservative therapy effectively rules out cancer as a cause (17). In addition, a patient without urinary retention is very unlikely to have cauda equine syndrome (<1 in 10,000) (17). Table 36.2 summarizes the accuracy of selected historical elements in diagnosing patients with LBP.

Physical Exam

A basic physical exam for LBP includes: assessing range of motion of the lumbar spine, palpation and inspection of the spinous processes and paraspinous muscles, assessing motor strength and deep tendon reflexes in the lower extremities and performing the straight leg raising test. Assessment of motor strength in the lower extremities, especially ankle dorsiflexion and extension of the great toe is important. Tables 36.3 and 36.4 summarize the accuracy of selected elements of the physical exam and the interpretation of common neurological deficits. Other good motor exam tests include having the patient walk on the heels and then the toes, or repeatedly lifting heels off the ground while standing. Asymmetry in strength when heel walking or toe walking may indicate a neuropathy. Similarly, fatiguing the muscle with repetitions may reveal asymmetric weakness. Additional tests may be indicated by the history such as an abdominal exam, pelvic exam or prostate exam.

The straight leg raising test (SLR) is performed with the patient supine to see if radicular pain occurs when the leg is elevated between 30 and 60 degrees. The SLR test is fairly sensitive for a herniated disk, but not very specific. It is considered positive when the maneuver causes pain to radiate down the leg—not when the SLR causes or increases LBP. The crossed SLR test (pain radiating down the leg on lifting the opposite leg) is more specific for a herniated disk, but less sensitive.

RECOMMENDED DIAGNOSTIC STRATEGY

Because the vast majority of causes of LBP are not due to a serious underlying condition and since most cases are self-limited, diagnostic testing can be used sparingly in the absence of red flag findings and usually only after patients have failed conservative

TABLE 36.2 Red Flags for Patients with Low Back Pain Indicating More Serious Disease

General	
	Failure to improve after 4–6 weeks of conservative therapy
	Unrelenting night pain or pain at rest
	Progressive motor or sensory deficit
Cancer	
	Age >50
	History of cancer or strong suspicion for current cancer
	Unexplained weight loss
Infection	
	Intravenous drug use
	Recent urinary tract infection or skin infection or decubitus ulcers
	Immunosuppression
	Fever or chills
Fracture	
	Age >50
	History of osteoporosis
	Chronic oral steroid use
	Substance abuse
	Significant trauma

TABLE 36.3 Diagnosis of Low Back Pain using the History and Physical Examination*

Diagnosis Suggested	Clinical Finding	Sn	Sp	LR+	LR−
Cancer	Age >50	0.77	0.71	2.7	0.32
	Previous history of cancer	0.31	0.98	14.7	0.70
	Failure to improve with 1 month of therapy	0.31	0.90	3.0	0.77
	Unexplained weight loss	0.15	0.94	2.7	0.90
	No relief with bedrest	>0.90	0.46	1.7	0.21
	Age >50 or history of cancer or unexplained weight loss or failure of conservative therapy	1.00	0.60	2.5	0.0
Compression fracture	Age >50	0.84	0.61	2.2	0.26
	Age >70	0.22	0.96	5.5	0.81
	Trauma	0.30	0.85	2.0	0.82
	Corticosteroid use	0.06	0.995	12.0	0.94
Spinal stenosis	Pseudoclaudication	0.60	N/A		
	No pain when seated	0.46	0.93	6.6	0.58
	Pseudoclaudication and age >50	0.90	0.70	3.0	0.14
Herniated disk	Sciatica by history	0.95	0.88	7.9	0.06
	Ipsilateral SLR	0.80	0.40	1.3	0.50
	Crossed SLR	0.25	0.90	2.5	0.83
	Ankle dorsiflexion weakness	0.35	0.70	1.2	0.93
	Great toe extensor weakness	0.50	0.70	1.7	0.71
	Sensory loss	0.50	0.50	1.0	1.0

Hx = history; LR+ = positive likelihood ratio; LR− = negative likelihood ratio; SLR = straight leg raising test; Sn = sensitivity; Sp = specificity.
*Data from Jarvik JG, Deyo RA. Diagnostic evaluation of low back pain with emphasis on imaging. *Ann Intern Med.* 2002;137(7):586–597; and Deyo RA, Rainville J, Kent DL. What can the history and physical examination tell us about low back pain? *JAMA.* 1992;268(6):760–765.

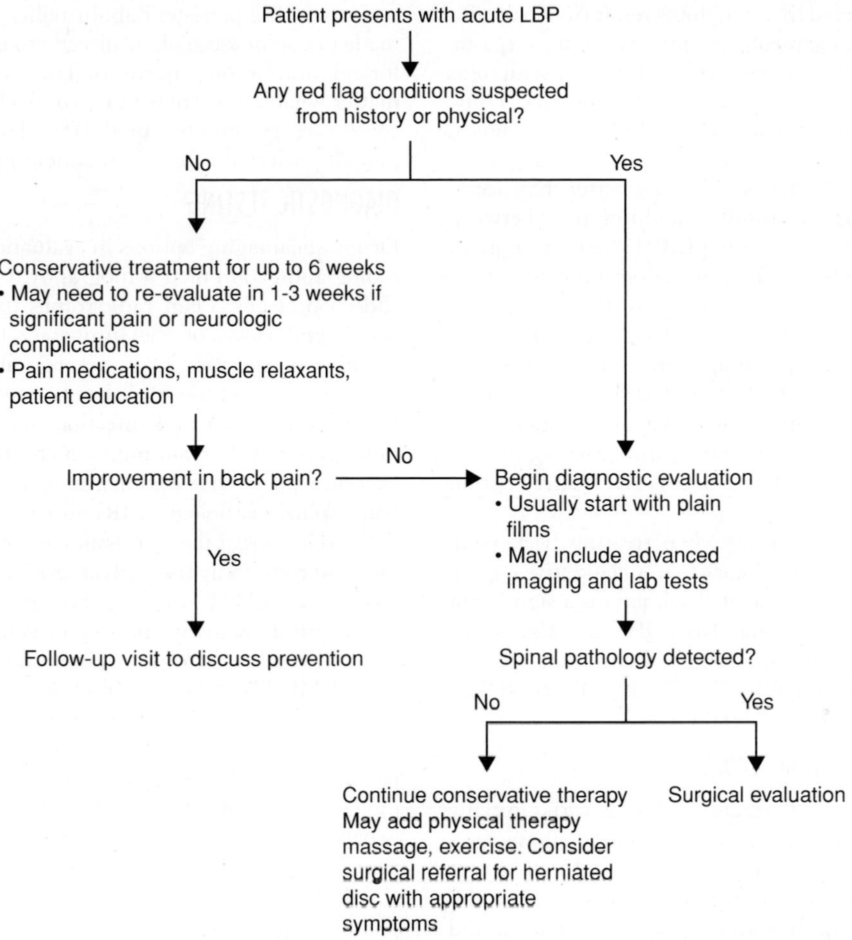
Patient presents with acute LBP
Any red flag conditions suspected from history or physical?
No
Yes
Conservative treatment for up to 6 weeks
• May need to re-evaluate in 1-3 weeks if significant pain or neurologic complications
• Pain medications, muscle relaxants, patient education
Improvement in back pain?
No
Begin diagnostic evaluation
• Usually start with plain films
• May include advanced imaging and lab tests
Yes
Follow-up visit to discuss prevention
Spinal pathology detected?
No
Yes
Continue conservative therapy May add physical therapy massage, exercise. Consider surgical referral for herniated disc with appropriate symptoms
Surgical evaluation

Figure 36.5 • An algorithm to guide management of low back pain.

management. Therefore for most patients, assuming they do not have any red flags, conservative management for the first 4 to 6 weeks is appropriate. This approach has been supported by many treatment studies and is considered the standard of care across almost all guidelines (18). Patients who have not recovered after 4 to 6 weeks should be re-evaluated, possibly with plain radiographs or advanced imaging. Patients who have worrisome findings on imaging or unresolving complications of a herniated disk (cauda equina syndrome, intractable pain, or progressive neurological deficits) should be referred to a spine specialist for surgical evaluation.

INITIAL MANAGEMENT OF ACUTE LOW BACK PAIN

Figure 36.5 outlines an approach to the management of LBP outlined in more detail below.

Acute Lumbar Strain

Acute lumbar strain, also previously called lumbago or nonspecific LBP, accounts for the bulk of back pain diagnoses, has a good prognosis, and can be treated conservatively. In this condition, no red flags are noted, there are no significant neurologic

TABLE 36.4 Neurological Findings on Physical Examination

Level of Disk Herniation	Nerve Root Affected	Sensory Loss	Motor Weakness	Exam Maneuver	Reflex Affected
L3–L4 disk	L4	Medial foot	Knee extension	Squat and rise	Patellar
L4–L5 disk	L5	Dorsal foot	Dorsiflexion ankle/great toe	Heel walking	None
L5–S1	S1	Lateral foot	Plantarflexion ankle/toes	Walking on toes	Achilles

findings and it is considered that symptoms result from a combination of inflammation, ligamentous injury, and muscle spasm. The goal of treatment is to provide pain relief until symptoms resolve rather than to "cure" anything. Acetaminophen, nonsteroidal anti-inflammatory drugs (NSAIDs), mild opioids, and skeletal muscle relaxants are all effective in treating acute LBP. There is no evidence that NSAIDs are better than acetaminophen or that there are significant differences between different types of NSAIDs in treating LBP (19,20) (strength of recommendation [SOR]=A). The most common side effect of NSAIDs is gastrointestinal toxicity. If this becomes a problem, acetaminophen can be used. Muscle relaxants, such as diazepam or cyclobenzaprine are effective in the short-term treatment of acute LBP (18,21–23) (SOR=A). If drowsiness is a problem with muscle relaxants, patients can take a lower dose, use them only at bedtime, or try metaxalone, which is less sedating. Local heat is an effective option for back pain.

Patient education is essential when treating back pain. There is some evidence for the theory that maladaptive coping (fear and pain avoidance) with acute back pain is a significant cause of progression to chronic LBP. Patients should be advised to stay active. There is strong evidence that bed rest does not decrease pain intensity or improve function and therefore should be avoided (18,24) (SOR=A).

HERNIATED DISK WITH RADICULOPATHY

Acute radiculopathy from a herniated disk (sciatica) is initially treated similarly to acute lumbar strain. Some of these cases may have mild neurological deficits (decreased reflexes or strength), but are still initially treated conservatively. Consider analgesics, including NSAIDs and/or muscle relaxants, and recommend physical activity as tolerated. Specifically, patients with sciatica who are advised to rest in bed have no significant difference in pain or functional status compared with patients advised to stay active (18,24) (SOR=A).

Most patients will improve over 4 to 6 weeks. Patients with severe or intractable pain or progressive neurologic deficits should be re-evaluated earlier and may need referral or imaging. Patients with radicular symptoms (such as lower extremity radiation of pain, numbness or absent reflexes) that are not improved at 6 weeks should probably have an MRI to determine whether there is a lesion that correlates with the symptoms. If a persistent abnormality is noted, referral can be made to a spine surgeon or directly to interventional radiology for epidural steroid injections. There is good evidence that no matter what treatment is pursued for the first 6 weeks the outcomes are essentially equal (18). Therefore, the treatment modality selected is based on patient preference.

DIAGNOSTIC TESTING

Diagnostic imaging options in evaluation of LBP include plain radiographs, computed tomography (CT), MRI, and radionuclide bone scans. Plain radiographs (typically anteroposterior and lateral views of the lumbosacral spine) are not highly sensitive or specific. They are reasonably useful to identify compression fractures and degenerative changes of the spine. Findings of cancer and infection may not show up on early radiographs. CT scanning, which involves more radiation exposure than other options, is relatively good for revealing bony spinal pathology. MRI, because it provides the most detailed images of the soft tissues of the disk and nerve roots, is the most commonly used advanced imaging modality for back pain. MRI and CT scanning, because they provide such good detail, also show many abnormalities that are not causing clinical symptoms, a factor that diminishes their specificity. In the case of MRI, studies in asymptomatic adults show herniated disks in about 30% to 40% of patients, bulging disks in about 50% of patients, and degenerative changes in up to 90% of patients (15). The diagnostic accuracy of common imaging modalities is shown in Table 36. 5. Radionuclide bone scanning is particularly helpful in detecting osteomyelitis, bony metastases, and occult fractures.

If the patient has any red flag symptoms or risk factors, a plain radiograph with or without a complete blood count and an erythrocyte sedimentation rate is an appropriate first step. If there is strong suspicion for serious underlying pathology and initial imaging is nondiagnostic, consider obtaining advanced imaging with MRI, CT, or a radionuclide bone scan.

CHRONIC LBP

LBP that is present for more than 3 months is considered chronic LBP. It is frequently a complicated and expensive condition that may prove difficult for the patient, their family, their employer, and the physician. It is important to maintain a positive therapeutic relationship with the patient. Monitoring

TABLE 36.5 Accuracy of Diagnostic Tests for the Patient with Low Back Pain*

Test	Sn	Sp	LR+	LR−	Approximate Cost ($)
Plain film (for cancer)	0.6	0.95–0.995	12–120	0.40–0.42	<150
CT (for HNP)	0.62–0.9	0.7–0.87	2.1–6.9	0.11–0.54	400–1,000
CT (for stenosis)	0.9	0.8–0.96	4.5–22	0.10–0.12	
MRI (for cancer)	0.83–0.93	0.90–0.97	8.3–31	0.07–0.19	750–1,500
MRI (for infection)	0.96	0.92	12	0.04	
MRI (for HNP)	0.6–1.0	0.43–0.97	1.1–33	0–0.93	

CT = computed tomography; HNP = herniated nucleus pulposus; LR+ = positive likelihood ratio; LR− = negative likelihood ratio; MRI = magnetic resonance imaging; Sn = sensitivity; Sp = specificity.
*Data from Jarvik JG, Deyo RA. Diagnostic evaluation of low back pain with emphasis on imaging. *Ann Intern Med*. 2002;137(7):586–597.

chronic analgesic use and occupational factors such as fitness for duty and return to usual work can be time consuming. Only a small percent of patients with acute LBP progress to chronic LBP, but the longer a patient is off work or disabled, the more likely that they will never return to work. There are significant psychosocial risk factors for chronicity that are not completely understood and not easily treated. These risk factors include: depressed mood, psychosocial distress, poor coping strategies, fear avoidance, somatization, workers compensation claims and litigation (4,25,26) (SOR=B). Many patients with chronic LBP do not have a demonstrable radiculopathy, neuropathy, or anatomic abnormality that explains their symptoms.

The treatment goals for patients with chronic LBP are largely functional: namely to optimize function, moderate or cope with pain, and decrease utilization of health care services. This typically requires a multidisciplinary effort. Complete eradication of pain is unlikely. Pain medicines such as acetaminophen, nonsteroidal anti-inflammatory drugs, and opioids are often used. Antidepressant drug therapy, particularly with tricyclic antidepressants, should be given a trial, even in patients without clinical depression (23,27,28) (SOR=A). Antidepressant therapy decreases pain, but does not have an impact on functional status.

Chronic pharmacologic therapy is usually not successful in relieving or curing chronic back pain. Adjunctive nonpharmacologic therapies have shown benefit in chronic back pain, though not necessarily in acute back pain. Exercise improves function and decreases pain in patients with chronic low back pain and is one of the most effective treatments (23,29,30) (SOR=A). Other nonpharmacologic treatments that may provide some benefit include spinal manipulation, massage, acupuncture, yoga, and intensive interdisciplinary rehabilitation (31–35).

PREVENTION

Strategies to prevent LBP, especially chronic LBP, have the potential to make a large impact given the prevalence of this symptom. Unfortunately, the multifactorial nature of back pain makes any single preventive strategy unlikely to account for much benefit. The most consistently identified risk factor for LBP is a history of back pain. Other risk factors include physical determinants such as heavy lifting, frequent bending, twisting and lifting, repetitive work with exposure to vibration, and the psychosocial issues mentioned previously.

The most effective prevention strategy seems to be physical exercise, which may decrease the incidence of new episodes, recurrences and lost work days (36) (SOR=C). Education in the form of back schools and instruction on proper lifting techniques does not seem to be helpful in preventing back problems and is not recommended. Education that assists in coping with back pain and encourages activity has a small benefit in preventing chronic or recurrent back pain (36,37) (SOR=C). There is strong evidence that back belts and lumbar supports are not effective in preventing back pain in workers and should not be recommended (36,37) (SOR=A). Overall, effective strategies for preventing initial or recurrent LBP are lacking. There are a variety of patient education materials that may be useful to help educate patients about prevention of back pain and management of common causes (37).

KEY POINTS

- Screen patients with new-onset low back pain for red-flag symptoms.
- Perform a focused exam: inspection, palpation, range of motion, straight leg raise, and neurologic exam of the lower extremities.
- Lumbar strain and most other causes of mechanical back pain, including herniated disks, can be treated conservatively with medications for the pain and advice to stay active.
- The goals of treatment for chronic back pain are to improve function and decrease pain while trying to prevent permanent disability and the chronic need for narcotic pain medicines.

CHAPTER

37

Neck Pain

Caryl J. Heaton and Rob Johnson

CLINICAL OBJECTIVES

1. Describe the prevalence of neck pain.
2. Describe the pathophysiology of neck injuries, including acceleration/deceleration injuries.
3. List the common sports-related neck injuries.
4. Understand the efficacy of various treatment options.

Nonspecific neck pain is very common; two thirds of people will have symptoms of neck pain at some time in their lives and 40% of adults report having had neck pain within the previous 6 months (1,2). The annual prevalence of neck complaints is reported to be 12% in women and 9% in men. One study of people engaged in a stressful occupation (salespeople) found the lifetime prevalence to be as high as 54% in men and 76% in women (3). The majority of neck complaints remit spontaneously within a few days, and medical care is not sought. Although neck pain is the primary complaint for only 1% to 2% of all adult visits to a family physician's office, the complex anatomy and physiology of the neck make these complaints difficult to specifically and rapidly diagnose. Neck pain that limits activities (both social and work) has a 1-month prevalence of 7.5% to 14% and a 12-month prevalence of 2% to 11% (4). Although there are many recommended treatments for neck pain that continue to be used as we will review in the following sections, the evidence for the effectiveness of many of these treatments is weak, conflicting, or, at times, nonexistent.

The prognosis of neck pain is generally very good. Most pain resolves within 2 weeks, and 90% of patients have resolution of their symptoms within 4 to 8 weeks (5). Patients who have had neck pain in the past have a much higher likelihood of having neck pain in any given year (odds ratio [OR]: 3.13 [1.29–7.58]). Other risk factors for neck pain include being female (OR: 1.63 [1.07–2.48]), increasing age (OR: 2.54 [1.39–4.62] for ages 40 to 49 years and OR: 2.46 [1.06–5.68] for age >50 years), presence of psychological stress (OR: 1.68 [1.10–2.57]), or headache (OR: 1.81 [1.18–2.76]) (5), prolonged talking on the telephone (OR: 1.4 [1.0–1.8]), or high amounts of twisting or bending at work (OR: 1.8 [1.2–2.7]) (6). Neck pain recurs within 1 year in 60% to 80% of those workers that get it, with white collar workers generally having shorter durations of disability than blue collar workers (4). Other factors affecting prognosis in the injured worker with neck pain include a more favorable outcome if the worker is a regular exerciser and a worse prognosis if the injured worker has a history of prior neck pain or prior sick leave (4).

Neck pain that produces severe disability occurs in approximately 5% of all patients with neck pain, the prognostic factors of which are not well defined. Even with severe disability and chronic neck pain, treatments may still be successful. One systematic review of six observational studies and 17 randomized controlled trials showed improvement in symptoms in 46% of patients with pain for 6 months or more (CI: 22%–79%) (7). More frequent long-term disability with acceleration/deceleration injury (previously known as "whiplash"-associated disorder) has been reported, but the factors associated with long-term disability from acceleration/deceleration injury vary from country to country and also are not well defined (8). A report from Saskatchewan indicates that a change to no-fault settlement of cases of whiplash associated disorder in that province had remarkable effects (5). In the 6 months after the legislative change, the incidence of whiplash claims decreased by 28%. The period from injury to settlement of the claim, which had been strongly associated with intensity of pain, level of physical functioning, and degree of depressive symptoms in whiplash patients, decreased by 43%.

DIFFERENTIAL DIAGNOSIS

The majority of neck pain seen in the family physician's office is nonspecific. Nonspecific neck pain is usually caused by the mechanical forces of daily movement, posture, sleep position, or neck tension. Whether aging in itself is a mechanical force is debatable, but the aging process most likely decreases the ability of the neck to withstand mechanical stress. With age, the disks become less resilient to compression and torsion. The disk spaces narrow, osteophytic impingement increases, and the facet (also known as zygapophyseal) joints become arthritic.

The differential diagnosis of neck pain (Table 37.1) includes multiple non-mechanical causes, such as bone pain (from tumor or infection) and pain from other inflammatory processes. Some causes of pain are not well understood. Cailliet (9) has reviewed the anatomic literature and proposed seven sites for mechanical pain in the structures of the lower cervical spine (Fig. 37.1). Irritation of, or injury to, the anterior longitudinal ligament, as occurs with an acute hyperextension injury or an anterior disc bulge, can cause neck pain without any irritation of the cervical nerve roots. The posterior longitudinal ligament similarly has pain receptors, and can be affected by a posteriorly protruding disc. A posterior disk extrusion, however, usually impinges on the nerve roots

TABLE 37.1 Differential Diagnosis for Neck Pain

Mechanical
- Nontraumatic
  - Neck strain
    - Postural
    - Tension
    - Torticollis (acquired)
  - Spondylosis* (degenerative arthritis)
  - Myelopathy*
  - Cervical fracture* (see neoplasm)
- Traumatic
  - Whiplash syndromes*
  - Disc herniation*
  - Cervical fracture*
  - Neck sprain
  - Sports (stinger*)

Non-mechanical
- Rheumatologic/inflammatory
  - Rheumatoid arthritis
  - Ankylosing spondylitis
  - Fibromyalgia
  - Polymyalgia rheumatica
  - Reiter syndrome
  - Psoriatic arthritis
- Neoplastic
  - Osteoblastoma
  - Osteochondroma
  - Giant cell tumor
  - Metastases
  - Hemangioma
  - Multiple myeloma
  - Chondrosarcoma
  - Glioma
  - Syringomyelia
  - Neurofibroma
- Infectious
  - Osteomyelitis
  - Discitis
  - Meningitis
  - Herpes zoster
  - Lyme disease
- Neurologic
  - Peripheral entrapment
  - Brachial plexitis
  - Neuropathies
  - Reflex sympathetic dystrophy
- Referred
  - Thoracic outlet syndrome
  - Pancoast tumor
  - Esophagitis
  - Angina
  - Vascular dissection
  - Carotidynia

Miscellaneous
- Sarcoidosis
- Paget disease

*With or without radiculopathy.

within the spinal canal. The outer annulus of the disc itself is thought to have nociceptive tissue, and this *discogenic* pain radiates to the paraspinous sites in the thoracic spine without dermatomal radiation.

Neurogenic pain, in contrast, is caused when the nerve roots exiting through the cervical foramina are involved. The sensory and motor nerve roots of the spinal cord join just after passing through the intervertebral foramen. Pressure on the nerve root causes paresthesia, hypesthesia (decreased sensation), or hypalgesia (decreased pain sense) but usually not direct pain. Ischemia or mechanical pressure to the capillaries or venules within the dural sheath of the nerve root is now considered the cause. Ischemia affecting the sensory (dorsal) nerve root produces pain in a dermatomal distribution. Stimulation of the motor (ventral) nerve root is thought to produce a deep unpleasant boring sensation in the region of the muscle group innervated by that specific root.

Pain receptors have also been found in the facet joints, spinous ligaments, and neck muscles. Degenerative changes within the cartilage of the facet joints are thought to cause pain, but these changes are usually asymptomatic until trauma has occurred. Injection of local anesthesia into the facet joints produces immediate relief that lasts for the duration of the anesthetic. The method by which mobilization or manipulation of these joints can relieve pain is unclear. The striated extensor and flexor muscles of the neck have pain receptors. Trauma from stretch or compression causes edema and may cause microscopic or even macroscopic hemorrhage. Pain at the myofascial periosteal junction can also cause pain when a muscle forcibly contracts. The mechanism of pain with sustained muscle tension, as in myofascial syndrome, is less well understood. Sustained isometric muscle contractions from stress, poor posture, or sleeping position are thought to occlude arterial flow. These contractions are associated with a buildup of metabolic products, causing further irritation, sustained contraction, and decreased vascular flow. The cycle of ischemia, muscle contraction, metabolic irritants, and further contraction produces pain. Trigger points are hyper-irritable palpable nodules in skeletal muscle and may be local specifically concentrated areas of this cycling phenomenon.

Conceptual Model to Approach Neck Pain

The Task Force on Neck Pain and Associated Disorders has proposed a four-grade classification of neck pain severity to assist clinicians and researchers in treating and studying this widespread problem (10):

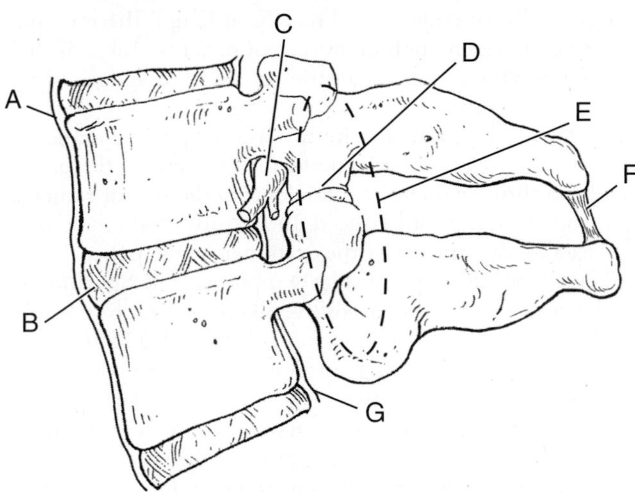

Figure 37.1 • Pain receptor sites of the lower cervical spine.

- Grade I: no signs or symptoms of significant structural abnormalities; minimal interference with normal activities; responds to minimal interventions; requires no diagnostic evaluation.
- Grade II: no signs or symptoms of significant structural problems; significant interference with daily activities; requires urgent attention and treatment to minimize prolonged disability.
- Grade III: no signs of symptoms of significant structural problems; neurologic signs present; may require diagnostic evaluation and more aggressive interventions.
- Grade IV: signs of structural problems; requires immediate diagnostic and treatment interventions.

This grading system has not yet been widely adopted for clinical use but nonetheless can serve as a useful clinical and prognostic guide.

Common Specific Causes of Neck Pain

CERVICAL SPONDYLOSIS

Cervical spondylosis refers to degenerative change in the intervertebral unit of the cervical spine. The term is used synonymously with degenerative disc disease or degenerative spondylosis. It is clear that degenerative changes are normal in the aging process. Autopsy studies report spondylosis in 60% of women and 80% of men by the age of 49. By the age of 79, 95% of both sexes have degenerative changes. These changes include disk space narrowing, osteophytes in the disc margins, and arthritic changes in the facet joints (11).

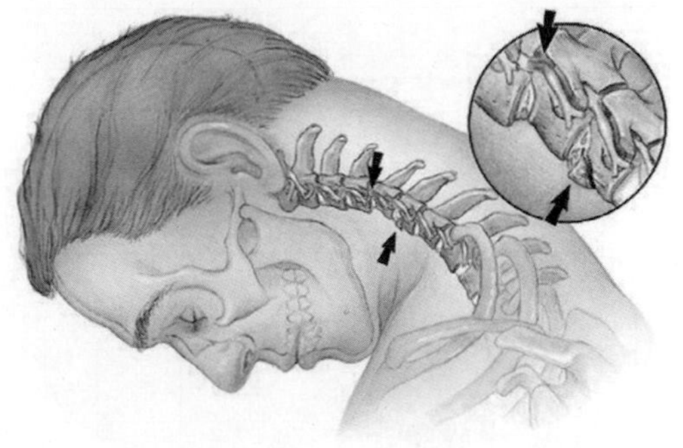

Figure 37.2 • Hyperflexion of the cervical spine.

CERVICAL SPONDYLOTIC MYELOPATHY

Cervical spondylotic (or spondylitic) myelopathy is a condition in which arthritic changes, primarily the development of osteophytes and thickening of the ligamentum flavum, cause direct compression of the spinal cord, resulting in myelopathy. Symptoms develop when the cord has been impinged by 30% or more. Motion can aggravate spinal cord damage by stretching the cord over protruding osteophytes in flexion or by pressure from a thickened bulging ligamentum flavum in extension.

ACCELERATION/DECELERATION INJURY (PREVIOUSLY KNOWN AS WHIPLASH-ASSOCIATED DISORDER)

The term *whiplash* was first coined in 1928 by Dr. Harold Crowe. It is typically defined as an acute injury to the cervical spine resulting from sudden acceleration (hyperextension) and subsequent deceleration (hyperflexion) of the head, often resulting from a rear impact motor vehicle accident (Figs. 37.2 and 37.3). However, any external force that results in a violent hyperextension/flexion stretch or tear in the paracervical muscles can cause the injury. It is estimated that a rear impact injury from a car traveling between 9 and 15 mph can generate a force to the neck of 5 times the gravitational force. A mild hyperextension of the lower cervical segment may cause strain without tear to the muscles of the neck. A more significant stress, however, can injure the anterior longitudinal ligament, the nerve roots, and the disk annulus, and most importantly, can force the facet joints to impact posteriorly on each other (see Fig. 37.3). Diagnostic blocks of the facet joints have confirmed that pain in these joints is the most common cause of chronic neck pain after an acceleration-deceleration injury (12). The symptoms often do not occur until 12 to 24 hours after the injury. The delay in symptoms may be because it takes time for edema to develop after microscopic hemorrhage and injury. Inflamed, edematous muscles will frequently undergo contraction, that is, spasm that results in decreased blood flow and ischemia (as above). There may be subjective or objective evidence of nerve root radiculopathy with whiplash associated disorder: this implies more significant injury. Because, by definition, the radiculopathy occurring in this context is a posttraumatic neurologic deficit, an acceleration-deceleration injury with radiculopathy requires imaging and consideration of referral.

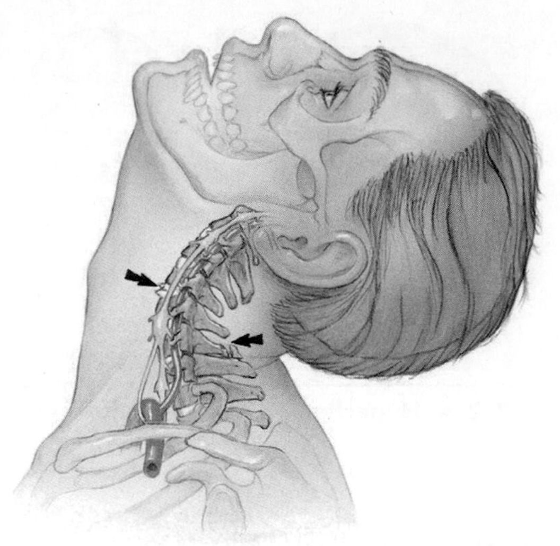

Figure 37.3 • Hyperextension of the cervical spine.

CLINICAL EVALUATION

Although the differential diagnosis of neck pain is broad and includes multiple serious causes, most cases of neck pain seen in the family physician's office are diagnosed using a basic patient-oriented history and physical examination. Learning to differentiate dangerous causes of neck pain by using red flag questions and a few diagnostic maneuvers should allow the examiner to identify those cases of neck pain requiring immediate imaging or referral.

History and Physical Examination

The history establishes the character of the pain (sharp, dull, boring, aching, radiating), location (neck, occiput, arm, upper back), mechanism and timing of onset (spontaneous, traumatic, after sleeping, after working), duration (<3 months = acute; >3 months = chronic), and clinical course (improving or worsening, the presence of aggravating or alleviating symptoms). Associated symptoms should be described. Is there radiation of pain, numbness, tingling, or weakness? Does the patient have functional limitations? Can he drive? Has she dropped things? Functional limitations that give the clinician useful information require questions about the impact of the injury on work, play, and sleep. What treatment measures have worked or failed in the past? And importantly, what psychosocial stresses or mental health problems may be present?

The physical examination should begin with an assessment of the patient's general appearance, posture, stance, and gait. The easiest way to assess the patient's range of motion in the cervical area is to position the patient so that he or she may easily observe the examiner's motions and ask the patient to then repeat the movements as they are performed: flexion, extension, side bending, and rotation. This is fast and simple, and allows for comparison with the examiner's own range of motion. The patient may remain seated for neurologic testing. Motor strength, deep tendon reflexes, sensory changes, and long tract signs of the upper and lower extremities should be checked. Cervical radiculopathy attributable to one nerve root can generally be diagnosed clinically, although there is some variation of presentation in individual patients (Table 37.2).

Three clinical tests can be used to aid the diagnosis of cervical disc herniation:

The Spurling test (also known as the Spurling maneuver or neck compression test) is performed by having the patient side bend (bring ear close to shoulder) to the side of radicular pain and extend his or her head. In a positive test result, pressure exerted downward by the examiner on the patient's head will create or intensify radicular symptoms. The Spurling test has been shown to have a positive likelihood ratio (LR+) of 4.3 and a negative likelihood ratio (LR−) of 0.75 for nerve impingement (13). This suggests it is useful when positive, but not so helpful if it is negative.

In the **axial manual traction test**, the examiner pulls up on the head to momentarily theoretically decrease the pressure on the cervical root. The **arm abduction test** is performed by elevating (full abduction of shoulder) the affected arm over the head of the seated patient. This, too, theoretically decreases the traction on the cervical root. The relief of pain with either test is considered a positive result for cervical root compression. The positive predictive value or likelihood ratios for these two tests are unknown. There is significant overlap between the physical examination of the neck and shoulder. Please see Chapter 38 for a discussion of the shoulder examination. Muscular atrophy of the shoulder, arms, or hands can suggest chronic nerve injury. Unsteady gait, lower extremity weakness, hyperreflexia, and the Lhermitte sign (shooting pain down the back with axial (straight down) head compression suggest cervical myelopathy.

DIAGNOSTIC TESTING

As already noted, many patients will not need blood work or imaging for short-lived neck pain without "red flags" (see the following section). Laboratory studies are indicated when the history and physical examination suggest systemic disease, inflammatory arthritis, or bone damage. Such patients with signs of infection or inflammation should have an erythrocyte sedimentation rate, complete blood count, and calcium/phosphate and other metabolic studies.

Most non-traumatic cervical problems (including prolapsed intervertebral disk) will improve within 4 weeks. Therefore, expensive tests (particularly imaging modalities) have little utility in the initial evaluation phase unless surgery is being considered. If there is no neurologic deficit, electrodiagnostic tests are not indicated because their main use is to assess neurologic function. If neurologic deficit is present, and a reasonable trial of non-surgical therapy has not been successful, specific anatomic testing in the form of imaging (computed tomography [CT] or magnetic resonance imaging [MRI]) are indicated, again especially if surgery is being considered. A reasonable trial of non-surgical therapy should be based on the patient's pain and functional limitations. Any discussion of surgery should be individualized to the patient, and it is important that the patient be fully informed of the poor evidence for long-term pain relief with surgery.

Table 37.3 lists red flags in the history and physical examination of neck pain. If red flags are present or if there is clinical deterioration, uncontrolled pain, progressive disability, or continual weakness for more than 4 weeks, the physician

TABLE 37.2 Clinical Findings of Neck Pain with Radiculopathy

Nerve Root	Level	Motor Weakness (Follows Myotomal Pattern)	Sensory Loss (Follows Dermatomal Pattern)	Paresthesia	Referred Pain	Reflex Loss	Subjective Pain
C5	C4/5	Deltoid, shoulder, biceps	Lateral upper arm	None in digits	Shoulder and upper lateral arm	Biceps	Shoulder (but relatively pain free)
C6	C5/6	Biceps, brachioradialis	Thumb and forearm proximal to thumb	Thumb	Radial aspect of forearm	Brachioradialis and biceps	Deltoid, rhomboid muscle areas
C7	C6/7	Triceps	Middle ring finger	Middle finger	Dorsal aspect of forearm	Triceps	Dorsolateral upper arm, superomedial angle of scapula
C8	C7/T1	Finger intrinsic	Inner forearm, little finger	Ring and little finger	Ulnar aspect of forearm and little finger	Triceps or none	Scapula, ulnar side of upper arm

The numbered cervical root passes through the foramen above the numbered cervical vertebra (e.g., the C6 spinal nerve exits in the foramen between the C5 and C6 vertebrae).

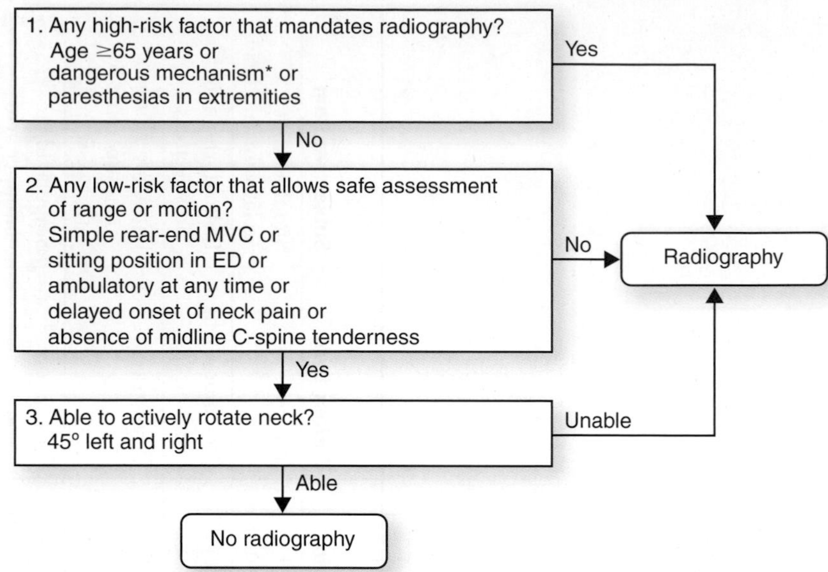

Figure 37.4 • The Canadian C-Spine rule. *A dangerous mechanism is considered to be a fall from an elevation of ≥3 feet or 5 stairs; an axial load to the head (e.g., diving); a motor vehicle collision at high speed (>100 km/hour) or with rollover or ejection; a collision involving a motorized recreational vehicle or a bicycle collision.

should consider further evaluation. Patients who are older, younger, or frail may deserve an evaluation sooner.

Radiographs are useful for detecting bony metastases, Paget disease, myeloma, and ankylosing spondylitis. A large prospective cohort trial compared two decision rules used to guide the ordering of cervical spine x-rays in patients with trauma (14). The Canadian C-Spine Rule (Fig. 37.4) was shown to be more sensitive and specific (99.4%, 45.1% respectively, with LR+ = 1.8 and LR− = .55). The rule was evaluated in emergency rooms, not the outpatient setting, so should be used with caution in primary care settings. Radiographs of the neck should include anteroposterior, lateral, and oblique views to show the foramina of the vertebrae. If occult fracture is ruled out, it may also be useful to request views in flexion and extension to show whether there is any spondylolisthesis (anterior shifting of one vertebral body onto the other) or instability. However, the significance of spondylolisthesis without neurologic signs or symptoms is unclear. CT and MRI are much more useful but are more costly tools in diagnosing nerve root compression, disc disease, and other soft-tissue pathology in the neck. MRI may be the study of choice in evaluating disc prolapse, but as in the lumbar spine, clinically insignificant abnormalities are not infrequently detected on imaging and therefore the role of imaging is to *confirm* a clinical diagnosis rather than to *make a diagnosis*. For example, in patients without neck complaints, MRIs show disk degeneration in 17% of all disks imaged. This finding occurred in at least one disk in 12% of women in their 20s, and in more than 80% of men and women older than age 60! Approximately 8% of pain-free subjects (most older than age 50) had posterior disc protrusion and evidence of foraminal stenosis (15).

TABLE 37.3 Red Flags for Patients with Neck Pain

Bowel/bladder or sexual dysfunction: Consider cervical myelopathy.
Unexplained fever/symptoms of infection: Consider infection related to recent previous neck surgery, immunosuppressed patient, intravenous drug use, or prolonged corticosteroid use.
Unexplained weight loss: Consider malignancy/metastatic lesions.
Psychosocial red flags: Non-physiologic pain distribution, non-organic physical signs, repetitive neck injuries, multiple failed treatments, litigation and/or disability claims, apparent secondary pain, substance abuse, depression or other psychiatric diagnosis.

MANAGEMENT

Initial Management

There is either unclear or conflicting evidence to support many of the commonly used therapies for uncomplicated neck pain (16–20). There is insufficient evidence of the effects of most treatments; heat or cold, traction, biofeedback, spray and stretch, acupuncture, and laser, to substantiate their effectiveness in patients with uncomplicated neck pain. Table 37.4 provides a long list of unproven treatments evaluated by systematic reviews (16). However, evidence of harm caused by these therapies is also clearly lacking. The critically thinking physician may therefore continue to prescribe these treatments while still acknowledging the lack of evidence of their efficacy.

A flow sheet outlining the management of neck pain is presented in Figure 37.5. This recommended management plan is based on a consensus guideline originally produced by the

TABLE 37.4 Treatments for Neck Pain of Unknown or Unconfirmed Effectiveness

Mechanical neck pain
Acupuncture
Biofeedback
Pharmacotherapy—nonsteroidal anti-inflammatory drugs, muscle relaxants, antidepressants
Heat or cold
Patient education
Pulsed electromagnetic field treatment (PEFT)
Soft collars or special pillows
Spray and stretch
Traction
Transcutaneous electrical nerve stimulation (TENS)
Acute flexion-extension injury
Pharmacotherapy
Exercise
Multimodal treatment
PEFT
Chronic flexion-extension injury
Multimodal treatment
Percutaneous radiofrequency neurotomy
Physical treatments
Neck pain with radiculopathy
Pharmacotherapy
Surgery versus conservative treatment

Florida Agency for Health Care Policy but no longer accessible (21). A list of evidence based treatment options is included in Table 37.5. In patients who are without red flag symptoms or physical findings, it is reasonable to continue symptomatic therapies for up to 4 weeks before further evaluation. If at that point cervical radiographs are negative or show only spondylosis, it is reasonable to continue nonoperative therapies for up to 8 weeks.

Strengthening exercises may continue to be helpful in chronic mechanical neck pain. Any course of physical therapy should include strengthening exercise as opposed to mobilization or stretching only.

Although the evidence based options for the practitioner are slim, our patients will continue to need our best advice. In the absence of contra-indications, certain non-operative therapies are reasonable to recommend. They include: (i) continuation of usual activity; (ii) physical therapy that includes strengthening exercises; (iii) analgesics (nonsteroidal anti-inflammatory drugs [NSAIDs] or acetaminophen) and/or topical analgesic medication (see Table 34.5); and (iv) exercise, combined with manipulation or mobilization. Muscle relaxants or short term use of opiates for severe pain may be prescribed in individual patients. In addition, very high-dose intravenous glucocorticoid (methylprednisolone) treatment has been shown to reduce pain (at 1 week) and sick days from whiplash-associated disorders if initiated within 8 hours of the injury (17).

The rationale for using NSAIDs for neck pain is based on the evidence that they are somewhat effective in treatment of low back pain and osteoarthritis of the knee and hip. NSAID medications, however, have not been shown to be of benefit compared to acetaminophen in neck pain in a systematic review. There were no high-quality studies that compared a NSAID to placebo in neck pain. Indeed, there is scant information on the effectiveness of any drug therapy for neck pain (20).

Manipulation of the cervical spine remains a controversial issue. Both clinicians who have been trained in manipulation and many patients attest to its value, but the evidence to support manipulation is inconclusive. The latest systematic review reports no significant difference between mobilization (supported range of motion) and manipulation (high- or low-velocity thrust movement through a limited range of motion), when compared to placebo or to each other. However there is good evidence from two systematic reviews that mobilization or manipulation *plus* exercise had significant benefit for patients with chronic mechanical neck pain (18,19).

The risks of manipulation may have been over-stated in the past. Serious adverse outcomes, including vertebral artery dissection, vertebrobasilar stroke, disc herniation, and even death, have been reported as a result of cervical manipulation, but these events are extremely rare. Prospective trials have never been done, but retrospective studies have suggested that the rate of stroke after cervical manipulation is from one in 400,000 to 1 in 2 million (22). One recent case control study suggests that the risk of vertebrobasilar stroke may increase as much as 6 times with chiropractic manipulation (23). However, that study may be flawed by the age of the patients' studied and recall bias. Still, the risk of harm caused by any intervention deserves attention and perhaps a discussion of risk with the patient is warranted by all who recommend cervical manipulation.

In chronic (usually defined as 3 months or more) mechanical neck pain more aggressive physical modalities have shown limited benefit. Two recent Cochrane reviews of electrotherapy for neck pain found poor-quality studies and could only conclude that pulsed electromagnetic field therapy (PEFT), repetitive magnetic stimulation, and transcutaneous electrical nerve stimulation (TENS) are more effective than placebo, but not more effective than other interventions (24,25). One small trial has shown botulinum toxin A (Botox) injections to be beneficial in patients with chronic whiplash-associated disorders (26).

NECK PAIN WITH RADICULOPATHY

Again, there is little credible evidence to support one best course of treatment for neck pain with radiculopathy. The only systematic review of this topic (which dealt with whiplash-associated disorders) could reach no conclusions (27). One non-blinded randomized trial (28) of patients with more than 3 months of radicular pain compared surgery with physical therapy or immobilization in a collar. The long-term result was no difference in pain, although the surgery group had a greater short-term reduction in pain, and a large proportion of patients in all groups eventually had surgery. Immobilization in a neck collar is no longer recommended as treatment for any causes of neck pain.

One very real problem in the study of the treatment of radicular symptoms is that the natural history of symptomatic radiculopathy is not known. The belief that untreated patients

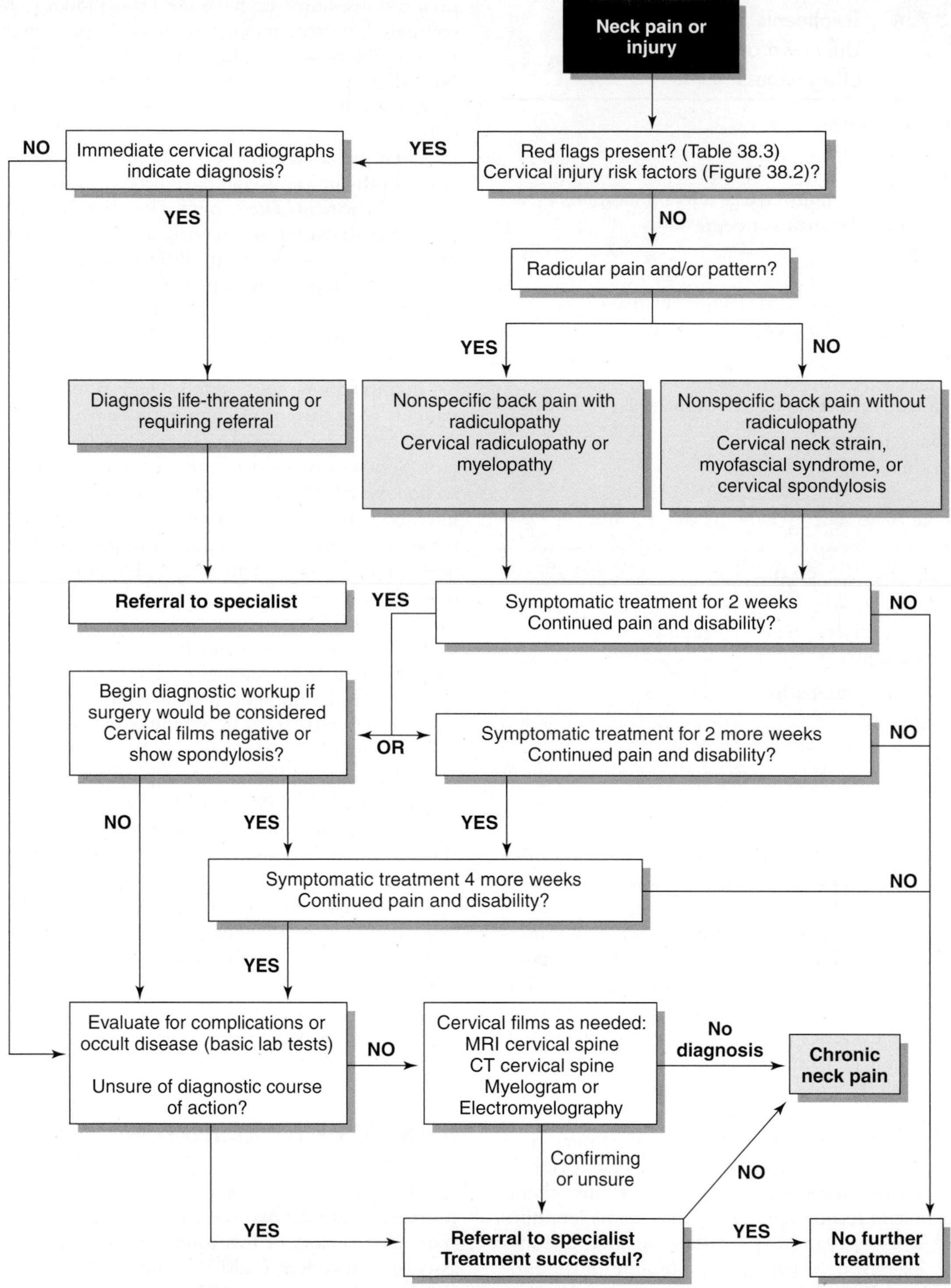

Figure 37.5 • General approach to the patient with neck pain.

will develop progressive disability is not supported by reliable evidence (27). The reported death rates from surgical procedures are 0% to 1.8%, and the rate of non-fatal complications is reported as 1% to 8% (29). Therefore, there are no clear indications for which patients with neck pain and radiculopathy should be referred for surgery and the choice of surgical procedure has not been established by appropriately designed studies (30).

CERVICAL SPONDYLOTIC MYELOPATHY

Although the course of cervical spondylotic myelopathy is variable, the conventional wisdom is that once frank myelopathy occurs, surgical intervention becomes necessary. The primary goal of surgery is to decompress the spinal cord, providing more room to the neural structures.

TABLE 37.5 Therapeutic Options for Management of Neck Pain

Condition and Treatment	Strength of Recommendation*	Amount of Benefit
Mechanical (nonspecific) neck pain—chronic		
Exercise—stretching and strengthening	B	Moderate to strong
Intramuscular injection of lidocaine versus placebo	B	Moderate
Manipulation or mobilization—plus exercise	A	Strong
Radiofrequency denervation/neurotomy	C	Limited
Mechanical (nonspecific) neck pain—acute		
Manipulation or mobilization alone	C	Limited
Mechanical (nonspecific) neck pain with headache—chronic		
Exercise—stretching and strengthening	B	Moderate
Manipulation or mobilization—plus exercise	A	Strong
Mechanical (nonspecific) neck pain with or without headache—chronic		
Multimodal care with mobilization or manipulation (chronic and subacute)	A	Moderate
Neck pain—chronic, with radiculopathy		
Epidural injection of methylprednisolone and lidocaine	C	Limited
Acute acceleration/deceleration injury (whiplash-associated disorder)		
Mobilization/usual activities	B	Limited
Intravenous methylprednisolone	B	Short term
Chronic neck pain from acceleration/deceleration injury (whiplash-associated disorder)		
Botulinum toxin A	C	Moderate

*A = consistent, good-quality patient-oriented evidence; B = inconsistent or limited-quality patient-oriented evidence; C = consensus, disease-oriented evidence, usual practice, expert opinion, or case series.
For information about the SORT evidence rating system, see *www.aafp.org/afpsort.xml*.

ACCELERATION/DECELERATION INJURY (WHIPLASH-ASSOCIATED DISORDER)

Early mobilization and early return to normal activities compared with immobilization is likely to be beneficial in acute whiplash-associated disorder patients, but the latest systematic reviews are actually less enthusiastic about the "rest makes rusty" concept (27,31,32). Only one trial compared an act-as-usual group (given advice plus NSAIDs) with an immobilization group (given advice, NSAIDs, and 14 days of sick leave) (33). The act-as-usual group had more improvement in pain during daily activities, neck stiffness, memory, concentration, and headache, but no significant differences in neck range of motion, total amount of sick leave, or resolution of their symptoms at 6 months.

One randomized double-blinded study (34) of percutaneous neurotomy has been performed in 24 patients with facet joint pain confirmed by diagnostic anesthetic block. The cause of this pain was described as a motor vehicle accident (although not all were classic whiplash), and this chronic pain had been uncontrolled by conventional therapy. The measured outcome of this study was the number of days it took for the pain to return to pre-operative (pre-neurotomy) level. By 27 weeks, 58% remained pain free in the treatment group, compared with only 8% in the control group ($p = 0.009$, ARR 50% to 95%, CI 3%–85%; NNT = 2, CI 1–29). Five patients in the treatment group had numbness or dysesthesias in the cutaneous area of the therapy, but none rated these changes as significant. The therapeutic effect of facet joint injection in the cervical spine has been shown to have short-term positive result for chronic whiplash-associated pain (28).

Sports-related Neck Injury

Management of neck injuries in athletes who play collision sports is similar to those in the general population with a few exceptions. The potential for re-injury is significantly higher for the injured athlete when she returns to her sport than in the general workforce. A discussion of catastrophic collision sport injuries is beyond the scope and purpose of this chapter. The content of this discussion is also directed to the typical outpatient management of neck pain separate from the acute sideline or event evaluation.

Management focuses on restoring normal, nearly pain-free range of motion with near normal strength. Once serious fractures of the cervical spine have been ruled out (clinically and radiographically), radiographic evaluation of the neck should include lateral flexion and extension radiographs to evaluate for ligamentous instability. Instability of the cervical spine is defined as >3.4 mm of anteroposterior displacement of one vertebral body compared with a subjacent vertebral body or >11 degrees of angulation (35) Angulation is determined by the angle formed by drawing a line from the bases of two adjacent vertebral bodies. Instability of the cervical spine is a contraindication to participation in collision sports.

Return to practice and play is dependent upon the athlete demonstrating normal strength accompanied by normal and pain-free range of motion and a readiness to return. The patient should be asymptomatic and have no x-ray or MRI changes, full range of motion, negative Spurling and axial compression tests (36). If the athlete is tentative about returning to play, the athlete should be held until he or she is confident about recovery from the injury.

A transient neurapraxia, (a "stinger" or "burner") is another form of neck injury unique to collision sports. The "stinger" is where the athlete complains of burning or tingling in an upper extremity after a collision. The distribution is usually in the upper arm or entire arm. Peri-scapular pain may also occur. Motor symptoms are less commonly present. The nerve roots most commonly affected are C5 or C6. The injury has been described as a traction injury to the brachial plexus or compression injury to the dorsal nerve root ganglion as it exits the neural foramen. Current research suggests compression as a result of neck extension and lateral bending is the more common cause (37). Symptoms associated with stingers last from minutes to hours. Usual return-to-play guidelines recommend the athlete have full, pain free range of motion and symmetric strength with the uninjured side. With resolution of the symptoms in this usual pattern, no radiographic evaluation is necessary. Special circumstances when this scenario does not apply include recurrent stingers (several a game or season) or persistent motor or sensory symptoms (37). Most of the athletes with recurrent stingers have cervical osteoarthritis with foraminal stenosis or cervical stenosis (narrowed cervical canal). These athletes require radiographs including flexion/extension views and MRI. The clinical picture of injury and recovery with the aid of imaging is necessary for proper counseling regarding return to play or withdrawing from future participation in collision sports. Bilateral symptoms of any kind suggest spinal cord involvement and must be managed with appropriate caution.

Long-term Management of Neck Pain

The long-term management of a patient with neck pain must include the support of an experienced specialist. A physiatrist (a specialist in physical medicine) can help determine the patient's degree of disability. Physiatrists emphasize rehabilitation and pain control, which can be extremely helpful to the patient (and to the referring physician). Electromyography continues to be the best test to use when considering nerve damage or impairment, and this test is performed by physiatrists and neurologists in most communities. A neurosurgical consultation for surgical options is warranted in most patients. Chapter 41 addresses management of chronic pain and reviews management modalities and options in chronic regional pain syndromes that will apply to neck pain. Attention to the role of stress and psychosocial factors is important to address.

PREVENTION

The accumulated evidence on prevention of neck pain is of poor quality. One systematic review that looked at prevention of neck or back pain found that exercise, but not "neck school" (provided by physical therapists) was an effective strategy to prevent acute episodes of neck pain (38). The role of exercise in preventing recurrent neck pain is unknown. As noted, certain occupations and sports are higher risk for neck injury and may be relatively contraindicated in certain patients.

KEY POINTS

- History and physical examination are important in assessing patients with acute neck pain.
- Many patients with neck pain without red flags do not need imaging and will improve with supportive treatments.
- There is little evidence to support the need for surgical treatment of acute neck pain.
- Many of the presently available treatments for neck pain are not evidence-based.

CHAPTER

38

Shoulder Problems

J. Herbert Stevenson

CLINICAL OBJECTIVES

1. List the most common shoulder problems and their relation to age, gender, and activity.
2. Describe the underlying anatomy and pathophysiology of rotator cuff disorders, adhesive capsulitis, shoulder osteoarthritis, and shoulder instability disorders.
3. Discuss an evidence-based evaluation for rotator cuff disorders, adhesive capsulitis, shoulder osteoarthritis, and shoulder instability disorders.
4. Apply the most up-to-date treatment recommendations for common shoulder problems with an emphasis on nonsurgical treatment options available to the family medicine provider.

Shoulder pain is defined as pain that is localized to the shoulder joint. It can have a primary (shoulder joint) or secondary (referred or systemic) etiology. Shoulder pain is responsible for approximately 16% of all musculoskeletal complaints (1) and has a yearly incidence of 15 new episodes per 1,000 patients seen in the primary care setting (2); an estimated 20% of the population will suffer an episode of shoulder pain during their lifetime (3). Shoulder pain is second only to low back pain in patients seeking care for musculoskeletal ailments in the primary care setting (4). Peak incidence of shoulder pain occurs during the fourth through sixth decades but can affect all patients, young and old, particularly athletes (2,5–7).

Assessing shoulder pain and determining the underlying etiology can be a challenge to the medical provider. A large component of the challenge is the numerous shoulder disorders that may present with similar shoulder pain characteristics. Furthermore, after a diagnosis is made, the primary care provider is faced with the challenge of what methods you should utilize in the treatment and how best to optimize nonsurgical treatment options in the care of the patient.

This chapter will review the four most common problems of primary shoulder pain that constitute more than 90% of primary shoulder pain seen in the ambulatory setting (2,8). These include: rotator cuff disorders (tendinopathy, partial tears, and complete tears), adhesive capsulitis, osteoarthritis (glenohumeral and acromioclavicular), as well as shoulder instability (subluxation, dislocation).

DIFFERENTIAL DIAGNOSIS

Shoulder pain can arise from multiple and, at times, overlapping etiologies. A sound understanding of the underlying anatomy is essential to understand the different conditions, pathophysiology, and potential treatment options for shoulder problems. Figure 38.1 highlights key parts of the shoulder joint anatomy.

The bony anatomy of the shoulder is composed of: the humerus, the clavicle and the scapula, which is further divided into the acromion, the coronoid, and the glenoid. The shoulder joint complex has four different articulations: the sternoclavicular, acromioclavicular (AC), glenohumeral, and scapulothoracic joints. The majority of osteoarthritis of the shoulder occurs at the acromioclavicular joint, particularly with repetitive overhead activities or a history of heavy weight lifting. Osteoarthritis of the glenohumeral joint is much more rare and generally occurs with a history of distant trauma/dislocation or a history of auto-immune arthritis involving the shoulder joint. Both conditions involve the degeneration of articular cartilage at the joint with associated synovitis, effusion, and osteophyte formation; all classic elements of osteoarthritis.

The soft-tissue support is essential for the stability of the shoulder and can be divided into static and dynamic stabilizers. The static stabilizers include: the bony support, joint capsule, glenohumeral ligaments, and glenoid labrum. The dynamic stabilizers include the rotator cuff muscles (supraspinatus, infraspinatus, teres minor, and subscapularis) along with the long head of the biceps tendon. The primary role of the dynamic stabilizers is to maintain the humeral head centered within the glenoid of the scapula during shoulder movement. When there is a disruption of the static and/or weakness of the dynamic stabilizers, athletes are at risk of sustaining a shoulder subluxation (transient dislocation) or frank dislocation. The combination of the tremendous range of motion at the shoulder joint, combined with overall ligamentous and joint capsule laxity found commonly in young athletes, makes the joint particularly susceptible to subluxation or dislocation. The majority of subluxation or dislocation occurs anteriorly due to a fall with the arm in an abducted and externally rotated position.

The labrum, although a small structure, deepens the glenoid surface area by approximately 50% (9). An acute shoulder subluxation or dislocation can result in an injury to the labrum and can be a chief reason for chronic recurrent instability or dislocations.

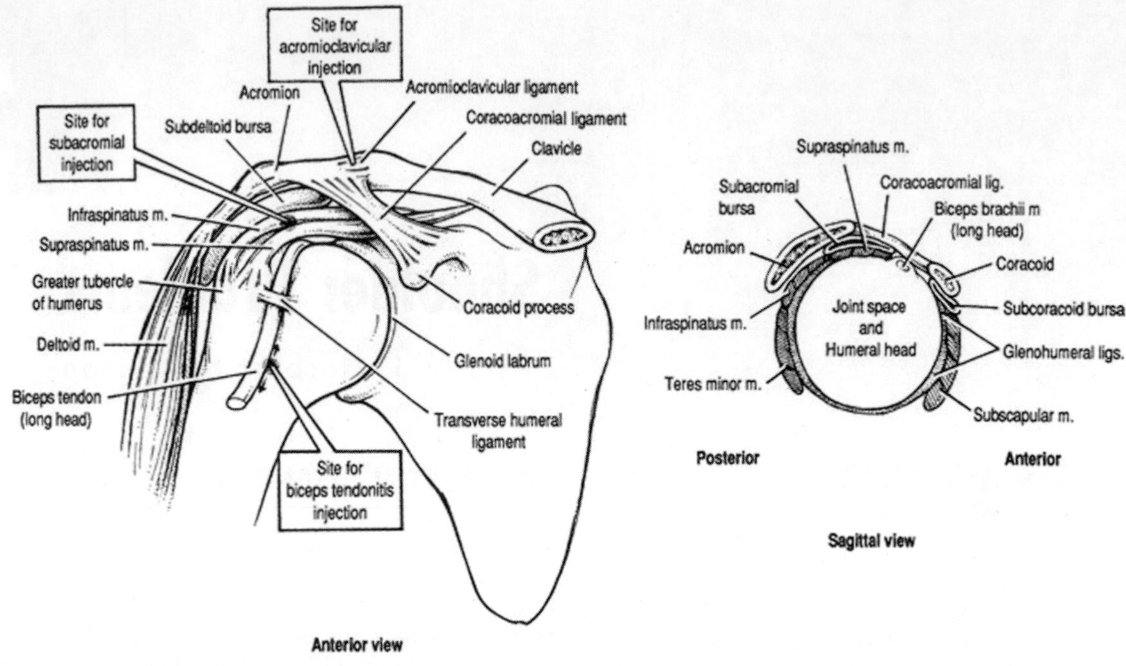

Figure 38.1 • Anatomy of the shoulder joint.

TABLE 38.1 Differential Diagnosis of the Patient with Shoulder Pain

Diagnosis	**Typical Features**	**Frequency in Family Medicine Clinic**
Rotator cuff disorders (tendinopathy, partial tears, complete tears)	• Often associated with repetitive overhead shoulder activities • Partial tears most common at older than age 40 years (10) • Complete tears most common at older than age 60 years (10) • Pain localized to the deltoid region • Pain worse with overhead activities and at night (11) • Pain and or weakness of the rotator cuff muscles on manual testing • Positive impingement tests	Very common
Adhesive capsulitis	• Pain with progressive loss of both active *and* passive range of motion • Associated with diabetes, females, and middle decades of life (40–60 years)	Common
Shoulder joint arthritis	Acromioclavicular joint arthritis: • All ages with history of repetitive overhead lifting or heavy weight training • Pain localized to superior aspect of shoulder (acromioclavicular joint) • Pain worse at night and with cross body movements • Tenderness at acromioclavicular joint on exam as well as with cross body adduction testing	Acromioclavicular joint arthritis: common
	Glenohumeral joint arthritis: • Most common over age of 60 years • History of trauma, rheumatologic disease • Deep, diffuse pain localized to shoulder region • Loss of passive range of motion in more advanced cases, can be confused for adhesive capsulitis	Glenohumeral arthritis: rare
Shoulder instability	• Most common in young patients and athletes • Often prior history of acute shoulder injury or fall with frank dislocation or sensation of "pop" or "shift" in the shoulder • Dislocation/subluxation most commonly occurs with arm in an abducted and externally rotated position • Positive apprehension test	Common, particularly young patients and athletes

TABLE 38.2 Key Elements in the History for Common Shoulder Disorders

History	Associated Condition
Age	<40 years: Instability (subluxation/dislocation), rotator cuff tendinopathy >40 years: rotator cuff tears, adhesive capsulitis, glenohumeral osteoarthritis (10,19,49)
Gender	Females higher risk for adhesive capsulitis
Pain location	Anterosuperior shoulder pain associated with acromioclavicular joint osteoarthritis Diffuse lateral/deltoid shoulder pain associated with rotator cuff disorders, adhesive capsulitis, glenohumeral osteoarthritis
Mechanism: history of repetitive overuse	Rotator cuff disease, acromioclavicular and glenohumeral arthritis
Mechanism: history of trauma	Younger than 40 years: shoulder dislocation/subluxation Older than 40 years: rotator cuff tear
Pain with overhead activity	Rotator cuff disorders
Limited passive range of motion	Adhesive capsulitis, glenohumeral osteoarthritis
Weakness	Rotator cuff disorders, glenohumeral osteoarthritis
Night pain	Rotator cuff disorders, adhesive capsulitis (11)
Numbness, tingling, radiating pain past elbow	Cervical spine radiculopathy
Diabetes or thyroid disorders	Adhesive capsulitis (50,51)
Occupation	Occupations requiring repetitive overhead activities: associated with rotator cuff disorders
Sports participation	Collision sports associated with shoulder instability (subluxation/dislocation) Weight lifting associated with acromioclavicular osteoarthritis (52)

*Adapted from Burbank K, Stevenson JH, et al. Chronic shoulder pain: Part I. Evaluation and diagnosis. *Am Family Phys* 2008;77(4):1–8.

The joint capsule plays a crucial role in adhesive capsulitis. The underlying mechanism of this condition is still being elucidated but involves the progressive fibrosis of the joint capsule, which results in a painful loss of shoulder range of motion. As the condition progresses through its stages, there is a gradual reduction in pain followed by eventual return of near normal range of motion.

The pathophysiology of rotator cuff disorders is often from repetitive overhead activity that causes recurrent impingement of the rotator cuff between the humerus and acromion. This is known as impingement syndrome (10). Rotator cuff injury can progress over time from tendinopathy (inflammatory changes in the tendon, also known as tendonitis or, more correctly, degeneration of the tendon known as tendinosis) to a partial tear followed by a complete tear of a rotator cuff tendon. There can be subacromial bursitis accompanying any of these stages, but bursitis is thought to occur secondarily to a primary rotator cuff injury. Throwing athletes, particularly those with microinstability, may present with rotator cuff tears on the undersurface of the supraspinatus and infraspinatus. These tears tend to present at a younger age and are felt to be due to the unique strain and torque on the shoulder from repetitive overhead throwing.

The differential diagnosis of shoulder pain is listed in Table 38.1.

CLINICAL EVALUATION

History-taking

A thorough history and examination are essential in making an accurate diagnosis for shoulder pain. Key parts of the history include demographic information: age, gender, occupation, and activity level. Location of the pain, associated symptoms, aggravating factors, as well as the mechanism of an injury are important components of the history to help you narrow the differential diagnosis. Table 38.2 highlights common historical findings and their associated conditions.

Red flags in the history are outlined in Table 38.3. Any history of trauma is also a red flag as fractures may present with shoulder pain and weakness similar to rotator cuff injury or shoulder subluxation/dislocation.

Physical Examination

The physical exam of the shoulder should proceed in a rational and orderly fashion to maintain consistency and develop an understanding of normal and abnormal findings. Challenges of the physical exam include the large number of exam maneuvers, relatively poor predictability of individual maneuvers, and the effect of pain on the ability to assess key findings such as strength and range of motion (ROM). Table 38.4 highlights

TABLE 38.3 Red Flags for Patients with Shoulder Pain Indicating More Serious Disease

Red Flags	Associated Conditions
Fever, chills, redness of joint, intravenous drug use, immune deficiency	Glenohumeral joint infection
Anorexia, Weight Loss	Malignancy (primary or metastatic)
Persistent shoulder pain in children <8 or in elderly without history of trauma or overuse	Malignancy, especially sarcoma in elderly (rare)
Profound shoulder weakness	Massive rotator cuff tear
Fall or trauma	Fracture or large rotator cuff tear (particularly in elderly)
Multiple joint involvement with effusion	Auto-immune etiology
Numbness, tingling or radiation of pain past elbow	Cervical etiology
Muscle atrophy	Peripheral nerve injury

TABLE 38.4 Diagnostic Accuracy of Selected Exam Findings and Tests of the Shoulder

Exam Maneuver	Associated Condition	Strength of Recommendation	Sensitivity (%)	Specificity (%)	LR(+)	LR(−)
AC tenderness	AC joint OA or chronic sprain	B (53)	96	10	1.07	0.4
Cross-body adduction	AC joint OA or chronic sprain	B (54)	77	79	3.50	0.29
Supraspinatus or infraspinatus weakness	Chronic rotator cuff tear	B (11)	56	73	2.07	0.60
Restricted active ROM	Rotator cuff disorder	B (11)	30	78	1.36	0.90
Restricted passive ROM	Adhesive capsulitis glenohumeral arthritis	C	NA	NA	NA	NA
Empty can supraspinatus test	Rotator cuff disorder involving supraspinatus	A (55)	44	90	4.4	0.62
External rotation/ infraspinatus strength test	Rotator cuff disorder involving infraspinatus	A (55)	42	90	4.2	0.64
Lift-off test of subscapularis	Rotator cuff disorder involving subscapularis	A (15)	62	100	>25	0.38
Hawkins impingement test	Impingement/ rotator cuff disorder	A (55)	72	66	2.1	0.42
Drop arm test	Large rotator cuff tear	A (55)	27	88	2.25	0.83
Apprehension test	Shoulder instability	A (56)	72	96	20.22	0.29

AC = acromioclavicular; NA = not available; OA = osteoarthritis; ROM = range of motion.
Strength of Recommendation A: very useful; B: moderately useful; C: of limited use.
*Adapted from Burbank K, Stevenson JH, et al. Chronic shoulder pain: Part I. Evaluation and diagnosis. *Am Family Phys* 2008;77(4):1–8.

key parts of the shoulder exam along with sensitivity, specificity, and likelihood ratios.

INSPECTION

The exam should commence with an inspection of the shoulder from anterior, lateral, and posterior perspectives. Observance of asymmetric atrophy or wasting of the suprascapular or infrascapular fossa may indicate a chronic rotator tear (11). Prominence of the AC joint may indicate arthritis or history of AC joint sprain.

PALPATION

Palpation of the AC joint for tenderness may be a sign of AC joint arthritis or acute sprain depending on the mechanism. Palpation overlying the subacromial bursa may reveal tenderness suggesting bursitis while palpation along the long head of the biceps will likely be tender in bicipital tenosynovitis.

RANGE OF MOTION

Range of motion (ROM) should be evaluated in flexion, abduction, internal rotation, and external rotation. If patient has full active range of motion then passive ROM need not be assessed. If, however, active ROM is impaired, it is critical to test passive (examiner, and not the patient, moves joint through various motions). Loss of active and passive ROM is the hallmark of adhesive capsulitis but can also be found with osteoarthritis of the glenohumeral joint. Loss of active ROM alone is often found with rotator cuff pathology. Pain with active ROM between 60 and 120 degrees is known as the "painful arc" and is associated with rotator cuff disease (12). The scapula can be held fixed as the patient abducts their arm, which prevents scapulothoracic movement and instead isolates movement to the glenohumeral joint.

MUSCLE STRENGTH TESTING

Strength testing isolates the individual muscles of the rotator cuff: abduction (supraspinatus), internal rotation (subscapularis), and external rotation (infraspinatus/teres minor). These maneuvers are best performed with the patient seated. Abduction strength should be tested with the arm abducted to 90 degrees and an inferiorly displaced force exerted by the examiner at the wrist. Internal and external rotation strength testing can be performed with the arms at the side and elbows flexed to 90 degrees. The patient will then exert external rotation followed by internal rotation against resistance. The examiner can manually test these motions by resisting at the patients wrist. Pain and weakness should be noted, as they are often associated with injury to the rotator cuff.

ADDITIONAL EXAM MANEUVERS

Special tests of the shoulder include impingement tests, AC joint tests, and tests of shoulder instability.

Impingement Tests

The underlying purpose with tests of impingement is, by certain movements, to trap the rotator cuff tendons (often supraspinatus) between the bony head of the humerus and the undersurface of the acromion. The Hawkins' impingement test is used to diagnose impingement of the rotator cuff: a positive result is when pain results reflecting rotator cuff injury (13). The test is performed by the examiner passively forward flexing the patient's arm to 90 degrees followed by passively internally rotating the arm to its end point (approximately 90 degrees). This is shown in Figure 38.2.

Rotator Cuff Tests

The "empty can test" isolates the supraspinatus more effectively than abduction and a painful result is often associated with rotator cuff disease (14). The empty can test is performed

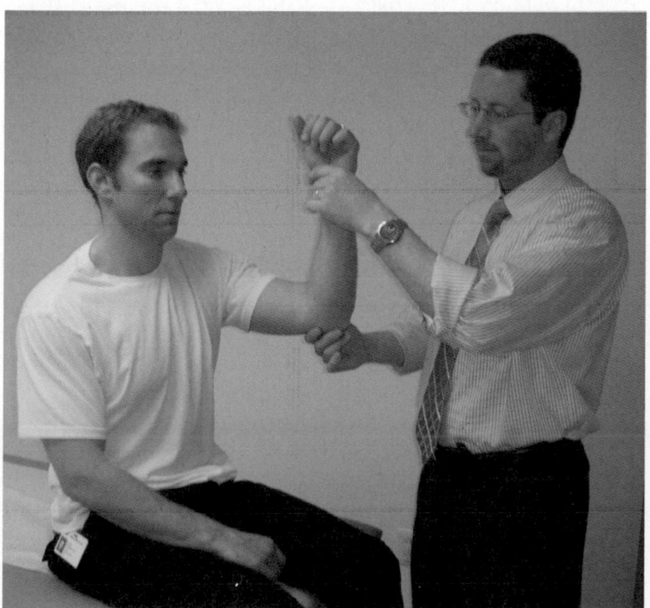

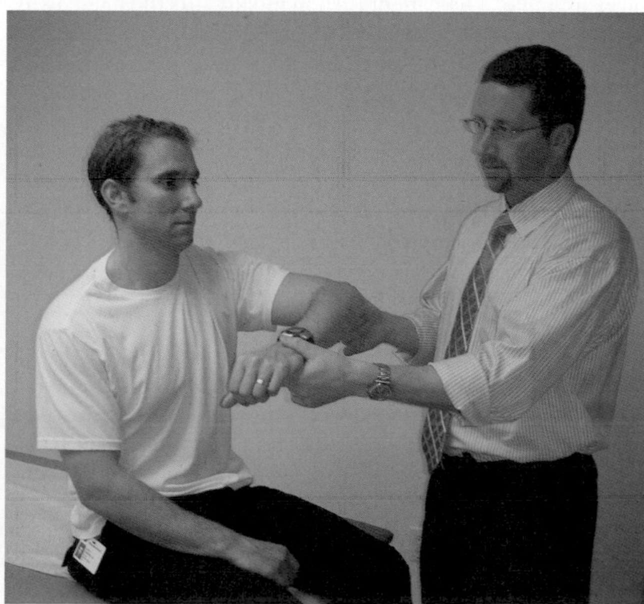

Figure 38.2 • The Hawkins' impingement test.

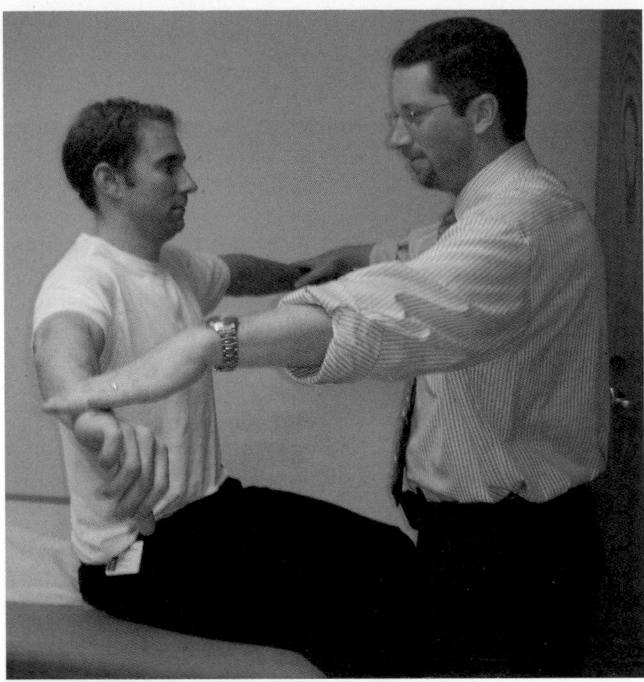

Figure 38.3 • The "empty can test".

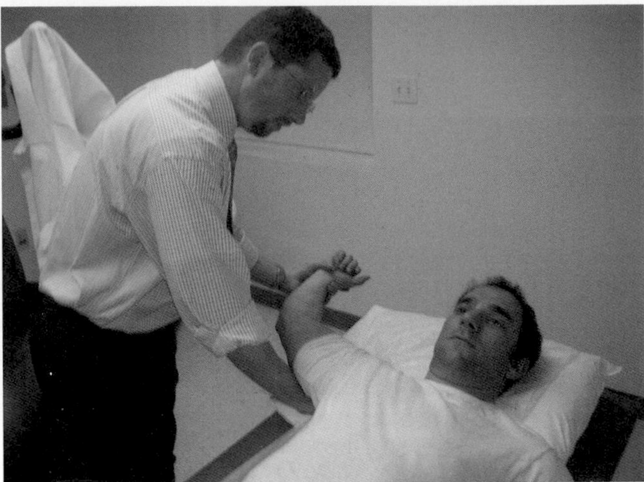

Figure 38.4 • The apprehension test.

by having the patient abduct their arm to 90 degrees, followed by forward flexing the arm 30 degrees to lie in the plane of the scapula. The patient is then instructed to "empty the imaginary can" he or she is holding with an internal rotatory movement. The examiner then places a downward force at the wrist, which the patient should resist. Pain and or weakness may signify a rotator cuff injury, particularly the supraspinatus (Fig. 38.3).

The subscapularis lift off test is designed to best isolate the subscapularis and is performed by having the patient place the dorsum of their hand against their low back while sitting on the exam table. The patient then manually lifts the hand away (mainly by forcible extension of the shoulder) from the low back while the examiner resists. Pain and/or weakness are considered a positive test and suggests injury to the subscapularis (15).

The drop arm test is performed by passively abducting the patients arm to 160 degrees then asking the patient to slowly lower the arm to their side. A positive test is when the arm cannot be lowered in a controlled fashion and "drops" to their side. When positive it is highly specific for a large or massive rotator cuff tear, often necessitating a surgical consultation (55).

AC Joint Tests

The AC joint is stressed with the cross-body adduction test, which can assist in the diagnosis of AC joint osteoarthritis (16). The test is performed by passively bringing the patient's arm across the body towards the contralateral shoulder. It is consider positive if patient has pain localized to the AC joint.

Tests of Shoulder Stability

Chronic anterior shoulder instability can be diagnosed with the apprehension test. This is performed by having the patient lie supine and in a relaxed state. The patient's arm is brought into 90 degrees of abduction with the elbow flexed to 90 degrees. The examiner then applies gentle external rotation with the arm still abducted at 90 degrees. If the patient becomes apprehensive, this is a positive sign of anterior instability. The examiner may augment the test by placing their contralateral hand behind the humeral head creating an anteriorly directed force (Fig. 38.4).

The sulcus sign is diagnostic of multidirectional instability (17). The test is performed with the patient's arm dangling at their side. The examiner then exerts an inferiorly directed force on the arm by pulling down on the patient's wrist. The test is positive if a sulcus or indentation is created between the acromion and proximal humeral head.

Various exam findings can be combined to develop a 'clinical decision rule' (18). A prospective analysis of 400 patients found that the triad of: (i) weakness on empty can test and (ii) external rotation along with a (iii) positive impingement test (i.e., Hawkins) had a 98% probability of a rotator cuff tear (partial or complete) (19). Further, in the subset of patients older than age 60 years two or more of these three findings had a 98% probability of a rotator cuff tear. A separate retrospective analysis of 191 subjects found that a combination of age >65, weakness on external rotation, and night pain resulted in a 91% probability of having a rotator cuff tear (partial/complete) (11).

Approach to Diagnostic Imaging

There are multiple imaging modalities available to aid in diagnosing shoulder pain. Plain radiographs are important in acute injuries to rule out fracture or dislocation. Plain radiographs can assess whether there is a hook or spur of the acromion, significant AC joint osteoarthritis, as well as a potential accessory os acromiale that might predispose patients to rotator cuff injury and impingement. Plain radiographs are also the preferred imaging modality for shoulder osteoarthritis and calcific tendonitis.

The majority of shoulder disorders can be diagnosed with history, physical exam, and plain radiographs. Generally the role of MRI is when a patient has failed 6 to 8 weeks of conservative management and the diagnosis remains uncertain. The diagnoses of shoulder OA, calcific tendonitis, and adhesive capsulitis generally do not require the use of an MRI unless an associated rotator cuff tear is suspected. MRI should be employed sooner if it will change management such as when suspecting a massive rotator cuff tear that would benefit from early surgical correction (positive drop arm test, profound weakness after a fall involving the shoulder). Another scenario to consider an early MRI is with a shoulder dislocation when one suspects an anterior labral tear (also known as a Bankart tear) in the young athlete younger than 20 years or a secondary rotator cuff tear that can be found in older athletes older than 40 years who sustain a shoulder dislocation.

MRI is the most often used device to image the soft tissue structures of the shoulder. A recent meta-analysis which looked at 29 different cohort studies found that for a full-thickness rotator cuff tear, MRI had a sensitivity of 0.89, and a specificity of 0.93. For partial-thickness tears, however, the sensitivity dropped to 0.44, and specificity remained high at 0.90 (20). However, the use of MRI arthrography increased the sensitivity to 0.84 and the specificity to 0.96 in another study on partial-thickness tears (21). The majority of partial thickness tears respond to conservative management, therefore the need to ever obtain an MRI arthrogram is for rare cases that have not responded to 6 to 8 weeks of conservative management and where a plain MRI is equivocal. MR arthrogram is also the preferred test when there is concern for a labral tear based on history and physical exam. The small size of the labrum makes diagnosing a tear on plain MRI challenging.

Ultrasound has also been described in the diagnosis of partial-thickness and full-thickness rotator cuff tears. It can offer an inexpensive alternative, but does not provide the same amount of information regarding possible concomitant pathologies of the shoulder. Results using ultrasound have also been found to be extremely dependent on the skills of the operator (22). A 2005 study found that the preoperative accuracy of ultrasound was similar to that of MRI, with 70% and 73% accuracy, respectively (23). Ultrasound, however, does offer the unique ability to perform functional imaging of the rotator cuff to assess for impingement. Table 38.5 summarizes the sensitivity, specificity, and likelihood ratios for both MRI and ultrasound in diagnosing rotator cuff tears.

Recommended Diagnostic Strategy

The diagnosis of shoulder disorders can be a challenge even to the most experienced clinician. Figure 38.5 outlines the best evidence based approach available to diagnose and manage acute shoulder pain. Figure 38.6 provides an algorithm for chronic shoulder pain.

MANAGEMENT

Rotator Cuff Disorders

Rotator cuff disorders span the spectrum from tendinopathy to partial and complete tears. Fortunately, short of a massive rotator cuff tear, the majority of rotator cuff pathology can be managed with nonsurgical treatment options (24,25). Unfortunately, there is limited and inconsistent data on the effectiveness of commonly used treatments for rotator cuff disorders. This is due to inconsistencies in diagnostic methods (clinical vs. MRI vs. diagnosis at time of surgery), the diagnosis studied (rotator cuff impingement not otherwise specified vs. specific description of rotator cuff injury [i.e., tendinosis, partial tear, complete tear]), treatment approaches, and outcomes measured. Additionally the quality of many studies is insufficient to draw firm conclusions. Table 38.6 highlights the best evidence for various treatment options for rotator cuff disorders.

The least invasive treatment options include relative rest with avoidance of overhead activity, anti-inflammatory medication, and physical therapy. There are no formal studies evaluating the benefit of activity modification. Clinically, patients who participate in sports or have occupations that involve repetitive overhead activities often will report decreased pain scores with activity modification (SOR=C).

TABLE 38.5 Diagnostic Accuracy of Imaging Tests for Rotator Cuff Tears

Imaging Test	Finding	Strength of Recommendation	Sensitivity (%)	Specificity (%)	LR(+)	LR(−)
Magnetic resonance imaging	Any rotator cuff tear	A (20)	83	86	4.85	0.22
	Partial-thickness rotator cuff tear	A (20)	44	90	3.99	0.66
	Full-thickness rotator cuff tear	A (20)	89	93	10.63	0.16
Ultrasound	Any rotator cuff tear	A (20)	80	85	5.09	0.27
	Partial-thickness rotator cuff tear	A (20)	67	94	8.90	0.36
	Full-thickness rotator cuff tear	A (20)	97	96	13.16	0.16

Strength of Recommendation A: very useful; B: moderately useful; C: of limited use.
*Adapted from Burbank K, Stevenson JH, et al. Chronic shoulder pain: Part I. Evaluation and diagnosis. *Am Family Phys* 2008;77(4):1–8.

often indicated as part of the assessment (44). Glenohumeral arthritis secondary to the initial injury or the surgical stabilization procedure is also possible (45). Posterior dislocations are much rarer than anterior dislocations but generally managed similarly.

Acromioclavicular (AC) Joint Arthritis

Shoulder pain from AC joint arthritis is a common condition and can be associated with hypertrophy of the AC joint. A hypertrophied AC joint can be associated with impingement and wear of the rotator cuff between the hypertrophied AC joint and the proximal humerus during repetitive arm abduction movements. The mainstay of treatment is pain control and activity modification. Pain control may be accomplished via NSAIDS or other analgesics in milder stages, while corticosteroid injections into the AC joint may be effective in short-term pain control for more severe cases (46). Failure to improve or maintain function with conservative measures warrants surgical referral. Resection of the distal clavicle is often ultimately effective in relieving pain symptoms from resistant AC arthritis (47).

Glenohumeral Joint Arthritis

Glenohumeral arthritis is a less common source of chronic shoulder pain but, when present, can result in significant pain and disability. The focus of treatment is to maintain overall function with adequate pain control. Initial attempts at pain control may be with anti-inflammatory or analgesic medications. If pain is inadequately controlled, an intra-articular steroid injection may be considered, although there is little evidence to support this intervention.

Physical therapy can be helpful to maintain function of the shoulder joint, but should be undertaken with caution as aggressive attempts at increasing ROM can be counterproductive. Control of comorbid conditions, such as rheumatoid arthritis, is imperative. Several potent oral and parenteral rheumatologic medications are available and discussed further in Chapter 35. Surgical referral is indicated for failure of conservative treatment. The time frame for referral varies depending on the level of disability. Capsular release and arthroscopic debridement, hemiarthroplasty, and total shoulder arthroplasty are surgical options (48).

KEY POINTS

- Shoulder pain is a very common complaint in the ambulatory setting with rotator cuff disorders comprising the majority of shoulder complaints.
- Pain medication, physical therapy exercises, and subacromial steroid injection have been shown to provide short-term improvements in rotator cuff disorders.
- Massive or retracted rotator cuff tears usually require prompt referral for surgical intervention.
- Systemic oral or glenohumeral joint steroid injections provide short-term improvement for adhesive capsulitis.
- Surgery has shown improved outcomes for shoulder dislocation in the young active athlete compared with conservative management.
- Relative rest, pain medication, and potential steroid injection will treat the majority of shoulder joint arthritis complaints.

CHAPTER

39

Skin Problems

Richard P. Usatine

CLINICAL OBJECTIVES

1. Describe skin rashes and lesions using the terms for primary and secondary morphologies.
2. Describe how to choose a topical corticosteroid for inflammatory skin conditions based on the skin lesion, the location, the severity, and the age of the patient.
3. Discuss diagnosis and treatment for the most common skin conditions.

Pattern recognition plays a large role in the diagnosis of skin problems. Experts who have seen countless cases of skin conditions can look at most lesions and make an immediate and accurate diagnosis through pattern recognition.

How does the novice get to this point? The first step is to learn the basic patterns of the primary and secondary lesions listed in Table 39.1. This will give you the proper vocabulary and conceptual model to observe and describe what you are seeing. Then, if you combine keen observation of the lesions (including type and distribution) along with a careful history, you will be able to create an informed differential diagnosis. The information you acquire from observation and history can be taken to a dermatology atlas, textbook, or consultant to complete the diagnosis. Sometimes further testing such as a biopsy or culture may be needed; however, you need to know enough about the possible diagnoses to appropriately plan a biopsy or laboratory evaluation.

FAMILY HISTORY

Understanding the family is important in the diagnosis, treatment, and prevention of skin problems. A number of skin diseases have a strong genetic component, including acne, atopic dermatitis, psoriasis, skin cancers, dysplastic nevi, and rare conditions such as neurofibromatosis and tuberous sclerosis. Taking a family history may help when these conditions are suspected.

PREVENTION EXAMINATION

The US Preventive Services Task Force concludes that the current evidence is insufficient to assess the balance of benefits and harms of using a whole-body skin examination by a primary care clinician or patient skin self-examination for the early detection of cutaneous melanoma, basal cell cancer, or squamous cell skin cancer in the adult general population (1). People at higher risk for melanoma include fair-skinned people older than 65 years, patients with many atypical moles, and those with more than 50 moles. Other risk factors for skin cancer include family history and a substantial history of sun exposure and sunburns (1). When a person has had a basal cell carcinoma (BCC), the risk of a second BCC is more than 40% in the next 3 years (2). Although the evidence to support screening skin exams is insufficient, it is still reasonable to perform a complete skin examination in people at highest risk for skin cancer. Such an examination also provides a good opportunity to discuss sun exposure, protective clothing, and use of sunscreens.

DIAGNOSIS

Although you are taught in medical school to perform the history before doing the physical examination, this is not the most efficient way to approach the diagnosis of a skin condition. When the patient has a skin complaint, take a look at the skin immediately and ask your questions while you examine the patient.

The first step is to look carefully at the lesions. Determine the type of primary lesions and whether any secondary lesions are present (see Table 39.1). Next touch the lesions. Use gloves if you think the lesions may be transmissible, as in scabies, syphilis, or herpes. For some lesions, such as actinic keratosis with scaling or the sandpaper rash of scarlet fever, feeling the skin lightly gives you a great deal of information. For deeper lesions, such as nodules and cysts, deep palpation is needed.

Observe the distribution of the lesions. Look at the local distribution first to determine if the primary lesions are arranged in groups, rings, lines, or merely scattered over the skin. For example, the vesicles of herpes simplex are usually grouped together because they follow a sensory nerve, whereas the vesicles of chickenpox are often scattered because the virus is bloodborne. Next, determine which parts of the skin are affected and which are spared.

Be sure to look at the remainder of the skin, nails, hair, and mucous membranes. Patients often only show you one small area and appear reluctant to show you the rest of their skin. With many skin conditions it is essential to look beyond the most affected area.

Think of yourself as a detective collecting clues. For example, it helps to look for nail pitting when considering a diagnosis of psoriasis (Color Plate Fig. 39.1). Patients may have lesions on their back or feet that they have not observed; for example, a patient may have an eruption on the hands that is an autosensitization to a fungal infection on the feet—if you do not look for the fungus on the feet, you will miss the diagnosis.

TABLE 39.1 Primary and Secondary Skin Lesions

Primary (Basic) Lesions	Description
Macule	Circumscribed flat discoloration (up to 5 mm)
Patch	Flat nonpalpable discoloration (>5 mm)
Papule	Elevated solid lesion (up to 5 mm)
Plaque	Elevated solid lesion (>5 mm) (often, a confluence of papules)
Nodule	Palpable solid (round) lesion, deeper than a papule
Wheal (hive)	Pink edematous plaque—round or flat-topped and transient
Pustule	Elevated collection of pus
Vesicle	Circumscribed elevated collection of fluid (up to 5 mm in diameter)
Bulla	Circumscribed elevated collection of fluid (>5 mm in diameter)
Secondary (Sequential) Lesions	
Scale (desquamation)	Excess dead epidermal cells
Crusts	A collection of dried serum, blood, or pus
Erosion	Superficial loss of epidermis
Ulcer	Focal loss of epidermis and dermis
Fissure	Linear loss of epidermis and dermis
Atrophy	Depression in the skin from thinning of epidermis and/or dermis
Excoriation	Erosion caused by scratching
Lichenification	Thickened epidermis with prominent skin lines

Some skin diseases (such as lichen planus) have manifestations in the mouth; finding white patches on the buccal mucosa may lead you to the correct diagnosis of lichen planus (Color Plate Fig. 39.2). Do not be shy about asking patients to remove their shoes and clothing and to show you all areas of the body needed to make an accurate diagnosis. A magnifying glass helps to distinguish the morphology of many skin conditions.

Once you begin looking at the skin, your history will be more focused and directed toward discovering the correct diagnosis. The following information will help you make a diagnosis and plan the treatment:

- Onset and duration of skin lesions—continuous or intermittent?
- Pattern of eruption—where did it start? How has it changed?
- Any known precipitants, such as exposure to medication (prescription and over-the-counter), foods, plants, sun, topical agents, or chemicals (occupation and hobbies)?
- Skin symptoms—itching, pain, paresthesias
- Systemic symptoms—fever, chills, night sweats, fatigue, weakness, weight loss
- Underlying illnesses—diabetes, HIV
- Family history—acne, atopic dermatitis, psoriasis, skin cancers, dysplastic nevi

Diagnostic Testing

The most important in-office tests in assessing skin disorders are the following.

1. Microscopy: In diagnosing a suspected fungal infection, scrape some of the scale from the skin lesion onto a microscope slide, add potassium hydroxide (KOH) (with a fungal stain if available). Now look for the hyphae of dermatophytes or the pseudohyphae of yeast forms of *Candida* or *Pityrosporum* species. Start on 10 power and confirm your findings on 40 power.
2. Wood's light examination: This examination is helpful in diagnosing tinea capitis and erythrasma. Tinea capitis caused by *Microsporum* species produce green fluorescence. Erythrasma has a coral red fluorescence.
3. Surgical biopsy: A shave, punch, or elliptical biopsy can be used as a diagnostic and treatment tool. Having a reasonable differential diagnosis will help you choose the appropriate biopsy type.

Treatment

Treatment of skin conditions and lesions can be divided into two categories—medical and surgical. Medical treatments include topical and systemic steroids, antibiotics, antifungal, and antiviral agents. Surgical treatments include shave, punch, elliptical, and scissor excisions. Cryosurgery, electrosurgery, and curettage are also important surgical techniques.

Topical corticosteroids are used to treat many skin conditions. Their most beneficial effects occur from their anti-inflammatory and antimitotic activity. Local adverse effects of topical steroids are common with regular use over weeks to months; the most common adverse effect of topical steroid use over time is skin atrophy, in which the epidermis becomes thin and the superficial capillaries dilate. Atrophy can be accompanied by hypopigmentation, telangiectasias, and striae. Although the atrophy is usually reversible in months, striae are irreversible. When fluorinated steroids (the strongest steroids) are continuously applied to the face, perioral dermatitis as well as rosacea-like and acneiform eruptions can occur.

Systemic adverse effects are rare and occur when large amounts of topical steroids are absorbed through the skin. The risk of such absorption increases with stronger steroids, thinner skin, younger patients, longer duration of therapy, and the use of occlusion in therapy. Prescribing the minimum strength needed for the shortest duration of time required helps prevent adverse effects.

CHOOSING AND DISPENSING TOPICAL CORTICOSTEROIDS

The art and science of choosing a topical steroid is one of maximizing benefit and minimizing adverse effects. The factors to consider include the following.

TABLE 39.2 Choosing Topical Corticosteroids

Vehicle
• If lesion is dry, use ointment or moisturizing lotion • If moist or weeping, use cream or gel • If in hair-covered area, consider lotion or liquid preparations
Strength (based on thickness of skin and severity and thickness of lesion)
• Face and genitals: thin skin—weakest strength, avoid atrophy • Soles of hands and feet: thickest skin—if lesion is severe and thickened (lichenified), may need most potent strength • Other areas: use strength appropriate to severity and thickness of lesions
Examples: (all available generically in multiple vehicles types)
• Low potency: 1% hydrocortisone (over the counter) • Low-moderate potency: 0.05% desonide • Moderate potency: 0.1% triamcinolone • High potency: 0.05% fluocinonide • Super-high potency: 0.05% clobetasol propionate

- Skin disorder: As the severity or chronicity of the disorder increases, the need for higher potency steroids increases. Thicker lesions (e.g., psoriatic plaques) need higher potency steroids.
- Site: Use only the weakest potency steroids on the face, genitals, and other intertriginous areas (skin folds) where skin is thin and/or moist, and skin atrophy and striae occur most rapidly. The skin on the palms and soles is so thick that the most potent steroids may be needed.
- Age: Avoid the use of high-potency topical steroids in infants and children because they have greater surface area per body mass than adults; they therefore have greater risk and consequences of systemic absorption.
- Steroid potency (strength and concentration): There are more than 50 types and brands of steroids. It is not necessary to memorize these lists, but you should know the names of at least one steroid from each of the four basic strengths; Table 39.2 lists several good choices. To save on costs, you can use generic agents from all the potency groups.
- Vehicle: The vehicle is the substance in which the steroid is dispersed. The most commonly used vehicles are creams, ointments, gels, solutions, and lotions (Table 39.3). The choice of vehicle is determined by the characteristics of the lesion (dry or moist), the site involved, and patient preference. The type of vehicle affects the potency of the steroid because it determines the rate at which the steroid is absorbed through the skin.

Most skin preparations can be applied two times a day, conveniently in the morning and evening. Try to estimate and prescribe an appropriate amount; many topical products are supplied in 15-, 30-, and 60-g sizes. To avoid adverse effects of steroid overuse, do not prescribe large quantities for small lesions, and specify duration of use. On the other hand, prescribing a small tube for a large area of involvement will be frustrating to the patient when the steroid runs out before the prescribed treatment duration is completed.

The duration of therapy should often be the time it takes for resolution of symptoms or lesions. To avoid adverse effects, the highest potency steroids should not be used continuously for longer than 2 weeks. However, they can be used intermittently for chronic conditions, such as psoriasis, in a pulse-therapy mode (e.g., apply every weekend, with no application on weekdays). For dry lesions, liberal use of emollients between steroid applications can minimize steroid exposure while maximizing the benefits of therapy.

TABLE 39.3 Commonly Used Vehicles for Steroids and Other Dermatologic Preparations

Creams
• Mixture of oil and water; may contain alcohol • White color; may be somewhat greasy • May cause stinging and irritation to broken skin • May be drying; best for moist or exudative lesions • Cosmetically most acceptable • Better in skin folds than ointments
Ointments
• Base is frequently petroleum jelly (petrolatum) • Translucent and very greasy • Best for dry lesions; lubricating • Greasy feeling persists after application • May get on clothes and be transferred from hands to surfaces at work • Cosmetically less acceptable in daytime (may be used at night and apply cream during the day) • Increased absorption of steroid and therefore enhances potency of the steroid • Too occlusive for exudative lesions and areas of skin folds (groin) • Too messy for hair-covered areas
Gels
• Greaseless mixtures of propylene glycol and water; may contain alcohol • Clear and jelly-like • Useful for exudative lesions; may be drying
Solutions and Lotions
• Water and alcohol base • Solutions usually clear; lotions have a milky appearance • Best for scalp and other hair-covered areas: penetrates easily and doesn't make hair greasy • May cause stinging and irritation to broken skin

Modified from Habif T. *Clinical Dermatology: A Color Guide to Diagnosis and Therapy*, 4th ed. St. Louis, MO: CV Mosby, 2003.

TABLE 39.4 Strength of Recommendation for Treatment of Bacterial Infections of the Skin*

Site	Infection	Treatment	Strength of Recommendation†
Epidermis	Impetigo Ecthyma (impetigo with ulceration) Bullous impetigo	Topical mupirocin or oral antibiotic that covers GABHS and *Staphylococcus aureus** (consider CA-MRSA coverage)	A A A
Dermis	Erysipelas Cellulitis (dermis and subcutaneous tissue also)	Oral or intravenous antibiotic* based on severity (consider CA-MRSA coverage)	A A
Dermal appendages (hair follicle, nail fold)	Folliculitis Carbuncle, furuncle Paronychia Abscess	Topical or oral antibiotic* I&D I&D I&D (consider antibiotic for CA-MRSA coverage)	C B B B
Subcutaneous tissue/ fascia	Necrotizing fasciitis	Hospitalize Intravenous antibiotic Debridement	B

CA-MRSA coverage = community-acquired methicillin-resistant *Staphylococcus aureus*; GABHS = Group A beta-hemolytic streptococci; I & D = incision & drainage; *S. aureus*.
*Oral antibiotics must cover *Group A Beta-hemolytic streptococci* and *S. aureus*: first line—dicloxacillin, cephalexin; second line—clindamycin for severe penicillin allergy.
†A = consistent, good-quality patient-oriented evidence; B = inconsistent or limited-quality patient-oriented evidence; C = consensus, disease-oriented evidence, usual practice, expert opinion, or case series.
For information about the SORT evidence rating system, see *www.aafp.org/afpsort.xml*.

MANAGEMENT OF SKIN INFECTIONS

Bacterial Infections

Bacterial skin infections can be classified by the portion of the skin involved (see Table 39.4). Most bacterial skin infections are caused by *Staphylococcus aureus*. Antibiotics that treat methicillin-sensitive *S. aureus* include cephalexin, dicloxacillin, and clindamycin. Community-acquired methicillin-resistant *S. aureus* (MRSA) is now an important cause of skin infections. In one large observational study in 11 emergency departments, adults with a purulent skin or soft-tissue infection of <1 week of duration were cultured. Of 422 patients, 249 had MRSA, 71 had methicillin-sensitive *S. aureus* infection, 64 had another bacterial infection, and 38 had no bacterial growth. Group A streptococcus was only rarely isolated. Among those with *S. aureus* infection, the percentage with MRSA ranged from 15% to 74%; in most cities, the percentage was between 50% and 70%. Independent risk factors for MRSA included non-Hispanic black race, use of an antibiotic in the past month, reported spider bite, history of MRSA infection, or close contact with a person with a similar infection. Antibiotic susceptibilities for MRSA were 100% to trimethoprim-sulfamethoxazole and rifampin, 95% to clindamycin, and 92% to tetracycline (3).

Topical antibiotics should only be used as monotherapy for the most mild and superficial bacterial skin infections. Mild cases of impetigo (see the following section) or minor wound infections can be treated with mupirocin (Bactroban) (4).

IMPETIGO

Impetigo is a superficial skin infection often characterized by "honey" crusts (Color Plate Fig. 39.3). It can also be vesicular or bullous. Impetigo in children often occurs around the nose and mouth. Homeless people are prone to impetigo because of sleeping on the streets and of lack of hygiene. Impetigo should be treated for 7 to 10 days with antibiotics that cover *S. aureus* and *S. pyogenes,* such as cephalexin or dicloxacillin (5) (strength of recommendation [SOR] = A).

Two variations of impetigo are ecthyma and bullous impetigo. Ecthyma has an ulcerated punched-out base and bullous impetigo is often caused by *S. aureus*. Community-acquired MRSA can present as bullous impetigo in children. Staphylococcal-scalded skin syndrome (SSSS) is a life-threatening, more severe variation of bullous impetigo. In SSSS, the bullae are caused by exfoliating toxin, and the patient is systemically ill. Patients who have SSSS need emergent hospitalization for intravenous antibiotics, fluids, and supportive therapy.

CELLULITIS AND ERYSIPELAS

Cellulitis is an acute infection of the skin that involves the dermis and subcutaneous tissues. Cellulitis is usually caused by β-hemolytic streptococci and *S. aureus*. Erysipelas is a specific type of superficial cellulitis with prominent lymphatic involvement causing lesions that are raised above the level of the surrounding skin with a clear line of demarcation between involved and uninvolved tissue. It is frequently caused by β-hemolytic streptococci and is seen most commonly on the extremities (6).

Cellulitis often begins with a break in the skin caused by trauma, a bite, or an underlying dermatosis (e.g., tinea pedis). It is usually seen on the legs and arms. The severity of the cellulitis, the systemic symptoms, and host factors determine whether oral or parenteral antibiotics are indicated.

FOLLICULITIS

Folliculitis is an infection or inflammation of the superficial portion of the hair follicle. Although it is usually caused by *S. aureus*, it can be caused by other bacteria, yeast, or occlusion. Its presentation can include perifollicular erythema, papules, or pustules. Magnification during the skin examination will reveal that the lesions are associated with hair follicles. Hot tub folliculitis is caused by pseudomonas; folliculitis also can be caused by *Pityrosporum* yeast or occlusion of hair follicles with tight fitting clothing. Treatment ranges from avoiding occlusive clothing and contaminated hot tubs to the use of topical or oral antibiotics or antifungals.

ABSCESS

An abscess is defined as a localized collection of pus; abscesses that occur in or directly below the skin include furuncles, carbuncles, and the abscesses around fingernails (acute paronychia). A furuncle or boil is an abscess that starts in a hair follicle or sweat gland. A carbuncle occurs when the furuncle extends into the subcutaneous tissue. Epidermal inclusion cysts often become inflamed and infected and form a skin abscess. Skin abscesses can occur anywhere on the body. Most skin abscesses are caused by *S. aureus* with MRSA becoming the predominant pathogen (3).

Incision and drainage is the preferred treatment for all types of abscesses. The pus must be drained so that the lesion can heal. Systemic antibiotics, whether parenteral or oral, do not adequately penetrate an abscess to cure the infection. If there is significant surrounding cellulitis, systemic antibiotics may be needed as an adjunct to incision and drainage.

NECROTIZING FASCIITIS

Necrotizing fasciitis, or "flesh-eating bacteria," is a deep infection of the subcutaneous tissues and fascia. It often presents with diffuse swelling of the arm or leg, followed by the appearance of bullae with clear fluid that may become violaceous in color. The patient has marked systemic symptoms such as pain out of proportion to the apparent skin lesion. Necrotizing fasciitis may be caused by a single organism or be polymicrobial.

Cases of necrotizing fasciitis that occur after varicella or minor injuries, such as scratches and insect bites, are almost always from *S. pyogenes*. In the polymicrobial form, there is an average of five pathogens in each wound, with most of the organisms originating from the bowel flora (e.g., coliforms, anaerobic bacteria) (6).

Necrotizing fasciitis, which at first may look like cellulitis, can lead to cutaneous gangrene, myonecrosis, shock, and death. It is crucial to not miss necrotizing fasciitis because it is life- and limb-threatening and requires surgical debridement along with intravenous antibiotics. Several clinical features suggest the presence of a necrotizing infection of the skin and its deeper structures: severe, constant pain; bullae; skin necrosis or ecchymosis (bruising) that precedes skin necrosis; gas in the soft tissues detected by palpation or imaging; edema that extends beyond the margin of erythema; cutaneous anesthesia; systemic toxicity, manifested by fever, tachycardia, delirium, and renal failure; and rapid spread, especially during antibiotic therapy (6).

Viral Infections

WARTS

Warts are caused by more than 100 subtypes of human papillomavirus (HPV). Warts commonly occur on the hands, feet, and genitals. The appearance of a wart is strongly related to its location. Warts on the hands (verruca vulgaris) are usually raised and hyperkeratotic. Warts on the soles of the feet (plantar warts) are flat, disrupt skin lines, have dark dots visible in them, and may be quite painful. Flat warts (verruca plana) are usually seen in groups on the face or legs. Genital warts (condylomata acuminata) often have a cauliflower appearance and are transmitted sexually. Ninety percent of genital warts are caused by HPV 6. High-risk HPV types (HPV 16, 18) generally do not cause visible genital warts but have been associated with cervical intraepithelial neoplasia and cervical cancer. New vaccines to prevent transmission of high-risk HPV types have shown promise in decreasing the incidence of cervical cancer. One of the two currently available vaccines immunizes against HPV types 6, 11, 16, and 18 (quadrivalent); the other immunizes against HPV types 16 and 18. For the quadrivalent vaccine, the estimated number needed to vaccinate to prevent an episode of genital warts is 8 and to prevent a case of cervical cancer is 324 (7).

The natural history for most warts is to eventually regress; and there are many treatments for warts. Some warts do not respond to treatment, or recur within a short period of time. In office practice, the following treatments are generally considered first-line therapy:

- Verruca vulgaris: salicylic acid or cryosurgery
- Plantar warts: salicylic acid or cryosurgery
- Flat warts: salicylic acid, topical tretinoin (Retin-A), cryosurgery, or imiquimod (Aldara)
- Condylomata acuminata: podophyllin resin, podofilox (Condylox), trichloroacetic acid, cryosurgery, or imiquimod (Aldara)

HERPESVIRUSES

The major herpesviruses that affect the skin are herpes simplex (HSV) types 1 and 2 and varicella-zoster virus (VZV). A major characteristic of herpes infection is that the virus lies dormant in dorsal root ganglia, leading to recurrences. All herpetic skin infections are characterized by vesicular eruptions with surrounding erythema, which progress to ulcers and/or crusts and then reepithelialize over the course of days or weeks. Infections caused by herpes viruses include:

- Herpes gingivostomatitis or labialis (cold sores): caused by HSV (most commonly type 1, but sometimes type 2). A primary episode can affect the entire mouth (gingivostomatitis) and can be accompanied by fever, chills, and malaise. Recurrent episodes often occur on the lips (labialis) and are milder, sometimes asymptomatic, but accompanied by viral shedding.
- Genital herpes: caused by HSV (most commonly type 2, but sometimes type 1). This sexually transmitted infection presents as herpetic lesions on the genitals, anus, or buttocks. As in gingivostomatitis, first episodes are often more severe; subsequent episodes range from moderate to asymptomatic but are accompanied by viral shedding and the possibility of

transmission to sexual partners. Genital herpes can be spread between active episodes of disease because infected people can shed the virus asymptomatically. Active ulcers create a higher risk of acquiring HIV during sexual contact with HIV-positive individuals (Color Plate Fig. 39.4).

- Chickenpox: This is the initial infection of VZV. It typically consists of a few days of fever and respiratory symptoms with the characteristic vesicles on a red base that begin on the trunk and over several days spreads to the extremities. Fortunately, the varicella vaccine has diminished the incidence of chickenpox.
- Herpes zoster (shingles): This is a reactivation of dormant VZV along a skin dermatome (Color Plate Fig. 39.5). The outbreak is usually unilateral and vesicular.

Most infections with HSV and VZV are acutely painful, uncomplicated, and resolve spontaneously in 1 to 2 weeks. Complications include encephalitis and disseminated infections; these occur especially in infants or immunosuppressed individuals. One prolonged and painful after-effect of the infection is postherpetic neuralgia (PHN) that presents as chronic pain in the dermatome previously infected with herpes zoster. The zoster vaccine that has been approved for adults older than age 60 decreases the incidence of zoster by approximately six cases per 1,000 person-years and PHN by approximately one case per 1,000 person-years (8).

There are no cures for HSV or VZV; the goals of therapy, therefore, are to diminish pain, viral shedding, and duration of symptoms, and to prevent recurrences. In HSV, prophylactic daily oral medication can prevent or reduce recurrences; in zoster, early antiviral treatment may prevent PHN.

Antiviral agents with proven effectiveness against herpes simplex and herpes zoster are acyclovir, famciclovir, and valacyclovir. These antiviral agents can be used to treat primary and recurrent herpes simplex and herpes zoster, and to prevent recurrent herpes simplex. Acyclovir is the only one also approved to treat acute varicella (chickenpox). Most importantly, the varicella vaccine is effective for primary prevention of varicella. In one large randomized clinical trial (RCT), male circumcision reduced the incidence of new HSV-2 infections and reduced the prevalence of infection with high-risk HPV subtypes (9).

Fungal Infections

Fungal infections of the skin occur at many sites and are most often caused by dermatophytes, *Candida*, or *Pityrosporum* species. The dermatophytes cause tinea infections that are commonly called ringworm, although no worm is involved in ringworm. The typical dermatophyte infection of the body (tinea corporis) has an annular appearance with central clearing, redness, and scale on the perimeter of this well-demarcated lesion (Color Plate Fig. 39.6). Tinea versicolor is caused by an inflammatory reaction to the yeast-like *Pityrosporum (Malassezia furfur)* rather than a dermatophyte (Color Plate Fig. 39.7). *Candida* thrives on wet mucosal surfaces but also affects the skin; it causes thrush, balanitis, vaginitis, and rashes in the groin and under the breast.

Common dermatophyte infections are tinea capitis, tinea corporis, tinea cruris, and tinea pedis. Tinea capitis (tinea of the head) causes patchy alopecia (hair loss) with broken hairs and scaling. Because the hair shaft and follicle are involved, topical antifungals are not effective. Oral antifungal medications include griseofulvin, itraconazole, and terbinafine, which are taken for 4 to 8 weeks. A meta-analysis found a 2- to 4-week course of terbinafine to be at least as effective as a 6- to 8-week course of griseofulvin for treating *Trichophyton* infections of the scalp. Griseofulvin was likely to be superior to terbinafine for the rare cases of tinea capitis caused by *Microsporum* species (10). In one RCT, 1 week of terbinafine was as effective as longer duration therapy for children with tinea capitis from trichophyton species (11).

Tinea corporis (tinea of the body) can occur on almost any part of the body. Small areas may respond well to topical antifungals. Topical over-the-counter (OTC) antifungals (miconazole, clotrimazole) should be first-line agents. Large areas may require treatment with oral antifungals (griseofulvin, terbinafine, itraconazole) for 2 to 4 weeks.

Tinea cruris (tinea of the groin) may be red and scaling without the central clearing seen in tinea corporis. It should be differentiated from candidal infection (which often is redder and has satellite lesions) and erythrasma (a superficial bacterial infection that may be pink or brown and may show coral red fluorescence under ultraviolet light). Topical or systemic antifungals may be used for tinea cruris depending on the severity of involvement. If you are uncertain if there is *Candida* involvement, it is best to choose an antifungal agent that covers both dermatophytes and *Candida* (e.g., not tolnaftate [Tinactin], nystatin, or naftifine [Naftin]). All other topical antifungal medications including the azoles and terbinafine (Lamisil) cover all superficial fungal skin infections.

Tinea pedis (tinea of the feet) may be seen as macerated white areas between the toes or as dry red scaling on the soles or sides of the feet (moccasin distribution). A third, less common presentation causes vesicles on the feet. It can be treated with the same topical or oral antifungals used for tinea corporis or cruris. Griseofulvin, terbinafine, or itraconazole may be used when the lesions are not responding to topical agents. A Cochrane review reports that oral terbinafine is more effective than oral griseofulvin for tinea pedis (12).

A skin scraping treated with KOH and analyzed using a microscope can be diagnostic when classic hyphae or yeast forms are detected. KOH with dimethyl sulfoxide will help to dissolve the cell membranes of the epithelial cells for easier viewing and eliminates the need to heat the slide. Using a fungal stain such as the Swartz-Lambkins stain will make the hyphae stand out better among the epithelial cells (Color Plate Fig. 39.8). False-negative results are common when specimen collection is inadequate, when the patient has started OTC antifungals, or when the slide is read by an inexperienced viewer. False-positive results occur when cell borders are misinterpreted to be hyphae. A KOH test for tinea on the skin (without fungal stains) has a sensitivity of 77% to 88% and a specificity of 62% to 95% (13). Fungal cultures are more expensive and need 1 to 2 weeks to grow, but they can provide the most definitive evidence of fungal infection while providing you with the identity of the fungus.

Onychomycosis (or tinea unguium) is a fungal infection of the nails. Topical antifungal agents do not work well, and oral antifungal agents may cause liver toxicity. These agents can be given continuously for 3 to 4 months for the toenails and 2 months for fingernails. It is important to establish a definitive diagnosis of onychomycosis before starting treatment with oral antifungals, because there are other causes for dystrophic nails such as psoriasis, lichen planus, and trauma. The three most useful methods for diagnosis are a KOH preparation from subungual scrapings, a nail culture, or a distal nail clipping sent in formalin for periodic acid-Schiff (PAS) staining by a pathologist. The sensitivities and specificities of each of the techniques are as follows: KOH: 80% and 72%; culture: 59% and 82%; PAS: 92% and 72% (14). A meta-analysis of RCTs found that continuous terbinafine of 250 mg daily for 16 weeks is the most effective treatment for onychomycosis (number needed to treat [NNT] = 3) (SOR=A) (15).

DERMATITIS

Dermatitis is a nonspecific term that means inflammation of the skin. The term eczema means to bubble up as in the vesicles of acute eczema. However, dermatitis and eczema are often used interchangeably. There are many causes and patterns of skin inflammation including atopic dermatitis, contact dermatitis, dyshidrotic eczema, and nummular eczema. Common forms of dermatitis are described in the following section.

- Atopic dermatitis is a type of eczematous eruption that is itchy, recurrent, and symmetric and often found on flexural surfaces (Color Plate Fig. 39.9). These patients often have either a personal or a family history of asthma and allergic rhinitis. In infancy, atopic dermatitis often appears on the face. After infancy, the dry, scaling, and red lesions are found in flexural areas such as the antecubital or popliteal fossa. Most atopic dermatitis is not caused by specific allergens, but develops from a number of trigger factors in patients who have a strong genetic predisposition to develop eczematous eruptions.
- Allergic contact dermatitis is an allergic response to an allergen such as the chemical found in the poison ivy or poison oak plant (rhus dermatitis). These lesions are often linear and vesicular. Other contact allergens include nickel in jewelry and belt buckles and chemicals in deodorants and cosmetics (Color Plate Fig. 39.10). There is also irritative contact dermatitis in which the contactant works as an irritant rather than an allergen. Diaper dermatitis secondary to feces and urine is an irritant contact dermatitis.
- Dyshidrotic eczema is seen on the hands and/or feet. Tapioca-like vesicles occur between the fingers or toes along with scaling. The scaling inflamed skin can proceed to develop painful cracks and fissures.
- Nummular eczema is coin-shaped (nummus = coin in Latin) with erythema and scale. It is found most often on the lower legs.

Treatment for all types of dermatitis or eczema shares basic principles. First, avoid skin irritants (e.g., drying soaps), and bathing in hot water, which will dry the skin and increase the pruritus. Second, use emollients or moisturizers to add needed moisture to the skin. Third, treat the inflammation with a topical steroid or another anti-inflammatory agent such as topical immunomodulators, choosing the strength and vehicle based on diagnosis, chronicity, and location. Fourth, because itching is a prominent feature of many types of dermatitis, efforts should be made to stop the scratch–itch cycle. Lichen simplex chronicus is a type of chronic eczema in which the skin gets thickened with prominent skin lines visible (lichenified). It often needs potent topical steroid ointments to penetrate the thick plaque and moisturize the cracked pruritic skin. There is little evidence that antihistamines improve the outcomes in atopic dermatitis but oral sedating antihistamines are often used to decrease itching, especially at night (16). Finally, a secondary bacterial infection may develop in any type of dermatitis. This may take the form of impetigo with weeping and crusting. Signs of infection should lead to treatment with an antibiotic that covers *S. pyogenes* and *S. aureus*.

Topical immunomodulators tacrolimus and pimecrolimus are indicated to treat atopic dermatitis and eczema for adults and children 2 years of age and older. These calcineurin inhibitors have similar effectiveness when compared with topical steroids without the risk of skin atrophy. However, concerns about risks for cancer has prompted the US Food and Drug Administration to publish an advisory that states tacrolimus and pimecrolimus should only be used as second-line agents for short-term and intermittent treatment of atopic dermatitis in patients 2 years and older unresponsive to, or intolerant of, other treatments.

Seborrhea

Seborrhea is a superficial inflammatory dermatitis. It is a common condition that is characterized by erythema and scaling on the scalp and face (Color Plate Fig. 39.11). The typical distribution of seborrhea includes the scalp (dandruff); eyebrows and eyelids; nasolabial creases; behind the ears; eyebrows; forehead; cheeks; around the nose; under the beard or mustache; over the sternum; and in the axillae, submammary folds, umbilicus, groin, and the gluteal creases. These areas are the regions with the greatest number of pilosebaceous units producing sebum.

The prevalence of seborrhea is approximately 3% to 5% in young adults. Its incidence increases with age, and it is especially common in people with Parkinson disease and in people who are HIV-positive. Although the cause of seborrhea is not entirely clear, it is thought to involve an inflammatory hypersensitivity to epidermal, bacterial, or yeast antigens. People with seborrhea have a profusion of *Pityrosporum (Malassezia)* on the skin. Although this yeast can be a normal skin inhabitant, people who have seborrhea appear to respond to its presence with an inflammatory reaction.

Seborrhea is characterized by remissions and exacerbations. The most common precipitating factors are stress and cold weather. The treatment of seborrhea should be directed at the inflammation and the *Pityrosporum*. Seborrhea is highly responsive to topical steroids, so a low-potency steroid is usually adequate. To avoid atrophy, it is especially important to use a low-potency steroid for the treatment of seborrhea on the face; 1% hydrocortisone cream or lotion or desonide cream or lotion works well (17,18) (SOR=B) . Prescribe lotion or solution for seborrhea in hair-covered areas because it is easier ad less messy to apply than a cream. If scalp seborrhea is severe, prescribe a high-potency steroid such as fluocinonide solution or clobetasol solution, as the risk of atrophy on the scalp is less than on the face.

To reduce the profusion of *Pityrosporum*, you should direct the patient to apply antifungals to the affected areas. For seborrhea of the scalp, the antifungal shampoos that are most effective contain selenium sulfide, zinc pyrithione, ketoconazole, or coal tar derivatives. For seborrhea of the skin, ketoconazole cream is one effective antifungal preparation.

Patients should understand that these treatments are not curative, and seborrhea may return when they are under stress or if they stop using the antiseborrheic shampoos. The antifungals can be used to prevent exacerbations, but the steroids should be applied only to active areas of inflammation.

Psoriasis

Psoriasis is a chronic condition characterized by alterations in the immune system that lead to epidermal proliferation and inflammation. The lesions of plaque psoriasis are well-circumscribed, red, scaling plaques, with white thickened scales (Color Plate Fig. 39.12). Areas affected can include the scalp, nails, and extensor surfaces of limbs, elbows, knees, the sacral region, and the genitalia. Psoriasis lesions may be guttate as in water drops, inverse when found in intertriginous areas such as the inguinal and intergluteal folds, or volar when found on the palms or soles. Psoriatic nail changes occur in 10% to 40% of people with psoriasis. These nail changes include pitting, onycholysis, and subungual keratosis (Color Plate Fig. 39.1).

Treatment options for psoriasis include emollients, topical steroids, topical vitamin D (calcipotriene or calcipotriol), topical tar and tar shampoo, intralesional steroids, ultraviolet light, and topical retinoids. Systemic treatment options include methotrexate, acitretin, cyclosporine, and the injectable biologics. The most common treatments of psoriasis involve using high-potency topical steroids. Combination therapies are helpful to patients with psoriasis. One RCT demonstrated that a topical combination product of calcipotriene and betamethasone is more effective than either agent used alone in the treatment of psoriasis (NNT = 2) (19). Tazarotene, a topical retinoid, is effective for treating plaque psoriasis but may cause local irritation. Combining tazarotene with topical steroids can increase the effectiveness of both agents and reduce the incidence of local adverse effects (20) (SOR=B).

Systemic steroids are contraindicated for the treatment of psoriasis; they can precipitate severe flares and generalized pustular disease. When using potent topical steroids for chronic therapy in psoriasis (or eczema), it helps to use pulse therapy on weekends to avoid side effects and loss of efficacy. Tacrolimus and pimecrolimus are effective in treating facial and intertriginous psoriasis and can be used to avoid steroid adverse effects (21) (SOR=B).

Acne

Acne is an inflammatory disease of the pilosebaceous unit (sebaceous glands and their associated small hairs). The glands produce sebum, which is a complex lipid mixture, to maintain hydration of the skin. Acne involves blockage of the pilosebaceous unit with sebum and desquamated cells, accompanied by an overgrowth of *P. acnes* in the follicle.

Noninflammatory lesions of acne are open comedones (blackheads) and closed comedones (whiteheads). When there is disruption of the follicle wall, *P. acnes*, sebum, hair, and cells extrude into the dermis. This causes inflammation and leads to the formation of papules, pustules, nodules, and cysts. The causes or exacerbating factors for acne are genetics; androgens; stress; excessive friction on the skin (e.g., with sweat bands and helmet straps); cosmetics; and medications, including corticosteroids, lithium, isoniazid, and hormonal contraception with increased androgenicity.

TABLE 39.5 Strength of Recommendation for Medications for Acne Therapy

Topical
Benzoyl peroxide: antimicrobial effect (gel, cream, lotion) (2.5%, 5%, 10%) B
Topical antibiotics: clindamycin and erythromycin B
Erythromycin: solution, gel
Clindamycin: solution, gel, lotion
Combination topicals
BenzaClin gel: clindamycin 1%, benzoyl peroxide 5%, B
Benzamycin gel: erythromycin 3%, benzoyl peroxide 5%, B
Retinoids
Tretinoin (Retin-A) gel, cream, liquid, micronized A
Adapalene (Differin) gel A
Tazarotene (Tazorac) gel A
Azelaic acid (Azelex) B
Systemic
Oral antibiotics—A
Tetracycline 500 mg qd–bid: inexpensive, need to take on an empty stomach; avoid within 2 hours of calcium or calcium containing products
Doxycycline 100 mg qd–bid: inexpensive, well tolerated, increases sun sensitivity
Minocycline 50–100 mg qd–bid: expensive, less resistance of *P. acnes*
Erythromycin 250–500 mg bid: inexpensive, frequent gastrointestinal disturbance
Estrogen-dominant birth control pills, women only: B
Isotretinoin (Accutane) for cystic and scarring acne that has not responded to other therapies: A

Table 39.5 summarizes the strength of evidence for acne treatments, and Table 39.6 summarizes treatments based on acne severity. Use morphology to distinguish between noninflammatory (comedonal, obstructive) and inflammatory acne (papules, pustules, nodules and cysts). Determine the distribution and severity of the case and base therapy on the type and severity of the acne. Mild comedonal acne responds to topical retinoids or azelaic acid. More severe inflammatory acne often requires oral antibiotics in combination with topical retinoids and benzoyl peroxide. If this fails, and acne is scarring, consider isotretinoin (Accutane). Isotretinoin is the most potent medication for acne but has many potential side effects, including birth defects. The medication should not be prescribed or dispensed to any woman without two negative pregnancy tests and two forms of birth control.

When starting topical retinoid therapy, it helps to begin with the formulations that cause the least inflammation. These include lower potency tretinoin (Retin-A) and adapalene

TABLE 39.6 Acne Therapy by Severity

Comedonal acne—obstructive acne • Retinoids • Azelaic acid • No place for oral antibiotics
Mild papulopustular • Topical antibiotics and benzoyl peroxide • Retinoids • Azelaic acid • May add oral antibiotics if topical agents are not working
Papulopustular or nodulocystic acne—moderate and inflammatory • May start with topical antibiotic, benzoyl peroxide, and oral antibiotic • Oral antibiotics are often essential at this stage • Retinoids • Consider stopping oral antibiotics when topical agents are working well
Severe cystic or scarring acne • Isotretinoin
Estrogen dominant birth control pills—can be used for any type of acne in women only, especially if the pill is desired for birth control too.

(Differin). For oily skin and more severe acne, it may help to use the strongest preparations, such as tretinoin gel, adapalene gel, or tazarotene gel. In a meta-analysis of five randomized trials, adapalene 0.1% gel was found to be just as efficacious as tretinoin 0.025% gel, worked faster, and was less irritating and less drying than tretinoin gel (22) (SOR=A). Tazarotene is a potent retinoid that demonstrated greater effectiveness in acne than adapalene in a number of measures (23) (SOR=B). However, tazarotene was associated with transiently greater levels of burning, pruritus, erythema, and peeling compared with adapalene. When prescribing topical tretinoin or tazarotene, explain to the patient that redness and scaling may occur, and that the acne may worsen during the first 2 to 4 weeks before an improvement is seen. Because retinoids increase sun sensitivity, the patient should be warned about sun safety measures.

Useful combination products for the treatment of acne combine benzoyl peroxide with clindamycin or erythromycin. Benzoyl peroxide has a direct toxic effect on *P. acnes* and defers development of *P. acnes* resistance to antibiotics. The least expensive prescription products for acne include oral tetracycline or doxycycline and topical erythromycin or clindamycin Patients who cannot afford the very expensive combination products can use these products with OTC benzoyl peroxide.

Sun Damage and Precancers

Sun damage to the skin can be seen in photoaging, which results in mottled hyperpigmentation and wrinkling. Sun damage can lead to precancers such as actinic keratosis and lentigo maligna.

The most common skin cancers are BCC (approximately 80% of all skin cancers), squamous cell carcinoma (SCC) (16%), and melanoma (approximately 4% of all skin cancers). Sun exposure is the most important risk factor; other risk factors include a positive family history and fair skin type. The incidence of these cancers increases with age, probably because of cumulative sun exposure.

BCCs are the most common skin cancer and occur 85% of the time on the head and neck. The three major morphologic types are nodular, superficial, and morpheaform (sclerosing). The typical nodular BCC is pearly and raised with telangiectasias (Color Plate Fig. 39.13). As it expands, its center may ulcerate, bleed, and become crusted. Superficial BCCs look like SCC—red or pink, flat, scaling plaques that may have erosions or crusts. Sclerosing BCCs are rare (1% of BCCs), flat, and scarlike. SCCs can look like a superficial BCC or can be more elevated and nodular; SCCs are frequently hyperkeratotic and bleed easily (Color Plate Fig. 39.14).

Actinic keratoses (AKs) are premalignant. The risk of progression of AK to primary SCC (invasive or in situ) was 0.60% at 1 year and 2.57% at 4 years in a prospective trial of a high-risk Veterans Administration population (24). Recognizing and treating AKs is a secondary method of skin cancer prevention. There is a spectrum of skin cancer disease—from actinic keratosis to Bowen disease (SCC in situ) to SCC. When a lesion is more thickened or indurated than a typical AK, a biopsy is suggested to determine a definitive diagnosis before initiating treatment. Otherwise, typical AKs can be treated with cryotherapy for small numbers of lesions or topical field treatment for areas with many lesions. The approved topical agents include 5-fluorouracil, imiquimod, and diclofenac. Photodynamic therapy is another option.

Melanoma in the United States has been increasing in the last few decades. Early detection and treatment can prevent deaths and morbidity. Table 39.7 presents "ABCDE" guidelines for the diagnosis of melanoma, and Color Plate Figure 39.15 provides a photograph of a melanoma that meets all the ABCDE criteria. Many benign growths can resemble melanoma, so a suspicious growth should be biopsied to make a definitive diagnosis.

TABLE 39.7 ABCDE Guidelines for Diagnosis of Melanoma

Asymmetry. Most early melanomas are asymmetrical—a line through the middle would not create matching halves. Common moles are round and symmetrical.
Border. The borders of early melanomas are often uneven and may have scalloped or notched edges. Common moles have smoother, more even borders.
Color. Common moles usually are a single shade of brown. Varied shades of brown, tan, or black are often the first sign of melanoma. As melanomas progress, the colors red, white, and blue may appear.
Diameter. Early melanomas tend to grow larger than common moles, generally to at least the size of a pencil eraser (about 6 mm or 1/4″ in diameter).
Evolving. Malignant melanoma changes over time with changes in color and size.

BENIGN GROWTHS THAT CAN BE CONFUSED WITH SKIN CANCERS

Some benign pigmented lesions that may be confused with melanoma include acquired nevi, congenital nevi, seborrheic keratoses, dermatofibromas, and lentigines. It is important to learn the appearance and characteristics of these benign lesions to differentiate them from melanoma. When there is a reasonable suspicion that the lesion is malignant and not one of these benign lesions, a biopsy should be performed.

Sebaceous hyperplasia may look like a BCC. These benign lesions are raised and can have pearly borders and telangiectasias like a BCC. When you are uncertain of the diagnosis, a shave biopsy can remove the lesion and determine whether it is malignant. Completely benign-appearing sebaceous hyperplasia is a cosmetic issue that can be treated electively if desired.

Seborrheic keratosis can mimic melanoma. These lesions develop with age and are often large and pigmented with irregular borders (Color Plate Fig. 39.16). Although they usually are verrucous and have a stuck-on appearance, they can be flat and irregular. When uncertain of the diagnosis, a biopsy is needed.

KEY POINTS

- Look beyond the primary rash for clues to diagnose skin disorders.
- Impetigo is the most superficial bacterial skin infection and often appears with honey-crusted lesions. Tinea capitis should be treated with oral antifungal agents.
- Atopic dermatitis is a common inherited childhood disorder that may occur with other atopic conditions such as allergic rhinitis and asthma.
- Seborrheic dermatitis is a common inflammatory disorder especially found on the scalp and face. Treating the Malassezia overgrowth and the inflammation helps to diminish the dermatitis.
- Do not treat psoriasis with oral or systemic steroids. This can precipitate a life threatening case of generalized pustular psoriasis.
- Topical retinoids are excellent to treat all types of acne and should be considered as the primary treatment in comedonal acne.

CHAPTER

40

Skin Wounds: Contusions, Abrasions, Lacerations, and Ulcers

Richard P. Usatine

CLINICAL OBJECTIVES

1. Describe the differences between contusions, abrasions, lacerations, and ulcers.
2. Discuss the benefits of using epinephrine combined with lidocaine for local anesthesia.
3. List methods to make local anesthesia less painful for the patient.
4. Discuss the use of nonabsorbable and absorbable sutures for laceration repair.

EVALUATION

Family physicians frequently treat skin injuries. This chapter discusses treatment of the most common skin wounds, including contusions, abrasions, lacerations, and ulcerations. For all skin injuries, begin with a good history and physical exam, including a pain assessment. If the skin injuries are secondary to trauma, start with an overall assessment of the patient before focusing on the skin wounds. Assure that the patient's circulatory and respiratory systems have been stabilized if they have been compromised, and control bleeding before any repair is initiated. (The assessment of major trauma is beyond the scope of this chapter, which focuses on the care of skin injuries in patients who are otherwise stable.) Figure 40.1 outlines a general approach to evaluation and treatment of skin injuries.

The key to evaluating skin wounds is to think carefully about the type of injury that occurred and the nearby structures that might be affected. Table 40.1 lists red flags that suggest a complicated wound. During your examination, palpate for a foreign body or fracture. Consider the possibility of injury to vital structures near the wound, such as nerves, tendons, or ducts (e.g., the parotid duct). Wounds involving electrical, thermal, or chemical injury require special evaluation and care, as do bites and puncture wounds. In limb injuries, rule out injury to peripheral motor and sensory nerves by performing and documenting a neurological exam of the involved extremities.

Examine the surrounding skin for evidence of preexisting pathology. For example, skin discoloration, edema, or atrophy may indicate venous, lymphatic, or arterial insufficiency. Loss of sensation, however, may allow the injury to go undetected at first. Muscle weakness or skeletal deformity may have contributed to the accident, and these problems can interfere with the healing process or produce recurrent injury. Explore the possibility of substance abuse or physical abuse if injuries are recurrent, or there are physical findings inconsistent with the history provided.

Plain radiographs or other imaging modalities should be used if deeper foreign bodies are suspected. Testing for immunity or exposure to communicable disease (e.g., HIV, hepatitis B) may be indicated if exposure to those conditions results from the injury. This is of particular concern for health care workers who sustain workplace injuries.

GENERAL MANAGEMENT

Pain

Keep in mind that patients who have had physical injuries and skin wounds are often in pain. Ask about pain and administer analgesics as needed to make the patient comfortable while you evaluate and treat the wounds. Often acetaminophen or a nonsteroidal anti-inflammatory drug (NSAID) may be adequate. If active bleeding is a problem, avoid use of aspirin and NSAIDs initially. For more painful injuries, discuss the benefits and risks of opiate analgesics, such as codeine or hydrocodone, which can be combined with acetaminophen. Patients may need to go home with a limited prescription for an opiate analgesic depending on the extent of the injury. If the patient is in recovery from a history of substance abuse, discuss the risks of relapse and develop a plan to help the patient avoid relapse while still providing adequate pain control. Do not withhold needed pain medication simply because the patient has an addiction history.

Tetanus Immunization

Any time you treat a patient whose skin has been injured, remember to inquire about tetanus immunization status and give any indicated immunization. For tetanus-prone wounds

Figure 40.1 • Wound treatment algorithm.

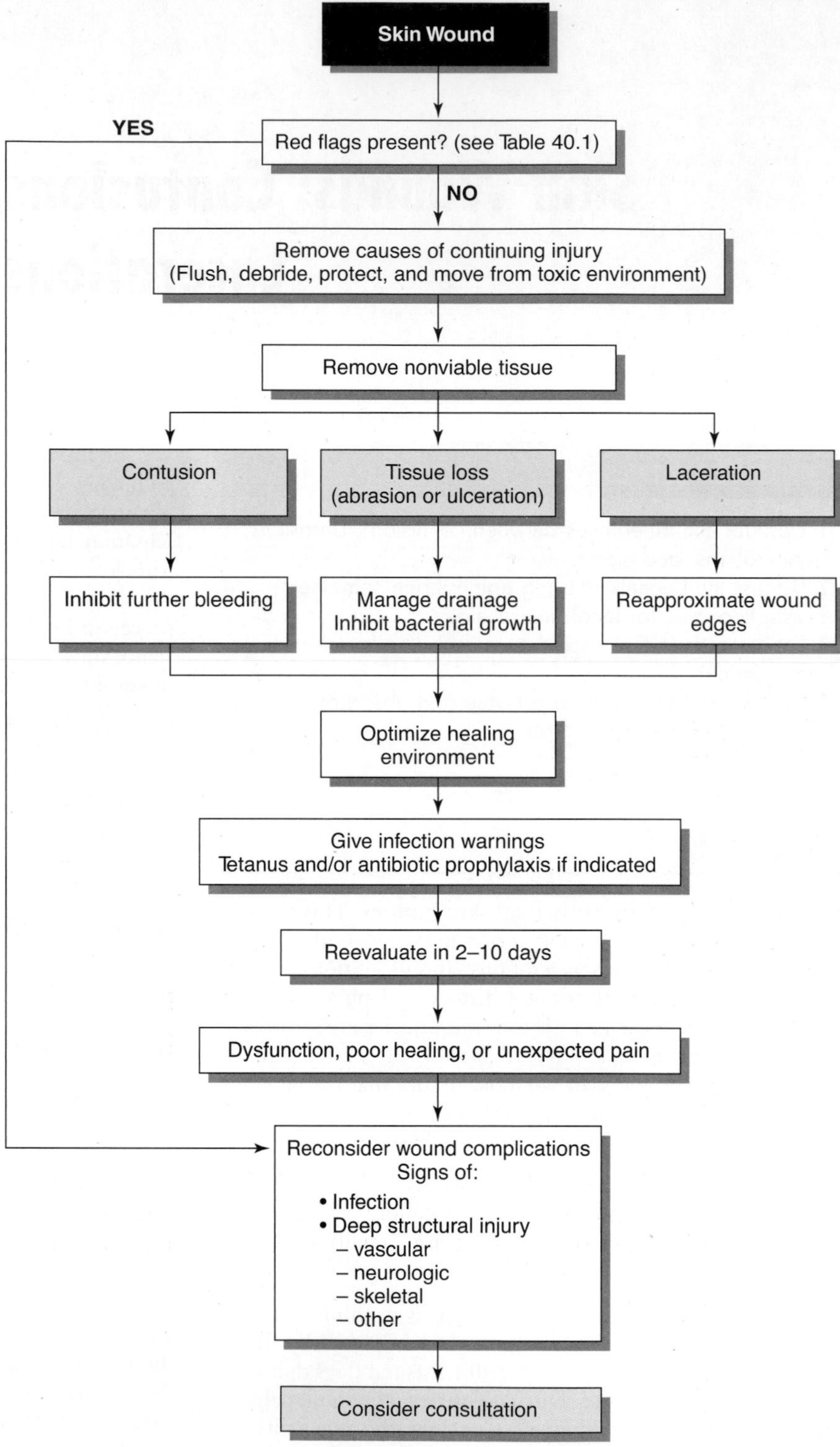

(characterized by the presence of contamination, devitalized tissue, puncture, muscle involvement, or more than 24 hours old), give a tetanus booster if the patient has not had one within 5 years; for clean wounds, the time allowance is 10 years. If the patient has not had a primary tetanus immunization series, also administer tetanus immune globulin for tetanus-prone wounds. Advise those patients lacking previous immunization (e.g., the elderly) to have a tetanus booster in 1 month and again in 6 to 12 months (1).

SPECIFIC INJURIES

Contusions

A contusion (bruise) results from trauma that injures underlying soft-tissue structures while leaving the epidermis intact. Cellular, vascular, and lymphatic damage causes blood and other fluids to leak into the tissue, producing swelling and

TABLE 40.1 Inspection of Red Flags in Skin Wounds

Sign	Check for
Deformity, severe swelling, increased pain on stressing bone	Fracture
Inability to visualize wound extent	Injury to deep structure
Difficulty controlling bleeding	Injury to large vessel
Altered function	Injury to nerve or musculoskeletal structures

discoloration (ecchymosis). A hematoma occurs when enough extravasated blood collects to produce a palpable knot.

Large bruises can take weeks to resolve, particularly if there is accompanying hematoma formation. The area of ecchymosis will gradually change from blue or purple to yellow-brown as the blood is converted to hematin and reabsorbed. These ecchymoses may travel to more dependent areas. Hematomas around the knee or calf, for example, will often lead to ecchymoses of the ankle or foot. Hematomas usually clot and become quite firm; they may become red, warm, and tender as the clot liquefies. At this stage they may appear to be infected, although this is seldom the case. To reduce patients' concerns during healing, instruct them about the sequential changes they can expect.

Initially, minimize hemorrhage and edema by elevating the affected part and applying pressure and ice. In general, do not aspirate or otherwise drain hematomas because they may recur, or you may introduce infection or both. Consider an underlying hemostatic disorder if the amount of bleeding seems out of proportion to the injury, but remember that tissue fragility normally increases as people age, and that many people take aspirin and NSAIDs on a regular basis; both aspirin and NSAIDs will inhibit platelet function.

Recommend applying cold for 5 to 30 minutes several times daily until swelling has stopped, usually for at least 48 hours after the injury (strength of recommendation [SOR] = C). Refreezable chemical gel ice packs are commercially available, but bags of crushed ice or frozen peas work equally well. Advise the patient that hematomas generally will be resorbed over several weeks if there is no reinjury. Rarely, hematomas in muscle will develop myositis ossificans with calcification of the involved tissue.

Abrasions

Abrasions are caused by scraping trauma that removes epidermis. For example, accidents that cause a person to slide on pavement are frequent causes of severe abrasions. These injuries tend to be quite painful because many nerve endings are exposed. As in a second-degree burn, the loss of epidermis causes the skin to lose water through weeping and evaporation. These injuries are often over joint surfaces, and the scab that forms tends to crack open when the joint moves.

All abrasions should be cleaned with soap and water or another cleansing agent. Adequate cleaning of more severe abrasions may require anesthesia. Apply topical anesthetic agents for superficial abrasions, and use an injectable anesthetic (e.g., lidocaine) for deep or dirty wounds. Next, irrigate with sterile saline or a mild antiseptic solution. Use forceps or gauze to remove ground-in dirt or asphalt to prevent tattoo formation. One method for preventing a "road-rash tattoo" is to wrap petrolatum (i.e., Vaseline) gauze or gauze with Bacitracin around the fingers and wipe off the asphalt and other foreign material embedded in the skin (2).

Once the abrasion is clean, your goal is to keep the wound moist and free of infection until it has reepithelialized. Instruct the patient to apply petrolatum or a topical antibiotic such as Bacitracin. The abrasion can be covered with any type of clean nonstick dressing (3). Alternatively, semiocclusive, transparent wound coverings that hasten reepithelialization by retaining moisture while allowing oxygen to reach the wound are available over-the-counter and in many office settings. If the abraded area is extensive, see the patient every day or two until infection seems unlikely. Systemic antibiotic prophylaxis is generally not indicated, but if the exudate becomes purulent or there is spreading erythema, obtain a culture and start an appropriate antibiotic.

Lacerations

The goals of laceration repair are to achieve hemostasis, prevent infection, preserve function, restore appearance, and minimize patient discomfort (2). When repairing a skin laceration, it is helpful to understand the three phases of wound healing. In **Phase 1** (initial lag phase, days 0 to 5), there is no gain in wound strength. A rapid increase in wound strength occurs in **Phase 2** (fibroplasia phase, days 5 to 14). At 2 weeks, the wound has achieved only 7% of its final strength. **Phase 3** (final maturation phase) begins around day 14 and continues until healing is complete. During this phase further connective tissue remodeling occurs, and the wound gains up to 80% of normal skin strength (2).

Nonabsorbable skin sutures or staples are used to give the wound strength during the initial two phases. After the nonabsorbable skin sutures are removed, wound closure tapes or previously placed deep, absorbable sutures may play an important role in the final phases of wound healing.

Indications for immediate wound closure include lacerations that are open and <18 hours old (<24 hours old on the face) as well as bite wounds in cosmetically important areas. Close follow-up is recommended in the latter situation. Contraindications to immediate wound closure include puncture wounds, wounds >18 hours old (>24 hours old on the face), and animal or human bite wounds (exceptions include facial wounds and large wounds from dog bites).

Each laceration needs to be evaluated to determine if it requires closure and which closure method will be work best. Choices include sutures, staples, tapes, or glue (tissue adhesive). Tapes such as Steri-Strips or a tissue adhesive may be adequate when the laceration is superficial and/or the patient is a child who would need sedation for a surgical repair. Table 40.2 lists the essentials for wound assessment.

A Cochrane systematic review found that tissue adhesives are acceptable alternatives to standard wound closure for repairing simple traumatic lacerations. They offer decreased procedure time and less pain compared with standard wound closure with sutures. A small but statistically significant

TABLE 40.2 Essentials of Wound Assessment (2)

Assessment	Comment or Example
Mechanism of injury	Sharp versus blunt trauma, bite
Dirty versus clean	Barnyard versus kitchen sink
Time since injury	Suture up to 18 hours after injury; 24 hours after injury on face
Foreign body	Explore and obtain radiograph for metal or glass
Functional examination	Check neurovascular, muscular, tendon functions
Need for prophylactic antibiotics	If needed, give as soon as possible and cover *Staphylococcus aureus*

increased rate of dehiscence (wound opening) with tissue adhesives is observed (4). Staples are also faster to place than sutures and are particularly good for closing scalp lacerations (5). Both staples and tissue adhesives are often more expensive than standard sutures and therefore may not be available in all medical settings.

Inspection, evaluation, cleaning, and treatment of larger lacerations require adequate anesthesia. Lidocaine in 1% (10 mg/mL) or 2% concentration is the most commonly used anesthetic solution. Using lidocaine with epinephrine is very helpful to decrease bleeding, minimize the risk of lidocaine toxicity, and prolong anesthesia. Epinephrine is generally avoided for digital blocks but there is no evidence that it needs to be avoided for local injection on the fingers, toes, earlobes, or penis in patients with normal circulation. Adequate anesthesia is generally obtained in a few minutes (the maximal epinephrine effect may take 10 minutes). Safe maximum dosage of plain lidocaine is 4 mg/kg of body weight and for lidocaine with epinephrine it is 7 mg/kg. The pain of injecting local anesthetic can be minimized by using a small-gauge needle (27 or 30 gauge), injecting slowly and directly into the dermis through the open wound (not through intact skin), using anesthetic warmed to body temperature, and buffering the anesthetic with sodium bicarbonate (9 parts lidocaine to 1 part bicarbonate) (2).

In some areas, a nerve block may be more effective than local injection. Circumferential blocks work well for injuries of the ear and nose. Block of the mental nerve produces good anesthesia to the lower lip and chin. For repairs on fingers or toes, usually a digital block is used. This is accomplished by anesthetizing the dorsal and ventral nerve branches on each side of the affected digit. To perform a digital block, use 3 mL 2% lidocaine without epinephrine, and a 27-gauge needle. Inject at the base of the digit and as you direct the needle toward the plantar surface inject 1 mL of lidocaine around both branches of the digital nerve and repeat with 1 mL on the other side (Fig. 40.2). It is helpful to add an additional 1 mL of lidocaine across the top of the digit to prevent pain carried by the smaller digital nerves that traverse this area.

After adequate anesthesia is obtained, the wound can be inspected and cleaned. An antiseptic solution, such as povidone-iodine (Betadine) or chlorhexidine (Hibiclens), may be used for initial cleaning of the surrounding skin, but not in the wound. If significant contamination with bacteria or chemicals is suspected, flush the wound profusely with sterile saline. Cleaning of the wound should be done by irrigation with normal saline. This can be accomplished by attaching an 18-gauge angiocatheter or a commercially available splash shield to a 30-mL syringe. At least 200 mL of irrigation is recommended (SOR=C). Alternatively, an intravenous bag with a compression device can be used to provide a high-pressure stream through an angiocatheter or needle. Debride severely contaminated or nonviable tissue, but be especially sparing on the face, where significant tissue loss can result in deformity. Clipping hair from around the laceration can make suturing easier, but avoid shaving the skin, which can increase the risk of infection.

After the initial assessment and administration of local or regional anesthetic, wounds should be thoroughly inspected for foreign bodies, deep tissue layer damage, and injury to nerve, vessel, or tendon. A radiograph should be obtained to look for remaining glass or metal in wounds sustained with broken glass or metal. Complex wounds, or those in cosmetically important areas, should be closed by an experienced clinician.

The timing of wound closure is important. The risk of infection is lowest if a laceration is repaired soon after injury, although cleaned wounds generally do well if closed within 18 hours (6). If the wound is more than 18 to 24 hours old, it

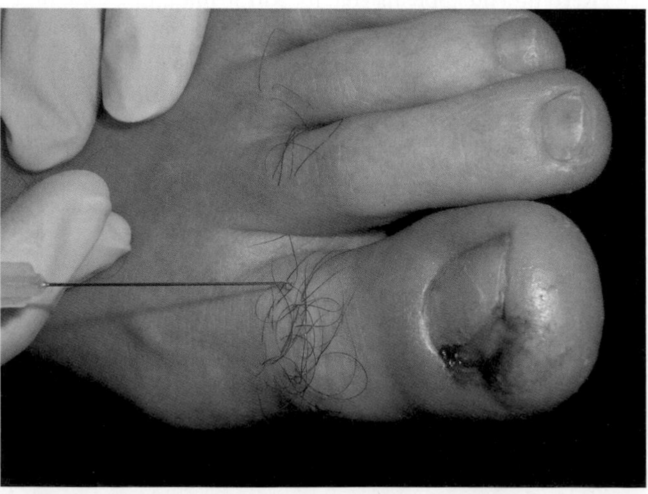

Figure 40.2 • Digital block being performed before partial resection of the toenail as treatment of an ingrown toenail. (Copyright Richard P. Usatine, MD).

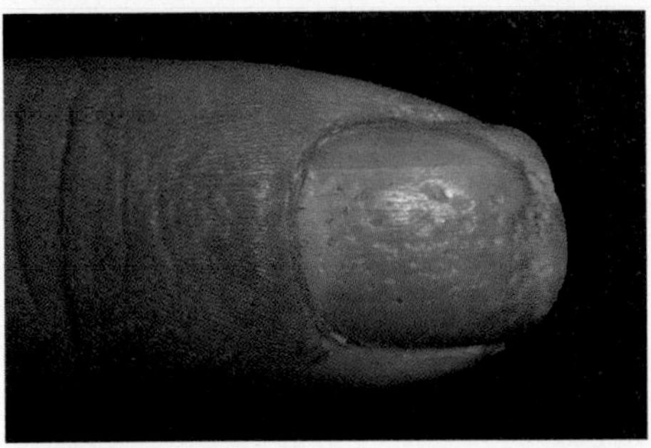

Figure 39.1 • Nail pitting found in a patient with psoriasis. (Copyright Richard P. Usatine, MD, and Courtesy of the Color Atlas of Family Medicine)

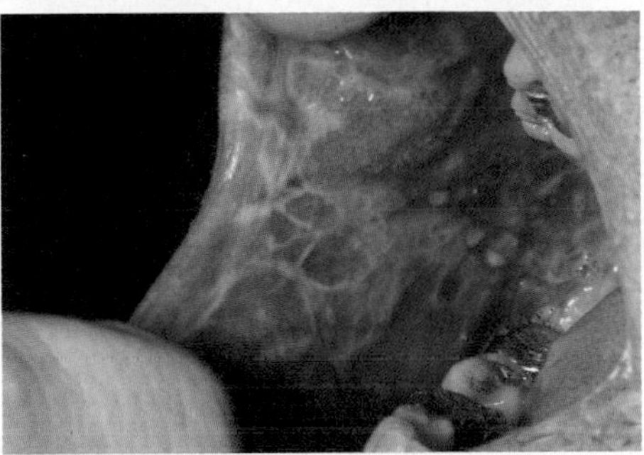

Figure 39.2 • Typical lacy white pattern on the buccal mucosa with lichen planus. (Copyright Richard P. Usatine, MD, and Courtesy of the Color Atlas of Family Medicine)

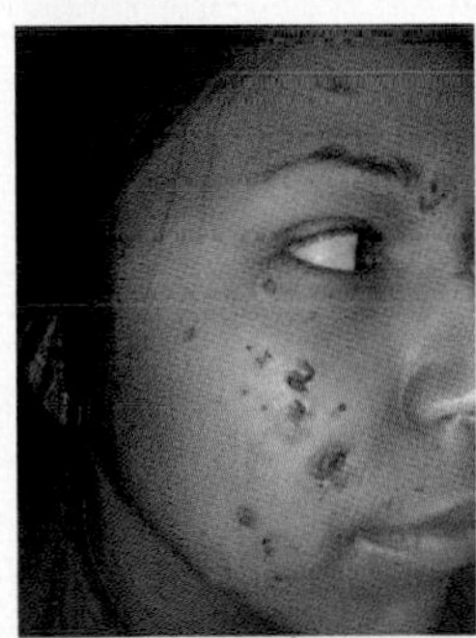

Figure 39.3 • Impetigo on the face with honey crusting. (Copyright Richard P. Usatine, MD, and Courtesy of the Color Atlas of Family Medicine)

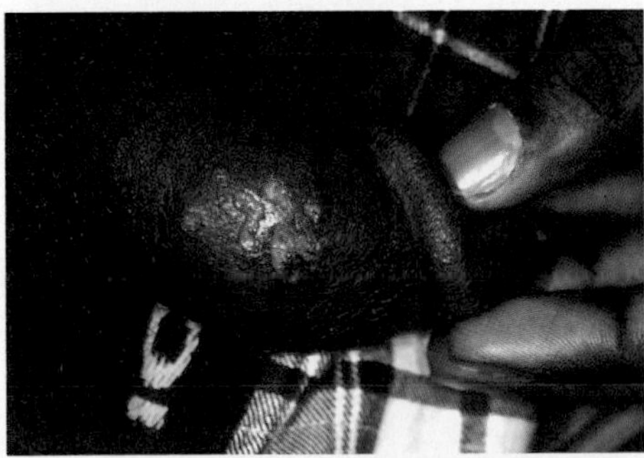

Figure 39.4 • Recurrent herpes simplex on the penis in the ulcerative stage. (Copyright Richard P. Usatine, MD, and Courtesy of the Color Atlas of Family Medicine)

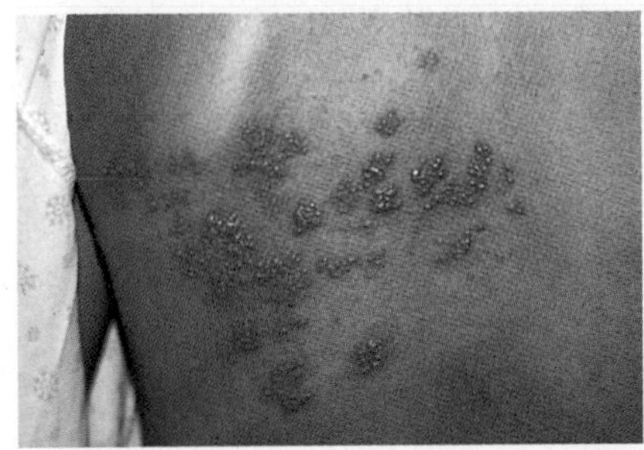

Figure 39.5 • Herpes zoster caused by the reactivation of the varicella zoster virus. Note the groups of vesicles in a unilateral dermatomal pattern. (Copyright Richard P. Usatine, MD, and Courtesy of the Color Atlas of Family Medicine)

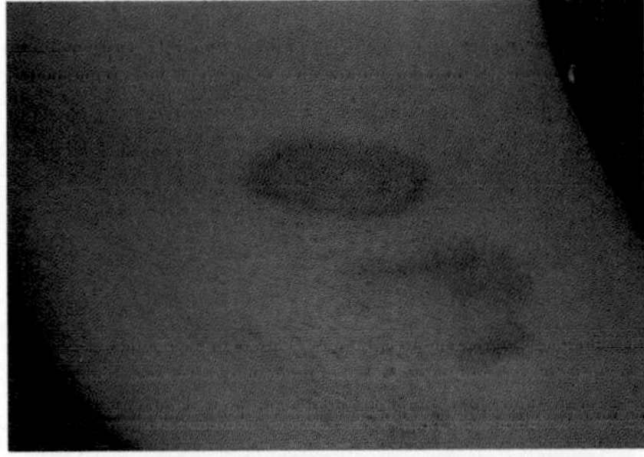

Figure 39.6 • Tinea corporis in the axilla of a young woman. Note the concentric circles, which is a very specific pattern seen with tinea corporis. (Copyright Richard P. Usatine, MD, and Courtesy of the Color Atlas of Family Medicine)

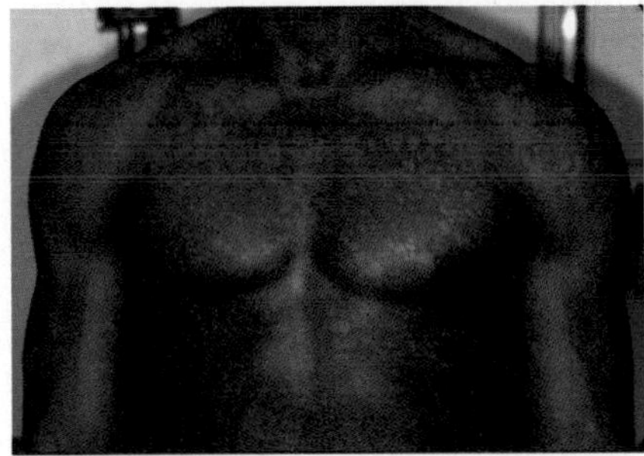

Figure 39.7 • Tinea versicolor causing hypopigmentation in a capelike distribution. (Copyright Richard P. Usatine, MD, and Courtesy of the Color Atlas of Family Medicine)

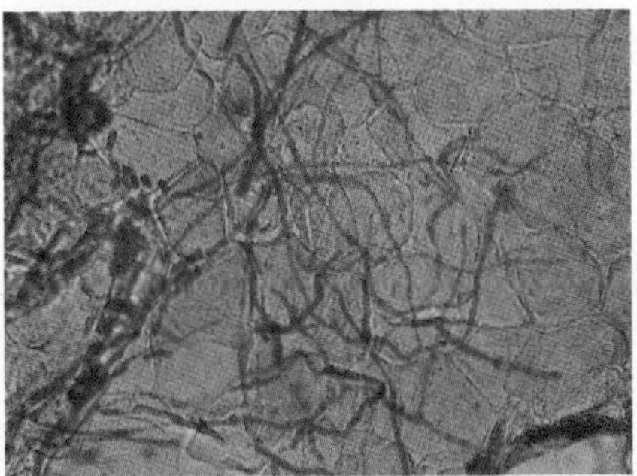

Figure 39.8 • Tinea corporis seen under high power after preparing with potassium hydroxide and a fungal stain. (Copyright Richard P. Usatine, MD)

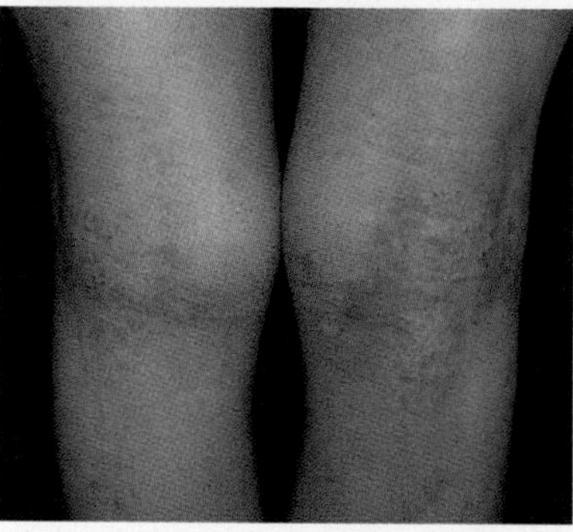

Figure 39.9 • Atopic dermatitis seen in the popliteal fossa of a young woman. Note the lichenification from years of scratching. (Copyright Richard P. Usatine, MD, and Courtesy of the Color Atlas of Family Medicine)

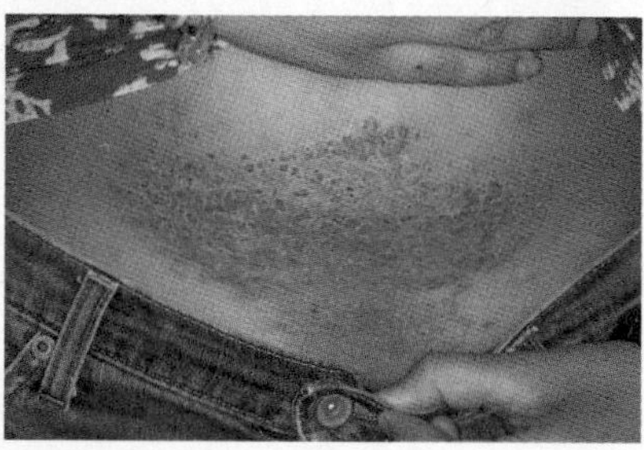

Figure 39.10 • Contact dermatitis to the metal of the pants' snap in a girl who also has atopic dermatitis. (Copyright Richard P. Usatine, MD, and Courtesy of the Color Atlas of Family Medicine)

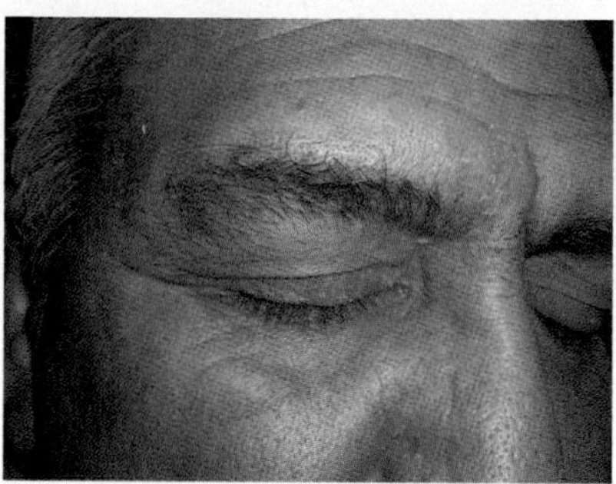

Figure 39.11 • Seborrheic dermatitis on the face in the typical distribution including the eyebrows, the glabella, and the alar crease. (Copyright Richard P. Usatine, MD)

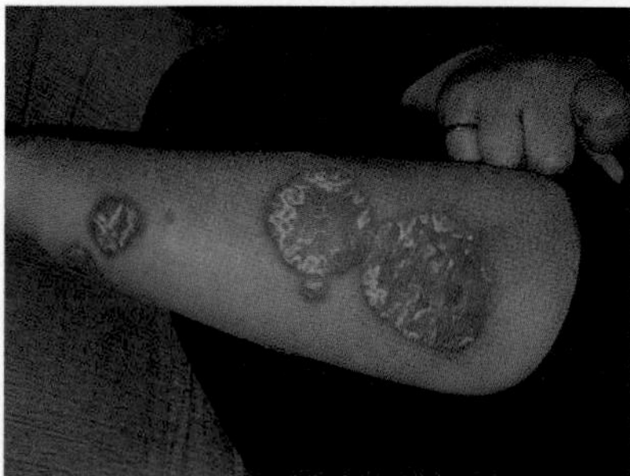

Figure 39.12 • Plaque psoriasis on the elbow and forearm. (Copyright Richard P. Usatine, MD, and Courtesy of the Color Atlas of Family Medicine)

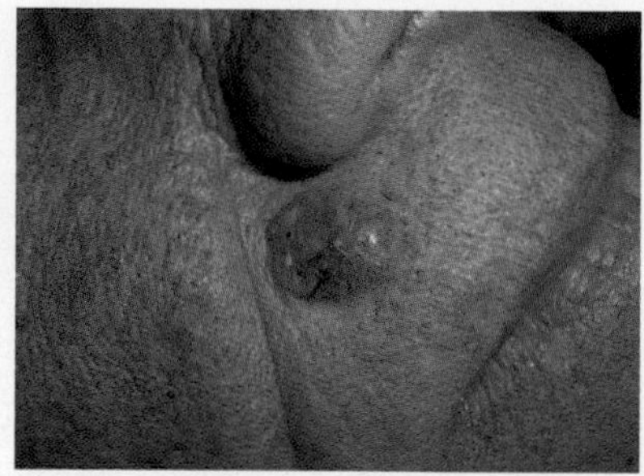

Figure 39.13 • Nodular basal cell carcinoma that appears pearly with telangiectasias. (Copyright Richard P. Usatine, MD)

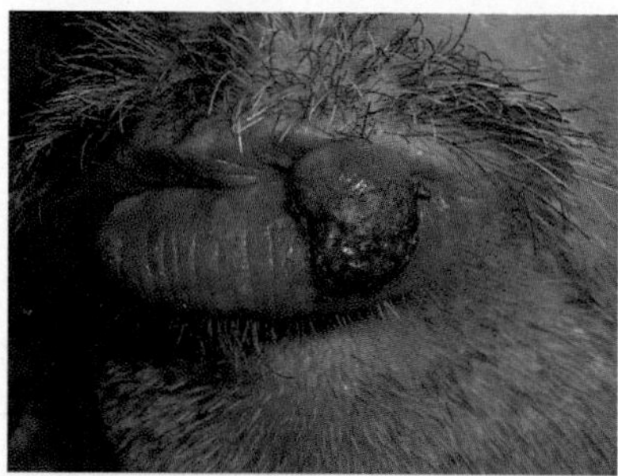

Figure 39.14 • A fast-growing squamous cell carcinoma on the lip of the patient who has had a transplant and is on immunosuppressive medication. (Copyright Richard P. Usatine, MD)

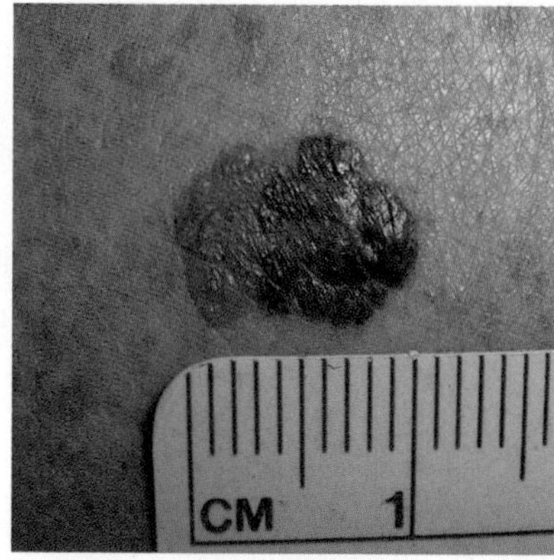

Figure 39.15 • Superficial spreading melanoma that is positive for all the ABCDE features. (Copyright Richard P. Usatine, MD, and Courtesy of the Color Atlas of Family Medicine)

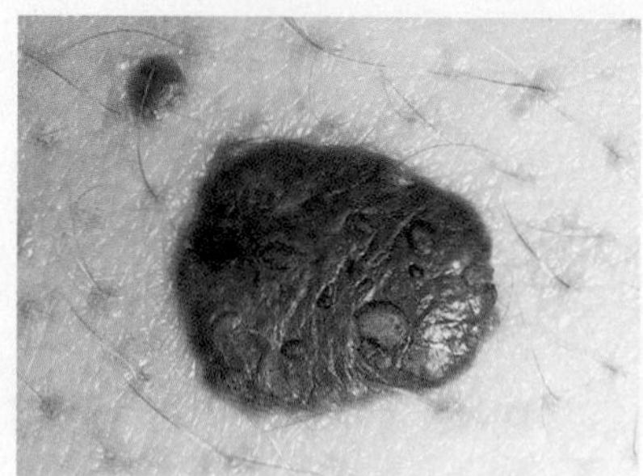

Figure 39.16 • Seborrheic keratosis with a stuck on appearance and typical horn cysts. (Copyright Richard P. Usatine, MD, and Courtesy of the Color Atlas of Family Medicine)

TABLE 40.3 Basic Supplies for Laceration Repair

Equipment	Uses
Gauze sponges	Absorbing blood and dressing wounds
Sterile gloves and eye protection	Protecting physician and patient from transfer of infectious organisms
Sterile drapes	Sterile field that sutures and instruments may contact
Adequate lighting	Complete visualization of wound
Toothed Adson forceps	Gentle grasp of tissues and foreign materials
Small hemostats	Closing bleeding vessels and grasping tissue
Smooth Adson forceps	Less traumatic grasp of tissues
Needle holder	Grasping the suture needle
Small Iris scissors	Cutting and undermining tissue
Scalpel with blade (no. 15)	Cutting tissue
Suture material and needle	Drawing wound edges together
Skin hooks (optional)	Pulling wound edges without damaging the surface

should simply be cleaned, inspected, and then dressed; suturing would promote infection by introducing foreign material and preventing drainage. If there is no sign of infection by the third to fifth day and approximation of wound edges is desirable, then the wound may be sutured at that time with the simultaneous use of prophylactic antibiotics (delayed primary closure).

WOUND REPAIR

Preparation

Having inspected and cleansed the wound and decided that it is appropriate to close the wound surgically, make certain that all potentially necessary instruments and supplies are at hand. Table 40.3 lists basic supplies for laceration repair. Table 40.4 suggests suture sizes for various body locations.

A number of suture materials are available, and each has its advantages. Monofilament nylon (Ethilon, Dermalon) or polypropylene (Prolene) sutures produce less skin reactivity and fewer infections. These are nonabsorbable and are used for closing most lacerations. Soft sutures (silk) cause less discomfort on mucosal surfaces (such as the lip or tongue) than the stiffer monofilaments. Absorbable materials chromic gut, polyglactin (Vicryl) are used for subsurface, deep, or mucosal repair.

Attached to the suture is a curved needle, the size and shape of which are generally shown on the package. A reverse-cutting, plastics grade needle (labeled P) is appropriate in most circumstances. Grip it with a needle holder approximately one third of the way from the blunt end. The proper grasp (Fig. 40.3) and following the curve of the needle when placing the suture will minimize needle bending.

After the wound is anesthetized and cleaned, and you have positioned the patient and your instruments, you are ready to put on sterile gloves and drape the wound. At this point, examine the wound carefully and plan your repair. Trim wound edges so that they are parallel, only if this can be done without removing essential tissue. Sharp scissors or a scalpel may be used to cut perpendicular to the skin surface when trimming is needed. Make excisions in hair-bearing skin parallel to the hair shafts to avoid damage to the follicles. After evaluating the wound, if you do not believe you can perform an optimum repair, consult a surgeon who has the necessary skills.

Suturing Techniques

Appropriate closure technique varies according to the depth of the laceration and the body area involved. Single-layer closure

TABLE 40.4 Guidelines for Suture Selection and Timing of Suture Removal

Location	Suture Size for Skin Closure	Days to Removal
Face	5-0 or 6-0	4–5
Scalp	3-0 or 4-0	5–7
Trunk and extremities	4-0 or 5-0	7–10
Over joint surfaces	3-0 or 4-0	10–14

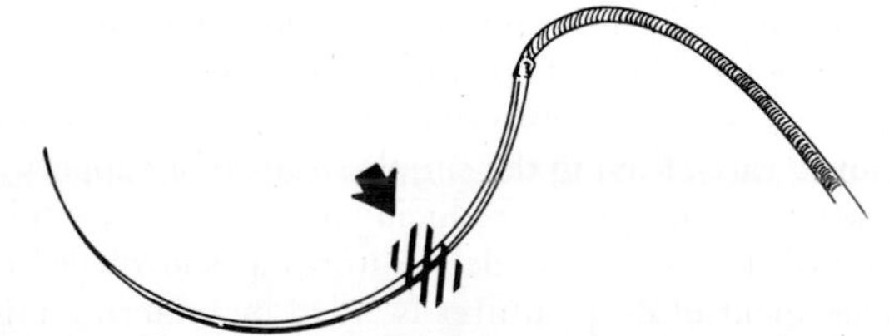

Figure 40.3 • Correct position for grasping a suture needle. This position provides enough length to rotate the needle through soft tissues, but is far enough forward to minimize bending.

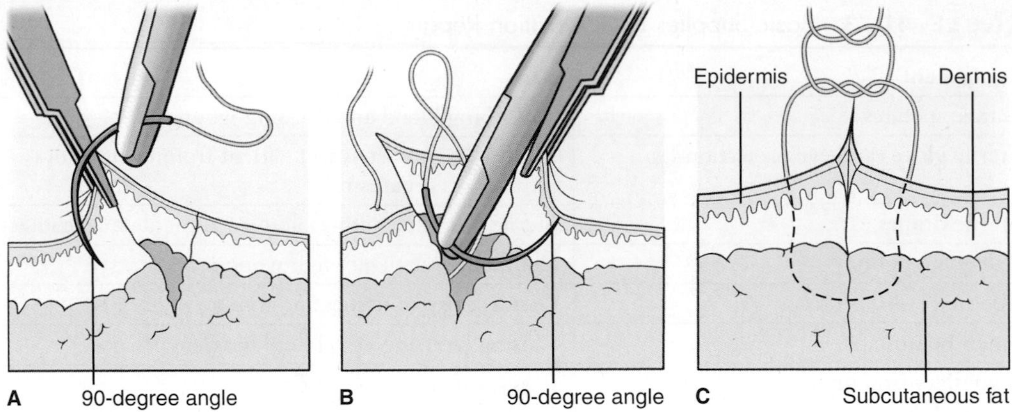

Figure 40.4 • Proper skin suture technique. **A.** Perpendicular insertion of the needle is aided by pulling back on the skin with the forceps. **B.** The reloaded needle is inserted upward through the fat and dermis to come out at a 90-degree angle to the epidermis. **C.** The final suture path has a modified flask shape to promote eversion of the skin edges and improved healing.

is used for superficial wounds and in areas with little subcutaneous tissue, such as the digits and backs of the hands. It is also useful on the scalp, where hemostasis can be a problem. Layered repair is better for deeper wounds, particularly in cosmetically sensitive areas such as the face. Also a two-layered closure is great to prevent dehiscence in areas in which there will be tension on the wound.

Principles of proper suture placement are shown in Figure 40.4. The goal is to gently evert the skin for better wound healing and cosmesis. This is done by creating a loop that is as wide at the bottom as near the skin surface. You can facilitate this by pulling back on the edge of the skin with forceps or skin hooks while pushing the needle through the skin at a 90-degree angle to the surface. Next, rotate your wrist to bring the needle up through the opposite wound edge, going wider in the deeper tissue. This can be facilitated by putting pressure on the skin with the tip of the forceps before puncturing up through the skin.

Usually sutures are placed as far apart as they are wide. In areas of skin tension, one may place sutures closer together and closer to the wound edge. Figure 40.5 shows this principle in the closure of an ellipse. A wound can be closed by halving it or starting at one end and working toward the other end.

A valuable method in lacerations with widely separated edges under tension is to place deep sutures first or use a vertical mattress suture (Fig. 40.6). The deep stitches will hold the dermis together for weeks, with suture that will dissolve over time. The alternative is to use vertical mattress sutures that provide greater strength and better approximation of tissue. Because they tend to heal leaving visible suture marks, alternate them with simple sutures. The mattress sutures can then be removed early, leaving the simple sutures for support.

The best technique for reducing tension on a wound is to place absorbable buried or deep sutures as shown in Figure 40.7. Placement of deep sutures is aided by undermining the tissue below the layer being closed. In part A of Figure 40.7, undermining has been performed in the fatty layer. It is best to use the scissors in a spreading motion to minimize vascular and nerve disruption, then place sutures so that the knots are buried. After the wound edges are brought together with the first layer of buried sutures the second layer of closure is accomplished with simple interrupted sutures or a running stitch.

V-shaped lacerations are repaired with the technique shown in Figure 40.8 or by using tissue adhesive, to minimize risk of compromise to the blood supply at the tip of the flap. The dog's ear deformity (standing cone) results when you have more skin on one side than the other toward the end of the wound, despite efforts to separate sutures by equal distances on both sides. The longer side tends to rise, making it difficult to approximate the edges without bunching on that side. Repair is performed as shown in Figure 40.9. Make the wound

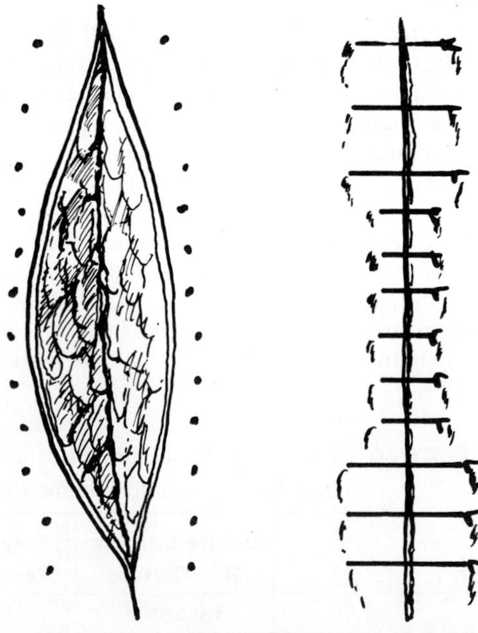

Figure 40.5 • Closure of an ellipse. Suturing is begun at one end of the wound. As the middle is approached, sutures are placed closer to each other and closer to the wound edge to minimize tension on each stitch.

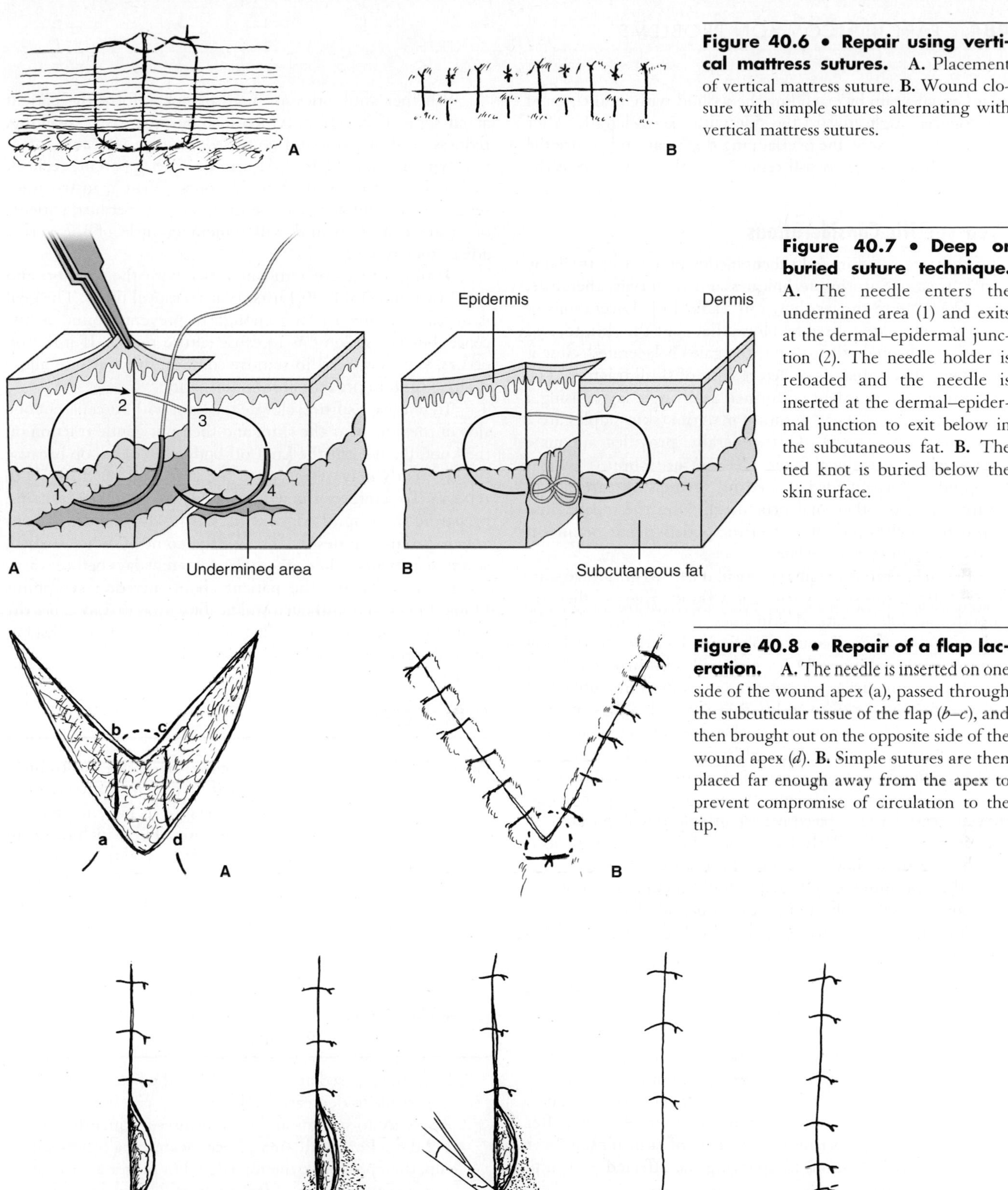

Figure 40.6 • Repair using vertical mattress sutures. **A.** Placement of vertical mattress suture. **B.** Wound closure with simple sutures alternating with vertical mattress sutures.

Figure 40.7 • Deep or buried suture technique. **A.** The needle enters the undermined area (1) and exits at the dermal–epidermal junction (2). The needle holder is reloaded and the needle is inserted at the dermal–epidermal junction to exit below in the subcutaneous fat. **B.** The tied knot is buried below the skin surface.

Figure 40.8 • Repair of a flap laceration. **A.** The needle is inserted on one side of the wound apex (a), passed through the subcuticular tissue of the flap (*b–c*), and then brought out on the opposite side of the wound apex (*d*). **B.** Simple sutures are then placed far enough away from the apex to prevent compromise of circulation to the tip.

Figure 40.9 • Repair of the "dog ear." **A.** Sometimes, as a wound is being sutured, one side ends up with more remaining tissue than the other, which creates an unsightly bulge called a dog ear. **B.** To begin repair of a dog ear, a marking incision is made 45 degrees from the end of the wound toward the longer side. **C.** Scissors are used to cut along the marking, and then used to undermine the shaded area. **D.** The longer skin edge is pulled across the incision line, and the resulting triangle of skin is excised along the line of overlap. **E.** The even skin edges can now be easily sutured.

edges equal again by extending the wound with an incision at a 45-degree angle toward the side with excess length. After undermining, excise the overlapping dog's ear and suture the incision. If some excess still remains on that side, repeat the process.

Area-specific Considerations

The character of skin and subcutaneous tissue over the body varies greatly. Suturing techniques and materials, therefore, vary from site to site, as shown in Table 40.4. Lacerations of the scalp often are caused by blows that split the skin to, and sometimes through, the galea. If the galea is lacerated, close it as a layer, after palpating to detect signs of skull fracture. The remaining closure is best performed as a single layer, using a large needle and 3-0 or 4-0 suture material (skin staples are a good alternative here). This generally provides adequate hemostasis if occasional large bleeders are clipped with a hemostat and coagulated or tied off (exercising care not to injure nerves or other vital structures). After the repair, rinse as much blood as possible out of the patient's hair because it can be difficult to remove later.

Facial lacerations require particular care to minimize scarring. Using tissue scissors trim the wound edges so they are smooth and follow natural skin lines, if this can be done by removing only a small amount of tissue. Use the layered skin closure shown in Figure 40.7, which will minimize tension on the surface. For surface suturing, use thin (6-0) monofilament sutures and remove them early, replacing with adhesive strips (Steri-Strips). Mark landmarks, such as the vermilion border of the lips, before they are obscured by injecting the anesthetic. The first suture can then be placed to assure correct alignment.

Lacerations of the tongue do not require repair, unless they are very large or bleed persistently despite application of ice and pressure. Similarly, lacerations of the oral mucosa usually heal well without suturing. Lacerations that penetrate from the skin into the oral cavity should include repair of the skin and muscle only, unless the mucosal defect is large. Leaving the mucosal surface open to heal secondarily reduces the chance of infection.

Aftercare

Petrolatum or antibiotic ointment is useful in wounds to promote healing by keeping the epithelium moist and reducing bacterial colonization (7). For draining wounds, apply a nonadherent material, such as Telfa, under a layer of cotton gauze. Tell patients to keep sutured wounds dry for 24 hours, after which showering is permitted. In areas of skin tension over joints, support lacerations by splinting the affected part until adequately healed.

Infection is the biggest threat to wound healing. As noted earlier, aggressive wound cleaning and tetanus prophylaxis are most effective at preventing infection. Antibiotics are not indicated for simple wounds (8), but many experts recommend their use when a bone, tendon, or joint space has been penetrated, and for heavily contaminated wounds (SOR=C).

When cosmetically important, selected animal bites may be closed after careful cleansing (9). Human bites require particularly careful cleaning and observation because of the large number of bacteria in saliva; generally these wounds should be treated as infected from the onset.

Whether antibiotics are used or not, inform the patient about signs of infection, which include progressive swelling, redness, heat or pain, and increased drainage. Because infection typically takes 1 to 3 days to become apparent, recheck high-risk lacerations at 48 to 72 hours. Written instructions regarding wound care can be quite helpful because patients often are distressed and will remember little of the verbal advice they receive.

Timing of suture removal varies with the location and type of wound. Table 40.4 lists suture removal times. The goal is to leave sutures in long enough to prevent wound dehiscence, but not so long as to cause suture marks. If infection occurs, you may need to remove some sutures early to allow drainage and to prevent abscess formation.

To remove a suture, elevate the knot with forceps, cut one side of the loop near the skin, and then put gentle traction on the knot. Do not cut the knot off both sides of a loop because the free ends may retract into the skin and be difficult to retrieve. To reinforce the wound, apply sterile adhesive strips, preparing the wound edges with Mastisol or tincture of benzoin to promote adhesion. These strips come off when soaked, so advise patients to keep them dry for a few days before washing them off. Warn the patient about infection symptoms (Table 40.5) and that the natural healing process may cause the wound to look red and swollen over the first few months, but within 6 months, it will have improved.

SKIN ULCERS

Acute skin ulcerations may be caused by accidental trauma, but also by excessive scratching in a patient with pruritus. Many skin ulcers are caused by pressure in patients that are immobilized or have impaired sensation. These include decubitus ulcers in the elderly and in patients with spinal cord injuries. Diabetic foot ulcers are caused by lack of protective sensation and occur in areas of wounds or increased pressure. Ulceration caused by systemic illness (e.g., ischemic emboli

TABLE 40.5 Injury Care Instructions for Patients

1. Keep the injured area raised above the heart as much as possible to decrease swelling.
2. Apply ice to sprains and deep bruises frequently for 1–2 days. For small areas, freeze water in a Styrofoam cup, then peel back the top edge. For larger areas, use an ice pack or a bag of frozen vegetables. A layer of cloth will prevent frostbite to the skin.
3. Inspect wounds daily for signs of infection (fever, swelling, or spreading redness and tenderness). If signs of infection develop or the wound starts to pull apart return for evaluation.
4. Keep any splints or pressure dressings on until instructed to remove them.
5. Return to our office to have your wound(s) checked in ____ days. Return to our office for suture removal in _____ days.

TABLE 40.6 Evidence for Treatment Recommendations for Venous Stasis Ulcers

Treatment Strategy	Strength of Recommendation*	Comments
Compression bandaging	A	Higher pressure is better, as long as arterial compression is avoided
Layered compression bandaging	B	No data to prove better than single-layer bandage
Oral pentoxifylline	B	No cost-effectiveness data
Cultured skin grafts	C	Very expensive
Recombinant growth factor (Regranex)	C	Indicated in diabetic ulcers, very expensive

*A = consistent, good-quality patient-oriented evidence; B = inconsistent or limited-quality patient-oriented evidence; C = consensus, disease-oriented evidence, usual practice, expert opinion, or case series.
For information about the SORT evidence rating system, see *www.aafp.org/afpsort.xml.*

from vasculitis or disseminated infection) is treated by addressing the underlying disorder.

Ulceration produces skin defects that are not amenable to simple surgical approximation; healing requires growth of epidermal tissue into the damaged area. This growth occurs most rapidly in oxygen-rich, moist environments where leukocytes are allowed to accumulate. Frequent cleansing, particularly with cytotoxic solutions such as povidone-iodine (e.g., Betadine) or chlorhexidine (e.g., Hibiclens), only delays healing.

Venous stasis dermatitis can result in particularly refractory ulcerations of the lower legs. Venous congestion results from damage to the deep veins draining the lower legs. It occurs after injury or, more commonly, after deep vein thrombosis. Treatment of these ulcers requires a huge expenditure of medical resources worldwide. Table 40.6 shows the evidence supporting various treatments.

Effective treatment of venous stasis ulcers requires limb elevation and compression to reduce tissue edema. Care must be taken to avoid wrapping so tightly that arterial circulation is compromised. Layered wraps have not been proven more effective than single-layer Unna wrappings using zinc paste–impregnated gauze (10); however, absorptive layers may be necessary to prevent frequent dressing changes caused by excessive exudate. Pentoxiphylline (Trental) has been associated with more rapid healing (11). Elastic compression stockings, elevation, and protection from trauma help to prevent recurrence after ulcers are healed.

KEY POINTS

- The key to evaluating skin wounds is to think carefully about the type of injury that occurred and the nearby structures that might be affected such as nerves, tendons, or ducts.
- The goals of laceration repair are hemostasis, prevention of infection, preservation of function, restoration of appearance and minimization of patient discomfort.
- Contraindications to immediate wound closure include wounds >18 hours old (>24 hours old on the face) and animal and human bite wounds (exceptions include facial wounds and large wounds from dog bites).
- A two-layered repair is better for deeper wounds, particularly in cosmetically sensitive areas such as the face and is great to prevent dehiscence in areas in which there will be tension on the wound.
- Effective treatment of venous stasis ulcers requires limb elevation and compression to reduce tissue edema.

ACKNOWLEDGMENT

I would like to acknowledge Wayne A. Hale, MD, for the work he did on the initial creation of this chapter.

CHAPTER

41

Chronic Nonmalignant Pain

Robert Jackman and Janey M. Purvis

CLINICAL OBJECTIVES

1. Describe and define chronic nonmalignant pain (CNMP).
2. Discuss the mechanisms underlying common chronic pain syndromes.
3. Outline a systematic approach to the patient with CNMP.
4. Discuss how to develop an appropriate treatment plan for CNMP.
5. Understand the benefits, risks, and appropriate use of opioid medications.
6. Address difficult issues arising during long-term CNMP management.

Chronic nonmalignant pain (CNMP) is one of the most common problems seen in family medicine, and one of the most difficult to manage (1). Surveys indicate that more than 50 million Americans suffer from chronic pain, at an economic burden of $85 to $90 billion annually (2). Concurrent with our aging population, we can expect a marked increase in the already overwhelming numbers of CNMP patients seeking treatment from family physicians and other primary care providers (3,4).

The past 10 years have witnessed a proliferation of pain guidelines, regulations, specialized clinics, research, pain journals, and the development of specialized training in pain medicine (3,5). Despite this, inadequate pain management in primary care persists, often because of physician barriers of lack of knowledge about treatment, inadequate pain assessment skills, and fears of regulatory scrutiny (6). It is imperative for family physicians to have a comprehensive, systematic approach to this complex and common issue.

General Approach to Treatment of Chronic Nonmalignant Pain

Common causes of CNMP that a family medicine physician will care for include: chronic neck and low back pain, migraine and other headache syndromes, osteoarthritis, fibromyalgia, chronic abdominal and pelvic pain, diabetic neuropathy, post-herpetic neuralgia, phantom pain secondary to disease or injury of the nervous system, post-stroke pain, multiple sclerosis, and mixed pain syndromes.

A systematic approach to CNMP includes a comprehensive evaluation, development of a treatment plan determined by the diagnosis and mechanisms, patient education and realistic goal setting (7,8). The main goal of treatment is to improve quality of life and increase function while decreasing pain. An initial comprehensive pain assessment is essential to the development of a treatment plan that addresses the physical, social, functional, and psychological needs of the patient (9). Successful treatment requires a fine balance between pain relief and improvement in quality of life on the one hand, and medication side effects and risks on the other.

Obstacles to appropriate pain management include diversion, abuse and addiction of opioid medications, lack of knowledge, concerns about opioid side effects, and fears of regulatory scrutiny (10–12). These may be overcome by adherence to the Federation of State Medical Boards guidelines for evaluating the physician's treatment of pain, including the use of controlled substances (available at *www.fsmb.org/grpol_pain_policy_resource_center.html*). Among the key components emphasized in these guidelines (Table 41.1) are: appropriate evaluation of the patient; development of a written treatment plan; informed consent and agreement for treatment (including use of urine/serum drug screening when requested, number and frequency of prescription refills, and reasons for which drug treatment may be discontinued); periodic review and monitoring for adherence, aberrant behaviors, and side effects; consultation when appropriate; accurate and complete medical records; and compliance with controlled substance laws and regulations (7,13).

When psychiatric comorbidities are present, risk of substance abuse is high, or pain management requires specialized treatments or consultation, referral to a pain management specialist can be helpful and is appropriate (11,14).

A Field in Evolution

Over the past 2 decades, perceptions of the public, of clinicians, and of regulators have shifted from treating too infrequently to treating too frequently. During the 1990s and beyond, advocates were increasingly vocal for better management of acute and chronic pain, with the goal of relieving suffering and improving quality of life (15). This movement manifested itself in such things as introduction of pain as a vital sign, routine questioning of patients about pain, and the promotion of pain management as a legal right (16).

In recent years, however, the pendulum has begun to shift. Reasons for this swing include belief that chronic long-term opioid therapy may not result in the return to function as expected, diversion of opioid prescriptions for nonmedical use, and untoward side effects such as hyperalgesia, hypogonadism in males, and constipation (15). Another serious concern is the increase in opioid-related overdoses and deaths. Between 1999 and 2006, the number of poisoning deaths in the United States nearly doubled, from approximately 20,000 to 37,000, largely because of overdose deaths involving prescription opioid

TABLE 41.1 Federation of State Medical Boards Criteria for Evaluating the Physician's Treatment of Pain, Including the Use of Controlled Substances (7)*

1. Evaluation of the patient
   Perform and document a medical history and physical that includes:
   - Nature/intensity of pain
   - Current/past treatment for pain
   - Underlying/coexisting disease or conditions
   - Effect of pain on function (physical/psychological)
   - History of substance abuse
   - Document if a controlled substance is indicated medically
2. Treatment plan
   A written treatment plan should:
   - State objectives to determine success
   - State if further diagnostic tests are indicated
   - Address psychosocial as well as physical function
   - Adjust therapy to meet needs of patient
   - Use treatment modalities in addition to medications
3. Informed consent and agreement for treatment
   - Discuss risks/benefits of drug therapy with patient or surrogate
   - Patient should receive prescriptions from one physician and pharmacy whenever possible
   - High risk patients should have a written agreement that includes:
     1. Urine drug screens when requested
     2. Written documentation of refill numbers and frequency
     3. Reasons for which drug therapy may be discontinued (violations of agreement)
4. Consultation
   Be willing to refer in order to achieve objectives. Special attention should be given to patients at risk for medication misuse, abuse, or diversion
   Consultation may be required in those with:
   - Psychiatric disorders
   - Substance abuse issues (past or present)
5. Periodic review
   The physician should:
   - Periodically review the course of pain treatment and any new information about the etiology of the pain
   - Evaluate and modify drug treatment based on:
     1. Patient's response
     2. Objective evidence of improved/diminished function
     3. If progress is unsatisfactory assess the appropriateness of continuing therapy, or modify therapy
6. Medical records
   Medical records should include:
   - Medical history and physical
   - Diagnostic tests and lab results
   - Evaluations and consultations
   - Treatment objectives and treatments
   - Informed consent and discussion of risks and benefits
   - Medication and refill documentation
   - Instructions and agreements
   - Periodic reviews

   Records are to be current and easily assessable for review
7. Compliance with controlled substances laws and regulations
   - State and federal regulations must be met
   - Refer to US Drug Enforcement Agency and state medical boards for relevant documents

*Adapted from Federation of State Medical Boards.

painkillers (17). This increase coincided with a nearly fourfold increase in the appropriate use of prescription opioids nationally (18). Given these recent findings, a call to temper prescribing patterns has emerged. Therefore, treatment of chronic pain must incorporate both the principles of prescribing as well as approaches to risk assessment and management that will withstand regulatory scrutiny (19).

Mechanisms and Pathophysiology

Tissue injury is thought to be the initial stimulus for development of chronic pain. The transformation to chronicity involves a cascade of alterations in pain processing, which results in the peripheral sensory neurons (nociceptors) becoming biochemically altered, leading to increased spontaneous neural activity (pain with no stimulus) and hyperresponsiveness to both noxious stimuli (hyperalgesia) and nonnoxious stimuli (allodynia). This process is known as "peripheral sensitization." From the nociceptors, whose cell bodies lie within the dorsal root ganglia, neural transmission proceeds through the cranial sensory ganglia, supraspinal nuclei, the thalamus, limbic and cerebral cortices, and diencephalic regions, where the perception of the pain and its meaning eventually occurs. As the message courses through each level, additional neurochemical modifications occur, resulting in a process known as "central sensitization." Central sensitization in chronic pain syndromes manifests as hyperexcitability, amplification, and self-perpetuation of pain (20,21). Many of the biochemical mechanisms in the process of peripheral and central sensitization are known, and provide sites for pharmacologic intervention (22).

Types of CNMP

CNMP is characterized as either nociceptive or neuropathic.

- *Nociceptive pain* arises from tissue injury and/or inflammation. Chronic nociceptive pain reflects alterations resulting in sustained pain and sensitization, with both peripheral and central components. Common conditions described as nociceptive pain include osteoarthritis, low back pain, and posttraumatic pain. Nociceptive pain often responds to opioid medications, implicating opioid receptors in this type of pain.
- *Neuropathic pain* occurs when a pathologic process causes damage or injury to nerve tissue either in the peripheral or central nervous system. Numerous medical disorders are associated with injury or toxic effects on neurons, resulting in alterations of neural processing. Neuropathic pain is often described as "burning, electrical, zinging, lightning, icelike, shooting, tingling, or lancinating." Some common examples include diabetic neuropathy, postherpetic neuralgia, trigeminal neuralgia, and possibly fibromyalgia. Neuropathic pain responds predominantly to medications used as adjuvant medications such as anticonvulsants, antidepressants, as well as opioids. Neuropathic pain also responds to medications that target specific neurochemicals such as N-methyl D-aspartate (23).
- Most CNMP syndromes are *mixed pain syndromes*, which have both nociceptive and neuropathic components. Thus, most CNMP syndromes involve multiple processing abnormalities, occurring at multiple sites along the complex journey through the peripheral and central nervous systems. For this reason, CNMP rarely responds to a single pharmacologic intervention. This concept provides the basis for using combinations of medications with differing mechanisms in pain management.

CLINICAL EVALUATION

Evaluating the patient with CNMP requires a systematic, biopsychosocial approach. Factors to consider can be found in Tables 41.1 and 41.2 and in Figure 41.1 (7,8).

History and Physical Examination

A comprehensive CNMP evaluation consists of a thorough pain history, medical history, social and psychiatric history, and complete physical examination. It is important to assess the pain's quality, type, timing, distribution, and relieving and exacerbating factors. In doing so:

- Identify the pain as nociceptive or neuropathic or both (Fig. 41.2).
- Quantify the pain using visual analogue scales such as Faces pain scale (Fig. 41.3) or the numeric rating scale (Fig. 41.4), which have been validated, are simple to administer, and can be used with young children, cognitively impaired individuals, and patients with language barriers (24,25). These scales are useful in both identifying the initial degree of suffering and in measuring changes after initiation of treatment (24,25).

The history should include prior investigations regarding the painful condition, prior surgical and nonsurgical treatments, all pharmaceutical and nonpharmaceutical treatments, and any comorbid and psychiatric conditions. Effects of the patient's pain on quality of life, activity, work, sleep, mood, and relationships should be documented. If a patient has already had a thorough CNMP evaluation and diagnosis by another physician, the new physician must review past records and documentation to determine if criteria for resuming and continuing any previous treatment are met. Establishing and confirming a legitimate chronic pain diagnosis is important; consider further investigations if indicated, rule out nonorganic conditions such as malingering, factitious disorder, drug seeking, or other aberrant behavior.

A thorough social and psychiatric history will alert the physician to issues such as current or past substance abuse, depression, anxiety, or other factors that may interfere with achieving pain treatment goals. Examination of work history, employment status, living situation, any pending litigation, or workman's compensation status is prudent. Current level of functioning and support network is also important.

Another important part of the assessment is evaluating the patient's risk of opioid abuse. This is important because approximately 2% to 35% of people with CNMP will take opioids at some point during their treatment course (26,27). Validated pain risk assessment tools, such as the Opioid Risk Tool, the Screener and Opioid Assessment for Patients With Pain, and a number of visual analog scales, can be found at the websites listed at the bottom of Figure 41.2 (24,28–31). By identifying patients at risk for possible opioid misuse, such as those with a history of prior or current substance abuse or those with psychiatric issues, one can choose to modify the treatment plan or refer to a pain specialist.

A complete physical examination provides an opportunity to evaluate objective findings in the area of the pain, determine neurological and musculoskeletal function, and observe any physical disability resulting from the chronic pain condition. Physical findings may serve as a baseline for comparison during

TABLE 41.2 Red Flags for Patients with Chronic Pain Suggesting the Need for Further Evaluation, Consultation, or Referral

Disease	Sign or Symptom Indicating Need for Further Evaluation
Neuropathic	
Diabetic neuropathy	Ulcers, fever, nonhealing wounds, escalating pain,* aberrant behavior†
CRPS#	Muscle atrophy, paresis, escalating pain
Phantom pain	Skin breakdown, intractable pain
Post-herpetic neuralgia	Skin infection, escalating pain
Multiple sclerosis	Constitutional symptoms‡, strokelike symptoms, escalating pain
Trigeminal neuralgia	Nontrigeminal nerve distribution of pain, intractable pain
Fibromyalgia	Constitutional symptoms, neurologic symptoms§, escalating pain
Post-stroke syndrome	Worsening or new stroke symptoms, change in quality of pain
Migraines	Neurologic symptoms, neurologic signs and symptoms when free of headache
Musculoskeletal	
Chronic headaches	Neurologic symptoms, vision changes, escalating pain
Osteoarthritis	Constitutional symptoms, joint destruction, inflammation of joints‖
Chronic back pain	Neurologic symptoms, constitutional symptoms, night pain, incontinence, saddle paresthesia, inflammatory changes, escalating pain
Fibromyalgia	(See above)
Mechanical/Compressive	
Chronic back pain	(See above)
Chronic abdominal pain	Constitutional symptoms, hematemesis, melena, hematochezia, signs of abuse¶
Chronic pelvic pain	Constitutional symptoms, vaginal bleeding or discharge, signs of abuse
Chronic neck pain	Neurologic symptoms, constitutional symptoms, night pain, inflammatory changes, dysphagia, escalating pain
Osteoarthritis	(See above)
Inflammatory	
Rheumatoid arthritis	Constitutional symptoms, escalating pain
Ankylosing arthritis	Constitutional symptoms, escalating pain

*Escalating pain: poor pain control may imply misdiagnosis, depression, malingering, drug seeking.
†Aberrant behavior: use of meds for other than pain control, selling, stealing, forging prescriptions, doctor shopping, reluctance to try nonpharmacologic therapies, calls for early refills, impaired control, compulsive use of medications despite harm to self.
‡Constitutional symptoms: fever, weight loss, anorexia, loss of function.
§Neurologic signs or symptoms: weakness, paresis, paresthesias, absent reflexes, release signs.
‖Unexpected inflammatory changes: extreme pain, persistent swelling, erythema.
¶Signs of abuse: physical, psychologic, or sexual.
#Complex regional pain syndrome.

the management process. The physical examination may also identify comorbid conditions that must be considered in the treatment plan. Signs of illicit drug use and other important issues may be noted during the examination.

Diagnostic Testing

Diagnostic testing may be performed to determine or verify the diagnosis, rule out more ominous disorders (Table 41.2) and identify comorbid medical conditions. This could include laboratory studies and radiological investigations, depending on the patient's presenting complaints. Occasionally, an interventional diagnostic test may help clarify the cause of a patient's pain. Diagnostic interventions include selective spinal nerve root block to determine the level of pathology if magnetic resonance imaging is inconclusive; discography to determine if an intervertebral disc is the "pain generator"; and nerve blocks done before radiofrequency lesioning to project efficacy of this treatment.

MANAGEMENT

Developing and Implementing a Management Plan

The first step in management of CNMP is to develop and document treatment plan, including setting realistic goals for treatment. The treatment plan should be multidisciplinary and have achievable goals, such as improvement of function and quality of

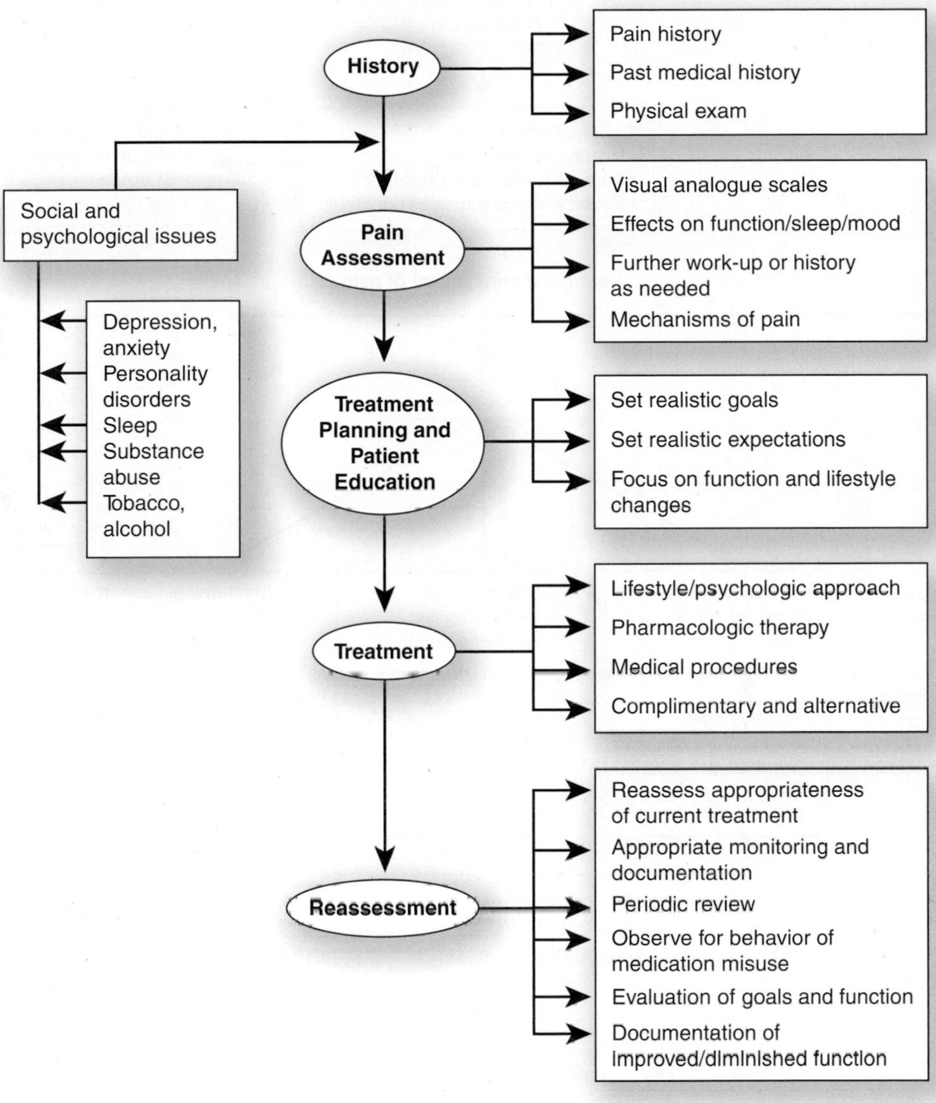

Figure 41.1 • Systematic approach to evaluation and treatment of chronic pain patient. Adapted from Pomm and Tenzer, 2005 (8).

life. Treatment options for CNMP should include nonpharmacologic and pharmacologic modalities. Nonpharmacologic modalities include lifestyle and psychologic approaches, complementary and alternative medicine, physical therapy, and interventional medical procedures. Pharmacologic treatments include use of adjunctive medications, nonopioid and opioid analgesics. When the choice to use opioids has been made, one should follow the guidelines of the Federation of State Medical Boards (FSMB) (7). The FSMB stresses appropriate patient selection by: assessment of risk factors for medication misuse, use of opioid agreements, choice of opioid medication, periodic review of treatment effectiveness, use of urine drug tests, addressing psychiatric issues, and minimizing medication side effects.

The character or mechanism of the pain, the specific pain disorder diagnosis, and the intensity of the pain determine appropriate treatment choices (Figs. 41.2 and 41.5) (32,33). Management guidelines for specific pain disorders, such as chronic musculoskeletal pain, neuropathic pain, chronic pelvic pain, fibromyalgia syndrome, and low back pain, have been developed by specialists in the respective fields and may be useful (23–36). After the pain disorder diagnosis is determined, an individualized treatment plan is developed and documented, and the diagnosis, management options, and goals of treatment are discussed with the patient.

The primary goal of CNMP management is to improve function and quality of life while decreasing pain. Improving the social, occupational, psychological, interpersonal, and physical disabilities, all which adversely affect the patient's quality of life, is the primary goal (9). Successful management begins with patient education and setting realistic goals (37). Completely eliminating pain is rarely a realistic goal, yet improving quality of life should be achievable.

Treatment options for CNMP include nonpharmacologic and pharmacologic modalities, as listed in Tables 41.3

Chronic pain

1st Step: Assessment
- History and physical
- Pain evaluation and description
- Functional/social assessment tools

Pain Scales/Tools
- Visual analogue*
- SOAAP†
- ORT‡

Determine mechanism of pain

Neuropathic (Burning, stabbing, shooting)
- Peripheral: CRPS, phantom pain, metabolic
- Central: Parkinson's, MS, myelopathies, stroke
- Fibromyalgia

Nociceptive

Musculoskeletal (Ache, soreness, stiff)
- Fibromyalgia
- Myofascial Pain Syndrome
- Trauma

Inflammatory (Ache, swelling, erythema, heat)
- Arthropathies (RA, AS)
- Infection
- Post-operative
- Tissue injury

Mechanical/Compression Pain (Ache, soreness, stiff)
- Low back pain
- Musculoskeletal
- Visceral
- Muscle, tendon, ligament

Mixed pain (Combination of pain patterns)
- various conditions

Key:

* = www.emergingsolutionsinpain.com/index.php?option=com_content&task=view&id=101&Itemid=100
† = www.painedu.com/soap.asp, and
‡ = www.painedu.com/tools.asp?Tool=5).

AS = Ankylosing spondylitis
CRPS = Chronic regional pain syndrome
MS = Multiple sclerosis
RA = Rheumatoid arthritis
ORT ‡ = Opioid risk tool
SOAAP† = Screener and opioid assessment for patients with pain

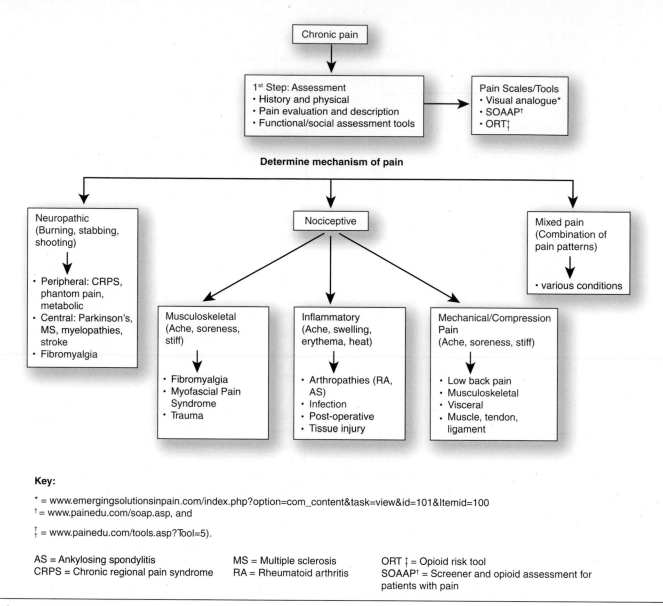

Figure 41.2 • Assessment of chronic pain (24,28,29,32).

and 41.4 and Figure 41.5. Evidence of the effectiveness of many of the treatment options is lacking or inconsistent, and further studies are clearly needed (38). Treatment with nonpharmacologic options, with or without medication should be tried initially. Nonpharmacologic treatments require patient participation and motivation, and hopefully result in improved physical mobility, fitness, mood, sleep, and general health.

Pharmacologic choices depend on the pain disorder diagnosis and whether the mechanism is characterized as neuropathic, nociceptive, or mixed. Rational polypharmacy is often employed, in that medication combinations target different

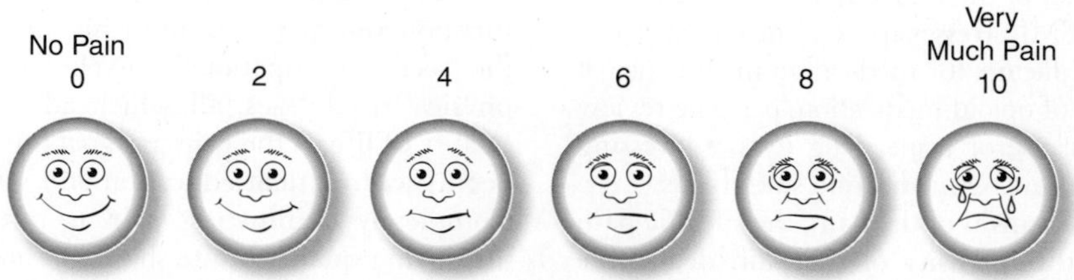

Figure 41.3 • The Faces pain scale for use in eliciting a patient's self-assessment of pain.

No pain		Mild		Moderate		High Moderate		Severe		Very Severe
0	1	2	3	4	5	6	7	8	9	10

Figure 41.4 • The numeric rating scale for use in eliciting a patient's self-assessment of pain.

locations along the pain pathways and to use their side effect profile to treat coexisting complaints (23,39). For instance, the use of NSAIDs and opioids in combination provide greater pain control than either medication alone. Initial pharmacologic choices should be nonopioids. If ineffective, opioid/nonopioid combinations may be required, but are limited by the maximum dose of the nonopioid component. The use of opioids has been shown to improve moderate to severe pain (33,40).

The use of opioid medications in the management CNMP, although currently standard of care, remains a subject

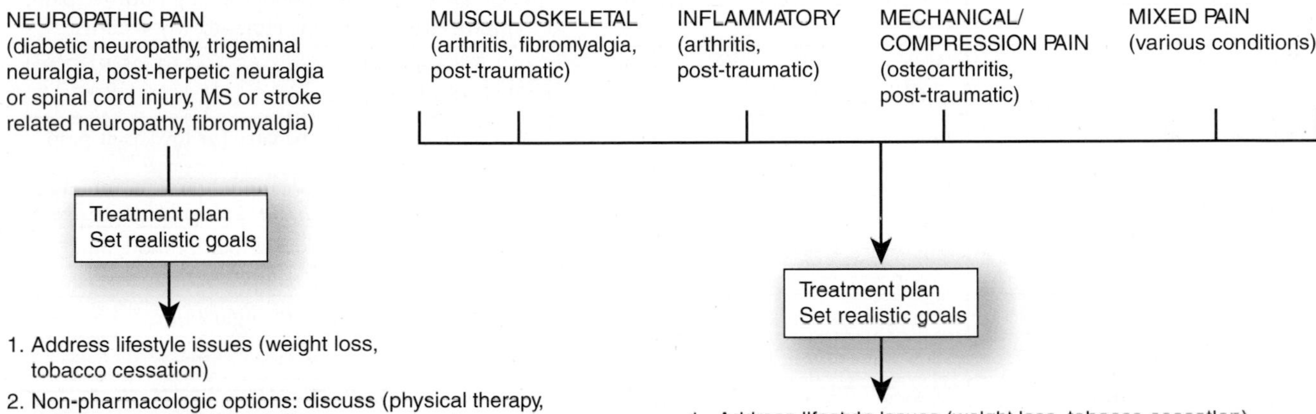

1. Address lifestyle issues (weight loss, tobacco cessation)
2. Non-pharmacologic options: discuss (physical therapy, exercise, manipulation, TENS, yoga, counseling, relaxation, cognitive behavioral therapy)
3. Initial pharmacologic treatment:
   1st line: Topical lidocaine, tricyclic antidepressants, dual reuptake antidepressants (i.e., venlafexine), gabapentin, pregabalin
   2nd line: opioid analgesics, tramadol (sign opioid agreement, anticipate side effects)
   3rd line: other anticonvulsant medications(carbamazepine or valproic acid), topical capsaicin, others
4. Periodic review: medication effectiveness, changes or additions, indications of opioid misuse (aberrant behaviors), UDS, goal revision.
5. Referral if management ineffective, drug abuse, or need advice.

1. Address lifestyle issues (weight loss, tobacco cessation)
2. Non-pharmacologic options: discuss (physical therapy, exercise, manipulation, TENS, yoga, counseling, relaxation, cognitive behavioral therapy)
3. Initial pharmacologic treatment: Non-opioids (acetaminophen, NSAIDs, salicylates–mild to moderate pain)
4. Change to non-opioid/opioid combination if ineffective or moderate to severe pain.
5. Sign opioid agreement, anticipate side effects.
6. Address mood and sleep.
7. Add adjuvant medication (antidepressants, anticonvulsants, topical lidocaine or others)
8. If ineffective, or severe pain, change opioid to "strong" or non-combination opioid. (Start with short acting, titrate upward to maximum effect with minimal side effects, change to long-acting)
9. Address breakthrough pain with short-acting opioids.
10. Periodic review: medication effectiveness, changes or additions, indications of opioid misuse (aberrant behaviors), UDS, goal revision.
11. Referral if management ineffective, drug abuse, or need advice.

Key

MS = multiple sclerosis
TENS = transcutaneous electrical nerve stimulation
UDS = urine drug screen

Figure 41.5 • Management of chronic pain by mechanism (1,6,10,12,32–37,40,54,57,65,66).

TABLE 41.3 Key Therapies for Chronic Pain and Evidence of Effectiveness per Cochrane Collaboration Review*

Intervention	Efficacy	SOR†	Comments and Cautions
Lifestyle and Psychological Approaches			
Weight loss			No reviews of efficacy in regard to chronic pain
Exercise	High quality evidence	A	Effective for Fibromyalgia symptoms[59]
	Slight effects	A	Osteoarthritis hip—limited conclusions, RCTs with small sample sizes[60]
	Good evidence	A	Osteoarthritis knee—short-term benefit: reduced knee pain and improved physical function[61]
	Slight effect	A	Effective for nonspecific chronic low back pain[62]
Tobacco and alcohol cessation			No reviews of efficacy in regard to chronic pain
Physical therapy			No reviews of efficacy in regard to chronic pain
Occupational therapy	Moderate evidence	B	Back schools in occupational setting improve pain, improve function and return-to-work status[63]
TENS	Available studies lack rigor	A	Insufficient evidence to recommend (25 RCTs) 99 ineligible studies[64]
Manipulation	Good evidence of effectiveness	A	As effective as standard care for low back pain[65]
Counseling			No reviews of efficacy in regard to chronic pain
CBT/BT	Maintained at 6 months	A	Weak effects on improving pain, mood, and disability[66]
Hypnosis			No reviews of efficacy in regard to chronic pain
Drug Therapy			
NSAIDS/acetaminophen	Modest effects	A	Superior to placebo for chronic pain[67]
Salicylates			No reviews of efficacy in regard to chronic pain
Opioid combinations			No reviews of efficacy in regard to chronic pain
Tramadol	NNT = 3.8, NNH = 8.3	A	Effective for neuropathic pain and small benefits for osteoarthritis[68,69]
Opioids—noncombination	Benefits still questionable	A	Effective for intermediate term (8–70 days), questionable for chronic low back pain[70]
	Variable study quality	A	Hydromorphone is as effective as morphine[71]
	Short-term—equivocal	A	Opioids effective for neuropathic pain[72]
Long-term opioids	Weak evidence	B	Clinically significant pain relief[73]
Adjunctive—antidepressants	Conflicting studies	A	No evidence for low back pain[74]
	NNT = 3	A	TCAs are effective for neuropathic pain[75]
Atypical antidepressants	NNT = 3	A	Venlafaxine effective for neuropathic pain,[74]
	Moderate evidence, 60 and 120 mg works	A	Duloxetine effective for diabetic neuropathy and fibromyalgia[75]
Adjunctive: anticonvulsants	NNT = 4.3	A	Gabapentin is effective for neuropathic pain[76]
	NNT = 1.8	A	Carbamazepine effective for neuropathic pain[77]
	More effective treatments available	A	Lamotrigine is not effective for neuropathic pain[78]
	NNT <6: neuropathic px, >7: fibromyalgia	A	Pregabalin is effective for neuropathic pain and fibromyalgia[79]
Adjuvant: topical	Compared with NSAIDS	A A	Non effective for salicylates[80] Limited data for capsaicin for chronic neuropathic pain
	NNT = 6.6, NNH = 2.5	A	Insufficient to recommend topical lidocaine for PHN[81]

TABLE 41.3 *(Continued)*

Intervention	Efficacy	SOR†	Comments and Cautions
Medical Procedures			
Injection therapy: epidural, facet joints, trigger point	Heterogenous studies	A	Insufficient evidence for or against (for low back pain)[82]
Radiofrequency denervation	Conflicting evidence	A	Inconclusive evidence for neck and back pain[83]
Sympathetic block		A	Unable to conclude; scarcity of studies for CRPS[84]
Sympathectomy	Low-quality studies	B	No evidence to recommend for neuropathic pain[85]
Botox injections			No reviews of efficacy in regard to chronic pain
Nucleoplasty/annuloplasty			No reviews of efficacy in regard to chronic pain
Intrathecal infusion pumps			No reviews of efficacy in regard to chronic pain
Deep brain stimulation			No reviews of efficacy in regard to chronic pain
Complementary/Alternative Terapies			
Touch therapies	Healing and therapeutic touch, Reiki	A	Modest effect in pain relief, more studies needed[86]
Biofeedback			No reviews of efficacy in regard to chronic pain
Yoga and stretching			No reviews of efficacy in regard to chronic pain
Music therapy	NNT = 5	A	Music reduces pain intensity levels and opioid requirements, but the magnitude of these benefits is small[87]
Herbal remedies	Convincing evidence	A	Evidence for avocado-soybean unsaponifiables in the treatment of osteoarthritis is convincing; evidence for other herbal interventions insufficient to either recommend or discourage their use[88]
		A	Reduces low back pain more than placebo[89]
Massage	Efficacy lasted at least 1 year after the end of the treatment	A	Might be beneficial for patients with subacute and chronic nonspecific low-back pain, especially when combined with exercises and education[90]
Acupuncture	No clear recommendations made about different techniques	A	Chronic low-back pain: more effective for pain relief and functional improvement than no treatment or sham treatment immediately after and short-term only, no more effective than conventional and "alternative" treatments, may be useful adjunctive[91]
		A	Useful and safe for migraine prophylaxis[92]
Reflexology			No reviews of efficacy in regard to chronic pain
Mindfulness meditation			No reviews of efficacy in regard to chronic pain

*The Cochrane Collaboration is an international nonprofit, independent organization focused on systemic reviews of health care interventions.
†A = consistent, good-quality patient-oriented evidence; B = inconsistent or limited-quality patient-oriented evidence; C = consensus, disease-oriented evidence, usual practice, expert opinion.
For information about the SORT evidence rating system, see *www.aafp.org/afpsort.xml*, SOR = strength of recommendation.
RCT = randomized controlled trial; TENS = transcutaneous electrical nerve stimulation; CBT/BT = cognitive behavioral; therapy/behavioral therapy; NNT = number needed to treat; NNH = number needed to harm; NSAID = nonsteroidal anti-inflammatory drug; PHN = postherpetic neuralgia; CRPS = complex regional pain syndrome.

of controversy. In the mid 1990s, physicians were reluctant to use opioids due to concerns of abuse, lack of knowledge and fears of regulatory scrutiny (19). The past 10 years has witnessed greater emphasis on opioids in CNMP, with much of the pain literature providing education, guidelines, and efforts to allay physician fears. As a result, the use of opioids has increased dramatically, but nonmedicinal use and abuse has also increased, with an alarming number of associated deaths (17). At the time of this writing, there is evidence of a movement toward increased regulations and attempts to control

TABLE 41.4 Six A's for Monitoring Patients with Chronic Nonmalignant Pain on Controlled Substances (36)

Analgesia (assess pain relief)
Affect (evaluate mood)
Activities (evaluate ADLs and function, quality of life)
Adjuncts (nonpharmacologic/nonopioid treatments)
Adverse effects (side effects of treatments)
Aberrant behavior (tolerance, dependence, and addiction)

ADL = activities of daily living.

opioid misuse (18). Recent debate among pain specialists on the treatment of CNMP with opioids acknowledges this issue and emphasizes the importance of appropriate patient selection and monitoring (41).

The evidence to support the long-term use of opioids to reduce pain and increase function in patients with CNMP is, at best, weak (12,42,43). However, consensus remains in favor of opioid use for moderate to severe CNMP, if used appropriately, on well-selected patients, with adequate supervision (41). Most patients with CNMP are eventually treated with opioid medications; therefore, it is essential that physicians that treat these challenging conditions are well educated about the use of opioids (36).

The decision to use opioids must be based on guiding principles, and justification for their use must be determined and documented. The FSMB provides a basic guideline for the use of controlled substances, which is augmented by individual state board regulators (see Table 41.1) (7). Prescribing physicians must consult the rules and regulations for opioid prescribing in their state. They must also have a clear understanding of opioid pharmacokinetics and the anticipated and unanticipated consequences of opioid use, including tolerance, dependence, addiction, pseudo-addiction, abuse, and adverse side effects (for discussion of these issues, see Chapter 47).

It is estimated that abuse issues arise in 9% to 50% of patients using opioids for pain (44). The currently known strongest predictors of abuse are personal or family history of substance abuse, younger age, and the presence of psychiatric conditions (41). Other known risk factors are age younger than 41 years, male gender, unemployed status, psychiatric comorbidity (personality, anxiety, depressive, or bipolar disorder), and social factors such as a history of legal problems or motor vehicle accidents (41). It is important to remember that patients at high risk for abuse or addiction may still suffer from intolerable pain. High-risk patients may, therefore, be treated with opioids, but may require a more regimented and strict monitoring program. This may include more frequent visits, increased random urine drug testing, and the provision of fewer medications at each visit. Advice from an addiction specialist or pain specialist may be necessary when the risks of abuse outweigh the benefits of opioid use.

It is essential for the patient to understand that opioids are "*one part* of a multimodal treatment plan to reduce pain intensity and improve quality of life, especially functional capacity" (36, 41). It is rare that CNMP completely resolves, and current guidelines suggest that an improvement of 2 to 3 on a 0 to 10 scale is a reasonable expectation (41). Setting small, but achievable goals, such as walking three blocks, going back to work, increasing outdoor activity, etc., will help the patient remain motivated and realistic.

Informed consent and agreement for treatment is accomplished by the use of "Opioid Agreements" (45). The agreement provides written documentation of the diagnosis, medications, the discussion between physician and patient about opioid use and the anticipated and unanticipated consequences of use. This agreement also includes the conditions that the patient must comply with to improve the safety of opioid use and limit the risk of abuse. Despite the common and recommended use of opioid agreements in CNMP, there is no evidence that their use decreases opioid abuse (45).

Choice of Opioid Medication

Pain management guidelines have historically claimed that long-acting opioid use is more effective and safer than the chronic use of short-acting opioids, but there is no good evidence to support this (46). Choice of drug delivery method depends on the condition of the patient, available sites for delivery, and on patient preferences and physician comfort.

The use of methadone, a synthetic opioid, deserves special mention. Methadone use has increased markedly over the past decade as revealed by a 933% increase in methadone sales from 1997 to 2006 (47). Methadone use gained popularity likely because of low cost and unique pharmacokinetics of longer half-life, increased bioavailability and its notable effect on opioid receptors as well as receptors found in neuropathic CNMP syndromes. In addition, it is speculated that methadone may help prevent central sensitization, opioid tolerance and the development of postopioid hyperalgesia (48). However, despite being considered a drug with less abuse potential due to a lack of euphoric effects, methadone has since become associated with drug abuse arrests, emergency department visits, and both intentional and unintentional fatal drug overdoses (49). Most deaths (72.3%) associated with methadone involve more than one drug (50). It is known, however, that when used in combination with other drugs, methadone toxicity is enhanced, with the combination of benzodiazepines and methadone creating the greatest risk of fatal overdose (50). Deaths are believed to be related to systemic accumulation of methadone, causing QT interval prolongation and torsades de pointes (51). The development of fatal arrhythmias may also be caused by the drug–drug interactions of methadone and other commonly used medications, such as fluoxetine. Consensus guidelines for the safe use of methadone were published in 2009, and contain suggestions such as advising patients of the potential for arrhythmias and using electrocardiogram monitoring (51,52).

Patient Monitoring

Periodic review (follow-up visits) provides a way to monitor treatment effectiveness, nonpharmacologic therapy compliance, and patient behaviors that may indicate violation of the opioid agreement or medication misuse. Follow-up visits also provide direction for further treatment and goal revision. All components of the six A's (Table 41.4) should be addressed at

Follow up Office Visit for Chronic Opioid Analgesia

Diagnosis:____

Pain Medications: _____________________________________

Pain Scale Rating: 0 1 2 3 4 5 6 7 8 9 10

Side effects: ☐ None ☐ Nausea ☐ Vomiting ☐ Confusion ☐ Sleepiness ☐ Fatigue ☐ Constipation

Treatment of Side Effects:____

Since the last clinic visit, how much RELIEF has pain treatments and medications provided? Please circle the one percentage that shows how much relief you have received.

0% 10% 20% 30% 40% 50% 60% 70% 80% 90% 100%

No relief Complete relief

Circle the one number that describes how, during the past 24 hours, PAIN HAS INTERFERED with your:

General Activity

0 1 2 3 4 5 6 7 8 9 10

Does not Interfere — Completely Interferes

Interactions with other people

0 1 2 3 4 5 6 7 8 9 10

Does not Interfere — Completely Interferes

Mood

0 1 2 3 4 5 6 7 8 9 10

Does not Interfere — Completely Interferes

Sleep

0 1 2 3 4 5 6 7 8 9 10

Does not Interfere — Completely Interferes

Ability to work (in or out of home)

0 1 2 3 4 5 6 7 8 9 10

Does not Interfere — Completely Interferes

Enjoyment of life

0 1 2 3 4 5 6 7 8 9 10

Does not Interfere — Completely Interferes

PHYSICIAN TO COMPLETE

Complaints/ROS____

Physical Exam: BP_____ HR_____ RR_____ Wt._____
HEENT:_______ Heart:_______ Lungs:_________ Focused Exam__________________

Impression:
1. Goals Attained? ☐ Yes ☐ No ☐ Working on 2. Progress?

Plan/Discussion:
1. Medication prescription provided? If yes what drug and amount__________________________

2. Urine drug screen ordered or due? ☐ Yes ☐ No If Male Check Testosterone periodically ☐ Yes ☐ No

3. Follow-up in ☐ 1 ☐ 2 ☐ 3 months__________________________________

Physician Signature____Date:_____________

Figure 41.6 • Sample monitoring template for follow-up visit for chronic nonmalignant pain. Form developed by Dr. Robert Jackman.

intervals of every 3 months or less depending on patient needs, stability, medication misuse risk, or as determined by state guidelines.

Urine drug testing (UDT) is not legally required but is recommended by many guidelines (7,36). The use of UDT, together with monitoring for aberrant behaviors results in the highest rate of identification of misuse of opioid medication in CNMP patients (53). The UDT can help solidify physician–patient trust by establishing the presence of the prescribed controlled substance in urine and thus alleviate any concerns about diversion or trafficking. Physicians must understand what medications are screened for in their specific laboratory, as pain panels and opioid screening tests vary between labs. It is important to understand the duration of substances present in urine, as patients may refrain from illicit substance use before office visits and provide misleading UDTs. Random UDT is therefore the preferred method of testing. Physicians using UDT should be familiar with opiate and opioid metabolites (13). Before urine drug-testing, physicians should anticipate actions that will be prompted when a UDT is positive for nonprescribed or illicit substances, or shows the absence of prescribed substances. All positive UDTs must be addressed and should result in some action: either dismissal, referral for substance abuse counseling or treatment, or refusal to prescribe further controlled substances.

Aberrant patient behavior often suggests medication misuse during follow-up visits. Aberrant behaviors include use of pain medications for reasons other than pain, impaired control (of self or use of medication), compulsive use of medication, continued use of medication despite harm (or lack of benefit), and craving or escalation of medication use (54). Selling, altering prescriptions, stealing or diverting medications, early refill requests, losing prescriptions, drug seeking behavior, doctor shopping, or reluctance to try nonpharmacologic interventions are other examples of aberrant behavior (54). To address these problems, practitioners should strictly follow the guidelines of the FSMB as outlined in Table 41.1, consider the routine use of random urine drug tests and appropriately write prescriptions to decrease the incidence of medication misuse (i.e., write out pill count and limit to one pharmacy) (13).

Psychiatric problems are common when dealing with CNMP. In one study, 77% of patients with CNMP secondary to low back pain have a lifetime psychiatric diagnosis, as compared with 46% of the general US population (11,55). Fifty-nine percent of those mentioned in the previous study have a current and active psychiatric diagnosis as compared with 26% of the general US population (11,56). Common psychiatric disorders in people with CNMP are mood, anxiety, somatoform disorders, substance abuse, and personality disorders (14). Given their high comorbidity, an understanding of their diagnosis and treatment is essential.

Monitoring for Medication Adverse Effects

Medication side effects, especially of opioids, need to be addressed and anticipated. The most common side effects encountered are somnolence, nausea, sedation, (tolerance or resolution usually develops within 10 days) and constipation (no tolerance or resolution develops) (12). As a preventative measure, start those taking opioids on a combination stimulant/ softener laxative to prevent constipation and provide an antinausea medication (for 10 days) (12). Avoid stool-bulking agents as they can worsen constipation in those taking opioids, for the main etiology of the constipation is slowing of stool transit time (57).

Several studies have demonstrated hypogonadism in association with chronic use of sustained release opioids (41). Evidence is not sufficient to recommend routine testosterone testing of asymptomatic patients, but it is prudent if symptoms such as decreased libido, sexual dysfunction, fatigue, or a poor sense of well-being are reported. Prolonged administration of opiates is associated with tolerance and possibly of increased pain sensitivity, otherwise known as opiate-induced hypernociception, a hyperalgesic response to prolonged exposure to morphine (58). This concept can include paradoxic pain in regions of the body unrelated to the initial pain stimulus and is thought to be mediated through cytokine disregulation (58).

Other potential problems commonly encountered in patients with CNMP include prolonged QT with methadone, NSAID-related peptic ulcer disease and dyspepsia, NSAID-related chronic renal insufficiency, hypertension, renal failure, and congestive heart failure exacerbations. Acetaminophen is associated with liver toxicity in high doses and should be avoided in people with liver dysfunction such as cirrhotics and alcohol abusers (41,57).

Referral and Pain Clinics

When chronic pain problems persist despite appropriate multidimensional management and ongoing opioid use, referral to a pain management specialist can be helpful (54,57). Consultation can help to assess the appropriateness of ongoing opioid prescriptions, to suggest alternate approaches to management of complex pain problems, or to consider interventional procedures. A history of substance abuse or interpersonal dynamics that seem to be complicating the treatment of pain may benefit from a consultation (11,14). Specifying exactly what is sought with the referral, either consultation or consideration of procedural intervention, is very helpful to the pain management specialist.

Pain specialists may provide suggestions for further evaluation (imaging studies, neurologic testing, surgical or physiatry consultation), any psychiatric consultation may be recommended. Interventional pain modalities have evolved significantly and include procedures to both further elucidate the diagnosis of CNMP and to provide treatment. Therapeutic interventions include epidural steroid injection for spinal nerve root inflammation, facet joint injection, radiofrequency lesioning, sacroiliac joint injection, sympathetic block (stellate or lumbar blocks) for complex regional pain syndrome, Botox injections for spasm, nucleoplasty or annuloplasty for discogenic pain, and implantation of devices such as spinal cord stimulators and intrathecal drug infusion pumps for refractory pain. Deep brain stimulation has also been attempted for intractable neuropathic pain (22). See Table 41.3 for a summary of available treatments for CNMP.

KEY POINTS

- The pathophysiology of chronic nonmalignant pain is entirely different than that of acute pain, indicating the need for a different management approach.
- A comprehensive pain evaluation is essential to establish a pain condition diagnosis before the development of a treatment plan.
- The management of chronic pain disorders is based on a multidisciplinary approach.
- A stepwise treatment approach includes nonpharmacologic and pharmacologic treatments.
- The use of opioids in chronic nonmalignant pain conditions introduces a complex array of issues that include: appropriate patient selection, concern for abuse and misuse, management of side effects, and special monitoring procedures.
- Careful documentation of goals, response to treatment and revisions of the treatment plan is essential for safe and effective chronic pain management.

CHAPTER 42

Dizziness

Philip D. Sloane, Otto R. Maarsingh, and Kathleen Klink

CLINICAL OBJECTIVES

1. Be able to vary one's clinical approach to patients with dizziness based on the age of the patient, the description of the dizziness itself, the onset and course of symptoms, and the presence or absence of other health conditions.
2. Be able to recognize the ways that neurological, cardiovascular, and psychological evaluations contribute to the differential diagnosis, evaluation, and treatment plan.

Dizziness is a term that includes many symptoms and presentations, none of which can be objectively measured. It is difficult for patients to describe and for clinicians to define, making the diagnosis challenging. Even with an accurate diagnosis, effective treatment can be elusive.

Patients may describe feelings such as a rotational or spinning sensation, giddiness, lightheadedness, instability or unsteadiness, imbalance, or near faint. The duration of symptoms may vary from short term (seconds or minutes) to long term (days, months, or years), or a combination of both. Symptoms may be acute in onset, chronic, new, or recurrent. Often, patients are able to identify provoking circumstances, such as getting up from a lying position, bending forward, turning of the head, exercise, standing still, or strong emotions. There may be associated symptoms such as nausea or vomiting, neurologic deficits, tinnitus, palpitations, anxiety, or other physical or psychological complaints (1–3). Life-threatening causes are relatively uncommon, but the astute clinician must be aware of them in order to intervene appropriately (4).

Dizziness is a common symptom in the community. About 20% of younger and middle-aged adults experience some form of dizziness (5–9), increasing to 30% in patients older than 65 years of age (1,7,10–12), and 40% to 50% in patients older than 80 years of age (10,11). Only a minority of people with dizziness actually seek help for their problem; 1% to 4% of younger and middle-aged adults visit a physician annually because of dizziness (6,13,14), increasing to 8% in patients older than 65 years of age, and 11% in patients older than age 85 (15).

Patients with dizziness are managed largely at the primary care level. Only 5% to 10% of dizzy patients are referred to medical subspecialties such as otolaryngology, cardiology, neurology, and psychiatry (13,14,16). Although medical specialists can be helpful during the evaluation and treatment of dizzy patients, many will overdiagnose conditions in their own specialty and be relatively inattentive to signs and symptoms suggesting a diagnosis outside their field (17). Consequently, generalist physicians are often in the best position to evaluate a dizzy patient and to make an accurate diagnosis, especially when multiple contributing factors are present.

DIFFERENTIAL DIAGNOSIS

It is instructive to begin to think about dizziness by reviewing the components of the body that contribute to a sense of stability. These include vision, the peripheral vestibular and auditory systems, proprioceptive receptors in joints of the spine and extremities, the cerebral cortex, the vestibular nuclei, the brainstem (including vestibular ocular and vestibular spinal reflex pathways), the cerebellum, and the cardiovascular system. Because the cerebral cortex is involved in perception of motion and stability, mental conditions can both cause and result from dizziness; so psychological factors are often important.

The character of the dizziness may give a clue to the body system that is most affected. There are four generally accepted subtypes or categories of dizziness: vertigo, presyncope, disequilibrium, and other dizziness (18–20).

- Vertigo is the false sensation that the body or the environment is moving, often described as spinning. It is due to an imbalance of tonic vestibular signals and usually arises from the inner ear, middle ear, brainstem, or cerebellum.
- Presyncope is a feeling of lightheadedness or faintness, as though one were about to pass out. It usually reflects cerebral hypoperfusion and has a cardiovascular origin, such as orthostatic hypotension (often from medication), arrhythmia, or congestive heart failure.
- Disequilibrium is a feeling of unsteadiness or imbalance that is primarily felt in the lower extremities, is most prominent when standing or walking, and is relieved by sitting or lying down. Any disturbance of the motor control system (vision, vestibulospinal, proprioceptive, somatosensory, cerebellar, or motor function) can lead to disequilibrium.
- Nonspecific dizziness is a feeling not covered by the above definitions. It may include swimming or floating sensations, vague light-headedness, or feelings of dissociation. This feeling may be difficult for the patient to describe. Virtually any type of dizziness can be responsible for such symptoms, but anxiety and depression are especially often expressed in this manner.

Unfortunately, many patients, especially older ones, do not fit neatly into the above typology and instead complain of more

TABLE 42.1 Common Causes of Dizziness in Primary Care

	Causes by Age Category	
Diagnostic Category	**Young and Middle-aged Adults**	**Older Adults**
Peripheral vestibular conditions	Benign paroxysmal positional vertigo Ménière disease Vestibular neuronitis	Benign paroxysmal positional vertigo Ménière disease Vestibular neuronitis
Cardiovascular conditions	Orthostatic hypotension (e.g., from a viral infection) Anemia or volume depletion (e.g., gastrointestinal bleed, pregnancy, menstrual disorders)	Cardiac arrhythmia Congestive heart failure Orthostatic hypotension (e.g., from dehydration) Valvular disease
Cerebrovascular conditions	Migraine	Transient ischemic attack Posterior circulation (including cerebellar) stroke
Neurologic conditions, excluding cerebrovascular conditions	Head injury	Head injury Multiple sensory deficits Parkinson's disease Peripheral neuropathy
Musculoskeletal conditions	Cervical spine disease	Cervical spine disease Physical deconditioning
Psychiatric conditions	Anxiety or panic disorder Depressive disorder Somatoform disorder	Anxiety or panic disorder Anxiety disorder, secondary to another cause of dizziness Depressive disorder Somatoform disorder
Metabolic conditions	Anemia Diabetes Thyroid disease	Anemia Diabetes Electrolyte disturbance
Impaired vision	Refractive changes	Cataract/postcataract surgery Diabetic retinopathy
Pharmacological conditions	Adverse drug effect Alcohol abuse Illicit drug use	Adverse drug effect Alcohol abuse Polypharmacy
Multifactorial	—	Multiple sensory impairments

than one type of dizziness. In such patients a system-oriented search for causes and contributing factors is more helpful.

Common Causes

In approaching the differential diagnosis of a patient with dizziness, it is useful to take a systematic approach. Thus, a mental list of the more common diagnoses in dizziness patients might proceed in this manner:

- Peripheral vestibular conditions
- Cardiovascular conditions
- Cerebrovascular conditions
- Neurologic (other than cerebrovascular) conditions
- Musculoskeletal conditions
- Psychiatric conditions
- Metabolic conditions
- Eye diseases and/or vision problems
- Drug adverse effects

Table 42.1 provides an overview of causes of dizziness commonly seen in primary care, by diagnostic category.

Potentially Life-threatening Causes

Relatively few causes of dizziness are life-threatening. The primary care clinician must, however, be especially vigilant to identify the small number of patients whose dizziness may represent an urgent need for treatment. Among the most prominent are the following four conditions, which should always be in the differential diagnosis of people with dizziness:

- Acute orthostatic hypotension from infection, acute cardiac failure, a gastrointestinal bleed, or any other cause of volume depletion or dehydration. A history of lightheadedness relieved by lying down, accompanied by tachycardia on sitting and standing, can usually be elicited. A general history will often reveal risk factors, such as melena, working long hours in the sun, or a history of fever.

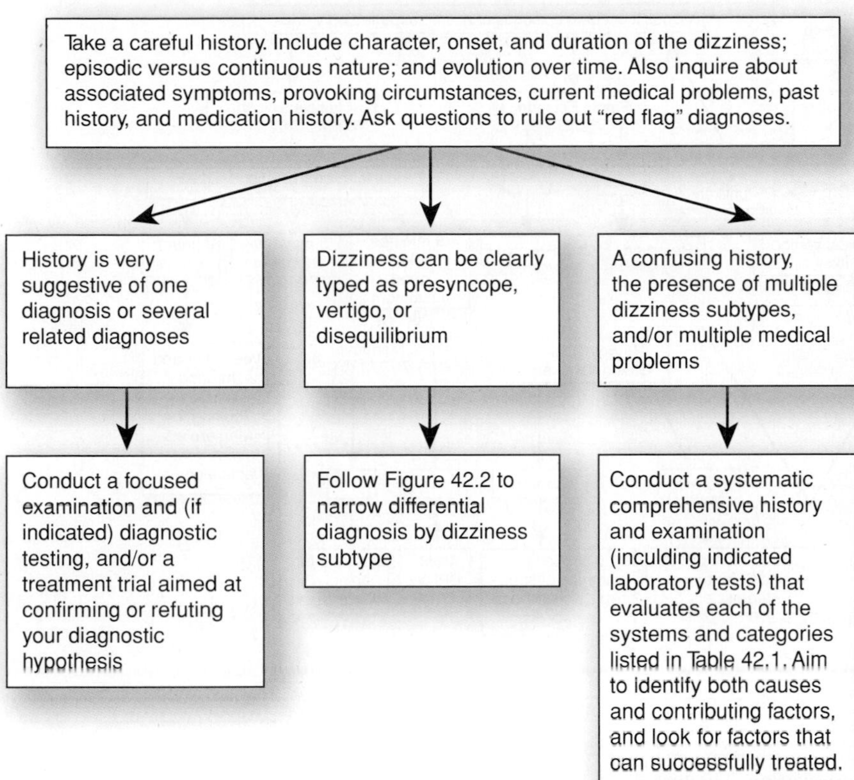

Take a careful history. Include character, onset, and duration of the dizziness; episodic versus continuous nature; and evolution over time. Also inquire about associated symptoms, provoking circumstances, current medical problems, past history, and medication history. Ask questions to rule out "red flag" diagnoses.
History is very suggestive of one diagnosis or several related diagnoses
Dizziness can be clearly typed as presyncope, vertigo, or disequilibrium
A confusing history, the presence of multiple dizziness subtypes, and/or multiple medical problems
Conduct a focused examination and (if indicated) diagnostic testing, and/or a treatment trial aimed at confirming or refuting your diagnostic hypothesis
Follow Figure 42.2 to narrow differential diagnosis by dizziness subtype
Conduct a systematic comprehensive history and examination (inculding indicated laboratory tests) that evaluates each of the systems and categories listed in Table 42.1. Aim to identify both causes and contributing factors, and look for factors that can successfully treated.

Figure 42.1 • General approach to the dizzy patient.

- Cardiac causes. Any disorder that compromises cardiac output, including atrial fibrillation or flutter, severe bradycardia, valvular disease (especially aortic stenosis), and heart block, can cause a feeling of lightheadedness or faintness. The symptom may be relieved by rest or lowering the head to allow improved cerebral perfusion.
- Stroke or transient ischemia of the vertebrobasilar system can present as vertigo. Usually (but not always) other neurological signs of a cerebellar or brainstem problem can be noted, such as diplopia, dysarthria, ataxia, or a central nystagmus (21).
- Posterior fossa tumors (i.e., acoustic neuromas or schwannomas). These typically present with vague, mild dizziness, and progressive hearing loss (22). In one series, 43% presented with total deafness on the affected side, and a large percentage with some hearing loss.

Most life threatening conditions are cardiovascular. For this reason, patients with risk factors for heart disease and/or stroke are at greatest risk for having serious and life-threatening causes of dizziness, and should receive an especially careful initial evaluation (23,24).

CLINICAL EVALUATION

The clinician caring for the dizzy patient must be prepared to deal with uncertainty. Empirical guidelines for diagnostic strategies do not exist and are unlikely to be developed in the near future, because of the complexity of the symptom and the lengthy differential diagnosis (20). Nevertheless, the primary care clinician must have a systematic approach to the clinical evaluation of the dizzy patient.

Clinical History

The clinical history plays a key role during the evaluation of dizzy patients and will provide crucial information to make a diagnosis in the majority of cases (25,26). Listen carefully to the way the patient describes the presenting complaint. Try to obtain this history in the patient's own words, preferably without the word "dizzy." Based on the history, we recommend proceeding down one of three decision-making pathways (Fig. 42.1):

- Sometimes the pattern of historical information strongly suggests one diagnosis or several related diagnoses, for example a drug reaction, a viral illness, a gastrointestinal bleed, or a panic disorder. If the history is highly suggestive in this way, use a focused physical examination, laboratory testing, other additional diagnostic testing, or (if indicated) a therapeutic trial to verify or refute your hypothesis.
- If the history clearly indicates one dizziness subtype (vertigo, presyncope, or disequilibrium) but is not pathognomonic of a single diagnostic entity, the differential diagnosis can be narrowed, and the clinician should proceed to systematically evaluate the causes of that dizziness subtype. Figures 42.2.a, 42.2.b, and 42.2.c provide guidance for this diagnostic process.
- If the history is confusing, then a more thorough, system-by-system approach is warranted. This applies particularly to

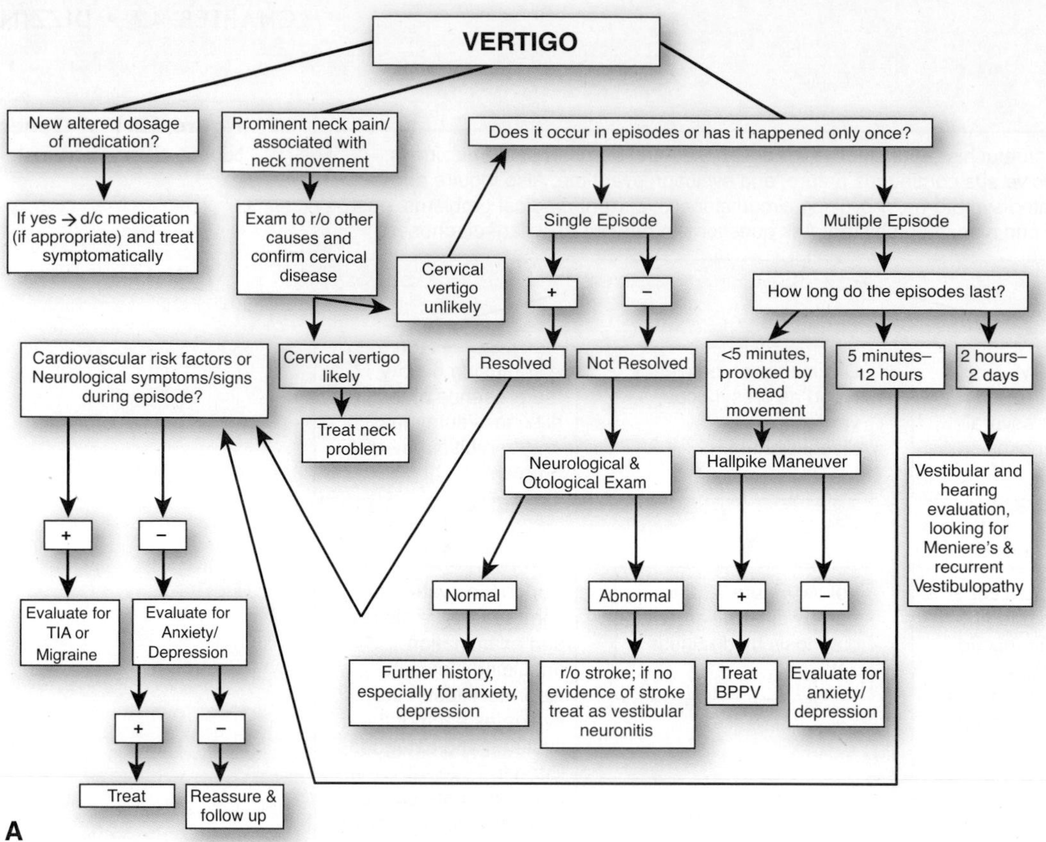

Figure 42.2 • **A.** Approach to the patient with vertigo. The history of onset, duration, accompanying symptoms, and episodic or continuous nature of the vertigo can be used to narrow your differential diagnosis.

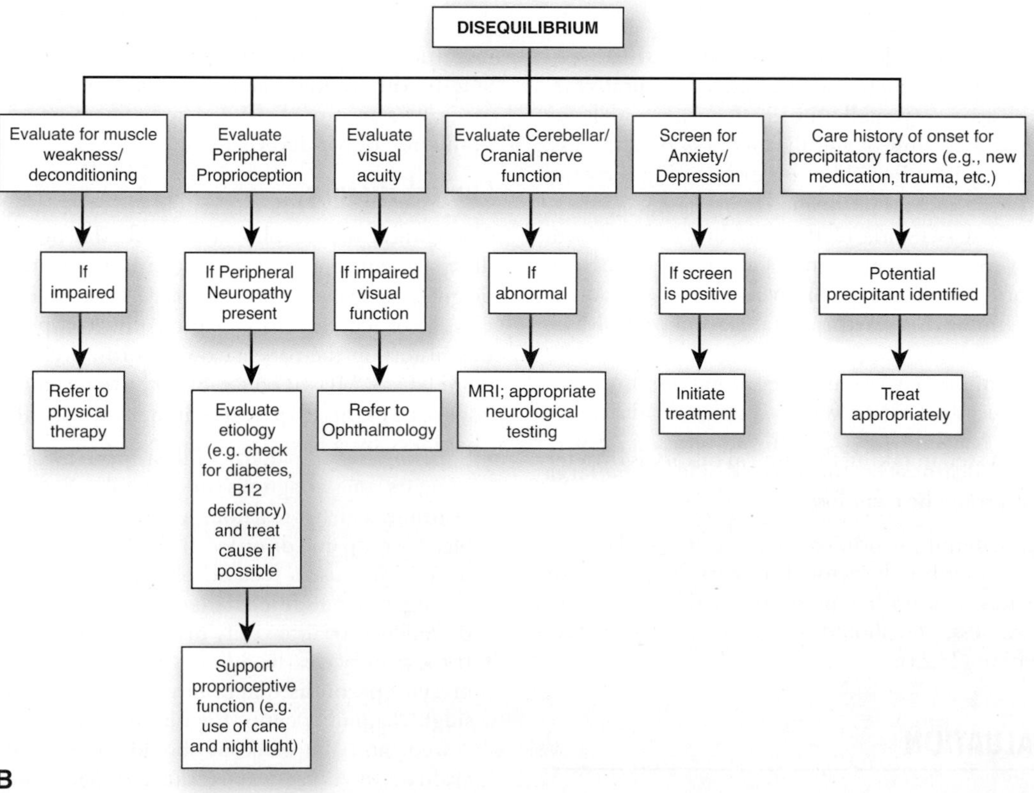

Figure 42.2 • **B.** Approach to the patient with disequilibrium (imbalance). Disequilibrium frequently has multiple causes or contributory factors; so a comprehensive evaluation of the balance system is generally warranted, with the management plan addressing each factor that you identify.

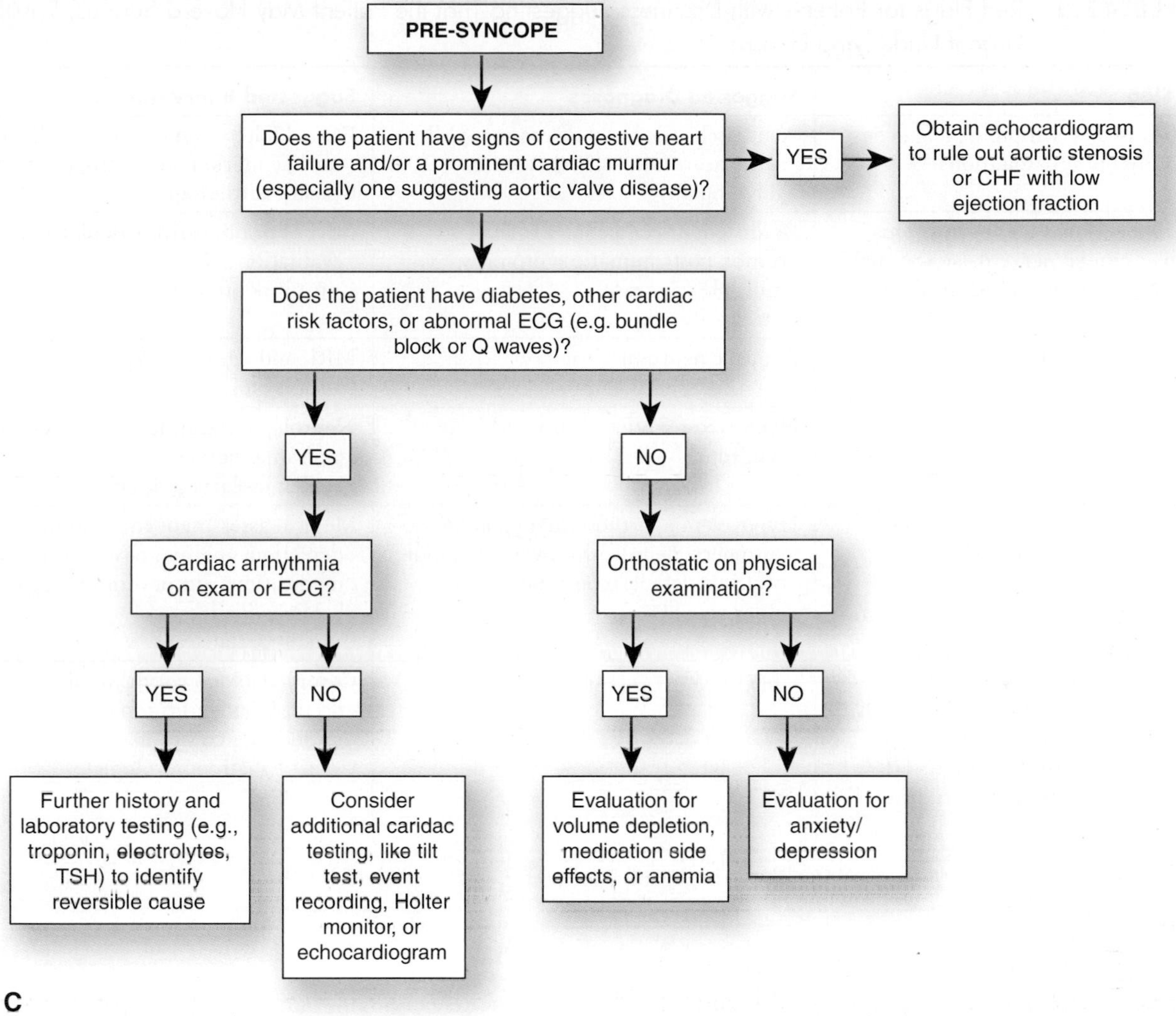
PRE-SYNCOPE
Does the patient have signs of congestive heart failure and/or a prominent cardiac murmur (especially one suggesting aortic valve disease)?
YES
Obtain echocardiogram to rule out aortic stenosis or CHF with low ejection fraction
Does the patient have diabetes, other cardiac risk factors, or abnormal ECG (e.g. bundle block or Q waves)?
YES
NO
Cardiac arrhythmia on exam or ECG?
Orthostatic on physical examination?
YES
NO
YES
NO
Further history and laboratory testing (e.g., troponin, electrolytes, TSH) to identify reversible cause
Consider additional caridac testing, like tilt test, event recording, Holter monitor, or echocardiogram
Evaluation for volume depletion, medication side effects, or anemia
Evaluation for anxiety/ depression
C

Figure 42.2 • C. Approach to the patient with presyncope. This symptom usually is caused by either cardiac disease, orthostasis, or anxiety, so the evaluation is directed toward these areas.

the majority of elderly patients with chronic dizziness (2); however, it also should be employed whenever a patient has multiple morbidities and/or has failed to be successfully diagnosed and treated using one of the other methods outlined above.

An important first step in taking the clinical history is to determine whether the problem is new or has been persisting for a few weeks or longer. If the problem is acute, then you can often narrow your potential diagnoses rapidly, using hypothesis generation and testing, combined with the dizziness subtype to aid your decision-making. If the problem is chronic, there is a higher likelihood that the problem is complex and involves multiple body systems, so a more systematic and thorough decision-making pattern is useful.

In taking the history, keep in mind that certain red flags suggest a progressive or life-threatening disorder. Among the serious disorders that can present as dizziness, and for which clinicians should be mindful, are cardiac disorders such as arrhythmias or heart failure, central nervous system disorders such as stroke or multiple sclerosis, eighth cranial nerve tumors, infections of cranial nerves such herpes zoster oticus, and orthostasis-related disorders such as hypovolemia or gastrointestinal bleeding. In addition, all patients with new dizziness should have a careful review of prescribed, over-the-counter, and herbal medications, because drugs can cause dizziness by a variety of mechanisms. Table 42.2 identifies and discusses key warning signs to screen for in patients with dizziness.

For people with chronic dizziness, standardized instruments such as the Dizziness Handicap Inventory can be useful for identifying patients with a high risk for persistent, disabling dizziness, and for monitoring the effect of therapeutic interventions (27–29).

Physical Examination

The purpose of the initial physical examination is to further identify and confirm the system or systems involved in the patient's complaint, and to plan further workup, referral, or treatment. The exam should be tailored based on the history; however, most exams should include a general assessment of

TABLE 42.2 Red Flags for Patients with Dizziness Suggesting That the Patient May Have a Serious, Possibly Urgent Underlying Disease

Red Flag	Suggested Diagnoses	Suggested Interventions
Cardiovascular symptoms (e.g., chest pain, dyspnea, palpitations)	Acute ischemic heart disease or AMI, acute heart failure, arrhythmia, valvulopathy	ECG, Holter monitor, echocardiogram, cardiac markers (e.g., troponin level) Consult cardiologist
Central nervous system symptoms, such as cranial nerve palsies, visual symptoms or vision loss, unilateral weakness	Brainstem or cerebellar stroke, TIA, tumor, posttraumatic symptoms, multiple sclerosis	MRI of brain, cardiovascular risk evaluation Consult neurologist
Gradual hearing loss and tinnitus	Acoustic neuroma	MRI, audiogram, BAER Consult otolaryngologist
Severe otalgia and vesicular eruption, usually of the external canal and pinna	Herpes zoster oticus/Ramsay-Hunt syndrome	Neurologic examination, especially of cranial nerves Consult otolaryngologist
Propensity to pass out and/or severe lightheadedness on standing	Hypovolemia, orthostatic hypotension, peripheral neuropathy, overmedication, multiple deficits (common in older people)	Medical assessment for volume depletion, anemia, new or multiple medications, deconditioning, gait or balance disturbance Consult geriatrician
Vomiting blood, black stools, or gradual increase in weakness with postural presyncope, especially in patients with risk factors for GI bleed (e.g., anticoagulation, prior bleed, or NSAID use)	Upper or lower GI bleed	Complete blood count, stool for occult blood, additional testing for underlying cause Consult gastroenterologist

AMI = acute myocardial infarction; BAER = brainstem auditory evoked response; CHF = congestive heart failure; ECG = electrocardiogram; GI = gastrointestinal; MRI = magnetic resonance imaging; NSAID = nonsteroidal anti-inflammatory drugs; TIA = transient ischemic attack.

vital signs, general health, and psychological status; a brief cardiovascular examination, including orthostatics if indicated; a screening neurological examination, including vision assessment; and a brief otological evaluation.

The empirical validation of commonly used diagnostic tests for the domain dizziness in primary care is poor (30). Table 42.3 summarizes data on (a selection of) previously studied diagnostic tests.

Certain aspects of the physical examination can be useful during the evaluation of specific subtypes of dizziness. Some of the more valuable diagnostic tests are discussed in the following section.

ORTHOSTATIC HYPOTENSION TEST (SUBTYPE PRESYNCOPE)

Orthostatic hypotension is defined by a 20 mm Hg decrease in systolic blood pressure or a systolic blood pressure below 90 mm Hg in response to standing from supine position, when accompanied by symptoms such as presyncope, weakness, feeling a need to sit down, and visual blurring with change of position.

BALANCE SYSTEM SCREENING EVALUATION (SUBTYPE DISEQUILIBRIUM)

People use three modalities to maintain balance: vision, the vestibular system, and proprioception. Two out of three are necessary to maintain posture. If there is sway with eyes open, consider a cerebellar problem. By closing the eyes (Romberg test), one system is removed; therefore, if a patient sways with eyes closed, the problem is either proprioceptive or vestibular in origin, and the test is considered positive. If the Romberg is positive and the complaint is vertigo, consider a vestibular origin; if vertigo is absent, examine proprioception further.

A complete peripheral sensory examination, including proprioception, is especially important for patients complaining of disequilibrium symptoms, as neuropathies are relatively common, especially in older people and diabetics. Keep in mind, however, that balance may be impaired with deconditioning or any neuromuscular disease of the lower extremities (31).

THE DIX-HALLPIKE MANEUVER (SUBTYPE VERTIGO)

This simple test is a cornerstone of diagnosis of benign paroxysmal positional vertigo (BPPV). With the patient in a sitting position, turn the patient's head 30 degrees to one side. Move the patient quickly to the supine position, keeping the head turned, until the patient's head is hanging 30 degrees off the table. This position places the lower ear's posterior semicircular canal—that most commonly involved in BPPV—in a plane relative to gravity, thereby causing the endolymph to spin and symptoms to be provoked. Because the two horizontal semicircular canals are aligned almost perpendicular to each other, the Dix-Hallpike maneuver must be done both with the head turned 30 degrees to the right, and then with it

TABLE 42.3 Characteristics of Selected Diagnostic Tests for the Evaluation of Patients Presenting with Dizziness

Diagnostic Test	Target Condition	Population/Setting	Test Characteristics
History includes: • absence of vertigo, or • age >69, or • neurological deficit[51]	"Serious" cause of dizziness	Dizzy, lightheaded, or "faint" patients; emergency department	Sensitivity 87%, specificity 43%; LR+ 1.5, LR− 0.3
History includes: • spinning sensation, • brief episodes, • brought on by head motion or position • associated with nausea/vomiting[52]	Benign paroxysmal positional vertigo	Dizzy patients; secondary care setting	*Spinning:* Sensitivity 60%, specificity 64%; LR+ 1.7, LR− 0.6 *Episodic:* Sensitivity 80%, specificity 27%; LR+ 1.1, LR− 0.8 *Positional:* Sensitivity 80%, specificity 36%; LR+ 1.3, LR− 0.6 *Nausea/vomiting:* Sensitivity 20%, specificity 64%; LR+ 0.6, LR− 1.3
Blood pressure and pulse after 0/1/2/3/5/10 minutes,[53] or 0/1/5/10 minutes[54]	Orthostatic hypotension	Patients with syncope,[53] or dizziness/vertigo[54]; secondary care setting	Sensitivity 51%–58%, specificity 72%–80%; LR+ 1.8–2.9, LR− 0.5–0.7
Dix-Hallpike maneuver[55,56]	Benign paroxysmal positional vertigo	Patients with vertigo; secondary/tertiary care setting	Sensitivity 59%–88%, specificity >90%
Head-shaking nystagmus[56–61]	Peripheral vestibular dysfunction	Patients from 5 studies with dizziness or vertigo; secondary/tertiary care setting	Sensitivity 35%–90%, specificity 51%–92%; LR+ 0.9–4.3, LR− 0.2–1.1
Head impulse test[60,62–64]	Peripheral vestibular dysfunction	Patients from 4 studies with dizziness or vertigo; secondary/tertiary care setting	Sensitivity 35%–93%, specificity 61%–97%; LR+ 2.3–12.5, LR− 0.1–0.7
Combination of head impulse test, cross-cover test, and nystagmus observation[33]	Differentiating stroke from vestibular neuronitis	101 patients with acute vertigo in an emergency department	Normal HIT plus direction-changing nystagmus or new gaze skew was 100% sensitive and 96% specific for stroke
PRIME-MD Patient Health Questionnaire[65]	Major depressive disorder (MDD), panic disorder (PD)	Dizzy patients; tertiary care setting	*MDD:* Sensitivity 73%, specificity 94%; LR+ 12.5, LR− 0.3 *PD:* Sensitivity 94%, specificity 96%; LR+ 25.1, LR− 0.06

turned 30 degrees to the left. The hallmarks of a positive response are:

- the occurrence of vertigo associated with a mixed torsional and vertical nystagmus
- a decline in the provoked vertigo and nystagmus within 30 seconds
- fatigability if the test is repeated several times

TESTS TO DIFFERENTIATE STROKE FROM ACUTE VESTIBULAR NEURONITIS (SUBTYPE VERTIGO)

Bedside neurological testing may be useful in distinguishing patients who are having stroke from those with vestibular neuronitis. Three tests are recommended (32,33):

- The horizontal head impulse test. The patient sits upright and is instructed to fix gaze on a central target (e.g., the examiner's nose) and to allow the examiner to passively move the head. The examiner rotates the patient's head slowly about 20 degrees to the left, and then rapidly moves it back to the midline, while observing the eyes. This maneuver is then repeated, this time turning the head to the right and bringing it back to midline. If the eyes deviate from forward gaze and then jump back to fix on the target, this is a positive result and indicates a vestibular injury on the side to which the head was turned rapidly. For a video illustration, see: *www.neurology.org/content/vol70/issue24_Part_2/images/data/2378/DC1/Video_e-1.wmv*.

- The prism cross-cover test for ocular alignment. With a patient fixating on a central target, the examiner should observe for eye misalignment and (to detect milder misalignment) ask the patient if he or she sees double. Next the examiner covers one eye and then rapidly removes the cover, observing to see if the eye is initially off center and jumps back into alignment. The *normal* response to alternately occluding each eye is for the eyes to remain motionless. In a patient who did not previously have a "lazy eye," an abnormal response is present if the eyes are misaligned when both are uncovered or if one eye jumps back into alignment after the cover is removed. For a video illustration see: *http://stroke.ahajournals.org/content/vol0/issue2009/images/data/STROKEAHA.109.551234/DC1/Kattah_Video3_LatMedullaStroke_SkewAltCover.wmv*
- Observation of nystagmus in different gaze positions. Have the patient look to the right, to the left, straight ahead, up and down. Nystagmus that changes direction indicates a central lesion such as stroke; nystagmus that is in only one direction indicates a peripheral problem such as vestibular neuronitis. For a video illustration, see *http://content.lib.utah.edu/cdm4/item_viewer.php?CISOROOT=/ehsl-dent&CISOPTR=2.*

When these three tests were performed together in evaluating 101 patients with acute vertigo in an emergency department, the presence of normal horizontal head impulse test, direction-changing nystagmus in eccentric gaze, or skew deviation (vertical ocular misalignment) was 100% sensitive and 96% specific for stroke, outperforming both head computed tomography and magnetic resonance imaging scanning in the acute setting (33).

TESTING FOR PSYCHOLOGICAL CONDITIONS

Formal testing can be useful in diagnosing anxiety disorders and depression in people with dizziness. These include:

- Formal instruments to screen for anxiety and/or depression. Numerous instruments are available to screen general medical populations; particularly useful are the various versions of the Patient Health Questionnaire. One approach would be to use the four-item version that screens for both depression and anxiety, and then to follow-up positive scores with a more detailed instrument (34).
- Hyperventilation provocation. If anxiety with hyperventilation is suspected, the patient should be instructed to breathe deeply and at a rapid rate for 60 seconds to attempt reproduction of the symptoms (35).

SEMMES-WEINSTEIN MONOFILAMENT TEST

People suspected of having a peripheral neuropathy should be tested with a monofilament, as is standard practice for diabetics (see Chapter 13 on diabetes) (36,37).

Additional Diagnostic Testing

Because only a small proportion of dizzy patients have life threatening illnesses, discretion should be used in deciding whether and when to perform laboratory testing. One study, for example, found no significant differences between 149 subjects with chronic dizziness and matched controls in results of laboratory testing, including complete blood count, erythrocyte sedimentation rate, blood urea nitrogen, electrolytes, glucose, cholesterol, liver function tests, and thyroid function tests (38). In a review of 4,538 patients, laboratory abnormalities that explained the dizziness were limited to 3 patients with electrolyte disturbances, 11 with glucose disorders, 11 with anemia, and 1 with hypothyroidism (39).

Diagnostic tests that can be helpful in specific situations include the following:

- Audiometry. Formal audiogram assessment is important in ruling out an acoustic neuroma (unilateral hearing loss is generally present) and in helping diagnose Ménière disease (unilateral or bilateral low frequency hearing loss is common).
- Electronystagmography. This refers to a combination of tests to evoke nystagmus and related eye movements, detected by electrodes placed on the skin surrounding the eyes. A key element is caloric testing by irrigating each ear with cool (30°C) and warm (44°C) water, which tests peripheral vestibular system function. A positive test (usually hyporeactivity) suggests a lesion somewhere between the vestibular end organ and the nerve root entry at the lateral medulla.
- Neuroimaging. Magnetic resonance imaging is the recommended modality to look for central disorders or those related to the internal auditory canal or vestibulocochlear nerve. Gadolinium enhancement may be useful to diagnose vestibular neuromas (i.e., schwannomas or meningiomas). Computed tomography is useful for middle ear disease, using thin sections for temporal bone assessment.
- Cardiac monitoring. A 12-lead electrocardiogram with a 1-minute rhythm strip will detect some arrhythmias, such as atrial fibrillation. A 24-hour Holter monitor or (better yet) an event monitor has better sensitivity for detecting arrhythmias.

MANAGEMENT

When a definitive cause is identified, treatment is directed at the cause. When multiple factors are present or the cause cannot be reversed, as is the case in many neurological disorders and in many older people, the best strategy is to treat contributing factors, with the goal of helping the person overcome or minimize the disabling aspects of the dizziness.

General Principles

Management of the patient with dizziness should follow these general principles:

1. If the patient has a clear diagnosis, treat the underlying cause.
2. If the problem is self-limited, provide reassurance. Symptomatic relief can be provided, but beware of using medications with significant side effects that may place the patient at risk for complications.
3. All patients, including those with permanent deficits, can be helped by approaches that focus on quality of life and improving function. Helpful strategies include strengthening compensatory mechanisms (vision, balance, muscle strength, proprioception), treating secondary symptoms (such as anxiety or neck pain), providing symptom relief when indicated and appropriate (e.g., meclizine for vestibular neuronitis), and giving appropriate reassurance.
4. There are patients whose histories and physical examinations do not fall neatly into a well-defined diagnosis.

In these cases the clinician should educate the patient about risks and benefits of various approaches to diagnosis and treatment and follow the patient closely as a therapeutic guide and partner.

Patients with dizziness are often suffering quite a bit, though they may not appear to be in distress. Furthermore, chronic dizziness symptoms, such as chronic pain, can be fatiguing and can lead to depression. These disabling aspects of dizziness are often not appreciated by the patient's family and friends. For these reasons, an empathic approach on the part of the physician is especially important. Since most cases of dizziness improve with time, usually days to weeks, the clinician should provide appropriate reassurance that symptoms will be ameliorated. If disability is persistent, then a rehabilitative approach should be taken, including referrals to a physical therapist familiar with balance and vestibular problems, and attention given to psychological status, medication, and general health issues such as nutrition and sleep.

Symptoms associated with chronic dizziness include persistent vertigo, chronic postural lightheadedness, unsteadiness, or a sensation of the environment bouncing when one walks (oscillopsia). Many patients with chronic dizziness are at increased risk for falls and have serious functional impairment, including anxiety and fear, sometimes leading to depression. Such dizziness-related symptoms can lead to loss of independence in self-care and activities of daily living. Management should be function-oriented, with improvement in quality of life as the major therapeutic goal. The clinician must address the multifactorial aspects contributing to the patient's symptoms, including such elements as vision, anxiety, and muscle strength (2,20). Many patients, particularly the elderly, are underreferred for specialty consultation and do not receive optimal treatment (40). Therefore, the clinician should consider consultation with a neurologist, otolaryngologist, or physical therapist for patients whose dizziness is chronic or recurrent (41).

Medications should be used judiciously, as there is no "dizziness medicine." The following classes of drugs can be helpful if the patient has vertigo: antihistamines, phenothiazines, anticholinergics, and benzodiazepines. However, all of these medications have significant side effects, and therefore, must be used with discretion, at the lowest effective dose, and for a short period (41). Furthermore, because they tend to make presyncope and disequilibrium worse, they are only indicated for vertiginous disorders. Finally, because the symptoms of BPPV are short-lived and intermittent, treatment with a high side effect profile drug is not appropriate for this diagnosis.

A word about meclizine (Antivert) is in order, because it is often used inappropriately. It is an antihistamine that dulls the normal vestibular response and is, therefore, especially useful in treating acute vestibular neuronitis. There is no place, however, for meclizine in patients who have dizziness secondary to disequilibrium of other etiologies, and it can cause harm to the elderly deconditioned patient who may also be taking other medications. Therefore, meclizine should be prescribed only for peripheral vestibular diseases, and with caution if at all in older people.

As in other chronic conditions, it is often helpful to track symptoms in a quantitative or semiquantitative manner. Several instruments have been developed to do this (42).

Treatment of Selected Diagnoses

Treatment will rely on the thoughtful and thorough evaluation needed in many cases to arrive at the appropriate diagnosis and to identify when treatment will help the patient, when referral is needed, and when watchful waiting is the best option. Because so many diagnostic possibilities exist in patients with dizziness, we cannot address all or provide in-depth recommendations. In the section that follows, we summarize key treatment recommendations for some of the more common diagnoses presenting as dizziness. Table 42.4 summarizes existing data on key therapies for selected dizziness diagnoses.

Benign paroxysmal positional vertigo (BPPV). Epley and Semont developed maneuvers to relocate loose particles from the utricular macula to the vestibule of the labyrinth where they do not cause symptoms. The Epley maneuver, as it has come to be known, has a success rate of 75% at 1 week, with the majority of patients being cured after one office visit (22). A literature review in 2004 concluded that the scientific evidence is adequate (strength of recommendation [SOR] = A) to support its value in providing symptom relief, but it is unknown if the effectiveness persists over a long period of time (43). An instructional video on the Epley maneuver is available on YouTube at *http://tw.youtube.com/watch?v=ZqokxZRbJfw&feature=related*. Additional treatment principles include symptom relief through vestibular habituation exercises (i.e., provoking the dizziness in a controlled setting, such as in bed, by rolling over or falling to the side) (44). Medication is usually not indicated; however, in severe or persistent cases, a vestibular suppressant medication such as meclizine or diazepam may be useful.

Vestibular neuronitis. Without treatment, the vertigo typically improves on a daily basis, such that within 7 to 10 days the individual is functioning fairly normally. During the acute phase, however, medication can be helpful. One series found methylprednisone more effective than placebo, with number needed to treat to improve symptoms being two. Dosage begins at 100 mg daily for 3 days, then tapers to 10 mg daily by 3 weeks (45). In the severely acute patient, the following medical therapies have been recommended, though in many cases the level of evidence supporting them is largely anecdotal: (i) metoclopramide 10 mg orally or intramuscularly once or twice daily, to decrease neurovegetative symptoms; (ii) diazepam 2 to 10 mg orally, intravenously or intramuscularly 2 to 4 times daily, to decrease oscillopsia, nystagmus, and activation of sensory substitution phenomena; (iii) magnesium sulfate solution twice daily, intravenously, to decrease vestibular damage; (iv) gabapentin 300 mg orally twice or three times daily, to stabilize visual fields and reduce nystagmus; (v) vestibular electrical stimulation by means of transcutaneous electrical nerve stimulation electrodes placed on the paravertebral muscles opposite the affected side and the trapezius of the affected side for 1 hour daily, to provide symptomatic relief; and (vi) lying on the healthy side with head raised to 20 degrees (46). After the acutely vertiginous stage, specific vestibular habituation exercises improve central nervous system adaptation and hasten rehabilitation (47). The exercises require about 30 minutes of instruction by either a vestibular physical therapist or someone who has been trained in vestibular rehabilitation.

Cerebrovascular ischemia or stroke. Patients whose dizziness is caused by a transient ischemic attack should have therapy aimed at preventing future occurrences. Since virtually all

TABLE 42.4 Key Therapies for Selected Dizziness Diagnoses

Diagnosis and Intervention	Strength of Recommendation*	Comment
Benign Paroxysmal Positional Vertigo (BPPV)		
Epley maneuver[44,66]	A	There is good evidence that the Epley maneuver is a safe, effective treatment for BPPV.
Modified Epley maneuver[67]	B	For patients at home, the modified Epley maneuver may be more suitable for self-treatment than conventional Brandt-Daroff exercises.
Vestibular rehabilitation[48]	B	Compared to repositioning maneuvers, there is less evidence for the use of vestibular rehabilitation as treatment for BPPV.
Vestibular Neuritis		
Vestibular rehabilitation[48]	A	There is moderate to strong evidence that vestibular rehabilitation (movement, exercise based) is a safe and effective approach to symptom mitigation in unilateral peripheral vestibular disorders.
Methylprednisone[46]	A	Methylprednisolone may improve the recovery of peripheral vestibular function in patients with vestibular neuritis. NNT = 2. Start with high dose and taper quickly.
Ménière Disease		
Diuretics[68]	C	There is no good evidence for or against the use of diuretics in Ménière disease.
Betahistine[69]	C	There is no evidence that betahistine is effective or ineffective in patients with Ménière disease or syndrome.
Migrainous Vertigo		
Medications used for migraine prophylaxis or treatment[70]	B	Prophylaxis, migraine abortive medicines and treatment for migraine are all effective along with vestibular rehabilitation exercises.
Vestibular rehabilitation[70]	B	

A = consistent, good-quality patient-oriented evidence; B = inconsistent or limited-quality patient-oriented evidence; C = consensus, disease-oriented evidence, usual practice, expert opinion, or case series.
For information about the SORT evidence rating system, see *www.aafp.org/afpsort.xml.*

transient ischemic attacks associated with dizziness are in the posterior circulation, carotid endarterectomy is generally not helpful, even if the person has carotid artery disease. Instead, therapy should include an antiplatelet agent or other agent that reduces thrombosis; it should address cardiac conditions, such as atrial fibrillation or congestive heart failure; and it should reduce risk factors such as hypertension, hyperlipidemia, and smoking. Patients who have had a stroke and experience dizziness will additionally benefit from postural and vestibular exercises, occupational and physical therapy, and home modification.

Migraine-associated dizziness. The first step in management of migrainous vertigo is the recognition of the overlying and complex relationship among migraine headaches, dizziness, and balance disorders. The natural history is benign, with spontaneous remission of four of five patients within 5 to 10 years (44). Treatment for migraine effectively treats the dizziness, when the diagnosis is correct. Physical therapy, though rarely used, has been found to be helpful in some series (48).

Anxiety and depression. Mood disorders are very common in people with dizziness, both as primary causes and as secondary effects. Because patients may have underlying vestibular, cardiovascular, or balance disorders and be anxious as a result, the clinician should not assume that anxiety is the only diagnosis, even when florid anxiety or depression is accompanied by dizziness. Instead, the patient should be evaluated thoroughly, in a similar manner to someone with any balance disorder. Selective serotonin reuptake inhibitors have been reported to be effective in reducing symptoms over time. Care should be taken in prescribing selective serotonin reuptake inhibitors, however, as they may cause nausea, sedation and dizziness—the same symptoms being treated. Slow titration to an effective dose should therefore be employed. Combined vestibular therapy with cognitive therapy has been shown to be useful for the dizziness but not the anxiety (49,50).

KEY POINTS

- Dizziness is usually not life-threatening, but it can cause considerable discomfort and disability.
- Because of the extensive differential diagnosis, the decision-making process should vary depending on the patient's symptoms and signs. In some instances, the presentation is classic, and pattern recognition can be used to arrive at a tentative diagnosis; at other times system-based or comprehensive strategies are more appropriate. For all cases, however, a systematic screen of the components of the balance system should be done, to rule out red flags for serious, life-threatening disorders.
- The approach to management should be individualized, aiming at treating underlying causes, providing reassurance when appropriate, educating the patient, and offering treatment that will minimize disability by supporting patient function.

CHAPTER

43

Fatigue

Thomas C. Rosenthal and Vinod Patel

CLINICAL OBJECTIVES

1. Describe four distinct types of fatigue: physiologic tiredness, secondary fatigue, chronic fatigue, and fatigue in the elderly.
2. Use screening tools, history, and physical exam to arrive at a diagnosis.
3. Guide patients to implement universally effective antifatigue strategies such as physical fitness, sleep hygiene, naps, and caffeine.
4. Use medication to treat fatigue as appropriate.

Fatigue is very common and has serious consequences. Fourteen percent of men, 20% of women, 25% of adolescents, and 98% of residents in long-term care facilities complain of fatigue (1,2). Overexertion, deconditioning, viral illness, upper respiratory infection, anemia, lung disease, medications, cancer, and depression are common contributing factors. Twenty percent of auto accidents are due to fatigue (3). In one of three cases, no etiology can be identified. The impact of fatigue on performance has resulted in rules limiting work hours in several professions (4).

In this chapter, we focus on fatigue and tiredness as a presenting complaint and differentiates among the four main categories of fatigue: (i) physiologic tiredness, which results from an imbalance of exercise, sleep, diet or other activity and is relieved by a structured program of rest; (ii) secondary fatigue, which accompanies and may follow for several weeks an acute illness such as influenza or cholecystitis; (iii) chronic fatigue, which lasts for more than 6 months and is unrelated to an identified medical condition (5); and (iv) fatigue associated with old age, which is often the earliest sign of frailty. The algorithm in the Figure 43.1 summarizes an evidence based approach to fatigue. For a discussion of sleep disorders, please see Chapter 44.

OVERVIEW

In evaluating a patient who complains of being tired or fatigued, the first clinical challenge is to differentiate between fatigue and sleepiness.

- *Sleepiness,* a form of physiologic tiredness, is characterized by a tendency to fall asleep. Sleepy people yawn and stretch because they are transiently aroused by movement (6). Sleepy patients desire a nap and often can be energized by physical activity. Sleepy patients fall asleep easily and are refreshed by napping.
- *Fatigue*, on the other hand, is characterized by a lack of energy, mental exhaustion, and poor muscle endurance. Fatigued patients feel worse and recover slowly after exercise and either cannot sleep or find sleep nonrestorative. Men are likely to use the word "tired" to describe fatigue. Women, on the other hand, may describe themselves as depressed or anxious (7,8). Fatigued patients have little strength or desire to perform. They lack energy, stamina, and ambition. Figure 43.2 provides a brief screening questionnaire to help differentiate fatigue from sleepiness.

Differential Diagnosis

The underlying causes of fatigue can be mental, physical, lifestyle, and idiopathic. Table 43.1 illustrates the broad differential diagnosis that should be considered when evaluating a patient with fatigue; Table 43.2 provides some guidance regarding which diagnoses are most common. During the evaluation, keep in mind that some patients will have more than one contributing factor. Among the common categories of etiology to consider are

- *Psychological factors*. Depression is the most common psychiatric illness associated with fatigue. Anxiety disorders also commonly present with fatigue (9).
- *Life transitions*. Adolescence, marriage, divorce, death of a spouse, and changes in work status can all present as fatigue. A significant increase or decrease in usual physical exertion, inadequate rest, sleep pattern disruption, and recent surgery or trauma may induce fatigue.
- *Substance abuse*. Caffeine, alcohol, and illicit drug use often masquerade as fatigue.
- *Environmental stresses*. Excessive noise, heat, or cold exposure can lead to a fatigue response (10).
- *Chronic disease*. Diabetes, acute infections, cardiovascular disease, and lung disease are examples.
- *Medications*. Common fatigue-associated drugs include narcotics, psychotropics, antihypertensives, and antihistamines. Even "nonsedating" antihistamines sedate 10% of people (11).
- *Toxins*. Carbon monoxide exposure and chronic poisonings (e.g., heavy metals) can present as fatigue.
- *Inflammatory and connective tissue disorders*. Fatigue is more common in rheumatoid arthritis and systemic lupus erythematosus than in osteoarthritis. Fibromyalgia patients present with fatigue and tender trigger points.

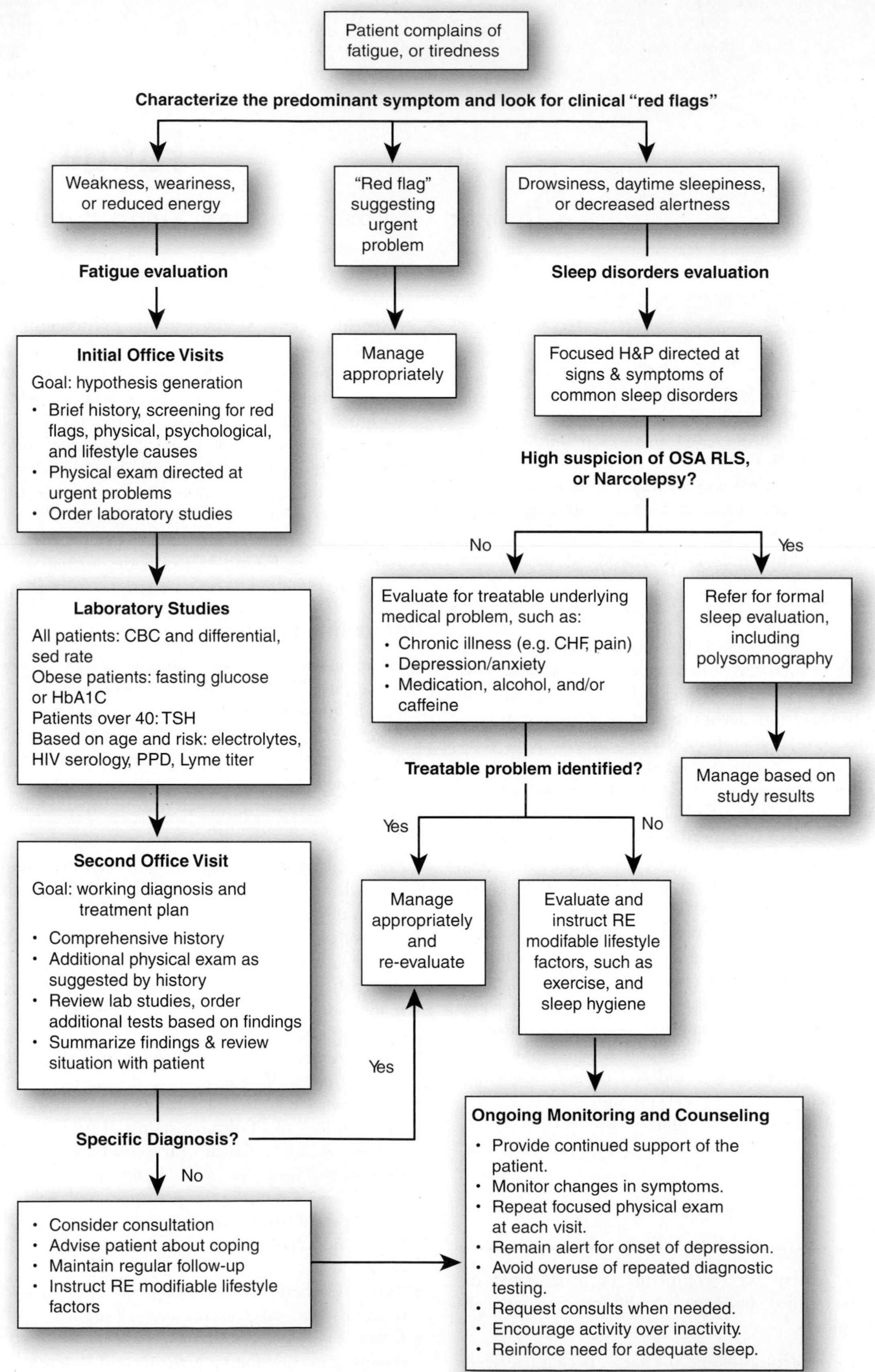

Figure 43.1 • General approach to patients with fatigue. OSA = obstructive sleep apnea; RLS = restless leg syndrome.

Sleepiness: How likely are you to doze off or fall asleep (as opposed to just feeling tired) in the following situations?	Never			Likely
1. Sitting and reading	0	1	2	3
2. Watching TV	0	1	2	3
3. Sitting inactive in a public place (theater, meeting)	0	1	2	3
4. As a passenger in a car for an hour when circumstances permit	0	1	2	3
5. Sitting and talking to someone	0	1	2	3
6. Sitting quietly after lunch without alcohol	0	1	2	3

Range 0–18: higher scores equate to greater sleepiness

Fatigue: Using a scale from 1 = strongly disagree to 6 = strongly agree, please indicate how much you agree or disagree with the following statements.	Strongly Disagree					Strongly Agree
1. Exercise brings on my fatigue	1	2	3	4	5	6
2. I start things without difficulty but get weak as I go on	1	2	3	4	5	6
3. I lack energy	1	2	3	4	5	6

Range 3–18: higher scores equate to greater fatigue

Interpretation: Scores for each section are compared and balanced. They should be used to inform clinical judgment and are not absolute.

Figure 43.2 • Questions differentiating between sleepiness and fatigue. Adapted from S Bailes, J Psychosomatic Res. 2006 (99).

- *Inactivity*. People who have a sedentary lifestyle are more likely to report fatigue than those who are physically active. This is probably because exercise has some inherent antidepressant and antianxiety effects, and improves sleep quality (12,13).

With careful follow-up, the number of undiagnosed patients should be quite small, but nonetheless some will remain chronically fatigued. Half of these patients will meet the criteria for chronic fatigue syndrome (CFS), a poorly understood syndrome that may represent more than one disease process. The diagnostic criteria for CFS are listed in Table 43.3. CFS patients must have unexplained persistent or relapsing fatigue that is not relieved by rest and is severe enough to significantly reduce daily activity levels. Although no specific treatment yet exists, making a diagnosis of CFS has several benefits. It reduces the need for continued investigation, provides an explanation to the patient, and helps support an application for disability benefits.

Patient evaluation should include a search for "red flags" that suggest a life-threatening problem. Because the differential diagnosis of fatigue, tiredness, and sleep complaints is extensive, the list of potential red flags can be quite broad. Table 43.4 lists the most prominent red flags and discusses the implication of each.

History

A detailed history should include information about the fatigue's duration and onset (sudden or progressive); whether it is a sleepy feeling, a physical lack of energy, or a mental fatigue; how long it takes to recover, and the patient's usual level of physical activity (sedentary or active). The patient should also be asked what aggravates their fatigue and if there are any modalities or activities that seem to relieve it. These questions will reveal that some patients are simply deconditioned, need little work up, and will respond to graded exercise therapy.

Unless the chief complaint clearly implicates a likely diagnosis, your history should include screening questions that touch on all the diagnostic categories listed in Table 43.2. A detailed review of all medications (prescribed and over the counter) is essential. Specifically ask about antihistamines, antidepressants, antihypertensives (e.g., clonidine, α-methyldopa, and β-blockers), corticosteroids, neuroleptics, antiarrhythmics (e.g., amiodarone), and complementary or herbal remedies. Toxic levels of medications such as digoxin or anticonvulsants often present as fatigue and are more likely in patients with renal or hepatic impairment. Acute and chronic environmental exposures (e.g., to carbon monoxide, lead, mercury, and arsenic) should also be considered.

TABLE 43.1 Differential Diagnosis of Tiredness and Fatigue

Category/Body System	Common Diagnoses	Findings
Disturbed sleep:	Sleep apnea, esophageal reflux, allergic/ vasomotor rhinitis, shift work, sleep hygiene.	Positive history of sleep problems.
Cardiopulmonary:	Congestive heart failure, chronic obstructive lung disease, peripheral vascular disease, angina pectoris.	Dyspnea, wheezing or crackles on auscultation, cyanosis, elevated jugular venous pressure, ankle edema, murmurs, extra heart sounds, diminished peripheral pulses.
Endocrine:	Diabetes mellitus, hypothyroidism, pituitary insufficiency, hypercalcemia, adrenal insufficiency, chronic kidney disease.	Polyuria, polydipsia, temperature intolerance, weight gain, goiter, thyroid nodule, skin and hair changes, constipation, pigmentation, delayed relaxation phase of reflexes.
Infectious:	Endocarditis, tuberculosis, mononucleosis, hepatitis, parasitic disease, malaria, HIV, cytomegalovirus.	History of injection drug use, unprotected sex, lymphadenopathy, hepatosplenomegaly, history of viral syndrome.
Gastrointestinal:	Malignancy, celiac disease, liver disease, GERD.	Blood in stool, anorexia, steatorrhea, weight loss, failure to thrive, jaundice, palmar erythema, Dupuytren's contractures, hepatosplenomegaly pruritus, excoriations, xanthelasma.
Hematologic:	Anemia, lymphoma, leukemia.	Pallor, tachycardia, systolic ejection murmur, night sweats, weight loss, lymphadenopathy.
Neurologic:	Multiple sclerosis, myasthenia gravis, Parkinson disease, amyotrophic lateral sclerosis.	Visual field defect, asymmetric deep-tendon or plantar reflexes, ataxia, nystagmus, muscle weakness, tremor, rigidity, bradykinesia, upper motor neuron impairment.
Inflammatory conditions:	Rheumatoid arthritis, systemic lupus.	Joint findings, rash.
Pharmacologic:	Hypnotics, antihypertensives, antidepressants, antihistamines, drug abuse.	Medication review including over the counter medications.
Psychologic:	Depression, anxiety, somatization disorder, dysthymia, partner abuse.	Positive screening.
Poisonings:	Carbon monoxide poisoning, arsenic, lead, mercury.	Shortness of breath, exposure to fumes, polyneuropathy.

Primary or secondary depression is present in about one quarter of patients presenting with unexplained fatigue. Patients experiencing grief or depression are more likely to have global complaints such as being unable to do "anything." Screening tests such as the Beck Depression Inventory can be helpful (14). Somatization disorder and panic disorder are also common. Some patients will have a history of a dysfunctional family setting or a previous history of functional health problems such as irritable bowel syndrome. In addition, ask the patient specific and probing questions regarding drug abuse and alcohol consumption.

Fatigued patients often do not sleep well. Sleep problems can be primary, such as sleep apnea or parasomnias, or secondary to other medical conditions. Interviewing the patient's bed partner is particularly critical in conducting a sleep disorders evaluation. The clinician should screen for sleep apnea by asking about daytime sleepiness, frequent snoring, choking, sudden awakening from sleep, or episodes of arrested breathing. For further details on sleep disorders, see Chapter 44.

THE HISTORY IN PHYSIOLOGIC TIREDNESS

Physiologic tiredness is initiated by inadequate rest or excessive physical and mental strain. The key history is that patient feels relief of their symptoms after rest and responds to realignment of their schedule or rearrangement of duties. The prevalence of physiologic tiredness is most common in adolescence, the elderly, shift workers, and people under stress. It is especially common in police officers, athletes, and medical residents (15–17). Key points about physiologic tiredness include:

- Sleep deprivation impairs concentration, judgment and triggers risk-taking behavior (18). The risk of an auto accident for sleep-deprived medical interns is equivalent to the risk of driving while intoxicated (19,20). Surgeons

TABLE 43.2 Common Causes of Fatigue in Primary Care

	Frequency in Primary Care		
Diagnosis	**As a Primary Diagnosis***	**In Patients with Recent-onset Fatigue**	**In Patients with Chronic Fatigue**
Depression	15.0%	Very common	Very common
Diabetes	10.6%	Very common	Very common
Acute infection	10.1%	Very common	Rare
Adjustment reaction	9.6%	Common	Uncommon
Cardiovascular disease	7.9%	Common	Common
Sleep disorders and lifestyle issues	7.8%	Very common	Common
Anxiety	6.1%	Common	Very common
Chronic pain	5%	Common	Very common
Lung disease (COPD, asthma)	4.9%	Common	Common
Connective tissue disease	4.7%	Uncommon	Common
Malignancy	3.2%	Uncommon	Common
Medication side effects	2.8%	Common	Common
Anemia	2.8%	Common	Uncommon
Hypothyroidism	2.6%	Uncommon	Uncommon
Substance abuse	2.2%	Common	Uncommon
Chronic infection (HIV, TB)	1.8%	Rare	Uncommon
GI causes: hepatitis, inflammatory bowel disease	1.6%	Rare	Rare
Neuromuscular disease (e.g., MS)	0.4%	Rare	Rare
Psychosis	0.1%	Rare	Rare
No diagnosis made	30%–40%	Very common	Common

COPD = chronic obstructive pulmonary disease; GI = gastrointestinal; HIV, human immunodeficiency virus; MS = multiple sclerosis; TB = tuberculosis.
*Note that patients often will have more than one disease contributing to the symptom of fatigue, and distinguishing the primary reason can be difficult.
†Previous studies of the causes of fatigue did not evaluate the extent to which other symptoms, such as pain and dizziness, may have been contributing factors.
(Adapted from Sloane, Essentials of Family Medicine, 5th ed, 2008)

who operate with inadequate sleep have higher complication rates. Similarly, tired farmers experience more injuries (21,22).

- Boredom, monotony, uninterrupted effort on a single task, and time of day or night all can engender fatigue (23).
- In adolescence the demands of rapid physical growth, frequent exposure to viral illnesses and pushing social limits makes fatigue almost routine (2).
- Obese patients who are deconditioned or patients suffering from peripheral vascular disease often describe their symptoms as fatigue (24).
- Stress is associated with fatigue (25). People in low-strain work environments experience the highest sleep quality and lowest level of fatigue.
- Irregular bedtime schedules, characteristic of shift work or college life, are associated with fatigue and a lower tolerance for exercise (26,27).

THE HISTORY IN SECONDARY FATIGUE

Secondary fatigue is due to illness. Patients with fatigue secondary to illness often describe specific activities they are unable to complete because they lack their former energy or stamina. Fatigue severity correlates more with the severity of illness than with age, psychological, or microbiological factors.

Viral infections are the most common cause of secondary fatigue. Twelve percent of patients report fatigue 6 to 12 weeks after Epstein-Barr and influenza infections (28). Forty-two percent of multiple sclerosis patients present with fatigue (29). In cancer, fatigue is the symptom most likely to interfere with daily routines, and 6 months after their last treatment 19% of disease-free cancer patients continue to report fatigue (30,31). Ninety-two percent of patients undergoing major abdominal surgery report fatigue that intensifies to day 14 and returns to baseline by day 45, with 10% continuing to report fatigue at 3 months. Fatigue after orthopedic surgery is less common but even minor surgery is frequently associated with postoperative fatigue (32,33).

THE HISTORY IN CHRONIC FATIGUE

Patients with fatigue lasting more than 6 months who have no discoverable etiology are termed chronically fatigued. Chronic fatigue is likely to be present all the time, acutely worsened by exercise, and unrelieved by rest. The highest prevalence of chronic fatigue is found among women,

TABLE 43.3 Diagnostic Criteria for Chronic Fatigue Syndrome[35]

Diagnosis requires
• At least 2 major plus 8 minor criteria; *or* • At least 2 major, 6 minor and 2 physical criteria
Major Criteria
• Six months' duration • Does not resolve with bed rest • Reduces daily activity by 50% • Other conditions excluded
Physical Criteria
• Low-grade fever • Nonexudative pharyngitis • Lymphadenopathy
Minor Criteria
• Description of initial onset as acute or subacute • Sore throat • Mild fever or chills • Lymph node pain • Generalized muscle weakness • Myalgia • Prolonged fatigue after exercise • New headaches • Migratory noninflammatory arthralgia • Sleep disturbance • Neuro-psychologic symptoms (photophobia, scotomata, forgetfulness, irritability, confusion, inability to concentrate, depression, difficulty thinking)

minority groups, and people with lower levels of education and occupational status.

A family physician with a typical practice will be following two patients with chronic fatigue (34). Two-thirds of these patients will fail to meet criteria to be classified as CFS, yet they will share many similarities and have only a slightly better prognosis than those who meet diagnostic criteria (35). Table 43.3 lists these diagnostic criteria. They are useful for defining disability or classifying a patient for inclusion in a study but may not be clinical helpful in all circumstances. Detailed psychiatric and sleep histories are helpful because many patients are relieved to know that their symptoms can be explained by psychosocial challenges.

Pre-morbid profiles of patients who develop chronic fatigue reveal that these patients had fewer responsibilities at home and at work than average and were more likely to use somatization when confronted with anxiety, depression, obsessions, substance use, and phobias (36,37). Childhood trauma is an important risk factor for CFS.

Negative feedback of the hypothalamus-pituitary-adrenal axis similar to that seen in other stress-related disorders seems to be the only consistent physiologic finding (38). Childhood trauma or abuse is associated with lifelong neuroendocrine dysfunction and correlates with adult vulnerability (39).

When fatigue has been present for more than 6 months, is debilitating, cannot be attributed to another condition, and does not meet criteria for chronic fatigue syndrome, it is termed idiopathic chronic fatigue. Obesity, sedentary lifestyle, and idiopathic chronic fatigue are so closely associated with one another that cause and effect are difficult to determine (24). Depression inventories help, but fatigued patients often have a depressed affect with a normal score on an objective screening tool (40).

A relationship between viral illness and chronic fatigue syndrome is unproven. Sixty-seven percent of patients with chronic fatigue syndrome test positive for a viral response. Epstein-Barr virus and a new retrovirus have been associated with many (but not all) patients with the syndrome (41). Patients with high stress scores experience viral infections more frequently, however, and evidence of cause and effect in chronic fatigue syndrome has been elusive (42). Focusing on a viral etiology is generally an unhelpful therapeutic strategy, because patients who believe they cannot get better until a virus is cured often fail to embrace aspects of recovery under which they do have control (43).

THE HISTORY IN FATIGUE IN THE ELDERLY

In the elderly, fatigue can be an independent early warning sign of imminent functional limitations and disability, predicting mortality and the need for additional services (44). Mortality rates at 10 years are 59% for older adults with fatigue versus 38% for those without fatigue (45).

Older people report greater fatigue after brief, intense physical exertion than do middle-aged subjects (46). Even temporary infirmities can compromise regular physical activity and lead to dependency, balance problems, and decreased quality of life (47,48). Deconditioning results in a rapid heart rate at lower exertion levels. A faster heart rate triggers the perception of fatigue and perpetuates the disability (49).

Physical Exam

The physical exam only occasionally identifies evidence of organ-based illness, but is useful in identifying some of the unusual causes of fatigue (Table 43.1) A complete detailed physical assures the patient that their complaints are being taken seriously, which is particularly important for the one third of patients in whom no cause is identified.

The exam should focus on the presence of lymphadenopathy (suggesting viral illness or cancer); cardiac rate, rhythm, and the presence of murmurs (congestive heart failure or, in the presence of fever, endocarditis); dyspnea and pulmonary abnormalities (chronic lung disease); goiter (thyroid imbalance), edema (heart or kidney failure, hypothyroidism, hypoproteinemia, or malnutrition), muscle tone (neurological condition), and neurologic abnormalities (stroke, brain metastases, dementia). If muscle fasciculation and/or atrophy and altered reflexes accompany fatigue, the patient may have a neuromuscular disease such as botulism, Guillain-Barré syndrome, multiple sclerosis, diphtheria or other myositis rather than pure fatigue. The clinician should also look for tender trigger points that may suggest fibromyalgia.

In children, the physical exam should include assessment of overall growth and development. If obesity is a problem, calculate an age-adjusted BMI. A careful head and neck exam

TABLE 43.4 Red Flags Suggesting Progressive or Life-threatening Disease in Patients with Fatigue

Red Flag(s)	Diagnosis Suggested
Suicidal ideation, marked social withdrawal	Major depressive episode; high suicide risk
History of alcohol, narcotic, or psychotropic drug abuse with recent discontinuation of use	Withdrawal syndrome; complications of drug use such as hepatitis, HIV, etc.
Fever >39.5°C, chills, hypotension, and/or neck stiffness	Life-threatening infection
Recent onset of severe or worsening fatigue, especially if accompanied by pallor, jaundice, or a history of recent blood loss, melena	Severe anemia due to blood loss or hemolysis
Gradual onset of fatigue in a patient with prominent risk factors for HIV exposure	AIDS
Orthopnea, edema, cardiomegaly, auscultatory crackles	Severe left-sided congestive heart failure
Polydipsia, polyuria	Poorly controlled diabetes
Lymphadenopathy	Lymphoma, leukemia, metastatic cancer
Peripheral edema, especially in the setting of chronic dyspnea and hypoxemia or hypercapnia	Pulmonary hypertension from severe obstructive sleep apnea with cor pulmonale
Recurrent falls	Multiple sclerosis, cerebrovascular disease
Falling asleep during activities, in conversation, or while driving	Significant accident risk; sleep disorder; possible narcolepsy

Adapted from Sloane, Essentials of Family Medicine, 5th ed, 2008.

should be conducted to look for craniofacial abnormalities such as micrognathia (Pierre Robin syndrome) and nasal obstruction. Tonsillar size should be assessed for hypertrophy, and the soft palate and uvula inspected for movement and tendency to collapse. Adenoidal hypertrophy may be assessed by nasopharyngoscopy or lateral neck radiographs. Neurologic assessment is also appropriate to look for evidence of hypotonia, which can be present in metabolic, primary neurologic or neuromuscular disorders (50).

For patients suspected of experiencing physiologic tiredness, the physical should concentrate on conditions that may interrupt sleep, such as arthritis, bursitis, neck masses, or spinal deformities.

In chronic fatigue the physical exam can be therapeutic, by communicating the physician's interest in and engagement with the patient's problems (40,51). Focused exams should be repeated at every visit.

With advancing age, skeletal muscle mass and strength decrease because of a phenomenon called sarcopenia. Strength may be normal but the speed with which maximum grip strength fatigues is one objective measure of fatigue. Patients can also be asked to grip a rubber ball as tight as possible and report when they feel they cannot maintain maximum strength. Any time less than 60 seconds is positive for fatigue and correlates well with activities such as carrying groceries (52). The physical exam should specifically look for the presence of other chronic disease and sources of inflammation, such as acute infections, immunologic disorders, deconditioning, and poor pulmonary function with hypoxia.

Diagnostic Testing

Laboratory testing has limited value in diagnosing fatigue. In a study of 325 patients with fatigue from 91 generalist physician offices, only 8% had a condition that was diagnosed by laboratory testing. Postponement of laboratory testing to a second visit did not affect outcomes (53). Indeed laboratory testing alters management in only 5% of patients (3).

Many physicians will order a complete blood count, erythrocyte sedimentation rate, chemistry screen, thyroid-stimulating hormone, and urinalysis as screening tests for patients with fatigue. Women of childbearing age should have a pregnancy test. If other studies are done, they should be ordered based on risks defined during the initial history and physical examination (Table 43.5). Examples include HIV serology, a skin test for tuberculosis, Lyme disease serology, oximetry, and spirometry. Testing for infectious mononucleosis is appropriate in selected patients younger than age 30; even with suggestive symptoms, however, the yield is no greater than 20% (54). Iron studies (including ferritin) should be considered in women, as some women with a normal hemoglobin and low ferritin experience relief of fatigue with iron supplementation (55).

Diagnostic Strategy Overview

When fatigue is a main complaint, a three-office visit evaluation is useful. Figure 43.1 outlines a general diagnostic strategy. The first visit should be used to: briefly assess elements of the history and physical examination that may indicate urgent problems (Table 43.4), establish if the patient is suffering from inadequate rest (physiologic tiredness) or true fatigue (40), order laboratory studies, emphasize need for a comprehensive assessment, and schedule a return visit of adequate length. Occasionally this initial evaluation will identify an obvious treatable cause, such as medication effect or a viral illness, and treatment will be started. If not, it is essential to introduce the differential diagnosis, including the role of stress.

TABLE 43.5 Laboratory Tests to Consider in Patient with Fatigue

Tests	Conditions being Considered	When to Order	Strength of Recommendation
Complete blood count	Anemia	Should be ordered on most patients with a 2-week history of fatigue. Results change management in 5% of patients. (Physical exam changes management in 2% of patients.)[59]	B
Sedimentation rate	Inflammatory state		
Chemistry panel	Liver disease, renal failure, protein malnutrition		
Thyroid panel	Hypothyroidism		
HIV antibodies	Chronic infection if not previously tested		
Pregnancy test if indicated	Pregnancy and breathlessness from progestins.		
CT Scan, TB test, echocardiogram	Adenopathy, cancer, tuberculosis, chronic infection, congestive heart failure	Rarely useful unless indications are present. Indicated in patients with physical findings or abnormal baseline blood tests.	C
ECG, ambulatory cardiac monitoring	Arrhythmia		
Pulmonary function tests	Chronic obstructive pulmonary disease		
Urine drug screen	Drug abuse		
Serologic studies (e.g. Lyme), cultures	Chronic infection		
Brain MRI	Multiple sclerosis	Rarely useful. Consider only if indicated by baseline testing.	C
Echocardiogram	Valvular heart disease, congestive heart failure		
Specialized blood testing such as ferritin, iron, iron binding capacity, B12, folate, Combs, etc.	Iron deficiency Addison disease, Celiac disease, myasthenia gravis, poisonings		

A = consistent, good-quality patient-oriented evidence; B = inconsistent or limited-quality patient-oriented evidence; C = consensus, disease-oriented evidence, usual practice, expert opinion, or case series.
For information about the SORT evidence rating system see *www.aafp.org/afpsort.xml*.
Original table using information from Fosnocht,[98] Fukada,[3] Lane,[54] and Koch.[53]

The second visit is used to gather additional information regarding the patient's social profile, medical history, family history, review of systems, current medications, and lifestyle issues, and to conduct a comprehensive physical examination and review the laboratory studies. At the end of this visit, findings should be summarized and treatment recommendations made based on the data. If sleep apnea or narcolepsy seems likely, referral to a sleep laboratory for polysomnography should be considered.

The third and subsequent visits are used to assess treatment, encourage adherence, and reassure the patient (and yourself) that nothing has been missed (40,56). Care should be taken to communicate your thoughts in a sensitive manner, and to develop a therapeutic partnership with the patient.

Management

Based on the history, physical exam, and laboratory studies, the clinician should make an effort to identify one or more medical, psychological, or lifestyle diagnoses for which specific treatment recommendations are available. Labels can be very comforting to patients.

Management of patients with persistent symptoms should follow the principles of chronic disease management: creation of a therapeutic partnership, involvement of a care team, appropriate use of medical therapy, careful monitoring, and active support. Table 43.6 provides key evidence-based recommendations. The clinician's challenge is to teach the patient about factors that can be modified and encourage optimism that a broad biopsychosocial approach leads to symptom improvement in most patients.

Generally, after the initial workup is complete, consultations from other physicians are more productive than further diagnostic testing. Consultations can clarify a diagnosis and reassure both the physician and the patient that tests have provided as much information as possible and that treatment is on the right track. For patients with sleep disorders, the specific approaches in Chapter 44 may be helpful, for anxiety see Chapter 48 and for depression see Chapter 50. In all cases, you should fully discuss plans and make a commitment to continuing care through follow-up visits.

MANAGEMENT OF PHYSIOLOGIC TIREDNESS

The treatment of choice for patients with physiologic tiredness is to rearrange schedules and practice good sleep hygiene. For those who must challenge normal sleep patterns, the judicious use of diet, naps, and caffeine can be helpful. Sedative hypnotics remain a last resort.

TABLE 43.6 Evidence-Based Therapeutic Recommendations for Practice

Clinical Recommendation	Strength of Recommendation	References	Comments
Studies have consistently shown exercise therapy benefits patients with fatigue, irregardless of etiology.	A	10,13,62,68, 70,84,85	There is no evidence that exercise therapy worsens outcomes.
Evidence favors the use of SSRI antidepressants such as fluoxetine or sertraline in patients with fatigue.	B	98,100	A 6-week trial is recommended to evaluate effectiveness.
Cognitive behavior therapy appears to be an effective and acceptable treatment for adult outpatients with chronic fatigue syndrome.	A	87–89	
Stimulants seldom return patients to predisease performance.	B	75,86	Stimulants are associated with headaches, restlessness, insomnia, and dry mouth.
In the elderly, long term β-alanine supplementation decreases fatigue.	B	92,93	Effect may take 3 months to manifest. Raises muscle carnosine.

A = consistent, good-quality patient-oriented evidence; B = inconsistent or limited-quality patient-oriented evidence; C = consensus, disease-oriented evidence, usual practice, expert opinion, or case series.
For information about the SORT evidence rating system see *www.aafp.org/afpsort.xml.*

A good night's sleep of generally 7 to 8 hours decreases tension and improves mood. Therefore, the patient with physiologic tiredness should be encouraged to practice good sleep hygiene as outlined in Table 43.7 and restructure their life to get the sleep they need, generally 7 to 8 hours (57). Naps help (58). When provided coverage for a 40-minute nap during overnight shifts, medical interns achieved morning fatigue scores equivalent to not being on-call (59). Once sleep-deprived, patients generally need two normal nights of sleep to achieve baseline function and stabilization of mood (60).

TABLE 43.7 Activities that Promote Better Nighttime Sleep

Maintain a regular morning rising time.
Avoid or limit napping to the early afternoon for less than an hour.
Increase activity level in the afternoon.
Avoid exercise in the evening or before bedtime.
Increase exposure to bright light during the day or early evening.
Take a hot bath within 2 hours of bedtime.
Avoid caffeine, nicotine, and alcohol in the evening.
Avoid excessive food or fluid intake at night.
Minimize light and noise exposure in the bedroom.
Use the bedroom only for sleep or sex.
Turn the television off when you are ready to go to sleep.

Fitness can combat physiologic tiredness. Truck drivers who engage in 30-minute exercise sessions more than once a week have fewer accidents (61). Ten weeks of supervised exercise increases energy levels among fatigued people regardless of medical condition (62).

A randomized double-blind crossover study in nighttime driving conditions confirmed that regular coffee (200 mg of caffeine or 8 oz. of coffee) resulted in fewer errors and was equivalent to a 30-minute nap (63). Modafinil, a prescription medication approved to modify fatigue induced by shift work, has the same impact on performance as 600 mg of caffeine. Caffeine and modafinil have fewer adverse cardiovascular effects and less abuse potential than amphetamines (63). Unfortunately, long-term use of all stimulant medications has been associated with dependency and depression (64). The combination of a 440-calorie meal and 200 mg of caffeine improves mood and cognitive performance (65).

Zolpidem has been used extensively to manage sleep and wake cycles in soldiers on extended combat assignment. Most soldiers found the medication useful to induce sleep; two-thirds reported no side effects or morning drowsiness; and one-third reported frequent awakenings or a morning "hang-over." There were no reports of abnormal sleep behaviors, but only one of six soldiers felt the medication was essential to maintaining performance (66).

MANAGING SECONDARY FATIGUE

Correcting physiologic parameters in secondary fatigue is often helpful. In cancer, renal disease, or other chronic diseases associated with anemia, patients report less fatigue if their hemoglobin is maintained at or above 10 g/dL, using erythropoietin injections if needed (30,67). Menstruating women with low ferritin may respond to 4 weeks of iron supplementation even if they have normal hemoglobin levels (55).

Performing some form of daily exercise, sustaining interpersonal relationships, and returning to work are consistently associated with improvement of fatigue regardless of its cause (10,68,69). Moderate aerobic activity (30 minutes of walking most days) reduces disease-related fatigue more effectively than rest. Yoga, group therapy, and stress management have been shown to diminish fatigue in cancer patients (70). Daytime napping should be discouraged as it interferes with a restorative night's sleep.

Patients who have features suggestive of depression can be offered a 6-week trial of a selective serotonin reuptake inhibitor, particularly the stimulatory selective serotonin reuptake inhibitor fluoxetine (71). Psychostimulants such as methylphenidates and modafinil have demonstrated short-term efficacy in patients with HIV, multiple sclerosis, stroke, renal failure, and cancer (72–74). Unfortunately stimulants are associated with headaches, restlessness, insomnia, and dry mouth (75). If used, stimulants work best for special events, on an as needed basis. Corticosteroids, anti-inflammatory drugs, and opiates should be titrated to alleviate pain without inducing fatigue.

MANAGING CHRONIC FATIGUE

The demanding nature of chronic fatigue has inspired multiple treatments and frustrations for over a decade (35). Although 64% of chronically fatigued patients will experience some improvement in symptoms, only 2% will report complete resolution of their fatigue. Patients who experience intensification of their symptoms lasting more than 24 hours after physical exertion have the worst prognosis (76,77). Although physicians often dispense medication or recommend tests, patients report greatest satisfaction with psychosocial management (51).

Patients do the best who receive a specific diagnosis from their doctor in the context of an empathetic relationship (78). A specific diagnosis assists the patient in discovery of relevant information, support groups, and access to disability benefits. Conditions such as fibromyalgia, somatization disorder, chronic fatigue syndrome, chronic back pain, chronic pelvic pain, and irritable bowel syndrome share many characteristics; so specific diagnostic criteria for CFS were developed to help separate the syndrome from some of these other entities (79). It is not uncommon, however, for patients not to fit diagnostic criteria.

Because medical treatment often has only modest success in CFS, there is a tendency for both the physician and the patient to try nontraditional sources of information and care (80). However, the Cochrane Database has reported that no high-quality studies yet show any nontraditional therapies to be effective in alleviating chronic fatigue (81). Still, constant searching is often engaged in by both physician and patient. Sharing findings and objectively evaluating evidence can contribute to the therapeutic relationship (82).

Referral to an occupational specialist, a psychiatrist, or another family physician is more helpful than repeating low-yield diagnostic tests (79). Patients who come to believe that their symptoms are influenced by modifiable factors, such as workload, stress, coping strategies, depression, or overcommitment, are much more likely to recover than are patients who maintain that their symptoms are due to external factors, such as a viral infection (83).

Meta-analyses confirm the efficacy of regular structured exercise. Four weeks of aerobic, strength, or flexibility training are associated with improved energy and decreased fatigue (84). A daily 30-minute walk has more consistently positive impact on fatigue than any other intervention studied (85). With the exception of antidepressant drug therapy, including stimulants, has only short-term impact (13,86). Cognitive therapy is also effective (87–89).

The clinician should consider a 6-week trial of a selective serotonin reuptake inhibitor such as fluoxetine or sertraline for fatigue patients for whom depression is possible (89). If the patient has difficulty getting restful sleep, trazodone, doxepin, or imipramine may be good choices (90). If pain is present, the patient may respond to venlafaxine, desipramine, nortriptyline, or a nonsteroidal anti-inflammatory drug.

Many patients perceive that physicians and other medical personnel are more responsive to physical or somatic complaints. As a result physical symptoms often become the ticket to see the doctor (91). Frequent visits (often every 2 weeks) allow the clinician to focus on fatigue as a central problem and circumvent the tendency for new symptoms to present as urgent appointments (79). Focusing on modifiable factors such as sleep, stress, and psychological health reduces reliance on medication and is ultimately effective (51).

MANAGING FATIGUE IN THE ELDERLY

In the elderly, fatigue does not correlate well with the severity of pathology; instead, it may be a final common distress call compelling an individual to reduce their level of activity. As with all other patients with fatigue, it is wise to attempt to identify biological, psychological, behavioral, social, cultural, or interpersonal factors that contribute to the symptom, and to encourage the maximum activity feasible.

Cognitive behavioral therapy can address the perception that fatigue is uncontrollable or a barrier to activity, and older adults tend to be more compliant with behavioral therapy than younger patients. Because exercise itself may help patients to focus less on their fatigue, graded exercise, and behavioral therapy share an overlapping impact.

Three months of supplementation with β-alanine, a naturally occurring β-amino acid, improved endurance by 30% of elderly in one study (92). β-alanine is the rate-limiting precursor of carnosine, a dipeptide and antioxidant concentrated in muscle and brain. β-alanine supplementation increases the concentration of carnosine in muscles and decreases fatigue (93). Typical doses are 400 mg or 800 mg gelatin capsules every 8 hours. Doses above 10 mg/kg of body weight can cause paraesthesias and painful neuropathy.

Comprehensive fatigue reduction programs after injury, surgery, or debilitation are proven effective in elderly patients. Program components include planned rest periods, activity, high-protein/high-carbohydrate diet supplements, and a 3-minute back rub at bedtime (94). Elderly who have more muscle strength need to engage less of their maximal strength in order to perform daily activities and report less fatigue; so strength training is an important component of treatment.

Yoga, tai chi, and walking all improve energy and vitality as measured by the SF-36 (95).

Disability

Working toward a diagnosis or label for the patient's symptoms can inform a decision about disability. A label will facilitate communication with other physicians and disability boards. Unfortunately some patients do not meet criteria for categorization and yet appear to be disabled.

Three pillars of a successful employer–employee work relationship are: (i) regular and consistent work hours and attendance; (ii) accurate and complete work; and (iii) an ability to respond appropriately to supervision, criticism, and the general public. When fatigue erodes these pillars of employment, disability should be considered. Thus, if it is anticipated that the patient will miss 5 or more days per month at random because symptoms render them physically or emotionally impaired, a finding of disability should be considered (96,97). When disability is disputed, consider referral to an occupational therapist for a second opinion.

Summary

Fatigue is a common presenting complaint. The therapeutic challenge is to combine a disciplined biomedical and diagnostic approach with the psychosocial support needed over time. Many patients will have a self-limited or reversible problem that can be identified, but many others will require a comprehensive, multivisit strategy.

Fatigue is a common denominator of a multiplicity of conditions and behaviors. Treatment includes evidence-based strategies as well as nonspecific tailored interventions that can be applied to improve symptoms and quality of life. A significant number of patients with chronic fatigue will have persistent symptoms despite application of the best diagnostic and therapeutic measures. These individuals need an empathic, broad psychosocial approach to care, with ongoing monitoring and support over time.

KEY POINTS

- One third of patients presenting to a family physician's office complain of fatigue.
- There are four general categories of fatigue: physiologic tiredness (relieved by rest), secondary fatigue (associated with illness), chronic fatigue (unrelated to illness and lasting more than 6 months), and fatigue in the elderly.
- Patients suffering fatigue commonly present with somatic complaints because physicians express greater comfort treating physical symptoms.
- All patients complaining of fatigue should be screened for depression.
- Physical fitness, sleep hygiene, naps (except in secondary fatigue), and caffeine are effective antifatigue strategies.
- Fatigue and tiredness are common expressions of frailty in the elderly.
- Secondary fatigue often responds to correction of laboratory parameters.

CHAPTER

44

Sleep Disorders

Parul Harsora and Jennifer Kessmann

CLINICAL OBJECTIVES

1. Identify the common causes of sleep disorders.
2. Identify the common presenting complaints associated with sleep disorders.
3. Discuss common methods for treating sleep disorders, including both pharmacologic and nonpharmacologic treatment options.

Sleep disorders are quite common in clinical practice. They are important because they contribute greatly to decreased quality of life and increased morbidity. Insomnia is likely the most common sleep disorder with an incidence of up to 30% in some studies (1,2). It results in high health care utilization with costs ranging from 77 to 92 million annually (2–4). It is important for physicians to be on the lookout for these conditions, because nearly 50% to 70% of patients will not discuss them without questioning (2–5). Improving sleep can be an invaluable way to improve the overall health and quality of life of your patients and their families.

Sleep disturbances often coexist with other conditions, making the search for a cause especially important. These underlying conditions are often chronic and linked to other serious health conditions such as hypertension, heart disease, and depression, and can be associated with polypharmacy. Consequences of poor sleep include a range of outcomes, including reduced sexual intimacy, increased accidents, decreased productivity, and reduced effectiveness in school or at work (5,6). These disorders are, therefore, potentially serious and should be approached in a systematic manner (7).

DIFFERENTIAL DIAGNOSIS

Difficulty sleeping can arise from numerous causes. In this section we will overview of common sleep disorders. Table 44.1 lists and classifies the common sleep syndromes.

Insomnia. This is defined as difficulty with initiating or maintaining sleep, or of experiencing nonrestorative sleep, with significant daytime impairment. Insomnia is categorized as either primary or secondary. Primary insomnia is not caused by another disorder, underlying psychiatric or medical condition (8,9). Secondary (or comorbid) insomnia implies an underlying cause such as depression or another sleep disorder.[2] Insomnia can be further classified as acute (i.e., lasting <4 weeks) or chronic (i.e., >4 weeks), with symptoms occurring on at least 3 nights per week. Regardless of duration, most studies have adopted a definition of insomnia as either: (a) a delay of more than 30 minutes in sleep onset, or (b) a sleep efficiency (i.e., the percentage of time in bed that is spent sleeping) of <85% (10). The evaluation of insomnia should include a search for a cause so one may tailor treatment appropriately for each individual patient. Nonpharmacologic treatment has been shown to be more long-lasting and cost-effective for most patients with primary insomnia (11–13).

Secondary sleep disorders. These are sleep problems that arise from psychological, medical, or lifestyle causes.

Psychosocial causes are especially common. They are typically either psychosocial or medical in origin. Anxiety can cause difficulty in maintaining sleep and difficulty in initiating sleep; depression typically causes early morning awakening with an inability to fall back asleep. Treating these conditions can improve sleep and therefore improve quality of life. Shift work can also be a reason for prolonged sleep onset. Adjustment to life changes such as the birth of a child or marriage changes can also affect a person's sleep.

Many people unknowingly affect their sleep quality through caffeine or alcohol use. Caffeine has a half-life of four hours; so, both the timing of the substance and the quantity can affect the ability to sleep. Diet pills—which often contain caffeine—can have a similar effect. Alcohol will initially induce sleep but produces activation as it wears off, often causing the patient to wake up in the middle of the night.

People with chronic medical illnesses are prone to a variety of sleep problems, often from alterations in their natural sleep cycle. Frequent nocturia or chronic pain can lead to full awakening and difficulty falling back asleep. Medications with sedating or activating properties can interfere with sleep also. There is a wide range of medications that may cause sleep problems (Table 44.1). Any of these factors may contribute to impairment in daily functioning and ultimately lead to a decreased quality of life.

Restless leg syndrome (RLS). This neurologic disorder affects approximately 10% of adults (14). It is characterized by an unpleasant urge to move the legs that is usually worse in the evening or at night. Patients often have difficulty describing the uncomfortable feeling and use words like "crawling" or "aching." The sensation subsides partially or totally with movement or stretching of the legs (15). It is now known to be associated with several medical conditions, including iron deficiency, anxiety and depression, Parkinson disease, pregnancy, chronic kidney disease, spinal cord injury, and rheumatoid

TABLE 44.1 Causes of Insomnia

Primary Sleep Disorders	Secondary	
	Disease-associated	**Medication-associated**
Primary insomnia	Anxiety	Alcohol
acute	Asthma	Antidepressants
chronic	Congestive heart failure	β-blockers
Obstructive sleep apnea	Chronic obstructive pulmonary disease	Caffeine
Restless leg syndrome	Depression	Chemotherapy agents
Narcolepsy	Fibromyalgia	Cimetidine
	Gastroesophageal reflux disease	Diuretics
	Hyperthyroidism	Herbal remedies
	Medications	Illicit drugs (selected)
	Menopause	Nicotine
	Pain	Phenytoin
	Pruritus	Pseudoephedrine
	Urinary incontinence	Steroids
	Nocturia	Stimulant laxatives
		Theophylline

Sources: Petit L, et al, 2003;[26] Kamel & Gammack.[27,28]

arthritis. Medications such as caffeine, antihistamines, neuroleptics, lithium, selective serotonin reuptake inhibitors, and tricyclic antidepressants can also cause RLS (14).

Obstructive sleep apnea (OSA). This is a fairly common disorder in family medicine as well. It often presents as a complaint of excessive daytime drowsiness and fatigue, causing the patient to sometimes fall asleep unexpectedly. People with OSA are often (but not always) overweight, and their bed partners frequently report loud snoring. Hypertension is commonly associated with this disorder, due to a physiological reaction to chronic hypoxemia. A sleep study or polysomnogram performed in a sleep laboratory can be helpful in making a diagnosis, determining the severity of this disease, and guiding the clinician's therapy. The severity of the condition is measured by the apnea-hypopnea index. This measures the number of apnea events (cessations of airflow) or hypopnea events (reduction of airflow) per hour that occur. Long-term mortality increases if patients have more than 20 respiratory events per hour, and so treatment is recommended (16). Although if patients are symptomatic, it is sometimes suggested to treat with greater than five events per hour.

Patients with mild OSA may respond to simple measures such as losing weight, avoiding sedatives and alcohol, and avoiding the supine position during sleep (17). Continuous positive airway pressure (CPAP) is a common method of treating moderate or severe cases of OSA. Other treatment options will be discussed later in this chapter.

Narcolepsy. This is a less common condition that causes patients to have disordered sleep cycles. It causes the patient to fall asleep, frequently without any notice. It can be extremely dangerous if sleep occurs during driving or operating heavy machinery. Patients usually will have abnormal sleep latency testing. Treatment includes medication such as modafinil and other sleep improvement measures.

CLINICAL EVALUATION

Many different illnesses and conditions can be associated with sleep difficulty; so your evaluation should be comprehensive (Table 44.2). Family member input can be helpful, because often they can contribute information; so it is useful to include them at the first or second visit. Initially, the history should focus on high-risk diagnoses such as depression, OSA, and narcolepsy. It should include a search for red flags that would identify problems that

TABLE 44.2 Key Elements of the History and Physical Evaluation for Sleep Disorders

Psychosocial history
Red flags
Medication use
Cough
Joint pains
Exertional dyspnea
Cardiopulmonary examination: screen for congestive heart failure, COPD, pneumonia, obstructive sleep apnea
Extremities: signs of edema (obstructive sleep apnea or congestive heart failure)

TABLE 44.3 Red Flags Suggesting Progressive or Potentially Life-threatening Disease in a Patient Complaining of Sleep Problems

Red Flag	Diagnosis Suggested
Depressed mood	Depression with suicidal risk
Substance abuse, recent discontinuation	Withdrawal syndrome
Falling asleep during activities	Narcolepsy, accident risk
Weight loss	Hyperthyroidism
Lower extremity edema	Cor pulmonale from obstructive sleep apnea
Polyuria, polydipsia	Diabetes
Orthopnea, paroxysmal nocturnal dyspnea, cardiomegaly, rales	Congestive heart failure

may be life-threatening (Table 44.3). Also, potential secondary causes should be evaluated for and corrected if possible.

The Clinical History

Because of the high prevalence of psychological and lifestyle causes, careful attention needs to be given to these aspects of the history. Depression, environmental stresses, and recent lifestyle changes should be specifically asked about. Understanding the patient's lifestyle, occupation and family life can contribute better to the understanding of their sleep complaints (7).

Family physicians should screen all patients for sleep problems with a question or two. Patients who screen positive should have a systematic history taken. The following are some suggested questions to help you in your evaluation with sleep disorders.

- Ask the patient how long it usually takes them to get to sleep. Also, evaluate the amount of time spent in bed divided by the amount of time spent sleeping. This would give you their sleep efficacy, which should be >85%.
- Inquire into whether the patient naps. If they do, this could be preventing them from sleeping well at night.
- Inquire into what is going on when the patient awakens. If they are busy thinking, then anxiety could be contributing to their insomnia. If they need to use the bathroom, then prostatic hyperplasia, congestive heart failure, or diabetes could be an issue. If pain is reported, then this could be causing insomnia.
- If noise or pets are awakening the patient, then a solution for this could be explored.
- Ask about medications, caffeine intake, alcohol use, and supplements (such as diet pills) that may be causing difficulty with sleep.
- Ask if they are falling asleep during the day. If they are then further evaluation for OSA and narcolepsy should be introduced.

Elements that suggest a psychological diagnosis include:

- a history of dysfunctional family setting or a previous history of functional health complaints;
- insomnia that is associated with increased stress and/or accompanied by multiple nonspecific symptoms;
- a recent life change, such as a job change, divorce, marriage, or a move;
- sadness associated with the insomnia, if your initial history suggests an underlying psychological issue. In such situations, you should consider screening with tests such as the Beck or Zung Depression Inventory (18); and
- request for an excuse from work, or associated domestic abuse[7].

When interviewing the patient's partner, ask about frequent snoring, choking, or sudden awakening from sleep, which are symptoms suggesting OSA. Also, ask about witnessed periods of apnea or spells where he or she is worried the patient may stop breathing. The patient may be unaware of these episodes, so it is important to have them ask anyone who might be aware of their sleeping. Note that snoring is not always associated with OSA, especially in children.

Screen for RLS by asking the patient about unusual sensations and an urge to move the legs while trying to get to sleep. Partners may witness frequent jerking of the legs that awakens them.

In children with sleep problems, parents should be questioned about not only snoring, but also apnea, mouth breathing, and frequent awakenings. Night terrors are an important condition that can be particularly scary for young children, causing them to not want to sleep.

The Physical Exam

The physical exam can be focused, as the history is often more contributory to the diagnosis. Key elements of the physical to include should be the following:

- Blood pressure should always be measured, as it is often elevated with patients with OSA.
- Measure the body mass index and neck circumference. Consider OSA in any obese patient with a body mass index of 30 or above or a neck circumference of 16.5 inches or more.
- Because longstanding OSA leads to chronic respiratory disease and right-sided congestive heart failure, pay special attention to the cardiovascular and respiratory exam, and look for lower extremity edema. Of course, physicians should strive to detect OSA before the development of the end-stage disease such as cor pulmonale, to prevent its development by proper treatment and counseling.
- Iron deficiency anemia can be evaluated by checking the conjunctivae and nail beds for pallor. However, it is often the case that iron deficiency associated with RLS is only detected via laboratory tests.

Diagnostic Testing

The laboratory evaluation should be tailored to each individual patient and tests ordered accordingly. If you suspect

Figure 44.1 • Epworth sleepiness scale. Source: Johns MW, 1991.[28]

How likely are you to doze off or fall asleep in the following situations, in contrast to just feeling tired? This refers to your usual way of life in recent time. Even if you have not done some of these things recently, try to work out how they would have affected you. Use the following **scale** to choose the most appropriate number for each situation:

0 = would never doze
1 = slight chance of dozing
2 = moderate chance of dozing
3 = high chance of dozing

Situation	Chance of Dozing (Circle your response)			
	Never	Slight	Moderate	High
1. Sitting and reading	0	1	2	3
2. Watching TV	0	1	2	3
3. Sitting inactive in a public place (theater or meeting)	0	1	2	3
4. As a passenger in a car for an hour without a break	0	1	2	3
5. Lying down to rest in the afternoon when circumstances permit	0	1	2	3
6. Sitting and talking to someone	0	1	2	3
7. Sitting quietly after lunch (without alcohol)	0	1	2	3
8. In a car, while stopped for a few minutes in the traffic	0	1	2	3
TOTAL	___ (out of a possible 24)			

depression, consider ordering a thyroid-stimulating hormone and complete blood count test to further screen for thyroid disorders and anemia. If RLS is present, then a serum ferritin should be ordered.

The most effective tool is often the sleep diary. Patients are asked to record their sleeping patterns over a 2-week period and bring this with them to their next appointment. The sleep diary should include such things as what the patient is doing as they attempt to sleep, how long it takes to fall asleep (sleep onset), any awakenings (with the reason for wakening), and any other sleep-related complaints. A sleep diary is available at *www.nhlbi.nih.gov/health/public/sleep/healthy_sleep.pdf*, (pages 56–57).

Another useful tool is the Epworth Sleepiness Scale (Fig. 44.1). It is a validated scale that allows determination of degree of sleepiness that the patient is experiencing. Based on the severity of the symptoms reported, the need for further testing or therapy can be determined.

The diagnosis of RLS is based primarily on the history, and further tests are usually not needed. If you suspect RLS, a search for iron deficiency should be conducted by ordering a serum ferritin.

Polysomnography and evaluation by a sleep specialist is recommended for patients you suspect have OSA or narcolepsy. Polysomnography measures a patient's airflow, abdominothoracic movements, oximetry, and electrocardiogram. Electroencephalogram readings are also monitored. The polysomnogram is extremely helpful in evaluating potential OSA patients. During this test, the patient can also be fitted for CPAP, which is one of the effective treatments for OSA. CPAP machines provide positive airway pressure that keeps the patient's airway open while sleeping. These apparatuses must be titrated to a pressure that reduces the number of events to fewer than 10 per hour. Usually this pressure is between 6 and 12 cm. Also, if the patient loses or gains weight, CPAP must be readjusted. A multiple sleep latency test is often needed if you suspect narcolepsy (Fig. 44.2).

General Approach to Evaluation of Sleep Complaints

Patients with sleep problems usually complain either of daytime sleepiness or trouble sleeping at night (insomnia). Daytime sleepiness is usually the result of insufficient sleep, with lifestyle issues and OSA being common causes. Insomnia is divided into acute and chronic. For acute insomnia, the physician's role is to try to identify a treatable cause and to help the patient overcome the problem; if self-limited, reassurance or medication can be helpful. For chronic insomnia, a detailed evaluation is warranted including a screen for common sleep disorders, a sleep diary, review of sleep hygiene, and a medication review. If the history suggests OSA, the patient should be referred for

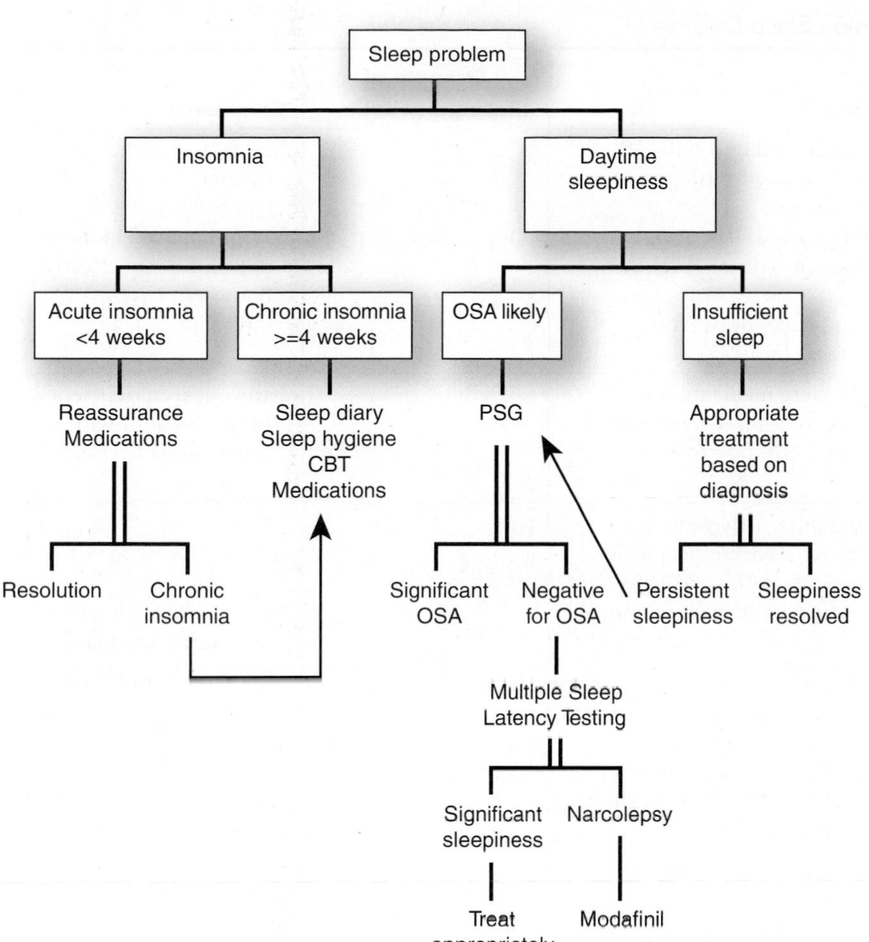

Figure 44.2 • Algorithm for the diagnosis of common sleep disorders. Source: Harsora & Kessman, 2009.[12] OSA = obstructive sleep apnea; PSG = polysomnography; CBT = cognitive behavioral therapy.

polysomnography; if the history suggests narcolepsy, a Multiple Sleep Latency test may be necessary. Numerous treatments are available for both acute and chronic insomnia, with the treatment needing to be tailored to the cause. Figure 44.2 displays the general approach to sleep problems.

MANAGEMENT

Management of sleep problems should be based on the available scientific evidence. This is a field for which many high quality studies exist, which can aid the physician and the patient in decisions regarding evaluation and treatment. Table 44.4 summarizes the evidence for common therapies for the major sleep disorders.

In patients with insomnia, sleep hygiene should be addressed (Table 44.5). A helpful strategy is to focus on one aspect of sleep hygiene that may be implicated in the patient's problem at a given visit. If the symptoms are acute, the cause is self-limited (e.g., death of a close family member), and immediate symptom relief is required, medication use is appropriate (19). Medications must be used with caution, however, because of safety issues and tolerance. For this reason, the newer generation nonbenzodiazepines are typically chosen instead of the older benzodiazepines. Elderly patients in particular may be prone to sedating side effects and withdrawal after discontinuing use.

For chronic insomnia, cognitive behavioral therapies are the initial step (3,4). These include stimulus control, sleep restriction, relaxation therapy, paradoxical intention, and cognitive psychotherapy with a therapist (Table 44.6). These therapies can be taught over 6 to 8 weekly sessions of 50 minutes in length. Underlying medical problems must be sought for and addressed.

In OSA, weight reduction (20) and lateral sleep position (21) may improve sleep disordered breathing. CPAP is well studied and is particularly effective for moderate to severe OSA (22). CPAP delivers positive airway pressure throughout the respiratory cycle. The positive airway pressure keeps the upper airway open, preventing upper airway collapse during sleep. The target airway pressure is determined by sleep studies and must be at a level that is acceptable to patient, achieves an open airway, maintains oxyhemoglobin saturation, and allows continuous sleep. Patients must, however, be fitted with a mask that is both comfortable and well fitting. Problems patients can encounter with CPAP include claustrophobia, nasal congestion, and mouth breathing. These may be

TABLE 44.4 Management of Common Sleep Disorders

Diagnosis	Recommended Intervention	Efficacy	Strength of Recommendation	Comments
Obstructive sleep apnea	CPAP	ESS improved by 1.8 (0–24); AHI decreases by 10 events/hour[29]	A	Screen for cardiac risk factors
	Weight loss	ESS improved; 10% weight reduction reduces AHI by 26%[20]	B	Weight control alone is not uniformly effective
	Oral appliances	ESS improves by 3; AHI decreases by 10[23]	B	not as effective as CPAP
Restless legs syndrome	Dopamine agonists (e.g., pramipexole, ropinirole)	Use of these medications results in reduced symptom severity. NNT = 6[24]	A	Rule out iron deficiency. High discontinuation rate from side effects
Narcolepsy	Provigil 200 mg daily	200 mg once daily reduces excessive daytime sleepiness in patients with narcolepsy[25]	A	
	Scheduled sleep	For patients with severe symptoms, significantly reduced unscheduled daytime sleep (p = .011)[26]	C	When used with stimulant medication and regular sleep schedules
Acute insomnia <4 weeks	Medications such as zolpidem or zopliclone	Nonbenzodiazepine sedative-hypnotic drugs are similarly effective and likely safer than benzodiazepines.[19]	C	Potential for tolerance to medications and side effects, especially in elderly patients
Chronic insomnia ≥4 weeks	Cognitive behavioral therapy	It is as good as pharmacologic therapy[12]	A	
	Exercise	Shortened time to fall asleep and longer time spent asleep[30]	B	Review of studies of elderly patients

SOR = strength of recommendation; CPAP = continuous positive airway pressure; ESS = Epworth sleepiness scale; AHI = apnea-hypopnea index; NNT = number needed to treat; A = consistent, good-quality patient-oriented evidence; B = inconsistent or limited-quality patient-oriented evidence; C = consensus, disease-oriented evidence, usual practice, expert opinion, or case series.
For information about the Strength of Recommendation Taxonomy evidence rating system, see *www.aafp.org/afpsort.xml*.

TABLE 44.5 Sleep Hygiene Recommendations for Patients with Insomnia

- Avoid caffeine and nicotine, especially late in the day
- Avoid exercise during the 4 hours before bedtime; daily exercise is beneficial to sleep, but can interfere if done close to bedtime
- Avoid large meals in the evening
- Avoid taking naps
- Go to sleep and wake up at the same times each day
- Keep the bedroom at a comfortable temperature
- Make the bedroom as dark as possible
- Set aside a time to relax before bed and use relaxation techniques

Adapted from Petit L, et al, 2003.[27]

mitigated by mask desensitization (wearing the mask during the day), air humidification, nasal steroids, and trial of facial (instead of nasal) mask. If CPAP flow is not tolerated by the patient, bilevel or auto titration of pressure may be tried. Oral appliances fitted by dentists are less effective than CPAP but are an alternative for patients who are unwilling to use CPAP (23). Surgery is also a treatment for OSA but there is less evidence to support its use.

RLS may be reduced by getting adequate sleep and exercise. It is also helped by limiting caffeine, alcohol, and medications with extrapyramidal side effects. Mild dopamine agonist medications are effective at treating RLS; these include pramipexole and ropinirole (24).

Narcolepsy is treated with stimulants such as modafinil, which reduces daytime sleepiness (25). In patients with moderate to severe narcolepsy, it is helpful to introduce scheduled sleep periods during the day in addition to regular sleep time (Table 44.6) (26).

TABLE 44.6 Cognitive Behavioral Therapy Approaches to Patients with Chronic Insomnia

Stimulus control	Helps patients to associate the bedroom with sleep and intimacy only, not other wakeful activities. Patients are instructed to leave the bedroom is unable to fall asleep after 20 minutes.
Sleep restriction	Consists of limiting time in bed to maximize sleep efficiency. Bedtimes are progressively increased as sleep efficiency improves.
Relaxation therapies	Techniques taught to patients to reduce high levels of arousal that interfere with sleep (e.g., meditation, progressive muscle relaxation, imagery training, biofeedback training, hypnosis).
Cognitive psychotherapy	Involves identifying a patient's dysfunctional beliefs about sleep, challenging their validity, and replacing them with more adaptive substitutes.
Paradoxical intention	Seeks to remove the fear of not being able to sleep by advising the patient to remain awake.

KEY POINTS

- The evaluation of sleep disorders includes focusing on the social and psychological contributors to sleep dysfunction.
- Identify OSA early and often, especially in your obese patients to help prevent the catastrophic complications of this disease.
- A sleep diary is often very helpful in the evaluation of the patient with insomnia or sleep complaints.
- Cognitive behavioral therapy has been shown to be beneficial for chronic insomnia. This treatment is further desirable because it often eliminates the need for treatment with potentially addicting medications.

CHAPTER

45

Headache

Stephen Gamboa

CLINICAL OBJECTIVES

1. List the three most common types of primary headache.
2. Describe warning signs that could indicate a life threatening cause of headache.
3. Apply evidence-based criteria in using imaging in diagnosis of headache.
4. Understand the primary therapeutic approaches to acute migraine, migraine prevention, tension-type headache, cluster headaches, and chronic daily headache.

Headache is the eighth most common outpatient diagnosis for family physicians and the 13th for general internists (1). Although headaches often interfere with daily activities at home or in the workplace, many people do not seek medical attention for their headaches. Consequently, many headache sufferers remain undiagnosed and possibly undertreated.

Family physicians have the opportunity and obligation to identify individual patients who have potentially treatable headache disorders, diagnose the likely cause of the headaches, recommend or prescribe appropriate interventions, and help patients find and implement changes in their lifestyle or environment that may prevent or reduce the severity of future headaches. Much of this can be accomplished by obtaining a thorough medical history and performing a focused physical examination (described in the following section), and by working with the patient on a longitudinal basis. Radiologic evaluation can sometimes be useful, and evidence-based guidelines can help the clinician determine their appropriate use.

DIFFERENTIAL DIAGNOSIS

The International Headache Society (IHS) published the first edition of its headache classification criteria in 1988 (2) and a revised edition in 2003 (3). Although these criteria can be useful for research purposes, they are too cumbersome to be useful in clinical practice.

Headaches can be considered either primary or secondary. Primary headaches result from processes that manifest themselves primarily as head pain, whereas secondary headaches are manifestations of another process. The most common primary headaches are migraine, tension-type, and cluster headaches; common causes of secondary headache include sinusitis, caffeine withdrawal, neck arthritis, and viral infections (see Table 45.1). Several of the most common headache types will be reviewed here.

Migraine

Migraine is a chronic, genetically linked primary headache that affects more than 10% of adults and is the most common headache seen in primary care (4). Migraines usually begin in late childhood or early adulthood, but the diagnosis may be delayed several years. The incidence is much higher in women than men among adults, but the ratio is equal in children.

The presentation of migraine is variable. Because neurologic symptoms may either precede ("aura") or accompany the headache, migraine can sometimes be confused with more serious causes of headache, such as a transient ischemic attack or stroke. Because patients with migraine often report pain in the face or around (or behind) one eye, they are sometimes misdiagnosed as having sinus headaches. Table 45.2 lists commonly accepted diagnostic criteria for migraine.

The frequency, severity, and associated symptoms of migraine can vary between patients and within a given patient's lifetime. Fluctuations in serum estrogen concentration in women (e.g., phase of the menstrual cycle, pregnancy) are often associated with onset, remission, or change in severity of migraine-related symptoms. Other known "triggers" include certain foods, caffeine, sleep deprivation, psychosocial stressors, or changes in weather or barometric pressure (Table 45.3). Daily pain diaries can help identify such triggers.

Tension-type Headache

Although migraine is the most common headache type encountered in the primary care setting, tension-type headache is the most common cause of headache overall, with a prevalence of between 30% and 80% in the general community (5–7). Tension-type headaches are usually mild or moderate in severity and are often self-treated. They are commonly episodic but can develop into daily or near-daily headaches. Many patients with tension-type headaches describe bilateral symptoms or a "headband-like" pain. Tension-type headache and migraine can occur concomitantly in the same patient.

Cluster Headache

Cluster headaches are not common, with a prevalence estimated at about 0.3% to 0.4% (8,9). Unlike the other two headache types discussed, cluster headaches are more prevalent in males. This primary headache type is named cluster because its classic presentation is described as a series of headaches occurring close together over 6 to 12 weeks. People

TABLE 45.1 Differential Diagnosis of the Patient with Headache

Diagnosis	Primary or Secondary	Typical Features	Percent of Headaches in Primary Care
Migraine	Primary	Intense facial pain, photophobia, variable presentation. Neurological complaints are common.	45–50
Tension-type headache	Primary	Bilateral headband-like pain. Mild to moderate symptoms.	20–25
Cluster	Primary	Male predominance. Series of several, intense, unilateral headaches with concurrent lacrimation, rhinorrhea, and ptosis possible.	5–7
Sinusitis	Secondary	Nasal purulence, obstruction and altered smell.	5–7
Withdrawal from caffeine, opiates, alcohol	Secondary	Associated with cessation of associated substance.	5–8
Arthritis/joint disease: osteoarthritis of cervical spine, temporomandibular joint disease	Secondary	Neck pain or tenderness common, pain on chewing or tenderness over temporomandibular joint.	2–4
Posttraumatic headache	Secondary	Preceding history of head trauma.	2–5
Viral syndrome	Secondary	Associated symptoms of influenza or other viral syndrome, such as fever and myalgias.	2–4
Ophthalmologic (glaucoma, eye strain)	Secondary	Vision loss or blurring, pain on eye movement, pain located on or around eye, conjunctival injection.	1–2
Meningitis	Secondary	Fever, stiff neck, and ill appearance are classic findings but presentation can be variable.	<1
Encephalitis	Secondary	Usually presents with headache, fever, and global mental status changes.	<1
Temporal arteritis	Secondary	Age >50, muscle aches (and/or history of polymyalgia rheumatica), pain in temporal artery. Temporal artery biopsy diagnostic.	<1
Subarachnoid hemorrhage	Secondary	Sudden onset, severe pain, sometimes with focal neurologic findings.	<1
Subdural hematoma	Secondary	More likely in older patients with new onset headache and history of trauma. Fluctuating cognitive status may accompany.	<1
Intracranial malignancy	Secondary	Isolated headache is unusual as presenting complaint. Neurologic impairments and seizures are common accompanying symptoms. Suspicion should be high if history of cancer (especially of lung).	<1
Disorders of cerebrospinal fluid circulation	Secondary	Can be iatrogenic (i.e., after lumbar puncture) or from idiopathic pseudotumor cerebri.	<1

TABLE 45.2 International Headache Society Criteria for the Diagnosis of Migraine

Diagnostic Criteria for Migraine without Typical Aura	
Headache Description (Any 2)	**Associated Symptoms (Any 1)**
• Unilateral • Pulsatile quality • Moderate to severe pain intensity • Aggravation by or causing avoidance of routine physical activity • Lasts 4–72 hours	• Nausea and/or vomiting • Photophobia and phonophobia
Diagnostic Criterion: Must have 5 attacks fulfilling the above criteria and no signs of a secondary headache disorder.	
Diagnostic Criteria for Migraine with Typical Aura	
Aura consisting of at least one of the following, but no motor weakness: • Fully reversible visual symptoms including positive features (e.g., flickering lights, spots, or lines) and/or negative features (i.e., loss of vision) • Fully reversible sensory symptoms including positive features (i.e., pins and needles) and/or negative features (i.e., numbness) • Fully reversible dysphasic speech disturbance	
Headache begins during the aura or follows the aura within 60 minutes	
Diagnostic Criterion: Must have at least 2 attacks fulfilling the above criteria and no signs of a secondary headache disorder.	

Adapted from International Headache Society (3).

with cluster headaches complain of severe, intense, unilateral pain lasting from several seconds to many minutes. Concurrent symptoms include ipsilateral lacrimation, rhinorrhea, and ptosis. The headache is also always on the same side, no matter how many months lapse between episodes.

Sinusitis and "Sinus Headache"

Many people with headache or facial pain incorrectly diagnose themselves with "sinus headache." Migraines and cluster headaches often have symptoms related to the nose and sinuses, such rhinorrhea, pain behind the eye (frontal sinus), and facial tenderness. Symptoms suggesting a nasal or sinus etiology (rhinosinusitis) include purulence in the nasal cavity, nasal obstruction, altered smell (hyposmia or anosmia), and/or fever.

Patients who self-treat presumed sinus headaches with decongestants often report incomplete resolution of their pain and present in the primary care office seeking antibiotics. One estimate is that 70% to 80% of patients presenting with "sinusitis

TABLE 45.3 Common Headache Triggers

Categories of Triggers	**Specific Triggers**	**Comments**
Alcoholic beverages	Tyramine in red wines, sulfites in white wines. Dehydration, "hangover."	Variable response
Caffeine and/or caffeine withdrawal	May be related to changes in vasomotor tone.	Headaches are worse on weekends in patients who drink a lot of caffeine at work
Food additives	MSG, aspartame, tyramine (found in aged cheeses, some red wines, smoked fish, etc.), sodium nitrite (found in processed meats).	Food diaries may be helpful, as may food challenges
Foods	Chocolate, fruits, dairy, onions, beans, nuts.	As above
Environmental changes	Light, odors (perfume, paint, etc.), travel, abrupt changes in weather or altitude.	May present as nasal "stuffiness" (sinus symptoms)
Lifestyle factors	Insufficient, excessive, disrupted, or irregular sleep; tobacco or alcohol use; fasting; physical activity; head injury; schedule changes; stress or release from stress; anger; or exhilaration.	Very common. Some people increase tobacco or alcohol use to try to alleviate headaches, thereby contributing to the problem.
Hormone changes, or addition of estrogen-containing medication	Timing of headache with menses or change/addition of hormones.	Headaches may worsen or improve

TABLE 45.4 Red flags Suggesting that a Headache May Indicate a Progressive or Life-threatening Disease

Red Flag	Possible Diagnosis
Sudden onset severe headache ("thunderclap" headache)	Subarachnoid hemorrhage
Headache first occurring with exercise	Ruptured aneurysm
New onset headache after age 50	Temporal arteritis, intracranial mass
Headache with fever, stiff neck, photophobia or other systemic signs	Meningitis, encephalitis
Headache hours to weeks after a history of trauma, especially in an older person	Subdural hematoma
Headache with focal neurologic signs or symptoms, or papilledema	Tumor, subdural hematoma, epidural bleed
Similar, new-onset of headaches in an acquaintance or family member	Environmental exposure such as carbon monoxide

Adapted from Clinch R. Evaluation of acute headache in adults. *Am Fam Physician*. 2001;63:685–692.

causing a headache" may actually have migraine or could be classified as having *probable migraine* based on the presence of most but not all of the IHS criteria for migraine (10).

Chronic Daily Headache

Between 3% and 5% of adults worldwide experience headaches daily or nearly daily (11–13). Paradoxically, the very medications commonly used to treat episodic headaches (including over-the-counter analgesics, especially acetaminophen, and migraine-specific medications such as triptans) are implicated in the transformation of episodic to chronic headaches, especially if consumed more often than 2 days per week over several months (14–17). Family physicians should be aware that this is a common condition associated with a significant burden of suffering, and that effective treatment of migraine and tension-type headache without the overuse of medication may help prevent the development of this difficult-to-treat condition.

CLINICAL EVALUATION

An important initial task for the family physician in the evaluation of a patient presenting with headache is to determine whether the patient's symptoms are a manifestation of a primary or secondary headache. Diagnosing a secondary headache usually involves looking for and investigating red flags that may serve as clues to the etiology of the headache (Table 45.4).

History and Physical Examination

A recently developed instrument adopted by the American Academy of Neurology to evaluate headache complaints, the brief headache screen, can be useful in guiding the history. It consists of four questions:

1. How often do you get severe headaches (i.e., without treatment it is difficult to function)?
2. How often do you get other (milder) headaches?
3. How often do you take headache relievers or pain pills?
4. Has there been any recent change in your headaches?

The presence of daily or intermittent severe headache has a 100% sensitivity for chronic migraine (18). Questions 2 and 3 may help to identify patients with medication overuse, and question 4 can identify patients with a possibly dangerous secondary cause of headache. Recent change in pattern or severity of headache can lead the clinician to suspecting a more serious cause of headache.

Additional questions that may help identify "red flags" are:

- When was the last time you had a headache of similar severity?
- Did your symptoms begin abruptly or slowly?
- What other symptoms or problems do you experience along with the headache, such as fever, rash, or neck stiffness?
- Are you experiencing any changes in your vision or do you have altered sensation or strength in any part of your body?

A patient experiencing sudden and severe headache raises suspicion for subarachnoid hemorrhage (SAH). SAH commonly presents with severe headache reaching maximal intensity within minutes and lasting an hour or more (19). SAH may be accompanied by focal neurologic signs or other symptoms such as nausea, vomiting, photophobia, neck stiffness, seizures, or altered level of consciousness. It is important to not miss SAH, because early diagnosis and treatment is essential to improving outcomes. Asking about headache severity in the context of previous headaches helps to ascertain the severity without suggestion or prompting of the patient with the words "worst headache of my life," which is not very sensitive or specific as a screening question for SAH. Cluster headache can have a sudden onset, too, but its unique, characteristic presentation should help in differentiating it from SAH.

Stroke or a transient ischemic attack can occasionally present with headache. If lateralizing neurologic findings or visual changes are present, a cerebrovascular diagnosis should be considered. Since migraine syndromes can also have associated neurologic findings, neurological symptoms or signs are not necessarily harbingers of stroke.

The presence of fever in conjunction with headache may indicate an infectious condition, thereby necessitating a more thorough physical exam. Headache is a common symptom of many infectious conditions including influenza, sinusitis, streptococcal pharyngitis, and many viral syndromes. The association

TABLE 45.5 Signs and Symptoms that Suggest Neuroimaging May be Indicated in Patients with Headache

Clinical Feature	Sensitivity	Specificity	LR+	LR−
Focal findings on neurologic examination	1.0	0.76	3.0–4.2	0.70
Abrupt onset of headache	0.55	0.79	2.5	0.57
Change or alteration in the characteristics of headache	0.67	0.67	2.0	0.49
Increased intensity and frequency of headaches	0.39	0.73	1.4	0.83
Persistence despite analgesics	0.6	0.56	1.4	0.71

LR+ = positive likelihood ratio; tests with higher values, especially >5, are good at ruling in disease.
LR− = negative likelihood ratio; tests with lower values, especially <0.2, are good at ruling out disease.
Modified from Aygun D, Bildik F. Clinical warning criteria in evaluation by computed tomography the secondary neurological headaches in adults. *Eur J Neurol.* 2003;10(4):437–442.

of fever with headache (especially occipital headache), photophobia, rash, and/or neck pain should raise the suspicion of a central nervous system infection, such as encephalitis or meningitis. An exam of the head, eyes, ears, nose, and throat is warranted if the history suggests vision change, ear pain, sore throat, or other symptoms in that region. Neck range of motion and palpation should be performed to evaluate for possible meningitis; neck stiffness is defined as an inability to touch the chin to the chest. In patients with suggested meningitis, the physical exam should also include attempts to elicit Kernig and Brudzinski signs. Caution is advised, however, in depending on the physical exam to evaluate for meningitis. Neither neck stiffness nor Kernig or Brudzinski signs achieve sufficient sensitivity to allow the clinician to exclude meningitis. If the diagnosis is suspected, antibiotic therapy should be initiated without delay, and a lumbar puncture with cerebrospinal fluid studies is indicated.

The neurologic evaluation should evaluate strength, sensation, cerebellar, and cranial nerve function. Any focal or lateralizing signs should be noted. Funduscopic exam should be performed to look for papilledema. Palpation of the temporal artery, spine and neck muscles, auscultation of the neck and orbit for bruit, and assessing the temporomandibular joint may provide useful clues, as with evaluation of gait and looking for lateralizing weakness.

Diagnostic Testing

A systematic review of the literature concluded that there was insufficient evidence to recommend any routine diagnostic testing (beyond a history and physical) for non-acute headache syndromes, with the possible exception of neuroimaging (20). In patients with suspected SAH and negative non-contrast computed tomography (CT) scan of the head, a lumbar puncture is indicated to look for xanthochromia or red cells.

The decision to obtain a CT scan should be informed by evidence-based guidelines, as CT provides enough radiation exposure to significantly increase the risk of cancer (21,22). Presence or absence of neurological findings on exam was the strongest predictor of an abnormal imaging study (Table 45.5). The likelihood ratio of an abnormal imaging study in patients with a normal neurological exam is estimated at 0.7 (95% confidence interval [CI]: 0.52, 0.93), whereas the likelihood ratio of finding a significant abnormality on an imaging study in the presence of an abnormal neurological examination is estimated to be 3.0 (95% CI: 2.3, 4.0). The authors concluded that the decision to use neuroimaging in a patient with nonacute headache (present for at least 4 weeks) should be made on a case-by-case basis (23,24).

Kumar and colleagues recommend that neuroimaging be considered in the following situations in patients with non-traumatic headache (25):

1. Recent significant change in the pattern, frequency or severity of headaches
2. Progressive worsening of headache despite appropriate therapy
3. Focal neurologic signs or symptoms
4. Onset of headache with exertion, cough, or sexual activity
5. Orbital bruit
6. Onset of headache after age 50 years

Headache diaries or headache questionnaires are often more useful than laboratory or radiological tests in helping the physician make a diagnosis. A sample headache diary can be downloaded free of charge from the American Headache Society at *www.achenet.org/tools/diaries/index.asp*. The information from these diaries may help both the patient and provider identify trends or triggers, which in turn may help prevent or treat the headaches.

MANAGEMENT

The management of headache depends on the diagnosis, frequency of symptoms, and surrounding circumstances. The discussion here will be geared toward primary headaches, as secondary headaches require a management plan tailored to the particular cause. Management can be grouped into abortive and prophylactic.

After a primary headache diagnosis has been made, discussion of treatment strategies can begin. Discussion points to cover include what interventions were attempted in the past, and concerns such as work impact, medication side effects, and expense of treatments. Table 45.6 summarizes evidence on key therapies; details are provided in the text below.

Migraine

Education about identifying and avoiding triggers (Table 45.3) should be the first treatment explored with the patient.

TABLE 45.6 Key Therapies for Chronic Headaches

Target Condition and Intervention	Strength of Recommendation	Comments and Cautions
Acute Migraine (47)		
Intranasal sumatriptan	A	Can use when patient unable to tolerate oral medications
Oral sumatriptan	A	Other triptan preparations available; all equally effective
APAP/ASA/caffeine	A	First line treatment for acute migraine.
Butorphanol nasal spray	A	Rescue treatment, higher abuse potential; PO opiate combinations are another alternative.
Dihydroergotamine nasal spray	A	For more severe migraine.
Migraine Prevention (47)		
Valproic acid	A	Weigh adverse effect risk vs. benefit in decision to treat.
Propranolol	A	Caution in asthma or COPD.
Amitriptyline	A	Titrate to effect and side effect tolerability
Tension-type Headache		
Amitriptyline (45)	A	Titrate dose as above.
Spinal manipulation (48)	C	Manual therapy with the best evidence. Low risk of side effects.
Cranial electrotherapy (48)	C	Less studied, but with low likelihood of side effects.
Cluster Headaches		
High-flow oxygen (49)	A	Can be used in combination with a triptan
Sumatriptan (50)	A	Administered PO or intranasal
Verapamil (51)	A	Used for prophylaxis in doses of 120–160 mg PO tid
Chronic Daily Headache		
Amitriptyline (45)	A	Start with 10 mg PO qhs; can titrate up to 75 mg PO qhs
Screen for medication overuse (46)	A	Medication overuse is a common cause of chronic headache

A = consistent, good-quality patient-oriented evidence; B = inconsistent or limited-quality patient-oriented evidence; C = consensus, disease-oriented evidence, usual practice, expert opinion; COPD = chronic obstructive pulmonary disease; PO = by mouth; q = every.
For information about the SORT evidence rating system, see *www.aafp.org/afpsort.xml*

TREATMENT OF AN ACUTE MIGRAINE ATTACK

Because of the debilitating nature of migraines for many patients, the goals of therapy for the acute episode should be clear to both the provider and the patient. They are to:

- Treat the headache rapidly
- Provide symptom relief or increased level of function within 2 hours.
- Minimize the use of second-line drugs (especially narcotics)
- Optimize in-home care
- Minimize the utilization of health care resources, including hospitalization
- Minimize the adverse effects from the therapies
- Prevent recurrence

Triptans are generally considered the first-line medications for moderate to severe migraine. Other medications that can provide relief include nonsteroidal anti-inflammatory drugs (NSAIDs), barbiturate and caffeine compounds, or, in rare occasions, narcotics, or migraine-specific medications such as ergotamine or isometheptene compounds. Behavioral strategies include resting in a dark, quiet place; meditation; massage; or heat or ice applied to the head or neck. Treatment in some cases may also be prescribed for accompanying symptoms (e.g., antiemetics for headache-associated nausea and vomiting). Migraines in children often respond well to NSAIDs such as naproxen, ibuprofen, or aspirin. Women with menstrual-related migraines also often respond well to the prostaglandin inhibition of NSAIDs.

There are two general approaches to medication use in migraine: stepwise and stratified. The stepwise approach starts with a simple treatment and gets more complex if it is not successful. For people whose headache pain is relieved by the early or first treatments, the stepwise approach is fine; good candidates for this approach are people with mild disability from the headache. However, the stepwise approach can result in patients suffering for longer than is necessary and, therefore, is not considered cost-effective for more severe headache.

The stratified approach uses as the first-line intervention the treatment that has been found previously to be most effective for the severity of headache the patient is experiencing

TABLE 45.7 Drugs Used in the Prophylaxis for Migraine Headaches

Medication	Dose	Onset of Action	Side Effects
Antidepressants: Tricyclic—amitriptyline or nortriptyline Most SSRI's	 10–150 mg/day 10–150 mg/day variable	 3–4 weeks (at appropriate dose) 3–4 weeks (at appropriate dose)	 Sedation, dry mouth, constipation caution with triptans or ergotamines
Anticonvulsants: Valproic acid (VA) Gabapentin (GBP) Topiramate (T) Pregabalin (PG)	 500–1,500 mg/day 900–1,800 mg/day 50–200 mg/day 150–300 mg/day	All require titration to effect 2–3 weeks 2–3 weeks: titrate to dose 2–3 weeks 2–3 weeks: titrate to dose	Nausea, tremor, hair loss Sedation-dizziness Weight—loss, memory (Topiramate) Similar to GBP-PG
β-blockers: Propranolol Timolol Nadolol Metoprolol	 80–240 mg/day (LA if possible) 10 mg BID-20 mg 1× a day 20–260 mg/day 200 mg/day	3–4 weeks (titrating up to effective dose)	Fatigue, drowsiness, may worsen asthma, impotence, may worsen depression (especially propranolol)
Calcium channel blockers: Verapamil Nimodipine	 120–240 mg/day 40 mg BID	3–4 weeks	A-V block (verapamil), constipation, edema, hypotension
Muscle relaxants: Tizanidine (Zanaflex) Botulinum toxin	 8 mg BID 25 to 75 mcg/injection	 Not well established After injections	 Drowsiness Very expensive, requires injections of trigger areas
Opioids—long acting: Methadone Morphine controlled release Oxycodone (OxyContin)	***Last resort*** 5–20 mg/day 20–50 mg/day 10–20 mg (or more)/day	Titrate to effect over weeks.	Drowsiness, impairment, withdrawal symptoms after chronic use. Constipation

Sources: Taylor F, Hutchinson S, Graff-Radford S, et al. Diagnosis and Management of Migraine; In Family Practice. Supplement to JFP Jan 2004 Woolhouse M. Migraine and tension headache—a complementary and alternative medicine approach. *Aust Fam Phys*. 2005;34(8):647–651.

based on attack-related disability and patient goals (26). For people reporting moderate or severe disability from a headache, such as inability to work or care for daily needs, the stratified approach is often preferable, and migraine-specific therapy should be employed at headache onset. If there is not rapid improvement (within 2 hours), the person may require "rescue" treatment, such as repeating a triptan dose, employing antiemetics (intramuscularly or per rectum), using intramuscular ketorolac, or even opioids. People with a known history of severe disability with the headache attack should always start with the most effective nonaddictive medications that abort the headache (27–29).

PREVENTING MIGRAINE ATTACKS

In addition to avoiding situations that trigger their headaches, people suffering from two or more headaches a week may benefit from prophylactic (preventive) therapy (30). Clinical criteria for migraine prophylaxis include:

- Headaches >2 days a week, on average
- Recurring migraines that, in the patient's opinion, significantly interfere with his or her daily routine
- Failure of, or contraindication to, acute therapies
- Patient preference
- Significant cost of acute therapies
- Presence of uncommon headache conditions including hemiplegic migraine, basilar migraine, migraine with prolonged aura, or migrainous infarction

Table 45.7 reviews prophylactic medications and the usual dosage ranges. Cognitive behavioral therapy, acupuncture, biofeedback, relaxation, and stress management training also have proven benefit (31,32).

Tension-type Headache

Tension-type headaches tend to not be debilitating, but patients often bring them to the attention of their health care providers. Medication treatment with acetaminophen

Question	Number of Days
1. On how many days in the past 3 months did you miss work or school because of your headaches?	______
2. How many days in the past 3 months was your productivity at work or school reduced by half or more because of your headaches?	______
3. On how many days in the past 3 months did you not do household work because of your headaches?	______
4. How many days in the past 3 months was your productivity in household work reduced by half or more because of your headaches?	______
5. On how many days in the past 3 months did you miss family, social or non-work activities because of your headaches?	______

Add up the numbers: there are four grades of severity for the MIDAS-
Grade I- minimal disability = 0-5
Grade II- mild or infrequent disability = 6-10
Grade III- moderate disability = 11-20
Grade IV- severe disability = 21+

Figure 45.1 • Migraine Disability Scale (MIDAS). This survey was developed by Richard B. Lipton, MD, Professor of Neurology, Albert Einstein College of Medicine, New York, NY, and Walter F. Stewart, MPH, PhD, Associate Professor of Epidemiology, Johns Hopkins University, Baltimore, MD.

1. When you have headaches, how often is the pain severe?

   Never Rarely Sometimes Very Often Always

2. How often do headaches limit your ability to do usual daily activities including household work, work, school, or social activities?

   Never Rarely Sometimes Very Often Always

3. When you have a headache, how often do you wish you could lie down?

   Never Rarely Sometimes Very Often Always

4. In the past 4 weeks, how often have you felt too tired to do work or daily activities because of your headaches?

   Never Rarely Sometimes Very Often Always

5. In the past 4 weeks, how often have you felt fed up or irritated because of your headaches?

   Never Rarely Sometimes Very Often Always

6. In the past 4 weeks, how often did headaches limit your ability to concentrate on work or daily activities?

Never	Rarely	Sometimes	Very Often	Always
______	______	______	______	______
I = 6 pts each	II = 8 pts each	III = 10 pts each	IV = 11 pts each	V = 13 pts each

Scores are calculated by summing the points from each column.

KEY

60 or >	High impact on quality of life
56–59	Substantial impact on life, missing work, school or family time
50–55	Some impact, but not losing time at work or with family
49 or <	Little impact, at present

Figure 45.2 • Headache Impact Test (HIT-6).

or NSAIDs is often successful (33). Complementary or alternative approaches such as nutritional supplements or acupuncture have been shown to be effective as well (34,35). In contrast, the data about the efficacy of manipulative treatments or Botox injections are inconclusive (36,37). Of nonpharmacologic options, biofeedback, and relaxation techniques have been shown to be most effective (38).

Prophylaxis should be considered for people who experience 15 or more tension-type headaches per month (39). Medications that have been shown to be of benefit in the prophylaxis of chronic tension-type headache are amitriptyline and mirtazapine. Cognitive behavioral therapy has also been shown to be of use (40).

Cluster Headaches

Cluster headaches are infrequently seen but are invariably debilitating. Treatment options for acute episodes include oxygen therapy (first-line treatment), triptans, ergot derivatives, and intranasal lidocaine. Verapamil may be used for prophylaxis (41).

Chronic Daily Headache

The mainstay of treatment of chronic daily headache is amitriptyline (42). Other tricyclic antidepressants may also be tried, but other medicines are less well studied. Chronic daily headache can be treated occasionally with acetaminophen or NSAIDs; however, as previously noted, overuse of these medications can induce chronic headache. Patients with chronic daily headache should be questioned about use of these medicines (43).

Long-term Monitoring

Headache questionnaires can be useful in monitoring patient's symptoms and response to treatment. The two most commonly used headache questionnaires are the Migraine Disability Assessment (MIDAS) Questionnaire (Fig. 45.1) and the Headache Impact Test (Fig. 45.2). These instruments may be used both to assess the level of disability associated with headaches at the time of initial evaluation and to monitor clinical change over time (44–46).

KEY POINTS

- Headaches can be characterized as primary or secondary.
- The three most common primary headache types are tension, migraine, and cluster.
- A change in quality, frequency, or intensity of headache merits further investigation.
- Imaging can be useful in evaluation of headache but should be used judiciously.
- Medication overuse is an important precipitant of headache.
- For patients with migraine, patients and providers should clearly discuss goals of therapy.

CHAPTER

46

Family Violence

Amy C. Denham and Adam J. Zolotor

CLINICAL OBJECTIVES

1. Describe conditions that should raise suspicion of child abuse, intimate partner violence, and elder mistreatment.
2. Discuss approaches to assessment for family violence.
3. List common risk factors for child abuse, intimate partner violence, and elder mistreatment.
4. Describe the adverse health consequences of family violence.
5. Discuss approaches to management of family violence.

Family violence includes child abuse, intimate partner violence, and elder mistreatment. Estimating the true prevalence of family violence is challenging, because it occurs in the privacy of the home and not all cases come to medical or professional attention, but it appears to be a common problem in the United States. All forms of family violence can have serious physical and mental health consequences. It is important that the family physician be alert to signs that might suggest family violence and understand approaches to managing the problem.

CHILD MALTREATMENT

Child maltreatment includes physical abuse, sexual abuse, psychological abuse, and neglect. Child maltreatment often presents with symptoms of inattention, school failure, disruptive symptoms, anxiety, depression, failure to thrive, and a broad range of somatic symptoms (ranging from the physical pain of a broken bone to psychogenic symptoms such as recurrent abdominal pain).

Estimates of child maltreatment rates vary widely by methodology. The most widely used method to estimate the incidence of child abuse is official reporting statistics. These statistics are biased, in that they only include those reports that come to the attention of protective services. Most public health and social service agencies count only substantiated reports, further undercounting real cases of abuse. In 2007, reports to protective services indicated that 794,000 children were found to be victims of abuse or neglect (10.6/1000) (1). An alternative method of ascertaining estimated of abuse is used in a periodic national incidence study. This study asks sentinel professionals who have regular involvement with children how many children they have seen in the past week who were harmed from abuse or neglect. This counts only children subjected of abuse or neglect that is known about by another adult who regularly and professionally has contact with children. In 2006, 1,256,600 (17/1000) children were estimated to be abused or neglected using this methodology (2). The true incidence of child maltreatment may be much higher (3). In many cases of abuse or neglect, only the victim and the perpetrator are privy to the abuse.

Physical Abuse

The family physician should suspect physical abuse in cases of childhood injury that are (i) unexplained, (ii) not plausible by the explanation offered, (iii) in a pattern suspicious for inflicted injury, (iv) developmentally inconsistent, or (v) from punishment with excessive force (4). In 2006 there were 85,800 substantiated cases of physical abuse according to social services (1). There were 323,000 victims of physical abuse in 2006 according to the National Incidence Study (2).

Sexual Abuse

Sexual abuse includes all forms of sexual contact (oral-genital, genital, anal) involving a child in which there is age or developmental discordance between the child and the perpetrator. It also includes noncontact abuse such as exhibitionism, voyeurism, and use of a child to produce pornography (5). In 2007 there were 60,300 substantiated cases of sexual abuse, according to social services (1). There were 135,300 victims of child sexual abuse in 2006, according to the National Incidence Study (2).

Child sexual abuse usually presents with child disclosure. However, presentations may vary and include acute sexual trauma, sexually transmitted diseases, pregnancy, extremes of sexualized behavior, and somatic symptoms such as dysuria and enuresis. Interviewing children for evidence of sexual abuse requires special skill and training. That does not preclude the family physician from taking a thorough medical history of a child, including open-ended and nonleading questions about various types of trauma and the etiology of specific findings. In this nonthreatening and familiar setting, a child may disclose abuse. These disclosures are admissible in court. When possible, medical history documentation of a disclosure should include direct quotations of questions asked by the provider and responses of the victim.

Neglect

Child neglect accounts for the vast majority of protective service cases with 468,500 substantiated cases in 2007 and 771,700 cases in 2006 according to the National Incidence Study (1,2). Neglect alone accounts for more than one third of the annual child maltreatment fatalities (1,760 in 2007) (1). Physicians caring for children need to understand the symptoms of neglect, be willing to report suspected neglect, and help families meet the needs of their children.

Neglect can be thought of as failing to meet the basic needs of a child. These needs include adequate supervision, food, clothing, shelter, medical care, education, and love. Neglect, unlike physical and sexual abuse, often manifests as a pattern of chronic unmet needs, sometimes along one domain, but often along multiple domains. Situations due to poverty are excluded from reporting laws in some states. However, the family physician should avoid this judgment if he or she recognizes inadequate care that may jeopardize the health or development of a child. The cause of neglect may not be malevolent, but the risk to the child remains the same. For example, a poor single father may leave his 2-year-old child home alone sleeping at night to work a second-shift job. Even though his circumstances drove him to this omission of care, the child is still at risk of significant harm.

Psychological Abuse

Psychological abuse of children is common; however, it is the least often substantiated type of abuse because of social norms and the challenges of proving both intent of the parent and harm to the child. In 2007, there were 52,900 children with substantiated reports for psychological maltreatment (1). The National Incidence Study reported 148,500 cases of emotional neglect in 2006 (2). Some states include emotional neglect as a type of neglect, whereas others include a separate category of psychological maltreatment, which may or may not include both commissions of abuse and omissions of love and nurturing care. Despite this low number of psychological abuse cases, primary surveys of parents reveal that this type of type behavior is far more common. In North and South Carolina in 2003, 12.8% of parents surveyed endorsed one or more of the following in the past year: (i) threatening to leave or abandon a child, (ii) threatening to kick a child out of the home, (iii) locking a child out of the house, or (iv) calling a name like stupid, ugly, or useless (6). It is difficult to determine when such behavior is abusive, as it is common, often chronic, and harm is difficult to measure or prove.

Assessment

PHYSICAL ABUSE

In considering an injury for suspicion of abuse, many physicians use the practical 24-hour rule. That is, if a mark lasts 24 hours, it is considered a significant injury. Red marks from spanking (with open hand, paddle, or switch) that resolve in <24 hours do not rise to the level of concern for injury by protective services in most jurisdictions (4). In evaluating any injury to a child, a detailed history should be obtained and carefully documented. In the case of suspicious injuries, detailed drawings or photographs can be helpful. The injury should be carefully matched to the reported mechanism. Does the skin mark resemble a known pattern of injury? Loops, teeth marks, and linear welts (from belts or switches) are common patterns in abusive injuries. Studies have shown that premobile children rarely bruise: fewer than 1% of children not yet cruising have bruises thought to be due to unintentional injury (7). Certain skeletal injuries are highly suggestive of abuse. Children younger than age 2 years with rib fractures (in the absence of a high impact trauma history or metabolic bone disease) are nearly always the result of abuse (8,9). Likewise, metaphyseal corner fractures of the long bones are usually from abuse in children younger than age 2 (10). Inflicted head injury is the most common cause of death from child physical abuse. Children younger than age 2 with other significant abusive injuries should be evaluated with brain imaging (computed tomography or magnetic resonance imaging) to identify occult brain injury and a skeletal survey to evaluate for bony injuries (10–12).

The most important factor in identifying physical abuse is a high index of suspicion. Clinicians with special training or experience in child abuse can be helpful in clarifying mechanisms in ambiguous injuries. These clinicians will also help search for alternative explanations for disease and injury patterns (e.g., coagulopathy, metabolic bone disease). Detailed documentation of history and physical exam is essential for protective service and legal investigation. Table 46.1 lists injuries that are suspicious for abuse and deserve careful history taking and documentation.

TABLE 46.1 Suspicious Injuries for Child Abuse

Bruises in non–weight-bearing child
Numerous bruises
Bruises over fleshy body parts (i.e., buttocks, thighs, cheeks)
Scalds (especially symmetric, perineal, clear margins)
Rib fractures
Metaphyseal fractures in children younger than age 2 years
Brain injuries (especially subdural hemorrhage)
Pattern skin injuries (i.e., iron, stove eye, loop, cigarette burn)
Oral injuries (especially labial frenulum laceration in non–weight-bearing child)

SEXUAL ABUSE

The physical examination for child sexual abuse should include visual inspection of the genitals and anus in supine frog-leg and knee-chest positions. This exam may be aided by the use of specialized instruments such as lighting devices and a colposcope for magnification. Instruments such as probes or specula should never be inserted into a prepubertal vagina without anesthesia or conscious sedation. Photodocumentation can be helpful for legal reference, but accurate pen and paper diagrams can be used when photocolposcopy is unavailable. Routine cultures for sexually transmitted diseases are not necessary in the absence of symptoms. Clinicians unskilled in the physical exam for sexual abuse should seek expert consultation. In the case of uncertain findings, photodocumentation or expert consultation can clarify equivocal findings. In the overwhelming majority of cases of chronic or past sexual abuse, physical exam findings will be either normal or nonspecific, making the history critical in determining sexual abuse victimization (13,14).

NEGLECT

Neglect may come to the family physician's attention in the form of medical nonadherence, failure or delay in seeking medical care, failure to thrive, unmanaged obesity, behavior problems, school failure, poor hygiene, or homelessness (15). In identifying a child suspected of being neglected, asking nonjudgmental questions about resources can help identify sources of problems and potential solutions. Because neglect often manifests as a chronic pattern, the physician must have a way to follow children over time. If a child failing to thrive does not return as scheduled, the physician should have a system in place to call the patient, reschedule the appointment, and identify barriers to follow through. When a pattern of omissions in care (or a single egregious episode) rises to the level of harm or significant risk of harm, the physician is obligated to report the case to protective services.

PSYCHOLOGICAL ABUSE

The diagnosis of psychological abuse is often made only through long-term observation of parent–child interaction. This can be facilitated by querying other adults involved in the life of the child (e.g., teachers, coaches). Symptoms of psychological abuse include: aggressiveness, impulsivity, depression, hyperactivity, school failure, inattention, disturbances of conduct, anxiety, eating disorders, and somatic symptoms. In the evaluation of children with disorders of behavior and development, parents may be witnessed belittling children in cruel ways ("he's stupid just like his daddy" or "she drives me crazy"). Discussing destructive behavior and role modeling positive behavior can help ameliorate a difficult visit and begin to help a parent identify problem parenting. However, in the setting of this type of abusive behavior, a child struggling at home or school will be very difficult to treat with any measure of success. When such behavior is observed over time or seems to be correlated with behavioral symptoms, the treating physician should consider a referral for family therapy or to protective services.

Management

All states, districts, and territories in the United States have child abuse reporting statutes that include physicians as mandated reporters for suspected child abuse and neglect. These laws include immunity from lawsuits for reports made in good faith. It is important for the parent involved to understand that the report is not placing blame or making judgment, but carrying out a legal responsibility. This helps to absolve some of the guilt that a physician may feel in making a report to child protective services. It is not required by law that a person reporting must inform the parent of the report to be made; however, this can set the stage for an open dialog and continued support of a family. How this is framed will depend on the nature of the suspected maltreatment and the suspected perpetrator.

Attention to careful documentation of history (both questions asked and responses in quotes) and careful documentation of injuries with drawings or photo documentation is critical. In many cases, a physician caring for a child suspected to be a victim of abuse or neglect may need to make a safety plan in conjunction with social services while the child is in the clinic, emergency room, or hospital. Ongoing evaluation will often include ancillary studies (i.e., skeletal survey, head computed tomography, coagulation studies). In many communities, the family physician will have access to a provider with special skill and training in the evaluation of children suspected to be maltreatment victims.

INTIMATE PARTNER VIOLENCE

Intimate partner violence (IPV), which includes physical, emotional and sexual harm by a current or former partner or spouse, is a common problem with serious physical and mental health consequences for victims and their children. Although women are most commonly affected, IPV affects both men and women and occurs in married and unmarried couples, affecting both heterosexual and same-sex couples. The Centers for Disease Control and Prevention defines IPV according to the following categories:

- **Physical violence** is the intentional use of physical force with the potential for causing death, disability, injury, or harm. Physical violence includes, but is not limited to, scratching; pushing; shoving; throwing; grabbing; biting; choking; shaking; slapping; punching; burning; use of a weapon; and use of restraints or one's body, size, or strength against another person.
- **Sexual violence** is divided into three categories: (i) use of physical force to compel a person to engage in a sexual act against his or her will, whether or not the act is completed; (ii) attempted or completed sex act involving a person who is unable to understand the nature or condition of the act, to decline participation, or to communicate unwillingness to engage in the sexual act (e.g., because of illness, disability, or the influence of alcohol or other drugs, or because of intimidation or pressure); and (iii) abusive sexual contact.
- **Psychological/emotional violence** involves trauma to the victim caused by acts, threats of acts, or coercive tactics. Psychological/emotional abuse can include, but is not limited to, humiliating the victim, controlling what the victim can and cannot do, withholding information from the victim, deliberately doing something to make the victim feel diminished or embarrassed, isolating the victim from friends and family, and denying the victim access to money or other basic resources (16).

IPV is a common problem: population-based estimates suggest that about 26% of women and 8% of men in the United States have been victims of IPV in their adult lifetimes (17). Although IPV affects all ages, races, ethnicities, and socioeconomic strata, young women and individuals with low incomes are at greatest risk (18,19). A prior history of IPV, child abuse victimization, or sexual assault are all associated with increased risk of IPV, as is a history of alcohol or other drug use and separated or divorced marital status (20). In addition to the toll that IPV takes on individuals and their families, the cost of IPV to society is large. It is estimated that IPV accounts for $4.1 billion in direct medical and mental health costs in the United States each year, with another $1.8 billion in lost productivity (21).

Because victims of IPV tend to have high rates of physical and mental health morbidity, they are frequent users of the health care system. For this reason, rates of IPV seen in primary care practices and emergency departments are even higher than those seen in the general population. One study of women enrolled in health maintenance organizations demonstrated that 44% of adult female patients reported IPV in their lifetimes and 8% had experienced IPV in the past year (22). Intimate partner violence is thus a condition that family physicians can expect to encounter frequently over the course of their careers.

Common Presentations

IPV influences multiple aspects of physical and mental health, affecting victims' health for many years, even after abuse has ended (23,24). Negative health effects occur whether abuse is physical, sexual, or emotional (24–26).

INJURIES

The most direct health effect of IPV is injury: partner violence causes about 2 million injuries in women and 600,000 injuries in men annually in the United States (19), although fewer than one in three IPV-related injuries are brought to the attention of health care providers (17). Certain patterns of injury, such as injuries to the head, neck, breast, or abdomen, should raise suspicion of intentional injury. Facial trauma, for example an orbital fracture or dental injury, is particularly suggestive (27,28). Fractures, sprains, or dislocations of the extremities account for about one quarter of IPV-related injuries (27). Victims of IPV also suffer long-term sequelae of injury, such as symptoms of traumatic brain injury or problems with swallowing and speech (29). The most serious direct consequence of IPV is mortality: more than 1,000 women are killed by intimate partners in the United States annually (18).

OTHER PHYSICAL HEALTH EFFECTS

Many of the health effects of IPV are not directly attributable to trauma. Concerns related to sexual health, such as sexually transmitted infections, cervical dysplasia, and unplanned pregnancy, are more common in victims of IPV (29,30). In addition, victims of IPV are at increased risk for cardiovascular disease and stroke (19). Functional gastrointestinal disorders such as irritable bowel syndrome (31,32) and a variety of chronic pain complaints, such as arthritis, migraine, fibromyalgia, chronic fatigue syndrome, and temporomandibular joint syndrome are all more common in victims of IPV (19,33). Patients with IPV may present with multiple somatic complaints, such as stomach pain, back pain, menstrual problems, headaches, chest pain, dizziness, fainting spells, palpitations, shortness of breath, constipation, generalized fatigue, and insomnia (33). The reason that IPV increases risk for such a wide range of conditions is unknown but may be related to the direct consequences of trauma, the long-term accumulated effects of chronic stress, and high prevalence of risky health behaviors.

IPV AND PREGNANCY

IPV often continues throughout pregnancy, increasing risk for complications such as spontaneous abortion, hypertensive disorders of pregnancy, vaginal bleeding, placental abruption, severe nausea and vomiting, dehydration, diabetes, urinary tract infection, and premature rupture of membranes (29,34). Victims of IPV are often delayed in seeking prenatal care, and the possibility of IPV should be considered in women who receive late or no prenatal care (29). IPV-related homicide is the leading cause of maternal mortality, accounting for 13% to 24% of all deaths in pregnancy (29). Infants of mothers who experience IPV during pregnancy also are at risk for medical complications, including low birth weight, prematurity, and perinatal death (34–39).

MENTAL HEALTH

IPV, whether it is physical, sexual, or emotional, also has mental health consequences (25). Victims of IPV commonly experience depression, suicidal thoughts and attempts, and posttraumatic stress disorder (31,34,40). Tobacco, alcohol, and illicit drug abuse are common (19,25,26,29), and victims of IPV are more likely to engage in risky sexual behaviors (19,29). Women who are abused are more likely to engage in disordered eating patterns (29). Adverse mental health consequences, such as depression, oppositional defiant disorder, developmental delay, school failure, or future violent behavior, are also seen in children who witness IPV (41).

Assessment

Assessing for IPV in the clinical setting can fall into one of two categories: clinicians may inquire about IPV in all patients at risk regardless of clinical suspicion (a universal screening approach), or they may confine inquiries to situations in which there is some suspicion that violence is occurring or in which knowledge of violence would be relevant to the presenting complaint.

Although routine screening for IPV is recommended by some organizations, the United States Preventive Services Task Force (USPSTF) states that there is insufficient evidence to recommend for or against routinely screening women for IPV (20). This recommendation was based on the lack of evidence regarding accuracy of IPV screening questionnaires, and more importantly, the lack evidence that primary care based interventions are helpful in preventing the negative consequences of IPV (41). Recent systematic reviews have confirmed that there is not yet strong evidence of effectiveness of any intervention, although some strategies show promise in mitigating the effects of IPV (42,43). After the USPSTF recommendation was published, a randomized controlled trial of screening for IPV in health care settings did not support a significant benefit from screening (44).

The USPSTF does state, however, that "all clinicians examining children and adults should be alert to physical and behavioral signs and symptoms associated with abuse or neglect. Patients in whom abuse is suspected should receive proper documentation of the incident and physical findings . . . ; treatment for physical injuries; arrangement for skilled counseling by a mental health professional; and the telephone number of local crisis centers, shelters, and protective service agencies" (20). In other words, although there may be weak evidence for *screening* for IPV, clinicians should still maintain an index of suspicion for IPV, remaining alert to situations suggestive IPV and providing appropriate treatment resources for patients in whom IPV is detected.

When patients present with issues consistent with IPV (Table 46.2), clinicians should consider inquiring about IPV, not only because intervention may be beneficial but also because knowledge of IPV could influence the treatment plan and help the clinician understand barriers to treatment adherence. Women with a history of IPV often have frequent primary care and emergency room visits and may be perceived to overuse the health care system. They often report strained relationships with their physicians. However, what physicians perceive as poor adherence to medical recommendations and lack of motivation may in fact be related to the abuse a patient is experiencing. Interference with receipt of health care may be part of the control that abusers exert in their partners' lives (29). Primary care physicians who diagnose IPV, and therefore begin to understand the barriers that their abused patients

TABLE 46.2 Situations that Should Raise Suspicion for Intimate Partner Violence

Injuries to the face or trunk
Pattern of injury not consistent with explanation given
Frequent somatic complaints
Chronic pain syndromes
Recurrent sexual health concerns
Late entry into prenatal care
Frequent late or missed appointments
Substance abuse
Frequent mental health complaints

face, may be able to form more effective therapeutic relationships. Identifying IPV also provides an important opportunity for providing the patient with empathic support and reassurance that the violence is not her fault; educating her regarding the dynamics of IPV and the future risks it poses to her and her children; and opening the door to future conversations.

Several questionnaires for assessing for IPV have been validated in a variety of populations and patient care settings and are practical for use in the primary care setting (Table 46.3). It must be kept in mind with each of these questionnaires, however, that what is considered a "positive" test depends on how IPV is defined, and sensitivity and specificity of the test depend on what criterion standard is used to define a true positive or negative test. Because it is difficult to objectively confirm the presence of IPV, determining accuracy of specific questions can be problematic.

Regardless of whether a clinician uses a structured instrument or simply asks questions informally in the context of a patient interview, several principles are important to follow. Physicians should ensure a private setting, without friends or family members (other than children under age three) present. They should assure patients of confidentiality, but notify them if any reporting requirements apply. Language should be direct and nonjudgmental. It is often helpful to preface questions about IPV with statements that normalize the inquiry; for example, "Because violence is a common problem, I routinely ask my patients about it," or "Many people with [condition] have worse symptoms if they have been physically, emotionally, or sexually abused in the past." If any language barriers are present, physicians should use the assistance of an interpreter, ideally one who has been trained to ask about IPV (45).

Management

When IPV is detected in the clinical setting, it is important that clinicians respond in a way that builds trust and sets the stage for an ongoing therapeutic relationship. Key components of an initial interaction should include validation of the patient's concerns, education regarding the dynamics and consequences of IPV, safety assessment, and referral to local resources. It is important to realize that IPV is usually a chronic problem that will not be solved in the one or two visits, but rather can be worked on over time. Because intervening on IPV is a complex and slow process, with outcomes that are often difficult to measure objectively, the evidence base for most health care–based interventions IPV is weak (42,43). Recommendations for management of intimate partner violence in the clinical setting are therefore largely based on expert opinion.

An initial response to a disclosure of IPV should include listening to the patient empathically and nonjudgmentally, expressing a concern for her health and safety, and affirming a commitment to help her address the problem. Women who have long been subjected to abuse may have very low self-esteem and may believe that the abuse is their fault. Physicians can help counter this belief, reassuring patients that although partner violence is a common problem, it is unacceptable and not the fault of the victim. It is also important to convey to victims of IPV a respect for their choices regarding how to respond to the violence. Taking control and attempting to steer a patient toward a specific course of action, for example leaving an abusive partner, can actually replicate a pattern of abuse, disempowering a patient who already has very little control over the circumstances of her life. Victims of IPV may have a clearer understanding than clinicians about the dynamics of their relationships and what courses of action may result in increased danger. If patients need to move slowly, scheduling frequent office visits can be helpful, providing ongoing support and addressing medical problems.

It is, however, important that clinicians provide patients with education on the dynamics of partner violence and potential effects on victims and their children. Patients should be helped to understand that once violent dynamics are established in a relationship, the violence generally continues and escalates over time. In a nonjudgmental way, physicians can convey concern to patients regarding the negative physical and mental effects that IPV may have on patients and their children.

Although addressing IPV is usually a long-term, ongoing process, physicians should be alert to potential crisis situations that could indicate imminent danger to patients' health or safety (Table 46.4). Even if none of these risk factors is currently present, assessing for them can help educate patients regarding what situations to be alert for that could indicate increased risk. It can be useful to offer patients a handout or brochure on safety planning and go over it with them. Examples can be found at the Family Violence Prevention website (*www.endabuse.org/*).

Finally, physicians should provide victims of IPV with referral to local resources that can provide advocacy and support. Family physicians should be familiar with the organizations in their communities that can provide assistance to victims of IPV, including organizations' capacity to accommodate specific populations such as immigrants; specific ethnic or cultural groups; teens; lesbian, gay, bisexual, or transgender clients; or people with disabilities. Resources might include community-based advocacy groups, shelters, law enforcement agencies, social workers, or support systems within the health-care setting. The National DV Hotline (800-799-SAFE) can serve as a resource. If immediate concerns for safety exist, the physician can offer for the patient to contact these resources from the office. A follow-up visit should be scheduled, and IPV should be readdressed at future visits.

TABLE 46.3 Tools to Assess for Intimate Partner Violence (46)

Test	Sensitivity (%)	Specificity (%)
Abuse Assessment Screen 1. Have you ever been emotionally or physically abused by your partner or someone important to you? 2. Within the last year, have you been hit, slapped, kicked, or otherwise physically hurt by someone? 3. Since you've been pregnant, have you been slapped, kicked, or otherwise physically hurt by someone? If YES, who? 4. Within the last year, has anyone forced you to have sexual activities? If YES, who? 5. Are you afraid of your partner or anyone you listed above? Any yes answer considered positive for abuse	93	55
HITS 1. How often does your partner physically **H**urt you? 2. How often does your partner **I**nsult or talk down to you? 3. How often does your partner **T**hreaten you with physical harm? 4. How often does your partner **S**cream or curse at you? Each question is answered on a 5-point scale: 1 = never, 2 = rarely, 3 = sometimes, 4 = fairly often, 5 = frequently Score ≥10 considered positive for abuse	86–96	91–99
Partner Violence Screen 1. Have you been hit, kicked, punched, or otherwise hurt by someone within the past year? If so, by whom? 2. Do you feel safe in your current relationship? 3. Is there a partner from a previous relationship who is making you feel unsafe now? Yes answer to question 1 if perpetrator is current or former partner, no answer to question 2 or yes answer to question 3 considered a positive test	65–71	80–84
WAST-short 1. In general, how would you describe your relationship? • A lot of tension • Some tension • No tension 2. Do you and your partner work out arguments with: • Great difficulty? • Some difficulty? • No difficulty? "A lot of tension" on question 1 or "great difficulty" on question 2 considered a positive test	92	100

Adapted from reference 46.

TABLE 46.4 Intimate Partner Violence Red Flags Indicating Increased Risk for Serious Injury or Homicide (45)

Increasing frequency or severity of violence
Recent use of or threats with a weapon
Homicide or suicide threats
Hostage taking or stalking
Alcohol or drug use
Recent separation from or threats to leave partner

INTIMATE PARTNER VIOLENCE AND CHILDREN

Partner violence and child maltreatment share many features and risk factors. They are often concurrent outcomes from family dysfunction, stress, and societal tolerance of violence. The best interest of children and parent victims may not be served in the same way.

Co-occurrence of Intimate Partner Violence and Child Maltreatment

IPV often occurs in households with child maltreatment. Studies that have screened for partner violence in a population of families affected by child maltreatment or for child maltreatment in families affected by partner violence have demonstrated that these types of violence often occur in the same homes. Between 26% to 73% of families reported to child protective services for child maltreatment are also affected by IPV (47–49). Conversely, families in which a woman is victimized by partner violence have rates of child maltreatment between 30% and 60% (47) with some studies reporting rates as high as 100% (50). More recent studies that used population-based samples and more appropriate comparison groups have demonstrated important relationships between partner violence and physical abuse, sexual abuse, and neglect (51–55).

Harmful Effects of IPV to Children

Partner violence can harm children physically and mentally. Children can be victims of "collateral damage" in an assault between intimate partners. Nearly half of homes with child maltreatment fatalities have reported IPV (47,50,55). One study of child injuries presenting to a pediatric emergency department demonstrates the range of these collateral injuries. Half of the child victims were younger than age 2, and 59% were being held by a caregiver when injured. Most of the child injuries were to the head (25%), face (19%), and eyes (12%). The child's father (50%), mother (13%), or mother's boyfriend (10%) were found responsible for the injuries in most cases (56). Children whose mothers have a history of partner violence have higher rates of emergency room utilization (57,58). Child reports of witnessed partner violence are associated with increased odds of suicidal ideation (59) and suicide attempt (60). Two reports from a high-risk cohort study have shown that witnessing partner violence during childhood leads to more mental health symptoms and more clinical depression, anxiety, and anger (61,62).

LEGAL RAMIFICATIONS

IPV is important to child welfare agencies because of the harm to children (physical and mental) and the risk it poses for subsequent or concurrent child maltreatment. At least 40 states, three territories, and the District of Columbia include children as a class of protected people in definitions of partner violence. In many states, an act of partner violence in the presence of a child confers a harsher penalty. Some states require the reporting of partner violence to child welfare agencies under some circumstances (63).

ELDER MISTREATMENT

Elder abuse is a less well-understood phenomenon than child abuse and IPV, but a growing body of research suggests that it is a common problem with potential for serious morbidity and mortality. A recent panel convened by the National Academy of Sciences to outline a research agenda in the field defined elder mistreatment as "(a) intentional actions that cause harm or create a serious risk of harm (whether or not harm is intended) to a vulnerable elder by a caregiver or other person who stands in a trust relationship to the elder or (b) failure by a caregiver to satisfy the elder's basic needs or to protect the elder from harm" (64). Elder mistreatment includes physical abuse, psychological abuse, sexual abuse, financial exploitation, and neglect. Elder self-neglect, or the failure of an elderly person to meet his or her own basic needs or protect his or her health and safety, is also sometimes considered to be a type of elder mistreatment.

Recent population-based studies suggest that between 2% and 11% of older adults report having been subject to some form of abuse in the past year (65–67). Neglect is most commonly reported, followed by emotional mistreatment, physical mistreatment, and sexual mistreatment (65). A minority of these events are ever brought to the attention of physicians or adult protective services agencies. Elder mistreatment, however, is difficult to measure, so the accuracy of prevalence estimates is unclear. Population-based research has generally relied on self-report of abuse from cognitively intact, community dwelling individuals and is therefore unable to accurately estimate the prevalence of mistreatment in vulnerable elders who suffer from dementia or live in long-term care facilities. Family caregivers and long-term care staff report even higher levels of abuse than do the elders themselves. In surveys of long-term care staff, 10% admit to physical abuse of residents, 40% admit to psychological abuse, and, impressively, 80% report having witnessed abuse (66,68). By any of these measures elder mistreatment is a common enough problem that any family physician who cares for elderly patients in outpatient, inpatient, or long-term care settings will encounter elder abuse frequently in clinical practice.

Although the causes of elder mistreatment are not well understood, several patient, caregiver, social, and environmental factors are markers of increased risk. Elders who live with their caregivers are more likely to be victims of mistreatment, probably simply from tensions that arise when there are greater opportunities for contact. Social isolation of both elders and their caregivers also appears to increase risk for mistreatment. Patients with dementia, in particular patients who have disruptive behavior or aggression, are at increased risk. Research on the role of physical frailty and dependence play in risk of abuse has been inconsistent. Caregiver factors that increase risk of mistreatment include mental illness, especially depression and alcohol abuse, and financial dependency on the elder. Factors that increase risk of abuse in long-term care facilities include inadequate staffing and staff training, staff burnout, and aggressive behavior by residents (64). Elder mistreatment has been linked to adverse health outcomes, including increased depression, hospitalizations, nursing home placement, and mortality (67,69).

Assessment

As with child maltreatment and intimate partner violence, the USPSTF states that there is insufficient evidence to recommend for or against routine screening for elder abuse, because of the lack of clear evidence that we can accurately identify and effectively intervene upon elder abuse in the clinical setting (20). The lack of evidence for universal screening, however, does not obviate the need for remaining alert to signs of elder mistreatment and appropriately treating when elder mistreatment is identified.

Unlike some of the patterns of injury that are clearly suggestive of child maltreatment—for example, the retinal hemorrhages and metaphyseal corner fractures of shaken baby syndrome—there is no clear constellation of symptoms that is suggestive of elder mistreatment. Falls and fractures are common in the frail elderly, and skin may be fragile and bruise easily. Weight loss may be a symptom of late stages of many illnesses seen in the elderly, but could also be a sign of neglect. Identification of elder mistreatment is also complicated by the fact that elderly individuals with cognitive impairment, who are particularly vulnerable, may not be able to give accurate accounts of abuse or neglect (64,67). Mistrust of caregivers can be part of the dementia process itself; it may be difficult to distinguish between financial exploitation and appropriate efforts by caregivers to take control of finances for an elder who is no longer able to manage independently.

Although there is no pattern of presenting symptoms that is specific to abuse, providers should remain alert to bruises or burns in unusual locations or injuries that are not consistent with the explanation offered. Injuries to wrists or ankles could be an indication of use of restraints. Genital or breast injuries should raise suspicion of sexual abuse. Findings that should raise suspicion for neglect include dehydration or malnutrition, pressure ulcers, poor hygiene, or medical nonadherence (70).

Several instruments have been developed to assess for elder mistreatment, but none have been well validated across different clinical settings and with different patient populations (41–64). In the absence of clear evidence for specific approaches to identifying elder mistreatment, several principles may guide clinicians who are attempting to determine whether abuse and/or neglect are occurring. If mistreatment is suspected, the patient should be questioned and examined in private, away from caregivers. General questions about home environment and safety can be followed with more direct questions about whether the patient has been hurt or threatened, food or medicines have been denied, the patient has been made to feel guilty about asking for help, personal belongings have been taken away, or unwanted touch has occurred. Any affirmative answers should be followed up with questions about details about the circumstances and frequency of potential abuse. Answers and physical findings should be documented carefully. For patients who have cognitive impairment, assessment of decision-making capacity is important, because it will guide an approach to intervention (67,70).

Caregivers may also be questioned directly about abuse or neglect, but physicians must be careful to avoid alienating caregivers, who could in turn restrict access to the elderly patient. It may be helpful to precede direct inquiries with permissive statements, such as "Caring for your father must be stressful. How do you manage?" If a caregiver does disclose abuse or neglect, the physician should be careful to refrain from passing judgment.

Management

There is a paucity of evidence to support any specific approach to intervening on elder mistreatment (64,71). Research on effective interventions is difficult for a number of reasons: elder mistreatment encompasses a heterogeneous group of problems with diverse causes; interventions for elder abuse are generally multifactorial and multidisciplinary and are difficult to standardize in the context of a controlled trial; elderly patients often have several serious comorbidities, including cognitive impairment, that make comparing outcomes across individual patients difficult; and access to patients may be limited by their caregivers. The most appropriate strategy for intervention will be determined by the nature of the abuse or neglect and the circumstances of the individual patient.

In most states, reporting of elder abuse and neglect is legally mandated. Adult Protective Services (APS) agencies exist in every state and are the point of first contact for reporting suspected elder mistreatment, including self-neglect. Each state also has a Long Term Care Ombudsman Program (LTCOP) that can provide assistance if abuse or neglect in a long-term care facility is suspected. State-level reporting requirements and a directory of APS and LTCOP contact information can be found at the National Center on Elder Abuse website (*www.ncea.aoa.gov*).

Strategies for managing elder mistreatment should be tailored to the specific situation. Lack of social support appears to be a risk factor for most types of abuse, so connecting elders with resources that can provide social support is likely to be beneficial in most situations. If abuse is thought primarily due to caregiver burden or mental health concerns, interventions can be targeted toward caregivers. These interventions might include caregiver education regarding what constitutes abuse, referral to respite care resources, connection with social support, and psychotherapy or pharmacotherapy to address mental health concerns. If abuse is a response to or is perpetrated by an aggressive patient with dementia, interventions to address behavior in the patient with dementia are indicated. If the abuse is a continuation of longstanding intimate partner violence, referral local IPV support organizations may be helpful. For patients who lack capacity for decision-making, pursuing guardianship may be necessary. Ideally, physicians should enlist the assistance of a multidisciplinary team (which might include physicians, nurses, government agencies, social workers, legal professionals, and law enforcement personnel) with expertise in various aspects of elder mistreatment (67).

KEY POINTS

- Child abuse, intimate partner violence, and elder mistreatment are all common problems in the United States.
- Child abuse, intimate partner violence, and elder mistreatment are all associated with substantial physical and mental health consequences.
- Current evidence does not support routine screening for family violence; however, clinicians should be familiar with common presentations of family violence and maintain a high index of suspicion.
- All states require physicians to report suspicion of child abuse. Elder mistreatment is required to be reported in most states.
- Referral to community-based organizations and enlisting the assistance of a multidisciplinary team of professionals with expertise in child abuse, intimate partner violence, or elder mistreatment are key components of management of family violence.

CHAPTER

47

Addictions

Carol E. Ripley-Moffitt, Adam O. Goldstein,
Robert E. Gwyther, and Katharine M. Patsakham

CLINICAL OBJECTIVES

1. Define addiction.
2. Identify signs of addiction and use brief screening instruments for assessing addiction.
3. Apply an algorithm to treat a patient with an addiction.
4. Describe comorbid conditions and their impact on addictions.
5. List support services to augment brief office interventions for addiction.
6. Justify the use of the chronic disease model for treating addiction.

The American Society of Addiction Medicine defines addiction to alcohol or another drug as "a disease process characterized by the continued use of a specific psychoactive substance despite physical, psychological, or social harm" (1). There are many terms that relate to substance use, some of which might be confused with addiction (Table 47.1). When a patient experiences negative consequences related to use of a substance, understands the association, and yet continues using the substance, that patient has an addiction. This chapter deals with addictions to tobacco, alcohol, and illicit and prescription drugs.

More than one quarter of US deaths are attributable to tobacco, alcohol, or drug abuse, which also cause staggering medical expenditures, borne largely by the public (2). Individuals who are addicted risk short- and long-term morbidity, job loss or instability, and isolation. Families of substance abusers experience higher rates of dysfunction and abuse in relationships. Communities are affected through intentional and unintentional injuries associated with inebriation, drug-related crime, and the early loss of elders to violence, injuries, and disease.

To treat addiction, health care providers must be able to identify the signs and symptoms of substance abuse, diagnose abuse using proactive assessments, and develop individual treatment plans. Several factors influence decisions about treatment, including the patient's willingness to undergo addiction treatment; his or her social support networks or living environment, health insurance status, and personal financial resources; programs available in the community; and the provider's skill in prescribing addiction medications. Caring for patients who have addictions involves treatment of underlying medical and psychiatric problems, as well as awareness of multiple potential drug interactions. Because addictions present challenges similar to those of chronic disease, perseverance and flexibility help facilitate positive outcomes.

Physicians see a higher percentage of people with tobacco, alcohol, and/or drug addiction than are found in the general population because these substances make people ill (Table 47.2). Patients with these disorders account for more than 15% of all outpatient visits, 25% to 40% of hospitalizations, nearly 50% of emergency department visits, and up to 80% of patients in some specialty units (e.g., burn units) (3). Approximately 70% of smokers see a physician each year (4).

With the exception of alcohol, most drugs of abuse have specific binding sites located in the limbic system (pleasure pathway) of the brain. Alcohol is active at GABA receptors and glutamate receptors in the brain and is thought to activate endogenous opioid receptors. Therefore, addiction is best thought of as a disease of the central nervous system (CNS). Addictive drugs provide users with positive reinforcement by altering the release, uptake, or metabolism of neurotransmitters such as dopamine and serotonin. Addiction does not involve higher cerebral function; the pleasure pathway is located in lower brain centers, which explains why models of addiction are available in mice and rats as well as in primates. Most people who struggle with substance abuse state that they do not want to be addicted; however, they feel unable to stop using drugs even though they know they should. There is evidence that genetic predisposition plays a role in addiction (5). Other factors include social norms, as well as tobacco and alcohol industry targeted marketing.

SCREENING AND DIAGNOSIS

Addiction often goes undiagnosed. Clinical practice guidelines recommend asking about tobacco use at every visit for every patient. One effective strategy is to include the questions, "Do you smoke or use other tobacco?" and if yes, "Do you plan to quit?" in the vital signs documentation. Clinics adopting this "vital sign" can significantly increase documentation rates for tobacco use status and provider counseling (6). The degree of tobacco dependence can be assessed with the abbreviated Fagerstrom tobacco test. The question that best predicts addiction is "How soon after you wake up do you smoke your first cigarette?" Table 47.3 presents this questionnaire and discusses its interpretation.

TABLE 47.1 Definitions of Common Terms Related to Substance Use

Term	Definition
Addiction	Chronic disease characterized by continued behavior or use of a substance, even after experiencing negative social, psychological, or physical consequences.
Misuse	Use other than as prescribed (e.g., taking the wrong dosage or at improper dosage intervals).
Abuse	Drug use that puts the user or others at risk (driving while intoxicated with alcohol; any tobacco use, no safe threshold exists); or use for a reason other than intended (e.g., taking oxycodone to get high rather than for pain); or use of an illicit drug (e.g., marijuana, heroin).
Tolerance	When the effect of a constant dose becomes diminished, or an increasing dose is required to achieve the desired result.
Dependence	When a withdrawal syndrome (psychological or physical symptoms) develops if a drug is discontinued. Most severe category of drug use disorder as defined by DSM IV.
Cross-tolerant drug	A drug which will relieve a patient's withdrawal symptoms because of similar actions to the drug on which patient is dependent (e.g., benzodiazepines are cross-tolerant with alcohol).
Withdrawal syndrome	Signs and/or symptoms resulting from abrupt removal or rapid decrease in use of a substance.
Detoxification	Process of eliminating a substance from a patient's body by slowly tapering or discontinuing intake. May require use of cross-tolerant drugs to facilitate patient comfort or safety.

TABLE 47.2 Adverse Effects of Common Recreational Drugs

Drug	Is Strongly Associated With or Directly Causes
Tobacco	Respiratory diseases including chronic obstructive pulmonary disease and pneumonia Cardiovascular diseases including coronary artery disease and stroke Cancer of the lung, head and neck, esophagus, cervix, kidney and bladder, pancreas, stomach, bone marrow, colon/rectum Reproductive effects including fetal death/stillbirth, low birth weight, pregnancy complications
Alcohol	Intoxication, leading to loss of judgment and inhibition that puts users and others at risk from dangerous behaviors (e.g., automobile crashes, drowning, suicide) Gastrointestinal diseases, especially gastritis, hepatitis, fatty infiltration of the liver, Laënnec cirrhosis, esophageal varices, and pancreatitis Hypertension and dilated cardiomyopathy Central nervous system diseases, secondary to vitamin deficiencies (e.g., Wernicke encephalopathy, Korsakoff syndrome) Oral and esophageal carcinoma (especially when used with tobacco), breast cancer Fetal alcohol syndrome, fetal alcohol effect
Cocaine	Seizures, acute psychoses Vasospasm of cerebral and coronary arteries, leading to ischemia, stroke, myocardial infarction, cardiac arrhythmias, and sudden death (especially in combination with alcohol, forming cocaethylene, which can cause necrotizing vasculitis, leading to stroke and myocardial infarction) Loss of appetite, weight loss Depression Financial deterioration Family and community violence and crime
Marijuana	Pulmonary diseases such as asthma and bronchitis Chronic underachievement Other drug use
Heroin	Overdose and respiratory depression Intravenous drug use sequelae, such as skin infections, endocarditis, hepatitis B and C, HIV, AIDS Violence and crime

TABLE 47.3 Fagerstrom Test for Nicotine Dependence

1. How soon after you wake up do you smoke your first cigarette?
   ○ After 60 minutes (0) ○ 31–60 minutes (1) ○ 6–30 minutes (2) ○ Within 5 minutes (3)
2. Do you find it difficult to refrain from smoking in places where it is forbidden?
   ○ No (0) ○ Yes (1)
3. Which cigarette would you hate to give up most?
   ○ The first in the morning (1) ○ Any other (0)
4. How many cigarettes per day do you smoke?
   ○ 10 or less (0) ○ 11–20 (1) ○ 21–30 (2) ○ 31 or more (3)
5. Do you smoke more frequently during the first hours after awakening than during the rest of the day?
   ○ No (0) ○ Yes (1)
6. Do you smoke even if you are so ill that you are in bed most of the day?
   ○ No (0) ○ Yes (1)

Total score: ______

Interpretation:

0–2	Very low dependence
3–4	Low dependence
5	Medium dependence
6–7	High dependence
8–10	Very high dependence

Recommended clinician response to the patient:

Scores under 5 "Your level of nicotine dependence is still low. You should act now before your level of dependence increases."

Score of 5 "Your level of nicotine dependence is moderate. Your level of dependence on nicotine will likely increase until you become seriously addicted. Act now to end your dependence on nicotine."

Score over 5 "Your level of dependence is high. You aren't in control of your smoking—it is in control of you! When you make the decision to quit, we can talk about nicotine replacement therapy or other medications to help you break your addiction."

Source: Heatherton TF, Kozlowski LT, Frecker RC, et al. The Fagerstrom Test for Nicotine Dependence: a revision of the Fagerstrom Tolerance Questionnaire. *Br J Addict.* 1991;86:1119–1127.

Screening, brief intervention, and referral for treatment for alcohol and drug use has become a recognized "best practice" for healthcare providers (7). Screening, brief intervention, and referral for treatment is mandated for certified trauma centers and transplant centers (8) and is being considered by the Joint Commission as a required service for inpatient facilities in the United States (9). The 2005 Clinician's Guide, *Helping Patients Who Drink Too Much,* recommends a single question about heavy drinking days: "How many times in the past year have you had 5 or more drinks in a day (for men) or 4 or more drinks in a day (for women)?" (10). Any number >0 indicates a positive screen. Two other screening tests for alcohol abuse useful to family physicians are the Cyr-Wartman and CAGE questions (Table 47.4). Screens for drug abuse include the CAGE-AID (Adapted to Include Drugs), modified from the alcohol screening. The CAGE-AID, as well as other alcohol and drug screening tests (e.g., Drug Abuse Screening Test and the Alcohol Use Disorders Identification Test) are readily available online (11).

Addiction is a clinical, rather than a laboratory diagnosis. All laboratory results for an addicted patient can be completely normal, although certain laboratory findings are suggestive of alcohol abuse, such as elevated transaminases (AST usually elevated more than ALT), macrocytic red blood cells, and thrombocytopenia. Intravenous drug abuse is associated with positive HIV, hepatitis B or hepatitis C titers. For tobacco, no safe threshold of use exists. So even if a patient is not addicted, any use is abuse.

COMORBIDITIES

Certain diagnoses and clinical situations are associated with a high incidence of substance abuse and addiction. Any patient presenting with cough, asthma, bronchitis, shortness of breath, chest pain, sinusitis, ear infection, stomach pain, pneumonia, or coronary artery disease should be assessed for use of or exposure to tobacco products. The gastrointestinal system is especially hard hit by alcohol, and patients with esophagitis, gastritis, hepatitis, and pancreatitis should be queried for excessive drinking behaviors. Trauma, especially single-car crashes and injuries sustained on the job, is highly correlated

TABLE 47.4 Screening Questions for Alcohol Abuse

Instrument	Questions	Interpretation
Single Question Screening	How many times in the past year have you had 5 or more (4 or more for women) drinks on a single drinking occasion?	Any number greater that 0 is a positive response and should prompt further questions about quantities and duration of alcohol use and any accompanying negative consequences of use.
Cyr-Wartman Alcoholism Screen*	1. When was your last drink of alcohol? (Positive = yesterday or today) 2. Have you ever had a problem with alcohol? (Positive = "yes")	A positive response to either question is a positive screen and should prompt further questions about quantities and duration of alcohol use and any accompanying negative consequences of use.
CAGE Alcoholism Screen†	1. Have you ever tried to *cut down* your use of alcohol? 2. Have you ever been *annoyed* by others criticizing your drinking? 3. Have you ever felt *guilty* because of your use of alcohol? 4. Have you ever needed an *"eye opener"* in the morning to settle your nerves?	A "yes" answer to two or more of these questions is a positive response and should prompt further questions about quantities and duration of alcohol use and any accompanying negative consequences of use.

*Adapted from Cyr MG, Wartman SA. The effectiveness of routine screening questions in the detection of alcoholism. *JAMA*. 1988;259:51–54. (Screen has a sensitivity of 91.5% and specificity of 89.7%)

†Adapted from Ewing JA. Detecting alcoholism. *JAMA*. 1984;252(14):1905–1907. Also see: Brown RL. Identification and office management of alcohol and drug disorders. In: Fleming MF, Barry KL, ed. *Addictive Disorders*. St. Louis, MO: Mosby-Year Book; 1992 (Screen has sensitivity of 85%–94% and specificity of 79%–88%)

with alcohol and other drugs of abuse. Physical violence, especially domestic violence and child abuse, is frequently linked to substance abuse, as are family disruption, marital discord, deteriorating financial status, and loss of employment. Patients with mental health issues, alcohol abuse, or drug abuse are more likely to smoke, with prevalence rates two to four times those of the general population (12).

LABORATORY TESTING

Testing for nicotine, though not routine, may be needed for certain insurance or employment records. A byproduct of nicotine, cotinine, can be measured in urine, serum, or saliva. Carbon monoxide monitors record the percentage of carbon monoxide in the breath, and will estimate corresponding levels in the hemoglobin as a result of recent smoking. Levels of alcohol can be measured in the blood and the breath; use may be documented by testing saliva or urine. Drug use may be documented by testing samples from urine, serum, or hair. Alcohol and drug screening can also be useful to confirm that a patient has taken a drug (e.g., cocaine use in a young stroke victim), or aid in the management of a disease process (e.g., blood alcohol level in a comatose patient). Patients who undergo a drug screen ordered by a physician are at no risk for criminal prosecution if positive for an illegal drug unless a chain of custody is initiated at the time an observed sample is taken and maintained until results are presented at trial (13). However, drug screen test results do become available when a court subpoenas medical records or when a patient signs routine insurance company release of medical information forms. In this manner, patients may experience negative consequences of drug testing, such as denial of health or life insurance or custody of dependent children. Physicians must be aware of these potential consequences when ordering drug testing and when sending results out of the office or hospital.

TREATMENT

Although physician advice to discontinue drug use will not cause most patients to become immediately abstinent, it can provide a starting point for entering the process of recovery. Providers who seek to understand a patient's desire to reduce or stop using, help increase motivation for change, and offer continuing support will greatly improve that patient's chances for successful abstinence.

Managing Tobacco Addiction or Dependence

Tobacco use treatment is one of the most cost-effective interventions available to a clinician. Most current tobacco users want to quit, and every user has the potential to do so successfully. The well-researched 2008 Clinical Practice Guideline for Treating Tobacco Use and Dependence recommends treatment options that are summarized in Table 47.5 (14). Clinicians are encouraged to use the "5 A's" as a guide (Figure 47.1):

1. **Ask** if patient uses tobacco. Treat tobacco use status as a vital sign and document at every visit.
2. **Advise** all patients who use tobacco to quit. Tailor messages to the current health concerns of patients when

TABLE 47.5 Therapeutic Options Available for the Treatment of Tobacco Use

Treatment Strategy	6–12 Month Abstinence Rates (%)	Estimated Odds Ratio	Strength of Recommendation*	Comment(s)
None (placebo)	3.1–13.8			Spontaneous quit rates vary depending on whether participants are enrolled in a clinical trial.
Counseling				
Physician advice to quit	10	1.3	A	Compared with no advice to quit.
Minimal counseling (<3 minutes)	13	1.3	A	Compared with no contact.
Low-intensity counseling (3–10 minutes)	16	1.6	A	
High-intensity counseling (>10 minutes)	22	2.3	A	
Quitline counseling	12.7	1.6	A	Compared with minimal or no counseling or self-help.
Medication				
Monotherapies				
Varenicline (2 mg/day)	33	3.1	A	Compared with placebo. Pharmacologic therapies assume clinician counseling in addition to drugs.
Nicotine nasal spray	27	2.3	A	
Nicotine inhaler	25	2.1	A	
Bupropion SR (Zyban)	24	2.0	A	
Clonidine	25	2.1	A	
Nicotine patch (6–14 weeks)	23	1.9	A	
Nortriptyline	23	1.8	A	
Nicotine gum	19	1.5	A	
Combination Therapies				
Patch (>14 weeks) + *ad libitum* NRT (gum or spray)	37	3.6	A	Compared to placebo. Pharmacologic therapies assume clinician counseling in addition to drugs.
Patch + bupropion SR	29	2.5	A	
Patch + inhaler	26	2.2	A	

*A = consistent, good-quality patient-oriented evidence; B = inconsistent or limited-quality patient-oriented evidence; C = consensus, disease-oriented evidence, usual practice, expert opinion, or case series.
For information about the Strength of Recommendation Taxonomy evidence rating system, see *www.aafp.org/afpsort.xml*.

possible. Physician advice to quit significantly increases quit rates, and interventions as brief as 3 minutes can be effective.

3. **Assess** patient's willingness to quit. Patients who express readiness to quit within the next 30 days should be offered treatments suggested in the next two steps. For patients who currently do not want to quit, use brief motivational techniques that will help patients identify ways in which continued smoking may be inconsistent with their values. Emphasize the "**5 Rs**"—**R**elevance, **R**isks, **R**ewards, **R**oadblocks, and **R**epetition (Fig. 47.1).
4. **Assist** patients in quitting. Counseling plus pharmacotherapy offers the best chance for success. *Counseling* may include educating patients about tobacco use, helping them identify reasons for quitting, brainstorming strategies for becoming tobacco-free and coping with triggers, and providing encouragement. Helpful strategies include: setting a quit date within the next 2 weeks; listing 10 to 20 activities that can serve as alternatives to tobacco use; making homes and vehicles tobacco-free; changing a routine (e.g., morning coffee and cigarette); and asking family and friends for support.

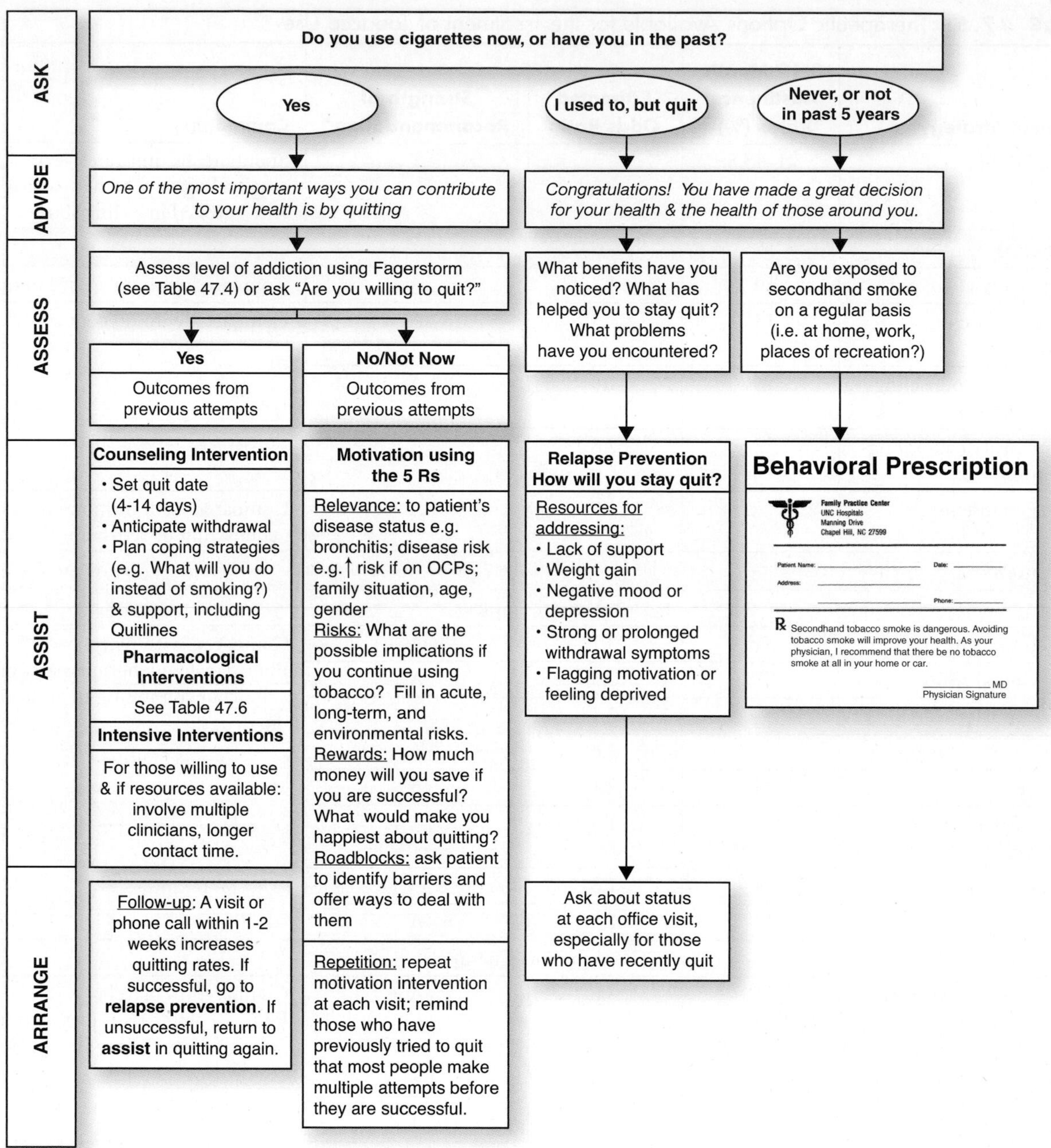

Figure 47.1 • Managing tobacco addiction or dependence. Brief Clinical Interventions for Smokers Using the 5As (Ask → Advise → Assess → Assist → Arrange) Framework.

Pharmacotherapy options include seven Food and Drug Administration–approved agents to assist patients who are trying to quit (Table 47.6). Through different mechanisms these medications act to decrease desire for tobacco, or to assist in the management of withdrawal symptoms, which include depressed mood, insomnia, irritability, frustration, or anger, anxiety, difficulty concentrating, restlessness, decreased heart rate, increased appetite or weight gain. In addition to becoming familiar with these products, consider the following in deciding the appropriate course of medication:

- Previous experience with smoking cessation medications: Rule out those that have not worked or caused adverse side effects. Check for appropriate use (e.g., patient may have continually chewed gum, instead of parking, or underdosed nicotine replacement therapy [NRT]), so patch plus gum may be recommended.
- Current medical conditions and medications (Table 47.6): Each medication has contraindications (i.e., chronic nasal disorders rule out use of NRT nasal spray); monoamine oxidase inhibitor therapy precludes use of bupropion; bupropion may be indicated for comorbid depression.
- Recommend medication with greatest potential for successful treatment (Table 47.5).
- Patient preference, if more than one course of pharmacotherapy is indicated: some patients will want to be free of

TABLE 47.6 First-line, FDA-approved Pharmacotherapy for Smoking Cessation

Drug	Cautions, Contraindications, Adverse Effects	Dosage	Relative Cost*
Varenicline	*Black box warning:* Advise patients to stop varenicline and contact medical provider immediately if any of following are experienced: agitation, hostility, depressed mood, atypical behavior or thinking, suicidal ideation, allergic or skin reactions. *Contraindications:* history of psychiatric illness, suicidal ideation/attempt Caution in Cl_{Cr} <30 mL/min or dialysis *Adverse effects:* nausea, sleep disturbance, vivid dreams, headache, impaired ability to drive or operate heavy machinery	Days 1–3: 0.5 mg once daily Days 4–7: 0.5 mg twice daily Day 8 to end of treatment: 1.0 mg twice daily	$$
Bupropion SR	*Black box warning:* Advise patients to stop bupropion and contact medical provider immediately if any of following are experienced: agitation, hostility, depressed mood, atypical behavior or thinking, suicidal ideation, allergic or skin reactions. *Contraindications:* history of seizure, eating disorder, use of monoamine oxidase inhibitor within 14 days; severe hepatic cirrhosis; excessive ETOH or abrupt discontinuation of ETOH or sedatives. *Adverse effects:* Insomnia, dry mouth	150 mg qAM × 3 days, then 150 mg BID Begin treatment 1–2 weeks prequit 7–12 weeks; maintenance up to 6 months May combine with NRT	$$
Nicotine gum	*Contraindications:* (***applies to all NRT***): within 2 weeks post-MI, serious arrhythmias, unstable angina pectoris *Adverse effects:* Mouth soreness, dyspepsia	**1–24 cpd**—2 mg gum (up to 24 pieces/day) **25+ cpd**—4 mg gum (up to 24 pieces/day) Up to 12 weeks	$$
Nicotine inhaler	*Adverse effects:* Local irritation of mouth and throat	6–16 cartridges/day Up to 6 months	$$
Nicotine lozenge	*Adverse effects:* nausea, hiccups, heartburn, headache, coughing	Smokes first cigarette >30 minutes after waking: 2 mg Smokes first cigarette within 30 minutes of waking: 4 mg	$$
Nicotine nasal spray	*Additional contraindication:* Severe reactive airway disease *Adverse effects:* Nasal irritation	8–40 doses/day 3–6 months	$$
Nicotine patch	*Adverse effects:* Local skin reaction, insomnia	**>10 cpd:** 21 mg/24 hours × 4–6 weeks, then 14 mg/24 hours × 2 weeks, then 7 mg/24 hr × 2 weeks. **≤10 cpd:** 14 mg/24 hours × 6 weeks, 7 mg/24 hours × 2 weeks	$$

FDA = Food and Drug Administration.
*The cost per day varies depending amount used. Average range for all of these methods is around $2.50 to $10 per day (spring 2010).

nicotine; others will not want to "use drugs," so work to find option with highest efficacy and greatest likelihood of adherence.

- Resources for obtaining medication: Medicaid currently (2010) covers all smoking cessation medications. Private insurance and Medicare Part D insurers vary in coverage. Patients with these plans or with no insurance may have difficulty purchasing recommended medications.
- Adjustment of current medications or drug use: stopping smoking and/or nicotine can affect the metabolism of other drugs (e.g., many psychotics, caffeine). Use of medications will need to be adjusted by original prescriber.

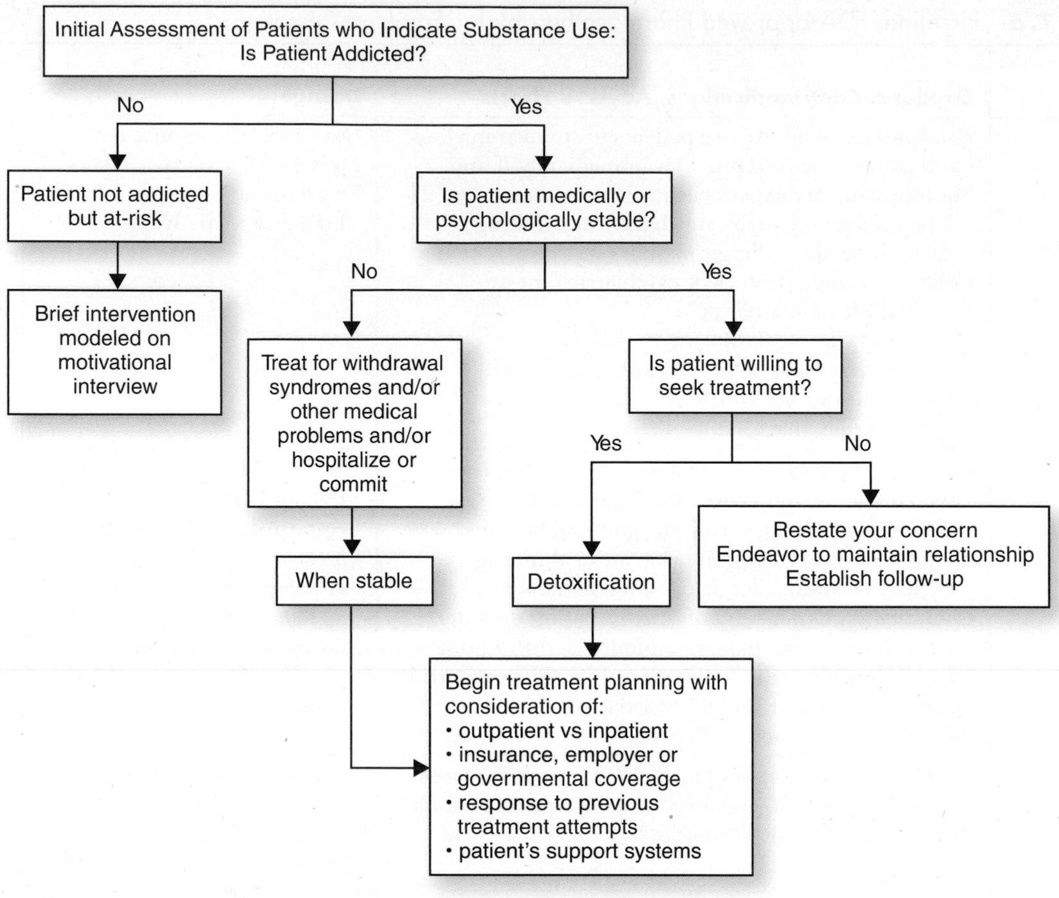

Figure 47.2 • Alcohol and other drug addiction screening algorithm.

Note that the effectiveness of smoking cessation medications has not been proven for pregnant women, smokeless tobacco users, light smokers, and adolescents.

5. **Arrange** follow-up. Contact patients on or around their quit date to offer encouragement and, if necessary, make adjustments to the quit plan. Give patients information about telephone quit lines, and if available in your state, fax a referral to initiate a proactive call to your patient. Quitlines increase success, provide additional support, and are available in every state (1-800-QUIT-NOW).

In addition to treating current tobacco users, physicians should offer support to recent quitters by congratulating them on their success and providing assistance to cope with the challenges they may face in remaining abstinent. Remember that more intensive interventions (frequency, duration, and number of clinicians involved) are associated with higher abstinence rates. If offering the 5As is not feasible, physicians should at a minimum follow the first two (Ask and Advise) with referral to community resources (classes or specialty clinics) or the Quitline.

Finally, it is critical to establish an office system that facilitates tobacco cessation for patients and staff that includes:

- A clear statement of the clinic's tobacco policy, to include establishment of tobacco-free clinic building and grounds; refusal to display magazines in the waiting room that carry tobacco advertisements; and, prominent display of pro–health, tobacco-free messages.
- Consistent documentation of tobacco use, such as a tobacco-use vital sign.
- Ongoing access to training and resources for clinicians in tobacco use and dependence.
- A plan for tracking outcomes and quality improvement.
- A designated staff person responsible for coordinating tobacco use and dependence treatment, including implementation and monitoring of these suggested system components.

Managing Alcohol and Other Drug Addiction

Managing alcohol or drug addiction depends on the severity of the addiction and of any concomitant medical or psychiatric problems. Prophylaxis and treatment of withdrawal syndromes may be indicated. An algorithm for decision making is presented in Figure 47.2.

ASSURING MEDICAL AND PSYCHOLOGICAL STABILITY

Initial management of alcohol and drug addiction depends on the medical acuity of the patient. The comatose heroin-addicted patient requires intubation and/or treatment with naloxone for a presumed overdose. An alcoholic known to have esophageal varices, who is in shock after a bloody emesis, should initially receive volume expanders, followed by blood transfusion. Patients in an acute care setting who might be chronic alcohol abusers should routinely be given 100 mg of thiamine to prevent Wernicke syndrome. Consider intramuscular or intravenous magnesium sulfate to prevent complications of alcohol withdrawal.

A patient's psychiatric status must also be evaluated. In all cases, but particularly in acute care settings, patients must be screened for potential to harm themselves or others before finalizing treatment plans. Patients who present a danger to themselves or others must be committed to protective custody. People admitted to hospitals for addiction treatment may need suicide precautions or physical restraints. In no case should an intoxicated patient be discharged to drive home alone.

BRIEF INTERVENTIONS FOR AT-RISK PATIENTS

Many patients see a physician when they begin using alcohol or addictive drugs, before serious medical or psychiatric sequelae have occurred. Sometimes patients are using risky quantities of alcohol (i.e., >14 drinks/week for men; >7 drinks/week for women) (15) and are unaware that these levels are associated with negative outcomes. Several brief intervention strategies tested with at-risk drinkers can reduce alcohol consumption to moderate levels (16). Even if the brief intervention is unsuccessful, it can provide motivation for more intensive interventions. Essential elements of the brief intervention are as follows:

- Inform the patient of your concern about his or her substance use. Using the historical and laboratory data at hand, attempt to link drug or alcohol use to negative physical, psychological, or social consequences. Avoid parental or accusatory phrasing.
- Encourage the patient to state his or her point of view.
- Assess the patient's readiness to change alcohol or drug use, and employ techniques (e.g., motivational interviewing) to encourage the patient to reduce or stop using.
- If the patient is willing, attempt to initiate planning toward reduction or discontinuation of alcohol or ceasing drug use. For moderate problems, this might include a visit to an open meeting of Alcoholics Anonymous (AA)/Narcotics Anonymous (NA).
- If the patient denies that a problem exists but is willing to consider exploration, attempt to negotiate a commitment for cutting down or eliminating use. Suggest keeping a drug-use diary, noting urges to use, situations in which urges occur, responses, and both positive and negative consequences of use. Schedule a return appointment, and attempt to include a spouse or significant other who can corroborate the diary and help you better understand the patient's problem.
- If the patient is unwilling to explore the problem, attempt to maintain a therapeutic relationship by expressing your concern for his or her well-being; convey your willingness to discuss the matter at a future date.
- Treat drug and alcohol use as a "chronic problem," such as hypertension or diabetes. Inquire about use at follow-up visit. Reinforce successes and be willing to change strategy if initial plans fail or if the problem should become more pronounced. Check for negative consequences of use.

WITHDRAWAL SYNDROMES AND DETOXIFICATION

Substance abusers must be evaluated for signs of withdrawal, usually seen in patients who are dependent on opiates or sedative-hypnotic drugs including alcohol (Table 47.7). All withdrawal syndromes are uncomfortable; sedative-hypnotic withdrawal is medically more dangerous. To treat a withdrawal syndrome, you should give a cross-tolerant drug in doses sufficient to alleviate the signs and symptoms of withdrawal (Table 47.8). Initial loading doses may be needed to increase patient comfort and, in the case of alcohol and sedative-hypnotic drugs, to prevent seizures and progression to delirium tremens, a potentially fatal complication.

Patients withdrawing from opiates may experience mydriasis, piloerection ("goose flesh"), abdominal cramps, myoclonic jerks, and rhinorrhea. Patients dependent on opiates are usually stabilized in the hospital with a sufficient daily dose of methadone to replace the amount of opiates that they were using before admission. Typically, patients addicted to opiates are maintained on this dose during the admission and subsequently discharged to methadone treatment programs or to physicians qualified to prescribe buprenorphine.

Patients withdrawing from alcohol (or any sedative-hypnotic drug) may experience tremor, tachycardia, nausea, diaphoresis, and fever. Decisions about when to use drug prophylaxis are based on the patient's blood alcohol level, previous withdrawal experiences, and clinical assessment of signs and symptoms. Assess the severity of the withdrawal syndrome by using a scale such as the revised Clinical Institute Withdrawal Assessment for Alcohol (CIWA-Ar) scale (17). The CIWA-Ar score can be used to decide whether the patient should be hospitalized and whether medications are required for safe detoxification (18). Loading doses of (preferably long-acting) cross-tolerant medication are used when CIWA-Ar scores exceed 25.

Detoxification is completed by tapering patients off cross-tolerant drugs over a time period that depends on the half-life of the drug of abuse. In the case of alcohol, detoxification is generally accomplished in <1 week; benzodiazepine detoxification can take months, however. After patients have withdrawn from the substance, and their cognitive ability has been restored, the underlying addiction must be addressed.

OUTPATIENT VERSUS INPATIENT INTERVENTIONS

Addictions can be treated on either an outpatient or inpatient basis. Inpatient treatment is more expensive and has similar outcomes. When being referred for any addiction treatment, patients are much more likely to show up for evaluation and treatment if the referring physician is actively involved in the process. Referrals most reliably occur when the physician contacts the treatment resource initially and, with the patient present, introduces the patient to the consultant by telephone or in person.

In recommending an alcohol or drug addiction treatment program for a patient, the following factors must be considered:

- If significant medical or psychiatric complications exist, addicted patients are best treated in programs prepared to handle both.
- Patients with previous addiction treatment may benefit from a change of venue or program philosophy.
- Patient financial resources often dictate what programs are available.
- For patients who are fortunate enough to have supportive families, programs that include a strong family treatment component increase the chance of successful treatment.

TABLE 47.7 Withdrawal Symptoms

Drug	Withdrawal Symptoms and Staging of Severity	
Alcohol and sedative/ hypnotic agents	Stage	Symptoms
	1 (minor)	Restlessness, anxiety, sleeping problems, agitation, tremor, tachycardia, low-grade fever, diaphoresis, elevated blood pressure
	2 (major)	Signs of stage 1 plus visual or auditory hallucinations, whole-body tremor, pulse exceeding 100 beats per minute, diastolic pressure exceeding 100 mm Hg, pronounced diaphoresis, vomiting
	3 (medical emergency: mortality 2%–5%)	Delirium tremens, temperature exceeding 37.8°C (100°F), disorientation to time, place and person, global confusion, inability to recognize familiar objects or people
	Notes: • Extreme care is required, as abrupt withdrawal can be life threatening. • Seizures from alcohol may occur 12–48 hours after last drink; seizures from barbiturates usually within 72 hours after last use. • Withdrawal from benzodiazepines may take a week or more to manifest.	
Stimulants (i.e., cocaine or methamphetamine)	Depression, hypersomnia, fatigue, headache, irritability, poor concentration, restlessness, suicide attempts in severe cases; drug craving is prolonged and intense; paranoia and acute psychosis	
Opiates	Grade	Symptoms
	0	Drug craving, anxiety, intense drug-seeking behavior
	1	Yawning, sweating, lacrimation, rhinorrhea
	2	Mydriasis, gooseflesh, muscle twitching, anorexia
	3	Insomnia; increased pulse, respiratory rate, and blood pressure; abdominal cramps, vomiting, diarrhea, weakness

- People living in drug-infested environments have better long-term outcomes if relocated to a drug-free location during treatment and after discharge.

Most treatment begins with detoxification. Outpatient detoxification requires the patient to make a commitment to the treatment program and abstain from using any substance other than physician-prescribed medications. The patient also must engage a responsible family member or friend who will: (a) discard any alcohol or drugs in the patient's home, (b) support the patient's participation in the treatment program; (c) monitor for symptoms of serious withdrawal; (d) assist with any medications; and, (e) ensure that the patient keeps appointments. The physician must have the ability to monitor the patient on a daily basis, especially on weekends, until risks are minimal (about 6 days for alcohol; about 10 days for methamphetamines, opiates, cocaine). When prescribing adjunctive pharmacotherapy, no more than a 2 to 3 day supply should be dispensed at a time.

Inpatient detoxification is required if the criteria for outpatient treatment cannot be met, if the patient is experiencing moderate to severe withdrawal from sedative drugs (alcohol, barbiturates, benzodiazepines), which can be life-threatening, or if the patient has a history of any of the following: (a) high tolerance for the substance; (b) seizures, delirium, or psychosis on previous withdrawal attempts; (c) recent head trauma; or (d) recent or current stroke, acute abdominal pain, jaundice, liver failure, electrolyte imbalance, pneumonia, sepsis, dehydration, AIDS, arrhythmias, angina, ischemic heart disease, severe hypertension, or severe respiratory disease. Inpatient detoxification is also recommended for patients older than 65 years of age.

Inpatient treatment is also required for patients with opiate addictions who want to try an abstinence goal, because federal law forbids prescribing opiate medication to addicts in an outpatient setting. Alternatively, referral can be made to a methadone program or to a physician qualified to prescribe buprenorphine for initial opiate substitution, which subsequently may be slowly tapered to achieve abstinence. For other addictions, outpatient interventions, combining detoxification with treatment, can be effective.

Inpatient detoxification allows patients to be monitored while they go through the withdrawal process, and treatment can be tailored to the individual. After detoxification, inpatient or outpatient addiction treatment programs further address the patient's understanding of consequences and risks of continued substance use, emotional issues (e.g., hopelessness and despair over addiction, grief and remorse over past behavior), barriers to recovery, and involvement with recovery groups.

ADDICTION TREATMENT MODALITIES

A summary of treatment programs, with rates of abstinence are summarized in Table 47.9.

TABLE 47.8 Regimens for Detoxification from Alcohol and Opiates

Drug	Suggested Regimen
Alcohol	Order for all patients: • Thiamine: 100 mg IM on admission • Phenergan: 50 mg IM q6h PRN nausea • Magnesium sulfate: 1 g IM q8h × 3 doses Provide one of these drug detox regimens: Diazepam regimen Loading dose: 10–20 mg/hr (slow) IV or PO (until symptoms abate) Supplement: 10 mg PO (for agitation, tachycardia, etc.) 24-hour maximum: 60 mg Subsequent taper: 0–10 mg qid (symptom dependent) Decrease by 10 mg/day Lorazepam regimen Loading dose: 2–4 mg/hr (slow) IV, IM or PO (until symptoms abate) Supplement: 2 mg PO tid (for agitation, tachycardia, etc.) 24-hour maximum: 12 mg Subsequent taper: 0–2 mg qid (symptom dependent) Decrease by 2 mg/day
Opiates	1. Methadone: • First day: 10 mg PO q2–4h, in first 24 hours (titrate to relief of symptoms); up to 80 mg total • Subsequent days: total dose PO from day 1 every morning • May taper methadone by 10% per day, starting on fourth day 2. Phenergan: 25–50 mg IM q6h, PRN nausea 3. May discharge to methadone maintenance program on methadone, 30 mg PO qd, or lower dose if tapered lower

Adapted in part from: Devenyi P, Saunders S. *Physicians Handbook for Medical Management of Alcohol- and Drug-Related Problems*. Toronto, Canada: Addiction Research Foundation and the Ontario Medical Association; 1986.

Self help Groups

There are a variety of self-help organizations in the United States that attempt to help patients who suffer from alcohol and drug problems. AA views alcoholism as a disease over which the sufferer (an alcoholic) has no control. Any alcohol use is said to lead to uncontrolled use, which in turn leads to further deterioration of the user's life. The group believes that there are 12 steps to recovery, which if followed, provide a plan of action that can help the alcoholic stay sober. Members believe that lifelong attendance at AA meetings is necessary to stay sober. AA is the largest and most widely available self-help movement in the world. Using similar precepts to AA, a number of other 12-step programs have grown as spin-offs of the organization (e.g., NA). Other self-help groups include Smart Recovery, Women for Sobriety, Rational Recovery, and Secular Organization for Sobriety. In addition, religious organizations often offer local support to help congregation members achieve and maintain sobriety.

Minnesota Model

The Minnesota Model, which is one of the most common inpatient addiction treatment techniques in the United States, begins with detoxified inpatients being enrolled in a 28-day program. Treatment consists of large group activities in which patients are educated about the effects of alcohol or drugs and given the explanation for addiction as conceived by AA or NA; indoctrination of the AA/NA philosophy is part of the treatment. Each patient is assigned an individual addiction counselor, frequently a recovering alcoholic/addict, and with the counselor's guidance, systematically works through the first five steps of the AA/NA program. Patients attend daily meetings, initially in the hospital and later in the community. After discharge, AA/NA meetings are used as support groups.

Variations on the Minnesota Model exist throughout the United States. Intensive outpatient treatment programs eliminate the "hotel costs" and staff expenses of inpatient programs. The outpatient programs allow patients to work during the day, and keep them away from high-risk environments in the evenings. These programs typically run four evenings per week for several months and use urine screens to uncover concurrent drug use.

Cognitive Behavioral Techniques

Cognitive behavioral therapy uses strategies to enable patients' higher cognitive function to overcome their addictions. Patients are asked to think about their drug use, weigh the pros and cons of using, and change their behavior. Patients set individual drug use goals (usually abstinence) and explore ways in which they can reduce or eliminate drug use. As part of the therapy, patients are taught relapse prevention techniques, such as realigning social networks, adjusting daily living, and learning to drink soft drinks while others drink alcohol. They

TABLE 47.9 Therapeutic Options Available for the Treatment of Alcohol and other Drugs

	Treatment Strategy	6–12 Month Abstinence Rates (%)	Strength of Recommendation*	Comment(s)
Alcohol	Alcoholics Anonymous	50–79	C	Anonymity makes research difficult.
	Minnesota model	38–59	B	Wide variation in severity of illness, demographics, and available services to clientele.
	Cognitive-behavioral therapy	20–79	B	Many techniques have been studied; reduction in use, rather than abstinence, is often the outcome measured.
	Aversion therapy	40–60	C	
	Disulfiram (Antabuse)	18–23	C	
	Naltrexone	54–60 use reduction	A	Outcome measures are usually reduction in use, rather than abstinence.
	Acamprosate (Campral)	18	A	Increases proportion of dependent drinkers who maintain abstinence.
Heroin	Methadone maintenance	50–70 use reduction	A	Abstinence is not usually measured. Improved outcomes: reduced incarceration, HIV conversion, cost; increased employment stability.
	Buprenorphine	50–70 use reduction	A	Decreased illicit drug use.
	Narcotics anonymous	23–46	C	Anonymity makes research difficult.
	Naltrexone	6–12 overall; ≥93 among health care professionals	C	High rate of success found only among health care professionals whose licenses were at risk; otherwise, Naltrexone treatment usually found equal to or slightly better than placebo in the United States.

*A = consistent, good-quality patient-oriented evidence; B = inconsistent or limited-quality patient-oriented evidence; C = consensus, disease-oriented evidence, usual practice, expert opinion, or case series.
For information about the Strength of Recommendation Taxonomy evidence rating system, see *www.aafp.org/afpsort.xml*.

may even practice their prevention skills by going to bars or restaurants without drinking alcohol.

PHARMACOTHERAPY

Drugs available to treat alcohol and drug addiction use several different strategies, including substitution, adverse reaction, and blocking effects. Selecting a pharmacotherapy depends on the patient's drug addiction (Table 47.10). Pharmacotherapy options include the following:

- Methadone is the classic example of a *substitution pharmacotherapy*. An opiate antagonist that causes relatively little euphoria, methadone is given to patients who are addicted to other opiates (e.g., heroin, oxycodone). Methadone programs often have waiting lists, and because daily visits are required, many patients must frequently drive long distances for treatment.
- Buprenorphine, a partial agonist at opioid receptors, can be prescribed in primary care offices by physicians who have received special accreditation. Physicians must be able to provide or refer to counseling, when indicated, and are limited to 100 patients (19,20). A combination of buprenorphine with the opioid antagonist naloxone (Suboxone) is most commonly prescribed.
- Disulfiram (Antabuse) is an example of *adverse reaction pharmacotherapy*. If taken in adequate dosage (125 to 500 mg/day) within 24 hours, disulfiram causes patients to experience flushing, tachycardia, and nausea if they drink alcohol. It is used with some success by patients who take disulfiram before they have an impulse to drink later in the day. However, because alcohol-addicted patients can simply avoid taking the drug if they decide to drink, it has fallen out of favor with prescribers.
- A number of drugs are competitive antagonists for binding sites (i.e., blocking agents). They bind to drug receptors in the brain, displacing the drug of abuse or blocking its effects, but providing no stimulation of the receptor. Pharmacotherapies using blocking drugs have two mechanisms of action in treating addicted patients. The first mechanism is to immediately reverse the respiratory depressant effects of an overdose in an emergency situation (i.e., naloxone). The second is to treat

Ship To:

Anna Mortzfeldt
1412 Zimmerman Rd
Carlisle, PA 170159248 USA

Ship From:

TXTBOOKSNOW.COM-HALF
8950 W PALMER ST
RIVER GROVE, IL 60171

Return Information (cut and attach to the outside of return shipment)

TXTBOOKSNOW.COM-HALF
8950 W PALMER ST
RIVER GROVE, IL 60171

(Attn: Returns)

Order #: 343499965137-88405139101

DI61363

Date: 07/01/2013

Order #: 343499965137-88405139101

SKU	Qty	Condition	Title	Price	Total
5462834U	1	Used	Essen of Family Medicine (w/Bind-in A 6 9781608316557 Refund Eligible Through= 8/2/2013	$ 19.81	$ 19.81

Sub Total	$	19.81
Shipping & Handling	$	3.49
Sales Tax	$	0.00
Order Total	**$**	**23.30**

Order #: 343499965137-88405139101

Refund Policy: All items must be returned within 30 days of receipt. Pack your book securely, so it will arrive back to us in its original condition. To avoid delays, please use the return section and label provided with your original packing slip to identify your return. Be sure to include a return reason. For your protection, we suggest using a traceable, insured shipping service (UPS or Insured Parcel Post). We are not responsible for lost or damaged returns. Item(s) returned must be received in the original condition as sold and including all additional materials such as CDs, workbooks, etc. We will initiate a refund of your purchase price including applicable taxes within 5 business days of receipt. Shipping charges will not be refunded unless we have committed an error with your order. If there is an error with your order or the item is not received in the condition as purchased, please contact us immediately for return assistance.

Reason for Refund/Return:
Condition Incorrect Item Received Incorrect Item Ordered Dropped Class Purchased Elsewhere Other

Contact Us: For customer service, email us at customerservice@textbooksNow.com.

Page 1 of 1

We are in the process of relocating to our new Aurora Illinois Distribution Facility. You may receive orders shipped from one or both River Grove and Aurora locations until our move is complete. Some orders may be split with a portion fulfilled from our two locations - generating two shipments, each having its own packing slip, but consolidated into a single invoice or charge to your account, whichever is applicable.

TABLE 47.10 Pharmacological Interventions to Assist in Medical Management of Drug Addiction Problems

Drug of Addiction	Contraindications/Cautions/Adverse Effects	Dosage	Relative Cost*
For Opiate Addiction			
Methadone	Respiratory depression, COPD, hypercarbia, sleep apnea, prolonged QT interval, cardiac conduction defect, acute head injury or abdominal pain, constipation	10–120 mg/day; lower dose for hepatic impairment	$
Buprenorphine + naloxone (Suboxone) [or less commonly, buprenorphine (Subutex)]	CNS sedation, respiratory depression; headache, pain, insomnia, anxiety, nausea, vomiting, constipation; infection	For dependence, start 2–8 mg of buprenorphine SL qd and titrate up per protocol Maintenance 4–24 mg of buprenorphine SL qd; lower dose for hepatic impairment	$$
Clonidine (Catapres) (when the above are unavailable)	Hypotension, syncope on first dose; dizziness; rebound hypertension; sedation, dry mouth, constipation	0.1–1.2 mg/day in divided dose	$
Naltrexone	Precipitates opioid withdrawal; sedation, insomnia; nausea, vomiting; headache, arthralgias; do not give with hepatitis or liver failure	25–50 mg daily	$$
For Alcohol Addiction			
Disulfiram (Antabuse)	Respiratory depression, CV collapse, arrhythmias, MI, CHF, seizures, coma, psychosis	250 mg daily (range 125–500 mg)	$
Naltrexone (ReVia)	Precipitates opioid withdrawal; sedation, insomnia; nausea, vomiting; headache, arthralgias; don't give with hepatitis or liver failure	25–50 mg daily	$$
Acamprosate (Campral)	Severe renal impairment; depression or suicidality, anxiety, diarrhea, depression Rare: acute kidney failure, heart failure, mesenteric arterial occlusion, cardiomyopathy, deep thrombophlebitis, shock	666 mg (two 333-mg tablets) three times daily or, for patients with moderate renal impairment (CrCl 30–50 mL/min), reduce to 333 mg (one tablet) three times daily	$$

COPD = chronic obstructive pulmonary disease; CNS = central nervous system; CV = cardiovascular; MI = myocardial infarction; CHF = congestive heart failure.
*The cost per day varies depending on how much each is used. In general, $ = $2 or less per day; $$ = $3–10 per day.

patients who agree to take the blocking agents regularly, thereby eliminating the potential for pleasurable effects of the drugs to which they are addicted (e.g., naltrexone). Patients who have much to lose if they relapse are good candidates for blocking pharmacotherapy. Naltrexone, an opiate antagonist, has been used successfully to treat addicted professionals, such as physicians and lawyers. Patients take 25 to 50 mg/day and are subjected to random urine testing. Relapse leads to the loss of their license to practice, a strong deterrent, and some success rates have been documented in excess of 93% (21).

- Naltrexone has also been approved to treat patients with alcohol addiction. It helps reduce alcohol consumption and is associated with more rapid reestablishment of sobriety after relapse, especially when combined with behavioral treatment.
- Beginning in 2004, the US Food and Drug Administration approved acamprosate to treat alcohol dependence. Its mechanism of action is unknown. It does interact at both glutamate and GABA receptors, perhaps stabilizing their neurotransmitters. It is thought to reduce symptoms of long-term abstinence (e.g., insomnia, anxiety, restlessness). Patients should be fully withdrawn from alcohol before starting acamprosate, though it may be continued if patients subsequently relapse (10).

The antiseizure drug topiramate (Topamax) and the muscle relaxant baclofen have shown some reduction in total amounts of alcohol consumed (22,23). Neither has been approved by the Food and Drug Administration for use with alcohol dependent patients.

For patients addicted to prescription drugs, treatment depends on the type of drug being abused. Painkillers, stimulants, and CNS depressants are the most commonly abused medications. Treatments for addiction to these medications are similar to those for illicit drugs (e.g., addiction to opioid pain medications can be treated with buprenorphine). For addiction to stimulants or CNS depressants, there is no current pharmacotherapy, though behavioral therapies can be effective (20).

LONG-TERM MONITORING

Treating Tobacco, Alcohol, and Drug Abuse or Addiction as a Chronic Disease

Addiction is more typical of a chronic problem than an acute one (20,24). Patients usually need to be abstinent from using the drugs to which they are addicted. They must be monitored for diseases that accompany their drug use, such as cirrhosis, HIV, chronic obstructive pulmonary disease, or cancer. They may take medications to help them remain abstinent, such as nicotine replacement, methadone, buprenorphine, or disulfiram. They often relapse and need to undergo further treatment or have their medications adjusted. These features are far more like the chronic diseases of hypertension, diabetes, or asthma, whose sufferers must have side effects monitored, drug doses monitored and/or changed, negative consequences treated, and encouragement given for maintaining a healthy lifestyle.

Changes in Treatment of Other Health Problems

Physicians must also learn to alter their usual regimens when treating addicted individuals for other health problems. For instance, patients addicted to alcohol must avoid elixirs containing alcohol, often found in cold and cough remedies. Medications used to treat sleep problems (e.g., benzodiazepines or barbiturates), should not be prescribed, as they act much like alcohol in the brain and are associated with relapse. Patients addicted to heroin or oxycodone should not be given medications such as Lomotil and other opioid-based antidiarrheal medications. Opioid-addicted individuals who are admitted to a hospital with severe pain, such as a fractured femur, may be treated with intrathecal medications or nonopioid analgesics. If they must be treated with opioid drugs, they should be offered detoxification before discharge.

After a patient has been diagnosed with an addiction problem, future treatment should differ from that of other patients. The following are important considerations:

- Avoid prescribing mind-altering substances, if possible, for patients who are in recovery. Drugs to avoid include elixirs, sedative-hypnotic drugs, opiates, and antihistamines.
- Establish treatment contracts with patients involved in AA or NA. Discuss how you will handle allergies, viral illnesses, anxiety, depression, insomnia, pain, and other problems that are commonly treated by prescribing mind-altering substances.
- Use opiates only if absolutely necessary for adequate relief of pain; detoxify the patient with methadone once the pain has resolved.
- Continue the current methadone dose when admitting an opiate-addicted patient to the hospital. This will prevent a withdrawal syndrome. If needed, add other opiate analgesics, starting with usual doses. High doses may be required because of tolerance to opioids.
- Do not prescribe methadone to opiate-addicted outpatients, which is a violation of Drug Enforcement Administration guidelines. Methadone, for continued abstinence or detoxification, may only be prescribed to outpatients in federally monitored clinics.

Family Interventions for All Substance Addictions

Family members and friends are invariably affected by the addicted patient's tobacco, alcohol, and/or drug use. Significant others may also be abusing these substances. By virtue of training and because they provide care for multiple family members, family physicians are in an excellent position to influence the dynamics between the people involved. For example, parents of pediatric patients should be counseled to quit smoking to avoid exposing their children to second-hand smoke and to eliminate negative role modeling.

Several offshoots of 12-step programs have been developed to fulfill family-related needs. These include: Al-Anon and Nar-Anon, for family members of alcohol and drug addicted individuals; and Alateen, for teenagers with addicted family members. These organizations subscribe to the precepts of AA and NA. They provide family members with support from others who face similar challenges, help them better understand the addiction of their own family member, learn to recognize and change behaviors that may be enabling the addiction, and hear strategies for dealing with difficult situations at home. The meetings are free, available almost everywhere, and have members who are sympathetic and willing to help.

Treatment programs that include a significant family component can increase effectiveness (25). The family component may include:

- Teaching members about the disease concept of addiction, especially that it is not the patient's fault that he or she cannot "drink like other people"
- Attempting to resolve old conflicts while the addicted patient is still in the program and professional counselors are available
- Planning for successful immersion into the family before the patient returns home.

COMMUNITY INTERVENTIONS FOR ALL SUBSTANCE ADDICTIONS

Physicians are encouraged to participate in community prevention and education efforts (e.g., school and media based programs that seek to reduce initiation of tobacco, alcohol, and drugs among schoolchildren). The Tar Wars program (*www.tarwars.org*), adopted by the American Academy of Family Physicians, provides one model for such programs. Physicians can also join or offer support to community-based coalitions working toward policy changes, which can have significant impacts on the entire population. Examples include:

- Strengthening regulations that eliminate secondhand smoke exposure in public places
- Adopting 100% tobacco-free and drug-free school policies
- Reducing alcohol and tobacco advertising and promotion, including organizational no sponsorship polices
- Raising the costs of tobacco and alcohol products
- After policies are adopted, continual work is needed to educate and advocate for sustained enforcement, especially in areas such as youth access to tobacco and alcohol products.

KEY POINTS

- Family physicians will regularly encounter the challenging problem of addiction in their patients. The position that "we have nothing to offer you" is incorrect and unethical.
- Many addiction treatment modalities are low-cost and effective (e.g., brief counseling for smoking cessation or brief interventions with problem drinkers can significantly reduce abuse).
- Multiple medications are available on an outpatient basis to assist patients who are trying to abstain from tobacco or alcohol and some drugs. Combining medication with counseling increases abstinence rates.
- Addiction, like diabetes and hypertension, must be assessed and treated as a chronic disease. Relapse does not indicate failure, but rather the opportunity to re-engage in counseling or medical regimens that facilitate abstinence.
- The National Institute on Drug Abuse (*www.nida.nih.gov*) and the National Institute on Alcohol Abuse and Alcoholism (*www.niaaa.nih.gov*) offer up-to-date treatment information.

CHAPTER

48

Anxiety

Peter Ham

CLINICAL OBJECTIVES

1. List the most common anxiety disorders encountered in primary care.
2. Name several groups of people at high risk for anxiety disorders.
3. Discuss treatment options for children with anxiety disorders.
4. List common classes of medications used to treat anxiety disorders.
5. List other professionals who treat anxiety.
6. Recognize anxiety in the differential diagnosis for insomnia, pain, or fatigue.
7. Know how to screen for anxiety disorders using one or two questions.

Anxiety disorders affect 15 to 19 million Americans each year and 30 million at some point in their lives (3% to 8% of the population) (1). Patients with anxiety symptoms are common in primary care settings, and symptoms are associated with poor health, mental distress, poor sleep, pain, depression, alcoholism, suicide, and limited activity (2,3). Whether or not anxiety *causes* poor health or is a *result* of poor health, the burden of anxiety is considerable in a public health sense. People with anxiety disorders consume more health care resources than those with other psychiatric disorders (4). In emergency department settings, 17% to 25% of patients presenting with chest pain meet the criteria for panic disorder (5,6). The economic costs of anxiety disorders were estimated at $42 billion per year in 1990. These costs included psychiatric ($13 billion), nonpsychiatric ($23 billion), prescription drugs ($0.8 billion), work place costs ($4.1 billion), and mortality ($1.2 billion) (7). More up to date estimates have not been published although clearly health care inflation (5% to 9% per year) has increased the medical costs of anxiety since that time.

ANXIETY DISORDERS IN PRIMARY CARE

Anxiety disorders occur in 19% of primary care patients (8), greatly diminish quality of life, and have well-proven therapies. Yet, recognition of anxiety disorders in primary care is low (23%); and, fewer than 30% of patients receive treatment (1,9). Why is anxiety so common, yet hard to detect and treat?

Anxiety disorders encompass a range of diagnoses, including: generalized anxiety disorder (GAD), panic disorder, post-traumatic stress disorder (PTSD), acute stress disorder, social anxiety disorder (social phobia), specific phobias (e.g., fear of heights), and obsessive-compulsive disorder (OCD). Anxiety often complicates other medical conditions and becomes lost amidst other diagnostic work up and treatment. For example, 50% to 80% of chronic obstructive pulmonary disease patients have an anxiety or depressive disorder, yet only 31% receive treatment (10,11). Patients themselves possess varying degrees of coping skills, and the level of anxiety physicians perceive as requiring medical treatment for one person may not be the same for another.

DIFFERENTIAL DIAGNOSIS

Although there are distinct diagnostic criteria in the *Diagnostic and Statistical Manual of Mental Disorders* (DSM-IV), memorizing the DSM-IV is not particularly helpful. A better approach is to recognize the patient's pattern of cognitive errors and connect them to dysfunction. For example, feeling like a complete loser after losing a softball game represents the cognitive error of all-or-nothing thinking. Avoiding softball games because of the potential for loss or embarrassment would be a dysfunction. When diagnosing a person with an anxiety disorder, the core criteria are: (a) that the anxiety symptoms disrupt normal function and (b) that worry or fear is out of proportion to the event or situation. Learning the art of discussing whether a mental disorder could be causing a patient's chief complaint requires practice. Improperly raised, this issue may leave patients feeling dismissed, as if the problem is "all in their head." The discussion may increase anxiety if patients feel the physician is not seriously considering other etiologies.

Panic Disorder

Panic disorder is a common, disabling condition that is difficult to diagnose because its symptoms, such as chest pain or shortness of breath, also suggest life-threatening etiologies. The hallmark of panic disorder is the panic attack, which is typically the rapid onset of symptoms listed in Table 48.1. Attacks occur suddenly and usually last more than 10 minutes. In addition to the attacks themselves, panic disorder includes a persistent fear of having another attack that disrupts the patient's ability to function. This "fear of fear" may lead to agoraphobia (avoiding public places because of the fear of an attack). If a person cannot leave the house, it is not surprising that depression lurks not far behind. In fact, depression complicates panic disorder in one third of all cases (12). A useful

TABLE 48.1 Typical Symptoms of Panic Attacks

Shortness of breath
Dizziness
Palpitations
Trembling
Sweating
Choking
Nausea
Feeling that your body is not real
Numbness or tingling
Hot flashes or chills
Chest pain
Fear of dying
Fear of going crazy

screening test for panic disorder is the single question, "In the past 4 weeks, have you had an anxiety attack-suddenly feeling fear or panic?" (13).

Generalized Anxiety Disorder

In primary care, only 28% of patients with GAD are diagnosed (4). The hallmark of GAD is long standing (6 months) of "excessive worry" that decreases an individual's ability to function. Everyone experiences stress about work, school, or family; but when worry occurs without specific stressors or when worry causes disproportionate dysfunction, physicians should consider GAD. This disorder occurs in 8% of primary care patients and is more common in women. The peak incidence occurs between ages 35 and 60 years (4). GAD does not generally occur in isolation; at the time of diagnosis, two thirds of patients with GAD have a coexisting mental disorder such as major depression (37%), panic disorder (23%), or alcohol abuse (11%) (14). As shown in Table 48.2, two questions can reliably be used to screen patients for GAD in primary care settings (8).

TABLE 48.2 Screening Questions for Generalized Anxiety Disorder

Over the past 2 weeks, how often have you been bothered by the following problems: feeling nervous, anxious, or on edge? (0 = not at all, 1 = several days, 2 = more than half the days, and 3 = nearly every day)

Not being able to stop of control worrying? (0 = not at all, 1 = several days, 2 = more than half the days, and 3 = nearly every day)

A total score of 3 or more has a sensitivity of 86% and a specificity of 83% for generalized anxiety disorder.

PTSD and Acute Stress Disorder

PTSD and acute stress disorder relate to distress from vivid recollections of a traumatic, threatening event experienced by the person. Acute stress disorder applies to the period from 2 days to 1 month after the event, and PTSD applies beyond 1 month; otherwise the criteria are similar. Although uncommon in the general population (<1%) and in primary care patients (1% to 2%), these disorders are more prevalent in certain groups such as veterans, sexual assault victims, or refugees. Therefore, screening for a history of a traumatic event (e.g., sexual abuse) may identify patients at risk. Physicians who provide trauma care and who serve as responders in the aftermath of natural disasters or violent conflict will encounter acute stress disorder more often.

Social Anxiety Disorder

Social anxiety disorder, also known as social phobia, is shyness so extreme that it causes dysfunction. As opposed to avoidant personality disorder—where the person does not mind being isolated—social anxiety disorder patients are painfully aware of the problem, yet avoid scrutiny by others and barely endure public situations. In the general population, it is estimated that 5.2% of women and 3.8% of men have this disorder (8). Social anxiety disorder typically begins in childhood or adolescence. Public exposure may trigger panic attacks, creating some overlap between social anxiety disorder and panic disorder. A three-question social anxiety disorder screening tool described in Table 48.3 has a sensitivity of 89% and specificity of 90% (15). Because this tool was developed in a population with high rates of psychiatric disorders, it is most useful at ruling out social anxiety disorder.

Specific Phobias

The main feature of specific phobias is an immediate fear or anxiety response (again, this can be a panic attack) to a specific object or situation. To meet the criteria for a disorder, the symptoms must persist for more than 6 months. As with other disorders, fear or avoidance of the stimulus must significantly interfere with the person's quality of life, and the person should know the fear is unreasonable. (A delusion, on the

TABLE 48.3 Screening Questions for Social Anxiety Disorder

Fear of embarrassment causes me to avoid doing things or speaking to people
I avoid activities where I am the center of attention.
Being embarrassed of looking stupid are among my worst fears

Score each question 0 = not at all, 1 = a little bit, 2 = somewhat, 3 = very much, and 4 = extremely; positive screen score of 6 or greater.
Score <6 in a population with prevalence of 5% gives a 0.05% chance of social anxiety disorder. A score >6 gives a positive predictive value of 32% (86% sensitive, 83% specific).

other hand, is an unreasonable belief that people themselves do not see as unreasonable.) Many people can avoid snakes, heights, or other feared stimuli without disruption of their lives. However, if the person must restrict their lifestyle significantly to avoid a phobia response, it becomes a disorder. In children, phobias are usually transient, and they warrant treatment only if they impair normal development (e.g., going to school). The prevalence of phobias in the general population ranges from 4% to 8% (16).

Obsessive Compulsive Disorder

OCD is characterized by either intrusive, inappropriate thoughts (obsessions) or intrusive repetitive behaviors (compulsions) that disrupt normal functioning. For OCD, ritualistic behaviors such as hand washing, checking locks, or arranging household objects create stress and do not generate pleasure. For example, a gambling addiction is not OCD because gambling generates gratification or excitement. In OCD, the patient knows the thoughts or actions are unreasonable, whereas depressive ruminations are not usually considered absurd. OCD is chronic yet seldom disclosed by the patient. The lifetime prevalence rate of OCD may be as high as 2.5%, with the average age of onset in the early twenties (17,18). When clinical suspicion suggests OCD, begin with the question, "Do you ever find that certain thoughts or images keep coming into your head even though you try to keep them out?"

INITIAL EVALUATION AND GENERAL APPROACH

Family physicians encounter anxiety disorders daily; yet, diagnosis is difficult. Patients will not generally complain about anxiety. Rather they will often complain about symptoms such as insomnia, pain, or fatigue. Patients with OCD seldom disclose their rituals and thoughts and may only present with eczema from repetitive hand washing. Often a valuable clue that anxiety is a major factor in a patient's illness is that multiple treatments have not worked for a particular problem. Patients who bounce from drug to drug or do not fit a clinical picture merit consideration for anxiety and depression. With hypertension, for example, patients who report side effects not related to the antihypertensive medications they are taking, or patients who have switched among many antihypertensives, are more likely to have anxiety, panic, or depression (19). The same characteristics that isolate anxious patients in their nonmedical lives (e.g., fear of being exposed) make it equally difficult to confide in doctors and interpret symptoms objectively.

After anxiety is suspected, broaching it with the patient is also difficult. Mental health terms are unfamiliar to most patients. Patients who tend to normalize or "explain away" their anxiety symptoms are harder to diagnose and treat (20). Yet, breaking through patient barriers to disclosure, and getting a thorough history is vital. Anxiety disorders seldom improve without interventions to reduce isolation. Finding a nonthreatening way to broach the subject (e.g., using the terms such as "worry," "stress," or "tension" instead of anxiety) is important.

Should physicians screen all patients for mental health disorders? Although the prevalence data presented above suggest physicians underdiagnose anxiety disorders, it is unclear whether screening all patients actually improves patient outcomes. A well-done evidence-based review of depression screening suggests general screening of all patients using questionnaires is not worthwhile (21), but formal screening for anxiety currently lacks a consensus statement. If you choose to screen, use a few brief questions (see Tables 48.2 and 48.3) or a brief questionnaire that screens for both anxiety and depression (22). However, until studies demonstrate the benefits of general screening in primary care, recommendations to do so are speculative.

Screening high-risk patients is worthwhile. GAD and OCD are more common in pregnancy and postpartum (23). Women who experience a stillbirth, neonatal loss, or a sudden infant death syndrome loss may have incidences of PTSD as high as 21% during a subsequent pregnancy (24). Refugees relocated to western countries also have higher rates of PTSD (9%) (25). Alzheimer patients exhibit clinically significant anxiety in 25% to 75% of cases (26). In contrast, the elderly in general have lower overall rates of anxiety disorders than younger age groups (27).

As stated previously, many medical conditions mimic anxiety. Accordingly, there are no easy-to-follow diagnostic algorithms. (Some common conditions are listed in Table 48.4.) For example, a patient with Parkinson disease may appear agoraphobic by avoiding public places because of embarrassment about a tremor. Many symptoms, such as dyspnea, chest pain, and palpitations directly overlap with panic symptoms. Red flags for patients needing separate or concurrent evaluation and treatment for other conditions are shown in Table 48.5. The importance of follow-up in the evaluation of anxiety cannot be overstated. Obtaining information from other people who know the patient well (e.g., family, coworkers, teachers) is always helpful, but it is essential in children. Children can describe their feelings of distress well whereas adults are better at assessing the dysfunction. In children, diagnosis should include evaluation using a DSM IV Child Version with attention to other conditions (e.g., attention deficit hyperactivity disorder and learning disabilities) that may mimic anxiety (28).

TABLE 48.4 Medical Conditions that Mimic Anxiety

Alcohol withdrawal
Angina
Asthma
Attention deficit hyperactivity disorder
Bipolar disorder
Bulimia
Cardiac arrhythmias
Hyperthyroidism
Medication side effects
Menopause
Neurologic disorders
Stuttering
Substance abuse
Transient ischemic attacks

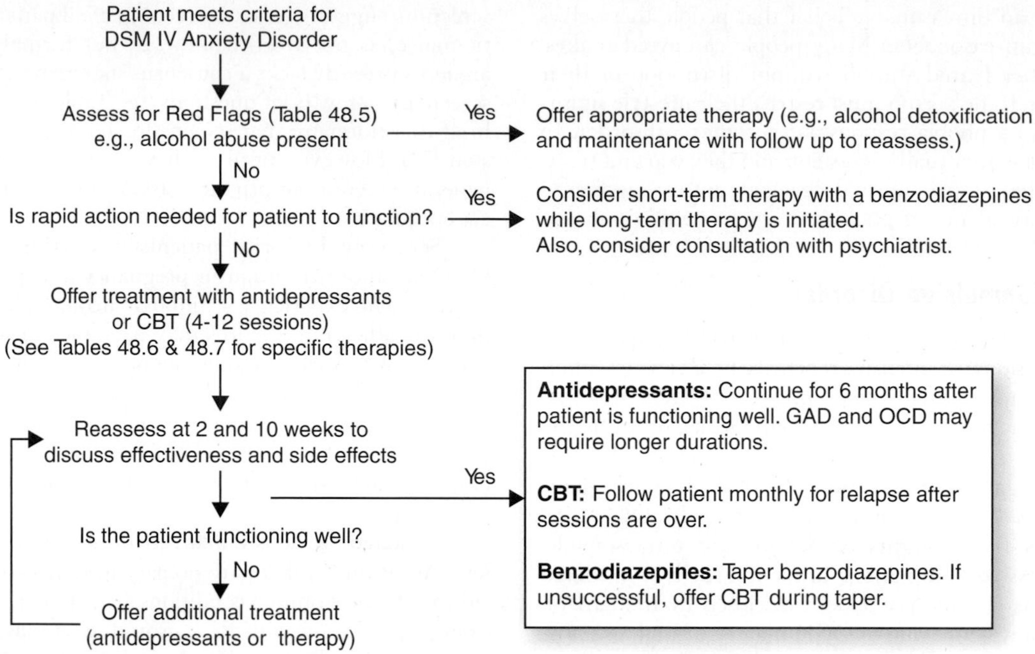

Figure 48.1 • General algorithm for the management of anxiety disorders.

One key element of treatment for any anxiety disorder is effective patient education. The possibility of an anxiety disorder should be mentioned to the patient early-on as part of a differential diagnosis. As a diagnosis of an anxiety disorder is discussed, it must be explained using terms and mechanisms that make sense to the patient. You should describe the course and prognosis as well as the effectiveness and side effects of therapies. Providing written resources, such as those available at *www.nimh.nih.gov/health* can be helpful.

TABLE 48.5 Clinical Red Flags Suggesting a Serious Additional Problem in Patients Presenting with a Suspected Anxiety Disorder

Alcohol abuse
Bulimia/anorexia
Delusions
Developmental delay
Focal, persistent weakness
Hallucinations—although reliving experiences in posttraumatic stress disorder can be very vivid
Neurologic physical exam findings
Sexual/physical abuse
Substance abuse
Suicidality
Syncope
Weight loss

MANAGEMENT

The goal of treatment in anxiety disorders is stabilization and improved function. Figure 48.1 shows one approach to managing anxiety disorders. It is important to recognize alcoholism initially. Even if patients are self-medicating their anxiety symptoms with alcohol, they should be referred for standard alcohol treatment before or during anxiety treatment (29). Sexual or physical abuse is another situation that requires a separate intervention to ensure safety while initiating antianxiety therapy. All patients with suspected anxiety should be asked about suicidal thoughts or plans. Coordination with other professionals should be considered depending on the skill and resources of the primary physician. These typically include cognitive behavioral therapists, psychotherapists, and psychiatrists.

Table 48.6 describes treatment options for each anxiety disorder and provides an evidence rating for each option. The therapeutic options for all anxiety disorders are remarkably similar, suggesting common pathophysiologic mechanisms. Cognitive-behavioral therapy (CBT), supportive psychotherapy, anti-depressants, and benzodiazepines are generally effective for most disorders. Patient choice in determining which therapy to use is important. Common features of anxiety management are described below, and therapies unique to individual disorders are provided under specific subject headings.

Antidepressants alone are highly effective in reducing symptoms and improving quality of life, with selective serotonin reuptake inhibitors (SSRIs) and tricyclic antidepressants

TABLE 48.6 Key Therapies for Treating Anxiety Disorders

Condition and Intervention	Efficacy	Strength of Recommendation*
Generalized Anxiety Disorder		
Antidepressants	Reduce anxiety symptoms (NNT 5) compared with placebo	A
Anxiolytics	Benzodiazepines, pregabalin, and buspirone effective in reducing anxiety measures compared to placebo	B
Insomnia meds	Eszopiclone added to escitalopram reduces anxiety symptoms	B
Cognitive behavioral therapy (CBT)	Effective in reducing anxiety measures compared with control groups. CBT is more effective than benzodiazepines in improving depression measures	B
Self-help manuals	Effective when combined with guidance or some contact with a professional	C
Panic Disorder		
CBT	Improves global functioning	B
Antidepressants	SSRIs and TCAs appear equally efficacious	A
Benzodiazepines	Reduce panic severity	A
β-Blockers	Pindolol reduces symptom severity in SSRI resistant PD	B
Self-help videos and books	These reduce panic severity when used with at least minimal (1–2 sessions) therapist contact	B
Exercise	Exercise reduces panic severity, but not as well as antidepressants	B
Social Anxiety Disorder		
β-Blockers for performance anxiety	Effective for subclinical "performance anxiety" but less evidence for use in true social anxiety disorder.	B
CBT	CBT with exposure or cognitive restructuring reduces distress and avoidant behavior	B
Antidepressants	SSRIs superior to placebo	B
Specific Phobias		
Benzodiazepines	Recommended for stabilization of symptoms if necessary	C
Antidepressants	Pilot studies of sertraline and paroxetine suggest effectiveness	C
CBT	Reduces phobic response	C
PTSD and Acute Stress Disorder		
Psychotherapy after event	Reduces PTSD	B
CBT	Reduces disability for 6 months	B
Antidepressants	Effective at reducing symptoms compared with placebo	A
Benzodiazepines	Effective compared with placebo. Use for stabilization (insomnia, agitation) and progress to other therapies	B
Antidepressants	Both SSRIs and TCAs (clomipramine) are effective compared with placebo	B
OCD		
Antipsychotics	Both risperidone and quetiapine reduce symptom severity in SSRI-resistant OCD	B
CBT	CBT especially using exposure techniques is effective at reducing symptoms in >80% of patients	B
Sertraline in children	Improves OCD rating scales (NNT 6 vs. placebo)	B

CBT = cognitive behavioral therapy; NNT = number needed to treat; OCD = obsessive-compulsive disorder; PD = panic disorder; PTSD = posttraumatic stress disorder; SSRIs = selective serotonin reuptake inhibitors; TCAs = tricyclic antidepressants.
*A = consistent, good-quality patient-oriented evidence; B = inconsistent or limited-quality patient-oriented evidence; C = consensus, disease-oriented evidence, usual practice, expert opinion, or case series.
For information about the SORT evidence rating system, see *www.aafp.org/afpsort.xml*.

(TCAs) generally showing equal efficacy. Each class of antidepressant has side effects, and patients' tolerance of any therapy may vary. Therefore, a follow-up appointment to assess response and to check for side effects is important. Patients should generally stay on an antidepressant for 6 months after the reduction of symptoms and be followed closely for recurrence after stopping antidepressants.

Anxiolytics (e.g., benzodiazepines) are effective in all anxiety disorders and may be used to stabilize patients over the short term. Symptoms such as extreme agitation or insomnia are indications for anxiolytics. Although long-term studies have shown that they are effective at reducing anxiety symptoms, benzodiazepines have long-term side effects (e.g., addiction, increased risk of falls, domestic violence) that make them inferior to CBT and antidepressants in improving overall patient quality of life, decreasing disability, and in measures of comorbid depression. Therefore, the goal should be to transition to a more appropriate long-term therapy. For patients on benzodiazepines, imipramine and buspirone are effective as adjuvant therapy to achieve a successful benzodiazepine taper (15 weeks of treatment tapering the benzodiazepines from weeks 4 through 10; number needed to treat [NNT] = 2) (30).

Family physicians may wish to refer patients with anxiety disorders to a therapist. In adults, there is evidence to support the benefits of nine to 12 sessions with a therapist skilled in CBT. Exposure technique (gradually placing patients into fearful situations) is one especially effective component of CBT (31). It is important to distinguish CBT (identifying cognitive errors and exercises to overcome fear) from generally supportive psychotherapy, which may be less effective in some anxiety disorders (31–33). Although long-term data are lacking as to whether CBT is more effective with or without simultaneous treatment with antidepressants, it is reasonable to combine CBT with antidepressant treatment. For patients who are having a difficult time weaning off antidepressants or benzodiazepines, CBT is an effective way to continue anxiety remission while tapering medications (34). CBT is especially useful in patients intolerant of medications. In elderly patients, both CBT and SSRIs (e.g., sertraline) reduce anxiety, with sertraline showing greater efficacy than CBT (35). Moreover, patients with dementia may not have the capacity to participate in CBT. Most children merit referral for 8 or more sessions of CBT which is effective (NNT = 3) both alone and with sertraline (36,37).

Generalized Anxiety Disorder

CBT reduces anxiety, worry, and depressive symptoms by 20% over 6 to 12 months in GAD (NNT = 3), although it is unclear whether CBT works any better than generally supportive psychotherapy (31). It is difficult to know which antidepressant should be first-line treatment for GAD without information from direct comparison trials; however, the antidepressants shown in Table 48.7 have been well studied (38). Benzodiazepines (e.g., clonazepam) are useful for stabilization and may be used long term. However, transition to other therapies such as CBT has been shown to be more effective (31). Pregabalin is effective in the short term (39). The anxiolytic buspirone is less effective compared to benzodiazepines for

TABLE 48.7 Medications for Treating Anxiety Disorders

Drug	Contraindications/Cautions/Adverse Effects	Relative Cost*
Selective Serotonin Reuptake Inhibitors		
Citalopram, escitalopram, fluoxetine, fluvoxamine, paroxetine, sertraline	Avoid with monoamine oxidase inhibitors (MAOIs), decreased libido	$–$$
Selective Norepinephrine Reuptake Inhibitors		
Venlafaxine	Same as citalopram, plus nausea and risk of increased blood pressure	$$
Duloxetine	Same as venlafaxine	$$ (61)
Benzodiazepines		
Alprazolam	Alcohol intoxication, sleep apnea, substance abuse, withdrawal seizures	$
Clonazepam	Same as for alprazolam	$
Tricyclic Antidepressants		
Clomipramine[†]	Same as for imipramine	$$
Imipramine	Avoid in heart block, cardiovascular disease, glaucoma, prostatic hypertrophy, and urinary retention	$
Miscellaneous Antianxiety Agent		
Buspirone	Decreased clearance in renal and liver disease, avoid with MAOIs	$
Pregabalin	Edema and dizziness	$$$
Eszopiclone	Headache	$$$

*$ Lowest cost to $$$ highest cost.
[†]Doses may be higher in obsessive-compulsive disorder.

GAD (40). The sleep aid eszopiclone added to SSRIs reduces anxiety in GAD patients with insomnia (41). Small studies have found that some alternative therapies, such as exercise and massage, are moderately effective; whereas reviews of meditation or herbal supplements either show no benefit or are inconclusive (42,43).

Panic Disorder

SSRIs and TCAs are two classes of antidepressants that have been well studied for treatment of panic disorder. Fifty percent of patients are panic free after 6 months of such therapy (NNT = 5) (44). There are no clear indications as to which antidepressant works most effectively, and the side effect profile should be considered when selecting which antidepressant to use. TCAs and benzodiazepines may be less well tolerated in the elderly. CBT remains an effective therapy alone or in combination with antidepressants or benzodiazepines. CBT may offer the best chance at long-term remission from panic attacks (32). In patients with noncardiac chest pain, CBT reduces severity and occurrences of pain (45). Where referral options to therapists skilled in CBT are limited, it appears that self-help treatment (book and video) is effective, but only when combined with at least one or two face-to-face or telephone sessions with a therapist (46).

PTSD and Acute Stress Disorder

Psychological debriefing with CBT during or after a traumatic event improves PTSD rates (NNT = 2) and anxiety symptoms at 6 months follow-up (33). In the immediate crisis setting, after addressing medical stabilization, safety, food, shelter, clothing, and family support concerns, responders may treat anxiety symptoms with pharmacotherapy, psychotherapy, or both. CBT beginning 2 to 3 weeks after the trauma exposure may speed recovery and prevent PTSD (47,48). In combat injuries, morphine use is associated with lower rates of PTSD (49).

The most important initial intervention after trauma and stabilization may be to arrange follow-up to evaluate for a stress disorder. After a diagnosis of ASD or PTSD is made, benzodiazepines and antidepressants, such as SSRIs and TCAs, have been shown to be effective first-line agents in doses equivalent to those used in other anxiety disorders (50). Antipsychotic or mood stabilizing medications may be helpful as second-line agents or for patients with comorbid psychotic disorders.

Obsessive Compulsive Disorder

Antidepressants such as SSRIs and TCAs are effective over 6 to 13 weeks in reducing symptoms by 25% (NNT = 6) compared with placebo in treating OCD (51). Of the SSRIs, fluvoxamine, sertraline, and fluoxetine have been extensively studied, and among TCAs, clomipramine has been studied the most in randomized controlled trials. The doses of antidepressants needed to treat OCD appear higher than those used with depression or other anxiety disorders (52). Referral of patients for 10 to 12 weeks of CBT, particularly with a therapist skilled in exposure and response prevention techniques, also is effective. It is reasonable to combine antidepressants with CBT, although long-term data on which therapy best maintains remission are lacking. Treatment responses occur in 40% to 60% of cases (53, 54). For OCD that does not respond to SSRIs, adding an antipsychotic medication such as risperidone or quetiapine reduces symptom severity (55). In children aged 6 to 16 years, sertraline is effective (56).

Social Anxiety Disorder

Medications and CBT improve measures of anxiety and social functioning in social anxiety disorder. CBT using exposure techniques in particular improves patients' distress and avoidant behavior. Combining CBT with antidepressants does not appear to add benefit when compared to psychotherapy or antidepressants alone (57). SSRIs are effective both short and long term (treatment for at least 1 year is recommended). Benzodiazepines are effective anxiolytics for social anxiety disorder. It should be noted that, although not necessarily meeting the criteria for social anxiety disorder, "performance anxiety" may respond to β-blockers (58).

Specific Phobias

It is unclear whether specific phobias are the exception to the rule suggested above that all anxiety disorders usually respond to the same therapies. CBT (with exposure technique) is effective in both adults and children and is the mainstay of therapy for debilitating specific phobias. Data on antidepressants are largely limited to pilot studies. However, pilot data from small trials show promise that antidepressants may also be broadly effective (16,59).

LONG-TERM MONITORING

There is no long-term evidence to suggest whether one particular therapy is better than another at maintaining remission in anxiety disorders. There are some data showing CBT is effective in preventing panic disorder relapse for up to 2 years (60). Until long-term data are available, follow-up at 3- to 6-month intervals, especially during periods of stress, to evaluate for relapse is warranted. Patients should be familiar with the signs and symptoms that indicate that anxiety is returning. CBT may be more effective than other treatments at sustaining remission because symptom education is part of the therapy. When patients discontinue anti-anxiety medication, they should be followed up by a physician within 2 months of stopping treatment to assess for symptoms. All follow-up visits provide opportunities to educate patients about relapse symptoms and therapeutic options.

KEY POINTS

- Anxiety disorders—generalized anxiety disorder, panic disorder, posttraumatic stress disorder, obsessive compulsive disorder, and acute stress disorder—are commonly encountered in primary care.
- An anxiety disorder should be considered in the differential diagnosis for insomnia, pain, or fatigue.
- Screening for anxiety disorders can be accomplished using one or two questions.
- Benzodiazepines may be needed to provide relief from anxiety symptoms in the short term, but most anxiety disorders can be managed over the long term with a selective serotonin reuptake inhibitor or cognitive behavioral therapy.

CHAPTER 49

Disorders of Behavior and Development

Adam J. Zolotor and Mollie Kane

CLINICAL OBJECTIVES

1. Describe some of the most common childhood behavioral and developmental challenges presenting to family physicians.
2. Demonstrate familiarity with common screening and diagnostic tests used to characterize developmental and behavior symptoms into diagnoses and syndromes.
3. Describe the role of the family physician in the multidisciplinary evaluation and treatment of children with behavioral and developmental problems.

Developmental delays and behavior disorders refer to disturbances in one or more developmental streams—motor, cognitive, or social-adaptive. Abnormalities of motor development may be reflected in abnormal fine or gross motor activity, such as in cerebral palsy. Cognitive delays may be language receptive, language expressive, problem solving, or visual-motor. Examples of cognitive delays are mental retardation, learning disorders, and communication disorders. Delays in the social-adaptive stream include attention deficit hyperactivity disorder (ADHD), autism, pervasive developmental delay, and age-specific issues such as sleep disorders or toileting problems.

Developmental delays and behavior disorders have numerous causes including genetics, temperament, illness, social environment, or intrauterine problems such as infection, trauma, or chemical exposure. Problems may also be intermixed, where one delay influences another area of development. Early skills that are needed to build higher-level skills may be absent.

Early identification and treatment of developmental delay and behavioral problems have been shown to improve outcomes significantly. The developing brain has a limited time window of malleability (1). Therefore, addressing problems during the preschool years, or earlier, has the greatest impact. Studies have found both short- and long-term benefits in children who receive early intervention. These children have improved intellectual, social, and adaptive behaviors, as well as higher rates of high school graduation and employment and lower rates of criminality and teen pregnancy (2,3).

The American Academy of Pediatrics recommends routine screening of all children for developmental delay and behavioral problems at each well child check. Should a child screen positive for a problem, further evaluation should be considered promptly (4).

Developmental delays and behavior disorders are common. Sixteen percent of American children have an impairment in speech or language, mental retardation, a learning disability, or an emotional or behavioral disturbance (5). However, between 70% and 80% of children with serious emotional and developmental disabilities are not diagnosed before entering school (6,7). Because the primary care provider is likely to be the only health professional that a young child visits, it is crucial that the primary care provider be able to identify developmental and behavioral problems. Because children with developmental delays or behavioral problems are likely to have frequent visits, many family physicians will see a patient with one of these problems almost every day.

The purpose of behavioral and developmental screening is to identify those children who require further evaluation. Studies have found that using clinical judgment alone, rather than screening tests, detects fewer than 30% of children with developmental delay. Similarly, clinical judgment alone will identify fewer than half of children with serious emotional or behavioral disturbances (5–7).

The best available screening tests have sensitivities and specificities of 70% to 80%. Achieving higher sensitivity and specificity is elusive because of the complexity of development (8). In addition, each screening is just a "snapshot" in time. New skills may be shown inconsistently until mastery is complete (9). A delay may not be noted until the age at which a milestone would normally be reached. Screening tests can help to identify precursors to milestones, resulting in earlier diagnosis (9).

Routine screening at well-child checks lets parents know that the physician places a priority on child development and behavior. Because most parents have questions and concerns about their child's behavior and development, they are often quite grateful for the physician's attention to this area. In addition, routine discussion of behavior and development may help parents to have more realistic expectations of their child (10). Parental concern has been found to be a strong predictor of developmental problems and should always trigger evaluation (11–14). Even when screening tests are normal, referral for further evaluation should be considered if parents remain concerned. See Table 49.1 for key recommendations for developmental screening and early intervention.

There are three types of screening tests (Table 49.2). Structured parent interviews and general checklists both rely on parental report of the child's skills and behaviors. Multiple studies have shown that parental report is accurate and can be used successfully for screening (15–17). The third type of screening test is direct examination screening. Direct examination testing should only be used for initial screening if a

TABLE 49.1 Key Recommendations for Developmental Screening and Treatment

Recommendation	Strength of Recommendation*	References
Developmental screening should be performed at all well-child checks, infancy through school age	A	4,8
Early treatment of developmental delays should be achieved, ideally in the preschool years, because it significantly improves outcomes	A	2,3
Parental concern about behavior or development should always trigger evaluation	A	11–14

*A = consistent, good-quality patient-oriented evidence; B = inconsistent or limited-quality patient-oriented evidence; C = consensus, disease-oriented evidence, usual practice, expert opinion, or case series. For information about the Strength of Recommendation Taxonomy evidence rating system, see *www.aafp.org/afpsort.xml*.

parent cannot give a report. This may be the case in situations of foster care or adoption, when the parent or caregiver does not yet know the child well. In addition, it may occur when a parent is significantly impaired.

The Individuals With Disabilities Education Act (IDEA) Amendments of 1997 require early intervention for individuals with developmental disabilities through the development of community based systems (19). Children younger than 3 years of age may receive services through the state's early intervention program. Those older than 3 years of age receive services through the local school district. The family physician will often need to put together an interdisciplinary team to optimize management.

FAILURE TO THRIVE

Failure to thrive occurs when growth is interrupted. Causes may be genetic, medical, nutritional, behavioral, psychological, or environmental. Whatever the underlying causes, the immediate cause of failure to thrive is malnutrition. This malnutrition may result because insufficient calories are offered, because of a child's inability to take or to retain sufficient calories, or because of increased caloric need secondary to increased metabolism (20). The diagnosis of failure to thrive should prompt an investigation for the underlying causes. Appropriate investigation may lead to the earlier diagnosis of medical or psychosocial problems.

Traditionally, failure to thrive has been considered to be organic in about 30% of cases and nonorganic in about 70% of cases. Instead, it is now understood that the causes of failure to thrive are usually intermixed and multifactorial. For example, an infant with gastrointestinal reflux disease may have decreased caloric intake because of discomfort. The infant may also have a decreased ability to retain sufficient calories secondary to emesis. As the parents watch their infant eating less, and possibly showing a growth disturbance, they will become anxious. The parents then coax or even force-feed their infant. This can lead to a power struggle with further decreased intake by the child and increasing frustration of the parent. The malnourished child will then become irritable and lethargic, escalating mealtime conflicts. After the diagnosis of failure to thrive is made the parent may feel a sense of failure, further complicating the parent–child relationship (20,21). As in this example, with any cause of failure to thrive behavioral complications related to feeding will usually develop and will often persist after the underlying disturbance has been corrected (22).

Failure to thrive is usually diagnosed by the primary care physician during well-child visits (23). Parents are often unaware of a growth disturbance. Eighty percent of children with failure to thrive are diagnosed by 18 months of age (24). The single greatest risk factor for failure to thrive is poverty. For children living in poverty, inadequate food availability, homelessness, and stress can lead to malnutrition (25,26). Children living in poverty are less likely to receive early diagnosis and intervention for medical and psychosocial problems, which can be precursors of failure to thrive.

Initial Evaluation

There is no single definition, measurement, or set of criteria that best diagnoses failure to thrive (27). Most clinicians will consider the diagnosis for children without weight gain in 2 months or children who have dropped 2 percentile curves in <6 months (24). The most common cause of an abnormal growth curve is measurement or plotting error. This should always been considered and ruled out before other action is taken.

Growth failure will initially be evident in weight alone, followed by height, and then head circumference. After height has been affected the malnutrition has become chronic. By the time head circumference is affected the child will be at increased risk for long-term neurological complications.

Failure to thrive must be distinguished from other causes of growth disturbance. In congenital, constitutional, familial, and endocrine causes of growth disturbance, length will decline before weight or proportionately to weight. Children with constitutional growth delay will be both short and thin. Those with endocrine related delays will be short and heavy. In familial short stature growth will remain parallel to the growth curve.

After the diagnosis of failure to thrive is established, the cause must be pursued. History is generally the most important diagnostic tool in finding the underlying cause of failure to thrive (24). Often several visits will be needed to obtain the full history. A thorough physical exam is also important. History and physical should be complete before any laboratory

TABLE 49.2 Developmental Screening Tools

Name	Age Range	Scoring	Sensitivity Specificity	Time	Number of Items	Cost
Tools with Information Obtained from Parents						
Ages and Stages Questionnaire (ASQ)	0–60 months	Pass/fail	70%–90% 76%–91%	10–15 minutes	30	~$4.60
Parents' Evaluations of Developmental Status (PEDS)	0–8 years	Low, medium, or high risk	74%–79% 70%–80%	2 minutes	10	~$1.19
Infant-Toddler Checklist for Language and Communication	6–24 months	Manual table of cut-off scores	78% 74%	5–10 minutes	24	~$3.60
Tools Requiring Direct Examination of Children						
Bayley Infant Neurodevelopmental Screener (BINS)	3–24 months	Low, medium, or high risk	Accuracy 75%–86%	10–15 minutes	10–13	~$10.45
Brigance Screens	0–90 months	Cutoffs, age equivalents, percentiles, and quotients	70%–82% 70%–82%	10 minutes		~$11.68
Battelle Developmental Inventory Screening Test (BDIST)	12–96 months	Cutoffs	70%–80% 70%–80%	15–35 minutes		~$20.55

Source: Glascoe FP, Commonly used screening tools, db.peds.org (18).

studies or radiographs are considered. There is no routine panel of tests for children with failure to thrive. History and physical should guide the choice of any diagnostic studies. Often, no diagnostic studies will be needed.

Almost any medical problem can lead to failure to thrive in young children. Inadequate intake of calories can occur from dysphagia, nausea, anorexia, or altered taste secondary to problems such as dental caries, enlarged adenoids, or medication side effects (22,28). A choking episode may result in food phobia. Cardiac or pulmonary disease may cause fatigue that interferes with intake. Malabsorption can occur in diseases such as cystic fibrosis, inflammatory bowel disease, and diarrhea. Increased caloric need can result from tumors, recurrent infections, or endocrine disorders.

Psychosocial factors leading to failure to thrive can be divided into three categories: interactions between the child and caregiver, psychosocial health of the caregiver, and infant characteristics (24). A caregiver suffering from an affective disorder or substance abuse may be unable to recognize a child's cues. This may lead to over- or underfeeding. An infant with special needs, prematurity, or a difficult temperament may be unable to adequately communicate his needs. Difficulty may arise from poor fit between the temperament of the child and the caregiver. For example, a baby who needs a firm, regular schedule may not do well with a caregiver who prefers an irregular schedule. Similarly, a calm caregiver may have difficulty meeting the needs of an energetic, crying baby.

Management

The management of children with failure to thrive must focus on the antecedents to the growth problem. Because the cause is usually multifactorial, the child may require nutritional, medical, psychological, and developmental treatment (29).

Even when the underlying cause of the malnutrition is not curable, nutrition can be optimized by working with the child and the family. The family should be educated in how to make mealtimes pleasant and minimize mealtime conflict. Parents can be taught to recognize infant cues and to understand normal toddler behavior.

Hospitalization is rarely needed for the child with failure to thrive. Hospitalization should be considered in cases of severe malnutrition, hypothermia, bradycardia, or hypertension. Hospitalization is also appropriate in the face of abuse or neglect, when there is an impaired caregiver, when there has been a lack of catch-up growth with outpatient treatment, or when there is a need to observe parent–child feeding.

Long-term Monitoring

Whether or not there are long-term sequelae from failure to thrive depends on the cause and the severity of the problem. When there are significant psychosocial problems involved children seem to have more long-term disturbances. Such disturbances are likely related to the underlying cause of the failure to thrive, rather than the malnutrition itself. In addition, failure to thrive in the first year of life, particularly the first

6 months, is more likely to affect brain development. Undernutrition during this time may cause persistent fine and gross motor problems and speech and language delay.

AUTISTIC SPECTRUM DISORDER

Autistic spectrum disorder (ASD) refers to a continuum of disorders of brain development involving impaired communication skills; impaired social interactions; and restricted, repetitive, or stereotypical patterns of behavior (30). The etiology of ASD remains poorly understood, although there is clearly a strong genetic component, which seems to be modulated by the child's environment. Each symptom of ASD may range from mild to severe in the individual child.

ASD, also referred to as pervasive developmental disorder, includes five subtypes including autistic disorder, Asperger syndrome, pervasive developmental disorder not otherwise specified, Rett syndrome, and childhood disintegrative disorder. On the severe end of the spectrum is autistic disorder. Higher functioning children may have the milder Asperger syndrome. Children with Asperger syndrome exhibit poor peer relationships, lack of empathy, and a tendency to over focus on specific topics. They often have normal intelligence and normal language skills. Pervasive developmental disorder-not otherwise specified refers to children who do not meet the criteria for autistic disorder but who have severe impairments.

Rett syndrome and childhood disintegrative disorder are very rare and very severe autistic spectrum disorders. Rett syndrome is a neurodegenerative disorder that affects girls ages 1 to 3 years after a period of normal development. Patients experience a loss of hand skills, gross motor and coordination skills, language and cognitive skills, and social interaction skills. Childhood disintegrative disorder occurs after age 24 months, following a period of normal development. It results in profound losses in play, language, social, and motor skills.

The prevalence of autistic disorder is thought to be about 1 in 1,000 children. Studies have found that at least 2 in 1,000 children, and possibly more, suffer from autistic spectrum disorder (31,32). Prevalence rates are increasing possibly due to changing inclusion criteria, increased awareness, or a true increase in prevalence (33,34). Recurrence rates in siblings are 3% to 7%, emphasizing the importance of genetic counseling for families that have a child with ASD (35).

Initial Evaluation

Early diagnosis and intervention is critical for optimal outcomes for children with ASD. Unfortunately, fewer than 50% are diagnosed before kindergarten entry. Parental concern about the development of social skills is fairly rare. Therefore, when it occurs it should be taken very seriously (36).

Concern should be raised when a child exhibits aberrant social skills, abnormal eye contact, aloofness, failure to orient to name, failure to use gestures to point or show, lack of interactive play, or lack of interest in peers (36). Several screening tools are available for use in the primary care office including the Checklist for Autism in Toddlers (i.e., CHAT) for 18 month olds, and the Pervasive Developmental Disorder Screening Test. When ASD is suspected based on history, clinical findings, or screening tests, referral should be made to a specialist who can confirm the diagnosis.

Management

There are no widely accepted guidelines or protocols for treatment of ASD. However, there is agreement that early and sustained intervention greatly improves outcomes. The effectiveness of most specific interventions remains unknown. For most children treatment should include parental education and support, community services, occupational therapy, physical therapy, structured play, behavior management, and, in some cases, medication.

CEREBRAL PALSY

Cerebral palsy (CP) is a disorder of movement and posture caused by injury to the motor areas of the brain. Motor abnormalities must be static, not progressive over time. Because of rapid developmental changes in the first year of life, a definitive diagnosis of CP should not be made until after 1 year of age. In most cases, muscle tone will be decreased in early infancy, with increased tone by 12 to 18 months of age.

CP has many different etiologies, all involving injury to the developing brain. The insult may occur during the prenatal period, during labor and delivery, or in the first few years of life. In 20% to 30% of cases no etiology is found despite a thorough workup. Congenital CP is present from birth, but may not be identified until later. Major causes of congenital CP include prenatal infection (particularly by rubella, cytomegalovirus, or toxoplasmosis), and Rh histoimmunoincompatibility syndrome. When CP occurs during labor and delivery it is usually from severe asphyxia leading to hypoxic–ischemic encephalopathy. This type of CP is much less common than previously believed, accounting for about 6% of cases. Postnatal CP may occur secondary to central nervous system infection (e.g., bacterial meningitis or viral encephalitis), injury (e.g., motor vehicle accidents, falls, or child abuse), or stroke from prematurity or coagulation disorders.

Initial Evaluation

The diagnosis of CP should be suspected if the child is older than 1 year of age and abnormalities occur in several of the following areas: posture, oropharyngeal problems (tongue thrusts, swallowing), strabismus, increased or decreased muscle tone, abnormal evolution of primitive reflexes, or abnormal deep tendon reflexes. Other conditions that often occur with CP include seizures, refractive errors, hearing loss, mental retardation, failure to thrive, learning disabilities, attention problems, and behavior problems.

There are four subtypes of CP: spastic, athetoid, ataxic, and mixed. For each type, severity can range from extremely mild to debilitating. Spastic CP is the most common, occurring in 70% to 80% of cases. It may occur as a diplegia involving only the bilateral lower extremities, a quadriplegia, or a hemiplegia. Muscles will often become stiffly contracted. Often legs will rotate inward and cross at the knees resulting in a scissors gait. Athetoid or dyskinetic CP occurs in 10% to 20% of cases and involves uncontrolled, slow, writhing movements. Dysarthria, drooling, and grimacing may also occur. Ataxic CP accounts for an additional 5% to 10% of cases and involves abnormalities of balance and depth perception. Children with ataxic CP will often have poor coordination, a wide-based gait, and an intention tremor.

Management

The prognosis for children with CP is extremely variable depending on the type and severity of the neurologic insult. Best outcomes will occur when an interdisciplinary team is involved early on in treatment. This team should include the primary care physician; a social worker; a psychologist; occupational, physical, and speech therapists; a communication therapist; and educational and vocational specialists.

MENTAL RETARDATION

Mental retardation (MR) refers to cognitive ability that is markedly below average for chronological age with a decreased ability to adapt to the environment. The diagnosis of decreased cognitive ability must be made via standardized testing. Because standardized testing is less predictive in young children, the term developmental delay is usually used for children younger than age 3.

MR occurs at four levels of severity. Mild MR refers to individuals with intelligence quotients (IQs) of 50 to 70. They are able to attain math and reading skills at a third- to sixth-grade level. Individuals with mild MR can conform socially, maintain employment, and integrate in society. Individuals with moderate MR have IQs of 35 to 49. They can perform simple activities and basic self-care. Individuals with severe MR have IQs of 20 to 34. They require supervision and support, but may participate in simple, repetitive self-care activities. Those with profound MR have IQs <20 and are not capable of self-care (30).

MR occurs in 2% to 3% of the general population. In 50% to 70% of cases, an etiology can be found. Acquired MR may occur in children from near-drowning, traumatic brain injury, central nervous system malignancy, or lead exposure. Prenatal MR can occur from infection, first trimester maternal fever, intrauterine alcohol or anticonvulsant exposure, or untreated maternal phenylketonuria. MR is more common in premature infants with very low birth weights. Mental retardation can also result from metabolic diseases (i.e., hypothyroidism), single gene mutations (i.e., fragile X syndrome or neurofibromatosis), or chromosomal abnormalities such as in Down syndrome, Klinefelter syndrome, or Prader-Willi syndrome (37,38).

ATTENTION DEFICIT/HYPERACTIVITY DISORDER

ADHD is the most common neurodevelopmental disorder of childhood and is characterized by inattention, hyperactivity, and impulsivity (30). Most studies on the prevalence of ADHD report between 4% and 8% of children have symptoms impairing function. Prevalence data are largely limited to children between 6 and 12 years of age (39). ADHD can lead to depression, low self-esteem, increased risk of injury, school failure, early school dropout, substance abuse, and increased risk of criminality. ADHD has been traditionally thought of as a disease of childhood; recent studies demonstrate that 60% to 80% of children with ADHD have symptoms with impairment into adulthood (40).

The American Academy of Pediatrics (AAP) recommends that primary care clinicians initiate an evaluation for ADHD in all children between 6 and 12 years of age presenting with symptoms of hyperactivity, inattention, impulsivity, academic underachievement, or behavior problems. The reliable diagnosis of ADHD requires the use of Diagnostic and Statistical Manual of Mental Disorders, Fourth Edition (DSM IV) diagnostic criteria (Table 49.3), collection of information from multiple sources, and a thorough clinical evaluation (41). Successful treatment requires: (i) establishing a management program, (ii) setting appropriate, behaviorally oriented treatment goals, (iii) the use of stimulant therapy and/or behavior therapy, and (iv) reassessment and monitoring (42).

Initial Evaluation

The evaluation should begin with the chief complaint. Why are the parents bringing this to the clinician's attention? Is this a routine exam? How is school? Has the teacher raised concerns with learning? Can the child complete tasks such as homework? Does she have problems with behavior at home or school? In setting the tone for the evaluation of ADHD, approach the parent as a partner. Recognize that many parents present with an agenda or opinion (often well informed), particularly with regard to medication. Describe the course, time frame, and contents of the evaluation.

DSM IV criteria should guide history taking (Table 49.3). Symptoms must be present for 6 months. There are three subtypes of ADHD: inattentive type, hyperactive type, and mixed type. A child must have six symptoms of inattention or six symptoms of hyperactivity and/or impulsivity as listed in the diagnostic criteria. Many children will meet criteria for both inattentive type and hyperactive-impulsive type ADHD (combined type). Symptoms of ADHD must be present before age seven and must be present in two or more settings (e.g., school and home). There must be clear impairment in functioning (social, academic, or occupational). Other disorders must be ruled out as the sole cause of symptoms (e.g., pervasive developmental disorder, schizophrenia, mood disorders, personality disorders) (30).

Many disorders co-occur with ADHD. In community-based samples of children with ADHD, oppositional defiant disorder is present in 35%, conduct disorder in 26%, anxiety disorders in 26%, and depressive disorders in 18% (41). The presence of these comorbid disorders does not preclude the effective evaluation or treatment of ADHD but special attention should be paid in the initial evaluation of patients for ADHD as the presence of these may complicate diagnosis and affect management plans. Children with more severe psychiatric disorders (e.g., conduct disorder and major depression) may be more appropriate for specialized care settings (42).

The AAP published evidenced-based guidelines on the diagnosis of ADHD in 2000. In addition to the use of DSM IV criteria, the guidelines recommend that information about the core symptoms of ADHD and the degree of impairment be obtained directly from both parents and teachers (or others responsible for the care of the child) (41). An interview with the parents should also include detailed information about pregnancy, birth, development, current or prior illnesses, injuries, or hospitalizations. A detailed family history of a child with ADHD will often reveal parents with ADHD, substance abuse, or job or marital instability. The AAP supports the use of ADHD specific checklists as one way of obtaining information from multiple settings (and multiple parents or

TABLE 49.3 DSM-IV Criteria for ADHD

I. Either A or B:
   A. Six or more of the following symptoms of inattention have been present for at least 6 months to a point that is disruptive and inappropriate for developmental level:
      Inattention
      1. Often does not give close attention to details or makes careless mistakes in schoolwork, work, or other activities.
      2. Often has trouble keeping attention on tasks or play activities.
      3. Often does not seem to listen when spoken to directly.
      4. Often does not follow instructions and fails to finish schoolwork, chores, or duties in the workplace (not from oppositional behavior or failure to understand instructions).
      5. Often has trouble organizing activities.
      6. Often avoids, dislikes, or doesn't want to do things that take a lot of mental effort for a long period of time (such as schoolwork or homework).
      7. Often loses things needed for tasks and activities (e.g., toys, school assignments, pencils, books, tools).
      8. Is often easily distracted.
      9. Is often forgetful in daily activities.
   B. Six or more of the following symptoms of hyperactivity-impulsivity have been present for at least 6 months to an extent that is disruptive and inappropriate for developmental level:
      Hyperactivity
      1. Often fidgets with hands or feet or squirms in seat.
      2. Often gets up from seat when remaining in seat is expected.
      3. Often runs about or climbs when and where it is not appropriate (adolescents or adults may feel very restless).
      4. Often has trouble playing or enjoying leisure activities quietly.
      5. Is often "on the go" or often acts as if "driven by a motor."
      6. Often talks excessively.
      Impulsivity
      1. Often blurts out answers before questions have been finished.
      2. Often has trouble waiting one's turn.
      3. Often interrupts or intrudes on others (e.g., butts into conversations or games).

II. Some symptoms that cause impairment were present before age 7 years.
III. Some impairment from the symptoms is present in two or more settings (e.g., at school/work and at home).
IV. There must be clear evidence of significant impairment in social, school, or work functioning.
V. The symptoms do not happen only during the course of a pervasive developmental disorder, schizophrenia, or other psychotic disorder. The symptoms are not better accounted for by another mental disorder (e.g., mood disorder, anxiety disorder, dissociative disorder, or a personality disorder).
   Based on these criteria, three types of ADHD are identified:
   1. ADHD, *Combined Type*: if both criteria 1A and 1B are met for the past 6 months
   2. ADHD, *Predominantly Inattentive Type*: if criterion 1A is met but criterion 1B is not met for the past 6 months
   3. ADHD, *Predominantly Hyperactive-Impulsive Type*: if Criterion 1B is met but Criterion 1A is not met for the past 6 months.

Reprinted with permission from the Diagnostic and Statistical Manual of Mental Disorders, Fourth Edition, Text Revision. (Copyright 2000). American Psychiatric Association.

guardians) in a time efficient and consistent manner (41,43). These checklists are not intended to be used as diagnostic or screening tests and lack the sensitivity for a good screening test and the specificity for a good diagnostic test. They facilitate the collection of information from multiple sources. Some of the available specific checklists include Connors, SNAP IV, ADHD IV, and ACTeRS (43). Other testing from the school such as psychological testing and reports from individualized education plan meetings should be reviewed when available (41).

Many diagnostic tests have been evaluated for routine or selected use during the evaluation of a child with suspected ADHD. These include thyroid testing, lead level, complete blood count, neuroimaging, electroencephalography, and continuous performance tests (computer-administered test of attention). None of these tests have been shown to have sufficient sensitivity or specificity for routine use in the evaluation of a child with suspected ADHD. However, some of these tests are appropriate in some contexts (41).

A complete history and physical is essential. Has the child had recent hearing and vision tests? A child with moderate sensory impairment is likely to have difficulty attending to task. Has there been a recent change in family structure (marriage, divorce, death, or serious illness)? Are there undiagnosed or undertreated medical conditions that affect a child's ability to pay attention? The initial visits for ADHD are also an opportunity to observe the child as well as the parents' response to the child. Is the child able to engage in a sustained conversion? Can he complete tasks? Is she fidgety? Does he respond appropriately to feedback? Do the parents have appropriate expectations? Are they firm and consistent yet fair? Many children struggling behaviorally at school and home are criticized frequently by parents. This often becomes the dominant or exclusive form of attention. These clues may or may not alter your diagnosis but often help lead treatment.

Management

The cornerstone of successful management of ADHD is the clinician's relationship with the child and family. At the time of diagnosis, it is important to set realistic treatment goals and to define these goals in behavioral terms (42). Attention to the specific behaviors that prompted the initial evaluation will ensure addressing the needs of the whole family. If the parent was concerned that the child was having trouble focusing on homework for 15 minutes each night, then using that as an initial, achievable, and measurable treatment goal for the child and parents.

ADHD is a chronic condition and as such a treatment plan should resemble that of a chronic disease. This should include a management plan with goals, and a plan for follow-up. Flow sheets can be helpful in monitoring progress (42).

There are essentially two distinct management strategies for ADHD: medication and behavior therapy. Both have proven success in treating the core symptoms of ADHD. The AAP guidelines on treatment recommend initiating treatment with a stimulant medicine and/or behavior therapy. Stimulants are well tolerated, inexpensive, and effective. Any given stimulant results in improvement in 70% of children with ADHD. Approximately 80% to 85% of children with ADHD will respond to at least one available stimulant. The AAP recommends that if a stimulant trial fails (inadequate improvement or intolerable side effects), another stimulant should be attempted. The mainstay of therapy for many years was short-acting methylphenidate. Short-acting dextroamphetamine also has been widely used (42,44,45). There has been a recent proliferation of novel drug delivery systems that have improved the once-daily dosing of methylphenidate, dextroamphetamine, and amphetamine-dextroamphetamine. These are usually about twice as expensive as short-acting generic products. However, they eliminate the need for in-school dosing and may eliminate some of the highs and lows of stimulant treatment (46,47). Generally, stimulants should be titrated to the highest tolerated dose with added gains in control of core symptoms and without intolerable side effects. In practice, this often means frequent visits with feedback from parents and teachers to establish a dose. After initial success, the dose should usually be titrated upwards. If there are no additional gains in symptom control or intolerable side effects occur, the dose should be lowered to the previous dose. Patients with hyperactive/impulsive type and combined type ADHD will often require higher doses of stimulants (47–49).

The tricyclic antidepressants, particularly desipramine and imipramine, have been used extensively for the treatment of ADHD. They have been subject to fewer, smaller, and shorter duration randomized controlled trials than the stimulants. However, they show similar efficacy. They have a different side effect profile and may be more difficult to tolerate with adequate doses. However, in children with intolerable weight loss or insomnia on stimulants, they are an excellent second choice (44).

Other antidepressants, especially the noradrenergic agonists bupropion and venlafaxine, have been used for the treatment of ADHD. Similarly, atomoxetine, a selective norepinephrine reuptake inhibitor, was recently developed and approved for the treatment of ADHD. Atomoxetine has been shown to improve the symptoms of ADHD, but has not been compared in direct trials against stimulants. In special cases, a variety of other drugs have been used in children with ADHD, including centrally acting alpha 2 blockers (clonidine and guanfacine), β-blockers, antiseizure medicines (e.g., carbamazepine and valproic acid), and antipsychotics (e.g., risperidone) (Table 49.4).

Behavior therapy is best delivered as a broad set of specific interventions with application to the home and school environment by parents and teachers. Behavior therapy emphasizes such techniques as positive and negative reinforcement, and token economies (e.g., child gets a star for each good day and after three good days gets a special reward). Behavior therapy is distinct from psychological therapy directed at insight into problems and thought patterns. Psychological therapy has not been shown to be helpful in the treatment of ADHD. Several studies have shown that behavior therapy is effective at managing the core symptoms of ADHD. However, studies usually involve extensive and expensive programs. Treatment effects of behavior therapy alone are slightly less impressive then a structured medication program alone. However, the combination of a structured medication program and a behavior therapy program leads to lower doses of medicines and higher parent satisfaction (44,49) (Table 49.5).

Long-term Monitoring

After stabilizing treatment, children with ADHD should be seen at regular intervals to monitor continued response to therapy, behavioral goals, academic progress, and side effects. The exact interval needed for each child is variable. In many states, this may be influenced by laws for prescribing controlled substances. Linear height and weight should be monitored every 3 to 6 months. Direct input from teachers should be solicited at least yearly. This can be easily accomplished by the repeat administration of ADHD specific checklists. Blood testing is not indicated in monitoring ADHD or treatment with the currently available medications. With significant weight loss, a clinician may also choose to screen for anemia periodically.

DISRUPTIVE BEHAVIOR

Disruptive behavior is the most common behavioral complaint presenting to a family physician. Disruptive behaviors represent a spectrum from normal disobedience and risk taking to severe conduct disorder. Oppositional defiant disorder (ODD) is characterized by negativistic, defiant, and hostile behavior towards authority figures. Conduct disorder (CD) is the persistent violation of the rights of others and societal, age appropriate norms. Both disorders persist over time and cause significant impairment in function (30).

The family physician's role in the evaluation of behavior disorders is to normalize age appropriate behavior (e.g., tantrums in toddlers, lying in preschoolers), offer appropriate

TABLE 49.4 Commonly Prescribed Medications for ADHD

Drug	Adverse Effects	Dosage	Relative Cost*
Methylphenidate (immediate release)	Anorexia, stomach ache, headache, weight loss, insomnia	5–20 mg BID to TID	$$
Methylphenidate (sustained release)	Anorexia, stomach ache, headache, weight loss, insomnia	20–60 mg daily	$$$
Dextroamphetamine (immediate release)	Anorexia, stomach ache, headache, weight loss, insomnia	2.5–10 mg BID	$$
Dextroamphetamine (sustained release)	Anorexia, stomach ache, headache, weight loss, insomnia	10–40 mg daily	$$$
Amphetamine/ dextroamphetamine (immediate release)	Anorexia, stomach ache, headache, weight loss, insomnia	2.5–10 mg daily to BID	$$$
Amphetamine/ dextroamphetamine (sustained release)	Anorexia, stomach ache, headache, weight loss, insomnia	10–40 mg daily	$$$
Atomoxetine	Nausea, vomiting, constipation, fatigue, dry eyes and mouth	40–100 mg daily	$$$
Tricyclics (desipramine and imipramine)	Sedation, constipation, dry eyes and mouth	10–50 mg BID (maximum daily dose 5 mg/kg)	$

*$ = inexpensive; $$ = moderate; $$$ = expensive; BID = twice daily; TID = three times daily.

parenting advice and resources in supportive and nonjudgmental ways, and refer children with more severe disorders or unclear diagnoses for early evaluation and treatment (50). Particularly with conduct disorder, referral for treatment should be made early in the course of disease.

The estimated prevalence of CD ranges from 1.5% to 3.4%. Boys are three to five times more likely to be affected (51). ODD is more common than CD, but estimates vary widely (52). CD is common among children in the juvenile justice system. Forty percent of children with CD will develop antisocial personality disorder (51).

Risk and causal factors for CD have been the subject of significant epidemiological, genetic, and environmental research. Genetics clearly plays a role but has been difficult to disentangle from the family environment. Poverty, male gender, increasing age (through adolescence), chronic illness, and

TABLE 49.5 Key Recommendations for Management of ADHD

Recommendation	Strength of Recommendation	References
In children presenting with behavior/school problems, initiate evaluation for ADHD	B	39,41
To diagnose ADHD, a child must meet DSM IV criteria	B	39,41
Direct information on the core symptoms of ADHD must be gathered from parents and caregivers in multiple settings	B	39,41
Evaluation should include assessment for coexisting conditions	A	39,41
Establish a management program treating ADHD as a chronic disease	B	42,44
Set goals with parents and teachers that are realistic and measurable	B	42,44
Recommend stimulant medicine and/or behavior therapy as first line treatment	A (stimulant) B (behavior)	42,44,49

A = consistent, good-quality patient-oriented evidence; ADHD = attention deficit hyperactivity disorder; B = inconsistent or limited-quality patient-oriented evidence; C = consensus, disease-oriented evidence, usual practice, expert opinion, or case series; DSM = Diagnostic and Statistical Manual of Mental Disorders. For information about the Strength of Recommendation Taxonomy evidence rating system, see *www.aafp.org/afpsort.xml*.

disability have been consistently shown to be risk factors. Temperament, hyperactivity, and early aggressive behavior are constitutional risk factors for later CD. The most important risk factors for CD are in the domain of the family: poor family functioning, substance abuse, psychiatric disease in a parent, marital discord, child abuse and neglect, and poor parenting. Child abuse is the strongest and most consistent risk factor for CD (51).

Initial Evaluation

With any behavior complaint, the family physician should listen to the parent in a supportive manner. What is the problem? In what settings does the problem occur? What has been tried to modify the behavior? What has worked? A comprehensive developmental, family, and social history is invaluable in the assessment of behavior problems. Acute stress, grief, acute disease, and chronic disease can cause and aggravate behavior problems. Specific evaluation of the level of impairment is important in helping develop an initial management plan. Has the child been arrested, in fights, or using weapons? Is the child taking risks that are extreme for age? How is he doing in school? Does she get along with peers (50)?

As with ADHD, comorbid disease is extremely common with CD and ODD. The family physician should consider both alternative and comorbid disorders including ADHD, depression, anxiety, personality disorders, learning disabilities, and substance abuse (51,52). Some clinicians find that broad band behavior rating scales such as the Child Behavior Checklist can help identify likely alternative or comorbid conditions (53). These scales lack sensitivity or specificity to be used for screening or diagnosis.

Management

The general approach to management will depend on the symptoms, severity, and differential diagnosis. The family physician is in an excellent position to offer supportive parenting advice and anticipatory guidance in a developmentally appropriate context from an early age. Parents should be reminded that the purpose of discipline is to teach a child to change, eliminate, or add a behavior. The parents should set the goals. A few simple principals can curb problem behaviors before they escalate to true disorders. Parents should be consistent, set limits, reward positive behavior, and use negative reinforcements, time out, and selective inattention for negative behaviors. Children often act out in an effort to get attention. Parents can shift the balance of positive and negative attention by selectively ignoring less bad behaviors like whining (selective inattention). Time-in is a principal in which parents use minimal physical contact to frequently reward positive behavior. This could be a pat on the head for patiently waiting for adults to finish a conversation. Positive reinforcement should include the lavish use of praise, small rewards, and special time with parents or loved ones. Time-out should involve a short (1 minute per year age) quiet time and space. This is less of a punishment and more of a way to defer negative attention giving in response to a behavior and allow a child to calm down. Token economies are a commonly used form of behavior modification in which a child will get a token (sticker, star, or chip) for a behavior. When the child gets a certain number of tokens (e.g., five) the child gets a deferred reward. Tokens are given for desirable behaviors and taken away for undesirable behaviors. The child should be clear on the rules of any set of behavior change efforts so that they understand the rewards and consequences of behavior. Parents should be consistent with one another and other caregivers, firm with rules, and frequently re-evaluate problems and solutions. Parents should select a limited number of behaviors to modify at any one time, and employ intermittent reinforcement to maintain new gains (50).

Children with more severe behavioral problems often require referral for diagnosis and management. The treatment of comorbid disease is very important in behavior disorders. A child with ADHD and CD will be more frustrated if he is having trouble staying on task. Adequate treatment of comorbid diseases will often result in improvement in symptoms of ODD and CD (51,52).

Family and parenting interventions have been consistently shown to reduce symptoms and morbidity from CD. Specifically, among delinquent youths with CD, a recent meta-analysis of randomized controlled trials showed that family and parenting interventions reduced the average number of days in an institution and future re-arrests for the following 1 to 3 years (54). Skill training for children is also helpful, but most helpful in the context of family or parenting interventions (51). Parent training programs have also been consistently shown to be decrease target behaviors in ODD (55). Parent and family training programs for both disorders focus on the same themes discussed previously, including positive and negative reinforcement, selective inattention, time-out, time-in, and token economies. These programs often combine group and family sessions, child age appropriate instruction, didactic and hands-on role playing or video examples (Table 49.6).

TABLE 49.6 Key Recommendations for Interventions for Behavioral Disorders

Target Disorder	Intervention	Strength of Recommendation	Comment
ODD	Parent training programs	A	Several systematic reviews of RCTs
CD	Family and parenting interventions	A	Meta-analysis of RCTs
CD	Child skill training	A	Most effective in addition to above

A = consistent, good-quality patient-oriented evidence; B = inconsistent or limited-quality patient-oriented evidence; C = consensus, disease-oriented evidence, usual practice, expert opinion, or case series; CD = conduct disorder; ODD = oppositional defiant disorder.
For information about the Strength of Recommendation Taxonomy evidence rating system, see *www.aafp.org/afpsort.xml*.

In well-designed trials drug therapy has not been shown to be helpful for ODD or CD, except when these disorders are present with comorbid ADHD. Most experts recommend treatment for other comorbid disorders to maximize success in the treatment of ODD or CD, especially depression and anxiety. A variety of drugs are commonly used for CD, including α-blockers (e.g., clonidine), mood stabilizers (lithium, carbamazepine, valproic acid), antipsychotics, and antidepressants (51,52,56).

LANGUAGE AND LEARNING DISORDERS

Language and learning disorders (LLD) very often co-occur with ADHD and disorders of conduct and should be considered in the differential diagnosis of any child with learning, behavior, or attention problems. Disorders of expressive (speaking) or receptive (understanding) language require delays in these areas not due to sensory or motor deficit or environmental deprivation. These delays must be in excess of those expected by nonverbal intelligence scores. Learning disorders (specific to reading or math) likewise require an IQ-achievement discrepancy (30). That is to say that a child with average intelligence who is reading several years behind grade level may have a reading disability. The diagnosis of any LLD requires significant impairment in school functioning. As with disorders of behavior, learning styles exist along a continuum. All people have learning strengths and weaknesses. Children not meeting criteria for disabilities often fail to receive the individualized attention required to meet their potential in school. Family physicians should encourage parents and children to understand a child's learning style, seek positive reinforcement for strengths, and help with weaknesses. Children at all levels of educational success can benefit from private tutoring and enrichment programs that meet the child's needs and strengths.

Children with LLD not only struggle to meet their academic potential, but may also have disorders of behavior, low self-esteem, and axis I psychiatric disorders. Half of children with LLD have axis I disorders, most commonly ADHD, anxiety, and depression (57). Three fourths of children with learning disabilities have social skill deficits (58). In the classroom, they have less on-task behavior, more off-task behavior, more conduct disorder, more distractibility, and more withdrawn behavior (59). As many as one in five children has a LLD, and 10% of US children receive special education services, over half for learning disabilities and one-fourth for language disabilities (57).

More than other disorders in this chapter, the diagnosis of LLD often requires specialized testing not commonly performed by a family physician. However, the family physician may be the first to consider the possibility of an LLD. She may be in the best position to make a referral or advocate for school-based testing. She may also manage other comorbid conditions (such as ADHD) and coordinate the overall mental health treatment plan for the child. Family physicians can assist families by teaching them about their rights under IDEA. Family physicians may assist families by attending individualized education plan meetings. Last, as mentioned previously, the diagnosis of all LLDs requires that the condition occur in excess of any sensory or motor impairment. For example, a child with hearing loss may have either an expressive or receptive delay in language because of the hearing condition alone. Correction of a hearing condition may improve the language disorder.

Initial Evaluation

In the context of school difficulty, the family physician should inquire about onset, severity, and context. What are the parents' concerns? Have they discussed these with the child's teacher? Teachers are often the first to notice and diagnose a specific disorder of learning. Records from school (report cards) and any prior psychological testing should be obtained. A thorough developmental, educational, social, and family history is important. A physical exam, with attention to sensory systems and a general neurological exam should be performed. Hearing and vision screening can identify sensory disorders early. Is there is a particular subject of difficulty (e.g., reading)? If a child is inattentive and the physician is considering a diagnosis of ADHD, asking about multiple settings is essential. LLDs often affect attention and behavior at school only.

The diagnosis of LLD is done predominantly through specialized testing by a speech pathologist and/or psychologist. Tests are normalized for age, include IQ tests and specialized testing of reading, mathematics, receptive, and expressive language. Tests must be culturally and linguistically appropriate.

Management

Children with a diagnosis of LLD qualify for specialized services in public schools including an individualized education plan. Parents and physicians may need to advocate for these services. Most treatment occurs in the school setting. There is an increasing evidence base about effective treatment strategies, including reading programs, summer school, one-on-one instruction, and self-concept interventions (60–64). The family physician can help parents identify local community resources to optimize the educational environment for a child.

EATING DISORDERS

Eating disorders are a group of conditions that involve dysfunctional eating habits, body image disturbance, and change in weight (65). The pathogenesis of eating disorders remains unclear. Environmental factors, social factors, psychological predisposition, and biological vulnerability may all play a role (66). Aggregation of eating disorders in families points to the possibility of a genetic predisposition as well (66). Eating disorders remain more common in industrialized countries where there is a cultural value placed on thinness. However, they are being seen in increasing rates in developing countries as well. Within the United States, eating disorders are being seen at increasing rates among very young patients, male patients, patients of color, and patients of low socioeconomic status.

Eating disorders include anorexia nervosa (AN), bulimia nervosa (BN), eating disorder not otherwise specified (EDNOS), and binge eating disorder. Patients with anorexia nervosa refuse to maintain even a minimally normal body weight, have intense fear of gaining weight or becoming fat despite being underweight, and exhibit disturbance in the perception of the shape or size of their bodies (30). Amenorrhea will be present in postmenarchal women. A minimally normal body weight is generally considered to be 85% of the normal weight for age and height. Weight loss is generally accomplished via restricted caloric intake. Some patients will lose weight by excess exercising purging behaviors (30).

Patients with BN exhibit recurrent episodes of binge eating with recurrent inappropriate compensatory behaviors to prevent weight gain. BN patients feel a sense of lack of control over their binge eating. Compensatory behaviors include vomiting; use of laxatives, diuretics, enemas, or diet pills; fasting; and excessive exercise. To meet diagnostic criteria for BN, the binge eating and compensatory behaviors must occur at least twice a week for at least 3 months. The patient's self-esteem must be excessively influenced by her body image (30).

EDNOS occurs when a patient has many eating disorder symptoms but does not meet criteria for classic AN or BN. This may occur when a patient meets criteria for AN but does not have amenorrhea (30). Similarly, a patient may meet criteria for anorexia nervosa but be above 85% of normal body weight if she started at a very high weight. Other individuals with EDNOS may meet criteria for bulimia nervosa, but with binge eating and compensatory behaviors less often than twice per week for 3 months. Others may perform compensatory behaviors after eating only small amounts of food. EDNOS should be considered a serious disorder that causes significant suffering and is potentially life threatening.

Binge eating disorder is a form of EDNOS that involves binge eating without regular compensatory behaviors. Binge eating disorder will result in varying degrees of obesity. Patients may report that their eating or weight has negatively affected their relationships, their work, and their self-esteem. Binge eating disorder is a newly recognized distinct entity without widely accepted diagnostic criteria.

The lifetime risk for AN is 0.3% to 1% for women (67). The rate of AN in men is about one-tenth of that seen in women. Eating disorders are most common in the adolescent age group, with 40% occurring between age 15 and 19 years (68). The prevalence of bulimia nervosa is about 1% for females and 0.1% for males. The prevalence of binge eating disorder is estimated to be about 1% for females and males. Because there are no clear diagnostic standards for EDNOS and there is a wide heterogeneity of symptoms, the prevalence remains unknown.

Initial Evaluation

A patient with disordered eating may present with symptoms related to almost any organ system. Occasionally, the patient or a family member may express concern about weight loss, weight gain, disordered eating, or purging. More often, presenting complaints are physical, such as abdominal pain or syncope, or psychological, such as irritability, depression, or sleep disturbance. Often the patient will have seen multiple providers and may have had significant medical work-ups for their symptoms.

History and physical is the cornerstone to making the diagnosis of an eating disorder. Appropriate history and physical exam can often spare the patient a potentially invasive workup for their medical complaints. There is no routine laboratory panel that will help to diagnose an eating disorder. In healthy young people, laboratory studies often remain normal until disease is advanced. Nevertheless, there are laboratory abnormalities that are often seen in the presence of disordered eating or purging behaviors as shown in Table 49.7.

TABLE 49.7 Laboratory Abnormalities Commonly Seen in Patients with Disordered Eating

Weight Loss
- Decreased white blood cell count
- Decreased red blood cell count
- Increased AST or ALT
- Hypercholesterolemia
- Hypernatremia
- Increased BUN and creatinine
- Normal albumin and protein

Purging

Vomiting
- Hypochloremic, hypokalemic, metabolic alkalosis
- Increased amylase

Laxatives
- Metabolic acidosis
- Hypocalcemia

Diuretics
- Hyponatremia
- Hypomagnesemia
- Increased or decreased potassium

AST = aspartate aminotransferase; ALT = alanine aminotransferase; BUN = blood urea nitrogen.

Gastrointestinal symptoms are often severe and may be an area of intense focus by the patient. Food restriction and/or purging can lead to gastroparesis, gastroesophageal reflux disease, severe constipation, cathartic colon syndrome, gallstone disease, and ruptured esophagus. Cardiovascular complications can include arrhythmia, prolonged QT interval, mitral valve prolapse, bradycardia, hypotension, and heart failure. Neurological complications that can be seen on magnetic resonance imaging include enlarged ventricles and decreased cortical substance. Although both white and gray matter decreases during severe weight loss, only white matter returns to premorbid levels after weight gain. Loss of gray matter can persist (69).

Disordered eating can affect the endocrine system in several ways. Hypothalamic activation occurs from a high stress state. Levels of ACTH, cortisol, growth hormone, prolactin, epinephrine, norepinephrine, interleukin-1, interleukin-2, and tumor necrosis factor all increase. Hypothalamic abnormalities in thermoregulation occur. As bone remodeling decreases, the risk of osteoporosis increases. The role of oral contraceptives in restoring bone density in patients with disordered eating remains unclear. Dual-energy x-ray absorptiometry of bone is generally recommended. Documentation of osteopenia may be helpful to motivate patients in their recovery (70).

Decreased gonadotropin releasing hormone leads to a decrease in leuteinizing hormone and follicle-stimulating hormone to prepubertal levels. Because these hormonal changes occur due to stress, up to 70% of patients with amenorrhea secondary to disordered eating lose their menstrual cycles before significant weight loss.

Management

Initial management of the patient with disordered eating should focus on correcting any immediate health risks. An electrocardiogram should be done to rule out prolonged QT interval. The remainder of the initial workup should be tailored to the findings in the history and physical exam. After the patient is stabilized, treatment should focus on weight restoration. Refeeding with electrolyte replacement will often be indicated. Hospitalization is indicated for refeeding in the face of severe malnutrition, as well as in the presence of any significant hemodynamic compromise or electrolyte abnormality. Hospitalization may also be necessary for patients with poor motivation, suicidal ideation, severe psychiatric disease, or a difficult home environment, especially if abuse is present (70).

After initial stabilization has occurred, a treatment team can be established. Such a team will often include a therapist, nutritionist, and primary care physician. Treatment requires the establishment of a trusting long-term relationship with the patient. Often the family needs to be involved, particularly for patients younger than 18 years of age.

There may be some role for psychopharmacology in the treatment of eating disorders. Selective serotonin reuptake inhibitors (SSRIs) may help to decrease binging behavior, particularly in high doses. Selective serotonin reuptake inhibitors have not been shown to improve or hasten weight gain in starved patients (71,72). Psychiatric symptoms often improve with weight gain, as the psychological effects of malnutrition decline. Thus, after some weight gain has occurred, it may be useful to treat remaining symptoms with psychotropic medications. Treatment of residual psychiatric symptoms may help to prevent relapse. Several small, open-label studies have shown that low dose atypical antipsychotic agents may improve weight gain and depression in patients with eating disorders (73–75).

Long-term Monitoring

For most individuals suffering from them, eating disorders tend to be long-term, chronic diseases. Mortality rates are 5% to 6% for both anorexia nervosa and bulimia nervosa. When death occurs it is usually due to frank starvation, purge-related arrhythmia, or suicide. In patients with anorexia nervosa, about half will recover and do well over time in regard to their body weight and nutritional status. Another 30% will do quite well but continue to have symptoms. Unfortunately the remaining 20% will do poorly. With bulimia nervosa 50% of patients achieve full recovery within 2 years. However, 20% to 46% will continue to have symptoms after 6 years of treatment (76).

KEY POINTS

- Broadly considered, disorders of behavior and development are among the most common conditions of childhood.
- Family physicians need to consider the developmental needs and goals of children at all stages to identify children likely to require follow-up or specialty referral.
- Many children with developmental and behavioral needs will have limited or no early access to school services and a yearly check up may be the only opportunity to identify these issues in early childhood.
- Children in school or childcare with parent expressed concerns regarding behavior or development will usually require data collection from multiple sources to establish a diagnosis.
- ADHD is the most common neurodevelopmental disorder of childhood.
- Treatment of behavioral and developmental disorders will often require referral and care coordination with the school system, mental health, occupational therapy, physical therapy, and other child health professionals.

CHAPTER

50

Depression

Donald E. Nease, Jr.

CLINICAL OBJECTIVES

1. Discuss the prevalence of depression in primary care.
2. Describe a strategy for initial assessment and treatment of a patient with possible depression.
3. Discuss commonly used antidepressants and their use.
4. Describe a strategy for long-term monitoring of patients being treated for depression.

More than just sadness, the clinical syndromes that fit under the grouping of depression are complex entities associated with significant impacts on quality of life. The various depressive or mood disorders are defined by diagnostic criteria set forth in the Diagnostic and Statistical Manual of Mental Disorders, Fourth Edition, Text Revision (DSM) of the American Psychiatric Association (1). The most common disorders and their diagnostic criteria are listed in Tables 50.1 through 50.5.

Depression is highly prevalent within the general population. In 1 year, mood disorders will be experienced by 9.5% of adults, major depressive disorder (MDD) by 6.7% and bipolar disorders by 2.6% (2). Depression is important in primary care not only because of its high prevalence, but also because primary care is often the only source of care for patients suffering from this condition (3). Depression substantially affects patient well-being and function. In addition, it is costly, responsible for an estimated $26.1 billion in direct medical costs and $51.5 billion in workplace costs in the year 2000 (4).

There is increasing evidence of the impact of depression on other chronic medical conditions such as coronary artery disease and diabetes (5–7). The high incidence of depression in the post-myocardial infarction (post-MI) patient and the negative effect of comorbid depression on post-MI outcomes prompted the American Academy of Family Physicians to develop and publish a specific guideline on the detection and management of post-MI depression (8).

Finally, although primary care patients are occasionally diagnosed and successfully treated for a single, limited episode of depression, the vast majority of patients with a diagnosis of depression seen by family physicians experience it as a chronic illness with periods of recovery and relapse.

Family physicians should maintain a high level of watchfulness for symptoms or functional impairment suggestive of depression. Unfortunately, recognizing depression in primary care is complicated because patients often present with somatic complaints (e.g., palpitations, abdominal pain, fatigue) (9). Other factors that may contribute to under-recognition of depression in primary care include concern about labeling with a mental health diagnosis (10), the burden of many competing demands in primary care (11–13), and patients' own attributions about the source of their symptoms (14). Tiredness or fatigue as a presenting complaint should trigger the clinician to suspect depression, whereas agitation or difficulty maintaining concentration may indicate the presence of an anxiety disorder. Prolonged somatic symptoms that do not appear to have a recognizable, physiologic etiology and do not resolve with several weeks of watchful waiting may indicate the presence of depression. Pursue any suspicion that depression may be present with careful, yet tactful, questioning to confirm or rule out the diagnosis.

In patients 18 to 65 years of age, depressive disorders ranked among the top 10 diagnoses by family physicians according to the 2002 National Ambulatory Medical Care Survey (15), and there is no reason to expect this has changed. Prevalence estimates of depression within primary care patients range from 6% to 9%, with up to 50% of these being unrecognized (16), indicating that in a busy practice of 20 to 30 patient visits a day, as many as 2 to 3 may be depressed, of which one or more may be undiagnosed. Therefore, the importance of clinical suspicion cannot be overemphasized.

DIAGNOSIS

Depression has been traditionally diagnosed on the basis of clinical suspicion and confirmation using DSM criteria. However, evidence of high rates of unrecognized depression has led experts to evaluate the effectiveness of routine screening. The US Preventive Services Task Force updated its recommendations for depression screening in 2009, recommending "screening adults for depression when staff-assisted depression care supports are in place to assure accurate diagnosis, effective treatment, and follow-up," but against *routinely* screening when staff-assisted depression care supports are not in place (17,18). The UK National Institute for Clinical Excellence also updated its recommendations in 2009, calling for alertness to "possible depression (particularly in people with a past history of depression or a chronic physical health problem with associated functional impairment)" (19). A 2005 Cochrane review concluded that general screening for depression did not improve outcomes, although that review excluded studies that included quality improvement or care management strategies (20). These somewhat conflicting recommendations highlight the importance of

TABLE 50.1 Diagnostic Criteria for Major Depression

Criteria for an Episode of Major Depression

A. Five (or more) of the following symptoms have been present during the same 2-week period and represent a change from previous functioning; at least one of the symptoms is either (1) depressed mood or (2) loss of interest or pleasure.
Note: Do not include symptoms that are clearly from a general medical condition, or mood-incongruent delusions or hallucinations.
  (1) Depressed mood most of the day, nearly every day, as indicated by either subjective report (e.g., feels sad or empty) or observation made by others (e.g., appears tearful).
  Note: In children and adolescents, can be irritable mood.
  (2) Markedly diminished interest or pleasure in all, or almost all, activities most of the day, nearly every day (as indicated by either subjective account or observation made by others).
  (3) Significant weight loss when not dieting or weight gain (e.g., a change of more than 5% of body weight in a month), or decrease or increase in appetite nearly every day.
  Note: In children, consider failure to make expected weight gains.
  (4) Insomnia or hypersomnia nearly every day.
  (5) Psychomotor agitation or retardation nearly every day (observable by others, not merely subjective feelings of restlessness or being slowed down).
  (6) Fatigue or loss of energy nearly every day.
  (7) Feelings of worthlessness or excessive or inappropriate guilt (which may be delusional) nearly every day (not merely self-reproach or guilt about being sick).
  (8) Diminished ability to think or concentrate, or indecisiveness, nearly every day (either by subjective account or as observed by others).
  (9) Recurrent thoughts of death (not just fear of dying), recurrent suicidal ideation without a specific plan, or a suicide attempt or a specific plan for committing suicide.

B. The symptoms do not meet criteria for a mixed episode.
C. The symptoms cause clinically significant distress or impairment in social, occupational, or other important areas of functioning.
D. The symptoms are not due to the direct physiological effects of a substance (e.g., a drug of abuse, a medication) or a general medical condition (e.g., hypothyroidism).
E. The symptoms are not better accounted for by bereavement (i.e., after the loss of a loved one), the symptoms persist for longer than 2 months, or are characterized by marked functional impairment, morbid preoccupation with worthlessness, suicidal ideation, psychotic symptoms, or psychomotor retardation.

Criteria for Major Depressive Disorder, Single Episode

A. Presence of a single major depressive episode.
B. The major depressive episode is not better accounted for by schizoaffective disorder and is not superimposed on schizophrenia, schizophreniform disorder, delusional disorder, or psychotic disorder not otherwise specified.
C. There has never been a manic episode, a mixed episode, or a hypomanic episode.
Note: This exclusion does not apply if all of the manic-like, mixed-like, or hypomanic-like episodes are substance or treatment-induced or are due to the direct physiological effects of a general medical condition.

Criteria for Major Depressive Disorder, Recurrent

A. Presence of two or more major depressive episodes.
Note: To be considered separate episodes, there must be an interval of at least 2 consecutive months in which criteria are not met for a major depressive episode.
B. The major depressive episodes are not better accounted for by schizoaffective disorder and are not superimposed on schizophrenia, schizophreniform disorder, delusional disorder, or psychotic disorder not otherwise specified.
C. There has never been a manic episode, a mixed episode, or a hypomanic episode.
Note: This exclusion does not apply if all of the manic-like, mixed-like, or hypomanic-like episodes are substance or treatment-induced or are due to the direct physiological effects of a general medical condition.

systems that ensure proper monitoring and follow-up. As will be discussed later, these are mainstays of proper depression treatment. Where screening is implemented, use of the Patient Health Questionnaire (PHQ)-2 (21), which assesses the first two DSM depression symptoms, is advantageous because of its brevity and ease of confirmation with a full PHQ-9 (22).

In all situations, maintaining a high index of suspicion, particularly in those at increased risk for depression, is vital. Significant risk factors include a history of depression, significant physical illness causing disability, substance abuse, and other mental health problems. Experienced clinicians use a variety of clinical clues to help them determine the presence of depression (23). The following clues suggest depression:

TABLE 50.2 Diagnostic Criteria for Dysthymic Disorder

A. Depressed mood for most of the day, for more days than not, as indicated either by subjective account or observation by others, for at least 2 years.
   Note: In children and adolescents, mood can be irritable and duration must be at least 1 year.
B. Presence, while depressed, of two (or more) of the following:
   (1) poor appetite or overeating
   (2) insomnia or hypersomnia
   (3) low energy or fatigue
   (4) low self-esteem
   (5) poor concentration or difficulty making decisions
   (6) feelings of hopelessness
C. During the 2-year period (1 year for children or adolescents) of the disturbance, the person has never been without the symptoms in Criteria A and B for more than 2 months at a time.
D. No Major Depressive Episode has been present during the first 2 years of the disturbance (1 year for children and adolescents); i.e., the disturbance is not better accounted for by chronic major depressive disorder, or major depressive disorder, in partial remission.
   Note: There may have been a previous major depressive episode provided there was a full remission (no significant signs or symptoms for 2 months) before development of the dysthymic disorder. In addition, after the initial 2 years (1 year in children or adolescents) of dysthymic disorder, there may be superimposed episodes of major depressive disorder, in which case both diagnoses may be given when the criteria are met for a major depressive episode.
E. There has never been a manic episode, a mixed episode, or a hypomanic episode, and criteria have never been met for cyclothymic disorder.
F. The disturbance does not occur exclusively during the course of a chronic psychotic disorder, such as schizophrenia or delusional disorder.
G The symptoms are not due to the direct physiological effects of a substance (e.g., a drug of abuse, a medication) or a general medical condition (e.g., hypothyroidism).
H. The symptoms cause clinically significant distress or impairment in social, occupational, or other important areas of functioning.

TABLE 50.3 Diagnostic Criteria for Mood Disorder from . . . [Indicate the General Medical Condition]

A. A prominent and persistent disturbance in mood predominates in the clinical picture and is characterized by either (or both) of the following:
   (1) depressed mood or markedly diminished interest or pleasure in all, or almost all, activities
   (2) elevated, expansive, or irritable mood
B. There is evidence from the history, physical examination, or laboratory findings that the disturbance is the direct physiological consequence of a general medical condition, such as myocardial infarction, stroke, or cancer.
C. The disturbance is not better accounted for by another mental disorder (e.g., adjustment disorder with depressed mood in response to the stress of having a general medical condition).
D. The disturbance does not occur exclusively during the course of a delirium.
E. The symptoms cause clinically significant distress or impairment in social, occupational, or other important areas of functioning.

- Complaints that involve multiple organ systems or are physiologically unrelated
- Emotional flatness, or worry that is not consistent with the severity of the presenting problem
- Sleep disturbance that is persistent or unrelated to obvious stressors
- Frequent office visits for unclear or seemingly minor complaints
- Frequent emergency room visits for unexplained physical symptoms
- Patients who are "difficult" for unclear reasons
- Patients who express thoughts or emotions that are inappropriate to the context
- Patients with a previous history of emotional disturbances or "nervous breakdowns"

In situations in which a specific DSM diagnosis is important for treatment or billing decisions, use the diagnostic criteria from the DSM as listed in Tables 50.1 through 50.5.

Differential Diagnosis

Because depression often presents as a manifestation of an underlying medical condition, the patient with depressive symptoms should undergo a careful medical evaluation. If the patient has recently suffered a major illness, consider whether the depressive symptoms are secondary. Medications should

TABLE 50.4 Diagnostic Criteria for Bipolar II Disorder

Criteria for Hypomanic Episode

A. A distinct period of persistently elevated, expansive, or irritable mood, lasting throughout at least 4 days, that is clearly different from the usual nondepressed mood.
B. During the period of mood disturbance, three (or more) of the following symptoms have persisted (four if the mood is only irritable) and have been present to a significant degree:
   (1) inflated self-esteem or grandiosity
   (2) decreased need for sleep (e.g., feels rested after only 3 hours of sleep)
   (3) more talkative than usual or pressure to keep talking
   (4) flight of ideas or subjective experience that thoughts are racing
   (5) distractibility (i.e., attention too easily drawn to unimportant or irrelevant external stimuli)
   (6) increase in goal-directed activity (either socially, at work or school, or sexually) or psychomotor agitation
   (7) excessive involvement in pleasurable activities that have a high potential for painful consequences (e.g., the person engages in unrestrained buying sprees, sexual indiscretions, or foolish business investments)
C. The episode is associated with an unequivocal change in functioning that is uncharacteristic of the person when not symptomatic.
D. The disturbance in mood and the change in functioning are observable by others.
E. The episode is not severe enough to cause marked impairment in social or occupational functioning, or to necessitate hospitalization, and there are no psychotic features.
F. The symptoms are not due to the direct physiological effects of a substance (e.g., a drug of abuse, a medication, or other treatment) or a general medical condition (e.g., hyperthyroidism).
   Note: Hypomanic-like episodes that are clearly caused by somatic antidepressant treatment (e.g., medication, electroconvulsive therapy, light therapy) should not count toward a diagnosis of Bipolar II Disorder.

Criteria for Bipolar II Disorder

A. Presence (or history) of one or more major depressive episodes.
B. Presence (or history) of at least one hypomanic episode.
C. There has never been a manic episode or a mixed episode.
D. The mood symptoms in Criteria A and B are not better accounted for by schizoaffective disorder and are not superimposed on schizophrenia, schizophreniform disorder, delusional disorder, or psychotic disorder not otherwise specified.
E. The symptoms cause clinically significant distress or impairment in social, occupational, or other important areas of functioning.

TABLE 50.5 Criteria for Seasonal Pattern Specifier

With Seasonal Pattern (can be applied to the pattern of major depressive episodes in bipolar I disorder, bipolar II disorder, or major depressive disorder, recurrent)

A. There has been a regular temporal relationship between the onset of major depressive episodes in bipolar I or bipolar II disorder or major depressive disorder, recurrent, and a particular time of the year (e.g., regular appearance of the major depressive episode in the fall or winter).
   Note: Do not include cases in which there is an obvious effect of seasonal-related psychosocial stressors (e.g., regularly being unemployed every winter).
B. Full remissions (or a change from depression to mania or hypomania) also occur at a characteristic time of the year (e.g., depression disappears in the spring).
C. In the last 2 years, two major depressive episodes have occurred that demonstrate the temporal seasonal relationships defined in Criteria A and B, and no nonseasonal major depressive episodes have occurred during that same period.
D. Seasonal major depressive episodes (as described previously) substantially outnumber the nonseasonal major depressive episodes that may have occurred over the individual's lifetime.

TABLE 50.6 Medications that often Cause or Worsen Depression

Category	Examples
Drugs of abuse	Alcohol Amphetamines Cocaine Marijuana
Steroid hormones	Prednisone (or any glucocorticoids) Oral contraceptives
Psychoactive drugs	Opiate analgesics (e.g., codeine) Sedative-hypnotics (e.g., triazolam) Barbiturates Anxiolytics (e.g., diazepam)
Antihistamines	Chlorpheniramine Diphenhydramine
Cancer chemotherapy	

TABLE 50.7 Red Flags Suggesting More Serious or Complex Disease in Patients Presenting with Depression

Red Flag	Significance
Personal or family history of mania, hypomania, or formal diagnosis of bipolar disorder	Consider a diagnosis of bipolar disorder
Personal or family history of substance abuse	Screen for co-occurring substance abuse disorder
Prominent anxiety symptoms	Consider co-occurring diagnosis of an anxiety disorder and/or management of anxiety symptoms as antidepressant is taking effect.

also be considered as a potential cause of depressive symptoms. Table 50.6 provides a list of medications frequently associated with depression. Note that β-blocker medications are no longer included in this list (24). If medications are suspected of contributing to depression, minimize their use. Be on the alert for substance abuse, mania, hypomania, or anxiety.

After reviewing underlying medical conditions and medications as potential causes, next consider whether the symptoms may be secondary to another psychiatric condition, particularly substance abuse. Although some guidelines suggest that treating depression is extremely difficult in the face of a substance abuse condition (16), several studies have shown that this is not necessarily the case (25–28).

In considering a specific diagnosis for your patient, remember that anxiety and depressive disorders overlap, with many patients meeting criteria for both. In fact, patients meeting criteria for a depressive disorder may have a symptom profile that favors an anxiety disorder (29). Finally, when considering a diagnosis of depression, assess for a personal or family history of mania and symptoms that may suggest bipolar disorder. This is important for two reasons. Patients with hypomania or bipolar disorder type I are at high risk for developing acute mania if treated with a selective serotonin reuptake inhibitor. Additionally, bipolar disorder type II patients may be resistant to more commonly prescribed antidepressants (30).

Common Depressive Disorders in Primary Care

MAJOR DEPRESSIVE DISORDER

An illness often experienced as chronic and relapsing, MDD may cause significant impairment over the lives of those who experience the illness. Initial episodes often occur in adolescence; however, MDD sometimes first develops late in life. Periods of exacerbation of MDD are marked by anhedonia, feelings of failure, inability to think positively about current life events or the future, and suicidal thoughts. Both genetic and environmental influences increase an individual's risk of MDD (31). Periods of remission can last years, during which patients lead quite normal lives. Stressful life events can be associated with relapse (32–34). Table 50.7 lists red flags suggesting more serious or complex disease in patients presenting with depression.

TABLE 50.8 Operating Characteristics of the PHQ-2 and PHQ-9 in Primary Care

Scale	Probability of Depression when Score is Above Threshold	
PHQ-2 (21)	MDD	Any Depressive Disorder
Score of 3 or greater (MDD LR+ 2.9)	38.4%	75%
PHQ-9 (22)		
Score of 10 or greater (MDD LR+ 7.1)	34.9%	67.9%

LR+ = positive likelihood ratio; tests with higher values, especially >5, are good at ruling in disease; LR− = negative likelihood ratio; tests with lower values, especially <0.2, are good at ruling out disease; MDD = major depressive disorder.

MOOD DISORDER SECONDARY TO A GENERAL MEDICAL CONDITION

Many chronic medical conditions have a significant impact on patients' affect and sense of well-being. Patients who have recently suffered an MI, stroke, trauma, hospitalization, or a diagnosis of cancer are at risk for development of depression. This can present in the same way as MDD, and is often difficult to distinguish from a primary depressive disorder. Although improvement of the underlying medical condition may be enough to resolve the depressive symptoms, specific treatment of the depressive symptoms is often needed.

DYSTHYMIA

This disorder is generally less severe than MDD, yet is more resistant to treatment. Patients with dysthymia experience a persistent, chronic depressed mood that is less likely to be relieved by periods of remission or by antidepressant treatment.

BIPOLAR DISORDER, TYPE II

Bipolar disorder has gained recent prominence because it appears to be more common in primary care than had been previously reported (35,36). The diagnosis of bipolar type II disorder is easy to overlook because it only requires the presence of one hypomanic episode along with features of a MDD diagnosis.

SEASONAL PATTERNS

The most recent revision of the DSM, DSM IV-TR, has subsumed the diagnosis of seasonal affective disorder under the *Seasonal Pattern Specifier* designation within MDD and bipolar disorder. A seasonal pattern should be suspected when patients present with depressive symptoms during winter months in regions that experience a marked decrease in ambient light during the winter. Symptoms of hypersomnia, hyperphagia, and psychomotor slowing are also part of the symptom complex. A history of remission during the summer months is helpful in making the diagnosis. These patients often respond to high-intensity light therapy; therefore, pharmacologic treatment is reserved for cases that are severe or are resistant to phototherapy.

History and Physical Examination

If initial clinical clues cause you to suspect depression, discuss it with the patient as part of the differential diagnosis. When the clinician fails to discuss concerns about depression, initially, proceeding instead with an intensive biomedical evaluation, the patient may assume there is a "physical" cause of his or her symptoms and later have difficulty accepting a diagnosis of depression. If, instead, you open the door early to considering depression or anxiety in a nonjudgmental fashion, patients will often admit to having a concern themselves. For this reason, it is helpful to develop a way of introducing the possibility early in the discussion of a patient's illness. For example, "Just as physical symptoms sometimes have what people think of as a 'medical' cause, physical symptoms are often caused by stress or other fears. It is important that we keep an open mind about the role these may play in your symptoms. Have you wondered about whether stress or similar issues might be causing your symptoms?"

This discussion can be effectively augmented by use of screening questions such as those contained in the PHQ-2, "Over the last 2 weeks, how often have you been bothered by any of the following problems: (i) little interest or pleasure in doing things, and (ii) feeling down, depressed, or hopeless?" A positive response to either of these items should be followed up by a full assessment for MDD (21).

Diagnostic Testing

After a depressive disorder is suspected and initially explored via discussion and the PHQ-2 questions, evaluation should proceed in a logical fashion. Unfortunately, laboratory evaluation is not usually helpful except to rule out suspected contributing or underlying medical conditions. However, a formal evaluation of the patient using the DSM criteria for depression should be performed. The DSM criteria may be rapidly assessed using the nine-item PHQ-9 (22). A downloadable version of the PHQ-9 with scoring instructions is available at the MacArthur Initiative on Depression in Primary Care website (*www.depression-primarycare.org/clinicians/toolkits/materials/forms/phq9/*). The PHQ-9 is particularly useful because it permits a simultaneous assessment of both DSM criteria and severity (37), and therefore can be used as a guide to treatment and management both in the initial assessment and for monitoring purposes. The questionnaire can be completed by most patients in 3 minutes or less (22) and quickly scored by adding up the responses. Table 50.8 displays the operating characteristics of both the PHQ-2 and PHQ-9.

TREATMENT

Effective management of a patient with depression should proceed through stages of discussion and shared agreement on the diagnosis, preferred treatment modalities, plans for follow-up, monitoring, and duration of treatment.

A strong, trusting relationship and a therapeutic alliance between the physician and patient is the foundation for managing depression. This has been shown in referral populations (38,39), and is reasonable to infer in family medicine. A strong therapeutic alliance facilitates discussion and development of a diagnosis, choice and monitoring of treatment modalities, discussion of referral if needed, and agreement on long-term treatment when necessary. In other words, it is important to emphasize early your commitment to see the patient through the treatment, even if you decide at some point that referral is necessary.

This initial discussion also lays the groundwork for the supportive counseling and education that is a cornerstone of treatment. Much of this activity is undocumented and, therefore, difficult to study in terms of its effectiveness (40). However, it is in this context that much of the primary care treatment of depression occurs.

If the depression is secondary to an underlying medical condition, supportive counseling in the context of treatment for the underlying condition is always appropriate. Beyond this, encouraging the patient to seek out a local support group for people suffering from the condition may also be helpful. If the depression is severe enough to interfere with the patient's daily life or ability to participate in treatment of the medical condition, specific pharmacologic treatment should be initiated. The PHQ-9 (mentioned previously) can be useful in guiding decisions about pharmacologic versus psychotherapeutic treatment modalities. Generally, initial PHQ-9 scores of 15 or above should steer the decision to include pharmacologic treatment.

Answer any questions patients may have about their diagnosis because a mental health diagnosis often carries with it fears of "losing one's mind" or "being crazy." Additionally, patients' beliefs about their depression and the need for medication shape their likelihood of adherence to treatment, and skepticism is strongest in younger patients (41,42). You should give reassurance and emphasize the effectiveness of treatment. Several books are available to help patients understand their condition. Two excellent ones are: *Feeling Good: The New Mood Therapy* by David Burns (43) and *How to Heal Depression* by Harold Bloomfield and Peter McWilliams (44). For patients with Internet access, the National Institute of Mental Health web site (www.nimh.nih.gov) has excellent information for patients about depression and its treatment. National Institute of Mental Health also has excellent patient education brochures that are available for download or purchase.

Finally, your initial discussions with patients should set the stage for self-management activities. Self-management is a cornerstone of chronic illness care (45) and depression is no exception. For patients with depression, self-management takes the form of encouraging patients to re-engage in activities that were formerly enjoyable or common parts of their daily routine (46). Patients should be encouraged to start reintroducing activities at a comfortable pace while also pushing themselves somewhat. These self-management activities are useful in goal setting and provide touch points for discussion at follow-up visits.

Assessment of Suicide Risk

Risk factors for suicide are listed in Table 50.9. An open discussion of suicidal thoughts does not increase the likelihood that patients will act on their thoughts, but does give you a chance to intervene if needed. Because the PHQ-9 includes a question on suicidal thoughts, this may facilitate identification and discussion of the topic. Patients may feel shame about having thoughts that they might be better off by ending their pain. When these thoughts are disclosed, you should remind them that most, if not all, patients with depression experience them. When several risk factors for suicide are present, consider referral to a mental health specialist.

Patients who have considered a specific plan for suicide or have made a suicidal gesture should be referred to a mental health specialist for rapid evaluation. Patients at high risk of suicide often experience suicidal thoughts as intrusive and express an inability to control them. Therefore, they may require escorting to an emergency room with mental health specialists on staff. Telephone contact between the family physician and the receiving specialist is essential to convey the specific statements of the patient that are eliciting concern.

Choice of Treatment Modality

The primary, proven modalities of depression treatment are prescription medication and formal psychotherapy. The choice of either single or combination therapy is one that should be made with your patient after considering the severity of the depression. Table 50.10 summarizes the evidence for the common treatments.

TABLE 50.9 Factors Increasing the Risk of Suicide in Depressed Patients*

1. Increased age (>70 years in men, 60 in women)
2. Gender (women make more attempts; men are more often successful)
3. Poor social support
4. Lack of marital support and absence of children
5. Chronic physical illness or chronic pain
6. Alcoholism or substance abuse
7. History of prior attempts
8. Specific plan or explicit communication about intent
9. Family history of successful suicide

*Several risk factors together are particularly significant; for example, a recently widowed, 70-year-old man who drinks excessively is an extremely high suicide risk and requires specific assessment.

Selecting an Antidepressant Medication

Medication should be initiated when:

- symptoms have been present for more than 1 month,
- symptoms result in significant interference with ability to function at work or home, or
- score on the PHQ-9 is 15 or greater.

Fortunately, your decisions about which medication to use do not need to be based on considerations of efficacy. Instead, you should base your choice primarily on adverse effects, potential for drug interactions and considerations of cost and insurer formularies. First-generation antidepressants include tricyclic antidepressants (TCAs) and monoamine oxidase inhibitors (MAOIs). TCAs and MAOIs are not commonly used due to their side-effect profile and consequent risk for discontinuation, and tricyclics have a relative contraindication in patients with cardiac disease. All available medications in the selective serotonin reuptake inhibitor (SSRI) classes have good rates of response to treatment for depression. Hypericum (St. John's wort) has shown evidence for efficacy in mild to moderate depression when compared with placebo (47), equal efficacy to paroxetine in one trial of moderate to severe depression (48), and may be an option for those who have a preference for a complementary substance. Finally, exercise should be encouraged for patients with depression as several studies suggest it confers additional benefit (49,50). A list of commonly prescribed antidepressants with their contraindications and/or adverse effects is provided in Table 50.11.

Points to consider when selecting a medication include:

- History of good response to previous use
- Successful use of an agent in a close relative (use by a parent or sibling may enhance compliance)
- Presence of chronic pain or severe sleep disturbance (if so, consider using a TCA)
- Coexisting medical conditions (e.g., avoid TCAs in patients with known cardiac conduction disturbances)
- Hypersomnia (if so, consider an SSRI)
- Cost

TABLE 50.10 Recommended Treatments for Depression

Intervention	Efficacy	Strength of Recommendation Taxonomy Rating*	Comment
Moderate to Severe MDD (PHQ-9 ≥ 10)			
Prescription antidepressants vs. placebo	69% of placebo users had worse outcomes than average antidepressant users over 6 weeks	A	
SSRIs vs. other antidepressants	No difference in efficacy	A	Some evidence exists that the lower side-effect profile reduces non-adherence in SSRIs
Formal psychotherapy in combination with medication	OR for improvement 1.86 (95% CI 1.38–2.52) vs. medication alone	A	
Mild to Moderate MDD (PHQ-9: 5–14)			
Cognitive therapy (CBT) and Interpersonal Therapy (IPT)	OR for recovery vs. usual care 3.4 (95% CI 2–6); IPT vs. usual care OR 3.45, (95% CI 1.91–6.51)	A	

*A = consistent, good-quality patient-oriented evidence; B = inconsistent or limited-quality patient-oriented evidence; C = consensus, disease-oriented evidence, usual practice, expert opinion, or case series.
For information about the Strength of Recommendation Taxonomy evidence rating system, see *www.aafp.org/afpsort.xml*.

Recently SSRIs have earned a "black box" warning for risk of suicidality in pediatric patients. However, although caution and close monitoring of pediatric patients taking SSRIs is certainly prudent, it should be noted that the meta-analysis of trials that raised this concern also failed to find any evidence of completed suicides in children taking SSRIs (51).

The Agency for Healthcare Research and Quality has published a comparative effectiveness guide for second-generation antidepressants, which provides a useful review of the relative efficacies and side effect profiles (*http://effectivehealthcare.ahrq.gov/index.cfm/search-for-guides-reviews-and-reports/?pageaction=displayproduct&productid=61*).

The Sequenced Treatment Alternatives to Relieve Depression (STAR*D) trial provided valuable information regarding treatment of depression in primary care (52). STAR*D was designed as a naturalistic trial, enrolling patients suspected by their treating clinicians to have depression. Patients who were indeed depressed were begun on initial treatment with citalopram and received routine monitoring. Clinicians were given feedback and coached on when to increase dosage. Roughly 30% of patients achieved remission with citalopram alone, and importantly, many required 12 to 14 weeks of treatment. Patients who did not achieve remission in the first level were enrolled in a complex randomization that also incorporated patients' own treatment preferences. At the second level, another 30% of patients experienced remission whether they were switched to a different medication (sertraline, venlafaxine, or bupropion), had another medication added (bupropion or buspirone), or were switched to or added cognitive therapy. Subsequent levels of randomization resulted in additional cumulative remission rates of 63% and 67%.

Lessons learned from STAR*D include the following. After a specific medication has been chosen, give enough time to adequately assess its effectiveness. Included in this is a willingness to increase the dose to a level at which the drug is effective. Allow 12 to 14 weeks of treatment at a maximum effective dose before abandoning the drug. If there is no response by 14 weeks, augment or switch medication and/or consider referral. It is important to emphasize to the patient that the failure of one medication does not mean that the condition is untreatable. Monitoring of patients was also key in STAR*D, and the trial demonstrated that measurement-based care is feasible in primary care. Finally, remission—not just improvement—as measured by a monitoring instrument should be the goal of treatment.

For initial episodes of depression after achieving remission, continue treatment for 9 to 12 months. At that point, consider discontinuance of the medication (via taper), but be aware that one third of MDD patients will relapse within a year. For those who do, consider chronic therapy in an effort to prevent or decrease the severity of relapses (53).

Role of Psychotherapy

Studies continue to show the effectiveness of psychotherapy in the treatment of depression (54,55). There is also evidence for enhanced relapse prevention when cognitive behavioral therapy (CBT) has been used in conjunction with medication (55,56). Occasionally, family physicians have obtained enough experience and training in brief psychotherapy to provide this to their patients, but time and poor insurance reimbursement

TABLE 50.11 Common Antidepressants

Drug	Contraindications/Cautions/ Adverse Effects	Dosage	Relative Cost*
Selective Serotonin Reuptake Inhibitors			
Fluoxetine	Initial nervousness/arousal/insomnia	20–80 mg once daily	$
Paroxetine	Drowsiness	10–50 mg once daily	$$
Sertraline	Insomnia	25–200 mg once daily	$$
Citalopram	Diarrhea	10–60 mg once daily	$$
Escitalopram		10–40 mg	$$
Other Agents			
Bupropion	Contraindicated with history of seizures, eating disorders or substance abuse	100–150 mg bid-tid	$
Mirtazapine	Drowsiness, marked weight gain	15–45 mg at bedtime	$$
Nefazodone	Black-box warning for liver disease	100–600 mg bid	$
Venlafaxine	Risk of hypertension (dose-dependant)	37.5–150 mg tid	$$
Tricyclics			
Amitriptyline	Contraindicated in patients with cardiac conduction abnormalities, benign prostatic hypertrophy, glaucoma, orthostatic hypertension and seizures/ marked sedation and anticholinergic effects	25–300 mg at bedtime	$
Nortriptyline	Contraindicated in patients with cardiac conduction abnormalities, benign prostatic hypertrophy, glaucoma, and seizures/marked sedation and anticholinergic effects	25–150 mg at bedtime	$
Trazodone	Marked drowsiness	50–600 mg at bedtime	$$
Complementary Therapy			
Hypericum	Contraindicated in conjunction with selective serotonin reuptake inhibitors	300 mg tid (0.3% standardized extract)	$$

*$ = inexpensive; $$ = moderate; $$$ = expensive.

often result in patients being referred for these treatments. It is helpful to have familiarity with therapy modalities, however. Two of the most studied therapies are briefly described below, as is problem-solving therapy that has been studied specifically in primary care.

INTERPERSONAL THERAPY

Interpersonal therapy (IPT) focuses on practical resolution of problematic interpersonal relationships or other stressful events. The therapist seeks to:

- Identify events or relationships that stimulate abnormal amounts of stress or grief
- Encourage discussions about the nature and origin of the stress reaction
- Move through strategies to resolve the stressful situation or relationship

For example, a common source of interpersonal stress is social isolation. Practical suggestions for such a situation might include calling a friend with whom the patient has lost contact, joining a social club specific to an interest the patient may have, volunteering for a community or religious group, or enrolling in adult education classes.

A common problem to which IPT is often directed is marital stress, which may be somewhat more complicated, but still benefits from engaging with an outside person (e.g., the primary care physician) in mutual problem solving. IPT may seem simplistic at times, but patients can be very appreciative of this problem-solving approach when they have lost the motivation or cognitive function to identify and resolve the source of their distress.

COGNITIVE BEHAVIORAL THERAPY

CBT is based on the observation that depressed patients suffer from an unrelenting and unjustifiably negative view of the world around them. CBT has been tested in both MDD and panic disorder patients and found to be as effective as antidepressant medication in mild to moderate disease (57). The main function of the therapist is to provide "homework" assignments to the patient. These assignments require the patient to gather and process information about his or her situation and relationships in a way that leads to new cognitive views of their surroundings, new relationships, or new social skills. This may require the therapist to provide basic information in a didactic way, such as knowledge about the origin of panic symptoms.

Therapists also teach patients new ways of self-talk—positive self-statements made before, during, and after stressful events that would normally provoke significant symptoms. Sometimes the therapist actually encourages the patient to seek stressful events, after much practice and preparation, as a way of testing new skills and achieving new levels of comfort in daily responsibilities. CBT is most successful if it is framed as exercises or assignments, the therapist is very specific about the assignments, the patient is seen frequently to provide appropriate feedback, and the patient is deeply engaged in the problem-solving process.

PROBLEM-SOLVING THERAPY

Problem-solving therapy is a recently developed therapy that is designed for the primary care setting (58). Patients are led through stages of identifying their main problems, generating solutions, and trying out these solutions. Trials show promising results in treatment of mild to moderate depression with use of this technique in the primary care outpatient setting (59–61).

Indications for Referral

Patients with a history of severe, chronic symptoms often benefit from referral. Also consider referring patients with a history of unresponsiveness to treatment, bipolar disorder, or those who are at high risk for suicide. Again, early establishment of a strong therapeutic alliance with the patient will greatly facilitate the referral process and enhance the likelihood that the patient will experience a successful result from the referral. When not restricted by a patient's health insurance plan, direct referral with close communication with the mental health specialist is desirable. Co-management with a mental health specialist is frequently promoted as a model for primary care; a survey of family physicians in Michigan found that collaborative treatment actually occurred in about 30% of their cases. Managed care carve-outs and lack of geographic proximity were seen as barriers to collaborative care by respondents (62).

LONG-TERM MONITORING

As discussed previously, once you have begun treating a patient with depression, monitoring his or her course is essential. The critical nature of systematic follow-up is evident from its inclusion in the USPFTF depression screening recommendations (17) and from the results of STAR*D (52). After beginning treatment schedule follow up in 1 to 2 weeks, even though response is not often seen that early. Early follow-up allows you to assess for side effects, reinforce the need for treatment, and assess for possible worsening. After patients are showing early improvement the frequency of monitoring can be extended to monthly. Monitoring the patient with a structured instrument such as the PHQ-9 allows you and the patient to review current and previous scores and make necessary adjustments to treatment. Some of the work of monitoring and follow-up can be performed over the telephone by office staff who are equipped with monitoring instruments and basic skills in care management.

At each office visit, assess current stressors, response to treatment, and the presence of suicidal thoughts. Patients under treatment often respond initially to questions about treatment response with a very general statement such as, "I'm doing better." It is useful to follow this up by eliciting a description of exactly what "doing better" means. Find out how the patient is responding to stressful situations, because these rarely go away just because treatment was started. This questioning will guide the patient into a discussion about how response to previously stressful situations has or has not changed after initiation of treatment or changes in treatment. Also ask patients whether spouses or significant others have noted changes. Any specific areas of improvement should be noted in the record and can provide useful markers of relapse for both the physician and patient.

It is also important to inquire about medication side effects. Patients may withhold mentioning these unless prompted, especially if they include sexual side effects such as erectile dysfunction or loss of libido. You can reassure patients with confidence that side effects are important to you, and that if they do not improve, a change in medication can be made.

Self-management activities set as goals at prior visits should also be discussed during follow up and monitoring. Where patients are successful in meeting their activity goals, help them to set new goals. If they have been unsuccessful, probe gently to elicit barriers to their successful achievement and work together to develop strategies for success.

Monitoring should be monthly during treatment; once a patient has returned to baseline functioning and symptoms are in remission, monitoring and visits may be performed at decreased intervals. Regular monitoring of patients helps to ensure that treatment remains matched to their symptoms and helps reinforce the importance of relapse prevention once recovery has occurred.

KEY POINTS

- Depression is highly prevalent in family medicine patients and a frequent comorbid condition with other chronic medical illness.
- Treatment for depression in family medicine is based on a strong therapeutic alliance between the patient and clinician.
- Treatment of depression to remission rather than symptom improvement is the goal.
- Routine monitoring of depression treatment using a standardized questionnaire is feasible and essential for guiding treatment.

CHAPTER

51

Allergies

Jennifer Keehbauch

CLINICAL OBJECTIVES

1. Describe the common causes and manifestations of allergies in children and adults.
2. Cite the most evidence-based treatment recommendations for allergies.
3. Assess when a patient should be referred to an allergist.

The patient with atopy may have one or many of the following conditions: allergic rhinitis, atopic dermatitis, asthma, and food allergy. These conditions are closely linked; they share many of the same precipitants, mechanisms, and treatments. Asthma is reviewed in Chapter 52 and atopic dermatitis is addressed in Chapter 39.

The following definitions are from the most recent clinical report from the American Academy of Pediatrics in 2008 (1).

- Allergy: a hypersensitivity reaction initiated by a cell mediated immune response
- Atopy: a personal or familial tendency to produce immunoglobulin E (IgE) antibodies after exposure to low levels of allergens
- Atopic disease: a clinical syndrome encompassing atopic dermatitis, asthma, allergic rhinitis, and food allergy

Allergies affect approximately 35 million Americans with the peak prevalence in childhood and young adulthood. The prevalence rate varies from 10% to 30% of adults to about 40% of children (2–4). Rhinitis (runny nose and nasal congestion), a prominent symptom of allergy, is classified as allergic or nonallergic. The majority of patients have mixed allergic and nonallergic rhinitis (44% to 87%) (4). Of the allergic subtype, 30% to 50% has seasonal allergies and the remainder has perennial symptoms. Seasonal allergies are associated with outdoor allergens such as pollens from trees, grasses, weeds, and fungi. Patients with the perennial form typically have symptoms year round in response to indoor allergens such as molds, dust mites, cockroaches, animal dander, or allergens in the workplace.

Nonallergic rhinitis is difficult to differentiate from allergic rhinitis. There are no diagnostic tests to distinguish between the two and the treatments are similar. There are many types of nonallergic rhinitis to including vasomotor rhinitis, infectious rhinitis, occupational rhinitis, nonallergic rhinitis with eosinophilia syndrome, atrophic rhinitis, and geriatric rhinitis. Some nonallergic types are physiologic such as hormonal rhinitis, which may occur with menses or pregnancy. Certain foods and alcoholic products may induce rhinitis through a vagally medicated mechanism. Drug-induced rhinitis may be caused by angiotensin-converting enzyme inhibitors, phophodiesterase-5-selective inhibitors (Viagra), phentolamine, alpha-receptor antagonists, aspirin, and nonsteroidal anti-inflammatory drugs (4). Geriatric rhinitis is a result of the physiology of the aging nose (5).

Risk factors for allergic rhinitis include serum IgE >100 international units (IU)/mL in children younger than age 6 years, family history of atopy, and positive allergy skin prick test (4). A high-risk child is defined as a child with at least one first-degree relative (parent/sibling) with allergic disease (1).

PATHOPHYSIOLOGY

Allergic symptoms are caused by a cascade of events after pollens or other allergens come in contact with the nasal mucosa. Allergenic molecules are processed by macrophages and dendritic cells, which present them to Helper T (T_H) cells and then to B cells. People with an allergic tendency have a large population of T_H2 cells, which stimulate B cells to secrete allergen-specific IgE. The IgE attaches to basophils and mast cells that, when exposed again to the same antigen, release histamine, leukotrienes, and cytokines. Eosinophils and additional T_H2 cells are recruited to the area; the allergic response is amplified for the original antigen and facilitated for new antigens, creating a positive feedback loop (6).

In people without an allergic tendency, a high proportion of T_H cells are T_H1 cells, which participate in cell-mediated immune responses. T_H1 cells produce substances that limit the allergic response. Conversely, T_H2 cells limit production of T_H1 cells. This suggests that exposure to infections that stimulate T_H1 responses might prevent allergic reactions. In fact, there is some evidence that early exposure to infections, by having older siblings or by attending day care in the first 6 months of life, results in lower rates of allergies and/or asthma in school-age children (7).

Allergen exposure may produce an early phase and a late-phase response. In the early phase, there is an immediate response of sneezing, watery eyes, and nasal discharge that resolves within an hour after removal of the stimulus. Symptoms may return 4 to 12 hours later, but with a predominance of congestion (4). The early-phase symptoms are associated with the initial histamine release, whereas the late-phase symptoms are related to the recruitment of additional inflammatory cells and mediators. Ongoing or recurrent exposure to

TABLE 51.1 Key Elements in the History and Physical Exam for Allergic Rhinitis and Conjunctivitis

Question/Maneuver	Purpose
Detailed history of runny nose, nasal congestion, sneezing, and character of mucus, including severity, time course, and precipitating factors	To determine severity and type of rhinitis, and potential allergens or irritants
Similar history regarding watering and itching eyes, swelling of eyelids	To characterize possible allergic conjunctivitis symptoms
Personal or family history of atopy (eczema, asthma, previous diagnosis of "allergies")	To identify increased risk for allergic rhinitis or conjunctivitis
Any particular exposure (e.g., cats, dogs, dust) or time of year when symptoms are worse	To identify possible allergens for avoidance or specific treatment
Any medications that have been tried and their effects	To identify potential treatments
Examination of lids and conjunctiva for color, irregularities, secretions, and any preauricular nodes	To determine extent of involvement and to differentiate between allergic, viral, and infectious causes (preauricular nodes suggest viral conjunctivitis)
Examination of nasal mucosa for color, swelling, secretions, blockage, or polyps	To identify signs of allergic rhinitis, polyps, or sinusitis
Visualization of tympanic membranes	To identify middle ear fluid or infection
Auscultation of lungs	To screen for asthma
Examination of skin	To identify evidence of eczema or urticaria

allergens can cause continuous symptoms. Irritants such as ozone, tobacco and wood smoke, perfumes, and cleaning chemicals can cause similar symptoms.

INITIAL EVALUATION

Allergic rhinitis results in sneezing, runny nose, nasal itching and congestion, and a sense of fullness in the head. Eye symptoms such as itching, watering, and blurred vision, with pink edematous conjunctiva, are common and indicate allergic conjunctivitis. Ask patients about these symptoms and those listed in Table 51.1. Patients whose symptoms recur at a particular time of year have seasonal rhinitis, usually related to specific pollens (Table 51.2). Other causes of rhinitis should be considered including irritants (e.g., ozone in smog, fumes from cleaning agents), medications (as noted previously), and hormones (from pregnancy or ingested hormones) (4).

The physical examination begins as you approach the patient from across the room, noting if the patient's eyelids appear swollen, if there are dark circles under the eyes ("allergic shiners"), and if the patient is mouth-breathing. Conjunctiva may be swollen and either erythematous or pale, sometimes with a cobblestone appearance. The nasal mucosa is often pale and swollen, but sometimes is erythematous. Pale glistening polyps may be present in the nose on the lateral wall. The position of the nasal septum should be noted, as deviation can cause obstruction and symptoms confused with or exacerbating allergic rhinitis. Nasal discharge is usually thin and clear or white, but may be thick and yellow or green especially with coexisting sinusitis.

The tympanic membranes may have fluid lines or be retracted if the eustachian tube is not functioning well (the generalized edema from inflammation can cause obstruction of their openings into the posterior pharynx) (Table 51.1). The lungs should be auscultated for wheezing, prolonged expiration, or decreased breath sounds suggesting coexisting asthma. Atopic dermatitis may be present.

DIFFERENTIAL DIAGNOSIS

More serious conditions should be considered when evaluating patients for allergies. Clear nasal discharge that begins after head trauma may be cerebrospinal fluid rhinorrhea. Unilateral nasal obstruction can be caused by foreign bodies (especially in children) or tumors. Tumors may also cause pain, facial swelling, decreased sense of smell, or decreased sensation on part of the face. More noticeable edema and erythema of eyelids in association with purulent discharge occur in bacterial conjunctivitis, which requires topical or occasionally systemic antibiotics. If the erythema and swelling are more pronounced, especially if unilateral and in a child, periorbital cellulitis may be present; this is usually treated initially with intravenous antibiotics.

Nasal polyps produce nasal congestion and loss of smell. They may occur in conjunction with rhinitis and worsen symptoms. There is no evidence that polyps are a result of allergies. Additional anatomic abnormalities that may also contribute to the patients symptoms include nasal septal deviation and hypertrophy of the nasal turbinates. Ciliary dysfunction may contribute to rhinitis and recurrent infection. The ciliary disturbance may be a result of primary ciliary dyskinesia or secondarily due to infection or tobacco use (4).

Normal physiologic reflexes may mimic allergic reactions. Common conditions that produce sneezing are sudden

TABLE 51.2 Triggers for Allergies and Suggested Management Strategies

Allergens	Comments and Management
Pollens • Tree pollen (early spring) • Grass pollen (late spring) • Weeds (late summer to autumn)	• During your "allergy season," keep windows closed when possible • Consider air conditioner, change air filter regularly or use special air filters or air purifiers
Animal dander (skin scales of furry or feathered animals)	• Keep pets outdoors, give them away, or at least keep them out of the bedroom • If visiting a home with pets, use a mast cell stabilizer (cromolyn or nedocromil nasal spray or inhaler) beforehand, if not already on daily anti-inflammatory medicines • Remove carpets if possible, because dander can collect in them and be hard to vacuum out
Dust mites (microscopic mites that live in bedding, carpets, cloth-covered furniture, etc.)	• "Dust-proof" covers on mattresses • Either use dust-proof pillow covers or wash pillows weekly in hot water • Wash sheets and blankets weekly in hot water (>130°F) • Keep indoor humidity <50% • Remove or avoid lying on overstuffed furniture, cushions and carpets • Wash stuffed animals weekly, or avoid their use
Cockroaches	• Do not leave food out where it will attract cockroaches • Use closed garbage containers and empty them frequently
Molds • Outdoor molds (summer and fall)	• Repair leaky faucets and other sources of moisture • Use a bleach-containing cleaner to remove mold

changes in temperature and sudden exposure to bright light. Congestion may occur with supine position, with pressure in the ipsilateral axilla or during the periovulatory period (8).

DIAGNOSTIC TESTING

Laboratory testing is needed only when the diagnosis and etiology are not clear or the patient does not respond to first-line therapy. A nasal smear is no longer recommended as part of the evaluation (4).

Skin testing can identify the specific allergen triggers. A drop of fluid containing the allergen is placed on the skin and a tiny puncture or prick is made through it. Several substances are usually tested at once, along with positive and negative controls. If IgE to the particular substance is present in skin mast cells, an area of swelling (wheal) and surrounding erythema (flare) will appear. Fifteen to 20 minutes after the test is placed, the diameter of any resulting wheal is measured. If the patient reacts, the wheal is compared with the controls. The results can be used both to identify what stimuli to avoid and also to determine what allergens should be included if immunotherapy is used. If the patient reacts strongly to several antigens in the test, allergic symptoms including urticaria, bronchospasm, and anaphylaxis can result. The clinician doing allergy testing must be prepared to immediately treat severe reactions.

Blood tests for specific IgE antibodies are less sensitive (sensitivity about 70% to 75% compared with the skin tests) and more expensive (4). They are used when the patient has a very high level of allergic response and the risk of anaphylaxis is great, or when the patient will not tolerate the discomfort of skin testing (9).

Testing can only be evaluated in context of the patient history. The sensitivity and specificity of these tests are far from ideal. Sensitization to one or more allergens is common in the general population of healthy people. Studies have found 50% to 60% of people have a positive skin test to foods and 26% have a positive skin test or an increased specific IgE level to 1 or more stinging insect venoms, yet most have never experienced an allergic reaction (10).

MANAGEMENT

The first step in treatment is to identify the allergens and irritants that trigger symptoms and minimize exposure to them. Specific suggestions are listed in Table 51.2. When environmental control does not adequately control the patient's symptoms, the next step is to provide medication that breaks the cycle in which increasing inflammation causes worsening symptoms and more inflammation. Table 51.3 presents a stepwise management plan.

Nasal Steroids

Nasal corticosteroids have consistently demonstrated superiority for allergy symptom control over oral agents in numerous meta-analysis and review studies and are considered the treatment of choice (2,11–14). Nasal steroids are better than antihistamines for use on an as-needed basis. Topical steroids, oral and topical antihistamines have similar efficacy in treating allergic conjunctivitis (4).

The combination of an intranasal steroid with an antihistamine was found to have a greater improvement in quality of life than either alone in two small randomized controlled

TABLE 51.3 A Stepwise Approach to the Management of Allergy

Step	Class	SOR*	Therapy	Adverse Effects	Comments
1	Nonpharmacologic	B	Allergen avoidance	N/A	• See specific avoidance measures in previous table
2	Topical steroids	A	Flunisolide (Nasarel) Fluticasone propionate (Flonase)	Nasal irritation and bleeding Perforation is rare	• Most effective treatment for allergic rhinitis
	Antihistamines First generation	A	Diphenhydramine (Benadryl) Chlorpheniramine	Sedation, constipation, dry mouth, dizziness	• Good efficacy for relief of nasal symptoms • Chlorpheniramine is not recommended in children <6 years
	Second generation	A	Loratadine (Claritin) Cetirizine (Zyrtec) Levocetirizine (Xyzal) Fexofenadine (Allegra)	Cetirizine may cause sedation at recommended dosage. Loratadine and desloratadine may cause sedation at higher doses.	• Similar efficacy to first generation with additional anti-inflammatory properties • Less effective for nasal congestion • Levocetirizine has also been shown to maintain symptom relief longer • Fexofenadine may improve watery eyes and nasal congestion better than loratadine • Levocetirizine and cetirizine have the quickest onset of action at 1 hour with others take up to 3 hours
3	Decongestants	A	Pseudoephedrine phenylephrine	Insomnia, irritability and palpitations Avoid in patients with cerebrovascular or cardiovascular disease, hypertension, BPH, glaucoma, and hyperthyroidism	• Decreases nasal congestion • Does not relieve sneezing, itching, and rhinorrhea • Use with caution in children and elderly • Contraindicated with MAO inhibitors
	Mast cell stabilizer	B	Cromolyn (NasalCrom)	Nasal dryness	• Most effective when used prior to exposure to allergen and used 4 times per day
	Leukotriene receptor antagonists	A	Montelukast (Singulair)	Headache, flulike symptoms, and abdominal pain	• Consider if unable tolerate other first-line agents or patient has coexisting asthma
	Intranasal antihistamines	A	Azelastine (Astelin)	Sedation	• No benefit over oral antihistamines or topical steroids
	Intranasal anticholinergics	A	Atrovent	Nasal dryness	• Only for rhinorrhea, does not control congestion or conjunctival symptoms
	Ocular preparations Anti-histamines Decongestants Mast cell stabilizers	 A A A	Naphthazoline/pheniramine (Naphcon-A) Ketotifen 0.025% (Zaditor, Alaway) Nedocromil sodium	Stinging, burning Rebound hyperemia Stinging, burning	• For patients who are not controlled with oral antihistamines • Use decongestants for short-term • Mast cell stabilizers have longer duration of action
4	Immunotherapy	A	"Allergy shots"	Local reaction, anaphylaxis	• Effective when symptoms correlate with allergen tests, used when fails oral medical management
	IgE antibody	A	Omalizumab (Xolair)	Anaphylaxis	• Monoclonal antibody directed against IgE • Recommended only with allergic asthma

Ig = immunoglobulin; BPH = benign prostatic hyperplasia.
*A = consistent, good-quality patient-oriented evidence; B = inconsistent or limited-quality patient-oriented evidence; C = consensus, disease-oriented evidence, usual practice, expert opinion, or case series.
For information about the SORT evidence rating system, see *www.aafp.org/afpsort.xml*

trials (15,16). A short course of oral corticosteroids for 5 to 7 days may be necessary in severe cases at the onset of treatment or for nasal polyposis. However, a single steroid injection is not recommended (4).

Antihistamines

Many patients are able to manage their symptoms with over-the-counter (OTC) remedies before seeking medical care. It is reasonable to try a first-generation antihistamine for those needing only intermittent relief and who do not develop significant anticholinergic side effects. However, because of the poor benefit to risk ratio, they are generally not recommended for long-term use (17).

Loratadine (Claritin) is the first-line choice to provide relief of itching, sneezing, and rhinorrhea for most patients. It is nonsedating, once-a-day regimen is convenient and cost-effective (11). Most of the negative anticholinergic side effects (e.g., sedation, constipation, dry mouth) are caused exclusively with first-generation agents (12). All of the second-generation antihistamines are equally effective in relieving rhinorrhea symptoms but are less effective for nasal congestion than nasal steroids (11).

Most of the superiority studies comparing second-generation antihistamines are industry supported and whether statistical differences translate into real-life improvement is unclear. Not all patients respond in the same way to the various antihistamines and patients may need to try a couple different ones to determine the best fit. There are no data to support continual use as superior to demand usage of oral antihistamines. However, it is recommended that all patients take their antihistamine at least 2 hours before exposure to the allergen if possible (12).

Use antihistamines with caution in patients with narrow-angle glaucoma, stenosing peptic ulcer, pyloroduodenal obstruction, symptomatic prostatic hypertrophy, bladder neck obstruction, bronchial asthma, increased intraocular pressure, hyperthyroidism, cardiovascular disease, and hypertension.

Leukotriene Receptor Antagonist

Systematic reviews of the effectiveness of leukotriene receptor antagonists when used alone have been conflicting. However, when used in combination with an antihistamine, relief of symptoms is greater than with either agent alone (13,18,19). This combination therapy may be comparable in efficacy to a nasal steroid, but at more than twice the cost of generic flunisolide nasal spray. Experts recommend leukotriene receptor antagonists be considered in allergic patients with comorbid asthma (17).

Decongestants

Decongestants decrease mucosal swelling and nasal congestion, but have little effect on secretions. Most OTC nasal sprays are topical decongestants that provide quick relief. If they are used more than 10 days in a row and then stopped they may result in rebound congestion (rhinitis medicamentosa) (20). Cromolyn nasal spray has a different mechanism of action. It is a mast cell stabilizer that blocks both early and late phase responses, prevents symptoms if used before exposure to allergens, and can decrease chronic symptoms when used regularly. Intranasal antihistamines (Astelin) are effective in treating nasal symptoms but have not been found to be more effective than the first-line alternatives (11).

Monoclonal Antibody

Omalizumab (Xolair) is a murine monoclonal antibody directed against circulating IgE. It has proven efficacy when compared with placebo but has not been compared with less expensive alternatives (21). Omalizumab is administered subcutaneously and is generally well tolerated. It is currently recommended only in patients with comorbid asthma (22).

Ocular Symptoms

Ocular symptoms can often be controlled by intranasal steroids or oral antihistamines (4). Allergic conjunctivitis management sometimes requires anti-inflammatory eyedrops containing cromolyn, an antihistamine, or a decongestant. In severe cases, topical corticosteroid drops can be used, but because of the risk of herpetic ophthalmitis, they should be prescribed only in consultation with an ophthalmologist.

Nasal Polyps

Nasal polyps sometimes shrink after treatment with nasal steroid sprays. If polyps persist or they are very large and obstructing the nasal passages, they may be surgically removed. Some patients have a syndrome of nasal polyps, aspirin allergy, and asthma, so if polyps are present the patient should be questioned about the other two conditions.

Immunotherapy

If a decision is made to use immunotherapy, the patient is given subcutaneous injections of a dilute solution of the offending allergens, usually twice a week, with a very slow increase in the dose. When the maximum dose is reached, injections are gradually spaced to every 3 to 4 weeks. Injections stimulate an increase in IgG "blocking" antibodies, a decrease in IgE, and a switch to predominantly T_H1 lymphocytes or to a modified T_H2 response.

Immunotherapy has been shown to be effective for some outdoor molds, ragweed, grasses, some trees, cat dander, cockroaches, and dust mites. It is also recommended for severe allergic responses to bees, wasps, hornets, and fire ants (23,24). A recent Cochrane review concluded that immunotherapy reduced symptoms and need for allergy medications without long-term complications (25). Treatment is usually continued for at least 3 years to maintain its benefits.

Referrals should be considered for failure of medical therapy to control symptoms, co-morbid asthma, consideration for immunotherapy, or history of anaphylaxis.

SPECIAL POPULATIONS

Pregnancy

First- and second-generation antihistamines are safe for use during pregnancy. Topical treatments such as intranasal steroids, cromolyn, and decongestants are also generally considered safe. Oral decongestants should be avoided in the first trimester. Immunotherapy may be continued during pregnancy, but is should not be started and the dosage should not be increased because of risk of anaphylaxis.

Children

In 2008, the Food and Drug Administration asked that OTC cough and cold medications product labels state "do not use" in children younger than 4 years of age. This recommendation was based on lack of scientific data showing efficacy and the demonstrated risk to this age group.

A randomized controlled trial of diphenhydramine and loratadine found no impairment in children's school performance with either medication when compared with placebo (26). Nasal steroids have not been found to cause growth suppression and can be safely used in children. The Food and Drug Administration has approved the use of fluticasone (Flonase) and Mometasone (Nasonex) from age 2 years and other nasal steroids from ages 4 to 6 years and older (17,27).

Elderly

Allergic rhinitis presents in the typical fashion in older people, with rhinorrhea and conjunctivitis. Unfortunately with other more pressing comorbidities in this age group, allergies are underrecognized and undertreated (5). First-generation antihistamines should be avoided in the elderly from drug interactions and potential side effects and adverse reactions. Second-generation antihistamines can be used with caution in selected patients (17).

Geriatric rhinitis presents with nasal congestion and thick postnasal drip. This is due to the normal physiologic aging of the nose. Nasal airway narrowing, glandular hypertrophy reduced submucosal glands, and restricted blood flow result in thicker, dryer secretions. These secretions are more difficult to clear and treatment with antihistamines and decongestants actually make them worse. Geriatric rhinitis is treated with increasing moisture via topical saline, humidifiers, and guaifenesin (up to 2,400 mg daily) (5).

FOOD ALLERGY

As with the other atopic conditions, food allergies also demonstrate a familial tendency. Infants born to families with an atopic history have a one in four chance of developing a food allergy.

Food allergies are classified as IgE-mediated and non–IgE-mediated. The IgE-mediated reactions are less common, rapid in onset, and result in urticaria and anaphylaxis. Non–IgE-mediated reactions are milder in nature and result in atopic dermatitis and gastrointestinal symptoms.

Food allergies have significantly increased across the world in the last decade. However, only one in 10 adults who report a food allergy (25%) actually have a true food allergy (2% to 3%). Often people confuse food intolerance with food allergies. Common adverse reactions to food include caffeine-induced irritable bowel, tyramine producing headaches and nausea, and lactose intolerance. Bacterial contamination and histamine released from stale fish will also produce gastrointestinal symptoms that mimic non-IgE mediated reactions.

Children have a higher prevalence rate of food allergy at 6%. Food allergies typically arise during infancy and peak by age 1 year. Eighty-five percent of children will outgrow their allergies to milk, egg, soy, and wheat. Allergies to peanut, nuts, and seafood typically persist through adulthood. The prevalence of peanut allergy has doubled in the last decade among children.

Diagnosis and Management of Food Allergy

The clinical features of food allergies vary from mild gastrointestinal symptoms to severe anaphylaxis and death. Peanut allergy is the most severe and the leading cause of fatal food-induced allergic reactions. Milk allergy is very common in infants and can produce IgE or non–IgE-related symptoms as described above. Nearly all infants allergic to cow's milk (98%) can tolerate extensively hydrolyzed milk-based formulas (Table 51.4).

Food allergies are a major cause of atopic dermatitis in children younger than 5 years of age. A food elimination diet or specific IgE levels may help in evaluating these children. A total of 30% to 40% of these children will improve with proper identification and removal of the offending foods.

Making the diagnosis of a food allergy requires an accurate history. A food diary, food-specific IgE measurements, skin testing, and elimination diets are keys to the diagnosis and management. A food diary will help identify the relationship between the offending food and the patient's symptoms. After the food item(s) are identified, specific IgE antibody testing of the patient's serum can be performed. This test is more reliable than RAST testing; however, false positives and negatives still occur.

Skin testing to the identified food antigens can also be performed. Testing patients with suspected food allergies to a standard panel is not recommended because of the high false-positive rate of 50%. However a negative test results in a 95% true-negative rate.

Elimination diets are helpful when skin testing and IgE antibody testing fail to confirm the suspected food. The suspected food or foods are withheld for 6 weeks. If symptoms resolve, then they are reintroduced one food at a time. Because there are many hidden ingredients in foods, careful instructions must be provided.

Observed oral food challenges are indicated when the above testing is negative and the history is consistent with a specific food or when anaphylaxis occurred. Skin testing and

TABLE 51.4 Infant Formulas for Use in Children with Cow's Milk Allergy

Extensively hydrolyzed casein (cow's milk protein)	Enfamil Nutramigen LIPIL (Mead Johnson) Enfamil Pregestimil (Mead Johnson) Similac Alimentum Advance (Ross)
Partially hydrolyzed whey (cow's milk protein)	Good Start Supreme (Nestle)
Partially hydrolyzed whey/casein (cow's milk protein)	Enfamil Gentlease Lipil (Mead Johnson)

Adapted from: Greer F, Sicherer S, Burks W. Effects of early nutritional interventions on the development of atopic disease in infants and children: the role of maternal dietary restriction, breastfeeding, timing of introduction of complementary foods, and hydrolyzed formulas. *Pediatrics*. 2008;121:183–191.

oral food challenges should be done by qualified personnel who are equipped to handle a possible anaphylactic reaction. These tests are often done by allergists.

The Food Allergy and Anaphylaxis Network has excellent information for physicians, patients, and caregivers (*www.foodallergy.org* or 1-800-929-4040) (28).

ALLERGY PREVENTION

Research does support several strategies to reduce the development of allergies in children at high risk (those with a first-degree relative with allergy). Dietary restrictions (e.g., peanuts, eggs, milk) during pregnancy or breast-feeding do not provide a protective effect from asthma or atopic dermatitis for the child (29). Authors of a Cochrane review found inconclusive evidence to support maternal dietary restriction to prevent allergic rhinitis, conjunctivitis, and urticaria (30). Prolonged delay in starting solid foods beyond 4 months of age and use of soy-based formulas also does not prevent allergies. House dust mite reduction is no longer recommended for primary prevention of allergies but can still be recommended for secondary prevention (1,29).

ANAPHYLAXIS

Anaphylactic reactions are an acute, emergent condition with life-threatening involvement of the respiratory and circulatory systems. Even when a patient presents with mild symptoms initially, there is the potential for rapid progression to a severe and even fatal outcome. Any delay in the recognition of the initial signs and symptoms of anaphylaxis worsens the prognosis.

The prevalence rate of anaphylaxis in the general population is unknown. However, research has shown that the rate is increasing, especially among the young. Common triggers include foods such as shrimp and peanut; medications such as penicillins, cephalosporins, and other β-lactam antibiotics; insect stings; and natural rubber latex. In children and adolescents, foods are the most common trigger. In adults, medications and stinging insect venoms are more common, as is idiopathic anaphylaxis (31).

Pathogenesis

Anaphylaxis usually occurs through a mechanism that involves cross-linking of IgE and aggregation of high-affinity receptors for IgE on mast cells and basophils. This results in basophil and mast cell membrane destabilization, allowing the release of cell mediators, which in turn causes a spiral of the inflammatory process (32).

Diagnosis

Diagnosis is based primarily on the clinical history of exposure to a potential trigger and the temporal relationship to the development of symptoms over minutes to hours. The clinical manifestations generally include skin or mucosal changes (hives, itching, flushing, swelling of lips, tongue, or uvula), respiratory symptoms (dyspnea, bronchospasm, or stridor), and less frequently the gastrointestinal (nausea, vomiting, abdominal cramping), circulatory (tachycardia, hypotension, syncope), and central nervous system symptoms (headache, confusion, altered level of consciousness). Angioedema and hives are the most common presenting signs of anaphylaxis. The severity of symptoms varies widely from a mild self-limiting event to death (32,33).

Acute anaphylactic symptoms typically begin within 30 minutes of exposure to an offending trigger. A repeat or biphasic reaction may occur 8 to 12 hours after the initial attack, but reactions have been reported to recur as remotely as 72 hours. These biphasic reactions are seen in up to 20% of cases. A protracted anaphylactic reaction may last for hours or days, despite aggressive treatment (33).

Anaphylaxis can be mistaken for numerous other medical conditions to include asthma exacerbation, generalized hives, syncope, pulmonary embolism, and panic attack. In infants, one should consider foreign body aspiration, congenital malformations of the respiratory and gastrointestinal tracts, and sudden infant death syndrome. In older adults, acute cardiovascular and cerebrovascular events should also be included in the differential. The vasovagal reaction is often confused for an anaphylactic reaction. It may occur after an injection or ingestion of certain foods that would also be suspicious as an allergic trigger. The vagal reaction produces a bradycardic heart rate without hives or wheezing (32,33). The "Chinese restaurant syndrome" can also masquerade as anaphylaxis. The reaction to monosodium glutamate may produce chest tightness, nausea, diaphoresis, and headache (28).

Laboratory testing is generally not needed. Currently, histamine and total tryptase are the only tests measured in clinical laboratories but these tests must be obtained as soon as possible after the onset of symptoms (within 3 hours) because of their transient elevations. Additionally neither test is ideally sensitive or specific. Therefore we must continue to rely on an accurate history. The history will further guide selection of allergens for skin testing or measurement of allergen-specific IgE levels in serum to help confirm the suspected trigger. These tests are optimally performed at least 3 to 4 weeks after the episode (32).

Treatment

The evidence for treatment of anaphylaxis consists largely of expert opinion due to the lack of well-designed randomized controlled trials. Treatment begins with assessment of the ABCs—airway, breathing, and circulation. Epinephrine is the medication of choice for anaphylaxis and there are no absolute contraindications for epinephrine in acute anaphylaxis (33,34). Epinephrine 0.3 to 0.5 mL or 0.01 mg/kg in children should be administered intramuscularly for symptoms of respiratory or circulatory compromise. The airway should be protected and maintained. The patient should be placed in the recumbent position with elevation of the lower extremities. Oxygen should be administered. Two large bore intravenous lines with infusion of normal saline should be initiated for fluid replacement and venous access. Anaphylaxis results in increased vascular permeability, which results in leakage of as much as 50% of the intravascular volume into the extravascular space within 10 minutes.

Adjunctive medications are given parenterally and include diphenhydramine (25 to 50 mg in adults and 1 to 2 mg/kg in children) and ranitidine (50 mg in adults and 1 mg/kg in children). Although there is no evidence from randomized controlled trials to support the use of antihistamines in the emergent management of anaphylaxis, they are both commonly administered for itching and hives (33,34). A systemic glucocorticosteroid is also frequently used for prevention of the delayed biphasic reaction and possible

Sample Action Plan

Name: ______________________ **Age:** ________

Allergy to: ______________________

Asthma: ☐ Yes *(high risk for severe reaction)* ☐ No

Other health problems besides anaphylaxis: ______________________

____

Concurrent medications, if any: ______________________

____

Symptoms of anaphylaxis include:

Mouth	Itching, swelling of lips and/or tongue
Throat*	Itching, tightness/closure, hoarseness
Skin	Itching, hives, redness, swelling
Gut	Vomitng, diarrhea, cramps
Lung*	Shortness of breath, cough, wheeze
Heart*	Weak pulse, idzziness, passing out

Only a few symptoms may be present. Severity of symptoms can change quickly.
****Some symptoms can be life-threatening! ACT FAST!***

What to do:

1. Inject epinephrine in thigh using (*check one*): ☐ EpiPen Jr (0.15 mg) ☐ Twinject 0.15 mg
☐ EpiPen Jr (0.3 mg) ☐ Twinject 0.3 mg

Other medication/dose/route: ______________________

IMPORTANT: Asthma puffers and/or antihistamines can't be depended on in anaphylaxis!

2. Call 911 or rescue squad (before calling contacts)!

3. Emergency contact #1: Home ________ Work ________ Cell ________
Emergency contact #2: Home ________ Work ________ Cell ________
Emergency contact #3: Home ________ Work ________ Cell ________

Do not hesitate to give epinephrine!

Comments: ______________________

____

____

____

Doctor's signature/Date **Parent's signature (for individuals under age 18 yrs)/Date**

 Further discussion of the Anaphylaxis Emergency Action Plan is available in: Simons, FER. Killer allergy: long-term management in the community. J Allergy Clin Immunol 2006; 117:367.

Figure 51.1 • Example of Anaphylaxis Emergency Action Plan.

protracted anaphylaxis (33). Patients with mild anaphylaxis who respond quickly to treatment can be discharged home after observation for a minimum of 2 to 8 hours (33).

Prevention of Recurrence

As with other allergies, avoidance of the offending trigger is the first step in prevention of recurrence of anaphylaxis. When the patient is discharged, they should leave with three essential items—epinephrine for emergency use, an action plan, and a referral to an allergy specialist for further testing and treatment.

Ideally, the patient will leave with an auto-injectable epinephrine pen and a prescription for an additional one. The patient and family should be instructed on its usage. An action plan should be personalized for each patient. An example can be found in Figure 51.1. Anaphylaxis emergency action plans are currently used by almost 40% of people at risk for anaphylaxis in the community, or their caregivers (32). Patients should also be advised to wear a medical alert identifier (i.e., bracelet or wallet card) (32).

KEY POINTS

- Allergic symptoms are caused by a cascade of events (involving helper T cells stimulating B cells to secrete allergen-specific IgE) beginning after pollens (e.g., trees, grass, weeds) or other allergens (e.g., animal dander, dust mites) come in contact with the nasal mucosa.
- Diagnostic testing is needed only when the diagnosis and etiology are not clear or the patient does not respond to first line therapy.
- Management of allergy begins with identifying the allergens and irritants that trigger symptoms and minimizing exposure to them.
- Evidence-based treatments include nasal corticosteroids (first-line) and oral antihistamines; for persistent symptoms a leukotriene receptor antagonist can be combined with the antihistamine (particularly if the patient has comorbid asthma or immunotherapy).
- Referrals to an allergist should be considered for failure of medical therapy to control symptoms, comorbid asthma, consideration for immunotherapy, or history of anaphylaxis.
- Food allergies are classified as IgE mediated, resulting in urticaria and anaphylaxis, and non–IgE-mediated resulting in atopic dermatitis and gastrointestinal symptoms; a food diary, food-specific IgE measurements, skin testing, and elimination diets are keys to the diagnosis and management.

ACKNOWLEDGEMENT

We would like to recognize Dorothy E. Vura Weis as the original author. Her contributed text from the original chapter was greatly appreciated.

CHAPTER

52

Asthma

Michelle A. Roett and Christina Gillespie

CLINICAL OBJECTIVES

1. Describe diagnostic criteria and clinical classification of asthma.
2. Describe key differential diagnoses for common presenting asthma complaints.
3. Discuss history and physical findings in patients with asthma.
4. Discuss diagnostic tests used in evaluating patients with suspected asthma and tools used for ongoing monitoring.
5. Describe clinically effective treatment interventions and long-term management for patients with asthma.
6. Describe tertiary preventive measures for asthma management such as patient or family strategies for managing exacerbations.

Asthma is a chronic inflammatory disease of the airways characterized by hyperresponsiveness and airflow limitation. According to the National Asthma Education and Prevention Program guidelines (1), asthma is defined as a chronic inflammatory disease involving mast cells, neutrophils, eosinophils, T lymphocytes, macrophages, and epithelial cells. This inflammatory process may lead to diffuse, variable airflow obstruction, manifested as recurrent episodes of coughing, wheezing, breathlessness, and chest tightness. Airway obstruction in asthma worsens in response to a number of stimuli (such as infection, allergies, and irritants), and improves either spontaneously, after withdrawal of the offending stimulus, or with treatment. Status asthmaticus is defined as severe continuous bronchospasm.

Children born in the United States are more likely to develop asthma than children born elsewhere (2). In 2009, 13.1% of all Americans older than 18 had been diagnosed with asthma (3). The prevalence of asthma increased from 30.7 per 1,000 in 1980 to 72.0 per 1,000 in 2002. Approximately 7.3% of the American population, or 20 million people, have asthma. Non-Hispanic black children are more likely to have ever been diagnosed with asthma (21%) or to still have asthma (16%) than Hispanic children (11% and 7%) or non-Hispanic white children (13% and 9%) (3). Emergency room (ER) visits, hospitalizations, and deaths from asthma are two to four times higher in African Americans than Caucasians (4). Independent predictors of more than six ER visits per year include non-Caucasian race, Medicaid insurance and uninsured status. Older age and lower socioeconomic status are also associated with more frequent ER visits (5).

In 2007, an estimated 9.4% of children (7 million) had asthma. Children in poor families or in fair or poor health were more likely to have ever been diagnosed or to still have asthma (3). Sixty percent of these children had experienced at least one asthma exacerbation in the previous year. In 2006, approximately 2% of all ambulatory care visits among children younger than age 18 were attributable to asthma. For every 1,000 children, there were 47 visits to physicians' offices and 6 visits to hospital outpatient departments for asthma (6). In 2006, 10.6 million visits to office-based physicians were for asthma (7). Approximately 3,600 deaths were attributable to asthma in 2006. Of note, death rates from asthma were twice as high for African Americans than for Caucasians (8).

ETIOLOGY

Asthma is characterized by widespread but variable pulmonary obstruction (1). A number of triggers, often allergic but also infectious, irritant, or emotional, can precipitate airflow obstruction in patients with asthma. Allergen-induced acute bronchoconstriction results from an immunoglobulin (Ig)E-dependent release of mediators from mast cells including histamine, tryptase, leukotrienes, and prostaglandins, which directly contract airway smooth muscle (9). Neutrophils are particularly involved for smokers, occupational asthma, and sudden-onset fatal asthma exacerbations (1). Mucosal swelling, mucus production, and constriction of smooth muscles encircling bronchioles lead to cough, wheezing, and shortness of breath.

Airway resistance normally follows a diurnal pattern with highest resistance at night and lowest resistance in early afternoon. Small airways under 2 mm in diameter lack supportive cartilage resulting in early and more severe effects. Airways in children are proportionately smaller, explaining greater susceptibility to asthma. Acute asthma symptoms usually stem from bronchospasm, requiring bronchodilator therapy. Acute and chronic inflammation can affect airway caliber and airflow as well as underlying bronchial hyperresponsiveness, enhancing susceptibility to bronchospasm (10). More persistent disease involves further limitation in airflow associated with airway edema, mucus hypersecretion, formation of inspissated mucous plugs, and airway smooth muscle hypertrophy and hyperplasia. Airway remodeling may result in decreased response to therapy. Remodeling includes thickening of the sub-basement membrane, subepithelial fibrosis, vascular proliferation, and dilation (11).

Viral infections play an important role in asthma exacerbations. The first episode of wheezing in children is often associated with bronchiolitis, commonly as a result of respiratory syncytial (RSV) or parainfluenza virus infection. A prospective study of infants tested at 1, 6, and 12 months of age suggested development of a symptomatic RSV infection is more likely in infants predisposed to asthma (12). Long-term prospective studies of children hospitalized for RSV-induced bronchiolitis show that approximately 75% wheeze in the first 2 years after initial illness, more than 50% still wheeze 3 years later, and 40% continue to wheeze after 5 years (13). Among school-aged children, allergies or atopic sensitization is a more prominent cause of wheezing, displacing respiratory infections as a main trigger of exacerbations (14). Among adults with asthma, 40% have other atopic conditions, and 10% have occupational asthma from workplace exposures (15).

Asthma symptoms are also commonly due to nonviral exposures. In patients with intrinsic asthma, psychological stress may precipitate an exacerbation. Extrinsic asthma symptoms, also referred to as allergic asthma, occur after exposure to allergens. Exercise-induced asthma features bronchospasm with exercise, which improves after ceasing exercise. Drug-induced asthma is associated with certain triggers, including aspirin and nonsteroidal anti-inflammatory drugs (NSAIDs), β-blockers, sulfites, and some foods and beverages. Aspirin and other NSAIDs may also cause a non–IgE-dependent response that involves mediator release from airway cells (16,17). Aspirin-induced asthma usually involves rhinorrhea, nasal polyps, rhinosinusitis, conjunctival edema, and dyspnea with wheezing after aspirin ingestion. Cross-reactivity may occur with other NSAIDs, including fenoprofen, ibuprofen, indomethacin mefenamic acid, naproxen, phenylbutazone, and salsalate.

RISK FACTORS

The newly discovered gene ADAM 33 (A Disintegrin And Metalloproteinase) is a member of the ADAM family of zinc-dependent metalloproteases, and may increase the risk of development of asthma and airway hyperresponsiveness (18). Metalloproteases may also have an effect on airway remodeling. However, the variation in phenotypic expression of ADAM 33 has yet to be established. Asthma is more likely to occur in people with a family history of asthma and allergies. Male children are more commonly affected than females, but by adolescence into adulthood women are more often and more seriously affected than men. First-born children are more likely to have asthma than third or fourth children (19,20).

Comorbid allergic conditions such as atopy or food allergies might play an important role in defining risk factors for developing asthma. More than half of children with asthma will cease symptoms by age 6 years, and those who continue wheezing are more likely those with symptoms of atopy (eczema, allergic rhinitis, or allergic conjunctivitis) and with a family history of allergy (21). Eighty-five percent of children older than 6 years of age with asthma have other evidence of atopy (22). In 2007, 29% of children younger than age 18 with food allergies also had asthma, compared to 12% without food allergies (23). This is particularly important because patients with both asthma and food allergies may be at greater risk of death from anaphylactic reactions (24). A causative link between allergies and asthma is yet to be proven.

There are several modifiable risk factors for asthma. In a cohort study including more than 88,000 participants, overweight women (body mass index [BMI] 25 to 29.9 kg/m^2) had a 40% higher risk of adult-onset asthma than normal-weight women. Obese women (BMI $\geq$30 kg/m^2) had more than three times the odds (odds ratio [OR] 3.3). Of note, women with waist measurements >35.2 inches had a higher likelihood of adult-onset asthma regardless of whether they were normal weight (OR 1.4), overweight (OR 1.7), or obese (OR 2.4) compared with those who had waist circumferences <35.2 inches (25). The authors did not account for family history or environmental exposures, but this study suggests truncal obesity in particular may play an important role in asthma risk for adults.

Atopy and tobacco smoking may increase the risk of occupational sensitization (26). Maternal use of tobacco during pregnancy and later exposure to environmental tobacco smoke (second-hand smoke) also increase the risk of development of asthma (27). Several other familial factors and exposure histories have been associated with developing asthma. These include an increased risk and a dose-response relationship with antibiotic use during the first year of life; and a decreased risk associated with having more siblings and earlier day care entry (19,28). Asthma severity for children may also be worse with fractured or time-limited parent–child relationships, suggesting an important role for specific social support mechanisms (29). A link between birth by cesarean section and asthma has also been suggested. In a study of more than 1.7 million Norwegian newborns, children delivered by cesarean section had a 52% increased risk of asthma compared with children born by spontaneous vaginal delivery (30). A causal relationship for these situational factors has yet to be established.

There is conflicting evidence for whether infant formula use is associated with asthma development. Exposure to cow's milk or soy protein in infant formula during the first 4 months of life is associated with a 25% increased risk of asthma by 6 years of age (31). In a meta-analysis, the use of hydrolyzed formula for 4 months in infants not exclusively breastfed, who also had a first-degree relative with atopy, was associated with reduced likelihood of asthma or wheezing in the first year of life (RR 0.40, CI 0.19–0.85) (32). Additionally, in a prospective cohort of 1,000 children, breastfeeding did not protect against development of asthma or allergies in adulthood (33). According to the American Academy of Pediatrics Committee on Nutrition, infants at high risk of developing atopic disease have decreased chances of developing atopic dermatitis and cow-milk allergy by being breastfed rather than using milk-based formula, but breastfeeding does not seem to prevent allergic asthma (34).

Exposures to a number of additional factors are associated with both the development of asthma and the possible onset of exacerbations. These include allergens from pollen types, dust mites, cockroaches, cats, dogs, rodents, and some fungi; irritants from tobacco smoke and outdoor air pollution (ozone, nitrogen oxides, sulfur dioxide, and diesel exhaust particles); infections caused by RSV; and occupational agents that might sensitize the lungs to allergens (27). Older age (OR per 10 years, 1.4, 95% CI 1.3 to 1.6), male gender (OR 4.5, CI 2.3 to 8.5), self-identified black race (OR 2.2, CI 1.3 to 3.8), current or past smoking (OR 3.9, CI 1.8 to 8.6; and OR 1.6, CI 1.2 to 2.3 respectively), aspirin sensitivity (OR 1.5, CI 1.0 to 2.4); and longer asthma duration (OR per 10 years 1.6, CI 1.4 to 1.8) have all been identified as risk factors for severe or difficult-to-treat asthma in adult patients with persistent airflow limitation (PAFL). PAFL was less likely associated with Hispanic race, higher education, family history of atopic dermatitis, pets in the home, or dust sensitivity (35).

DIAGNOSIS

Differential Diagnosis

Multiple diagnoses can be characterized by presenting complaints similar to those seen in patients with asthma. Allergic rhinitis, postnasal drip, sinusitis, and gastroesophageal reflux disease (GERD) can cause a chronic cough with or without triggering wheezing. Other causes of wheezing and shortness of breath include congestive heart failure, chronic obstructive pulmonary disease (COPD), airway obstruction, and pulmonary embolus. A chronic, nonproductive cough may also result from an angiotensin-converting enzyme inhibitor. These factors should be considered in the initial evaluation of a patient suspected of having asthma or if the patient fails asthma treatment. Some patients wheeze during an acute respiratory infection and for several weeks afterward, but do not have persistent symptoms or any evidence of obstruction on spirometry with or without provocation tests. These patients may or may not eventually develop asthma.

Isolated inspiratory wheezing is likely to indicate upper airway obstruction from mucus, a foreign body, epiglottitis, or croup. Many conditions can cause cough and wheezing in infants including GERD, allergic rhinitis and sinusitis, foreign body aspiration, vocal cord dysfunction, bronchiolitis, cystic fibrosis, heart disease, laryngeal abnormalities, tracheomalacia, bronchopulmonary dysplasia, enlarged lymph nodes or tumor, primary immunodeficiency or parasitic disease (1). COPD, which includes chronic bronchitis and emphysema, shares a number of features with asthma, including similar symptoms, physical findings, and treatments (see Chapter 55). Asthma symptoms are usually completely reversible while COPD by definition is not completely reversible. The two diagnoses may also coexist in the same patient. If a patient describes symptoms consistent with asthma related to work exposure and demonstrates improvement or resolution of symptoms on weekends or while on vacation, occupational asthma should be suspected.

History and Physical Examination

Asthma is diagnosed by a combination of history, physical findings, and pulmonary function test (PFT) results. A chronic cough lasting several months primarily occurring at night may be the only symptom. More typical symptoms of asthma include difficulty breathing, wheezing, and cough, either in combination or alone. Parents may report that their children have rapid or labored breathing, often with wheezing. In children and adolescents, chest pain with exercise may be the presenting symptom. Adults with asthma may describe difficulty in getting enough air, tightness in the neck or chest, or having to work harder or concentrate more in order to breathe (36). Exposure to allergens or workplace irritants may cause symptoms immediately or several hours later as a late-phase reaction, which might complicate identification of triggers. Tables 52.1 and 52.2 provide a guide for history and physical examination findings associated with asthma.

Exercise may precipitate asthma symptoms by increased ventilation, resulting in the irritation of airways secondary to loss of heat and moisture. Several factors distinguish exercise-related asthma symptoms from those due to poor physical conditioning. Exercise-induced asthma typically begins more than 5 to 15 minutes after starting exercise and continues more than 10 minutes after stopping. Shortness of breath from poor physical conditioning may start within 5 minutes of initiating activity but resolves in <5 minutes after stopping (37). Exercise-related symptoms may be the only manifestation of asthma. Pretreatment with a bronchodilator usually prevents significant symptoms and confirms the diagnosis.

Keep in mind that people of different ethnic or cultural backgrounds may describe asthma exacerbations or associated signs or symptoms differently. For example, African Americans may make rare mention of standard terms such as "shortness of breath" or "wheezing" (38). Instead, terms such as "tight throat," "tough breath," "scared," or "agitated" may be used to describe similar symptoms. Most people with asthma recognize a rapid worsening of obstruction more accurately than a slow deterioration or the absolute degree of obstruction. As an attack is resolving, patients might perceive normalization despite persistent presence of significant obstruction. Nevertheless, it is important to ask patients what they have noticed about the time course of symptoms and any exacerbating and alleviating factors (39,40).

Up to 25% of asthma patients have normal physical examinations even when obstruction can be demonstrated by pulmonary function tests (41). Limited data exist on sensitivity and specificity of physical findings at the time of initial diagnosis. During an acute episode, the patient may look anxious, have rapid or labored breathing, and be sitting upright or standing to maximize efficiency of thoracic muscles. Use of accessory muscles, with intercostal and supraclavicular retractions and tightening of the sternocleidomastoid muscles, often accompanies moderate-to-severe disease, especially in children with asthma. Vital signs are important. Respiratory rate and heart rate may be increased, and a fever may be present if infection is the trigger. Pulsus paradoxus (when the difference between systolic blood pressure in inspiration and in expiration is increased > 10 mm Hg) may be present with significant airway obstruction. Cyanosis is rare, but if present indicates a critically ill patient.

Auscultation is the most useful technique for evaluating obstructive airway disease. Decreased intensity of breath sounds is the most common finding in asthma, present in 33% to 65% of patients (41). Wheezes during expiration are characteristic of obstructive airway disease, especially when they dominate the expiratory phase or if also heard in inspiration. Wheezing is heard in 21% to 70% of patients with obstructive lung disease, and is present more often with more severe illness. However, during a severe exacerbation minimal airflow might result in no audible wheezing,

TABLE 52.1 Key Elements in the History and Physical Examination for Asthma

Question or Maneuver	Purpose
Detailed history of wheezing, shortness of breath, frequent cough, and character of sputum if present	To identify patterns related to time of day, activity, or infection
History regarding time of year, place, pet or pollen exposure associated with symptoms	To determine if allergens likely contributing to asthma
Does the patient wheeze with viral respiratory infections?	To identify whether infection is a common trigger for this patient
Personal or family history of atopy (allergic conjunctivitis, rhinitis, or eczema) or family history of asthma	To identify increased risk for asthma
Previous diagnosis of asthma or use of inhalers	To determine duration and to help differentiate between transient wheezing and true hyperresponsive airways
History of smoking by either patient or by other household members	To identify a trigger for asthma and to begin the process for helping the patient or household members stop smoking
Assessment of heart rate, respiratory rate, cyanosis, and use of accessory muscles	To identify patients needing prompt intervention Respiratory rate >30 breaths/minute and/or tachycardia with heart rate >120 beats/minute may indicate severe asthma
HEENT and skin examination	To identify sinusitis, URI, allergic rhinitis or conjunctivitis, and eczema, which may precipitate or accompany asthma
Lung examination for wheezing, prolonged expiration, increased resonance to percussion, and low diaphragm	These findings support a diagnosis of obstructive airway disease
Lung examination for basilar or other localized rales, decreased resonance	These findings would suggest infection with consolidation or effusion, CHF, or mass

CHF = congestive heart failure; HEENT = head, eyes, ears, nose, and throat; URI = upper respiratory infection.

suggesting a need to closely monitor patients and limit assumptions regarding improvement based on diminished wheezing. Wheezing on forced expiration suggests asthma but may be a normal finding, especially if it is short, monophonic, and present only at the end of a maximal forced expiration (42).

TABLE 52.2 Physical Examination Findings in Status Asthmaticus (85)

Tachycardia and tachypnea: heart rate >120 beats/minute and/or respiratory rate >30 breaths/minute may indicate ensuing cardiorespiratory failure
Use of accessory respiratory muscles
Pulsus paradoxus (inspiratory decline in systolic blood pressure >10 mm Hg): pulsus paradoxus >18 mm Hg may be indicative of impending cardiorespiratory failure
Wheezing: absence of wheezing or decreased wheezing can indicate worsening obstruction
Mental status changes: generally secondary to hypoxia and hypercapnia and constitute an indication for urgent intubation
Paradoxical abdominal and diaphragmatic movement on inspiration: indicates diaphragmatic fatigue, important sign of impending respiratory crisis

Rhonchi are low-pitched breath sounds similar to snoring, often present during exacerbations. Wheezes have a higher pitched, hissing sound in comparison. Inspiratory crackles may indicate either pneumonia or atelectasis from secretions and bronchospasm. A prolonged expiratory phase compared to the duration of the entire respiratory cycle is indicative of an obstructive process in adults but may be normal in children. Chest percussion may disclose hyper-resonance from increased lung volume, a low diaphragm from increased residual volume, or decreased diaphragmatic excursion during respiration from a smaller inspiratory reserve volume in about 25% of patients with asthma (41). A palpable cardiac point of maximal impulse in the subxiphoid area correlates with obstructive disease and is specific but not sensitive. Nasal examination may disclose pale boggy mucosa or nasal polyps, suggesting atopy in asthmatic patients with accompanying allergic rhinitis. Skin examination may show eczematous dermatitis. Clinical findings suggesting impending respiratory failure include altered mental status, inability to speak, intercostal retractions, worsening fatigue, absence of wheezes, and bradycardia. Pulsus paradoxus will initially be present but in respiratory failure may be lost due to respiratory muscle fatigue.

Diagnostic Testing

PULMONARY FUNCTION TESTS

Spirometry is recommended to confirm diagnosis and define the severity of asthma. Basic tests are forced vital capacity (FVC), forced expiratory volume in 1 second (FEV_1), and the ratio of the two (FEV_1/FVC). Obstructive disease is defined by an FEV_1/FVC ratio of <70% in adults (or <80% in children). In asthma, both the FEV_1 and FEV_1/FVC ratio are decreased, and the FEV_1 improves at least 12% (and at least 200 mL) with bronchodilators such as inhaled albuterol (43). If the FEV_1 does not increase by at least 12% after albuterol, the diagnosis is more likely COPD. Because the assessment might occur in the midst of varying stages of obstruction, a 12% increase may not be demonstrated until after a course of oral corticosteroid therapy.

Closely related to the FEV_1 is the peak expiratory flow rate (PEF), which occurs at the time of the steepest slope of the spirogram curve, near the beginning of the forced expiration. As with the FEV_1, PEF is reduced significantly by bronchospasm. PEF can also be measured with peak-flow meters, which are portable and relatively inexpensive. In a study comparing percent-predicted PEF with percent predicted FEV_1 before, during, and after treatment of asthma exacerbations, the correlation coefficients were approximately 0.8 each (42). An exercise challenge test may be used to establish the diagnosis of exercise-induced bronchospasm. This can be performed in a formal laboratory setting or by simply having the patient reproduce the previously inciting physical activity. A 15% decrease in FEV_1 or PEF after exercise is compatible with exercise-induced bronchospasm (1).

When asthma is suspected despite normal office spirometry, or if spirometry is not available immediately, patients can record PEF at home twice daily for 2 weeks (in the morning and the early afternoon to detect the exaggerated diurnal variation of asthma), and during episodes of wheezing or shortness of breath. If albuterol has been prescribed as a therapeutic trial, peak flows can be recorded before and after use. Three measurements are needed each time, and the highest is recorded. A peak-flow variation of 20% or more is consistent with asthma. The severity classification of asthma is determined by a combination of (i) symptoms; (ii) the FEV_1 or PEF compared with the predicted value for the person's age, height, and sex; and (iii) the variability of PEF at different times of day or over several days.

If neither spirometry nor peak-flow diary results are diagnostic, the patient may be referred to a pulmonologist for provocative tests. Methacholine is given in progressively higher concentrations to determine the dose causing a 20% reduction in FEV_1. Reaction to a concentration <10 mg/mL is diagnostic of asthma. Children younger than age 5 years are usually unable to effectively perform pulmonary function tests. In these children diagnosis is based primarily on history (including the parents' reports of symptoms at home), physical examination, and response to inhaled albuterol.

OTHER TESTS FOR PATIENTS WITH ASTHMA

Pulse oximetry is useful during an exacerbation to assess patients with rapid respiratory rate, cyanosis, or any respiratory distress. Laboratory evaluation is needed only for specific indications. Initial findings on arterial blood gas analysis in an asthma exacerbation typically include hypoxemia and hypocapnea. The patient hyperventilates to maintain a normal pO_2, and the pCO_2 drops. Primary hypocapnea, with its resulting acute (cellular) and chronic (renal) compensation, produces a respiratory alkalosis. Respiratory acidosis or a failure to reduce pCO_2 indicates respiratory muscle fatigue and impending respiratory failure (44). A complete blood count and differential is sometimes useful to help differentiate infectious versus atopic etiology. Eosinophilia may be seen with allergies, and increased neutrophils may be seen with infection. In a cross-sectional study of 47 patients, the presence of more than 3% eosinophils in the sputum was 86% sensitive and 88% specific for asthma. In the same study exhaled nitric oxide concentration exceeding 20 parts per billion was 88% sensitive and 79% specific (45). If supported with additional studies, exhaled nitric oxide and sputum eosinophil concentration may become routine features of conventional testing for asthma.

Chest x-rays show hyperinflation in about 45% of patients with asthma, but are needed only if other processes are suspected (e.g., pneumonia), in patients who do not respond to standard therapy, as a baseline in patients with severe asthma, and in very young or old patients who are at higher risk for other causes of dyspnea such as congenital heart disease or congestive heart failure. In patients with preexisting pulmonary disease, B-type natriuretic peptide (BNP or pro-BNP) testing in the emergency department is effective at distinguishing an exacerbation due to heart failure from that caused by pulmonary disease. As a result of initiation of more appropriate therapy in the emergency department, hospitalizations are fewer, duration of hospitalization is shorter, and costs are lower when BNP testing is employed (46). Electrocardiogram and continuous cardiac monitoring might be appropriate for severe exacerbations, especially for patients older than 50 years of age or with known cardiac or pulmonary disease. Right ventricular strain may be demonstrated in some severely obstructed patients, which may resolve with successful therapy (47).

MANAGEMENT

The National Heart Lung and Blood Institute Expert Panel Report suggests four components of asthma management:

1. Control factors that contribute to asthma severity (such as allergens and irritants) to improve baseline respiratory status and decrease the frequency of exacerbations.
2. Monitor respiratory status with objective measures of lung function for diagnosis, for classification of severity, and to assess response to treatment.
3. Use pharmacologic therapy to address the inflammatory nature of asthma.
4. Provide education for a partnership in asthma care, so that the patient and family understand the disease well enough to be motivated to make changes, use medications wisely, and work collaboratively with the physician.

With asthma, as with many chronic diseases, effective self-management by patients or parents is essential for controlling the disease. Self-management requires fundamental

Asthma Action Plan

For: ______ Doctor: ______ Date: ______

Doctor's Phone Number ______ Hospital/Emergency Department Phone Number ______

GREEN ZONE

Doing Well

- No cough, wheeze, chest tightness, or shortness of breath during the day or night
- Can do usual activities

And, if a peak flow meter is used,

Peak flow: more than ______ (80 percent or more of my best peak flow)

My best peak flow is: ______

Take these long-term control medicines each day (include an anti-inflammatory).

Medicine	How much to take	When to take it

Before exercise ■ ______ ■ 2 or ■ 4 puffs ______ 5 to 60 minutes before exercise

YELLOW ZONE

Asthma Is Getting Worse

- Cough, wheeze, chest tightness, or shortness of breath, or
- Can do some, but not all, usual activities

–Or–

Peak flow: ______ to ______ (50 to 79 percent of my best peak flow)

First → **Add: quick-relief medicine–and keep taking your GREEN ZONE medicine.**

______ (short-acting beta$_2$-agonist) ■ 2 or ■ 4 puffs, every 20 minutes for up to 1 hour ■ Nebulizer, once

Second → **If your symptoms (and peak flow, if used return to GREEN ZONE after1 hour of above treatment:**

- Continue monitoring to be sure you stay in the green zone.

–Or– ______

If your symptoms (and peak flow, if used) do not return to GREEN ZONE after1 hour of above treatment:

- Take: ______ (short-acting beta$_2$-agonist) ■ 2 or ■ 4 puffs or ■ Nebulizer
- Add: ______ (oral steroid) mg per day For ______ (3–10) days
- Call the doctor ■ before/ ■ within ______ hours afer taking the oral steroid.

RED ZONE

Medical Alert!

- Very short of breath, or
- Quick-relief medicines have not helped, or
- Cannot do usual activites, or
- Symptoms are same or get worse after 24 hours in Yellow Zone

–Or–

Peak flow: less than ______ (50 percent of my best peak flow)

Take this medicine:

■ ______ (short-acting beta$_2$-agonist) ■ 4 or ■ 6 puffs or ■ Nebulizer

■ ______ (oral steroid) mg

Then call your doctor NOW. Go to the hospital or call an ambulance if:

- You are still in the red zone after 15 minutes AND
- You have not reached your doctor.

DANGER SIGNS
- **Trouble walking and talking due to shortness of breath**
- **Lips or fingernails are blue**

→

- **Take ■ 4 or ■ 6 puffs of your quick-relief medicine AND**
- **Go to the hospital or call for an ambulance** ______ (phone) **NOW!**

Figure 52.1 • Asthma action plan. From National Heart Lung and Blood Institute. Asthma Action Plan. NIH pub no 07-5251, 2007. Bethesda, MD: National Institutes of Health.

understanding of the disease, triggers, recognition of worsening status, and appropriate interventions. An asthma action plan (Fig. 52.1) provides a written set of instructions. Asthma action plans usually use a "zone" system, patterned after the red-yellow-green lights of a traffic signal, to describe the severity of an exacerbation and to determine the appropriate intervention. The green zone has a peak flow of 80% to 100% of the target value and few if any symptoms; the yellow or "caution" zone has a peak flow of 50% to 80% of the target value and symptoms that are mild to moderate; and the red or "danger" zone has a peak flow <50% of predicted and/or severe symptoms such as shortness of breath with most activity levels.

Many studies have evaluated the effectiveness of self-management education. PEF and symptom monitoring are equally effective and both play an important role in effective self-management (strength of recommendation [SOR] = A). Long-term daily PEF may help detect exacerbations requiring treatment, response to therapy or provide a quantitative measure of impairment. Unfortunately, a 30% decrease in PEF often goes unnoticed by both the patient and treating physician. In one study, a 30% drop was detected only retrospectively during data analysis rather than being associated with symptoms sufficient to require medical attention (48). According to a systematic review, education involving self-monitoring by either PEF or symptoms, along with regular medical review and a written action plan (especially if two to four decision points are specified on medication adjustments) resulted in improved quality of life, decreased urgent medical care visits, and decreased hospitalizations (49,50). The asthma action plan also lists the controller medications for daily use and the steps to take if an exacerbation occurs (Figs. 52.1 and 52.2). Written action plans and/or home PEF monitoring during exacerbations are particularly recommended for patients who have poorly controlled asthma, moderate or severe persistent asthma or a history of severe exacerbations (SOR=B).

Controlling Factors that Affect Asthma Severity

The primary mode of prevention for allergen- or irritant-induced asthma is to avoid exposure. If the family is renting their home, the landlord could correct environmental problems contributing to asthma symptoms. Comprehensive control of allergens and irritants (see Chapter 51), matched to an individual's triggers has been found to be more effective for decreasing asthma exacerbations than control of single factors (51,52). Skin allergy testing and a serum radioallergosorbent test for allergens are helpful for patients with moderate to severe asthma. Results on indoor and outdoor allergens could help guide decisions about immunotherapy. Positive tests for indoor allergens could also help to guide housekeeping

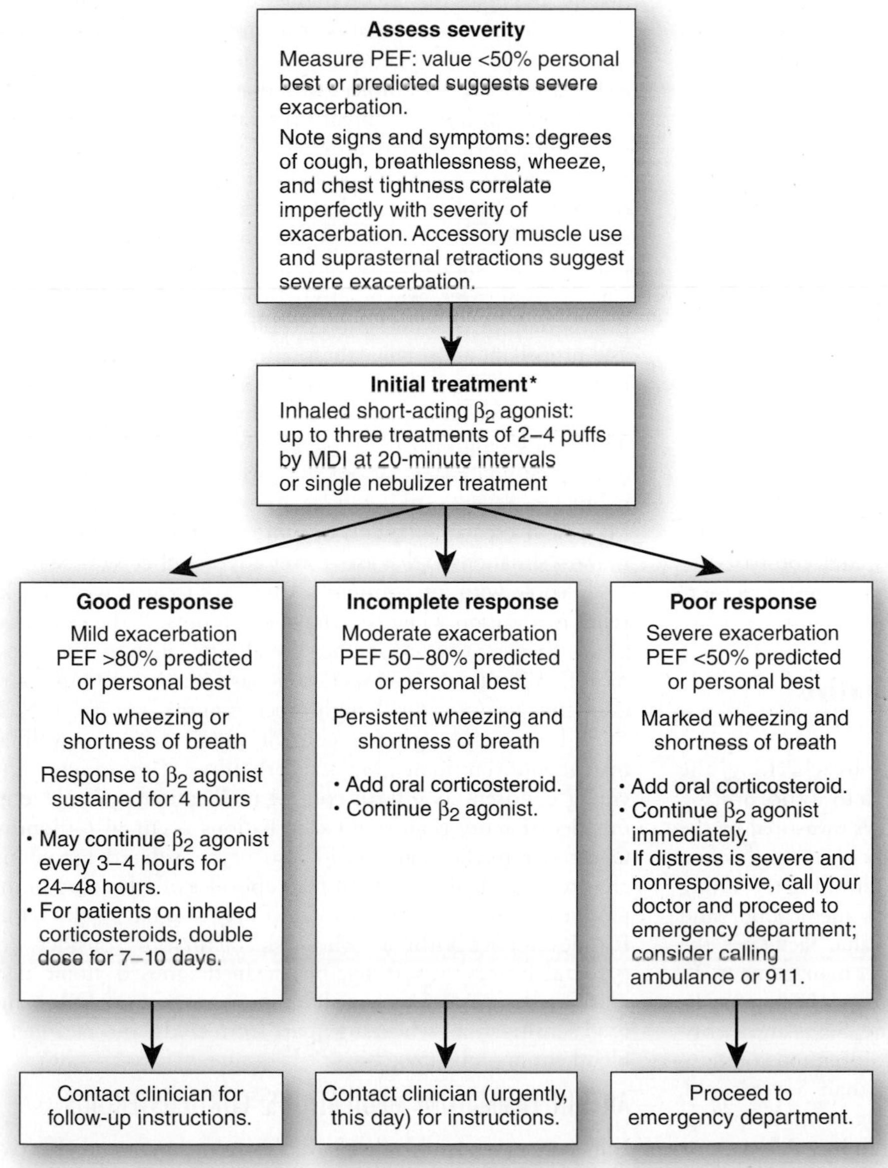

Figure 52.2 • Home management of asthma exacerbations. *Patients at high risk of asthma-related death (see Table 52.7) should receive immediate clinical attention after initial treatment. Additional therapy may be required. From National Asthma Education and Prevention Program. Expert Panel Report II: guidelines for the Diagnosis and Management of Asthma. Washington, DC: US Department of Health and Human Services, 1997.

measures. Two meta-analyses demonstrated the effectiveness of specific immunotherapy in patients with asthma and allergies to dust mites, pollen, animal dander, and mold (53,54). Asthma triggered by worksite exposures presents special challenges if a patient has only a late-phase reaction and symptoms do not occur until the patient is at home. Improvement on weekends and vacations suggests this etiology, and carefully kept diaries might prove useful. After a patient is sensitized to airborne particulate irritants or allergens, improved worksite ventilation is unlikely to provide adequate relief. If occupational exposures are triggering asthma, the physician could formally recommend a change in work assignment for the patient.

Conditions associated with asthma exacerbations should be controlled or treated. Treatment of some comorbid conditions is associated with improved response to asthma therapy: allergic bronchopulmonary aspergillosis (SOR=A), GERD (SOR=B), obesity (SOR=B), obstructive sleep apnea (SOR=C), and rhinitis or sinusitis (SOR=B) (1). Respiratory viruses, including rhinovirus, coronavirus, and influenza, can trigger asthma exacerbations. Patients should be advised on routine preventive measures such as hand washing. Annual influenza immunization is recommended, although there is no definite evidence that this decreases the number of asthma exacerbations. Pneumococcal vaccine is indicated for patients with asthma older than 19 years of age.

Psychosocial stress and negative family dynamics may affect asthma control. If exacerbations are frequently triggered by emotional reactions, individual or family counseling can be very useful with improved asthma treatment responses associated with treatment of comorbid chronic stress or depression (SOR=C) (1). In a study of 60 children with chronic asthma over a period of 18 months using daily symptom diaries, PEF measurements and interview assessments of life events, participants reported significant increases in asthma exacerbations within 48 hours of negative life events (OR 4.69) and up to twofold increase 5 to 7 weeks after the event (55). In a study of patients with asthma, those who wrote about stressful experiences for 20 minutes 3 days in a row had improved FEV_1 up to 4 months later compared to those who wrote about neutral experiences, suggesting a therapeutic benefit (56).

Monitoring Asthma Status with Objective Measures of Lung Function

Baseline asthma severity is determined by checking the patient's FEV_1 and FVC or PEF measured in the office or PFT lab, determining the variability in peak flows measured by the patient at home, and reviewing the patient's symptom history. Establishing the baseline severity is important in determining the intensity of initial long-term control medication, and knowing the "personal best" peak-flow value facilitates the classification of exacerbations and determines management. To evaluate severity of an exacerbation, the patient checks a peak-flow value to compare with the target value. Signs and symptoms are used to assess asthma status in children too young to use a peak-flow meter, usually younger than 5 years old. Parents are instructed to note the frequency of coughing, wheezing, retractions, and rate of breathing. All asthma patients should be advised on the signs and symptoms of severe exacerbations because patients with intermittent asthma might still have life-threatening exacerbations.

Pharmacotherapy

Pharmacotherapy for asthma is guided initially by classification of asthma severity (Tables 52.3 and 52.4). Medications are divided into two groups: those used for long-term control (anti-inflammatory medications and long-acting bronchodilators) and those that provide quick relief of exacerbations (fast-onset bronchodilators and short courses of systemic corticosteroids). They are shown with SOR ratings in Table 52.5 and specific medication dosages are listed in Table 52.6. Whenever possible, medications are given by inhalation to increase delivery to the lungs and decrease systemic adverse effects. Metered-dose inhalers (MDIs) are small and very portable, but are difficult for some patients to use effectively. Adding a large-volume spacer (e.g., AeroChamber) is helpful. The MDI is inserted in one end of the spacer, and the patient puts the other end in or near his or her mouth, presses down on the MDI to release the medication into the spacer, breathes in deeply, and holds the breath in the lungs until the count of ten. After a few normal breaths, the process is repeated. Most patients, even young children, can use this successfully with either a standard mouthpiece or a mask (Fig. 52.3).

Some inhalers are "breath-activated" and do not release medication until the patient takes a breath in with the inhaler in the mouth (a spacer is not used). These inhalers use a powder form of medication and are called "dry-powder inhalers" or DPIs. MDIs were developed using chlorofluorocarbon (CFC) propellants. Because of concerns that CFCs deplete the earth's ozone layer, a switch to hydrofluoroalkane (HFA) propellant took place. Medication droplets from MDIs with HFA as a propellant are smaller than with CFC's, which may result in medication reaching the smaller airways more effectively. Inhaled medications can also be delivered using a nebulizer. This is most appropriate for patients who become very anxious during asthma exacerbations and are accustomed to using a nebulizer. Several studies have shown that a properly used MDI with a spacer is equally or more effective than a nebulizer in most situations and causes fewer adverse effects (57,58).

People with intermittent asthma are treated with quick-relief medication when they have symptoms. If the exacerbation is persistent or severe, they are also given an oral corticosteroid. All patients with persistent asthma (symptoms more than twice a week or 2 nights per month) (see Table 52.2) should receive long-term control medications as well as instructions on managing exacerbations. For infants and young children, long-term control medication is also recommended if more than two exacerbations occur in 6 months. Controller medication should also be considered for young children who had more than four episodes of wheezing in the past year lasting more than 1 day if they also have risk factors for developing asthma. The risk factors to consider are parental history of asthma, physician-diagnosed atopic dermatitis, sensitization to aeroallergens, or two of the following: food sensitization, wheezing apart from colds, and peripheral blood eosinophilia (59).

ANTI-INFLAMMATORY MEDICATIONS: CORTICOSTEROIDS

Inhaled corticosteroids (ICS) are the most potent and effective medication for long-term control of asthma (SOR=A). As

TABLE 52.3 Classification of Asthma in Adults

Severity Classification	Pretreatment Symptoms	Pretreatment Lung Function (Between Exacerbations)
Intermittent	Daytime symptoms ≤ twice a week Nighttime symptoms ≤ twice a month Between exacerbations, no symptoms and normal FEV_1 No interference with normal activity	• FEV_1 normal between exacerbations • FEV_1 >80% of predicted • FEV_1/FVC normal
Mild Persistent	Daytime symptoms > twice a week but less than daily Nighttime symptoms 3–4 times a month Minor limitation in normal activity	• FEV_1 ≥80% of predicted • FEV_1/FVC normal
Moderate persistent	Daily daytime symptoms Daily use of inhaled β_2 agonists Nighttime symptoms > once a week but not nightly Some limitations in normal activity	• FEV_1 60%–80% of predicted • FEV_1/FVC reduced 5%
Severe persistent	Continual daytime symptoms Nighttime symptoms frequent Extremely limited activity	• FEV_1 <60% of predicted • FEV_1/FVC reduced >5%

FEV_1 = forced expiratory volume in 1 second; FVC = forced vital capacity.
Adapted from National Asthma Education and Prevention Program. Expert Panel Report: Guidelines for the Diagnosis and Management of Asthma – Update on Selected Topics 2002. Washington, DC: US Department of Health and Human Services.

anti-inflammatory medications, ICS block late-phase reactions to allergens, reduce airway hyperresponsiveness, and inhibit inflammatory cell activation. ICS should be considered as daily treatment for all patients with persistent asthma. The dose-response relationship to ICS varies in individual patients. The majority of evidence shows that increasing the dose of ICS may have only a modest benefit in patients with mild-moderate asthma. Addition of a long-acting beta agonist (LABA) is preferred in these patients. A few well-designed

(text continues on page 620)

TABLE 52.4 Long-term Control Medications for Managing Asthma in Adults

Intermittent Asthma	**Persistent Asthma** Assess control, step up when needed, step down if possible.				
Step 1	**Step 2**	**Step 3**	**Step 4**	**Step 5**	**Step 6**
No long-term control medications needed: β_2 agonists as needed for symptoms. Note: Severe exacerbations may occur separated by long periods of normal lung function and no symptoms. A course of systemic corticosteroids is recommended for more severe exacerbations	Preferred: low-dose ICS Alternative*: cromolyn, leukotriene modifier, nedocromil, OR sustained-release theophylline	Preferred: Low-dose ICS and LABA OR medium dose ICS Alternative*: Low dose ICS and either leukotriene modifier, theophylline or Zileuton	Preferred: Increase ICS within medium-dose range and add LABA. Alternative*: Increase ICS within medium-dose range and add either leukotriene modifier, theophylline, or Zileuton	Preferred: High-dose ICS and LABA AND consider Omalizumab for patients with allergies	Preferred: High-dose ICS and LABA and, oral corticosteroid AND consider omalizumab for patients with allergies

ICS = inhaled corticosteroids; LABA = long-acting inhaled β-agonist.
Adapted from National Asthma Education and Prevention Program. Expert Panel Report: Guidelines for the Diagnosis and Management of Asthma – Update on Selected Topics 2002. Washington, DC: US Department of Health and Human Services.

TABLE 52.5 Management of Asthma

Treatment Strategy	Efficacy	Strength of Recommendation*	Comments
Prevention			
Exclusive breastfeeding for at least 3 or 4 months decreases risk of developing asthma	OR of asthma up to age 6: 1.25 if not exclusively breastfed for 4 months (31); OR of developing asthma 0.70 if exclusively breastfed at least 3 months (86)	A	Note: This does not imply a shortening of the standard recommendations for exclusive breast-feeding for 6 months.
Avoid exposure to tobacco smoke, including prenatally	Fourfold increase in wheezing illness in infants whose mothers smoke (87)	A	Although wheezing illnesses increased, no increase in atopic sensitization. Tobacco smoke is also a trigger for those who already have asthma.
Education and Monitoring			
Self-management education programs including written asthma management plan and regular physician review	Compared with "usual care," RR 0.64 for hospitalization, RR 0.82 for emergency room visits, RR 0.79 for missed work or school (49,50)	A	
Action plans based on symptoms or peak flow equally effective in adults (88)		B	
Routine peak expiratory flow monitoring useful for patients with moderate and severe asthma (1)		C	Although difficult to separate from other program components, peak-flow monitoring beneficial in several studies and recommended
Controlling chronic home environmental triggers may reduce asthma symptoms	In comprehensive individually tailored programs, days with symptoms were 3.2 per 2 weeks in control group and 2.6 per 2 weeks in treatment group (52).	B	Comprehensive interventions appear effective but expensive: $750–$1,000 for 34 fewer days of symptoms per year. Single interventions not as effective.
Long-term Control			
Inhaled corticosteroids most effective as long-term controller	RR of exacerbation 0.46 compared with placebo (89)	A	Effective in children and adults. Appears to prevent structural changes in airways that would cause chronic obstruction.
Inhaled LABA effective as add-on medicine when ICS don't provide adequate control	When added to ICS, RR of exacerbation 0.76 compared with addition of placebo (89)	A	Most effective therapy to add to ICS. (Note: Initial treatment with ICS/LABA no better than ICS alone) (90)
Leukotriene antagonists are second-line as single agent.	Less effective than ICS (RR for exacerbations 1.65) (91) but more effective than placebo (RR for exacerbations 0.59) (89)	A	LTRAs decrease β_2 agonist use.

(*continued*)

TABLE 52.5 *(Continued)*

Treatment Strategy	Efficacy	Strength of Recommendation*	Comments
LABA better than leukotriene antagonists as add-on to ICS	LABA more effective (RR for exacerbations 0.83 compared with LTRA) (64)	A	
Specific immunotherapy (allergy shots) effective for high IgE asthma patients with positive skin tests	Meta-analysis shows NNT = 5 to prevent need for increased meds	A	Useful in patients whose symptom pattern and allergen tests match. Risk of anaphylaxis needs to be balanced.
Anti-IgE effective for mild-severe asthma in patients with high IgE	Decreased risk of exacerbation - OR 0.49; More likely to be able to reduce steroids by 50% compared with placebo—OR 2.50 (66)	A	Requires subcutaneous injection every 2–4 weeks, very expensive.
Treatment of Acute Symptoms and Exacerbations			
MDI with spacer at least as effective as nebulizer for albuterol delivery	RR hospitalization 0.42 compared with nebulizer in children younger than age 5 (57,92)	A	At least as effective with fewer side effects for most patients.
Ipratropium bromide added to albuterol for moderate to severe exacerbations	RR 0.68–0.75 for hospitalization if multiple doses ipratropium given with albuterol in ED (93,94)	A (93,94)	Effectiveness seen for both children and adults.
Systemic corticosteroids for exacerbations	7–10-day courses of systemic steroids reduce admissions and decrease relapse rates (95)	A	
ICS for acute exacerbations	OR for hospitalization 0.30 compared with placebo (73)	B	Meta-analysis on studies done in emergency departments.

ED = emergency department; FH = family history; ICS = inhaled corticosteroids; LABA = long-acting β_2 agonist; LTRA = leukotriene antagonist; MDI = metered dose inhaler; NNT = number needed to treat; OR = odds ratio; RR = relative risk.

*A = consistent, good-quality patient-oriented evidence; B = inconsistent or limited-quality patient-oriented evidence; C = consensus, disease-oriented evidence, usual practice, expert opinion, or case series. For information about the SORT evidence rating system, see *www.aafp.org/afpsort.xml*

TABLE 52.6 Medications Used for Asthma

Generic Name (Trade Name)	Usual Adult Dosing Range	Main Adverse Drug Events	Approximate Retail Cost Per Month, Usual Dose*	Pediatric Dosing/ Comments
Inhaled corticosteroids (usually split BID)[†] *Children's doses are usually ~ 2/3 of adult dose in each dosage range*				
Beclomethasone HFA (QVAR), 40 or 80 mcg/puff	Use BID Max 640 mcg/day	Sore throat, dry mouth; oropharyngeal candidiasis (gargle afterwards)	$	5–11 years Maximum 160 mcg/day >12 years Maximum 640 mcg/day
Budesonide (Pulmicort Flexhaler) DPI—dry powder inhaler—90, 180 mcg/dose	Use BID Maximum 1,440 mcg/day	Same	$$	>6 years Maximum: 720 mcg/day
Budesonide (Pulmicort Respules) solution for inhalation—0.25, 0.5, 1 mg/2 mL nebulizer	Use BID Age 1–8 Maximum 1 mg/day	Same	$$$	12 months to 8 years Not approved for adult use
Flunisolide (AeroBid) 250 mcg/puff	Use BID Maximum 2000 mcg/day	Same	$	6–15 years Maximum 1,000 mcg/day
Fluticasone (Flovent HFA)—44, 110, or 220 mcg/puff MDI	Use BID Maximum 880 mcg/day	Same	$$	4–11 years Maximum 176 mcg/day >12 Maximum 880 mcg/day
Fluticasone (Flovent Diskus)—100, 250 mcg/blister DPI	Use BID Maximum 2,000 mcg/day	Same	$$	4–11 years Maximum 200 mcg/day >12 years Maximum 2,000 mcg/day
Fluticasone-salmeterol combination (Advair)—100/50, 250/50, 500/50 mcg/blister DPI	Use BID Maximum 500/50 mcg BID	Same	$$	4 years and up
Budesonide-formoterol (Symbicort)—80/4.5, 160/4.4 mcg/spray MDI	2 puffs BID Maximum 640/18 mcg/day	Same	$$	12 years and up
Triamcinolone (Azmacort) 75 mcg/puff	Use TID–QID Maximum 1,200 mcg/day	Same	$$	6–12 years Maximum 900 mcg/day >12 years Max: 1200 mcg/day
Mometasone (Asmanex) 110, 220 mcg/puff DPI	Use QD-BID Maximum 880 mcg/day	Same	$$$	4–11 years Maximum 110 mcg/day >12 years Maximum 880 mcg/day
Leukotriene Antagonists				
Montelukast (Singulair)—10-mg tabs 4, 5 mg chewable 4 mg granule packet	10 mg QHS (adults)	None common. Rare itching or tingling, sinus inflammation	$$	1–5 years 4 mg qpm 6–14 years 5 mg qpm >15 years 10 mg qpm
Zafirlukast (Accolate)—10, 20 mg	20 mg BID	Rare headaches, nausea	$$	5–11years 10 mg BID >12 yrs 20 mg BID

(*continued*)

TABLE 52.6 *(Continued)*

Generic Name (Trade Name)	Usual Adult Dosing Range	Main Adverse Drug Events	Approximate Retail Cost Per Month, Usual Dose*	Pediatric Dosing/ Comments
5-Lipoxygenase Inhibitor Zileuton CR (Zyflo)—600 ER tablets	1,200 mg BID Maximum 1,200 BID	Hepatotoxicity and behavior disturbances		Extended release form only approved in the United States
Long-acting β_2 Agonists				
Salmeterol Xinafoate (Serevent)—50 mcg/ blister DPI	50 mcg BID	Occasional tachycardia, tremor, nervousness	$$	4 years and up
Formoterol fumarate (Foradil)—12 mcg/cap DPI	Use BID Maximum 2 caps/day	Same	$$	5 years and up
Albuterol (VoSpire ER)—4, 8 mg tablets	Use q12h Maximum 32 mg/day	Tachycardia, tremor, nervousness—more systemic effects than inhaled β2 agonists	$–$$	6–12 years Max: 24 mg/day >12 years Max: 32 mg/day
Mast Cell Stabilizers				
Cromolyn[‡]—20 mg/ 2 mL nebulizer	20 mg neb QID	Cough	$	2 years and up
Nedocromil—1.75 mg/puff	2 puffs QID	Same as above, unpleasant taste		6 years and up
Methylxanthines				
Theophylline—multiple PO and IV strengths available	Use QD–BID Maximum 600 mg/day	Nausea, tremor, tachycardia, nervousness, seizures at high doses	$	Adjust dosage by blood levels. Other medications may raise level.
Anti IgE				
Omalizumab (Xolair)—150 mg/injection site SQ	Dose determined by serum IgE and weight. May need to be given q2–4wk	Injection site reactions. Risk for anaphylaxis	$$$	12 years and up
Short-acting β_2 Agonist				
Albuterol[‡] (multiple brand names available)—90 mcg/spray MDI	2–4 puffs q4–6h or as directed in asthma management plan	Tachycardia, tremor, nervousness	$	>4 years Maximum 12 puffs/day
Levalbuterol[‡] (Xopenex)—45 mcg/puff HFA	2 puffs q4–6h	Same	$	4 years and up
Anticholinergic				
Ipratropium bromide[‡] (Atrovent)—17 mcg/ spray MDI	2 puffs with albuterol prn exacerbations	Cough, sore throat, rare palpitations; if sprayed in eye can precipitate glaucoma	$$	Used for severe asthma exacerbations

*Relative cost: $ = <$100; $$ = $100–$200; $$$ = $200.
[†]Inhaled corticosteroid dosages in "high dose" range are higher than US Food and Drug Administration–approved levels, but are recommended in major guidelines such as National Asthma Education and Prevention Program and Global Initiative for Asthma.
[‡]Also available as solution for nebulizer.

How to position the inhaler:

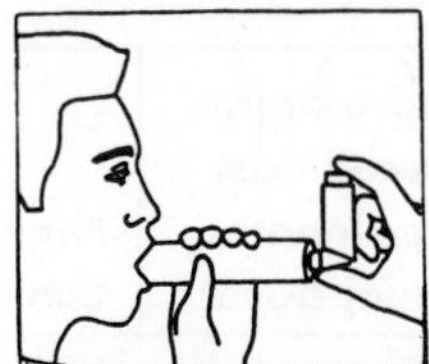

A. Use spacer. This is especially recommended for young children, for others who have difficulty coordinating inhaler use, and for all corticosteroid inhalers.

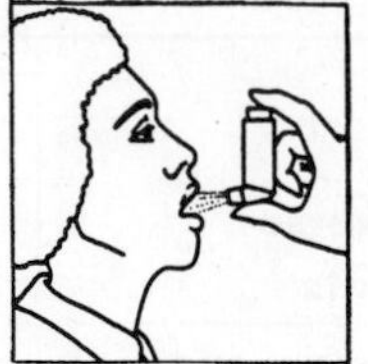

B. Open mouth with inhaler 1–2 inches away.

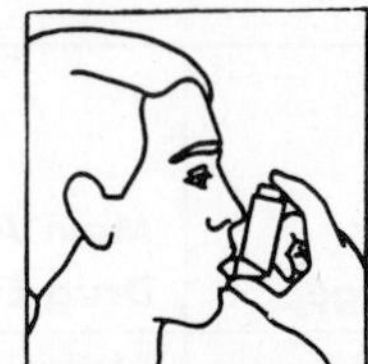

C. In the mouth. Do not use with inhaled corticosteroids. Use this position for breath-activated inhalers.

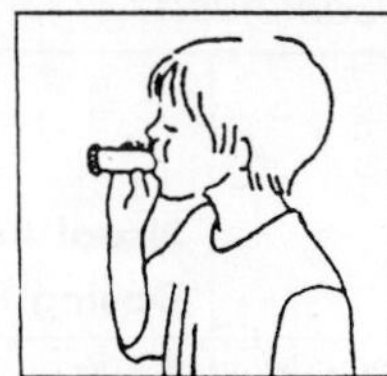

D. Dry powder inhalers (DPIs) require a different inhalation technique. To use a dry powder inhaler, it is important to close the mouth tightly around the mouthpiece of the inhaler and to inhale rapidly.

Figure 52.3 • How to use the inhaler. Adapted from National Asthma Education and Prevention Program. Expert Panel Report II: guidelines for the diagnosis and management of asthma. Washington, DC: US Department of Health and Human Services, 1997.

How to Use Your Inhaler

A. With a spacer (this is the preferred method for most inhalers):
1. Remove the cap, hold the inhaler upright, and shake it.
2. Insert the inhaler into one end of the spacer.
3. Breathe out slowly.
4. Put the other end of the spacer in your mouth.
5. You can press the inhaler to release the medication either just before or right as you begin to *breathe in slowly* all the way. Hold your breath for 10 seconds.
6. Wait a minute, and then repeat if using more than one puff.

B, C. If you use your inhaler without a spacer:
1. Remove the cap, hold the inhaler upright, and shake it.
2. Tilt your head back slightly and *breathe out slowly.*
3. Position the inhaler as in sketches A or C.
4. As you start to breathe in (or within a second after starting the breath) press down on the inhaler to release the medication.
5. Continue to *breathe in slowly* (over 3 to 5 seconds), then hold your breath for 10 seconds to allow the medicine to reach deeply into your lungs.
6. Wait a minute, and then repeat if using more than one puff.

D. Using a breath-activated inhaler (or DPI):
1. Follow the instructions for your inhaler to prepare it for use.
2. *Breathe out slowly.*
3. Put the inhaler in your mouth with your lips making a tight seal.
4. *Breathe in rapidly to activate the inhaler.*
5. Hold your breath for 10 seconds to allow the medicine to reach deeply into your lungs.
6. Wait a minute, and then repeat if using more than one puff.

trials have suggested that patients with mild persistent asthma may not need daily ICS. This group appears to have equally good outcomes whether using ICS or β_2 agonists only when needed for exacerbations (60,61).

Patients with severe persistent asthma do seem to benefit from increasing doses of ICS (1). Adverse effects of inhaled corticosteroids include hoarseness and candidiasis of the posterior pharynx, which can be decreased by using a spacer and by rinsing the mouth and gargling with water and spitting it out after each dose. Low and medium doses have been found to be safe in most studies of adrenal function. Higher doses may cause suppression of the hypothalamic-pituitary-adrenal axis and also increase the risk of cataracts. Studies on the impact of ICS on growth in children have shown a short-term decrease in growth velocity but no difference in height at age 20 years compared with controls (62). Many effective inhaled corticosteroids are available, and the choice for a particular patient is based on a combination of convenience of dosing schedule, ease of use of delivery device, insurance coverage, and cost (Table 52.6).

In severe persistent asthma, oral corticosteroids may be needed to deliver a higher total dose and to reach small airways inaccessible to inhaled medications in the presence of obstruction. In view of the serious adverse effects of long-term systemic steroids, they should be replaced by inhaled forms as soon as possible or reduced to the lowest effective dose (e.g., 5 to 10 mg of prednisone) given in the morning to decrease adrenal suppression. Oral corticosteroid therapy is associated with acceleration of bone loss, with fractures occurring in up to 30% to 50% of chronically treated patients. There is also a dose-related reduction in hip bone mineral density associated with ICS treatment in premenopausal women (63).

OTHER ANTI-INFLAMMATORY MEDICATIONS

Leukotriene modifiers block the airway inflammatory response, preventing smooth muscle contraction and airway edema. They are alternative, but not preferred treatment for mild persistent asthma (SOR=A). Because leukotriene modifiers are not as effective as ICS they are not first-line therapy, and are less effective as adjunct therapy than inhaled LABA (SOR=A) (64). When used as adjunct therapy, the ICS dosage needed for effective control can sometimes be reduced. Leukotriene modifiers come in oral formulations, which some patients prefer, and they are helpful for some patients with coexisting allergic rhinitis. Montelukast (Singulair) is given once a day in the evening, and is available for children older than age 1 year as well as adults. Zafirlukast (Accolate) is given twice a day and is indicated for patients older than 5 years of age. It has minor adverse effects (e.g., headache, nausea, diarrhea), but has several drug interactions (e.g., it increases the effect of warfarin and may cause bleeding, and increases erythromycin and theophylline levels). Leukotriene modifiers are often useful for asthma triggered by aspirin and NSAIDs. Zileuton (Zyflo) is a 5-lipoxygenase pathway inhibitor approved only for adults. Its use is limited by the need for liver function monitoring and limited efficacy data.

The mast cell stabilizers Cromolyn (Intal) and nedocromil (Tilade) are considered alternative anti-inflammatory medications for the treatment of mild persistent asthma (SOR=A). They are less effective than inhaled corticosteroids and might be useful as pretreatment before exposure to known allergens and before exercise (65). The subcutaneous immunomodulator omalizumab (Xolair) is an anti-IgE antibody that binds free IgE, inhibiting IgE from binding to basophils and mast cells, causing their degranulation. Omalizumab is a subcutaneous injection administered every 2 to 4 weeks, and is used for patients 12 years of age and older with severe persistent allergic asthma uncontrolled with ICS and other medications (SOR=B). Omalizumab has been reported to cause anaphylactic reactions even after 12 months of regular treatment. Clinicians administering this agent should be prepared to identify and treat anaphylaxis if it occurs. Omalizumab is also very expensive, and is typically reserved for patients with severe asthma (66).

Pregnant women with asthma can be treated according to the same protocols as other patients. All of the inhaled asthma medications may be used in pregnancy. Montelukast and zafirlukast both have Category B safety indications for pregnancy. Because very little prednisone crosses the placenta, it is also considered safe in pregnancy. Poorly controlled asthma during pregnancy is a known risk factor for intrauterine growth retardation.

LONG-ACTING BRONCHODILATORS

Long-acting bronchodilators are used as controller medications that induce sustained relaxation of airway smooth muscle. They are indicated in combination with ICS for management of moderate or severe persistent asthma. Several trials have reported greater benefit with the addition of LABA compared with increasing the dose of ICS (SOR=A) (67). Long-acting β_2 agonists should not be used without an ICS because such use has been associated with increased risk of severe asthma exacerbations leading to death (SOR=A) (68). Asthmatic patients homozygous for the variant resulting in arginine at the 16th amino acid position of the β2-adrenergic receptor (Arg/Arg genotype), may experience reduced airflow and worsening asthma control when using β2 agonists to treat their asthma. This genotype occurs in one sixth of the American population and appears to be disproportionately present in some ethnic groups, including African Americans. Consequently, African Americans may be vulnerable to the potential long-term adverse effects associated with the use of inhaled LABAs (69).

Inhaled forms of LABA are preferred over systemic versions because they have fewer side effects. Salmeterol (Serevent) or formoterol (Foradil or Perforomist) are available commercially in combination with fluticasone (Advair) and budesonide (Symbicort), respectively. Adverse effects may include tachycardia, QTc prolongation, hypokalemia, and hyperglycemia. Sustained-release albuterol in tablet form can improve control, especially for nighttime symptoms, but it is more likely to cause systemic adverse effects such as tremor and palpitations than inhaled long-acting bronchodilators. Sustained-release theophylline can be used as adjunctive therapy with ICS (SOR=A). It is much less expensive than salmeterol or formoterol, but its use is limited by adverse effects such as tremors, palpitations, nausea, and rarely seizures at high serum concentrations. Serum theophylline levels should be monitored periodically with a target range of 5 to 15 mcg/mL.

Managing Acute Exacerbations

Oxygen should be administered to maintain oxygen saturation >90%. Three types of quick-relief medications are commonly used to control acute symptoms. The short-acting β_2 agonist albuterol acts directly on the smooth muscle of the bronchioles to oppose the bronchoconstriction caused by inflammatory mediators. Onset of action is rapid, and it can be repeated as often as every 20 minutes during an exacerbation if needed, or used continuously in a monitored setting. Ipratropium bromide (Atrovent) is an inhaled anticholinergic medication that blocks the bronchoconstriction caused by cholinergic stimulation of the more proximal bronchioles. It is effective in decreasing the need for hospitalization when used with albuterol in urgent care/emergency settings for severe acute asthma exacerbations in both children and adults (70,71). Levalbuterol, the R-isomer of albuterol, can be used for patients with intolerable side effects from albuterol. It is available as a solution for a nebulizer (Xopenex) or as an MDI (Xopenex HFA), and is more expensive than albuterol.

Corticosteroids are used to treat exacerbations that do not respond adequately to the short-acting bronchodilators. Either an oral steroid (most commonly prednisone or prednisolone) or intravenous (IV) corticosteroid (e.g., methylprednisolone) is commonly used. A typical adult dose is 40 to 60 mg of prednisone per day for 3 to 10 days, or until the peak flow has returned to more than 80% of the patient's personal best. It can be stopped abruptly without danger of adrenal suppression if it has been used for <2 weeks. For children, 1 to 2 mg/kg/day of prednisolone liquid is used. Alternatively, a patient's dose of ICS can be doubled to quadrupled for 1 to 2 weeks to regain control. This approach has been effective in both emergency department settings and as part of instructions in asthma action plans (72,73). Patients with severe acute asthma exacerbations may benefit from IV magnesium sulfate in the ER. A meta-analysis showed that treatment with IV magnesium sulfate decreased rates of hospital admission and improved PEF and FEV1 when combined with routine asthma care (74).

Patients can manage most asthma exacerbations themselves if they have medication (albuterol MDI and spacer), a peak-flow meter, instructions in the form of an asthma action plan, and the ability to interpret symptoms or peak-flow measurements. See Figures 52.1 and 52.2 for standard regimens. A well-educated patient might use albuterol, adjust doses of ICS, and if needed begin an oral corticosteroid at home in coordination with a physician. When patients come to the office or ER with a more severe acute exacerbation, higher or more frequent doses of β_2 agonists, often with ipratropium bromide, are given either by MDI and spacer or by using a nebulizer with a mouthpiece or mask.

Oral corticosteroids are prescribed to break the cycle of inflammation and airway hyper-responsiveness. If the patient's symptoms fail to respond adequately, hospitalization may be necessary. In status asthmaticus, intubation might be difficult, and is often initiated before respiratory arrest when a patient fails to respond to bronchodilators and systemic corticosteroids. Intubation may be avoided with the use of adjunctive therapy such as heliox-driven albuterol nebulization and intravenous magnesium sulfate therapy (47), but should not be delayed once deemed necessary. Frequent asthma exacerbations signify the long-term management plan is inadequate. The physician should review the environmental exposures to decrease asthma triggers, and add or increase the dosages of long-term control medications.

Achieving Long-term Control of Persistent Asthma

The most important part of asthma management is to develop a chronic treatment regimen allowing the patient to maintain a normal activity level preventing exacerbations. Inhaled corticosteroids decrease the inflammatory response of the airways to various stimuli and are first-line therapy because of their proven effectiveness in controlling symptoms. The initial choice and dose of controller medications is determined by the patient's baseline asthma severity. β_2-agonists can be used three to four times per day with the initiation of controllers until the anti-inflammatory medication takes effect (2 to 4 weeks), and then can be withdrawn and saved for use during exacerbations. Several studies have shown that "personal best" PEF or FEV_1 measurements improve with continued use of inhaled corticosteroids for 6 months, followed by a slowed rate of age-related decline compared to before starting steroids (75). If asthma remains well controlled for 3 months based on symptoms and peak-flow measurements, it is reasonable to try reducing medications, assessing the patient's degree of impairment and underlying risk status before and after the change is made.

Many of the environmental triggers for asthma are beyond the control of the individual patient and can only be controlled by changes in public policy. Family physicians can have a significant impact in these areas by advocating for laws to limit both environmental tobacco smoke exposure and outdoor air pollution, and programs providing assistance to schools, landlords, and families to improve indoor air quality. Family physicians can manage asthma in the majority of their patients. Consultation with a pulmonary or allergy specialist is indicated if a patient's diagnosis is in doubt, the history suggests that immunotherapy may be beneficial, the asthma remains uncontrolled within 3 to 6 months of appropriate treatment, or the patient has severe asthma. If the patient has any red flags indicating increased risk of death (Table 52.7), management should be coordinated with appropriate specialists, health educators, and home health or school nursing clinicians.

TABLE 52.7 Red Flags for Increased Risk of Death from Asthma

History of previous life-threatening exacerbation with
- sudden onset
- intensive care unit admission
- intubation

Frequent unscheduled care manifested as
- two or more hospitalizations in past year
- three or more emergency visits in past year
- emergency visit or hospitalization within past month
- lack of a written asthma action plan

High medication need, as evidenced by
- use of two or more MDIs of β_2 agonists per month
- current use or recent withdrawal from systemic corticosteroids

Behavioral issues
- serious psychiatric disease (including depression and psychosis)
- illicit drug use

Social factors
- low socioeconomic status
- urban residence
- limited access to ongoing medical care

Cognitive problems
- difficulty perceiving changes in airflow obstruction
- inability of patient or caretaker to understand instructions

Adapted from National Asthma Education and Prevention Program Expert Panel Report 3: Guidelines for the Diagnosis and Management of Asthma, NIH pub no 07–4051, 2007. Bethesda, MD: National Institutes of Health.

PATIENT EDUCATION

Multiple educational interventions have been developed to reduce absent days from school or work and emergency room visits for children and adults. In a meta-analysis including 3,076 patients, formally teaching children and adolescents how to manage their asthma in multiple-session programs focusing on individualized responses to changes in peak-flow measurements was associated with improved perceived self-efficacy; 10% increase in peak-flow measurement; and decreased ER visits, absent days from school and number of days with restricted activity (76). A Cochrane review found similar benefits of asthma self-management education programs (77). An inpatient multiphasic educational intervention focused on improving asthma care and addressing psychosocial support reduced hospital readmission rates for all causes in a randomized trial of 96 adults with asthma who had at least one prior hospitalization. School and work absenteeism were also reduced (78).

Several factors are associated with frequent emergency room use. In a survey-based study, maternal symptoms of depression, maternal age 30 to 35 years, and higher asthma morbidity were all associated with increased emergency department use for children in kindergarten through fifth grade (79). According to a randomized controlled trial with 184 children, school-based asthma care is effective in decreasing absenteeism in children ages 3 to 7 years with persistent and severe categories of asthma, provided they did not experience environmental tobacco smoke exposure at home (80). One intervention of advice to quit smoking targeting parents of children with asthma demonstrated no difference in parental smoking in the presence of (or at an increased distance from) their asthmatic children (81). Nevertheless, parents who smoke and have children with asthma should be informed that they place their children at increased risk, should be advised to quit smoking and offered assistance to help them become smoke free (see Chapter 47). A Cochrane review suggested that culture-specific programming for minority adults and children with asthma might be more effective than generic programs for improving quality of life, asthma knowledge, decreasing asthma exacerbations and improving asthma control (82).

Asthma differs from most other chronic diseases in that the exacerbations may be dramatic and even terrifying, thus posing a true challenge to the patient to respond calmly and appropriately. Several points deserve special mention.

- The difference between dosage schedules for chronic versus acute management is confusing to patients. An asthma action plan needs clear instructions identifying the controller medicines that should be taken daily, both when asthma is controlled and during exacerbations, and listing the steps to follow during exacerbations with addition of quick relief medication and adjustment of controller medications. Make photocopies for the patient to keep in several locations.
- Few asthma patients use their MDIs or peak-flow meters correctly on a regular basis. Have patients demonstrate them at every visit and review their technique.
- Similarly, reinforce use of the peak-flow meter and the importance of keeping a diary when patients have moderate or severe asthma. If patients realize that a decrease in peak-flow value or an increase in symptoms can predict an asthma attack, they may be motivated to check their peak flow and use medication more appropriately.
- Remind patients to bring their peak flow diary to each visit for review. They should measure and record peak flow twice per day for 1 to 2 weeks when medications are changed. In addition, patients with moderate-to-severe asthma should maintain a record of their peak-flow readings for early detection of deterioration.
- Parents become understandably frantic if their child does not respond to quick-relief medications in his or her usual manner. It is important to let them know ahead of time that each attack is likely to be a little different, that the written instructions will indicate the proper response, and that a phone consultation with the physician is encouraged whenever they are unsure how to proceed.
- Asthma has a major impact on family relationships, especially when the patient is a child. Parents often need to be encouraged to be consistent in their expectations and their response to any unacceptable behavior and to provide frequent positive feedback to the child separate from dealing with the asthma. Providing education and clear-cut guidelines for the asthma management can help to reduce their anxiety level. They should be reassured that most children with asthma can maintain normal activity levels and keep up with their peers.
- Environmental measures to decrease exposure to allergens and irritants should be reviewed every 6 to 12 months to reinforce their importance. If asthma is difficult to control, the possibility of environmental tobacco smoke should be reassessed (83,84).
- Health educators, nurses, respiratory care practitioners, and community workers can reinforce and expand on the education done in physicians' offices, both in classes and in individual sessions, in an office setting or in the patient's home.

KEY POINTS

- Asthma is a common, chronic inflammatory disease of the airways characterized by hyperresponsiveness and airflow limitation. It is diagnosed by history, physical exam, and spirometry.
- Pharmacotherapy for asthma should be guided by classification of asthma severity.
- Patients with intermittent asthma are treated with fast-acting β2-agonists (e.g., albuterol) via metered dose inhaler for relief of symptoms.
- Patients with persistent asthma of any severity should use inhaled corticosteroids daily, with the addition of a long-acting β-agonist as "step-up" therapy when warranted.
- Self-management by patients (or their parents), including measurement of peak flows in those older than 5 years, is essential for controlling asthma.
- Asthma exacerbations are usually treated with inhaled fast-acting β2-agonist along with ipratropium and a course of systemic corticosteroids when needed.

CHAPTER

53

Acute Respiratory Infections in Adults

Arch G. Mainous III and William J. Hueston

CLINICAL OBJECTIVES

1. Distinguish respiratory tract infections likely caused by viruses from those caused by bacteria.
2. Discuss when antibiotics are indicated as treatment of acute respiratory tract infections.
3. Differentiate the signs and symptoms of serious lower respiratory tract infections from those associated with self-limited respiratory infections.

Acute respiratory infections range from self-limited conditions such as uncomplicated upper respiratory infections (URI, common cold) to serious life-threatening conditions such as pneumonia. URIs and acute bronchitis are among the most common reasons for visits in ambulatory care; they account for significant morbidity and absenteeism from work and school. The majority of antibiotics prescribed in ambulatory settings are for respiratory tract infections (1). The injudicious use of antimicrobial agents is costly, causes adverse drug effects such as diarrhea and rarely more serious infections, and creates an environment for developing resistance. Consequently, appropriate treatment of acute respiratory tract infections has become a challenge to the clinician. This chapter reviews the common infections of the upper and lower respiratory tract (sore throat is covered in Chapter 18).

Bacterial or viral pathogens can invade the respiratory tract and grow rapidly and aggressively. The physiological responses to viral or bacterial pathogens in respiratory tract infections tend to be similar, resulting in similar signs and symptoms. It is important to be aware that the majority of colonized bacteria found in the respiratory tract do not cause any problems for individuals with normal immune systems, until there is a breakdown in the immune system. For example, a significant proportion of children are colonized by *Streptococcus pneumoniae*, the leading cause of pneumonia, otitis media, and bacteremia. Yet *S. pneumoniae* bacteria tend not to cause illness in people with normally functioning immune systems; treating children with antibiotics, therefore, to eradicate *S. pneumoniae* has been effective in preventing illness.

DIFFERENTIAL DIAGNOSIS

Many diagnoses used for respiratory tract infections have significant symptom overlap with others (e.g., acute sinusitis and common cold; common cold and acute bronchitis). It may be useful to conceptualize these entities in more general terms (2). For example, infections localized in respiratory structures above the larynx can be conceptualized as URIs, and correspondingly those below the larynx as lower respiratory tract infections. An advantage to focusing on different primary sites of infection is that different pathogens are more common at certain sites than others thereby providing a guide for treatment.

Before discussing infectious causes, it is important to briefly review noninfectious causes of respiratory symptoms. The most common causes of noninfectious nasal discharge include allergic rhinitis and foreign bodies. Key historical findings that suggest causes other than infection for a runny nose include unilateral nasal discharge (as seen with a foreign body or necrotic tumor) or a clear nasal discharge that has persisted for several weeks (suggesting allergy).

For lower respiratory symptoms such as cough, additional noninfectious causes should be considered (Table 53.1). Congestive heart failure, aspiration of gastric contents or foreign bodies, lung neoplasms, asthma, and other inflammatory pulmonary conditions can produce a cough and shortness of breath. Congestive heart failure and pulmonary embolism also can cause pulmonary infiltrates and effusions that can be confused with pneumonia. Medications, most notably angiotensin-converting enzyme inhibitors, may cause a cough as well.

If a lower respiratory infection is suspected, it is important to differentiate acute bronchitis, a self-limited condition, from pneumonia. In addition to pneumonia, pulmonary abscesses may produce undulating fevers, shortness of breath, and cough. Abscesses are associated with certain types of pneumonia-causing organisms such as *Staphylococcus* sp. Bronchiectasis is a bronchial wall disease that allows accumulation of large amounts of secretions in the diseased bronchus. The copious secretions result in a chronic productive cough. Furthermore, these pooled secretions often become infected and can produce a fever, shortness of breath, and purulent sputum production consistent with pneumonia.

Uncomplicated URI/Common Cold

Adults typically have two to four URIs or "common colds" annually, and children in day care have as many as six or seven (3,4). Although URIs are mild, self-limited, and of short duration, (5) each year, they account for 170 million days of restricted activity, 23 million days of school absence, and 18 million days of work absence. And although colds may be viewed as benign, the impact of URIs on quality of life is similar in magnitude to such chronic illnesses as chronic lung disease, depression, or osteoarthritis (6).

TABLE 53.1 Causes of Cough

Upper respiratory tract
Acute rhinitis/pharyngitis (common cold)
Allergic rhinitis
Sinusitis
Tracheolaryngitis (croup)
Epiglottitis
Lower respiratory tract
Infectious causes
Acute bronchitis
Pneumonia
Tuberculosis
Pneumocystis carinii
Bronchiectasis
Lung abscess
Noninfectious causes
Asthma
Chronic bronchitis
Allergic aspergillosis
Bronchogenic neoplasms
Sarcoidosis
Pulmonary fibrosis
Chemical or smoke inhalation
Cardiovascular causes
Congestive heart failure/pulmonary edema
Enlargement of left atrium
Gastrointestinal tract
Reflux esophagitis
Esophageal-tracheal fistula
Other causes
Medications, especially angiotensin-converting enzyme inhibitors
Psychogenic cough
Foreign body aspiration

Reprinted with permission from Hueston WJ. Cough. In: Weiss BD, *20 Common Problems in Primary Care*. New York, NY: McGraw Hill; 1999:181–206.

URIs can be spread through contact with inanimate surfaces (7) as well as direct hand-to-hand contact (8). They have a seasonal variation, with an increased prevalence in the United States between September and March. It is unclear why this variation exists although it may be related to increased crowding of indoor populations in the colder months. Temperature is not the key to seasonal variation without the presence of a pathogen. Evidence from Antarctica showed that spacious well-ventilated rooms reduced transmission of URIs compared with crowded poorly ventilated rooms regardless of temperature (9).

One study of 200 young adults in the ambulatory setting was able to identify the specific virus believed to cause a URI in 69% of all episodes (10). Rhinoviruses were the most common virus (52%), followed by coronaviruses (8.5%), and influenza A or B virus (6%). Identified bacterial pathogens were *Chlamydia pneumoniae*, *Haemophilus influenza*, *Streptococcus pneumoniae*, and *Mycoplasma pneumoniae*. None of the patients had β-hemolytic group A *Streptococcus*. In terms of bacterial pathogens, infections without evidence of a viral infection occurred in only 0.05% of the cases.

Uncomplicated URIs are characterized by rhinorrhea, nasal congestion, sneezing, sore or "scratchy" throat, and cough (11). The incubation period varies between 48 and 72 hours. In some cases a low-grade fever is present, but temperature elevation is rare in adults. The early symptoms may be minimal and limited to malaise and nasal symptoms. The nasal discharge is initially clear and watery. There is a subsequent transition period where the nasal discharge becomes viscous, opaque, and discolored (white, yellow, green) (11). The color of the secretions alone is not predictive of a bacterial infection. The clinical presentation is similar in both adults and children. The episode tends to be self-limited; the median duration of a cold is 1 week, with most patients improving by day 10, but lingering symptoms may last up to 2 weeks.

Acute Rhinosinusitis

Because sinusitis usually is a complication of upper respiratory viral infections, the incidence peaks in the winter. Among children, sinusitis is frequently found as a comorbidity with otitis media (12). Children are also more likely to have posterior ethmoidal and sphenoid inflammation, whereas adults have mainly maxillary and anterior ethmoidal sinusitis (13). Some medical conditions may increase the risk for rhinosinusitis. These include cystic fibrosis, asthma, immunosuppression, and allergic rhinitis (13). Cigarette smoking may also increase the risk of bacterial sinusitis during a cold because of reduced mucociliary clearance.

Sinus inflammation can be caused by viral, fungal, and bacterial infections as well as allergies. Most acute sinusitis is caused by viral infection. The inflammation associated with viral infections clears without additional therapy. Cultures from patients with sinusitis show that the most common organisms are *S. pneumoniae* and, especially in smokers, *H. influenza*. These two organisms are present in 70% of bacterial acute sinusitis cases (14). When antibiotics are used to treat acute bacterial rhinosinusitis (ABRS), selection criteria should include sufficient coverage of these two organisms. Fungal rhinosinusitis is very rare and usually occurs in immunosuppressed individuals or those with diabetes mellitus.

Acute rhinosinusitis has considerable overlap in its constellation of signs and symptoms with URIs. Most patients with sinus symptoms seen in primary care do not have rhinosinusitis, and acute bacterial rhinosinusitis is even less common (15). URIs are often precursors of sinusitis, and symptoms from each condition overlap. Sinus inflammation from a URI without bacterial infection is common. In a series of 60 children undergoing computed tomography (CT) for non–sinus-related diagnoses, 47% had evidence of sinus inflammation with no clinical signs of sinusitis, and with complete resolution after their viral illness (16).

Rhinosinusitis starts with a URI that leads to sinus ostial obstruction. The resulting obstruction leads to symptoms of pain and pressure along with purulent drainage. Several clinical decision tools have been proposed to clinician's differentiate rhinosinusitis from common cold. The signs and symptoms that increase the likelihood that the patient has acute sinusitis are a "double sickening" phenomenon (patients who say they started with cold symptoms, but a few days later "got sicker"), maxillary toothache, purulent nasal discharge, poor response to decongestants, and a history of discolored nasal discharge (17–19). Relying simply on facial pain or swelling has a low sensitivity for rhinosinusitis (18). While these signs and symptoms are indicative of rhinosinusitis, they do not necessarily predict whether this is a viral rhinosinusitis or ABRS.

Differentiating rhinosinusitis from viral causes and ABRS is difficult. The gold standard remains sinus puncture with bacterial culture yielding $>10^5$ organisms per milliliter, which is unreasonable to perform in every patient (20). No office-based test is available that can help distinguish ABRS from viral rhinosinusitis. However, based on a consensus conference, it is recommended that the diagnosis of ABRS and antibiotics therapy should be restricted to patients who have had symptoms for more than 10 days (21). Patients with symptoms of shorter duration often experience spontaneously resolution of their rhinosinusitis and do not require treatment (20).

Acute Bronchitis

Acute bronchitis in the otherwise healthy adult is one of the most common medical problems encountered in primary care. The prevalence of acute bronchitis peaks in the winter and is much less common in the summer.

Viral infection is the primary cause of most episodes of acute bronchitis. A variety of viruses have been shown as causes of acute bronchitis including influenza, rhinovirus, adenovirus, coronavirus, parainfluenza, and respiratory syncytial virus (22). Nonviral pathogens including *Mycoplasma pneumoniae* and *Chlamydia pneumoniae* have also been identified as causes (23,24).

The etiologic role of bacteria such as *H. influenza* and *S. pneumoniae* in acute bronchitis is unclear because these bacteria are common upper respiratory tract flora. Sputum cultures for acute bronchitis are therefore difficult to evaluate since it is unclear whether the sputum has been contaminated by pathogens colonizing the nasopharynx.

Cough begins early in the course of the illness and is the most prominent feature of the condition. An initially dry cough may later result in sputum production, which characteristically changes from clear to discolored in the later stages of the illness. Thus, discolored sputum does not reliably predict a bacterial etiology. The cough may last for a significant time. Although the duration of the condition is variable, one study showed that 50% of patients had a cough for more than 3 weeks, and 25% had a cough for more than 4 weeks (25).

Patients with acute bronchitis usually have a viral respiratory infection with transient inflammatory changes that produce sputum and symptoms of airway obstruction. Acute bronchitis is essentially a diagnosis of exclusion. The history should include information on cigarette use, exposure to environmental toxins (e.g., dust, beryllium, volatile organic compounds, asbestos), as well as medication history (e.g., use of angiotensin-converting enzyme inhibitors). The chronicity of the cough should be established to distinguish acute bronchitis from chronic bronchitis since they have different treatments.

Both acute bronchitis and pneumonia can present with fever, constitutional symptoms, and a productive cough. Although patients with pneumonia often have rales, this finding is neither sensitive nor specific for the illness. Prospective studies of patients with cough have found that a chest x-ray should be performed for any patient with a fever of more than 100°F, tachypnea greater than 20 breaths/minute, tachycardia higher than 100 beats/minute, or if a patient has any two of the following: rales, decreased breath sounds, or no history of asthma (26). Patients without this constellation of findings are very unlikely to have pneumonia and chest x-ray is not needed unless they are not improving, worsening, or have other worrisome symptoms such as hemoptysis.

Asthma and allergic bronchospastic disorders can mimic the productive cough of acute bronchitis. When obstructive symptoms are not obvious, mild asthma may be misdiagnosed as acute bronchitis. Further, because respiratory infections can trigger bronchospasm in asthma, patients with asthma that occurs only in the presence of respiratory infections may present as patients with acute bronchitis.

Asthma should be considered in patients with repetitive episodes of acute bronchitis. Patients who repeatedly present with cough and wheezing can be given pulmonary function testing with and without a bronchodilator. For patients for whom routine pulmonary function testing is equivocal but asthma is highly suspected, further or provocative testing with a methacholine challenge test may help differentiate asthma from recurrent bronchitis. Finally, nonpulmonary causes of cough should always be considered (Table 53.1).

Bronchiolitis

Acute bronchiolitis is a distinct syndrome occurring in young children with a peak incidence at 6 months of age. It is an acute respiratory illness resulting from inflammation of small airways and characterized by wheezing. Children generally acquire the infection from family members or other children in day care who are infected with an upper respiratory tract infection. Bronchiolitis is not uncommon, with approximately 15% of children experiencing this illness during the first 2 years of life.

Respiratory syncytial virus (RSV) is the most common cause of bronchiolitis accounting for between 50% and 90% of cases. The majority of the cases occur during the winter and early spring mirroring the prevalence of the viral pathogens in the community.

The diagnosis of bronchiolitis is based on clinical findings and on the knowledge of the prevalence of viral pathogens prevalent in the community. The classic signs of bronchiolitis are wheezing and hyperexpansion of the lungs. Bronchiolitis begins as a URI, but soon the patient develops a cough, audible wheezing, irritability, listlessness, dyspnea, and cyanosis. Chest radiographs may reveal atelectasis, hyperinflation, or both. Untreated, infants with bronchiolitis can die from hypoxemia, dehydration, or apnea; $<1\%$ of affected infants die, however. Most recover but suffer recurrent wheezing episodes, usually precipitated by viral infections.

Influenza

Approximately 10% to 20% of the population in the United States develops influenza annually, with influenza season usually peaking between late December and early March. In recent influenza seasons, especially when influenza A type H3N2 predominated, 80% to 90% of influenza-related deaths occurred in individuals older than 65 years of age. It is the fifth leading cause of death in individuals older than 65, and the most common infectious cause of death in this country. Rates of disease are increased in individuals 65 years of age or older and in those with underlying health problems, such as diabetes mellitus and coronary artery disease (27,28).

Influenza is caused by highly infectious RNA viruses of the orthomyxovirus family. Influenza A viruses are classified into subtypes based on two surface antigens—hemagglutinin (H) and neuraminidase (N). Changes in the H or N antigen account for the epidemiologic success of these viruses. Infection with one subtype, however, provides little protection against infection with other subtypes, and infection or vaccination with one strain does not result in immunity to distantly related strains of the same subtype because of antigenic drift. Consequently, major epidemics of respiratory disease are caused by influenza virus strains not represented in that year's vaccine.

Occasionally, there are major shifts in the antigenic composition of the influenza virus. Such shifts are believed to be associated with the deadly pandemic of influenza in 1917–1918 as well as pandemics in 1957, 1968 (29,30), and most recently with the novel H1N1 (swine) flu pandemic in 2009. What made the 1918 influenza pandemic so remarkable was the high fatality rate in young to middle-aged adults. Concerns about emerging antigen shifts associated with avian flu viruses compare possible consequences to the 1918 pandemic, although there is no evidence that an avian strain was associated with this prior epidemic.

Influenza is extremely contagious and is transmitted from person to person through small particles of virus-laden respiratory secretions that are propelled into the air by infected people during coughing, sneezing, and talking. The abrupt onset of fever, myalgia, sore throat, and a nonproductive cough characterize the typical influenza infection. Symptoms usually last 1 to 5 days. Unlike other common respiratory illnesses, influenza viruses cause severe malaise lasting several days. The symptoms vary by age, with children commonly presenting with cough, rhinorrhea, and croup, whereas adults present with cough, myalgia, sore throat, and headache. The elderly usually complain of cough alone or in combination with headache. A key to diagnosis is being aware of influenza outbreaks in the community at the time of presentation. Respiratory syncytial virus, parainfluenza, adenovirus, enterovirus, *Mycoplasma*, *Chlamydia*, and streptococcal disease can also cause influenza-like illness, but these patients do not benefit from antiviral therapy.

The availability of rapid tests to identify influenza has made it possible to evaluate patients quickly for this disorder. However, the cost-benefit of this approach is questionable (31). Most studies show that during flu season when influenza is highly likely, it is best to simply treat the patient empirically. The value of office-based testing is probably during the "shoulders" of flu season when the probability of influenza is lower.

Community-acquired Pneumonia

Pneumonia is one of the most common reasons for hospitalization and is the sixth leading cause of death in the United States. It occurs in about 12 people/1,000 per year, but is much higher in the elderly population (32). In the United States, hospitalizations for pneumonia in adults older than age 65 rose by 20% between 1990 and 2000 (33). Pneumonia is even more common in the very elderly. One of every 20 individuals older than the age of 85 will be hospitalized for pneumonia in a given year (33). In addition to age, the chronic use of acid suppressants or steroid inhalers, institutionalization, and debilitation all increase the risk for acquiring pneumonia (34). Smokers and patients with chronic respiratory diseases are more likely to require hospitalization for pneumonia (35).

Patients with underlying comorbidities such as congestive heart failure, cerebrovascular diseases, cancer, diabetes mellitus, and poor nutritional status are more likely to die from pneumonia if they are infected. Thus, age and comorbidities are important factors to consider when deciding whether to hospitalize a patient with pneumonia.

In the past, more than 80% of confirmed pneumonia cases were caused by *Streptococcus pneumoniae* with mortality rates between 20% and 40% (36). More recent data from a number of North American studies estimate that pneumococcal pneumonia now represents about 20% to 60% of documented cases. Atypical agents such as Legionella and *Mycoplasma* are identified in 10% to 20% of infections, whereas less common causes include viruses (2% to 15%), *Haemophilus influenza* (3–10%), *Staphylococcus aureus* (3% to 5%), and gram-negative organisms (3% to 10%) (36).

The most common presenting complaints for patients with pneumonia are fever and a cough, which may be either productive or nonproductive. In one study, 80% of patients with pneumonia had a fever (32). Other symptoms that suggest pneumonia include dyspnea and pleuritic chest pain. However, none of these symptoms is specific for pneumonia.

Symptoms of pneumonia may be very nonspecific in older patients. Elderly individuals who suffer a general decline in their function, become confused or have worsening dementia, or experience frequent falls should receive a chest radiograph even if no pulmonary symptoms or physical findings are present (37). Elderly patients who have preexisting cognitive impairment or depend on someone else for support of their daily activities are at highest risk for not exhibiting typical symptoms of pneumonia (37).

The most consistent sign of pneumonia is tachypnea. In one study of elderly patients, tachypnea was observed to be present 3 to 4 days before the appearance of other physical findings of pneumonia (38). Rales or crackles are often considered the hallmark for pneumonia, but these may be heard in only 75% to 80% of patients (32,34). Other signs of pneumonia, such as dullness to percussion or egophony, which are usually believed to indicate consolidation, occur in less than one third of patients with pneumonia (36).

Chest radiography is the diagnostic standard for pneumonia. In rare cases, the chest radiograph may be falsely negative. This generally occurs in profound dehydration, early pneumonia (first 24 hours), infection with *Pneumocystis*, and severe neutropenia (36). Not every infiltrate is an infectious pneumonia, however. Other conditions such as postobstructive pneumonitis, pulmonary infarct from an embolism, radiation pneumonitis, and interstitial edema from congestive heart failure may produce infiltrates that are indistinguishable from an infectious process.

Blood or sputum cultures are not generally recommended for ambulatory patients. For patients admitted to the hospital, sputum cultures may be useful because when the results are positive, they can help guide initial therapy (39). However, even for those who can produce sputum that is sufficient for culture, 30% to 65% of specimens do not grow out a predominant organism. Procalcitonin is another tool under investigation to help clinicians distinguish bacterial from viral pneumonias.

TABLE 53.2 Red Flags in the History and Physical Examination

Red Flag	Other Conditions to Consider
Unilateral purulent nasal drainage	Occult nasal foreign body
Severe sore throat with deviation of the uvula laterally	Peritonsillar abscess
Difficulty swallowing with stridor	Epiglottitis
Hoarseness persisting more than 30 days	Laryngeal cancer or nodule
Cough persisting more than 30 days	Lung cancer
Hemoptysis	Bronchial lung cancer
Cough with unilateral wheezing	Bronchial foreign body
Early morning cough with hoarseness	Reflux esophagitis
Shortness of breath with unilateral decreased breath sounds	Spontaneous pneumothorax

In one study evaluating treatment based on serum procalcitonin levels compared with standard care, no increased risk was noted when antibiotic therapy was stopped based on procalcitonin levels (40). Studies to date suggest that a cutoff of 0.25 ng/mL and above should be used as to consider using antibiotics with a level of 0.50 ng/mL strongly indicating antibiotics should be used (41). Although this test is not yet widely available in clinical laboratories, if these results are confirmed in future studies, it is anticipated that this test will reduce antibiotic use in cases of pneumonias.

Blood cultures are controversial for patients with pneumonia. Even in hospitalized patients, the clinical usefulness and cost-effectiveness of blood cultures in otherwise healthy nonimmunosuppressed patients is controversial (42). For patients in whom hospitalization is considered, serum electrolytes, blood urea nitrogen/creatinine, and arterial oxygen saturation should be determined. For patients who appear well and for whom hospitalization is not expected, assessment of oxygen saturation with a pulse oximeter may be sufficient.

CLINICAL EVALUATION

Patients with acute respiratory infections need a focused history that includes current and recent symptoms, duration of episode, prior episodes and treatment, other family members affected, risk factors, and smoking history. In addition, several red flags in the history and physical examination may alert the clinician to noninfectious or life-threatening emergencies (see Table 53.2).

History and Physical Examination

Fever is a nonspecific sign, but can be used to discriminate mild, self-limited problems, such as acute bronchitis, from more significant infections such as pneumonia. Both the height of the temperature and the pattern of its development can give clues to the diagnosis. For example, URI ("colds") generally cause little or no fever in older children and adults. However, a child with symptoms of a common cold but who also has a high fever might be suspected of having otitis media, rhinosinusitis, or another bacterial infection. Fever also can be used to discriminate between different types of virally mediated illnesses such as the common cold and influenza, because influenza generally produces a high fever.

Rhinorrhea, either watery or purulent, indicates inflammation in the nasal cavities from either an infectious or noninfectious source. Although viral illnesses commonly cause runny noses, noninfectious conditions such as allergic rhinitis (hay fever) and a foreign body in the nose can also present with rhinorrhea. In viral illnesses, the nose is usually red and swollen with patchy areas of exudates. In contrast, in allergic rhinitis, the mucosa usually is swollen (boggy) and often pale with a clear, glistening surface and little exudate. With foreign bodies, generally only one nostril is affected and the drainage is usually purulent and foul smelling.

Headache is another symptom that can arise from respiratory and nonrespiratory structures. Frontal headache, particularly if it gets worse by bending over, suggests sinus inflammation from either a cold or rhinosinusitis. Facial pain is another symptom of sinus disease, because portions of the sinuses, the ear, and the skin of the face are all supplied by the trigeminal nerve. However, as noted below, facial pain alone is not a good predictor of bacterial rhinosinusitis since many patients with common colds also have sinus inflammation. Sinus inflammation also can cause maxillary toothache because the superior alveolar nerve passes through that sinus.

Hoarseness generally indicates narrowing of the airway in the region of the larynx. Typically, the cause is inflammation of the vocal cords from laryngitis. In small children, narrowing of the same air passage leads to stridor. (Sore throat is addressed in Chapter 18).

Cough is the most common symptom observed in lower respiratory tract infections, but is common in URIs as well; Table 53.1 lists causes of cough; inflammation of the trachea, bronchi, bronchioles, or alveoli causes cough regardless of the etiology of the inflammation. Infections also cause hypersecretion of and production of infectious exudates that are cleared with coughing. Some infections, such as mycoplasma influenza and other viral infections, produce inflammation without a great deal of exudate and are typified by a nonproductive or dry cough. The degree of cough provides little indication of disease severity; many viral respiratory infections cause severe, persistent cough, even when they are largely resolved.

Chest pain can occur with some respiratory infection, but it is a rare symptom in isolation. Usually chest pain is present with coughing, shortness of breath, fever, or some other sign of infection. Chest pain with infection is usually pleuritic in nature and represents pleural inflammation from the infectious process. The pleuritis can be mild as seen in some cases of acute bronchitis, severe as with some Coxsackie B virus infections, or associated with significant pleural effusions and respiratory compromise in pneumonias. Because other conditions, such as a pulmonary embolism, can cause chest pain and low grade fever, clinicians should consider noninfectious causes as well as respiratory infections when patients complain of chest discomfort. Finally, cough can lead to chest pain by straining or otherwise injuring the muscles and bones of the chest wall or by irritating an inflamed trachea or bronchi. Red flags in the history that suggest other disorders are shown in Table 53.2.

When evaluating a patient with a potential respiratory infection, a first step is to assess the overall appearance of the patient, and his or her vital signs. Patients who are comfortable, breathing easily, and afebrile are unlikely to have a life-threatening disease. However, tachycardia, tachypnea, and alterations in mental status are ominous signs that are associated with much higher death rates from respiratory infections such as pneumonia.

After initial assessment, careful attention should be paid to the ears, nose, throat, neck, and chest. As noted earlier, the appearance of the nasal mucosa may be helpful in determining if rhinorrhea is caused by infection as opposed to allergy. Palpation of the sinuses is sometimes performed, but since this maneuver offers little value in differentiating rhinosinusitis from a common cold and is likely to be highly operator-dependent, it is of little value. Transillumination of the sinuses has a much higher value in differentiating a sinusitis from a cold (18), but, as indicated earlier, does not distinguish between viral rhinosinusitis and acute bacterial rhinosinusitis.

Cervical adenopathy, which is common with streptococcal pharyngitis and mononucleosis, should be searched for during the neck examination. Palpation of the neck also may be useful in detecting an enlarged thyroid or other mass that may be compressing the trachea and producing stridor. A complete lung examination is crucial in patients with suspected lower respiratory infections. Auscultation over all areas of the lungs is important to detect rales or a rub from pleuritis. Percussion of the lower lung fields may be useful in detecting pleural effusions.

Diagnostic Testing

Routine laboratory testing is not indicated for the vast majority of respiratory infections (43). Sinus radiographs or CT scans offer little benefit over clinical criteria for rhinosinusitis and should be reserved only for patients with very confusing clinical pictures or fever without a clear origin.

For lower respiratory infections, the most common test is a chest radiograph, although according to a Cochrane review on the use of chest imaging in lower respiratory tract infections there is little value in obtaining a chest x-ray in ambulatory patients where pneumonia is already considered to be the most likely diagnosis. The chest x-ray is useful in differentiating pneumonia from acute bronchitis or other causes of shortness of breath and cough. It is recommended for patients with where there is a clinical suspicion of pneumonia. As noted earlier, a chest x-ray should be performed for any patient with a fever higher than 100°F, tachypnea higher than 20 breaths/minute, tachycardia >100 beats/minute or if a patient has any two of the following: rales, decreased breath sounds, or no history of asthma (26). The appearance of the infiltrate on the chest radiograph is sometimes helpful in predicting the etiologic agent as well (see Table 53.3). However, clinicians should be wary of false negative chest radiographs, which can occur in patients who are dehydrated or neutropenic.

Sputum cultures and blood cultures are less helpful; they are often unreliable or contaminated. Many studies have found that only about one third of hospitalized patients with pneumonia are able to produce adequate specimens for culturing. Blood cultures also rarely produce a finding that results in a change of antibiotics or any other clinical outcomes, but add significant cost to the care of the patient. Empiric treatment based on the age of the patient, severity of illness, and other risk factors is the most cost-effective strategy.

MANAGEMENT

Patient management and treatment is based on the condition. Table 53.4 summarizes the evidence for treatment options for most acute respiratory infections.

Uncomplicated URI/Common Cold

The most effective symptomatic treatments are over-the-counter decongestants (44). Preparations containing pseudoephedrine are effective in treating the nasal congestion associated with the common cold. However, several states have begun regulating the purchase of pseudoephedrine because of its integral role in the illicit manufacture of methamphetamine.

Despite the viral etiology of common colds, several studies have shown that the majority of common cold cases seen by physicians are treated with antibiotics (45,46). Controlled trials of antibiotic treatment of URIs have consistently demonstrated no benefit (47–53). One trial attempted to isolate "bacterial colds," for which antibiotics might be effective treatments (54). Although there was some indication of patient improvement at day 5, the differences were gone by day 10. It is important to emphasize to patients that the normal duration of a URI is 1 to 2 weeks. In addition, it is important to emphasize that the use of antibiotics for URIs does not prevent bacterial complications such as otitis media (55).

Despite the lack of any evidence that antibiotics are useful in viral respiratory infections, clinicians continue to prescribe them anyway. One rationale for the use of antibiotics is that it takes less time to write a prescription than to explain why one is not needed. Also, physicians believe that withholding an antibiotic will reduce patient satisfaction. However, neither of these appears to be true (56). The only result of prescribing antibiotics for upper respiratory tract infection is that patients are more likely to seek care in the future and expect to receive antibiotics for subsequent URIs.

Many alternatives to antibiotics for URIs have been investigated and have their advocates, if not strong evidence of effectiveness. Zinc gluconate lozenges are available without a prescription and have been suggested as effective in decreasing the duration of the common cold (57). However, one meta-analysis of eight randomized trials and another of seven trials concluded that zinc lozenges were not effective in reducing the duration of cold symptoms (58,59).

TABLE 53.3 Appearance of Infiltrates on Chest Radiograph

Immunocompetent Host	Immunosuppressed Host
Focal opacity	Focal opacity
Streptococcus pneumoniae	Same as immunocompetent plus:
Haemophilus influenzae	*Cryptococcus neoformans*
Mycoplasma pneumoniae	*Nocardia*
Chlamydia pneumoniae	Kaposi sarcoma
Staphylococcus aureus	
M. tuberculosis	
Gram-negative bacteria	
Anaerobic bacteria	
Interstitial/miliary pattern	*Interstitial/Miliary pattern*
Viruses	Same as immunocompetent plus:
Mycoplasma pneumoniae	*Pneumocystis carinii*
M. tuberculosis	*Leishmania donovani*
Fungi	Cytomegalovirus
Hilar adenopathy ± infiltrate	*Hilar adenopathy ± infiltrate*
Epstein-Barr virus	Same as immunocompetent plus:
Chlamydia psittaci	*Cryptococcus neoformans*
Mycoplasma pneumoniae	Fungi
M. tuberculosis	Lymphoma
Fungi	Kaposi sarcoma
Atypical rubella	

Reprinted with permission from Bartlett JC. Approach to the patient with pneumonia. In: Gorbach SL, Bartlett JG, Blacklow NR. *Infectious Disease*, 2nd ed. Philadelphia, PA: WB Saunders. 1998:554–557.

Echinacea has shown mixed results as a treatment for URIs in both children and adults. Although several smaller studies have observed some benefit, larger studies have tended to find no significant benefit for using echinacea (60). Several recent studies have found echinacea beneficial when compounds are used that mix echinacea with other treatments such as vitamin C or tea (61,62).

Vitamin C also has been advocated for URIs; systematic reviews of the literature, however, provide only weak support for its effectiveness (63). Antihistamines, with a few exceptions, have not been shown to be effective treatments (64–66).

Other treatments also are being evaluated for use in URIs. Ipratropium bromide has demonstrated use in controlling congestion and rhinorrhea (67,68), but its cost has limited its usefulness to date. Other treatments that are being investigated for URIs include acupuncture (69), nitric oxide (70), vitamin E (71), and North American ginseng (72). Some appear promising, but it is premature to recommend them as treatments because of limited evidence of their benefits.

Acute Rhinosinusitis

Antibiotics are commonly prescribed for adult patients who present with complaints consistent with acute rhinosinusitis. Four recent placebo-controlled, double-blind, randomized trials of antibiotics for acute rhinosinusitis encountered in general practice settings have yielded mixed results (5,73–75). Two of these trials showed no benefit of antibiotics, but two demonstrated significant effects of penicillin and amoxicillin. The trials demonstrating benefit suggested that patients with more severe signs and symptoms, as well as radiographic or CT confirmation, may benefit from an antibiotic. A meta-analysis of 32 randomized trials of antibiotics versus placebo and antibiotics of different classes found that acute maxillary rhinosinusitis may benefit from treatment with penicillin or amoxicillin for 7 to 14 days (76).

If an antibiotic is used, short duration treatment (e.g., 3 days) is likely as effective as longer treatment (77). Further, a meta-analysis indicates that narrow spectrum agents are as effective as broad-spectrum agents (78), and cause less antibiotic resistance.

Acute Bronchitis

Antibiotic treatment for acute bronchitis is quite common, and 60% to 75% of adults visiting a doctor for acute bronchitis receive an antibiotic (79). Three meta-analyses of antibiotics for otherwise healthy people with acute bronchitis were recently conducted (80–82). In one meta-analysis, neither resolution of cough nor clinical improvement at reexamination

TABLE 53.4 Evidence Supporting Management of Common Respiratory Tract Infections

Treatment Strategy	Strength of Recommendation*	Recommendations/Conclusions
Upper Respiratory Tract Infections		
Pelargonium sidoides	B	Meta-analysis found that it may be effective for bronchitis, sinusitis, or common cold.
Antibiotic therapy	A	No benefits seen and complications higher in treated group
Use of decongestants	A	Assist in symptom control, no effect on duration of illness
Echinacea products	B	Early trials demonstrated modest benefit, better controlled trials show no benefit
Zinc lozenges	A	Effectiveness in adults not shown; one randomized trial showed no benefit in children
Antihistamine therapy	A	No benefit at relieving symptoms or altering duration of disease
Acute Bronchitis		
Use of routine antibiotics	A	Meta-analyses show weak/modest benefit; no evidence of effectiveness in single trials of individual drugs
Use of short-acting bronchodilators	A	Cochrane review showed effectiveness only in patients with wheezing illness
Influenza		
Use of amantadine/rimantadine	A	Not recommended because of widespread resistance
Use of neuraminidase inhibitors	A	Useful in influenza A and B and works best if started in first 30–36 hours Beneficial in preventing complications in high-risk patients
Acute Sinusitis		
Antibiotic therapy	A	Useful, but benefit limited to small number of patients; highly dependent on accurate diagnosis
Community-acquired Pneumonia		
Routine use of antibiotics	C	Antibiotic selection depends on situation and patient risks
ATS/ISDA guidelines for antibiotic selection	B	ATS guideline adherence decreased morbidity and hospitalizations

ATS/IDSA = American Thoracic Society and Infectious Disease Society of America.
*A = consistent, good-quality patient-oriented evidence; B = inconsistent or limited-quality patient-oriented evidence; C = consensus, disease-oriented evidence, usual practice, expert opinion, or case series.
For information about the SORT evidence rating system, see *www.aafp.org/afpsort.xml.*

was affected by antibiotic treatment. Importantly, side effects were more common in the antibiotic groups compared with placebo. The meta-analyses concluded that antibiotics may be modestly effective for acute bronchitis resulting in about a half-day decrease in cough and sputum production on average. Meta-analyses agreed that the benefits of antibiotics should be weighed against the impact of excessive use of antibiotics on the development of antibiotic resistance.

Data from clinical trials suggest that bronchodilators may provide effective symptomatic relief to patients with acute bronchitis (83,84). Treatment with bronchodilators demonstrated significant relief of symptoms including faster resolution of cough, as well as return to work. However, one study evaluated the effect of albuterol in a population of patients with undifferentiated cough and found no beneficial effect (85). A subsequent Cochrane review did not find benefit from β-2 bronchodilators except when patients have some evidence of wheezing (86). Based on this, it is reasonable to provide albuterol or other β-2 agonists to patients who are wheezing, but not to prescribe this for patients without evidence of wheezing or undifferentiated coughs.

Recent attention has been focused on *Pelargonium sidoides* for treatment of acute bronchitis. This extract, which is used in many eastern European countries, has been examined in three heterogeneous studies that were the topic of a Cochrane review. Although the review stated that *Pelargonium* may be

TABLE 53.5 Pharmacotherapy Treatment for Influenza

Drug	Dosage	Adverse Effects	Cost per Course ($)*	Comments
Zanamivir	• 2 inhalations q12h for 5 days • Approved in children ≥7 years of age	Cough	$$$	Start within 30 hours; Types A & B shorten symptoms by 1 to 1.5 days
Oseltamivir	• 75 mg BID for 5 days • Approved in children ≥1 years of age, ≤15 kg, 30 mg BID; >15–23 kg, 45 mg BID; >24–40 kg, 60 mg BID; >40 kg, 75 mg BID	Nausea and vomiting; insomnia; vertigo; bronchitis	$$$	Initiate treatment within 36 hours of symptoms; Types A & B shortens symptoms by 1 to 1.5 days

*$ = <$33; $$ = $34–$66; $$$ = >$67.

effective in reducing symptoms of acute bronchitis, the authors acknowledged that because of the scarcity and quality of the evidence there is still some doubt to this conclusion (87).

Bronchiolitis

The mainstay of therapy consists of respiratory support, nutrition, and hydration. Bronchodilators have been suggested as treatments for bronchiolitis, but a meta-analysis of eight trials of bronchodilators versus placebo indicated that bronchodilators produce only limited short-term improvement in clinical scores (88). This small benefit must be weighed against the costs of these agents.

The use of antivirals in the treatment of RSV infections remains controversial. Ribavirin is the only antiviral agent licensed for the treatment of RSV infections and should be considered in severely affected or immunosuppressed children. Patients undergoing therapy should be placed in negative pressure rooms with frequent air exchanges and scavenging systems to decrease ribavirin exposure of health care providers and to minimize release into the surrounding environment. Uncontrolled trials show that early therapy with ribavirin aerosol may be beneficial (89). In a systematic review of 10 trials of ribavirin for RSV, it was concluded that the trials lack sufficient power to provide reliable estimates of the effects (90). The cumulative results of three small trials show that ribavirin reduces length of mechanical ventilator support, and may reduce days of hospitalization. Vaccines against RSV are under development but not yet available. Hand washing is currently the most effective preventive measure.

Influenza

Treatment of influenza infection is targeted toward symptoms, with spontaneous recovery within 5 to 7 days. Therapy includes bed rest, oral hydration, acetaminophen or nonsteroidal anti-inflammatory drugs to reduce fever, headache, and myalgias, and over-the-counter throat lozenges. Preventative measures along with antiviral drugs are used to shorten the disease course and decrease secondary complications (91).

Selected patients with influenza may benefit from antiviral agents (Table 53.5). Two neuraminidase inhibitors, zanamivir and oseltamivir, are useful to treat both influenza A and B. An analysis of six randomized placebo-controlled trials of zanamivir indicated a decrease in illness duration ranging from 1 to 2 days in different populations (92). The greatest benefit was found in patients >50 years of age. Randomized trials of oseltamivir have also demonstrated reduced duration of illness (93,94). The treatments must be given within 36 hours, and preferably within 24 hours, of onset to be effective.

PREVENTION

Vaccination for influenza is the most common and effective way to prevent influenza. Each year's vaccine contains three virus strains representing the viruses that are predicted to circulate in the United States during the upcoming influenza season. Unfortunately, sometimes the supply of influenza vaccine is delayed or insufficient to cover all patients recommended for immunization (95).

According to the 2010 recommendations of the Centers for Disease Control and Prevention, all persons 6 months and older should receive the influenza vaccine. A special effort should be made to include the following high risk groups:

- All children between the ages of 6 months and 18 years;
- Children or adults who have a chronic lung condition (including asthma), heart disease (except hypertension), diabetes, liver disease, cognitive, neuromuscular/neurologic, hematologic, or metabolic disorder;
- Children or adults who are immunosuppressed;
- Pregnant individuals;
- Health care personnel;
- Children or adults who reside in long-term care facilities.
- Children who are receiving long-term aspirin therapy;
- Household contacts and caregivers of adults older than age 50 or children younger than the age of 5 with particular attention to those caring for infants younger than 6 months of age;
- Household contacts and caregivers of individuals with medical conditions that would put them at higher risk for complications from influenza.

Because of the decline of immunity during the year and antigen variation from year to year within the influenza virus, individuals should receive the vaccine every year. The optimal time for vaccination is October to mid-November.

TABLE 53.6 Oral Pharmacotherapy for Ambulatory Management of Community-acquired Pneumonia in Adults

Drug	Dosage	Cost ($)*	Dosing Instructions†
Azithromycin	500 mg day 1, then 250 mg for 4 days	$$	
Doxycycline	100 mg twice daily for 10–14 days	$	Contraindicated in children and pregnancy. May cause photosensitivity. Do not give calcium or dairy products within 2 hours of dose.
Cefuroxime axetil	250–500 mg twice daily for 10 days	$$$	May cause elevated liver enzymes.
Amoxicillin-clavulanate potassium	875 mg twice daily for 10–14 days	$$	Use reduced dose if impaired renal function.
Levofloxacin	250–500 mg once per day for 10–14 d	$$	Do not give to children or pregnant women; if renal impairment, reduce dose. Do not give calcium, iron, or magnesium within 2 hours of dose.
Moxifloxacin	400 mg once per day for 10 days	$$$	Do not give to children or pregnant women.

*$ = <$33; $$ = $34–$66; $$$ = >$67.
†All of these medications can cause diarrhea or nausea.

Community-acquired Pneumonia

A Centers for Disease Control and Prevention working group on drug-resistant *S. pneumoniae* released recommendations on management of community-acquired pneumonia (CAP) (97) (see Table 53.6). These recommendations are similar to more recent recommendations from the American College of Chest Physicians (98). For outpatient treatment of CAP, suitable empiric oral antimicrobial agents include a macrolide (e.g., erythromycin, clarithromycin, azithromycin), doxycycline (or tetracycline) for children age 8 years or older, or an oral β-lactam with good activity against pneumococci (e.g., cefuroxime axetil, amoxicillin, or a combination of amoxicillin and clavulanate potassium). As an alternative a respiratory fluoroquinolone (e.g., levofloxacin, maxifloxin) can be used. Although expert opinion usually advises 10 to 14 days of antibiotic treatment for community-acquired pneumonia, one study showed that antibiotic courses as short as 3 to 5 days were equally effective (99).

In addition to appropriate antibiotic management, several other factors influence whether the patient with pneumonia should be cared for at home or in the hospital (100). The decision whether the patient should be hospitalized versus treated at home can be assisted by some simple decision tools such as the CURB-65 Severity score (101). The CURB-65 relies on three clinical criteria (confusion, hypotension, tachypnea), one laboratory value (blood urea nitrogen), and patient age to computer a score that reflects the overall risk to the patient (Table 53.7) If the decision is made to treat the patient at home, the patient's primary caregiver(s) should be instructed in the management plan and be capable of carrying out the plan. Additionally, the patient should be able to carry on with their usual activities of living and have adequate oxygenation either on room air or with supplemental oxygen. Suitable follow-up should be arranged, and the patient should be reliable about returning for subsequent care or if problems arise.

If patients are at high risk for mortality based on their age, clinical condition, or pre-existing comorbidities, the patient should be hospitalized for treatment. Empiric antimicrobial regimens for inpatient pneumonia depend on the patient's severity of illness and the risk for pseudomonas (102). For lower risk patients who are not severely ill, therapy can include an intravenous β-lactam, such as cefuroxime, ceftriaxone sodium, cefotaxime sodium, or a combination of ampicillin sodium and sulbactam sodium, plus a macrolide. New fluoroquinolones with improved activity against *S. pneumoniae* can also be used to treat adults with CAP. To limit the emergence of fluoroquinolone-resistant strains, the new fluoroquinolones should be limited to adults for whom one of the above regimens has already failed, who are allergic to alternative agents; or who have a documented infection with highly drug-resistant pneumococci (e.g., penicillin mean inhibitory concentration 4 μg/mL). Studies examining the effectiveness of fluoroquinolones compared to two-drug regimens have confirmed that a respiratory fluoroquinolone alone is equally effective and may be more effective in patients with severe pneumonia (102). Vancomycin hydrochloride is not routinely indicated for the treatment of CAP or pneumonia caused by drug-resistant *S. pneumoniae*.

PREVENTION

Multivalent pneumococcal vaccine is recommended for individuals older than age 65, and those 2 years of age or older with diabetes mellitus, chronic pulmonary or cardiac disease, and those without a spleen. Additionally, vaccination is recommended for people in certain high-risk populations, such as Native American, Alaska Native populations, and those people older than age 50 living in chronic care facilities should be vaccinated. Despite these recommendations, the evidence that pneumococcal pneumonia is successful in preventing pneumonia or death from pneumonia is weak; a meta-analysis that

TABLE 53.7 The CURB-65 Decision Rule to Guide Hospitalization for Pneumonia

Factor		Score
Confusion		1 point
Blood urea nitrogen >19		1 point
Respiratory rate ≥30 per minute		1 point
Systolic blood pressure ≤90 or diastolic blood pressure ≤60		1 point
Age ≥65		1 point
CURB Score	**Risk of Death (%)**	**Clinical implications**
0	0.6	Consider home care
1	2.7	Consider home care
2	6.8	Hospitalization or home care with close observation
3	14.0	Hospitalization
4 or 5	27.8	Hospitalization, consider intensive care

Note: If omitting the blood urea nitrogen, only a score of 0 should be used for home care.
Data from Aujesky D, Auble TE, Yealy DM, et al. Prospective comparison of three validated prediction rules for prognosis in community-acquired pneumonia. *Am J Med* 2005;118:384–392; Ebell MH. Point of Care Guide: Outpatient vs. inpatient treatment of community-acquired pneumonia. *Am Fam Physician*. 2006;73(8):1425–1428.

included more than 100,000 people found that for older patients and those with chronic illnesses, pneumococcal pneumonia vaccination was not effective at preventing presumed pneumococcal pneumonia (RR = 1.04, 95% confidence interval 0.78–1.38) or all-cause pneumonia (RR = 0.89, 95% CI 0.69–1.14) (103). Immunosuppressed patients including those with HIV, alcoholism, cirrhosis, chronic renal failure, sickle cell disease, or multiple myeloma may benefit from immunization, but the evidence is less convincing.

In addition to initial vaccination, clinicians should advise patients that the duration of protection is uncertain. For those at particularly high risk of mortality from pneumococcal pneumonia, such as patients older than age 75 and those with chronic pulmonary disease or lacking a spleen, revaccination every 5 years may be appropriate.

For children, pneumococcal conjugate vaccination is recommended starting at 2 months of age. For previously unimmunized children, catch-up vaccination is recommended for those still younger than 59 months old.

PATIENT EDUCATION

Patients need to be educated that most viral illnesses are short-lived and will resolve without any treatment. In particular, patients should be counseled about the lack of benefit of antibiotics and the potential for harm from using these drugs. Physicians also may be able to reshape patient expectations by relabeling illnesses. For example, rather than calling a problem "acute bronchitis," clinicians can tell patients they have a "chest cold." This reinterpretation of their disease may lead to improved satisfaction at not receiving antibiotics as expected (104).

Rather than prescribe antibiotics for viral syndromes, some clinicians have examined the use of "delayed" or "safety net" prescriptions, by which they provide the patient with an antibiotic prescription but advise them not to fill it right away. In one study focusing on otitis media, only 38% of the parents of children who received "safety net" antibiotics filled the prescription (105). Another study examining the use of a backup prescription in patients with acute respiratory illnesses found that only about half of these were filled despite the observation that 76% of patients thought that an antibiotic would be necessary for their illness (106). With appropriate guidance for patients about not filling the prescription right away, this approach is another strategy to reduce unnecessary antibiotic use.

In addition to counseling regarding treatment options, patients need to be reminded to practice careful hand sanitation to reduce spread of their infection and to cough into the crook of their arm rather than create a viral "fog" that spreads 3 to 6 feet in front of them.

KEY POINTS

- Most acute respiratory tract infections, including most episodes of acute bronchitis, are viral and do not benefit from antibiotics.
- A chest x-ray should be performed for any patient with acute RTI and a fever higher than 100°F, tachypnea more than 20 breaths/minute, tachycardia higher than 100 beats/minute, or if a patient has any two of the following: rales, decreased breath sounds, or no history of asthma.
- Use the CURB-65 clinical decision rule to determine the prognosis and best location of treatment for adults with pneumonia.
- Consider antibiotics for patients with acute rhinosinusitis of at least 10 days' duration.

CHAPTER

54

Acute Respiratory Infections in Children

Vince Winkler Prins and William Wadland

CLINICAL OBJECTIVES

1. Describe and differentiate between common upper and lower respiratory tract illnesses in children.
2. Use evidence-based principles to assist in the assessment and management of common respiratory illnesses in children.
3. Discriminate serious from less serious respiratory illnesses in children.

Respiratory illness is the most common acute reason that children visit their primary care physicians. Although common, approaches to assessment and management differ widely and are not uniform. There is, however, a considerable body of evidence that suggests best practices that can aid in diagnosis and management of the child acutely sick with a respiratory illness.

This chapter will focus on the most common acute respiratory illnesses in children and will offer best practices to assessment and management. We have divided this topic into sections on initial triage with assessment for severity of illness, and then disease entities organized by upper versus lower respiratory disease. The assessment of the very young infant, 3 months of age or younger, requires a higher index of suspicion for serious bacterial illness. This topic is well covered in pediatric texts and will not be the subject of this chapter.

INITIAL TRIAGE OF RESPIRATORY ILLNESS

The Institute for Clinical Systems Improvement has issued an evidence-based health care guideline that addresses the assessment of respiratory illness in children and adults (1). A modification of this with a focus on children is shown in Figure 54.1. Table 54.1 addresses assessment for potentially serious illness.

UPPER RESPIRATORY ILLNESSES

For the purposes of this chapter, clinical entities that encompass acute upper respiratory tract illness include acute viral upper respiratory tract infection (AVURI) or common cold, pharyngitis, acute rhinosinusitis (sinusitis), and acute otitis media. Clinical entities that encompass acute lower respiratory tract illness will include acute bronchitis, croup, bronchiolitis, influenza, and pneumonia.

Acute Viral Upper Respiratory Tract Infections (Common Cold)

HISTORY

AVURIs are very common in children, averaging between five and eight per child per year. Children in day care are more likely to get more frequent infections early on but fewer as they get older (2).

Common causative organisms include rhinoviruses (most common cause), parainfluenza viruses, adenoviruses, coronaviruses, influenza viruses, respiratory syncytial virus (RSV), and enteroviruses. Symptoms commonly include some combination of sore throat, sneezing, headache, nasal congestion, rhinorrhea, cough, conjunctival injection, mild irritability or fussiness, decreased appetite, sleep disturbance, and mild eye redness or drainage of relatively acute onset. Symptoms usually peak in 3 to 5 days and usually resolve in 7 to 14 days with a mild residual cough that may last up to a few weeks (3,4).

PHYSICAL EXAMINATION

Children with AVURI should not appear very ill and should not have signs of more serious toxicity listed in Table 54.1. Low-grade fever rhinorrhea, mild conjunctival injection, cough, and mild pharyngeal erythema are common clinical findings on exam. Nasal drainage begins clear and usually becomes yellow or green toward the end but this does not signify the need for antibiotic treatment (5).

DIAGNOSTIC TESTING

The diagnosis of an AVURI is a clinical one after the other diagnoses under consideration have been reasonably excluded. No testing is indicated.

TREATMENT

The goal with treatment is to provide the child and family with education about the natural course of the illness and comfort measures that may assist during recovery. Symptoms should improve over the course of 10 days and should not worsen after 5 days. Parents may benefit from education about differences between viral and bacterial illness and problems and concerns about use and overuse of antibiotics (5). Strategies to prevent further spread may include: handwashing more than 10 times daily (number needed to treat [NNT] = 4), wearing masks (NNT = 6), wearing N95 masks (NNT = 3), wearing gloves (NNT = 5), wearing gowns (NNT = 5), and handwashing, masks, gloves, and gowns combined (NNT = 3) (6). Breast-feeding may also offer some protection to the infant exposed to children with AVURI (7). Some evidence

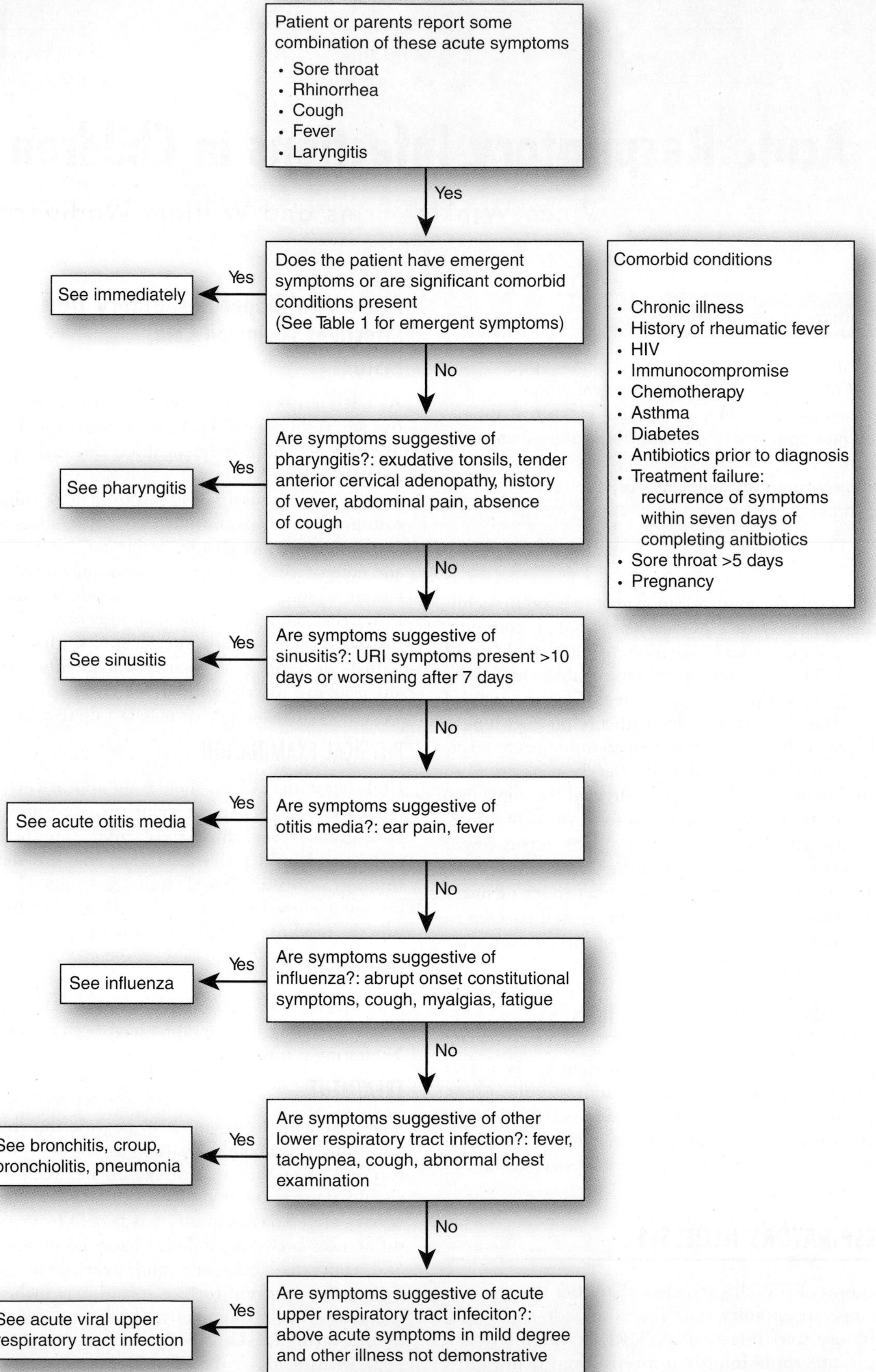

Figure 54.1 • Triage and diagnosis of respiratory illness in children. (Adapted from Institute for Clinical Systems Improvement. Health Care Guideline: Diagnosis and Treatment of Respiratory Illness in Children and Adults.)

TABLE 54.1 Emergent Symptoms or Signs of Potentially Serious Illness

	Younger than 3 Months of Age	3 Months to 3 Years of Age	Age 4 years Old and Older
Respiratory distress	• Grunting • Retractions • Cyanosis • Stridor with croup symptoms not relieved by conservative measures	• Retractions • Cyanosis • Marked dyspnea • Rapid respiratory rate • Shallow respirations • Difficulty swallowing • Choking • Foreign body inhalation • Stridor with croup symptoms not relieved by conservative measures	• Retractions • Cyanosis • Moderate to severe dyspnea • Rapid respiratory rate • Shallow respirations • Difficulty swallowing • Choking • Foreign body inhalation • Drooling • Dysphonia • Feeling that throat is closing
Responsiveness and activity	• Flaccid • Lethargic • Cannot awaken or keep awake • Weak cry or weak suck • Inconsolable • Refuses feedings	• Unresponsive • Decreased level of consciousness • Cannot awaken or keep awake • Markedly decreased activity • Very lethargic • Sleeps excessively • Inconsolable • Weak suck or weak cry (infant) • Refuses feedings	• Altered mental state • Decreased level of consciousness • Markedly decreased activity • Refuses to eat • Very lethargic • Sleeps excessively • Cannot awaken or keep awake • Unresponsive
Dehydration and vomiting	• Reduced wet diapers over a period greater than 8 hours	• No urine over 6–8 hours if younger than 1 year • No urine in more than 12 hours if older than 1 year	• No urine in more than 12 hours
Meningeal signs		• Stiff neck • Persistent vomiting	• Stiff neck • Persistent vomiting • Severe headache
Other	• Petechial or purpuric rash	• Petechial or purpuric rash	• Increased urination with decreased intake • Petechial or purpuric rash

(Adapted from: Institute for Clinical Systems Improvement. Health Care Guideline: Diagnosis and Treatment of Respiratory Illness in Children and Adults. Available at: *www.icsi.org/respiratory_illness_in_children_and_adults_guideline_/respiratory_illness_in_children_and_adults_guideline_13116.html.* Accessed 3.10.2010)

suggests that vitamin C may decrease the duration and severity of symptoms and ginseng when used regularly may reduce the duration of AVURIs. Probiotics may also reduce the incidence and duration of AVURIs (8–10).

Evidence to support treatment with humidifiers or vaporizers, either hot or cold, is mixed (11). Humidifiers increase the probability of mold in the home and are common breeding grounds for microorganisms. Hot humidifiers increase the risk for burns (12). Nasal bulb syringes with soft rubber tips, often given to parents of newborns in the hospital may be used to gently clear the nostrils of very young infants and may provide comfort, but there is otherwise no proof of improved outcomes with their use. Acetaminophen is effective for fever and headache as are ibuprofen and naproxen (13). Extra fluids, elevating the head of the bead, and warm liquids (e.g., chicken soup) are also often cited comfort measures without obvious proof of improved outcomes for children. In fact the adage of "pushing fluids" was evaluated in a meta-analysis in 2004 with no evidence found to support its effectiveness (14). More concerning was that the authors found evidence of theoretic risk for harm from this practice (14). The US Food and Drug Administration discourages use of cough suppressants in children younger than age 2 and proof of utility for the older child is also lacking, although there may be some evidence of effectiveness of honey for cough suppression in children 2 years and older (15,16). Honey should not be used in the younger child. Antihistamines may help relieve nasal symptoms in older children (17).

Pharyngitis

HISTORY

Pharyngitis is the third most common acute respiratory illness in children after AVURIs and otitis. Most pharyngitis is of viral origin with many potential pathogens that include: adenovirus, parainfluenza, rhinovirus, herpes simplex type 1 and 2 (especially gingivitis and stomatitis), respiratory syncytial virus (hoarseness and wheezing more common), Epstein-Barr virus (infectious mononucleosis), influenza, coxsackievirus A (herpangina—summer/fall predominantly), enterovirus (diarrhea), HIV, coronavirus, and cytomegalovirus (18).

Mononucleosis is classically associated with adolescence although not exclusively and should be suspected in patients 10 to 30 years of age who present with sore throat, prominent fatigue, fever, adenopathy (especially posterior cervical), and hepatosplenomegaly. Fatigue may persist and slowly resolve over months (19).

Differentiating between pharyngitis of viral etiology (including infectious mononucleosis) and bacterial illness with streptococcus is often the major concern for the clinician. Group A beta hemolytic strep (GABHS) is classically a disease of school-aged children and adolescents, is very uncommon in children younger than 3 years and is more common during the winter and spring. It accounts for 15% to 30% of bacterial cases of acute pharyngitis in children. With the exception of gonococcal pharyngitis, which would more likely present in adolescence and often be associated with fever, arthralgias, rash and dysuria, most other bacterial pathogens are not normally virulent and do not normally require treatment. Classic GABHS symptoms include odynophagia, high fever, lethargy, and absence of other AVURI symptoms. Abdominal pain may also be part of the presenting picture in younger children. Potential complications of GABHS pharyngitis include peritonsillar abscess, retropharyngeal abscess, cervical lymphadenitis, acute poststreptococcal glomerulonephritis, and rheumatic fever. Pharyngitis often precedes other symptoms associated with AVURI, and this feature often helps discriminate viral from bacterial illness.

PHYSICAL EXAMINATION

Findings on exam may include fever, pharyngeal erythema, tonsillar enlargement, tonsillar exudates, palatal petechiae, anterior and/or posterior cervical lymphadenopathy (more common with mono), bad breath, and possibly a rash. A sandpaper-like "scarlatiniform" rash is classic for scarlet fever—strep throat with a rash.

DIAGNOSTIC TESTING

Physicians are not very good at differentiating viral from bacterial illness (20). Use of a validated clinical decision rule helps clinicians decide the likelihood of viral versus bacterial pharyngitis and when testing is appropriate prior to making a decision about treatment. The Centor/McIsaac clinical decision rule for diagnosis of Group A beta-hemolytic strep pharyngitis is shown in Figure 54.2.

If suspicion is higher for infectious mononucleosis then testing for this should be considered. Immunoglobulin M antibody for Epstein-Barr viral capsid antigen has the most sensitivity and specificity in the acute setting (21). Note that the commonly used "monospot" test for heterophile antibodies has poor sensitivity in children younger than 13 years of age.

TREATMENT

Management of pharyngitis is primarily supportive and educational unless GABHS is identified. Treatment of GABHS infection with antibiotics reduces the risk of suppurative complications and rheumatic fever, although the latter is extremely uncommon nowadays. Recommended treatment options for this infection include penicillin for 7 to 10 days orally or via single intramuscular injection. Macrolides are alternatives for penicillin allergic patients, as are cephalosporins for those whose penicillin allergy warrants consideration of cephalosporins as an

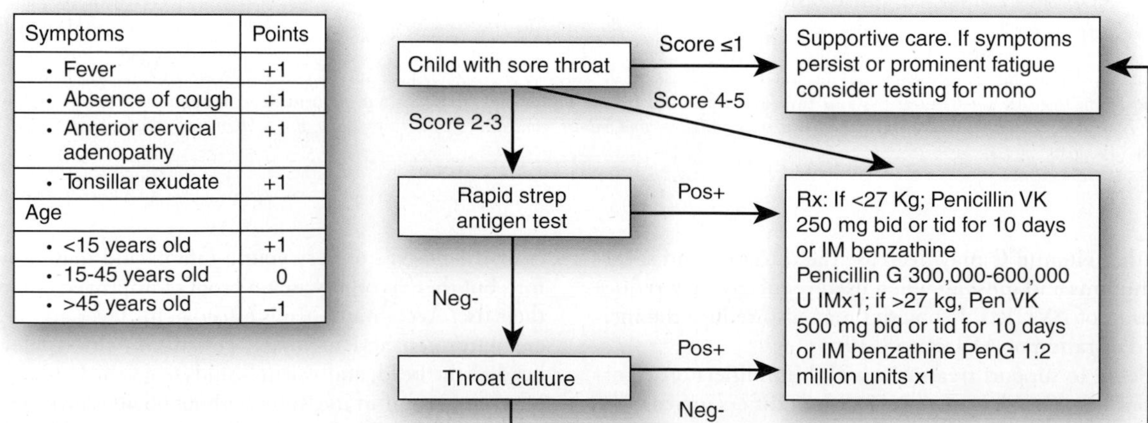

Symptoms	Points
• Fever	+1
• Absence of cough	+1
• Anterior cervical adenopathy	+1
• Tonsillar exudate	+1
Age	
• <15 years old	+1
• 15-45 years old	0
• >45 years old	−1

Figure 54.2 • Assessment and management of the child with pharyngitis. Adapted from: Willies-Jacabo L. Sore throat and pharyngitis. In *Essential Evidence, 2009*. John Wiley and Sons, Inc; 2009.

TABLE 54.2 Common Antibiotics for Treatment of Bacterial Sinusitis in Children

Name	Concentration	Frequency and Duration
First-line unless allergic		
Amoxicillin	80/90 mg/kg/day	BID, 10 days
Cephalosporin alternatives		
Cefdinir	14 mg/kg/day	BID, 10 days
Cefuroxime	30 mg/kg/day	BID, 10 days
Cefpodoxime	10 mg/kg/day	BID, 10 days
Clarithromycin	15 mg/kg/day	BID, 10 days
Macrolide alternative		
Azithromycin	10 mg/kg/day on day 1, 5 mg/kg/day on days 2–4	Once per day for 5 days

BID = twice daily.

alternative. It is not known, however, if cephalosporins reduce the risk of rheumatic disease (22). Acetaminophen is usually sufficient to reduce the pain of pharyngitis in children. In GABHS-negative children with severe pharyngitis pain, corticosteroids can significantly reduce pain in strep-negative pharyngitis as can acetaminophen (23). GABHS carriers are unlikely to be vectors for spread and are at little risk for complications. Referral to an otolaryngologist for consideration of tonsillectomy is indicated for children who develop more than six episodes of GABHS pharyngitis in a 12-month period (24).

Acute Rhinosinusitis

HISTORY

Acute rhinosinusitis, often simply called sinusitis, is inflammation of the mucosa of the paranasal sinuses and nasal epithelium. When considering the diagnosis of sinusitis, it is helpful to remember that the ethmoid sinuses are pneumatized at birth, the maxillary sinuses at 4 years, sphenoidal at 5 years, and frontal at age 7 or 8 years (25). Although the term *sinusitis* often connotes bacterial infection, most illnesses of this type do not require antibiotics. Complications of sinusitis include orbital cellulitis, periorbital cellulitis, or other intracranial infections, but these are rare. Acute sinusitis incidence peaks during the fall and winter, generally mirroring the AVURI season (26). It is most commonly seen after an AVURI, but allergic rhinitis also increases risk. Sinusitis develops in 6% to 13% of children by the age of 3 years (27), and although viral isolates are common, the most common bacterial isolates in those with bacterial superinfection are *Streptococcus pneumoniae*, *Haemophilus influenza*, and *Moraxella catarrhalis* (26). The most common symptoms suggestive of sinusitis are rhinorrhea, cough, fever, postnasal drip, and face pain.

PHYSICAL EXAMINATION

Normally the child with acute sinusitis will present with signs of a viral upper respiratory tract infection. Additional findings may include nasal and pharyngeal mucosal erythema with purulent yellow or green rhinorrhea. Physical findings that may increase the probability of sinusitis for which antibiotics would more likely be useful include more severe illness and fever, unilateral purulent drainage, and signs and symptoms of orbital or meningeal infection.

DIAGNOSTIC TESTING

Diagnostic imaging is not needed, as sinusitis is primarily a clinical diagnosis. Air fluid levels in the sinuses are not uncommonly noted on paranasal sinus x-rays, but this finding alone may not require treatment. Transillumination is not useful in children, and computed tomography scanning should be generally reserved for those in whom surgery is being considered for chronic disease (28).

TREATMENT

Judicious use of antibiotics is indicated in certain circumstances. Consider antibiotics in children when symptoms of AVURI persist beyond 10 days or when symptoms are more severe than usual after several days of improvement (26). Antibiotics may be indicated in situations of severe illness especially with concomitant fever and purulent rhinorrhea (26,29). When antibiotics are indicated, high-dose amoxicillin for 10 days remains the initial recommendation (Table 54.2). If the patient is allergic and the reaction is not a type 1 hypersensitivity reaction, then the cephalosporins listed in the table are appropriate options. In cases of severe allergic disease the macrolides provide good alternatives. If the patient does not improve within 48 to 72 hours, has recently been treated with antibiotics, has an illness that is more severe, or attends day care, initiate therapy with high-dose amoxicillin-clavulanate or the cephalosporins listed in Table 54.2 (28). Parenteral ceftriaxone may be used for a child who cannot tolerate oral antibiotics (e.g., because of vomiting).

Nasal washing with saline can improve and eliminate nasal sections and reduce edema. The effectiveness of intranasal corticosteroids remains uncertain in children but may improve symptoms in some patients who are also receiving antibiotics (30). There is no good evidence that topical or oral decongestants or decongestant-antihistamine combinations are effective.

Acute Otitis Media

HISTORY

Acute otitis media (AOM) remains one of the most frequent reasons for acute visits to pediatric providers and a major cause of missed school by children and missed work by parents. Children with AOM usually present with the acute onset of fever and/or ear pain. Most AOM is associated with AVURIs, but allergies and exposure to smoke and particulates increase risk. Pathophysiologically, the net effects are eustachian tube swelling, negative middle ear pressure, and serous fluid accumulation. This serous fluid may then become infected by bacteria or viruses. Although middle ear fluid is sterile in 30% of children with AOM, the most commonly isolated bacteria are *Streptococcus pneumonia* (30%), *H. influenza* (25%), *M. catarrhalis* (10%), Group A streptococcus, (10%) and *Staphylococcus aureus* (10%) (31).

Preventive strategies may include breast feeding, reducing pacifier use, elimination of smoke exposure, eliminating supine feedings in infants, and decreasing day care exposure (32). Influenza immunization reduces risk of AOM, but pneumococcal vaccination does not seem to confer the same benefit (33,34).

PHYSICAL EXAMINATION

Although only the combination of high fever and vomiting identify those most likely to benefit from antibiotics (35), specific exam findings that best rule in AOM include middle ear fluid on exam or testing (pneumatic otoscopy) and signs of middle ear inflammation, which may include erythema or purulent middle ear fluid.

DIAGNOSTIC TESTING

The diagnosis of AOM remains a clinical one without need for laboratory studies or x-ray. Pneumatic otoscopy or tympanometry should be used to aid in the diagnosis.

TREATMENT

A recommended protocol for the management of AOM is shown in Figure 54.3. Pain can be treated with appropriate doses of acetaminophen or ibuprofen, and children older than age 2 years with mild illness can be observed without antibiotics for 24 to 48 hours as long as follow-up is available (36,37). Children younger than 2 years will have symptoms for a median of 8 days. Regardless of antibiotic treatment, some children will have fever, ear pain, or both for several days. Complications such as mastoiditis are rare in the antibiotic era.

Antihistamines, decongestants, intranasal steroids and topical analgesic ear drops are not effective for treatment of AOM (38,39). Myringotomy and tympanostomy tubes reduce the recurrence of AOM in children with three or more episodes within 6 months and four or more episodes within a year (40). Adenoidectomy and tonsillectomy are of minimal benefit in preventing recurrences (41). Additional information on AOM can be found in Chapter 16, Ear Pain.

LOWER RESPIRATORY ILLNESSES

Acute Bronchitis

HISTORY

Children with acute bronchitis typically present with an acute respiratory infection with cough as the predominant symptom, with or without fever and sputum production. The symptoms can last for 3 to 4 weeks. Nighttime cough or wheezing may be the only sign of bronchial obstruction. Repetitive episodes of acute bronchitis may be symptomatic of reactive airway disease or underlying asthma. There may be a social history for secondary smoke or toxic inhalant exposures. There may be reported exposure to other children or family members with similar symptoms. Common causes of acute bronchitis are the typical respiratory viruses, including parainfluenza, respiratory syncytial virus, influenza A, and influenza B. Bacteria such as *Mycoplasma pneumoniae*, *Chlamydia pneumoniae*, *Bordetella pertussis*, and *Bordetella parapertussis* cause <10% of cases (42). Close contact with a confirmed case of pertussis would be strongly suggestive of the same diagnosis, especially if the cough lasts for more than 2 weeks, accompanied by paroxysms, vomiting, and whooping (42).

PHYSICAL EXAMINATION

Children often but not always present with a low-grade fever and a predominant cough, without acute respiratory distress. Exam may show rhinitis or pharyngitis, conjunctivitis, or otitis media. Neck exam may have lymphadenopathy. Lung exam may show mild wheezing, rhonchi, or prolonged expiratory phase but no acute obstructive findings.

DIAGNOSTIC TESTING

There are no clear diagnostic criteria for acute bronchitis. Chest x-ray would be merited to rule out pneumonia in children presenting with high fever (>38°C), toxic appearance, respiratory distress, or increased heart rate for age. Clinicians have not been able to accurately distinguish viral from bacterial causes of acute bronchitis based on clinical findings (20). A procalcitonin level of >2 ng/mL or a C-reactive protein level >6.5 mg/dL can help distinguish bacterial from viral infections in children, but these tests are not routinely done in the outpatient setting because of added cost and time. Cultures for pertussis have low sensitivity (25% to 50%), giving high false-negative rates (43).

TREATMENT

Antibiotics should not be prescribed for acute bronchitis unless there is a high suspicion for pertussis. Even fever and green sputum do not increase the probability that an antibiotic will help those with a negative chest x-ray (44–46). Tactics that can be used to provide appropriate care for acute bronchitis include giving parents an information sheet explaining the lack of efficacy of antibiotics, referring to the condition as a "chest cold," and using delayed prescription filling for persistent or worsening symptoms. Perhaps contrary to many clinicians' impressions, using these strategies does not increase the duration of the office visit. Aggressive forcing of fluids in children is not warranted and may provoke hyponatremia. Cough suppressants should not be used in children younger than age

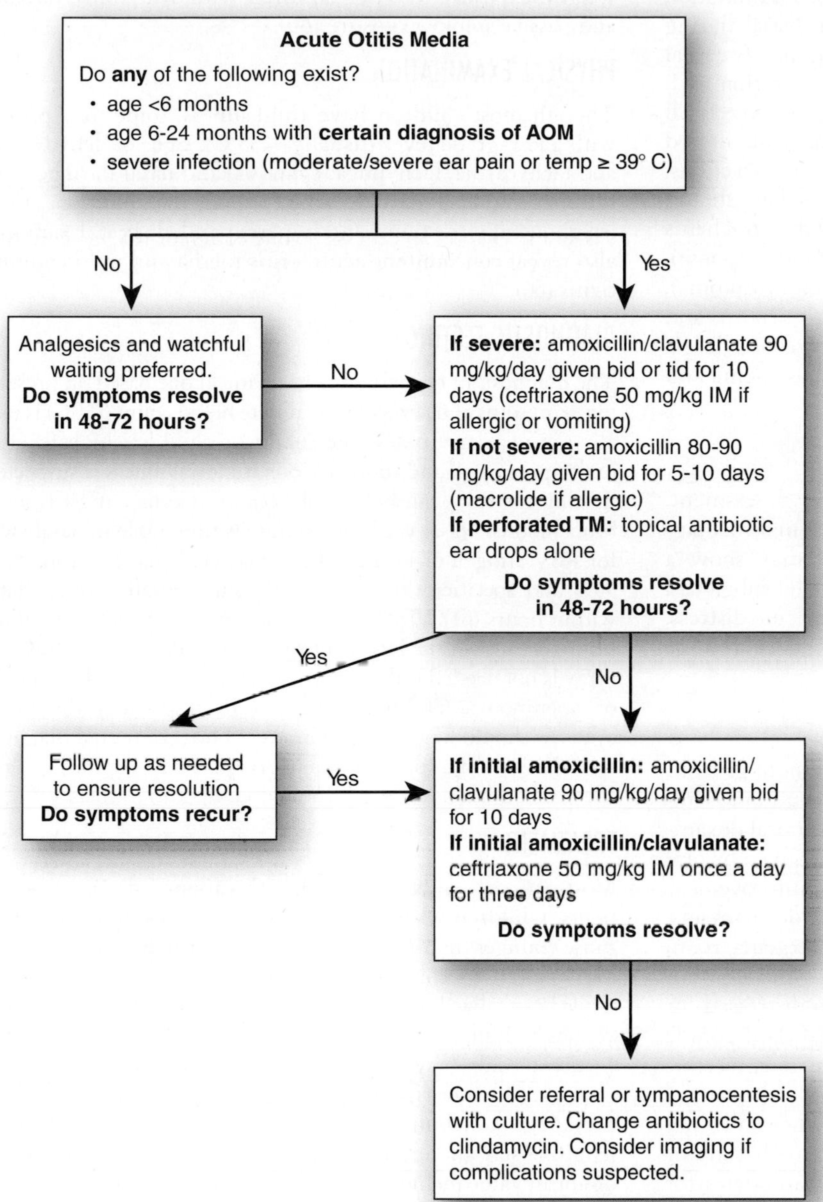

Figure 54.3 • Management of acute otitis media. Adapted from Cooke JM, Shaughnessy AF. Otitis media (acute). In *Essential Evidence Plus 2009*. John Wiley & Sons, Inc. and based on AAFP/AAP Practice Guidelines. American Academy of Pediatrics Subcommittee on Management of Acute Otitis Media. Diagnosis and management of acute otitis media. *Pediatrics*. 2004;113(5):1451–1465.

6 years and are no more effective overall than placebo in decreasing cough (47–53).

Croup

HISTORY

Children with croup typically are age 5 years or younger and present with a harsh barking seal-like ("croupy") cough with gradually increasing respiratory stridor and hoarseness. There may be a 2- to 5-day prodrome of fever, rhinorrhea, wheezing, sore throat, malaise, and more frequent coughing at night (54). The most common causes of croup are parainfluenza virus (types 1, 2, and 3) and influenza A and B (54). Less common causes are respiratory syncytial virus, mycoplasma pneumoniae, adenovirus, rhinovirus, enterovirus, and herpes simplex (54). Stridor is triggered by edema and swelling of the subglottic region.

PHYSICAL EXAMINATION

Children may present with a fever and have varying degrees of illness. There may be tachycardia and tachypnea with loud stridor and barking cough. There are four levels of severity: level 1 (mild)—occasional barky cough, no stridor at rest, and mild retractions; level 2 (moderate)—frequent barky cough, stridor at rest, retractions at rest, and with minimal agitation; level 3 (severe)—frequent barky cough, prominent stridor, significant retractions, marked distress, and agitation; and level 4 (impending respiratory failure)—barky cough, stridor at rest, retractions, lethargy or decreased level of consciousness, often dusky without supplemental oxygenation (55). Examination may show mild inflammation of the pharynx. Nasal flaring may imply severe croup or pneumonia. Lung exam may reveal wheezing, inspiratory stridor, and prolonged inspiration with mild suprasternal and chest wall retractions. A severely ill child with impending respiratory arrest may have an altered mental state, pallor, cyanosis, severely increased retractions, and decreased stridor and breath sounds. Clinicians should consider other possible diagnoses, such as bacterial tracheitis (high fever, toxic appearance, and poor treatment response), foreign body (choking history without viral symptoms), epiglottis (sudden high fever, drooling, sitting upright), and retropharyngeal abscess (throat pains and fever), or allergic reaction (wheezing without stridor; also often has edema and rash).

DIAGNOSTIC TESTING

The diagnosis of croup is made by clinical assessment. Laboratory and radiologic tests are not needed to make a diagnosis. An anteroposterior x-ray of the neck may show a "steeple sign," with cone-shaped narrowing of the subglottis. The study should not be done when a child is in acute distress. Viral and rapid antigen testing does not enhance routine management.

TREATMENT

It is important to make the child comfortable without provoking agitation. Blow-by oxygen without humidification to children with hypoxia is appropriate. A single dose of oral dexamethasone (0.6 mg/kg up to a maximum of 10 mg given by oral or parenteral route) usually brings about clinical improvement in 6 hours, reduces length of stay in emergency departments, and reduces hospital admissions and return emergency room visits (56,57). It should be considered even in children with mild croup. Children who are vomiting or too distressed for oral medication will benefit from nebulized budesonide (58,59). For children with severe respiratory distress, racemic epinephrine delivered via nebulizer may provide short-term improvement for 1 to 2 hours. Children who have not improved within 4 hours after receiving dexamethasone or who have little family and social support are candidates for hospitalization. Children with impending respiratory failure may require intubation and intensive care. Most mild croup will resolve in 48 to 72 hours and require little follow-up care.

Bronchiolitis

HISTORY

Seen predominantly in infants and children younger than 2 years of age, bronchiolitis (inflammation of the small airways) usually presents with wheezing after a prodrome of upper respiratory symptoms of rhinorrhea, nasal congestion, and cough. Respiratory syncytial virus (RSV, with 2 major subtypes A and B) is the most common cause of bronchiolitis. Other etiologies listed in decreasing frequency are parainfluenza, adenovirus, influenza virus, and rhinovirus. *Mycoplasma pneumoniae* may be present in some cases. The infection causes inflammation and reactivity of bronchial/bronchiolar smooth muscle with mucus production and plugging. Potential for complications is greatest in children younger than 1 year of age. Risk factors for bronchiolitis include male sex, low birth weight, exposure to other children with symptoms, daycare, and passive smoke exposure (60).

PHYSICAL EXAMINATION

Though most children have mild illness, some may present with a low-grade fever (usually <38°C), signs of dehydration, and tachycardia, tachypnea, cyanosis, and nasal flaring. Lung findings may include wheezing, prolonged expiration, crackles, rhonchi, retractions, and hyperexpanded chest. Exam may also reveal concomitant acute otitis media and mild conjunctivitis (60).

DIAGNOSTIC TESTING

The diagnosis of bronchiolitis is a clinical one based on presenting symptoms and severity. Complete blood count (CBC) is usually not necessary unless the infant or child has high fever or toxic appearance and more serious bacterial illness is suspected. Testing for RSV can be useful because it causes most cases of bronchiolitis. Nasal wash or aspirate is preferable to nasal swab for RSV antigen or immunofluorescence. It has a sensitivity of 90% and specificity of 95%, and results usually are available within hours (61). Viral culture and serology have little clinical utility because of the length of time needed to get results. Chest x-ray is not needed unless there are clinical signs and symptoms of pneumonia. Children with severe respiratory disease or cyanosis should have pulse oximetry. The differential diagnosis includes asthma, pneumonia, foreign body aspiration, and chronic conditions such as bronchopulmonary dysplasia (62).

TREATMENT

Most patients can be managed with supportive care as outpatients. Children with a pulse oximetry measurement <90%, those younger than 3 months of age, or with ill or toxic appearance should be considered for hospitalization. Management while hospitalized may include warm, humidified oxygen; intravenous hydration; and respiratory isolation. Bronchodilators and corticosteroids may be beneficial but are also controversial, requiring further rigorously designed studies to evaluate efficacy (62–64). Nebulized 3% saline may significantly reduce the length of stay and improve clinical severity (65). Treatments of doubtful value include antibiotics, aerosolized ribavirin, nebulized furosemide, intravenous RSV immunoglobulin, or inhaled interferon (66). Prophylaxis with palivizumab has not been proven to be cost effective as yet (66).

Follow-up within 1 to 2 days to reevaluate clinical status is appropriate, depending on the severity of the illness and age of the child. Children with RSV are at fivefold greater risk for reactive airway disease one year after infection, with recurrent risks decreasing over time. General precautions of limiting daycare exposure, hand washing, avoiding smoke exposure, and exposure to sick children are recommended. Influenza vaccine is recommended for children ages 6 months of age and older and household contacts.

Influenza

HISTORY

Common symptoms of influenza include fever, myalgias, arthralgias, malaise, dry cough, fatigue, weakness, chest discomfort, and mild upper respiratory symptoms. Diarrhea and vomiting may be present in children. The signs most useful for ruling in influenza include: rigors (LR+ = 7.2), the combination of fever and onset of symptoms <3 days before the office visit (LR+ = 4.0), and sweating (LR+ = 3.0). Symptoms useful in ruling out influenza include: no systemic symptoms (LR− = 0.36), absence of coughing (LR− = 0.38), being able to cope with daily activities (LR− = 0.39), and not needing to be confined to bed (LR− = 0.50) (67). Complicated or severe influenza may present with dyspnea, tachypnea, hypoxia, severe dehydration, and altered mentation meriting hospitalization in young children. There are two types of influenza viruses that cause epidemic disease in humans—influenza A (with two subtypes-HIN1 and H3N2) and influenza B. Influenza C has been described in Japan and France. Young children have increased risk of transmission in households and daycare (68). Duration of symptoms can range from several days to over 2 weeks.

PHYSICAL EXAMINATION

Children may have fever higher than 38°C. Exam shows mild pharyngeal erythema and possibly associated otitis media. Lung findings may reveal occasional wheezes, rhonchi, and crackles. Though most cases are mild and managed as outpatients, children may have signs of toxicity with cyanosis, pallor, dehydration, and respiratory distress (68).

DIAGNOSTIC TESTING

Tests available to confirm influenza include rapid antigen testing, viral culture, serology, reverse transcriptase-polymerase chain reaction, and immunofluorescence assays. The rapid antigen tests have greater yield, if taken by nasopharyngeal or nasal sampling, than throat swabs (69). Routine testing, however, is not recommended, even during epidemic periods. The predictive value of testing will vary, depending on the baseline prevalence of influenza in the community. Testing should be considered for hospitalized patients, severely toxic patients, and the management of close contacts with a person who died of suspected influenza. Other tests, such as a CBC or chest x-ray, are of limited value except when serious concurrent bacterial illness is suspected.

TREATMENT

Treatment of influenza is largely supportive. Recommend rest, fluids, close observation, and use of nonaspirin antipyretics. There is an increased risk for Reye syndrome with aspirin products. Oseltamivir (Tamiflu) can be given to children older than age 1 year. If begun with acute onset of symptoms and taken for 5 days, it may decrease severity of symptoms and secondary complications (70). Zanamivir (Relenza) is an alternative antiviral medication with similar efficacy (71). Antiviral resistance patterns should be monitored to determine the selection of drug and appropriate usage.

For close contacts, chemoprophylaxis with amantadine can be used in high-risk children who have not been immunized, vaccinated children waiting for immunity, immunodeficient persons with poor antibody response to vaccine, and those with a history of anaphylaxis to eggs or with previous influenza vaccine use. Amantadine is associated with possible increased seizure activity. Prophylaxis with antivirals (oseltamivir or zanamivir) for high-risk asymptomatic children with household contacts has some benefit in both symptom reduction and prevention with 1 person not getting influenza for every 14 to 15 people who receives the drug, but at considerable cost (72). Gastrointestinal effects, headaches, and dizziness are reported with antivirals. Monitoring for secondary respiratory infections is important, particularly in children at high risk such as those younger than 6 months of age, those with chronic conditions such as asthma, and those who are immunocompromised. Limiting contacts during febrile illness and maintenance of good hand hygiene and respiratory protection are recommended precautions to prevent transmission. Children age 6 months and older should receive annual vaccinations for influenza if there are no contraindications (73–75).

Pneumonia

HISTORY

Combinations of clinical symptoms are more predictive of pneumonia than any single symptom or sign. Symptoms include fever, cough, shortness of breath, and malaise. Children may also present with poor feeding and chest pains. Pneumonia often follows a previous upper respiratory infection, allowing invasion of the lower tract by pathogens that trigger inflammation.

Common causes of pneumonia vary by age. In children from age 1 to 3 months, common causative organisms include *Chlamydia trachomatis*, RSV, and *Bordetella pertussis*. Among children ages 1 to 5 years, RSV, influenza, parainfluenza, *Staphylococcus aureus*, *Streptococcus pneumoniae*, *Chlamydia trachomatis*, and *Mycoplasma pneumoniae* are common. In older children and adolescents, *M. pneumoniae*, *S. pneumoniae*, *C. pneumoniae*, and respiratory viruses predominate. Eight to 40% of cases of community-acquired pneumonia are mixed infections (76–79). Other diagnoses such as bronchiolitis (if wheezing, younger than age 2 years, and hyperinflation), asthma (recurrent wheezing), aspiration pneumonia (history of choking), and hospital-acquired pneumonia (if recent hospitalization) should be considered.

PHYSICAL EXAMINATION

Pneumonia in children is suggested by the presence of tachypnea, hypoxia, or nasal flaring. Tachypnea is a major sign for identification of pneumonia in infants. Respiratory rates >60 per minute if younger than 2 months of age, >50 per minute if 2 to 12 months of age, and >40 per minute if older than 12 months are of concern. Fever higher than 38.5°C and chest retractions also are markers of potential concern. Nasal flaring is a key indicator for younger children. Lung exam may reveal dullness on percussion, rales, wheezes, crackles, and coarse breath sounds (80).

DIAGNOSTIC TESTING

A chest x-ray showing an infiltrate in the child who has suggestive symptoms and signs is diagnostic of pneumonia. A CBC (looking for an elevated white blood cell count) may be helpful in differentiating viral from bacterial pneumonia. Procalcitonin and C-reactive protein may also be helpful to make this distinction but are not routinely used at present (43). Cultures of sputum or blood have shown to be of little to no benefit.

TREATMENT

Ambulatory, nontoxic children older than age 12 months can be treated as outpatients, with close monitoring and reliable follow-up care. Children younger than age 12 months or who are toxic appearing require hospitalization and close inpatient monitoring. Hypoxic patients should receive oxygen (81). Poor fluid intake may merit intravenous fluids. Antipyretics with non-aspirin products will help maintain comfort. There is no evidence supporting the use of antitussives in children (82). If bacterial pneumonia is suspected, children should be treated with antibiotics. Young infants should be treated with a macrolide to cover *C. pneumonia*. Children age 4 months to 5 years should be treated with high-dose amoxicillin to cover *S. pneumoniae*, and children older than 5 years should be treated with a macrolide to cover *M. pneumoniae*. Typical durations of treatment are 14 days for erythromycin, 5 days for azithromycin, and 7 to 10 days for amoxicillin in uncomplicated infections. Chest physiotherapy has no proven efficacy in children (83).

KEY POINTS

- Most acute respiratory illnesses in children are clinical diagnoses that do not involve diagnostic testing. However, clinical decision tools should be used for otitis media and pharyngitis.
- Antibiotics are often overprescribed for otitis media, AVURIs, pharyngitis, and acute bronchitis. Decision tools can reduce this rate, ensure good outcomes, and maintain patient and family satisfaction.
- Antitussives have almost no place in the care of the young child.
- Influenza vaccine for the child 6 months of age and older should strongly be encouraged.
- Dexamethasone is the treatment of choice for the child with croup.
- A diagnosis of bronchiolitis increases the probability of asthma in the future.
- Procalcitonin and C-reactive protein are evolving tests that may assist the clinician in discriminating viral from bacterial illness.
- Triage for more serious illness and special vigilance for the very young are vital to ensure good outcomes.

CHAPTER

55

Chronic Obstructive Pulmonary Disease

Caroline J. LeClair and David L. Gaspar

CLINICAL OBJECTIVES

1. Identify strategies to reduce the burden of chronic obstructive pulmonary disease (COPD).
2. Describe objective measures for COPD diagnosis and how disease severity is classified.
3. Describe clinical interventions used to achieve optimal patient-centered outcomes.
4. Develop an appropriate treatment plan for patients with COPD to maximize patient function and reduce symptoms.
5. Describe the management of an acute exacerbation of COPD.

COPD is a chronic inflammatory respiratory disease primarily caused by tobacco smoke. It is characterized by progressive airflow obstruction that is not fully reversible, and there are important systemic manifestations that contribute to the severity of COPD.

COPD is a common and costly medical condition. It is a large public health problem in the United States and also has become an epidemic world wide. It is one of the few chronic diseases in which mortality increased instead of decreased between 2000 and 2005 (1). During this time the death rate from COPD increased by 8%, whereas the death rate from other conditions such as cardiovascular disease and stroke decreased (1). In 2005, approximately 1 of 20 deaths in the United States had COPD as the underlying cause, and smoking was estimated to be responsible for 75% of COPD deaths (1). The monetary and societal costs of COPD include consumption of health care resources, caregiver burden, reduced quality of life, and lost workplace productivity because of disability.

COPD is incurable, and the long-term prognosis has been considered poor. Interventions for patients with COPD are aimed at improving quality of life and decreasing symptoms rather than simply improving objective tests of lung function. Thus, a patient-centered orientation is crucial. In addition, because the disease is linked closely with smoking and air pollution, public health strategies to improve air quality and to encourage smoking cessation and avoidance of tobacco can do much to reduce the burden of disease. Family physicians play a key role not only in the management of this condition but in providing family support, advocating for public policy changes to reduce air pollutants and encouraging smoking cessation.

Patients with COPD have a poorer quality of life as their breathing difficulties progress, and disease progression significantly affects the ability to perform activities of daily living. The disease progresses slowly, and patients modify their activities and life in ways to compensate for their respiratory symptoms. They often attribute symptoms to aging or deconditioning. It is common for COPD patients to have significant comorbidities along with their pulmonary difficulties. These additional health problems add to the overall burden of disease that the patient and his family experience and to the cost and complexity of treatments. Some comorbid diseases, such as ischemic heart disease and congestive heart failure have risks that overlap with COPD. COPD patients are known to have evidence of systemic inflammation, which may also contribute to the development or worsening of comorbid diseases (2–4). Extrapulmonary systemic inflammation with activation of circulating inflammatory cells and increased levels of proinflammatory cytokines is associated with skeletal muscle dysfunction, nutritional abnormalities, and weight loss further contributing to morbidity (4). As with many chronic diseases, there is an increased risk of concurrent depression that can cause further deterioration in quality of life. As COPD progresses other nonrespiratory manifestations contribute to a reduction in exercise tolerance and a worsening quality of life. COPD patients experience acute exacerbations of COPD that can vary in severity from mild worsening that requires only a change in medication regimen to a severe exacerbation that requires hospitalization, intubation, or can result in death.

The only intervention that changes the course of the illness is smoking cessation, and targeting smokers to encourage them to quit is an important element of COPD management. Although rehabilitation programs and pharmacologic treatments can improve symptoms and quality of life, none of the existing treatments has been shown to stop disease progression. Exacerbations need to be managed promptly with the goal to avoid hospitalization and serious respiratory compromise. Chronic disease management principles apply to COPD, and a partnership with patients needs to be established so they may take an active part in the decisions involved in the management of their disease (5). In addition to negotiating goals of therapy, advanced directives should be discussed and documented.

Worldwide, the most common risk factor for COPD is smoking. Other risk factors include air pollution, occupational dusts and chemicals, and the burning of biomass fuels in poorly ventilated dwellings. Biomass fuels are used for cooking and heating and pose a risk factor common to women, especially in developing countries such as China and India. It is important to recognize people with risk factors for COPD and ask about symptoms. Because symptoms tend to develop gradually in COPD, people may be unaware of them or may have adapted to them. Many people present to their physician only when their symptoms impact lifestyle and they have to modify activities. By this time, however, many patients are in the later stages of COPD. Most people seek medical attention when they have chronic respiratory symptoms and already have moderate COPD. Many patients are diagnosed at hospitalization when they have an exacerbation of disease. A major goal of the Global Initiative for Chronic Obstructive Lung Disease is to increase health care providers' and the general public's awareness of the significance of COPD symptoms. Chronic cough and sputum are not normal, and their presence should trigger a search for an underlying cause (6). Earlier diagnosis allows for earlier intervention, modification of risk factors, and treatments, which can improve quality of life.

There is a high prevalence of known COPD and a family physician is likely to encounter patients with COPD at least weekly in clinical practice. COPD is on the rise and is now the fourth leading cause of death in the United States. COPD is projected to become the third leading cause of chronic disease related morbidity and mortality worldwide by the year 2020 (1,7). This increase is largely because of alarming smoking rates in the United States and developing countries, especially among women. Approximately 16 million people currently live with a diagnosis of COPD worldwide. However, this number is likely an underestimate of the true prevalence of COPD because it is underdiagnosed and patients often do not present to their doctor until they are in the later stages as mentioned above. An estimated 10 million US adults reported physician-diagnosed COPD in 2000 (1). However, data from the third National Health and Nutrition Examination Survey suggest that approximately 24 million US adults have evidence of impaired lung function (1).

The burden of suffering caused by COPD is substantial. COPD is known to have a sizeable impact on the frequency of disability as well as the cost of disability (8). COPD accounted for 8 million physician office visits, 1.5 million emergency department visits, 726,000 hospitalizations, and 119,000 deaths in the United States in 2000 (1,8). The number of deaths increased to 126,000 in 2005. The direct and indirect costs of COPD have been estimated at $32.1 billion in 2003 (1,8). Of that, direct costs for hospital care, physician and other professional services, home care, nursing home care, and pharmacy accounted for $18 billion, whereas indirect costs for lost earnings because of illness and lost future earnings resulting from death comprised $14.1 billion (9–11). Although there is inconsistent reporting of COPD across countries, overall estimates of COPD prevalence are 4% to 10% (12).

DIAGNOSIS

Most COPD occurs in smokers. The incidence and severity increase with longer duration of smoking and higher number of packs smoked per day. The diagnosis of COPD is based on clinical suspicion and is confirmed by spirometry. History and physical exam alone are not sufficient to establish the diagnosis. COPD should be suspected when symptoms of cough, sputum production, and dyspnea occur in smokers or former smokers. Symptoms may precede airflow obstruction by many years. Airflow obstruction may also develop without significant symptoms. The symptoms of COPD overlap with other diseases and it is important to differentiate their cause. For example, asthma and COPD have many of the same symptoms. Asthma is characterized by reversible airflow obstruction, whereas airflow obstruction in COPD is incompletely reversible. Making the correct diagnosis is imperative for early intervention and in the selection of appropriate therapy. Spirometry must be done to confirm the diagnosis of COPD and differentiate reversible causes and restrictive lung disease. COPD responds differently to medications and has many associated extrapulmonary manifestations that contribute to the complexity of disease. Symptoms and spirometry should be taken into consideration when developing an individualized treatment plan for patients diagnosed with COPD.

Differential Diagnosis and Comorbidities

The evaluation of a COPD patient presenting for the first time or presenting with worsening symptoms of breathlessness may pose challenges because it may initially be difficult to determine if the symptoms are because of COPD or whether they are caused by other common conditions or comorbid diseases. Asthma, coronary artery disease, congestive heart failure, pulmonary vascular diseases such as thromboembolic disease, and other lung diseases all can be in the differential diagnosis. Clues pointing to alternative cardiac or pulmonary diagnoses are presented in Table 55.1.

COPD is often associated with multiple comorbidities that can affect functional capacity, level of dyspnea, quality of life, and mortality. Comorbidities increase the risk of hospitalization and mortality, especially in later stages of COPD. Further, comorbid disease significantly increases healthcare costs and health resource utilization. Physicians should be aware of common comorbidities in COPD (Table 55.2) and they should be addressed in the overall management as they complicate the morbidity and mortality of COPD.

The functional capacity of patients with COPD is diminished. Decreased exercise capacity actually predicts mortality better than other measures of lung function in COPD (2). Patients also commonly have skeletal muscle weakness and cachexia. Several studies suggest that systemic inflammation is an important factor involved in the pathogenesis of weight loss and low muscle mass (2). This muscle weakness in turn affects respiratory function, exercise tolerance, health status, mortality, and use of health care resources. Muscle wasting has been identified as a significant determinant of mortality in COPD, which is independent of lung function, smoking, and body mass index (2).

COPD increases the risk of cardiovascular disease by two- to threefold (2,3). A small number of COPD patients (1% to 3%) develop severe pulmonary hypertension. Progression of pulmonary hypertension can lead to cor pulmonale and further increased mortality. Normocytic anemia occurs in 15% to 30%, whereas polycythemia is relatively rare (2).

There is a high prevalence of osteoporosis in patients with COPD. This may be because of several common risk factors such as advanced age, poor mobility, smoking, poor nutrition, low body mass index, and high doses of inhaled corticosteroids as well as courses of oral steroids. COPD itself may also be a risk factor for osteoporosis, possibly related to systemic

TABLE 55.1 Differential Diagnosis of Chronic Respiratory Symptoms

COPD	• Mid-life onset • Slowly progressive symptoms • Smoking history • Dyspnea with exertion • Largely irreversible airway obstruction
Asthma	• Early onset • Symptoms vary day to day • Atopic conditions often present • Family history of asthma • Airflow obstruction is largely reversible
Congestive heart failure	• Fine basilar crackles on exam • Dilated heart, pulmonary edema on chest radiograph • Volume restriction on pulmonary function tests • Brain natriuretic peptide elevated
Bronchiectasis	• Large volume of purulent sputum • Commonly associated with bacterial infection • Coarse crackles and clubbing on exam • Bronchial dilatation and bronchial wall thickening on imaging
Tuberculosis	• Onset at all ages • Lung infiltrate or granulomata (nodular lesions) on chest film • Acid fast bacilli–positive
Sarcoidosis	• Dry cough • Fever present • Symptoms and signs of systemic inflammation present
Obliterative bronchiolitis	• Onset at younger age and in nonsmokers • History of rheumatoid arthritis or fume exposure • Computed tomography on expiration shows hypodense areas

inflammation (2). Bone mineral density testing should be done in later stages of COPD, and those found to have osteoporosis should be treated appropriately.

Every clinician caring for COPD patients should have a high index of suspicion for the presence of anxiety and depression. Anxiety and depressive symptoms are common in patients with COPD because of a heightened feeling of anxiety associated with dyspnea, as well as grief, loss, and social isolation associated with disability from COPD (13). Left untreated, depression leads to increased hospital length of stay and increased frequency of hospitalization, impaired quality of life, and premature death (2,13). Exercise training and carefully selected pharmacotherapy are often effective in treating anxiety and depression.

TABLE 55.2 Common Comorbidities in Patients with COPD

Anemia
Anxiety
Cachexia
Congestive heart failure
Depression
Diabetes
Ischemic heart disease
Lung cancer
Metabolic syndrome
Obstructive sleep apnea
Osteoporosis
Pulmonary hypertension
Skeletal muscle wasting

Patients with COPD are three to four times more likely to develop lung cancer than smokers with normal lung function, and lung cancer is a common cause of death in COPD patients (2). Of note, smoking cessation does not appear to reduce the risk of lung cancer (2). Lung cancer is also shown to be more common in patients with COPD who are lifetime nonsmokers (2).

COPD patients who also have sleep apnea are said to have "overlap syndrome." Such patients have a higher chance of developing hypercapnic respiratory insufficiency and pulmonary hypertension than patients with sleep apnea alone or COPD alone (14,15). COPD patients therefore should be assessed for signs and symptoms of sleep apnea. If the diagnosis of sleep apnea is confirmed by polysomnography, it should be appropriately treated.

History and Physical Examination

The history in patients suspected to have COPD should include assessing exposure to risk factors such as smoking or occupational exposures. Occupational exposure to a variety of dusts and chemicals can cause both obstructive and restrictive lung disease. Ask about a history of respiratory diseases such as asthma, sinusitis, allergy, or nasal polyps. Alpha-1 anti-trypsin (AAT) deficiency is the most commonly known genetic cause of COPD. A strong family history or onset of COPD at a young age (<45 years old) should prompt screening for AAT deficiency. Include assessment of the timing of symptom development. COPD typically develops in adulthood, whereas asthma typically develops in childhood. Patients with COPD are aware of increased breathlessness, more frequent "winter colds" and restriction of social activities for a number of years before seeking medical attention (6). Attention should be paid to identify possible comorbidities and other systemic manifestations that are common in COPD (discussed previously). It is important to determine how symptoms affect the patient and his family's lifestyle. Ask about limitation of activities, missed work, family routines, and feelings of depression and anxiety. It is also important to determine what social and family support is available to the patient.

The most common complaint that leads patients with COPD to see a physician is dyspnea (12,16). Dyspnea worsens over time, and patients may describe an "increased effort to breathe," "heaviness," "air hunger," or "gasping" (6). A method to quantify the impact of breathlessness on a patient's health status is the Medical Research Council Questionnaire (Table 55.3). This scale helps identify patients with a poor quality of life and provides prognostic information on survival with COPD (17). In addition, it can be used to help determine response to treatment. Chronic cough with or without sputum production may occur and is usually the first symptom. Other symptoms reported in COPD include chest tightness, wheezing, insomnia, general malaise, weakness, depression or mood change, weight loss, and nocturnal awakenings. In advanced COPD, people may exhibit signs of respiratory failure or cor pulmonale (right heart failure) such as hypoxia, leg edema, or jugular venous distention. Even if mild symptoms occur and the patient has exposure to risk factors, COPD should be considered and testing should be done.

Physical exam is neither sensitive nor specific in the diagnosis of COPD. However, the exam might provide clues to the diagnosis and need for spirometric confirmation of COPD. Some exam findings might include cyanosis, barrel chest, protruding abdomen, paradoxical in-drawing of lower rib cage on inspiration, tachypnea, pursed lip breathing, accessory muscle use in breathing, and ankle edema, which may indicate right heart failure. Key elements in the history and physical exam for COPD are listed in Table 55.4.

TABLE 55.3 Medical Research Council Grading of Functional Limitation from Dyspnea

1. "I only get breathless with strenuous exercise."
2. "I get short of breath when hurrying on the level or walking up a slight hill."
3. "I walk slower than most people of the same age on the level because of breathlessness or have to stop for breath when walking at my own pace on the level."
4. "I stop for breath after walking about 100 yards or after a few minutes on the level."
5. "I am too breathless to leave the house" or "I am breathless when dressing."

Diagnostic Testing

Pulmonary function tests are the best objective measurement of respiratory impairment. They are used to identify airway obstruction, classify the severity of the disease, and establish baseline lung function. The basic test is spirometry, which can be performed either in the office or in a pulmonary function laboratory. The patient takes a full inspiration and then forcibly exhales into a spirometer that is connected to sensors that measure and record air flow. Expiratory flow volume is measured over 6 seconds, and volume versus time graphs are produced. The test is repeated after administration of an inhaled bronchodilator such as albuterol. Results are compared with normal predicted values for people of the same age, height, and gender. Volume/time graphs comparing asthma and COPD are presented in Figure 55.1.

Spirometric measurement of forced vital capacity (FVC), forced expiratory volume in 1 second (FEV_1), and the ratio of FEV_1/FVC are used in the diagnosis of COPD. Obstructive diseases cause limitation of expiratory flow. There is a decreased ability to forcibly exhale because of air trapping and the speed with which this occurs is slower. Thus, the FEV_1 and FEV_1/FVC are lower than expected. In COPD, the FEV_1/FVC ratio is <0.7 when measured after administration of an inhaled bronchodilator. If after administration of an inhaled bronchodilator, measured values return to normal or near normal then the obstruction or airflow limitation is reversible. This would be indicative of asthma. Although indices of airway obstruction can fluctuate over time, testing must show persistent obstruction that is not fully reversible in order to make the diagnosis of COPD. Thresholds for the diagnosis and severity of COPD have been set by the Global Initiative for Chronic Obstructive Lung Disease (GOLD) consensus guidelines and are based on post-bronchodilator FEV_1 and FEV_1/FVC ratio (Table 55.5).

Chest x-rays (CXRs) and computed tomography (CT) imaging are not routinely used to diagnose COPD and are reserved for ruling out other lung and chest conditions. They may be performed in patients who have acute exacerbations in the emergency department, hospital, or clinic setting. There are some changes that typically occur on CXRs of a COPD patient, but these changes can be variable. In early COPD, the CXR be normal, but later it may show hypertransparency and hyperinflation of lung fields, diminished height of phrenic dome, enlarged retrosternal space, small droplet-shaped heart, barrel chest, and bullae or blebs that would indicate more severe disease. CT scans are done in patients considered for lung reduction surgery as the distribution of emphysematous lung tissue at the apices of the lungs determines a more favorable outcome (18). A complete blood count (CBC) is not always needed, but may show evidence of infection (elevated white blood cell count) or chronic hypoxia (elevated hematocrit) which also raises the possibility of pulmonary hypertension. A CBC is also helpful in diagnosing anemia in COPD patients. The level of hemoglobin is strongly and independently associated with functional dyspnea, decreased exercise capacity, as well as quality of life and in some studies is an independent predictor of mortality (2).

TABLE 55.4 Key Elements in the History and Physical Examination for Chronic Obstructive Pulmonary Disease

Question or Maneuver	Purpose
Detailed history of shortness of breath, wheezing, cough, and character of sputum	To identify symptoms and their time patterns, including aggravating factors such as tobacco smoke, pollution, or infection, and to identify frequent mucus production
Smoking history—by either patient or household members	To identify contributing factors and to begin the process for helping the patient to stop smoking
Family history of chronic obstructive pulmonary disease, including age at onset and whether any family member smoked	To determine probability of α_1-antitrypsin deficiency
History of atopy (allergic rhinitis, sneezing) or asthma in patient or family members	To assess likelihood of a significant reversible (asthmatic) component
History of exposure to asbestos, silica, and other dusts or chemicals that damage lungs	To determine risk for restrictive disease as coexisting or alternative diagnosis
History of hypertension, palpitations, chest pain, hyperlipidemia	To determine likelihood of cardiac disease as cause of symptoms
Assessment of heart rate, respiratory rate, cyanosis, and use of accessory muscles	To identify patients needing prompt intervention
Lung examination for decreased breath sounds, wheezing, prolonged expiration, increased resonance to percussion, or low diaphragm	These findings support a diagnosis of obstructive airway disease
Lung examination for fine basilar or other localized rales, decreased resonance	These findings would suggest congestive heart failure, infection, tumor, or pleural effusion

Arterial blood gases (ABGs) are measured in patients with more severe disease to determine the need for oxygen therapy. Oxygen has been shown to decrease mortality (19), when used at least 15 hours daily. ABG testing is reserved for patients with an FEV_1 <50% or who show signs of respiratory failure (cyanosis) or right heart failure (ankle edema or increased jugular venous distension). Measurement of ABGs also has value in identifying "CO_2 retainers." These are people with longstanding, severe COPD whose respiratory drive is stimulated only by low blood oxygen levels and not by increased carbon dioxide levels. If they are given enough supplemental oxygen to achieve normal blood oxygen levels, they have no stimulus to breathe and progressively retain more carbon dioxide. They become acidotic and stuporous. Thus, when oxygen therapy is used it is recommended to titrate the liters used to a pulse oximetry at or around 90%.

Sputum Gram stain is sometimes used to guide antibiotic therapy during exacerbations, although most often antibiotics are chosen empirically. Sputum culture and sensitivity are indicated only in patients who are severely ill and require hospitalization, especially if pneumonia is suspected.

Approximately 1% of people with COPD have a severe deficiency of α_1-antitrypsin (AAT), an inhibitor of neutrophil elastase; without adequate amounts of AAT, the elastase destroys alveolar tissue. COPD tends to occur earlier in these patients, often without smoking exposure, and it progresses

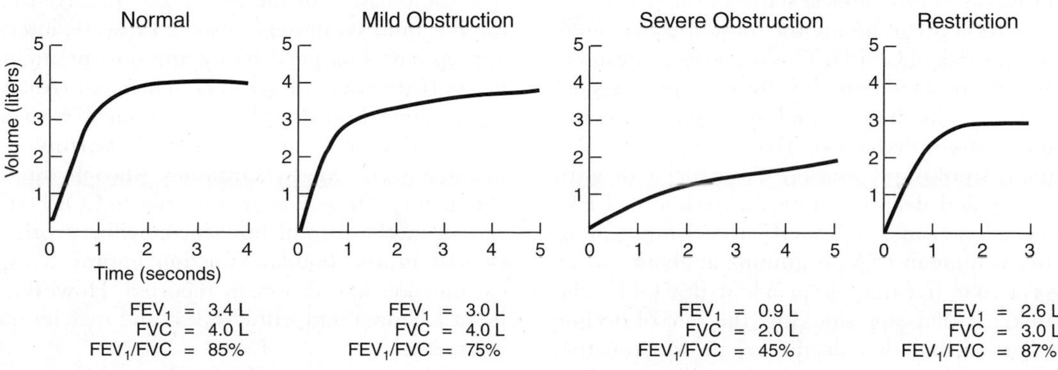

Figure 55.1 • Flow volume loops.

TABLE 55.5 Stages of Chronic Obstructive Pulmonary Disease (GOLD Report Classification 2008 Update)

Stage	Symptoms	Spirometry
I—Mild	With or without chronic symptoms: cough, sputum production.	$FEV_1/FVC < 0.7$ $FEV_1 \geq 80\%$ predicted
II—Moderate	With or without chronic symptoms: cough, sputum production, SOB on exertion.	$FEV_1/FVC < 0.7$ $50\% \leq FEV_1 < 80\%$ predicted
III—Severe	With or without chronic symptoms: cough, sputum production, SOB on exertion, decreased exercise capacity, fatigue, repeated exacerbations.	$FEV_1/FVC < 0.7$ $30\% \leq FEV_1 < 30\%$
IV—Very severe	With or without chronic symptoms: cough, sputum production, SOB on exertion, decreased exercise capacity, fatigue, repeated exacerbations, chronic respiratory failure, cor pulmonale.	$FEV_1/FVC < 0.7$ $FEV_1 < 30\%$ predicted OR $FEV_1 < 50\%$ predicted plus presence of chronic respiratory failure

FEV_1 = forced expiratory volume in 1 second; FVC = forced vital capacity; SOB = shortness of breath.

more rapidly. Screening by testing AAT serum levels is indicated only if a patient has unusually severe disease compared with age and smoking history (before age 45 years in smokers and in any nonsmoker) or has a positive family history of AAT deficiency. Only patients with severe deficiency, consistent with homozygous disease, benefit from AAT replacement therapy.

MANAGEMENT

COPD management requires a multifaceted approach. The overall goals are to relieve symptoms, improve quality of life, and reduce mortality. None of the medications used to treat COPD modify the overall decline in lung function, but an additional goal is to prevent disease progression. An approach to managing COPD is presented in Figure 55.2. Therapy is increased at each stage in a stepwise manner. Pharmacotherapy tends to be cumulative. The decision to add therapy depends on the stage of disease and the clinical status of the patient.

Smoking cessation programs are the most effective intervention to reduce the risk of COPD. This is also the only intervention that has been shown to slow disease progression. Smoking cessation results in decreased symptom frequency including cough, sputum production, dyspnea, and wheezing (20). Maintained smoking cessation is associated with decreased mortality and decreased rates of decline in FEV_1 (8,21,22). A normal nonsmoker loses 15 to 30 mL/year of forced expiratory volume in FEV_1 beginning at about age 20; the rate of loss is two to five times in people with COPD who continue to smoke. If they stop smoking, the rate of decline will return to normal, but they do not regain lost function (21,22). The standard of care for promoting smoking cessation includes behavioral therapy and counseling in conjunction with pharmacologic therapy. Brief intervention and advice on quitting smoking from health care providers has been shown to increase quit rates (23). Pharmacologic interventions include nicotine replacement therapy, bupropion, and more recently varenicline. Overall, these agents have been shown to increase smoking cessation rates, but many patients are unable to maintain sustained cessation (8,24,25).

Patients with COPD should receive an annual influenza vaccine, and GOLD guidelines recommend the use of pneumococcal vaccination for COPD patients age 65 or older. Serious illness and death is reduced by 50% in COPD patients when vaccinated against seasonal influenza (5). Additionally, pneumococcal vaccine has been associated with a decreased incidence of community acquired pneumonia in COPD patients younger than 65 years of age with an $FEV_1 < 40\%$ of predicted and should be considered in this patient population (6).

Bronchodilators are the mainstay of treatment, and they improve patient symptoms. Short-acting bronchodilators such as β-agonists (albuterol), anticholinergics (ipratropium), or a combination of the two (e.g., Combivent) are used first (6). For mild symptoms or stage I disease, intermittent use is appropriate. For persistent symptoms or night awakenings (stage II disease and greater), scheduled treatment with the short acting bronchodilators combined with a long acting bronchodilators (e.g., salmeterol, tiotropium) is recommended (2,3). Methylxanthines (theophylline) have bronchodilatory effects that are effective in COPD treatment. The precise mechanism of how theophylline works is unknown. Besides its bronchodilatory action, improved respiratory muscle function has also been reported. However, theophylline has a narrow therapeutic index, and toxicity limits common use today.

Despite the role that inflammation plays in COPD, inhaled corticosteroids have little or no effect on the rate of

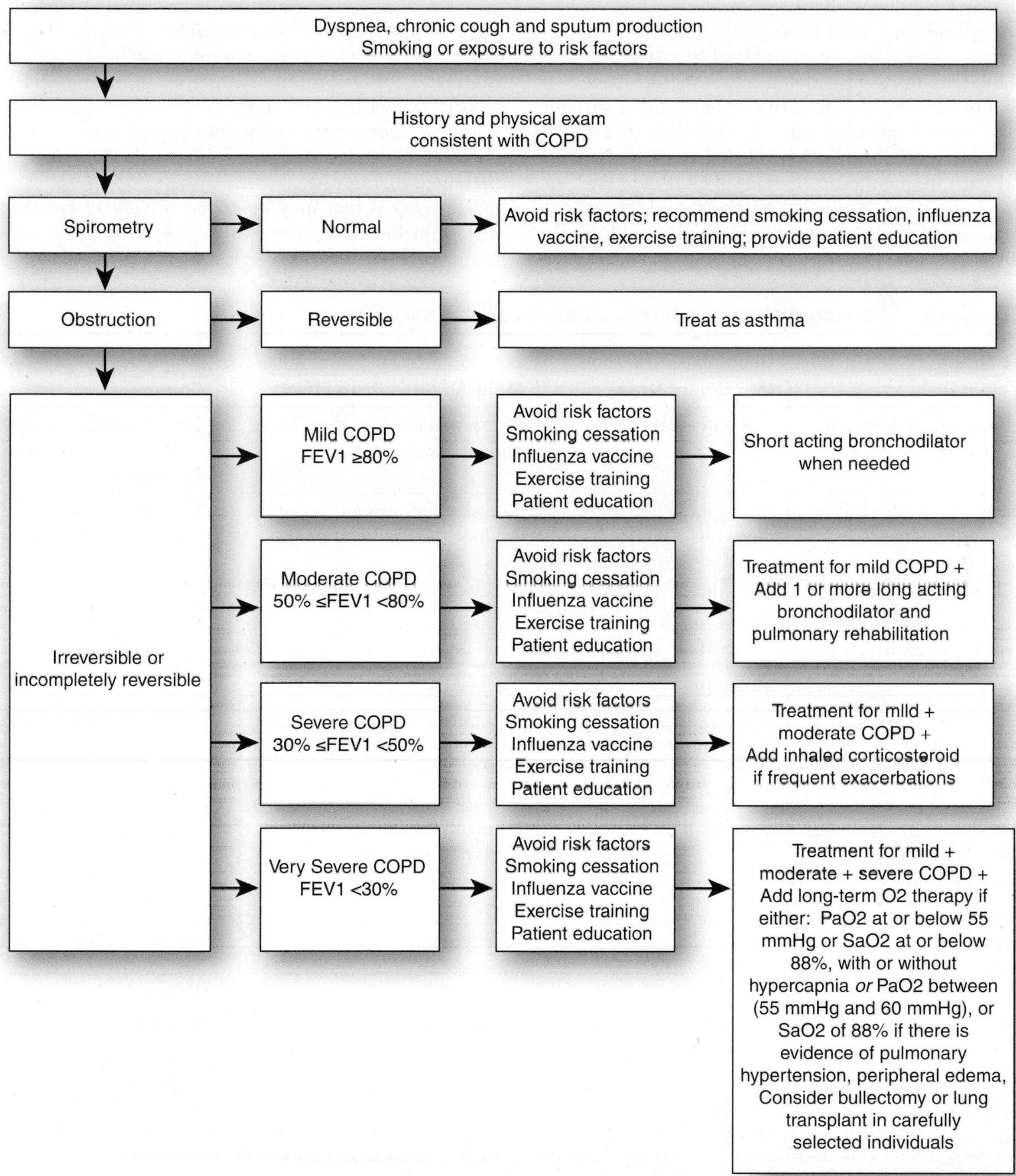

Figure 55.2 • Diagnosis and management of chronic obstructive pulmonary disease (COPD). Modified from the National Heart, Lung, and Blood Institute and World Health Organization. Global initiative for chronic obstructive lung disease: global strategy for diagnosis, management, and prevention of chronic obstructive pulmonary disease. 2009 update. National Institutes of Health, Bethesda, MD.

decline of lung function or all cause mortality (26). However, treatment with inhaled corticosteroids does result in significantly fewer exacerbations, improved health status, and lung function (26). Patients using inhaled corticosteroids have also been shown to have an increased risk of pneumonia without an increased risk of mortality (26,27). This should be taken into consideration when initiating inhaled steroids. Patients in stage III with frequent exacerbations of COPD likely benefit from the addition of inhaled corticosteroids. Frequent exacerbations are defined as at least one acute exacerbation a year for 3 years. Combination of an inhaled steroid with a long-acting β-agonist is more effective than either component alone (26). Oral corticosteroids also have been shown to improve COPD symptoms, but the significant side effects associated with oral steroids preclude long-term use. Response to oral steroids does not predict response to inhaled corticosteroids. A summary of commonly prescribed drugs is presented in Table 55.6.

Therapies that may be added in very severe (Stage IV) disease include long-term home oxygen therapy, which has

TABLE 55.6 Pharmacotherapy of Chronic Obstructive Pulmonary Disease

Generic Name (Trade Name)	Usual Dosing Range (Maximum Dose)	Main Adverse Drug Effects	Comments
Ipratropium bromide 0.03% MDI (Atrovent)	2–4 puffs TID-QID	Occasional dry mouth, cough, nausea; rare palpitations	If accidentally sprayed in eyes, acute narrow-angle glaucoma
Ipratropium bromide 0.02% solution (Atrovent)	0.5 mg in nebulizer every 4–8 hours	Occasional dry mouth, cough, nausea; rare palpitations	If accidentally sprayed in eyes, acute narrow-angle glaucoma
Albuterol MDI (outside United States: salbutamol) (Proventil, Ventolin)	2–4 puffs TID-QID (maximum 12 puffs/day)	Palpitations, tremors, nervousness	Can be used either for acute symptoms or as scheduled medication
	(6–8 puffs every 1/2–2 hours acutely)		
Albuterol nebulizer solution	2.5–5 mg in nebulizer every 1/2–2 hours acutely	Palpitations, tremors, nervousness	
Combination ipratropium and albuterol MDI (Atrovent or Combivent)	2 puffs QID	Palpitations, tremors, nervousness	Some studies show increased effectiveness compared with separate MDIs
Salmeterol Diskus (Serevent)	1 puff BID	Palpitations	Should not be used for acute symptoms Expensive
Formoterol (Foradil)	1 puff BID	Palpitations	Should not be used for acute symptoms Expensive
Tiotropium (Spiriva Handihaler)	1 inhalation QD	Dry mouth	Expensive
Theophylline, sustained release (Theo-Dur)	200–400 mg BID	Nausea, GERD, tremor, palpitations	In toxic doses, causes seizures; desirable serum level 5–12 μg/L
Albuterol, sustained-release tablets	4–8 mg every night or BID	Palpitations, tremors, nervousness	
Inhaled corticosteroids inhaler (e.g., beclomethasone)	For most, 2–4 puffs BID	Irritation of throat, thrush, increased risk of pneumonia	If used in high doses, can increase risk of cataracts and adrenal suppression
Prednisone, short-term	40–60 mg daily for 5–10 days	Increased BP, hyperglycemia, hypokalemia, irritability or euphoria	If used for less than 14 days, can be stopped without taper

BP = blood pressure; GERD = gastroesophageal reflux disease; MDI = metered-dose inhaler; QID = four times daily; TID = three times daily.
Based on prices at *www.drugstore.com*.

been shown to decrease mortality in people with severe daytime hypoxemia (19). It is recommended to initiate oxygen therapy in stage IV or very severe COPD if the partial pressure of arterial oxygen (PaO_2) is ≤55 mm Hg or the arterial oxygen saturation (SaO_2) is ≤88%. Oxygen may be initiated if the PaO_2 is between 55 and 60 mm Hg or SaO_2 of 88% and there is evidence of pulmonary hypertension, peripheral edema, or polycythemia (hematocrit >55%). Lung volume reduction surgery may benefit selected patients with predominantly upper lobe bullae or blebs (18). A summary of the strength of recommendation for COPD therapies is presented in Table 55.7. Pulmonary rehabilitation plays a significant role in management of COPD, and it should include exercise training targeted at the muscles of the upper extremities (28). All patients with stage II disease or greater should be referred for formal pulmonary rehabilitation. Benefits include improved exercise capacity, decreased dyspnea, decreased skeletal muscle dysfunction, improved quality of life, decreased hospitalizations, and reduced anxiety and depression associated with COPD (6,29). This benefit is lost after 6 months unless patients continue their exercise program.

End-of-life care and discussion of advance directives are important in the later stages of COPD. Patients with moderate to severe COPD deserve a discussion surrounding personal preferences regarding their care. Specific discussion might include treatment preferences related to intubation in the unfortunate event of respiratory failure. It is often very difficult to wean COPD patients off of a ventilator, and determining the patient's preference in advance is very helpful to the patient and their family.

There is not sufficient evidence to support the use of mucolytics, antitussives, antioxidants (such as N-acetylcysteine), morphine, leukotriene inhibitors, or continuous antibiotics in managing stable COPD. Antibiotic use is only recommended in treating acute infectious causes of COPD exacerbations (6). Although trimethoprim-sulfamethoxazole, doxycycline, and amoxicillin are commonly used a Cochrane review showed a decrease in short-term mortality regardless of antibiotic choice (30). Exacerbations of COPD are common and are defined by a change in the baseline dyspnea, cough, or sputum that is beyond usual day-to-day variations (6). The most common causes of COPD exacerbations are tracheobronchial tree infections and air pollution. Unidentified causes occur in as many as one third of severe exacerbations. Mild exacerbations may be treated on an outpatient basis, whereas moderate to severe flares may require hospitalization and possibly admission to the intensive care unit. Moderate exacerbations of COPD are treated by increasing the frequency of inhaled bronchodilator therapy to decrease bronchospasm. If symptoms do not resolve or improve at reassessment (within hours) a course of oral corticosteroids at 40 mg of prednisone per day for 7 to 10 days is considered reasonable and safe (16). The inhaled medications should be decreased to baseline as soon as possible. Prednisone can be stopped abruptly, without tapering, if given for fewer than 2 weeks. Many clinicians provide 5 days of prednisone and then stop it; others prefer to taper it after the patient's disease has stabilized in order to decrease the likelihood of recurrence.

Infections can cause COPD exacerbations by causing mucus production and bronchoconstriction. Although many of the infections are viral, consideration can be given to providing antibiotics for patients to keep at home so they can initiate treatment when mucus production increases and changes to a yellow or green color (31). Antibiotics are recommended if three cardinal symptoms are present: increased dyspnea, increased sputum volume, increased sputum purulence. If two cardinal symptoms are present and one is increased sputum purulence, antibiotics are recommended. Finally, antibiotics are recommended if the exacerbation is severe requiring mechanical ventilation. Common pathogens are *Haemophilus influenzae, Streptococcus pneumoniae, Moraxella catarrhalis*, and viruses. Appropriate antibiotic coverage is given depending on the patient risks and comorbidities.

If these measures are not effective or the patient's condition deteriorates rapidly, hospitalization may be necessary to give more intensive bronchodilator therapy, intravenous antibiotics, steroids, and oxygen therapy. Be aware of red flags suggestive of progressive or more severe disease (Table 55.8). Take into consideration that the patient's symptom exacerbation may not be due solely to COPD, and look for other causes such as heart failure. Intubation and mechanical ventilation may be necessary, but should be avoided if possible. It should be noted that guidelines related to management of acute exacerbations refer to patients who present to hospital emergency departments or those who require hospitalization.

LONG-TERM MONITORING

As COPD progresses, the frequency of physician visits by patients will increase. Ongoing monitoring and assessment of COPD includes asking about continued exposure to risk factors such as smoking and offering cessation assistance. Determine disease progression and development of complications by asking about symptoms and any change from baseline. Discuss effectiveness of pharmacotherapy and other medical treatments and determine compliance with medications or possible side effects. Monitor exacerbation history and numbers of self-treated exacerbations versus clinical or emergency department visits for exacerbations. Hospitalizations as well as use of critical care or intubation should be documented. Comorbidities such as ischemic heart disease, bronchial carcinoma, osteoporosis, anemia, and depression are more common in patients with COPD. Being aware of the common comorbidities will allow for their discovery and treatment of them as they contribute significantly to the severity of COPD.

Periodic spirometry is recommended, but not likely of benefit more than annually (6). Spirometry should be performed if there is a change in health status or a substantial increase in symptoms. Consider arterial blood gas testing if there are clinical signs of respiratory failure (cyanosis, hypoxia with pulse oximetry <92%) or cor pulmonale (ankle swelling, increased jugular venous pressure). ABGs will help determine the need for oxygen therapy and whether hypercapnia is present. Suspected cor pulmonale can be confirmed with echocardiography. CT scanning is not routinely done and is reserved for a small group of patients considered candidates for surgery such as lung volume reduction surgery. A blood count may reveal either anemia or polycythemia. A low hematocrit indicates a poor prognosis in COPD patients receiving long-term oxygen therapy (6).

TABLE 55.7 Strength of Recommendation for Management of COPD

Indications	Treatment Strategy	Strength of Recommendation*	Comments
For all patients	Influenza immunization	A	Reduces rate of hospitalization
For patients older than 65 years of age and consider for patients younger than 65 years with FEV_1 <40%	Pneumococcal immunization	B	Reduces rate of serious illness from pneumonia
For all patients	Patient education and self-management information	A	Reduces health costs, improves quality of life
For all patients	Smoking cessation	A	Improves long-term outcome Use of nicotine substitutes and bupropion doubles cessation rate
Chronic Management			
Stage I COPD:	Inhaled β-agonist (albuterol) or anticholinergic (Ipratropium) as needed for symptoms up to 2–4 puffs four times daily	A	Improves dyspnea, exercise tolerance No consistent effect on quality of life
	Consider combined ipratropium and albuterol metered-dose inhaler (Combivent)	C	Easier to use, improves adherence but not superior for dyspnea, exercise tolerance or quality of life compared with individual components
Stage II COPD	Add long-acting bronchodilator Salmeterol (long-acting inhaled β-agonist)	A	Improves dyspnea and quality of life but not shown to improve exercise tolerance
	or tiotropium bromide (Spiriva) a long-acting anticholinergic	A	Improves dyspnea and quality of life Decreases the number of acute exacerbations
Stage II–IV	Pulmonary rehabilitation	A	Improves dyspnea, exercise tolerance, and quality of life
Stage III–IV COPD	Consider trial of inhaled corticosteroid if frequent exacerbations	A	No improvement in dyspnea, exercise tolerance or quality of life Reduces severity but not the frequency of exacerbations
	Combination inhaled corticosteroid and long-acting bronchodilator (e.g., fluticasone and salmeterol [Advair])	C	Use for convenience if on both a long-acting β-agonist and inhaled corticosteroid
	Consider long-acting theophylline	B	Improves dyspnea and exercise tolerance

(*continued*)

TABLE 55.7 *(Continued)*

Indications	Treatment Strategy	Strength of Recommendation*	Comments
Stage IV COPD	Long-term oxygen therapy (>15 hours per day) if $PO_2 \leq 55$ mm Hg with or without hypercapnia or If PO_2 56–60 mm Hg if pulmonary hypertension, CHF, or polycythemia	A	Improved survival Improved sense of well-being
Management of Exacerbations			
For all exacerbations	Add inhaled β-agonist or ipratropium	A	Improves symptoms more than the small improvements in FEV_1 seen
Moderate-severe Type II	Systemic glucocorticoids	A	Reduce severity of exacerbation and shorten recovery
If purulent exacerbation	Antibiotics (trimethoprim-sulfamethoxazole, doxycycline, amoxicillin, and others)	A	Symptomatic improvement

CHF = congestive heart failure; COPD = chronic obstructive pulmonary disease; FEV_1 = forced expiratory volume in 1 second.
*A = consistent, good-quality patient-oriented evidence; B = inconsistent or limited-quality patient-oriented evidence; C = consensus, disease-oriented evidence, usual practice, expert opinion, or case series.
For information about the Strength of Recommendation Taxonomy evidence rating system, see *www.aafp.org/afpsort.xml*.

TABLE 55.8 Red Flags in Patients with Congestive Pulmonary Obstruction Disease

Red Flag	Condition of Concern	Comments
Hemoptysis	Pulmonary neoplasm, pulmonary embolus, congestive heart failure	Further pulmonary imaging warranted
Hypoxia	Impending respiratory failure	Usually a determinant of need for hospitalization in the setting of acute exacerbations
Peripheral edema	Heart failure, thromboembolic disease	Consider pulmonary embolism if exacerbation occurs associated with unilateral lower extremity edema and congestive heart failure with bilateral edema
Hypercapnia	Impending respiratory failure	Rising hypercapnia may occur with oxygen treatment, cautious titration is advised
Hypotension, confusion, lethargy, coma	Sepsis	Usually a determinant of need for hospitalization in the setting of acute exacerbations

KEY POINTS

- COPD is preventable and treatable but is still progressive and not fully reversible.
- Smoking is still the primary cause of COPD, and every attempt should be made to help patients stop smoking.
- The diagnosis of COPD should be considered in patients with dyspnea, chronic cough, sputum production, and exposure to risk factors.
- Spirometry is the gold standard test to confirm the diagnosis of COPD.
- Management aims to reduce risk factors, prevent and control symptoms, reduce frequency of exacerbations, improve health status, and improve exercise tolerance.

CHAPTER

56

Tuberculosis

Steven W. Harrison, Frank Ganzhorn and Allen Radner

CLINICAL OBJECTIVES

1. Cite risk factors for tuberculosis (TB).
2. Summarize an approach to a patient with a positive TB skin test (TST).
3. Describe the evidence-based treatment recommendations for active and latent TB.

Tuberculosis (TB) is the second-leading cause of death from infection in the modern world. Despite effective treatment, the potential for vaccination, and knowledge of improved sanitation techniques which prevent spread, the only infection that kills more people is HIV. World Health Organization data from 2005 demonstrate that approximately 9 million people worldwide develop active TB every year and more than 2 million die from the disease (1).

The number of people estimated to have latent tuberculosis (LTBI) worldwide is approximately 2 billion. LTBI is found in people who had exposure to and brief infection with TB, but resolved the infection. These individuals are no longer contagious, but the rate of reactivation to active TB is 5% to 10% per lifetime in most individuals and 7% to 10% per year in HIV-positive individuals (2).

There has been a significant resurgence of TB in the third world, primarily associated with the HIV epidemic. In comparison, US data from the Centers for Disease Control and Prevention (CDC) show that there were 14,097 reported cases of active TB in 2005 with 640 deaths, for a death rate of 0.2% (3). This is considerably reduced from the 1953 death rate of 12.4% (4).

TB was described by Hippocrates as consumption around 460 BC (5). At the time, it was the most widespread disease in the world and almost always fatal. His advice to his fellow physicians was not to visit patients in the later disease stages because they would inevitably die and damage the reputation of the treating physician.

TB remained a leading cause of death in the developed world until the early 20th century. Public health measures decreased spread of disease. Sanitariums were established in the 1850s as the first real step in TB treatment. BCG vaccine, which can prevent up to 50% of TB cases (6), was first released in 1921 and came into widespread use in 1945. In 1943, the first effective medication (streptomycin) was discovered (6).

Treatment and eventual eradication of TB is complicated by lack of resources in less developed countries, specifically in sub-Saharan Africa where there are more than 300 cases per 100,000 annually (1). Political unrest and armed conflict contribute to making available treatment almost impossible to implement in some areas.

RISK FACTORS

Most cases of tuberculosis in the United States are diagnosed in minority and foreign-born populations. The more dangerous multidrug-resistant (MDR) strains tend to come from endemic areas such as Southeast Asia and Africa. In addition to ethnic and immigrant status, risk factors for infection or progression include: HIV, other immunocompromised states (e.g., cancer, treatment with tumor necrosis factor antagonists), chronic diseases such as diabetes mellitus, bariatric surgery recipients, injection drug users, personnel who work or live in high-risk settings (e.g., prisons, long-term care facilities, hospitals), and children younger than 4 years of age who are exposed to high-risk individuals (7).

DIAGNOSIS

In primary care, we see individuals who have undiagnosed TB in many settings. Although routine physical exams of children and adults no longer include automatic TB testing, TB surveillance is still performed as part of pre-employment exams in many work settings. Most cases found in this manner will be LTBI. We must also be alert to the sometimes obvious, but frequently subtle findings that lead to the diagnosis of active TB.

The accurate diagnosis of active TB becomes more difficult among patients with HIV because of the presence of nontuberculous mycobacteria. In addition, HIV infection can cause anergy and therefore a false-negative TST. Nucleic acid amplification testing (NAAT) can be used in an attempt to differentiate TB from other mycobacterial infections (8), although AFB culture is considered the gold standard. The CDC recommends repeat TST or chest x-ray (CXR) in HIV-positive individuals after beginning highly active anti-retroviral therapy (HAART), because these tests may turn positive after the individual's immune function improves with treatment (9).

Latent Tuberculosis Infection

LTBI is distinguished from active TB by history and test results (Fig. 56.1). Positive TST or interferon gamma release assay (screening blood testing) combined with a negative CXR

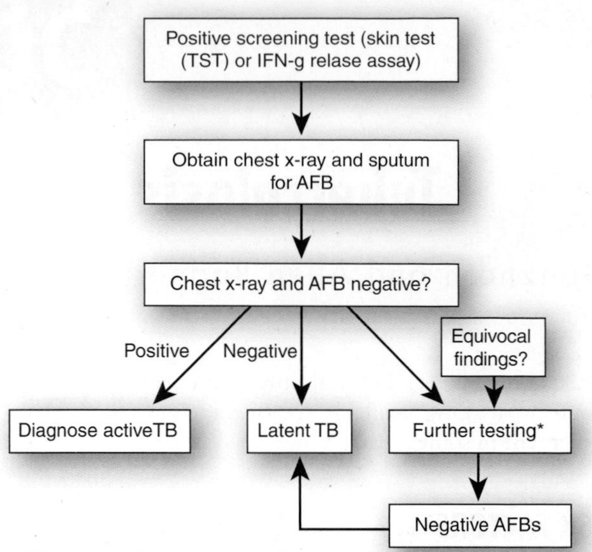
Positive screening test (skin test (TST) or IFN-g relase assay)
Obtain chest x-ray and sputum for AFB
Chest x-ray and AFB negative?
Positive
Negative
Equivocal findings?
Diagnose activeTB
Latent TB
Further testing*
Negative AFBs
*Can include CT scan, induced sputums or gastric aspirates, bronchoscopy with biopsy and or washings among others. Consultation and/or referral should be considered (e.g., Infectious Disease and Pulmonology).

Figure 56.1 • Workup of patients with a positive screening test for tuberculosis.

and lack of symptoms establishes the diagnosis of LTBI (10). In patients with a positive CXR or computed tomography (CT) scan or suggestive symptoms, three negative AFB cultures are required before diagnosing and treating a patient for LTBI rather than active TB.

Differential Diagnosis

The diagnosis of TB requires a high index of suspicion. Manifestations of active TB can be classified as pulmonary (about 80% of cases) or extrapulmonary. Clinical features of pulmonary infection are described under the history and physical examination section in this chapter.

The differential diagnosis for pulmonary TB includes bacterial or viral pneumonia, nontuberculous mycobacterium, sarcoidosis, aspiration pneumonia, lung abscess, fungal infections such as coccidiomycosis and histoplasmosis, Wegener granulomatosis, actinomycosis, and cancer. The clinical exam is inadequate for differentiating between these possibilities and further testing must be performed. Table 56.1 lists some clinical and laboratory features for differentiating these conditions.

Extrapulmonary TB results from blood borne (hematogenous) spread from primary disease or reactivation of latent infection. In order of decreasing frequency, sites for active TB infection include: lung, lymph nodes, pleurae, genitourinary tract, bone, brain (meningitis and other central nervous system involvement), and peritoneum (2). Disseminated or miliary TB involves the lung or multiple sites.

History and Physical Examination

Primary active TB may present as atypical pneumonia with fever, nonproductive cough, and positive CXR findings (see Fig. 56.2). Reactivation TB, however, is more common; symptoms include fever, chills, night sweats, anorexia, weight loss, hemoptysis, and malaise. Later in the disease course, patients may develop a nonproductive cough or cough with purulent sputum. Cough lasting more than 2 or 3 weeks with one additional symptom as previously mentioned should trigger suspicion for TB. TB should also be suspected in a patient who falls into a high-risk group with unexplained illness, including respiratory symptoms of more than 2 to 3 weeks' duration (11).

Pulmonary TB is generally accompanied by symptoms of chest pain, weight loss, fatigue, and anorexia. Examination of the lungs can reveal crackles and rhonchi. Hemoptysis, seen later in the disease course, usually accompanies cavitary disease (Fig. 56.2) (2). Dyspnea and hypoxia are signs of significant pulmonary involvement. Patients with extensive disease may develop acute respiratory distress syndrome.

Miliary TB (now considered synonymous with disseminated TB) refers to the classic finding of diffuse (millet) seedlike appearing (reticulonodular) patterns on plain CXR (Fig. 56.3). This results from hematogenous spread of infection; multiple sites are potentially involved. Pulmonary involvement is common but not universal (12).

TB can also invade other organ systems. Most lymph node disease is manifested as enlarged cervical nodes and accounts for approximately 40% of non-pulmonary cases. Genitourinary disease (kidneys, ureters, bladder, or genitals) accounts for about 15% of non-pulmonary disease. Patients with bone and joint disease (about 10% of extrapulmonary cases) present with pain in the affected area. Spinal column disease (commonly known as Pott disease) causes back or neck pain as vertebra and discs are destroyed by infection. Patients with Pott disease often have constitutional symptoms such as fever or weight loss and sometimes neurologic symptoms (spinal cord compression). Plural and pericardial disease can also be seen but are infrequent.

TB meningitis has a high mortality rate (about 40%) and significant morbidity. Unlike bacterial forms of meningitis, TB meningitis often begins with vague symptoms of fatigue, irritability, and anorexia for weeks, followed by stiff neck, vomiting, and headache (13). Young children (4 years and younger) and immunocompromised individuals are at increased risk. This form of the disease is fatal without treatment.

Laboratory Testing

Laboratory investigation for TB usually begins with TST with purified protein derivative (PPD). This test does not distinguish between LTBI and active TB, but is used to detect both in exposed or high-risk individuals. The interpretation of the test (induration or size of the wheel at the inoculation site) depends on the patient's underlying risk status (Table 56.2).

After a patient has a positive TST or a positive blood test by interferon gamma release assay (IFN-g), sputum tests for acid fast bacilli (AFB) and/or body fluid/biopsy analysis by polymerase chain reaction (PCR)/NAAT are obtained (14,15). The test characteristics for these studies are shown in Table 56.3. Both AFB culture or PCR /NAATs are highly specific, and when positive rule in disease (LR+ 10 or higher). A tissue diagnosis by bronchoscopy or pleural biopsy may be needed if noninvasive testing does not lead to a definitive diagnosis (10,13,16,17).

If the patient is from a country that administers BCG vaccine, a false-positive skin test result may have occurred. Interestingly, even if the subsequent CXR is negative, the patient could have LTBI and should be treated as such, per CDC guidelines.

TABLE 56.1 Differential Diagnosis of Active Pulmonary Tuberculosis

Diagnosis	Typical Features	Frequency (US Data)	Distinguishing Features	Mortality
Pulmonary TB (80% reactivation) (20% primary)	Abnormal chest x-ray Cough, fever, anorexia Pneumonia	4.4/100,000 nationwide	Positive PPD Positive AFB (smear, culture, or biopsy) Positive PCR or IFN-γ assay	0.2/100,000
Coccidiomycosis	Location in Southwest Fatigue Pneumonia *E. Nodosum*	91/100,000 in Arizona	Positive serology or culture Lung biopsy PCR	Mostly self-limited
Cryptococcosis	Productive cough Hemoptysis Weight loss if HIV infected	Rare (96% of cases in those with HIV) nationwide	Positive serology or culture CSF studies Lung biopsy	12%–28%
Histoplasmosis	Pneumonia Dysphagia Cavitary disease Cough Enlarged mediastinal nodes	22% of population have positive antibodies nationwide	Positive serology or culture Immunodiffusion test Lung biopsy	7%–23% (disseminated disease)
Neoplasm (lung cancer)	Smoker Cough Hemoptysis Shortness of breath Chest pain	219,000 new cases per year 0.06% nationwide	Sputum cytology Lung biopsy PET/CT scan	10% 5-year survival, overall Up to 35%–40% survival with successful complete resection
Sarcoid	Shortness of breath, cough Skin lesions Hilar adenopathy Diffuse lung disease	10–20/100,000 nationwide	Biopsy (non-caseating granulomas) Serum ACE level PET scan Diagnosis of exclusion	5–10%
Wegner granulomatosis	Fatigue Sinus pain Cough Rhinorrhea	<1/200,000 nationwide	c-ANCA/p-ANCA Lung biopsy	80% survival at 6–24 months
Actinomycosis	Cough Hemoptysis Sinus drainage Chronic soft-tissue swelling of the head and neck	1/60,000 nationwide	Culture Lung biopsy Sulfa granules in nasal discharge	Treatment prevents mortality

ACE = Angiotensin Converting Enzyme; AFB = acid-fast bacilli; c-ANCA = classical anti-neutrophil cytoplasmic antibodies; p-ANCA = Perinuclear Anti-Neutrophil Cytoplasmic Antibodies; CT = computed tomography; PET = positron emission testing; PPD = purified protein derivative; TB = tuberculosis.

Patients who are immunosuppressed may not produce a delayed type hypersensitivity reaction on PPD testing; these patients should undergo initial TST. If the TST is negative, particularly if HIV-positive, it may still be reasonable to pursue further screening using NAAT and standard sputum testing to rule out active TB (2,18).

TST and sputum analysis also play a major role in the diagnosis of extrapulmonary TB, if positive. Spinal fluid analysis and culture/NAAT are suggested for the evaluation of TB meningitis. Pleural biopsy and thoracentesis are recommended for diagnosing pleural TB. CT-guided needle biopsy is used to diagnose internal organ disease (e.g., adrenal glands) and osteomyelitis. A simple culture can be used to diagnose renal disease, suggested by "sterile pyuria." There are many published protocols that guide evaluation and treatment including the NICE is National Institute for Health and Clinical Excellence (NICE), CDC guidelines (includes the American Thoracic Society recommendations), and Canadian guidelines (13,15,19).

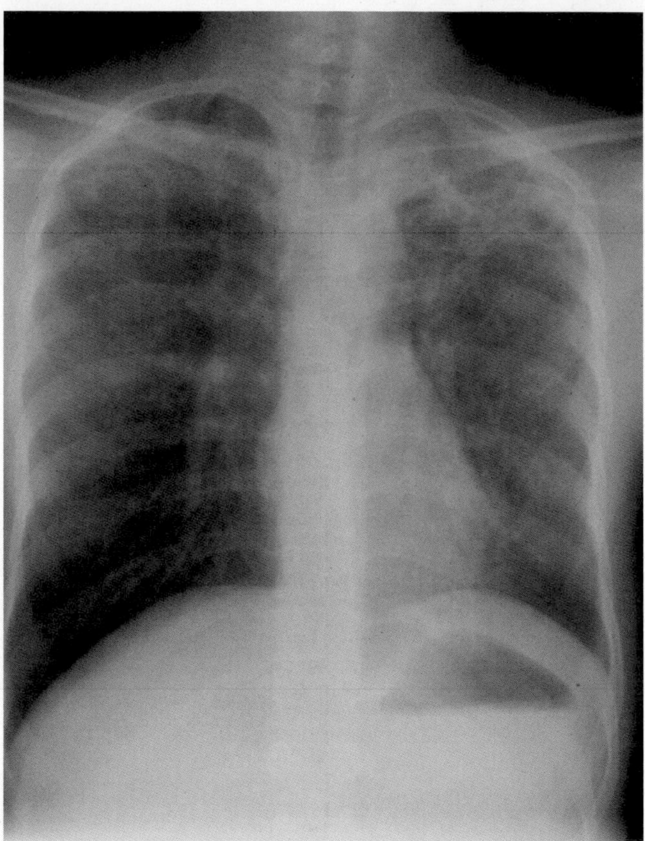

Figure 56.2 • Chest x-ray showing cavitary lesion and surrounding infiltrate (seen with reactivation disease).

TABLE 56.2 Defining a Positive Tuberculosis Skin Test by Risk Status

Risk Status	Positive Purified Protein Derivative Reading (Elevation of Wheel)
High Risk HIV infection Recent contacts of infectious tuberculosis cases People with chest x-ray findings of prior tuberculosis Organ transplant recipients Immunosuppressed for other reasons Taking ≥15 mg of prednisone daily Taking tumor necrosis factor-α antagonists	≥5 mm
Moderate Risk Recent immigration from high prevalence area Residents or employees of health care facilities or shelters/prisons, etc. Children younger than 4 years of age Children or adolescents exposed to adults at high risk of disease Injection drug users	≥10 mm
Low Risk No risk factors	≥15 mm

Information from: *www.cdc.gov/tb/publications/factsheets/testing/skintesting.htm*

Imaging

A CXR is the imaging test of first choice (9). This test is widely available and associated with markedly less radiation exposure than CT (Fig. 56.4). The sensitivity and specificity vary depending on the setting and pretest probability. CT scans provide significantly more detail, but don`t always obviate the need for a tissue diagnosis and should be reserved for cases when the diagnosis is unclear by CXR alone.

The CXR classically shows upper lobe infiltrate with cavitation (Fig. 56.2), but any pattern may be seen ranging from a solitary nodule to diffuse infiltrates representing bronchogenic spread. The CXR pattern in children often shows an infiltrate with hilar and paratracheal lymphadenopathy.

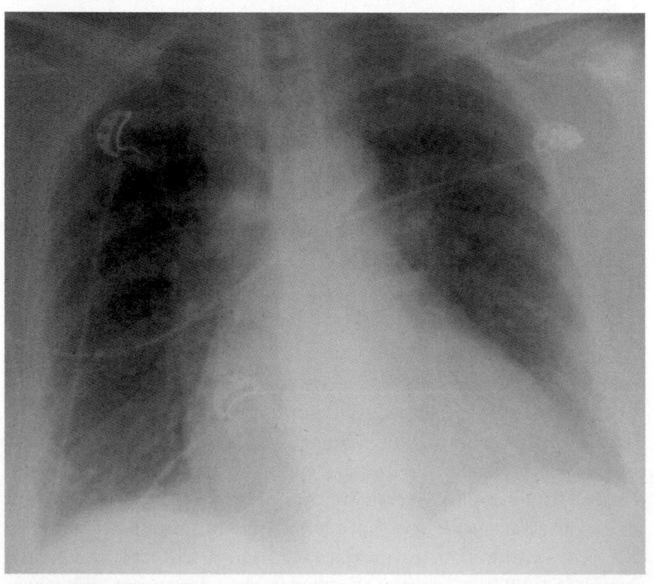

Figure 56.3 • Chest x-ray showing miliary tuberculosis.

TREATMENT

The most common presentation in a primary care office is a patient who has a positive TST and a negative CXR. This patient most likely has LTBI; however, single drug treatment should not begin until active TB disease has been excluded. For those suspected of having active TB, the recommended multidrug regimen should be started as described below until the correct diagnosis is established. Directly observed therapy (DOT) is the standard of care in many areas and is generally supervised by the local health department. Unfortunately,

TABLE 56.3 Available Tests and Test Characteristics for Diagnosing Active Pulmonary Tuberculosis

Test	Common Abbreviation	Sensitivity	Specificity	LR+	LR−
Tuberculin skin test	PPD	59%–100%	44%–100%	1.8 to high[†]	0.9 to low[†]
Chest x-ray	CXR	38–67%	59%–74%	0.9–2.6	1.1–0.5
Computerized tomography	CT	96%	50%	1.9	0.08
Acid-fast bacillus smear	AFB (smear)	50%–96%	98%	25–48	0.51–0.04
Acid-fast bacillus culture and sensitivity	AFB (culture)	93%–97%	98%	46.5–48.5	0.07–0.03
Polymerase chain reaction assay	PCR*	95%	98%	47.5	0.05
Interferon gamma release assay	Quantiferon Gold/TB spot	70%–90%	93%–99%	10.0–90.0	0.3–0.10
Bronchoscopy	Bronc	73%–94%	92%–100%	9.1 to high[†]	0.29 to low[†]

LR+ = positive likelihood ratio; tests with higher values, especially >10, are good at ruling in disease; LR− = negative likelihood ratio; tests with lower values, especially <0.1, are good at ruling out disease.
*Some nucleic acid amplification testing falls into this category.
†Ratio includes a zero in the denominator; undefined.
Information from: Escalante P. In the clinic. Tuberculosis. *Ann Intern Med* 2009;150(11):ITC61–614; Canadian Tuberculosis Standards. 6th Edition. 2007. Available at *www.phac-aspc.gc.ca/tbpc-latb/pubs/pdf/tbstand07_e.pdf*.

although DOT is frequently recommended as a method for improving adherence, a Cochrane review did not find DOT superior to self-administration of treatment with respect to cure or treatment completion (20).

TB is a reportable disease and the public health department (PHD) is tasked with its diagnosis and treatment nationwide. The PHD is a great resource and can guide or take over the treatment of any patient with TB, especially complicated patients. In all cases, the PHD is ultimately responsible for ensuring availability of appropriate diagnostic and treatment services and for monitoring the results of therapy. The other resources available to you vary by location, patient`s insurance and citizenship, and specialty availability; but include the local and regional infectious disease and pulmonary specialists.

You should obtain a list of the patient's current medications to avoid drug interactions. Some interactions to note include (16):

- Isoniazid (INH) increases blood levels of phenytoin (Dilantin) and disulfiram (Antabuse)
- Rifampin decreases blood levels of oral contraceptives, warfarin, sulfonoureas, and methadone
- Rifampin is contraindicated in HIV-infected individuals treated with protease inhibitors and most nonnucleoside reverse transcriptase inhibitors

LTBI

To determine whether an individual who has a positive TST or IFN-γ assay result is a candidate for treatment of LTBI, the CDC recommends determination of the benefits of treatment by evaluating individual's risk for developing active TB in addition to his or her commitment to complete a course of treatment and the resources available to ensure adherence; in

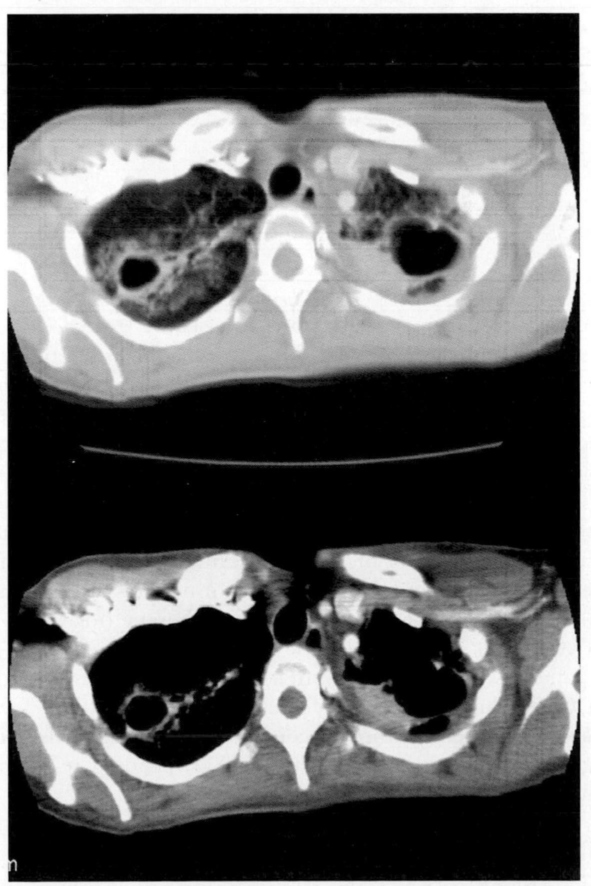

Figure 56.4 • Computed tomography scan showing upper lobe disease and mediastinal adenopathy.

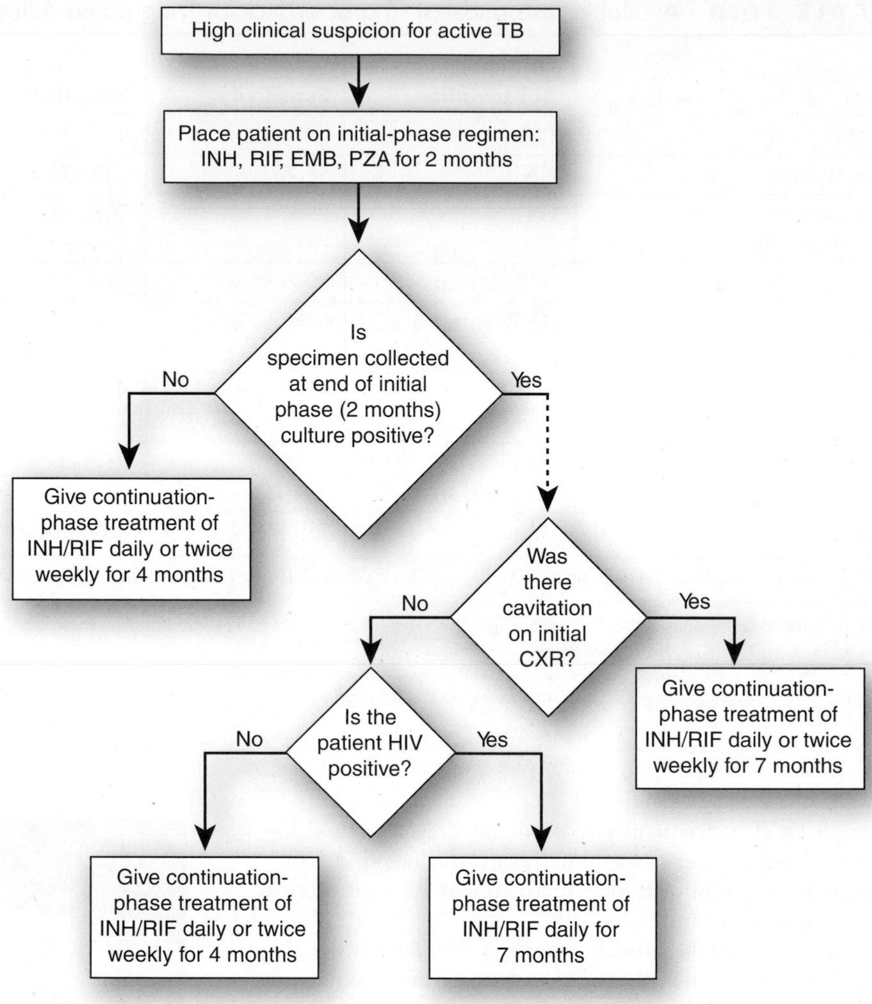

Figure 56.5 • Algorithm to guide duration of continuation-phase treatment for culture-positive tuberculosis patients. TB = tuberculosis; INH = isoniazid; RIF = Rifampin; EMB = ethambutol; PZA = pyrazinamide; CXR = chest X-ray; HIV = human immunodeficiency virus.

general, most patients with positive tests are treated (21). In patients who may have a false-positive TST because of prior BCG vaccination, treatment for LTBI is recommended because the vaccination is only effective in up to 50% of cases and only lasts approximately 15 years. There is no way to reliably distinguish false from true-positive tests.

Treatment for a variety of conditions is often deferred until therapy for LTBI (or active TB) is in progress. Specific examples are deferral of HAART until latent or active TB therapy is started and deferral of tumor necrosis factor antagonists in RA until near completion of therapy (for LTBI or active TB) (9). A Cochrane review supports treatment of LTBI in patients with HIV to prevent active disease (22). Finally, the CDC recommends therapy for children younger than age 5 years and severely immunocompromised individuals with high-risk exposures and negative TSTs, pending re-evaluation by sequential testing in 8 to 10 weeks (9).

For adult patients with LTBI, the CDC recommends the following options:

- Isoniazid for 9 months; twice-weekly regimens or 6-month therapy (daily or twice weekly) may be considered. Pyridoxine (B6) is usually given at 25 mg orally daily to prevent neuropathy.
- Rifampin daily for 4 months; primarily considered for patients who have isoniazid-resistant TB or allergy.

Active TB

For adult patients with active TB, there are four drugs used for initial treatment, with different options for dosing duration in a continuation phase as follows:

- Two-month initial treatment phase: INH, rifampin (RIF), pyrazinamide, and ethambutol.
- Four-month continuation phase with INH and RIF (daily or twice weekly); treatment is extended to 7 months (daily or twice weekly) for patients with cavitary pulmonary TB who remain sputum-positive after initial treatment, if pregnant, if HIV-positive, or in patients with concurrent silicosis to prevent relapse. An algorithm to guide treatment of patients with high clinical suspicion of active TB is shown in Figure 56.5.
- Two months' continuation therapy with INH and RIF is given for patients who remain culture negative and evaluation at

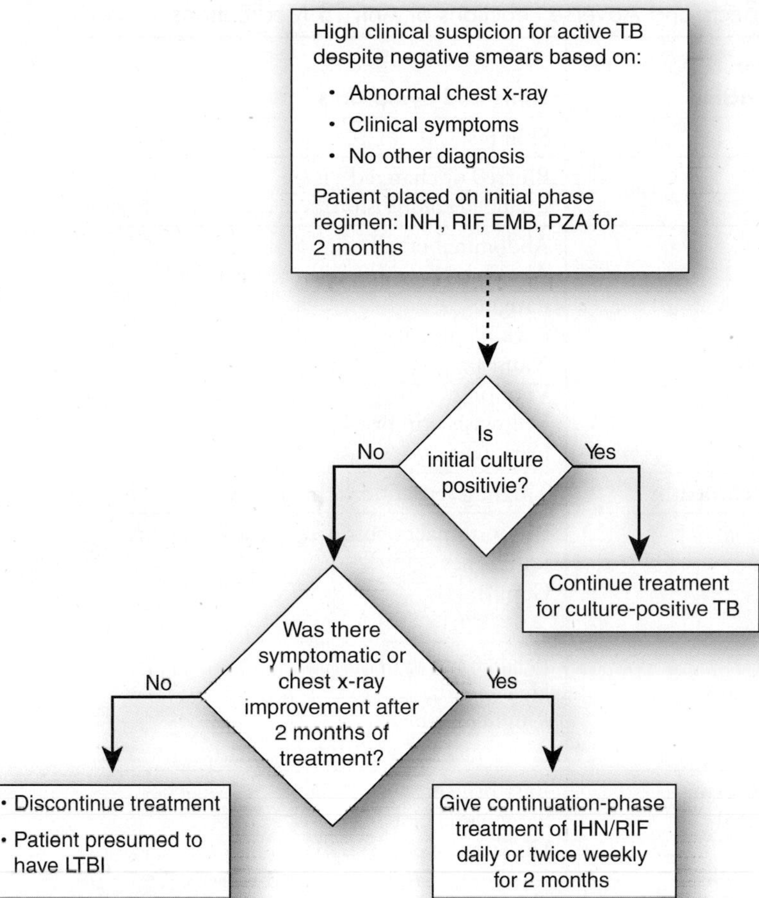

High clinical suspicion for active TB despite negative smears based on:
• Abnormal chest x-ray
• Clinical symptoms
• No other diagnosis
Patient placed on initial phase regimen: INH, RIF, EMB, PZA for 2 months
Is initial culture positivie?
No
Yes
Continue treatment for culture-positive TB
Was there symptomatic or chest x-ray improvement after 2 months of treatment?
No
Yes
• Discontinue treatment
• Patient presumed to have LTBI
Give continuation-phase treatment of IHN/RIF daily or twice weekly for 2 months

Figure 56.6 • Algorithm to guide treatment of culture-negative tuberculosis. TB = tuberculosis; INH = isoniazid; RIF = Rifampin; EMB = ethambutol; PZA = pyrazinamide

2 months reveals clinical and CXR response to antituberculosis drug therapy. An algorithm to guide treatment for culture-negative TB is displayed in Figure 56.6.

- To prevent isoniazid-related neuropathy, pyridoxine 10 to 25 mg/d is given, especially to those at risk for vitamin B6 deficiency (e.g., alcoholic, malnourished, pregnant or lactating women, HIV-positive patients, and those with chronic diseases).

Drug-resistant TB disease is caused by *Mycobacterium tuberculosis* organisms that are resistant on susceptibility testing to at least one first-line anti-TB drug. MDR TB is resistant to more than one anti-TB drug and at least INH and RIF. MDR TB is treated with a variety of injectable drugs including streptomycin, kanamycin, and amikacin or oral drugs including fluoroquinolones, ethionamide, cycloserine, and para-aminosalicylic acid PAS (23). In a Cochrane review of 11 small trials on the use of fluoroquinolones in TB regimens, investigators found no difference in trials substituting ciprofloxacin or ofloxacin for first-line drugs in relation to cure, treatment failure, or clinical or radiological improvement; however, substituting ciprofloxacin into first-line regimens in drug-sensitive tuberculosis led to a higher incidence of relapse in HIV-positive patients (24).

Extrapulmonary TB

The basic principles underlying pulmonary TB treatment also apply to extrapulmonary forms of the disease. Although relatively few studies have examined treatment of extrapulmonary TB, evidence suggests that 6- to 9-month regimens that include INH and RIF are effective. The exception to this is infection of the meninges for which a 9- to 12-month regimen is recommended. Prolongation of therapy is considered for any patient with TB in any site that is slow to respond to treatment (15).

OUTPATIENT INFECTION CONTROL

The CDC has published consensus-based recommendations to prevent spread of disease (19). It states that people with TB should not be routinely admitted to the hospital for diagnostic tests or care and that those with respiratory TB should be separated from immunocompromised patients (25).

TABLE 56.4 Potential Side Effects and Adverse Reactions of Anti TB Medications

Medication	Side Effect or Adverse Reaction	Signs and Symptoms
Any drug	Allergy	Skin rash
Ethambutol	Eye damage	Blurred or changed vision Changed color vision
Isoniazid, pyrazinamide, or rifampin	Hepatitis	Abdominal pain Abnormal liver function test results Fatigue Lack of appetite Nausea Vomiting Yellowish skin or eyes Dark urine
Isoniazid	Peripheral neuropathy	Tingling sensation in hands and feet
Pyrazinamide	Gastrointestinal intolerance Arthralgia Arthritis	Upset stomach, vomiting, lack of appetite Joint aches Gout (rare)
Streptomycin	Ear damage Kidney damage	Balance problems Hearing loss Ringing in the ears Abnormal kidney function test results
Rifamycin • Rifabutin • Rifapentine • Rifampin	Thrombocytopenia Gastrointestinal intolerance Drug interactions	Easy bruising Slow blood clotting Upset stomach Interferes with certain medications, such as birth control pills, birth control implants, and methadone treatment

Patients who have suspected or confirmed TB should be considered infectious if they are coughing or have positive sputum smears for AFB and are not receiving adequate antituberculosis therapy, have just started therapy, or have a poor clinical or bacteriologic response to therapy (25). The most contagious forms of TB are those that cause airborne spread. TB of the larynx and tuberculosis with cavitary disease (Fig. 56.2) and hemoptysis tend to be the most contagious. Patients are considered contagious until they have been on adequate chemotherapy for a minimum of 2 weeks, have three negative AFB sputum cultures (collected in 8- to 24-hour intervals with one early morning specimen), and show clinical improvement.

TB is not spread through direct contact, sharing food, or kissing. It is not necessary to separate an infectious person on treatment from other household contacts. Young children, however, who are close contacts can be given chemoprophylaxis to avoid separation from a parent. During the first 2 weeks of treatment for patients with smear positive pulmonary, laryngeal or respiratory tract disease patients should avoid unnecessary contact with people from outside the household. This will include exclusion from work, day care facilities, or schools.

Patients should remain noninfectious if regular, adequate chemotherapy is continued, even though bacilli might still be seen in sputum smears.

TREATMENT MONITORING

Baseline and routine laboratory monitoring, such as liver function tests, during treatment of LTBI are indicated only for patients with a history of liver disease, HIV infection, pregnancy (or within 3 months after delivery), or regular alcohol use (16). Clinical monitoring, including a brief physical examination, should occur at monthly visits to assess adherence and identify signs or symptoms of adverse drug reactions (Table 56.4).

The following tests should be obtained to monitor treatment effect in people with active pulmonary TB (15):

- Monthly sputum for AFB smear and culture (until two consecutive negative cultures)
- Serial sputum smears every 2 weeks to assess early response
- Additional drug-susceptibility tests if culture-positive after 3 months of treatment
- Repeat CXR obtained at completion of initial treatment phase for patients with initial negative cultures and at end of treatment for patients with culture-negative TB. CXR is not necessary for patients with culture-positive TB
- Follow-up laboratory testing for renal function, liver function, and platelet count if abnormalities were noted at baseline.
- Visual acuity and color vision monthly if ethambutol is used >2 months or in doses >15 to 20 mg/kg

KEY POINTS

- Limit TB screening to those at higher risk of disease including minority and foreign-born populations, HIV infection or other immunocompromised states, chronic diseases, bariatric surgery recipients, injection drug users, personnel who work or live in high-risk settings, and children younger than 4 years of age who are exposed to high-risk individuals.
- TB skin testing and interferon gamma release assays (IFN-γ) are equivalent screening tests, although IFN-γ may be more accurate in discriminating patients who have TB from those who have a positive skin test for other reasons.
- Obtain a CXR and sputum for AFB after a positive TB skin test result to distinguish LTBI from active TB before beginning treatment; a negative CXR and lack of symptoms establishes the diagnosis of LTBI.
- For patients with LTBI, the CDC recommends isoniazid for 6 to 9 months and pyridoxine (B6) to prevent neuropathy OR rifampin daily for 4 months (primarily considered for patients who have isoniazid-resistant TB or allergy).
- For patients with active TB, four drugs (isoniazid, rifampin, pyrazinamide, and ethambutol) are used for initial treatment for 2 months, with different options for dosing duration in a continuation phase based on risk factors for relapse.
- Tuberculosis is reportable to the PHD in your area; the PHD is charged with TB treatment and eradication nationwide and is an excellent resource. Local and regional pulmonology and infectious disease specialists are also excellent resources for consultation and numerous online resources are available to assist in the diagnosis and management of TB.

INDEX

Note: Page numbers followed by *f* indicate figures; those followed by a *t* indicate tables and those followed by a *b* indicate a box.